AMA
AMERICAN MEDICAL
ASSOCIATION

T0111865

ICD-10-PCS 2024

The Complete Official Codebook

AMA publications fund initiatives that drive improvements in
patient health, practice innovation and medical education.

Notice

ICD-10-PCS: The Complete Official Codebook is designed to be an accurate and authoritative source regarding coding and every reasonable effort has been made to ensure accuracy and completeness of the content. However, the American Medical Association (AMA) makes no guarantee, warranty, or representation that this publication is accurate, complete, or without errors. It is understood that the AMA is not rendering any legal or other professional services or advice in this publication and that the AMA bears no liability for any results or consequences that may arise from the use of this book.

Our Commitment to Accuracy

The AMA is committed to producing accurate and reliable materials. To report corrections, please call the AMA Unified Service Center at (800) 621-8335.

To purchase additional copies, visit the AMA store at amastore.com. Refer to product number OP201124.

Acknowledgments

Marianne Randall, CPC, *Product Manager*
Anita Schmidt, BS, RHIA, AHIMA-approved ICD-10-CM/PCS Trainer, *Subject Matter Expert*
Laura M. Anderson, RN, BSN, CCDS, *Subject Matter Expert*
Stacy Perry, *Manager, Desktop Publishing*
Tracy Betzler, *Senior Desktop Publishing Specialist*
Hope M. Dunn, *Senior Desktop Publishing Specialist*
Katie Russell, *Desktop Publishing Specialist*
Kate Holden, *Editor*

Anita Schmidt, BS, RHIA, AHIMA-approved ICD-10-CM/PCS Trainer

Ms. Schmidt has expertise in ICD-10-CM/PCS, DRG, and CPT with more than 15 years' experience in coding in multiple settings, including inpatient, observation, and same-day surgery. Her experience includes analysis of medical record documentation, assignment of ICD-10-CM and PCS codes, and DRG validation. She has conducted training for ICD-10-CM/PCS and electronic health record. She has also collaborated with clinical documentation specialists to identify documentation needs and potential areas for physician education. Most recently she has been developing content for resource and educational products related to ICD-10-CM, ICD-10-PCS, DRG, and CPT. Ms. Schmidt is an AHIMA-approved ICD-10-CM/PCS trainer and is an active member of the American Health Information Management Association (AHIMA) and the Minnesota Health Information Management Association (MHIMA).

Laura M. Anderson, RN, BSN, CCDS

Ms. Anderson is a Registered Nurse and CDI Specialist/Educator with more than 20 years of experience in the healthcare profession. She obtained her BSN at the University of Minnesota and spent most of her bedside nursing career on Medical-Surgical care units. Her clinical documentation experience began in 2007, covering CDI specialist training, education development, and physician engagement. She has served as a CDI Team Lead and consultant, working with senior leadership to incorporate CDI work into documentation compliance and quality metrics. Ms. Anderson also has a BS degree in Biology (Winthrop University), with research experience in liver cancer and radiation-induced leukemia. She has presented at the state and national levels for the Association of Clinical Documentation Integrity Specialists (ACDIS) and serves as a co-lead for the Minnesota state chapter.

Product Updates

Any changes and updates for this codebook, including the updates for April 1, 2024, will be provided on the AMA's product-updates page at ama-assn.org/product-updates.

Contents

What's New for 2024

The Centers for Medicare and Medicaid Services is the agency charged with maintaining and updating ICD-10-PCS. CMS released the most current revisions, a summary of which may be found on the CMS website at https://www.cms.gov/medicare/icd-10/2024-icd-10-pcs.

Due to the unique structure of ICD-10-PCS, a change in a character value may affect individual codes and several code tables.

Change Summary Table

2023 Total	New Codes	Revised Titles	Deleted Codes	2024 Total
78,530	78	14	5	78,603

ICD-10-PCS Code Totals, By Section

Medical and Surgical	68,058
Obstetrics	304
Placement	861
Administration	1,271
Measurement and Monitoring	422
Extracorporeal or Systemic Assistance and Performance	54
Extracorporeal or Systemic Therapies	46
Osteopathic	100
Other Procedures	88
Chiropractic	90
Imaging	2,978
Nuclear Medicine	463
Radiation Therapy	2,056
Physical Rehabilitation and Diagnostic Audiology	1,380
Mental Health	30
Substance Abuse Treatment	59
New Technology	343
Total	78,603

Table Addenda Highlights

- Device value Short-term External Heart Assist System was added to the root operation tables Insertion, Removal, and Revision in the Heart and Great Vessels body system for the body part Thoracic Aorta, Descending.
- Approach value Open was added to the root operation table Occlusion in the Heart and Great Vessels body system for the body part Thoracic Aorta, Descending.
- Approach value Open was added to the root operation table Occlusion in the Lower Arteries body system for the body part Abdominal Aorta, device value Intraluminal Device, and qualifier values Temporary and No Qualifier.

- Body part value Larynx was added to root operation table Reposition in the Mouth and Throat body system.
- Device value Magnetic Lengthening Device was added to the root operation table Insertion in the Gastrointestinal System body system for body part values Esophagus, Upper; Esophagus, Middle; and Esophagus, Lower.
- Qualifier value Laser Interstitial Thermal Therapy was added to root operation table Destruction in the Upper Bones body system for body parts Cervical Vertebra and Thoracic Vertebra.
- Qualifier value Laser Interstitial Thermal Therapy was added to root operation table Destruction in the Lower Bones body system for body parts Lumbar Vertebra and Sacrum.
- Device value Defibrillator Lead was added to the root operation tables Insertion, Removal, and Revision in the Anatomical Regions, General body system for the body part value Mediastinum.
- New row was added to the root operation table Transfusion to capture transfusion of whole blood, serum albumin, frozen plasma, fresh plasma, red blood cells, frozen red cells, and platelets into bone marrow.
- New row was added to the root operation table Assistance to capture ventilation of patients who are intubated in a prone position.
- New qualifier value Pafolacianine was added to the root operation table Other Procedures for the body region values Female Reproductive System and Trunk Region.
- Five new tables were added to the New Technology section:
    - X05   Nervous System, Destruction
    - X2H   Cardiovascular System, Insertion
    - X2U   Cardiovascular System, Supplement
    - XNR   Bones, Replacement
    - XX2   Physiological Systems, Monitoring
- Root operation table XV5 Male Reproductive System, Destruction was deleted from the New Technology section

Definitions Addenda

Section 0 – Medical and Surgical
Body Part Definitions

ICD-10-PCS Value	Definition	
Appendix	Add	Appendiceal Orifice
Intracranial Artery	Add	Middle meningeal artery, intracranial portion
	Add	Vertebral artery, intracranial portion
Pelvic Cavity	Add	Space of Retzius
Subcutaneous Tissue and Fascia, Face	Add	Chin

Section 0 – Medical and Surgical Device Definitions

ICD-10-PCS Value		Definition	
Add	Defibrillator Lead in Anatomical Regions, General	Add	EV ICD System (Extravascular implantable defibrillator lead)
	Internal Fixation Device, Sustained Compression for Fusion in Lower Joints	Delete Add	DynaNail® (Hybrid)(Mini) DynaNail® (Helix)(Hybrid)(Mini)
	Internal Fixation Device, Sustained Compression for Fusion in Upper Joints	Delete Add	DynaNail® (Hybrid)(Mini) DynaNail® (Helix)(Hybrid)(Mini)
Add	Intracardiac Pacemaker in Heart and Great Vessels	Add	Aveir™ VR, as single chamber
Add	Magnetic Lengthening Device in Gastrointestinal System	Add	Flourish® Pediatric Esophageal Atresia Device
	Short-term External Heart Assist System in Heart and Great Vessels	Add	Aortix™ System
	Stimulator Generator, Multiple Array for Insertion in Subcutaneous Tissue and Fascia	Add	Vanta™ PC neurostimulator
	Stimulator Generator, Multiple Array Rechargeable for Insertion in Subcutaneous Tissue and Fascia	Add	Intellis™ neurostimulator

Section 3 – Administration Substance Definitions

ICD-10-PCS Value		Definition	
	Other Anti-infective	Add	Plazomicin
Add	Vasopressor	Add Add Add	Angiotensin II GIAPREZA™ Human angiotensin II, synthetic

Section X – New Technology Device/Substance/Technology Definitions

ICD-10-PCS Value		Definition	
Add	Anacaulase-bcdb	Add Add	Bromelain-enriched Proteolytic Enzyme NexoBrid™
	Betibeglogene Autotemcel	Add	ZYNTEGLO®
Delete	Bromelain-enriched Proteolytic Enzyme	Delete	NexoBrid™
Add	Conduit through Femoral Vein to Popliteal Artery in New Technology	Add	DETOUR® System
Add	Conduit through Femoral Vein to Superficial Femoral Artery in New Technology	Add	DETOUR® System
Add	Conduit to Short-term External Heart Assist System in New Technology	Add	Impella® 5.5 with SmartAssist® System

ICD-10-PCS Value		Definition	
Add	COVID-19 Vaccine	Add Add	COMIRNATY® SPIKEVAX™
Add	COVID-19 Vaccine Booster	Add Add	COMIRNATY® SPIKEVAX™
Add	COVID-19 Vaccine Dose 1	Add Add	COMIRNATY® SPIKEVAX™
Add	COVID-19 Vaccine Dose 2	Add Add	COMIRNATY® SPIKEVAX™
Add	COVID-19 Vaccine Dose 3	Add Add	COMIRNATY® SPIKEVAX™
Add	Exagamglogene Autotemcel	Add	CTX001™
Delete	Interbody Fusion Device, Customizable in New Technology	Delete	aprevo™
Add	Interbody Fusion Device, Custom-made Anatomically Designed in New Technology	Add	aprevo™
Add	Internal Fixation Device, Open-truss Design in New Technology	Add	Ankle Truss System™ (ATS)
Add	Intracardiac Pacemaker, Dual-Chamber in New Technology	Add Add	Aveir™ AR, as dual chamber Aveir™ DR, dual chamber
Add	Intraluminal Device, Bioprosthetic Valve in New Technology	Add Add	TricValve® Transcatheter Bicaval Valve System VenoValve®
Add	Melphalan Hydrochloride Antineoplastic	Add	HEPZATO™ KIT (melphalan hydrochloride Hepatic Delivery System)
Add	Mosunetuzumab Antineoplastic	Add	LUNSUMIO™
Add	Sulbactam-Durlobactam	Add	SUL-DUR
Delete	Synthetic Human Angiotensin II	Delete Delete Delete	Angiotensin II GIAPREZA™ Human angiotensin II, synthetic
Add	Synthetic Substitute, Extraluminal Support Device in New Technology	Add	VasQ™ External Support device
Add	Synthetic Substitute, Talar Prosthesis in New Technology	Add	Total Ankle Talar Replacement™ (TATR)
Add	Synthetic Substitute, Ultrasound Penetrable in New Technology	Add Add	Longeviti ClearFit® Cranial Implant Longeviti ClearFit® OTS Cranial Implant
Add	Tibial Extension with Motion Sensors in New Technology	Add	Canturio™ te (Tibial Extension)
Add	Vein Graft Extraluminal Support Device(s) in New Technology	Add	VEST™ Venous External Support device

List of Updated Files

2024 Official ICD-10-PCS Coding Guidelines

- Guidelines B5.2b and B6.1a revised in response to public comment and internal review.

- Downloadable PDF

2024 ICD-10-PCS Code Tables and Index (Zip file)

- Code tables for use beginning October 1, 2024.

- Downloadable PDF, file name is pcs_2024.pdf

- Downloadable xml files for developers, file names are icd10pcs_tables_2024.xml, icd10pcs_index_2024.xml, icd10pcs_definitions_2024.xml

- Accompanying schema for developers, file names are icd10pcs_tables.xsd, icd10pcs_index.xsd, icd10pcs_definitions.xsd

2024 ICD-10-PCS Codes File (Zip file)

- ICD-10-PCS Codes file is a simple format for non-technical uses, containing the valid FY 2024 ICD-10-PCS codes and their long titles.

- File is in text file format, file name is icd10pcs_codes_2024.txt

- Accompanying documentation for codes file, file name is icd10pcsCodesFile.pdf

- Codes file addenda in text format, file name is codes_addenda_2024.txt

2024 ICD-10-PCS Order File (Long and Abbreviated Titles) (Zip file)

- ICD-10-PCS order file is for developers, provides a unique five-digit "order number" for each ICD-10-PCS table and code, as well as a long and abbreviated code title.

- ICD-10-PCS order file name is icd10pcs_order_2024.txt

- Accompanying documentation for tabular order file, file name is icd10pcsOrderFile.pdf

- Tabular order file addenda in text format, file name is order_addenda_2024.txt

2024 ICD-10-PCS Final Addenda (Zip file)

- Addenda files in downloadable PDF, file names are tables_addenda_2024.pdf, index_addenda_2024.pdf, definitions_addenda_2024.pdf

- Addenda files also in machine readable text format for developers, file names are tables_addenda_2024.txt, index_addenda_2024.txt, definitions_addenda_2024.txt

2024 ICD-10-PCS Conversion Table (Zip file)

- ICD-10-PCS code conversion table is provided to assist users in data retrieval, in downloadable Excel spreadsheet, file name is icd10pcs_conversion_table_2024.xlsx

- Conversion table also in machine readable text format for developers, file name is icd10pcs_conversion_table_2024.txt

- Accompanying documentation for code conversion table, file name is icd10pcsConversionTable.pdf

Introduction

ICD-10-PCS: The Complete Official Code Set is your definitive coding resource for procedure coding in acute inpatient hospitals. In addition to the official ICD-10-PCS Coding System Files, revised and distributed by the Centers for Medicare and Medicaid Services (CMS), Optum's coding experts have incorporated Medicare-related coding edits and proprietary features, such as coding tools and appendixes, into a comprehensive and easy-to-use reference.

This manual provides the most current information that was available at the time of publication. For updates to official source documents that may have occurred after this manual was published, please refer to the following:

- **CMS International Classification of Disease, 10th Revision, Procedural Coding System (ICD-10-PCS):**

  https://www.cms.gov/medicare/icd-10/2024-icd-10-pcs

- **CMS Inpatient Prospective Payment System (IPPS) and v41 MS-DRG Data Files, FY 2024**

  https://www.cms.gov/medicare/acute-inpatient-pps/fy-2024-ipps-proposed-rule-home-page

  https://www.cms.gov/Medicare/Medicare-Fee-for-Service-Payment/AcuteInpatientPPS/MS-DRG-Classifications-and-Software

- **American Hospital Association (AHA) Coding Clinics**

  https://www.codingclinicadvisor.com/

ICD-10-PCS Code Structure

All codes in ICD-10-PCS are seven characters long. Each character in the seven-character code represents an aspect of the procedure, as shown in the following diagram of characters from the main section of ICD-10-PCS, called the Medical and Surgical section.

	Section	Body System	Root Operation	Body Part	Approach	Device	Qualifier
Characters:	1	2	3	4	5	6	7

One of 34 possible alphanumeric values—using the digits Ø–9 and letters A–H, J–N, and P–Z—can be assigned to each character in a code. The letters O and I are not used so as to avoid confusion with the digits Ø and 1. A code is derived by choosing a specific value for each of the seven characters, based on details about the procedure performed. Because the definition of each character is a function of its physical position in the code, the same value placed in a different position means something different; the value Ø as the first character means something different from Ø as the second character or as the third character, and so on.

The first character always determines the broad procedure category, or section. The second through seventh characters have the same meaning within a specific section, but these meanings can change in a different section. For example, the sixth character means "device" in the Medical and Surgical section but "qualifier" in the Imaging section.

ICD-10-PCS Manual

Index

Codes may be found in the index based on the general type of procedure (e.g., resection, transfusion, fluoroscopy), or a more commonly used term (e.g., appendectomy). For example, the code for percutaneous intraluminal dilation of the coronary arteries with an intraluminal device can be found in the Index under *Dilation*, or a synonym of *Dilation* (e.g., angioplasty). The Index then specifies the first three or four values of the code or directs the user to see another term.

Example:

> **Dilation**
> Artery
> Coronary
> One Artery Ø27Ø

Based on the first three values of the code provided in the Index, the corresponding table can be located. In the example above, the first three values indicate table Ø27 is to be referenced for code completion.

The tables and characters are arranged first by number and then by letter for each character (tables for ØØ-, Ø1-, Ø2-, etc., are followed by those for ØB-, ØC-, ØD-, etc., followed by ØB1, ØB2, etc., followed by ØBB, ØBC, ØBD, etc.).

Note: The Tables section must be used to construct a complete and valid code by specifying the last three or four values.

Tables

The tables in ICD-10-PCS provide the valid combination of character values needed to build a unique procedure code. Each table is preceded by the first three characters of the code, along with their descriptions. In the Medical and Surgical section, for example, the first three characters contain the name of the section (character 1), the body system (character 2), and the root operation performed (character 3).

Listed underneath the first three characters is a table comprising four columns and one or more rows. The four columns in the table specify the last four characters needed to complete the ICD-10-PCS code. Depending on the section, the labels for each column may be different. In the Medical and Surgical section, they are labeled body part (character 4), approach (character 5), device (character 6), and qualifier (character 7). Each row in the table specifies the valid combination of values for characters 4 through 7.

Table 1: Row from table Ø27

Ø **Medical and Surgical**
2 **Heart and Great Vessels**
7 **Dilation**   Definition: Expanding an orifice or the lumen of a tubular body part
       Explanation: The orifice can be a natural orifice or an artificially created orifice. Accomplished by stretching a tubular body part using intraluminal pressure or by cutting part of the orifice or wall of the tubular body part.

Body Part Character 4	Approach Character 5	Device Character 6	Qualifier Character 7
Ø Coronary Artery, One Artery 1 Coronary Artery, Two Arteries 2 Coronary Artery, Three Arteries 3 Coronary Artery, Four or More Arteries	Ø Open 3 Percutaneous 4 Percutaneous Endoscopic	4 Intraluminal Device, Drug-eluting 5 Intraluminal Device, Drug-eluting, Two 6 Intraluminal Device, Drug-eluting, Three 7 Intraluminal Device, Drug-eluting, Four or More D Intraluminal Device E Intraluminal Device, Two F Intraluminal Device, Three G Intraluminal Device, Four or More T Intraluminal Device, Radioactive Z No Device	6 Bifurcation Z No Qualifier

For instance, table 1 above shows the first row from table Ø27 in ICD-10-PCS. The values Ø27 specify the section *Medical and Surgical (Ø)*, the body system *Heart and Great Vessels (2)*, and the root operation *Dilation (7)*. As shown, the root operation (Dilation) is also accompanied by its corresponding definition and explanation. Note, a definition of the root operation is provided for every table in ICD-10-PCS; however, an explanation may not always be applicable.

In total, this single row can be used to construct 240 unique procedure codes. The valid codes shown in table 2 (below) are constructed using the body part (character 4) value of Ø, Coronary artery, one artery, combined with all valid approach (character 5) values, device (character 6) values, and a qualifier (character 7) value of Z, No Qualifier.

Table 2: Code titles for dilation of one coronary artery (Ø27Ø)

Code	Title
Ø27004Z	Dilation of Coronary Artery, One Artery with Drug-eluting Intraluminal Device, Open Approach
Ø27005Z	Dilation of Coronary Artery, One Artery with Two Drug-eluting Intraluminal Devices, Open Approach
Ø27006Z	Dilation of Coronary Artery, One Artery with Three Drug-eluting Intraluminal Devices, Open Approach
Ø27007Z	Dilation of Coronary Artery, One Artery with Four or More Drug-eluting Intraluminal Devices, Open Approach
Ø2700DZ	Dilation of Coronary Artery, One Artery with Intraluminal Device, Open Approach
Ø2700EZ	Dilation of Coronary Artery, One Artery with Two Intraluminal Devices, Open Approach
Ø2700FZ	Dilation of Coronary Artery, One Artery with Three Intraluminal Devices, Open Approach
Ø2700GZ	Dilation of Coronary Artery, One Artery with Four or More Intraluminal Devices, Open Approach
Ø2700TZ	Dilation of Coronary Artery, One Artery with Radioactive Intraluminal Device, Open Approach
Ø2700ZZ	Dilation of Coronary Artery, One Artery, Open Approach
Ø27034Z	Dilation of Coronary Artery, One Artery with Drug-eluting Intraluminal Device, Percutaneous Approach
Ø27035Z	Dilation of Coronary Artery, One Artery with Two Drug-eluting Intraluminal Devices, Percutaneous Approach
Ø27036Z	Dilation of Coronary Artery, One Artery with Three Drug-eluting Intraluminal Devices, Percutaneous Approach
Ø27037Z	Dilation of Coronary Artery, One Artery with Four or More Drug-eluting Intraluminal Devices, Percutaneous Approach
Ø2703DZ	Dilation of Coronary Artery, One Artery with Intraluminal Device, Percutaneous Approach
Ø2703EZ	Dilation of Coronary Artery, One Artery with Two Intraluminal Devices, Percutaneous Approach
Ø2703FZ	Dilation of Coronary Artery, One Artery with Three Intraluminal Devices, Percutaneous Approach
Ø2703GZ	Dilation of Coronary Artery, One Artery with Four or More Intraluminal Devices, Percutaneous Approach
Ø2703TZ	Dilation of Coronary Artery, One Artery with Radioactive Intraluminal Device, Percutaneous Approach
Ø2703ZZ	Dilation of Coronary Artery, One Artery, Percutaneous Approach
Ø27044Z	Dilation of Coronary Artery, One Artery with Drug-eluting Intraluminal Device, Percutaneous Endoscopic Approach
Ø27045Z	Dilation of Coronary Artery, One Artery with Two Drug-eluting Intraluminal Devices, Percutaneous Endoscopic Approach
Ø27046Z	Dilation of Coronary Artery, One Artery with Three Drug-eluting Intraluminal Devices, Percutaneous Endoscopic Approach
Ø27047Z	Dilation of Coronary Artery, One Artery with Four or More Drug-eluting Intraluminal Devices, Percutaneous Endoscopic Approach
Ø2704DZ	Dilation of Coronary Artery, One Artery with Intraluminal Device, Percutaneous Endoscopic Approach
Ø2704EZ	Dilation of Coronary Artery, One Artery with Two Intraluminal Devices, Percutaneous Endoscopic Approach
Ø2704FZ	Dilation of Coronary Artery, One Artery with Three Intraluminal Devices, Percutaneous Endoscopic Approach
Ø2704GZ	Dilation of Coronary Artery, One Artery with Four or More Intraluminal Devices, Percutaneous Endoscopic Approach
Ø2704TZ	Dilation of Coronary Artery, One Artery with Radioactive Intraluminal Device, Percutaneous Endoscopic Approach
Ø2704ZZ	Dilation of Coronary Artery, One Artery, Percutaneous Endoscopic Approach

Table 3: Rows from table ØØH

Ø **Medical and Surgical**
Ø **Central Nervous System and Cranial Nerves**
H **Insertion**   Definition: Putting in a nonbiological appliance that monitors, assists, performs, or prevents a physiological function but does not physically take the place of a body part
        Explanation: None

Body Part Character 4	Approach Character 5	Device Character 6	Qualifier Character 7
Ø Brain Cerebrum Corpus callosum Encephalon	**Ø Open**	**1** Radioactive Element **2** Monitoring Device **3** Infusion Device **4** Radioactive Element, Cesium-131 Collagen Implant **M** Neurostimulator Lead **Y** Other Device	**Z** No Qualifier
Ø Brain Cerebrum Corpus callosum Encephalon	**3** Percutaneous **4** Percutaneous Endoscopic	**1** Radioactive Element **2** Monitoring Device **3** Infusion Device **M** Neurostimulator Lead **Y** Other Device	**Z** No Qualifier
6 Cerebral Ventricle Aqueduct of Sylvius Cerebral aqueduct (Sylvius) Choroid plexus Ependyma Foramen of Monro (intraventricular) Fourth ventricle Interventricular foramen (Monro) Left lateral ventricle Right lateral ventricle Third ventricle **E Cranial Nerve** **U Spinal Canal** Epidural space, spinal Extradural space, spinal Subarachnoid space, spinal Subdural space, spinal Vertebral canal **V Spinal Cord** Dorsal root ganglion	**Ø Open** **3** Percutaneous **4** Percutaneous Endoscopic	**1** Radioactive Element **2** Monitoring Device **3** Infusion Device **M** Neurostimulator Lead **Y** Other Device	**Z** No Qualifier

Table 3 is split into three rows; values of characters must all be selected from within the same row of the table. Rows 1 and 2 have the same body part (character 4) value of Ø Brain and the same qualifier value (character 7) of Z No Qualifier. However, the approach (character 5) values are not the same for these two rows, and there is one additional device (character 6) value in row 1 that is not included in row 2. As shown in row 1, body part value Brain (Ø) with device value Radioactive Element, Cesium-131 Collagen Implant (4) can only be used with approach value Open (Ø). In other words, code ØØHØ34Z would be invalid as the approach value 3 is only applicable to row 2 and the device value 4 is only applicable to row 1. It would be inappropriate to build a code for body part Ø if all of the values are not contained in its own row.

Note: In this manual, there are instances in which some tables due to length must be continued on the next page. Each section must be used separately and value selection must be made within the same row of the table.

Character Meanings

In each section, each character has a specific meaning, and this character meaning remains constant within that section. Character meaning tables have been provided at the beginning of each body system in the Medical and Surgical section (Ø) and the Obstetric section (1) to help the user identify the character members available within that section. These tables have purple headers, unlike the official code tables that have green headers and **SHOULD NOT** be used to build a PCS code. Following is an excerpt of a character meaning table.

Table 4: Rows from Central Nervous System and Cranial Nerves - Character Meanings Table

Operation–Character 3	Body Part–Character 4	Approach–Character 5	Device–Character 6	Qualifier–Character 7
1 Bypass	Ø Brain	Ø Open	Ø Drainage Device	Ø Nasopharynx
2 Change	1 Cerebral Meninges	3 Percutaneous	1 Radioactive Element	1 Mastoid Sinus
5 Destruction	2 Dura Mater	4 Percutaneous Endoscopic	2 Monitoring Device	2 Atrium
7 Dilation	3 Epidural Space, Intracranial	X External	3 Infusion Device	3 Blood Vessel
8 Division	4 Subdural Space, Intracranial		4 Radioactive Element, Cesium-131 Collagen Implant	4 Pleural Cavity
9 Drainage	5 Subarachnoid Space, Intracranial		7 Autologous Tissue Substitute	5 Intestine
B Excision	6 Cerebral Ventricle		J Synthetic Substitute	6 Peritoneal Cavity
C Extirpation	7 Cerebral Hemisphere		K Nonautologous Tissue Substitute	7 Urinary Tract
D Extraction	8 Basal Ganglia		M Neurostimulator Lead	8 Bone Marrow
F Fragmentation	9 Thalamus		Y Other Device	9 Fallopian Tube
H Insertion	A Hypothalamus		Z No Device	A Subgaleal space
J Inspection	B Pons			B Cerebral Cisterns

Sections

The first character of the procedure code always specifies the section. There are 17 sections within the PCS manual, listed below.

Medical and Surgical Section
Ø   Medical and Surgical

Medical and Surgical-related Sections
1   Obstetrics
2   Placement
3   Administration
4   Measurement and Monitoring
5   Extracorporeal or Systemic Assistance and Performance
6   Extracorporeal or Systemic Therapies
7   Osteopathic
8   Other Procedures
9   Chiropractic

Ancillary Sections
B   Imaging
C   Nuclear Medicine
D   Radiation Therapy
F   Physical Rehabilitation and Diagnostic Audiology
G   Mental Health
H   Substance Abuse Treatment

New Technology Section
X   New Technology

Medical and Surgical Section (0)

The Medical and Surgical section contains codes for the vast majority of procedures typically reported in an inpatient setting.

Character Meaning

The seven characters for Medical and Surgical procedures have the following meaning:

Character	Meaning
1	Section
2	Body System
3	Root Operation
4	Body Part
5	Approach
6	Device
7	Qualifier

Section (Character 1)

Medical and Surgical procedure codes all have a first character value of Ø.

Body Systems (Character 2)

The second character represents the body system—the general physiological system or anatomical region where the procedure is being performed.

Body Systems

Ø   Central Nervous System and Cranial Nerves
1   Peripheral Nervous System
2   Heart and Great Vessels
3   Upper Arteries
4   Lower Arteries
5   Upper Veins
6   Lower Veins
7   Lymphatic and Hemic Systems
8   Eye
9   Ear, Nose, Sinus
B   Respiratory System
C   Mouth and Throat
D   Gastrointestinal System
F   Hepatobiliary System and Pancreas
G   Endocrine System
H   Skin and Breast
J   Subcutaneous Tissue and Fascia
K   Muscles
L   Tendons
M   Bursae and Ligaments
N   Head and Facial Bones
P   Upper Bones
Q   Lower Bones
R   Upper Joints
S   Lower Joints
T   Urinary System
U   Female Reproductive System
V   Male Reproductive System
W   Anatomical Regions, General
X   Anatomical Regions, Upper Extremities
Y   Anatomical Regions, Lower Extremities

Root Operations (Character 3)

The third character represents the root operation, or the primary objective, of the procedure. There are 31 different root operations in this section, each with its own precise definition.

- *Alteration:* Modifying the natural anatomic structure of a body part without affecting the function of the body part

- *Bypass:* Altering the route of passage of the contents of a tubular body part

- *Change:* Taking out or off a device from a body part and putting back an identical or similar device in or on the same body part without cutting or puncturing the skin or a mucous membrane

- *Control:* Stopping, or attempting to stop, postprocedural or other acute bleeding

- *Creation:* Putting in or on biological or synthetic material to form a new body part that to the extent possible replicates the anatomic structure or function of an absent body part

- *Destruction:* Physical eradication of all or a portion of a body part by the direct use of energy, force, or a destructive agent

- *Detachment:* Cutting off all or a portion of the upper or lower extremities

- *Dilation:* Expanding an orifice or the lumen of a tubular body part

- *Division:* Cutting into a body part without draining fluids and/or gases from the body part in order to separate or transect a body part

- *Drainage:* Taking or letting out fluids and/or gases from a body part

- *Excision:* Cutting out or off, without replacement, a portion of a body part

- *Extirpation:* Taking or cutting out solid matter from a body part

- *Extraction:* Pulling or stripping out or off all or a portion of a body part by the use of force

- *Fragmentation:* Breaking solid matter in a body part into pieces

- *Fusion:* Joining together portions of an articular body part rendering the articular body part immobile

- *Insertion:* Putting in a nonbiological appliance that monitors, assists, performs, or prevents a physiological function but does not physically take the place of a body part

- *Inspection:* Visually and/or manually exploring a body part

- *Map:* Locating the route of passage of electrical impulses and/or locating functional areas in a body part

- *Occlusion:* Completely closing an orifice or lumen of a tubular body part

- *Reattachment:* Putting back in or on all or a portion of a separated body part to its normal location or other suitable location

- *Release:* Freeing a body part from an abnormal physical constraint by cutting or by use of force

- *Removal:* Taking out or off a device from a body part

- *Repair:* Restoring, to the extent possible, a body part to its normal anatomic structure and function

- *Replacement:* Putting in or on biological or synthetic material that physically takes the place and/or function of all or a portion of a body part

- *Reposition:* Moving to its normal location or other suitable location all or a portion of a body part

- *Resection:* Cutting out or off, without replacement, all of a body part

- *Restriction:* Partially closing an orifice or lumen of a tubular body part

- *Revision:* Correcting, to the extent possible, a portion of a malfunctioning device or the position of a displaced device

- *Supplement:* Putting in or on biological or synthetic material that physically reinforces and/or augments the function of a portion of a body part

- *Transfer:* Moving, without taking out, all or a portion of a body part to another location to take over the function of all or a portion of a body part

- *Transplantation:* Putting in or on all or a portion of a living body part taken from another individual or animal to physically take the place and/or function of all or a portion of a similar body part

The standardized level of specificity designed into ICD-10-PCS restricts the use of broadly applicable "not otherwise specified (NOS)" or "unspecified code" options in the system. A minimal level of specificity is required to construct a valid code. "Not elsewhere classified (NEC)" options are provided in ICD-10-PCS but only for specific, limited use. The root operation Repair in the Medical and Surgical section functions as a "not elsewhere classified" option. Repair is used only when the procedure performed is not one of the other specific root operations in the Medical and Surgical section.

Appendixes B and C provide additional subcategorization, explanations, and representative examples of the Medical and Surgical section root operations.

Body Part (Character 4)
The fourth character represents the body part, or specific anatomical site where the procedure was performed. The body system (second character) provides only a general indication of the procedure site. The body part and body system values, together, provide a precise description of the procedure site.

Approach (Character 5)
The fifth character represents the approach, or the technique used to reach the procedure site. There are seven different approach values in this section.

- *Open*: Cutting through the skin or mucous membrane and any other body layers necessary to expose the site of the procedure

- *Percutaneous*: Entry, by puncture or minor incision, of instrumentation through the skin or mucous membrane and any other body layers necessary to reach the site of the procedure

- *Percutaneous Endoscopic*: Entry, by puncture or minor incision, of instrumentation through the skin or mucous membrane and any other body layers necessary to reach and visualize the site of the procedure

- *Via Natural or Artificial Opening*: Entry of instrumentation through a natural or artificial external opening to reach the site of the procedure

- *Via Natural or Artificial Opening Endoscopic*: Entry of instrumentation through a natural or artificial external opening to reach and visualize the site of the procedure

- *Via Natural or Artificial Opening with Percutaneous Endoscopic Assistance:* Entry of instrumentation through a natural or artificial external opening and entry, by puncture or minor incision, of instrumentation through the skin or mucous membrane and any other body layers necessary to aid in the performance of the procedure

- *External*: Procedures performed directly on the skin or mucous membrane and procedures performed indirectly by the application of external force through the skin or mucous membrane

Appendix A provides definitions and comparisons of the components (access location, method, and type of instrumentation) for each approach and provides an example and illustration.

Device (Character 6)
The sixth character represents a device. Broad categories of devices found in this section include:

- Grafts (e.g., skin)

- Prostheses (e.g., hip joint)

- Implants (e.g., internal fixation device, mesh)

- Simple or Mechanical Appliances (e.g., drainage device, IUD)

- Electronic Appliances (e.g., pacemaker, monitoring device)

Depending on the procedure performed, there may or may not be a device left in place at the end of the procedure. For procedures that do not utilize a device, the value of *No Device* is available. For devices that cannot be categorized into one of the current values, many tables also have a device value of *Other Device*. This value is intended to be used temporarily until a more specific value can be added to the classification. No categories of medical or surgical devices are permanently classified to *Other Device*.

Instruments used to visualize the procedure site are specified in the fifth-character approach, not the sixth-character device value. Materials that are incidental to a procedure such as clips, ligatures, and sutures are not specified in the device character.

Appendix F compares the general device types and provides examples of each.

Appendix G provides an aggregation table that crosswalks specific device character values used for specific root operations to more general device character values used when the root operation represents an entire family of devices.

Qualifier (Character 7)

The seventh character is a qualifier that captures additional attributes of the procedure, where applicable.

Medical and Surgical Section Principles

In developing the Medical and Surgical procedure codes, several specific principles were followed.

Composite Terms Are Not Root Operations

Composite terms such as colonoscopy, sigmoidectomy, or appendectomy do not describe root operations, but they do specify multiple components of a specific root operation. In ICD-10-PCS, the components of a procedure are defined separately by the characters making up the complete code. The only component of a procedure specified in the root operation is the objective of the procedure. With each complete code the underlying objective of the procedure is specified by the root operation (third character), the precise part is specified by the body part (fourth character), and the method used to reach and visualize the procedure site is specified by the approach (fifth character). While colonoscopy, sigmoidectomy, and appendectomy are included in the Index, they do not constitute root operations in the Tables section. The objective of colonoscopy is the visualization of the colon and the root operation (character 3) is *Inspection*. Character 4 specifies the body part, which in this case is part of the colon. These composite terms, like colonoscopy or appendectomy, are included as cross-reference only. The index provides the correct root operation reference. Examples of other types of composite terms not representative of root operations are *partial* sigmoidectomy, *total* hysterectomy, and *partial* hip replacement. Always refer to the correct root operation in the Index and Tables section.

Root Operation Based on Objective of Procedure

The root operation is based on the objective of the procedure, such as *Resection* of transverse colon or *Dilation* of an artery. The assignment of the root operation is based on the procedure actually performed, which may or may not have been the intended procedure. If the intended procedure is modified or discontinued (e.g., excision instead of resection is performed), the root operation is determined by the procedure actually performed. If the desired result is not attained after completing the procedure (i.e., the artery does not remain expanded

after the dilation procedure), the root operation is still determined by the procedure actually performed.

Examples:

- Dilating the urethra is coded as *Dilation* since the objective of the procedure is to dilate the urethra. If dilation of the urethra includes putting in an intraluminal stent, the root operation remains *Dilation* and not *Insertion* of the intraluminal device because the underlying objective of the procedure is dilation of the urethra. The stent is identified by the intraluminal device value in the sixth character of the dilation procedure code.

- If the objective is solely to put a radioactive element in the urethra, then the procedure is coded to the root operation *Insertion*, with the radioactive element identified in the sixth character of the code.

- If the objective of the procedure is to correct a malfunctioning or displaced device, then the procedure is coded to the root operation *Revision*. In the root operation *Revision*, the original device being revised is identified in the device character. *Revision* is typically performed on mechanical appliances (e.g., pacemaker) or materials used in replacement procedures (e.g., synthetic substitute). Typical revision procedures include adjustment of pacemaker position and correction of malfunctioning knee prosthesis.

Combination Procedures Are Coded Separately

If multiple procedures as defined by distinct objectives are performed during an operative episode, then multiple codes are used. For example, obtaining the vein graft used for coronary bypass surgery is coded as a separate procedure from the bypass itself.

Redo of Procedures

The complete or partial redo of the original procedure is coded to the root operation that identifies the procedure performed rather than *Revision*.

Example:

A complete redo of a hip replacement procedure that requires putting in a new prosthesis is coded to the root operation *Replacement* rather than *Revision*.

The correction of complications arising from the original procedure, other than device complications, is coded to the procedure performed. Correction of a malfunctioning or displaced device would be coded to the root operation *Revision*.

Example:

A procedure to control hemorrhage arising from the original procedure is coded to *Control* rather than *Revision*.

Examples of Procedures Coded in the Medical Surgical Section

The following are examples of procedures from the Medical and Surgical section, coded in ICD-10-PCS.

- Suture of skin laceration, left lower arm: ØHQEXZZ

- Laparoscopic appendectomy: ØDTJ4ZZ

- Sigmoidoscopy with biopsy: ØDBN8ZX

- Tracheostomy with tracheostomy tube: ØB11ØF4

Obstetrics Section (1)

The Obstetrics section includes codes for procedures performed on the products of conception only. Procedures on pregnant females are coded in the Medical and Surgical section (e.g., episiotomy). The term "products of conception" refers to all physical components of a pregnancy, including the fetus, amnion, umbilical cord, and placenta. There is no differentiation of the products of conception based on gestational age. Thus, the diagnosis code, not the procedure code, specifies the products of conception as a zygote, embryo, or fetus, or of the trimester of the pregnancy.

Character Meanings

The seven characters in the Obstetrics section have the same meaning as in the Medical and Surgical section.

Character	Meaning
1	Section
2	Body System
3	Root Operation
4	Body Part
5	Approach
6	Device
7	Qualifier

Section (Character 1)

Obstetrics procedure codes have a first character value of *1*.

Body System (Character 2)

The second character represents the body system. There is only one value used in this section: *Pregnancy*.

Root Operation (Character 3)

The third character represents the root operation, or the primary objective, of the procedure. There are 12 values available in this section. Ten of these values specify root operations as defined in the Medical and Surgical section and include *Change, Drainage, Extraction, Insertion, Inspection, Removal, Repair, Reposition, Resection,* and *Transplantation.* The other two values are specific to this section only and are defined as follows:

- *Abortion*: Artificially terminating a pregnancy
- *Delivery*: Assisting the passage of the products of conception from the genital canal

A cesarean section is not a separate root operation because the underlying objective is *Extraction* (i.e., pulling out all or a portion of a body part).

Body Part (Character 4)

The fourth character represents the body part, which in this section is specific to the products of conception. The three values available are as follows:

- *Products of conception*
- *Products of conception, retained*
- *Products of conception, ectopic*

Approach (Character 5)

The fifth character represents the approach, as defined in the Medical and Surgical section.

Device (Character 6)

The sixth character represents a device used during the procedure, where applicable.

Qualifier (Character 7)

The seventh character is a qualifier that captures additional attributes of the procedure, where applicable.

Placement Section (2)

The Placement section includes codes for procedures that put a device in an orifice or on a body region, without making an incision or a puncture.

Character Meanings

The seven characters in the Placement section have the following meaning:

Character	Meaning
1	Section
2	Body System
3	Root Operation
4	Body Region
5	Approach
6	Device
7	Qualifier

Section (Character 1)

Placement procedure codes have a first character value of *2*.

Body System (Character 2)

The second character contains two values specifying either *Anatomical Regions* or *Anatomical Orifices*.

Root Operation (Character 3)

The third character represents the root operation, or the primary objective, of the procedure. There are seven values available in this section. Two of the values specify root operations as defined in the Medical and Surgical section and include *Change* and *Removal*. The other five values are specific to this section only and are defined as follows:

- *Compression*: Putting pressure on a body region
- *Dressing*: Putting material on a body region for protection
- *Immobilization*: Limiting or preventing motion of an external body region
- *Packing*: Putting material in a body region or orifice
- *Traction*: Exerting a pulling force on a body region in a distal direction

Body Region (Character 4)

The fourth character represents the specific body region or orifice. The body system (second character) provides only a general indication of the procedure site. The body region values and body system values, together, precisely describe the procedure site.

Approach (Character 5)

The fifth character represents the approach. Since all placement procedures are performed directly or indirectly on the skin or mucous membrane, the approach value is always *External*.

Device (Character 6)

The sixth character represents a device placed during the procedure, where applicable.

Except for devices used for fractures and dislocations, devices in this section are off the shelf and do not require any extensive design, fabrication, or fitting.

Qualifier (Character 7)

The seventh character is a qualifier. Because there are currently no specific qualifier values in this section, the value is always *No Qualifier.*

Administration Section (3)

The Administration section includes infusions, injections, and transfusions, as well as other related procedures, such as irrigation and tattooing. All codes in this section define procedures in which a diagnostic or therapeutic substance is given to the patient.

Character Meanings

The seven characters in the Administration section have the following meaning:

Character	Meaning
1	Section
2	Body System
3	Root Operation
4	Body System/Region
5	Approach
6	Substance
7	Qualifier

Section (Character 1)

Administration procedure codes have a first character value of *3*.

Body System (Character 2)

The second character can represent the general physiological system, anatomical region, or device to which a substance is being administered. The three values available in this section are *Indwelling Device, Physiological Systems and Anatomical Regions,* and *Circulatory System.*

Root Operation (Character 3)

The third character represents the root operation, or the primary objective, of the procedure. There are three values available in this section.

- *Introduction*: Putting in or on a therapeutic, diagnostic, nutritional, physiological, or prophylactic substance except blood or blood products
- *Irrigation*: Putting in or on a cleansing substance
- *Transfusion*: Putting in blood or blood products

Body/System Region (Character 4)

The fourth character represents the body system/region. The fourth character identifies the site where the substance is administered, not the site where the substance administered takes effect. Sites include *Skin and Mucous Membranes, Subcutaneous Tissue,* and *Muscle.* These differentiate intradermal, subcutaneous, and intramuscular injections, respectively. Other sites include *Eye, Respiratory Tract, Peritoneal Cavity,* and *Epidural Space.*

The body systems/regions for arteries and veins are *Peripheral Artery, Central Artery, Peripheral Vein,* and *Central Vein.* The *Peripheral Artery* or *Vein* is typically used when a substance is introduced locally into an artery or vein. For example, chemotherapy is the introduction of an antineoplastic substance into a peripheral artery or vein by a percutaneous approach. In general, the substance introduced into a peripheral artery or vein has a systemic effect.

The *Central Artery* or *Vein* is typically used when the site where the substance is introduced is distant from the point of entry into the artery or vein. For example, the introduction of a substance directly at the site of a clot within an artery or vein using a catheter is coded as an introduction of a thrombolytic substance into a central artery or vein by a percutaneous approach. In general, the substance introduced into a central artery or vein has a local effect.

Approach (Character 5)

The fifth character represents the approach, as defined in the Medical and Surgical section. The approach for intradermal, subcutaneous, and intramuscular introductions (i.e., injections) is *Percutaneous.* If a catheter is placed to introduce a substance into an internal site within the circulatory system, then the approach is also *Percutaneous.* For example, if a catheter is used to introduce contrast directly into the heart for angiography, then the procedure would be coded as a percutaneous introduction of contrast into the heart.

Substance (Character 6)

The sixth character represents the substance being introduced. Most of the values capture broad categories of substances to which several specific substances may be categorized.

Qualifier (Character 7)

The seventh character is a qualifier. The substance value (second character) provides the broad category to which a substance is classified. The qualifier and substance values, together, precisely describe the substance administered. Not every substance administered has its own unique qualifier.

Measurement and Monitoring Section (4)

The Measurement and Monitoring section represents procedures for determining the level of a physiological or physical function.

Character Meanings

The seven characters in the Measurement and Monitoring section have the following meaning:

Character	Meaning
1	Section
2	Body System
3	Root Operation
4	Body System
5	Approach
6	Function/Device
7	Qualifier

Section (Character 1)

Measurement and Monitoring procedure codes have a first character value of *4*.

Body System (Character 2)

The second character represents the body system or device being measured or monitored. There are two values available in this section, *Physiological Systems* and *Physiological Devices*.

Root Operation (Character 3)

The third character represents the root operation, or the primary objective, of the procedure. There are two values available in this section.

- *Measurement*: Determining the level of a physiological or physical function at a point in time
- *Monitoring*: Determining the level of a physiological or physical function repetitively over a period of time

Body System (Character 4)

The fourth character represents the specific body system measured or monitored.

Approach (Character 5)

The fifth character represents the approach, as defined in the Medical and Surgical section.

Function/Device (Character 6)

The sixth character represents the physiological or physical function, or the device function being measured or monitored.

Qualifier (Character 7)

The seventh character is a qualifier, which captures additional attributes of the procedure, where applicable.

Extracorporeal or Systemic Assistance and Performance Section (5)

The Extracorporeal or Systemic Assistance and Performance section describes procedures performed in a critical care setting, such as mechanical ventilation and cardioversion. It also includes other procedures, such as hemodialysis and hyperbaric oxygen treatment.

The procedures described in this section are meant to be temporary; that is, the equipment is used only for the duration of the procedure. The equipment resides primarily outside the body, though it may interface with the body via a tube or other means. Although parts of the equipment may be attached or inserted into the patient, such as lines or catheters, these are not coded as separate device insertion procedures.

Character Meanings

The seven characters in the Extracorporeal or Systemic Assistance and Performance section have the following meaning:

Character	Meaning
1	Section
2	Body System
3	Root Operation
4	Body System
5	Duration
6	Function
7	Qualifier

Section (Character 1)

Extracorporeal or Systemic Assistance and Performance procedure codes have a first character value of *5*.

Body System (Character 2)

The second character represents the body system. There is one value available in this section, *Physiological Systems*.

Root Operation (Character 3)

The third character represents the root operation, or the primary objective, of the procedure. There are three values available in this section.

- *Assistance*: Taking over a portion of a physiological function by extracorporeal means
- *Performance*: Completely taking over a physiological function by extracorporeal means
- *Restoration*: Returning, or attempting to return, a physiological function to its natural state by extracorporeal means

The root operation *Restoration* contains a single procedure code that identifies extracorporeal cardioversion.

Body System (Character 4)

The fourth character represents the body system for which support of a physiological function is required.

Duration (Character 5)

The fifth character specifies the duration of the procedure.

Function (Character 6)

The sixth character represents the physiological function assisted or performed (e.g., oxygenation, ventilation) during the procedure.

Qualifier (Character 7)

The seventh character is a qualifier, which captures additional attributes of the procedure, where applicable, such as the type of equipment used to support or assist a physiological function.

Extracorporeal or Systemic Therapies Section (6)

The Extracorporeal or Systemic Therapies section describes procedures in which equipment outside the body is used for a therapeutic purpose that does not involve the assistance or performance of a physiological function. For procedures such as hypothermia, for which the therapy is not applied to a specific body system but the entire body, a fourth character for *None* is used.

Character Meanings

The seven characters in the Extracorporeal or Systemic Therapies section have the following meaning:

Character	Meaning
1	Section
2	Body System
3	Root Operation
4	Body System
5	Duration
6	Qualifier
7	Qualifier

Section (Character 1)

Extracorporeal or Systemic Therapy procedure codes have a first character value of *6*.

Body System (Character 2)

The second character represents the body system. There is one value available in this section, *Physiological Systems.*

Root Operation (Character 3)

The third character represents the root operation, or the primary objective, of the procedure. There are 11 values available in this section.

- *Atmospheric Control*: Extracorporeal control of atmospheric pressure and composition

- *Decompression*: Extracorporeal elimination of undissolved gas from body fluids

  Decompression involves only one type of procedure: treatment for decompression sickness (the bends) in a hyperbaric chamber.

- *Electromagnetic Therapy*: Extracorporeal treatment by electromagnetic rays

- *Hyperthermia*: Extracorporeal raising of body temperature

  The term hyperthermia is used to describe both a temperature imbalance treatment and also as an adjunct radiation treatment for cancer. When treating the temperature imbalance, it is coded to this section; for the cancer treatment, it is coded in the Radiation Therapy section.

- *Hypothermia*: Extracorporeal lowering of body temperature

- *Perfusion*: Extracorporeal treatment by diffusion of therapeutic fluid

- *Pheresis*: Extracorporeal separation of blood products

  Pheresis may be used for two main purposes: to treat diseases when too much of a blood component is produced (e.g., leukemia) and to remove a blood product such as platelets from a donor, for transfusion into another patient.

- *Phototherapy*: Extracorporeal treatment by light rays

  Phototherapy involves using a machine that exposes the blood to light rays outside the body, recirculates it, and then returns it to the body.

- *Shock Wave Therapy*: Extracorporeal treatment by shock waves

- *Ultrasound Therapy*: Extracorporeal treatment by ultrasound

- *Ultraviolet Light Therapy*: Extracorporeal treatment by ultraviolet light

Body System (Character 4)

The fourth character represents the body system on which the extracorporeal or systemic therapy is performed (e.g., skin, circulatory).

Duration (Character 5)

The fifth character specifies the duration of the procedure. There are two values available in this section, *Single* or *Multiple.*

Qualifier (Characters 6 and 7)

The sixth and seventh characters are qualifiers. The qualifier captures additional attributes of the procedure, where applicable.

Osteopathic Section (7)

Character Meanings

The seven characters in the Osteopathic section have the following meaning:

Character	Meaning
1	Section
2	Body System
3	Root Operation
4	Body Region
5	Approach
6	Method
7	Qualifier

Section (Character 1)

Osteopathic procedure codes have a first character value of *7*.

Body System (Character 2)

The second character represents the body system. There is one value available in this section, *Anatomical Regions.*

Root Operation (Character 3)

The third character represents the root operation, or the primary objective, of the procedure. There is one value available in this section.

- *Treatment*: Manual treatment to eliminate or alleviate somatic dysfunction and related disorders

Body Region (Character 4)

The fourth character represents the body region. The body system (second character) indicates only the anatomical region involved in the procedure. The body region values and body system value, together, precisely describe the procedure site.

Approach (Character 5)

The fifth character represents the approach. There is only one value available in this section, *External.*

Method (Character 6)
The sixth character represents the method used to carry out the osteopathic treatment.

Qualifier (Character 7)
The seventh character is a qualifier. Because there are currently no specific qualifier values in this section, the value is always *None*.

Other Procedures Section (8)
The Other Procedures section contains codes for procedures not included in the other medical and surgical-related sections, including computer- and robotic-assisted procedures.

Character Meanings
The seven characters in the Other Procedures section have the following meaning:

Character	Meaning
1	Section
2	Body System
3	Root Operation
4	Body Region
5	Approach
6	Method
7	Qualifier

Section (Character 1)
Other Procedures section codes have a first character value of *8*.

Body System (Character 2)
The second character represents the body system/region or a device. There are two values available in this section, *Physiological Systems and Anatomical Regions* and *Indwelling Device*.

Root Operation (Character 3)
The third character represents the root operation, or the primary objective, of the procedure. There is one value available in this section.

- *Other Procedures*: Methodologies that attempt to remediate or cure a disorder or disease.

Body Region (Character 4)
The fourth character contains specified body-region values, and also the body-region value *None*.

Approach (Character 5)
The fifth character represents the approach, as defined in the Medical and Surgical section.

Method (Character 6)
The sixth character specifies the method (e.g., *Acupuncture, Therapeutic Massage*).

Qualifier (Character 7)
The seventh character is a qualifier. The qualifier is used to capture additional attributes of the procedure, where applicable.

Chiropractic Section (9)

Character Meanings
The seven characters in the Chiropractic section have the following meaning:

Character	Meaning
1	Section
2	Body System
3	Root Operation
4	Body Region
5	Approach
6	Method
7	Qualifier

Section (Character 1)
Chiropractic section procedure codes have a first character value of *9*.

Body System (Character 2)
The second character represents the body region. There is one value available in this section, *Anatomical Regions*.

Root Operation (Character 3)
The third character represents the root operation, or the primary objective, of the procedure. There is one value available in this section.

- *Manipulation:* Manual procedure that involves a directed thrust to move a joint past the physiological range of motion, without exceeding the anatomical limit.

Body Region (Character 4)
The fourth character represents the body region on which the chiropractic manipulation is performed.

Approach (Character 5)
The fifth character represents the approach. There is only one value available in this section, *External*.

Method (Character 6)
The sixth character represents the method by which the manipulation is accomplished.

Qualifier (Character 7)
The seventh character is a qualifier. Because there are currently no specific qualifier values in this section, the value is always *None*.

Imaging Section (B)
The Imaging section contains codes for procedures such as plain radiography, fluoroscopy, CT, MRI, and ultrasound.

Procedures such as PET, uptakes, and scans are in the Nuclear Medicine section. Therapeutic radiation, for the treatment of cancer, is in the Radiation Therapy section.

Character Meanings

The seven characters in Imaging procedures have the following meaning:

Character	Meaning
1	Section
2	Body System
3	Root Type
4	Body Part
5	Contrast
6	Qualifier
7	Qualifier

Section (Character 1)

Imaging procedure codes have a first character value of *B*.

Body System (Character 2)

The second character represents the general body system where the imaging is being performed. The available values mimic those that are found in the Medical and Surgical section but may not be exact matches.

Root Type (Character 3)

The third character represents the root type. The section title, *Imaging,* essentially identifies the root operation, while the values for the third character describe the type of imaging being performed. There are six root types in this section.

- *Computerized Tomography (CT Scan)*: Computer reformatted digital display of multiplanar images developed from the capture of multiple exposures of external ionizing radiation

- *Fluoroscopy*: Single plane or bi-plane real time display of an image developed from the capture of external ionizing radiation on a fluorescent screen. The image may also be stored by either digital or analog means

- *Magnetic Resonance Imaging (MRI)*: Computer reformatted digital display of multiplanar images developed from the capture of radiofrequency signals emitted by nuclei in a body site excited within a magnetic field

- *Other Imaging*: Other specified modality for visualizing a body part

- *Plain Radiography*: Planar display of an image developed from the capture of external ionizing radiation on photographic or photoconductive plate

- *Ultrasonography*: Real time display of images of anatomy or flow information developed from the capture of reflected and attenuated high frequency sound waves

Body Part (Character 4)

The fourth character represents the body part, or specific anatomical site where the procedure was performed. The body system (second character) provides only a general indication of the procedure site. The body part and body system values, together, precisely describe procedure site.

Contrast (Character 5)

The fifth character represents the type of contrast or enhancing material utilized to facilitate the procedure, when applicable.

Qualifier (Character 6)

The sixth character is a qualifier. The most common qualifier, *Unenhanced and Enhanced,* describes an image taken without contrast (unenhanced) followed by an image with contrast (enhanced). Other qualifier values describe other noncontrast material or technology used to facilitate the imaging.

Qualifier (Character 7)

The seventh character is a qualifier. The qualifier is used to capture additional attributes of the procedure, where applicable.

Nuclear Medicine Section (C)

The Nuclear Medicine section is organized like the Imaging section. Procedures captured in this section describe the introduction of radioactive material into the body to create an image, to diagnose or treat pathological conditions, or to assess metabolic functions.

The introduction of encapsulated radioactive material for the treatment of cancer is included in the Radiation Therapy section.

Character Meanings

The seven characters in the Nuclear Medicine section have the following meaning:

Character	Meaning
1	Section
2	Body System
3	Root Type
4	Body Part
5	Radionuclide
6	Qualifier
7	Qualifier

Section (Character 1)

Nuclear Medicine procedure codes have a first character value of *C*.

Body System (Character 2)

The second character represents the general body system or anatomical region to which the nuclear medicine procedure is performed.

Root Type (Character 3)

The third character represents the root type. The section title, *Nuclear Medicine*, essentially identifies the root operation, while the third character value describes the type of nuclear medicine being performed. There are seven root types available in this section.

- *Nonimaging Nuclear Medicine Assay:* Introduction of radioactive materials into the body for the study of body fluids and blood elements, by the detection of radioactive emissions

- *Nonimaging Nuclear Medicine Probe:* Introduction of radioactive materials into the body for the study of distribution and fate of certain substances by the detection of radioactive emissions; or alternatively, measurement of absorption of radioactive emissions from an external source

- *Nonimaging Nuclear Medicine Uptake:* Introduction of radioactive materials into the body for measurements of organ function, from the detection of radioactive emissions

- *Planar Nuclear Medicine Imaging*: Introduction of radioactive materials into the body for single-plane display of images developed from the capture of radioactive emissions

- *Positron Emission Tomography (PET) Imaging*: Introduction of radioactive materials into the body for three dimensional display of images developed from the simultaneous capture, 180 degrees apart, of radioactive emissions

- *Systemic Nuclear Medicine Therapy:* Introduction of unsealed radioactive materials into the body for treatment

- *Tomographic (Tomo) Nuclear Medicine Imaging*: Introduction of radioactive materials into the body for three dimensional display of images developed from the capture of radioactive emissions

Body Part (Character 4)
The fourth character represents the specific body part or region being studied, imaged, or treated. The body system (second character) provides only a general indication of the procedure site. The body part and body system values, together, provide a precise description of the procedure site.

Radionuclide (Character 5)
The fifth character represents the type of radioactive material utilized to facilitate the procedure, when applicable. The *Other Radionuclide* value is used for radioactive material that has been newly approved but does not yet have its own unique value in the coding system.

If more than one radioactive material is given to perform the procedure, more than one code is used.

Qualifier (Characters 6 and 7)
The sixth and seventh characters are qualifiers. Because there are currently no specific qualifier values in this section, the value is always *None*.

Radiation Therapy Section (D)
The Radiation Therapy section contains procedures performed for cancer treatment.

Character Meanings
The seven characters in the Radiation Therapy section have the following meaning:

Character	Meaning
1	Section
2	Body System
3	Modality
4	Treatment Site
5	Modality Qualifier
6	Isotope
7	Qualifier

Section (Character 1)
Radiation therapy procedure codes have a first character value of *D*.

Body System (Character 2)
The second character represents the general body system or anatomical region to which radiation therapy is being applied.

Modality (Character 3)
The third character represents the type of radiation, or modality, being used. There are four values available in this section.

- *Beam Radiation*
- *Brachytherapy*
- *Stereotactic Radiosurgery*
- *Other Radiation*

Treatment Site (Character 4)
The fourth character represents the specific body part or region being irradiated. The body system (second character) provides only a general indication of the procedure site. The treatment site and body system values, together, precisely describe the procedure site.

Modality Qualifier (Character 5)
The fifth character represents specific methods or materials unique to a particular type of radiation therapy. The modality (third character) and modality qualifier values, together, precisely describe the therapy performed.

Isotope (Character 6)
The sixth character represents the specific radioactive isotope introduced into the body, if applicable.

Qualifier (Character 7)
The seventh character is a qualifier. Besides the value of *None*, this section contains two other values, *Intraoperative* and *Unidirectional Source*.

Physical Rehabilitation and Diagnostic Audiology Section (F)

Character Meanings
The seven characters in the Physical Rehabilitation and Diagnostic Audiology section have the following meaning:

Character	Meaning
1	Section
2	Section Qualifier
3	Root Type
4	Body System/Region
5	Type Qualifier
6	Equipment
7	Qualifier

Section (Character 1)
Physical Rehabilitation and Diagnostic Audiology procedure codes have a first character value of *F*.

Section Qualifier (Character 2)
The second character qualifies which of the two services described in the section (character 1) is being represented. Therefore, only two values are available, *Rehabilitation* or *Diagnostic Audiology*.

Root Type (Character 3)
The third character represents the root type. The section qualifier (second character) identifies the root operation, while the

third-character value describes the type of rehabilitation or diagnostic audiology being performed. There are 14 root types available in this section, each classified into four general categories.

Assessment: Used to evaluate a patient's level of function to determine the type and timing of treatment required. Assessment procedures focus on the faculties of hearing and speech, on various aspects of body function, and on the patient's quality of life, such as muscle performance, neuromotor development, and reintegration skills.

There are six root type values available for assessment.

- *Speech Assessment:* Measurement of speech and related functions

- *Motor and/or Nerve Function Assessment:* Measurement of motor, nerve, and related functions

- *Activities of Daily Living Assessment:* Measurement of functional level for activities of daily living

- *Hearing Assessment:* Measurement of hearing and related functions

- *Hearing Aid Assessment:* Measurement of the appropriateness and/or effectiveness of a hearing device

- *Vestibular Assessment:* Measurement of the vestibular system and related functions

Treatment: Use of specific activities or methods to develop, improve, and/or restore the performance of necessary functions, compensate for dysfunction and/or minimize debilitation. Procedures include swallowing dysfunction exercises, bathing and showering techniques, wound management, gait training, and a host of activities typically associated with rehabilitation.

There are six root type values available for treatment.

- *Speech Treatment:* Application of techniques to improve, augment, or compensate for speech and related functional impairment

- *Motor Treatment:* Exercise or activities to increase or facilitate motor function

- *Activities of Daily Living Treatment:* Exercise or activities to facilitate functional competence for activities of daily living

- *Hearing Treatment:* Application of techniques to improve, augment, or compensate for hearing and related functional impairment

- *Cochlear Implant Treatment:* Application of techniques to improve the communication abilities of individuals with cochlear implant

- *Vestibular Treatment:* Application of techniques to improve, augment, or compensate for vestibular and related functional impairment

Caregiver Training: Educating a caregiver with the skills and knowledge needed to interact with and assist the patient.

There is only one root type value available for caregiver training.

- *Caregiver Training:* Training in activities to support patient's optimal level of function

Fitting(s): Design, fabrication, modification, selection, and/or application of splint, orthosis, prosthesis, hearing aids, and/or other rehabilitation device. The fifth character used in Device Fitting procedures describes the device being fitted rather than the method used to fit the device. Definitions of devices, when provided, are in the definitions portion of the ICD-10-PCS tables and index, under section F, character 5.

There is only one root type value available for fittings.

- *Device Fitting:* Fitting of a device designed to facilitate or support achievement of a higher level of function

Body System/Region (Character 4)
The fourth character represents the body system and body region, where applicable, that requires rehabilitation. For diagnostic audiology procedures, this value is always *None*.

Type Qualifier (Character 5)
The fifth character represents a type qualifier. The root type (third character) and type qualifier values, together, precisely describe the procedure performed.

Equipment (Character 6)
The sixth character represents any equipment used to facilitate the procedure. The values provided are broad categories that may capture several specific types of equipment.

Qualifier (Character 7)
The seventh character is a qualifier. As there are currently no specific qualifier values in this section, the value is always *None*.

Mental Health Section (G)

Character Meanings
The seven characters in the Mental Health section have the following meaning:

Character	Meaning
1	Section
2	Body System
3	Type
4	Qualifier
5	Qualifier
6	Qualifier
7	Qualifier

Section (Character 1)
Mental health procedure codes have a first character value of *G*.

Body System (Character 2)
The second character is always represented by the value of *None*. As mental health care manages the psychological aspects of a patient's health, there is no specific body system or region that can be represented in this section.

Type (Character 3)
The third character represents the type of procedure. There are 12 values available in this section.

- *Psychological Tests:* The administration and interpretation of standardized psychological tests and measurement instruments for the assessment of psychological function

- *Crisis Intervention:* Treatment of a traumatized, acutely disturbed, or distressed individual for the purpose of short-term stabilization

- *Medication Management:* Monitoring and adjusting the use of medications for the treatment of a mental health disorder

- *Individual Psychotherapy:* Treatment of an individual with a mental health disorder by behavioral, cognitive, psychoanalytic, psychodynamic, or psychophysiological means to improve functioning or well-being
- *Counseling:* The application of psychological methods to treat an individual with normal developmental issues and psychological problems in order to increase function, improve well-being, alleviate distress, maladjustment, or resolve crises
- *Family Psychotherapy:* Treatment that includes one or more family members of an individual with a mental health disorder by behavioral, cognitive, psychoanalytic, psychodynamic, or psychophysiological means to improve functioning or well-being
- *Electroconvulsive Therapy:* The application of controlled electrical voltages to treat a mental health disorder
- *Biofeedback:* Provision of information from the monitoring and regulating of physiological processes in conjunction with cognitive-behavioral techniques to improve patient functioning or well-being
- *Hypnosis:* Induction of a state of heightened suggestibility by auditory, visual, and tactile techniques to elicit an emotional or behavioral response
- *Narcosynthesis:* Administration of intravenous barbiturates in order to release suppressed or repressed thoughts
- *Group Psychotherapy:* Treatment of two or more individuals with a mental health disorder by behavioral, cognitive, psychoanalytic, psychodynamic, or psychophysiological means to improve functioning or well-being
- *Light Therapy:* Application of specialized light treatments to improve functioning or well-being

Qualifier (Character 4)

The fourth character is a qualifier. This value represents the specific technique used to evaluate or treat a patient's mental health. In conjunction with the type (third character), the qualifier value precisely describes the procedure.

Qualifier (Characters 5, 6, and 7)

The fifth, sixth, and seventh characters are qualifiers. As there are currently no specific qualifier values in this section, the value is always *None*.

Substance Abuse Treatment Section (H)

Character Meanings

The seven characters in the Substance Abuse Treatment section have the following meaning:

Character	Meaning
1	Section
2	Body System
3	Type
4	Qualifier
5	Qualifier
6	Qualifier
7	Qualifier

Section (Character 1)

Substance Abuse Treatment codes have a first character value of *H*.

Body System (Character 2)

The second character is always represented by the value of *None*. As the substance abuse treatment section describes management of the psychological aspects of a patient's health, there is no specific body system or region that can be represented in this section.

Type (Character 3)

The third character represents the specific type of treatment. There are seven values available in this section.

- *Detoxification Services:* Detoxification from alcohol and/or drugs
- *Individual Counseling:* The application of psychological methods to treat an individual with addictive behavior
- *Group Counseling:* The application of psychological methods to treat two or more individuals with addictive behavior
- *Individual Psychotherapy:* Treatment of an individual with addictive behavior by behavioral, cognitive, psychoanalytic, psychodynamic, or psychophysiological means
- *Family Counseling:* The application of psychological methods that includes one or more family members to treat an individual with addictive behavior
- *Medication Management:* Monitoring and adjusting the use of replacement medications for the treatment of addiction
- *Pharmacotherapy:* The use of replacement medications for the treatment of addiction

Qualifier (Character 4)

The fourth character is a qualifier. The qualifier value further characterizes the type (character 3) of treatment being rendered, where applicable.

Qualifier (Characters 5, 6, and 7)

The fifth, sixth, and seventh characters are qualifiers. As there are currently no specific qualifier values in this section, the value is always *None*.

New Technology Section (X)

General Information

Section X New Technology is a section added to ICD-10-PCS beginning October 1, 2015. The new section provides a place for codes that uniquely identify procedures requested via the New Technology Application Process or that capture other new technologies not currently classified in ICD-10-PCS.

Section X does not introduce any new coding concepts or unusual guidelines for correct coding. In fact, Section X codes maintain continuity with the other sections in ICD-10-PCS by using the same root operation and body part values as their closest counterparts in other sections of ICD-10-PCS. For example, the codes for the infusion of Sarilumab, use the same root operation (Introduction) and body part values (Central Vein and Peripheral Vein) in section X as the infusion codes in section 3 Administration, which are their closest counterparts in the other sections of ICD-10-PCS.

Character Meanings

The seven characters in the new technology section have the following meaning:

Character	Meaning
1	Section
2	Body System
3	Root Operation
4	Body Part
5	Approach
6	Device/Substance/Technology
7	Qualifier

Section (Character 1)

New technology procedure codes have a first character value of *X*.

Body System (Character 2)

The second character values for body system combine the uses of body system, body region, and physiological system as specified in other sections in ICD-10-PCS.

Root Operation (Character 3)

The third character utilizes the same root operation values as their counterparts in other sections of ICD-10-PCS.

Body Part (Character 4)

The fourth character represents the same body part values as their closest counterparts in other sections of ICD-10-PCS.

Approach (Character 5)

The fifth character represents the approach, as defined in the Medical and Surgical section.

Device/Substance/Technology (Character 6)

The sixth character represents the key feature of the new technology procedure. It may be specified as a new device, a new substance, or other new technology. Examples of sixth character values are *Robotic Waterjet Ablation, Interbody Fusion Device, Customizable,* and *Nafamostat Anticoagulant.*

Qualifier (Character 7)

The seventh character qualifier is used exclusively to specify the new technology group, a number or letter that changes each year that new technology codes are added to the system. For example, Section X codes added for the first year have the seventh character value 1, *New Technology Group 1*, and the next year that Section X codes are added have the seventh character value 2, *New Technology Group 2*, and so on. Changing the seventh character value to a unique letter or number every year that there are new codes in the new technology section allows the ICD-10-PCS to "recycle" the values in the third, fourth, and sixth characters as needed.

New Technology Coding Instruction

Section X codes are standalone codes. They are not supplemental codes. Section X codes fully represent the specific procedure described in the code title, and do not require any additional codes from other sections of ICD-10-PCS. When section X contains a code title which describes a specific new technology procedure, only that X code is reported for the procedure. There is no need to report a broader, non-specific code in another section of ICD-10-PCS.

For example, code XW033G5 Introduction of Sarilumab into Peripheral Vein, Percutaneous Approach, New Technology Group 5, would be reported to indicate that Sarilumab was administered via peripheral vein. A separate code from table 3E0 in the Administration section of ICD-10-PCS would not be reported in addition to this code. The X section code fully identifies the administration of the sarilumab, and no additional code is needed.

The New Technology section codes are easily found by looking in the ICD-10-PCS Index or the Tables. In the Index, the name of the new technology device, substance or technology for a section X code is included as a main term. In addition, all codes in section X are listed under the main term New Technology. The new technology code index entry for sarilumab is shown below.

Sarilumab XW0

New Technology
   Sarilumab XW0

ICD-10-PCS Index and Tabular Format

The *ICD-10-PCS: The Complete Official Code Set* is based on the official version of the International Classification of Diseases, 10th Revision, Procedure Classification System, issued by the U.S. Department of Health and Human Services, Centers for Medicare and Medicaid Services. This book is consistent with the content of the government's version of ICD-10-PCS and follows their official format.

Index

The Alphabetic Index can be used to locate the appropriate table containing all the information necessary to construct a procedure code, however, the PCS tables should always be consulted to find the most appropriate valid code. Users may choose a valid code directly from the tables—he or she need not consult the index before proceeding to the tables to complete the code.

Main Terms

The Alphabetic Index reflects the structure of the tables. Therefore, the index is organized as an alphabetic listing. The index:

- Is based on the value of the third character
- Contains common procedure terms
- Lists anatomic sites
- Uses device terms

The main terms in the Alphabetic Index are root operations, root procedure types, or common procedure names. In addition, anatomic sites from the Body Part Key and device terms from the Device Key have been added for ease of use.

Examples:

> *Resection* (root operation)
>
> *Fluoroscopy* (root type)
>
> *Prostatectomy* (common procedure name)
>
> *Brachiocephalic artery* (body part)
>
> *Bard® Dulex™ mesh* (device)

The index provides at least the first three or four values of the code, and some entries may provide complete valid codes. However, the user should always consult the appropriate table to verify that the most appropriate valid code has been selected.

Root Operation and Procedure Type Main Terms

For the *Medical and Surgical* and related sections, the root operation values are used as main terms in the index. The subterms under the root operation main terms are body parts. For the Ancillary section of the tables, the main terms in the index are the general type of procedure performed.

Examples:

> **Biofeedback** GZC9ZZZ
> **Destruction**
> > Acetabulum
> > > Left ØQ55
> > > Right ØQ54
> > Adenoids ØC5Q
> > Ampulla of Vater ØF5C

> **Planar Nuclear Medicine Imaging**
> > Abdomen CW1Ø

See Reference

The second type of term in the index uses common procedure names, such as "appendectomy" or "fundoplication." These common terms are listed as main terms with a "see" reference noting the PCS root operations that are possible valid code tables based on the objective of the procedure.

Examples:

> **Tendonectomy**
> > *see* Excision, Tendons ØLB
> > *see* Resection, Tendons ØLT

Use Reference

The index also lists anatomic sites from the Body Part Key and device terms from the Device Key. These terms are listed with a "use" reference. The purpose of these references is to act as an additional reference to the terms located in the Appendix Keys. The term provided is the Body Part value or Device value to be selected when constructing a procedure code using the code tables. This type of index reference is not intended to direct the user to another term in the index, but to provide guidance regarding character value selection. Therefore, "use" references generally do not refer to specific valid code tables.

Examples:

> **CoAxia NeuroFlo catheter**
> > *use* Intraluminal Device
> **Epitrochlear lymph node**
> > *use* Lymphatic, Left Upper Extremity
> > *use* Lymphatic, Right Upper Extremity
> **SynCardia Total Artificial Heart**
> > *use* Synthetic Substitute

Code Tables

ICD-10-PCS contains 17 sections of Code Tables organized by general type of procedure. The first three characters of a procedure code define each table. The tables consist of columns providing the possible last four characters of codes and rows providing valid values for each character. Within a PCS table, valid codes include all combinations of choices in characters 4 through 7 contained in the same row of the table. All seven characters must be specified to form a valid code.

There are three main sections of tables:

- Medical and Surgical section:
  - *Medical and Surgical* (Ø)
- Medical and Surgical-related sections:
  - *Obstetrics* (1)
  - *Placement* (2)
  - *Administration* (3)
  - *Measurement and Monitoring* (4)
  - *Extracorporeal or Systemic Assistance and Performance* (5)
  - *Extracorporeal or Systemic Therapies* (6)
  - *Osteopathic* (7)

— *Other Procedures* (8)

— *Chiropractic* (9)

• Ancillary sections:

— *Imaging* (B)

— *Nuclear Medicine* (C)

— *Radiation Therapy* (D)

— *Physical Rehabilitation and Diagnostic Audiology* (F)

— *Mental Health* (G)

— *Substance Abuse Treatment* (H)

• New Technology section:

— *New Technology* (X)

The first three character values define each table. The root operation or root type designated for each table is accompanied by its official definition.

Example:

Table ØØF provides codes for procedures on the central nervous system that involve breaking up of solid matter into pieces:

Character 1, Section	Ø: Medical and Surgical
Character 2, Body System	Ø: Central Nervous System and Cranial Nerves
Character 3, Root Operation	F: Fragmentation: Breaking solid matter in a body part into pieces

Tables are arranged numerically, then alphabetically.

When reviewing tables, the user should keep in mind that:

• Some tables may cover multiple pages in the code book—to ensure maximum clarity about character choices, valid entries do not split rows between pages. For instance, the entire table of valid characters completing a code beginning with 4A1 is split between two pages, but the split is between, not within, rows. This means that all the valid sixth and seventh characters for, say, body system *Arterial* (3) and approach *External* (X) are contained on one page.

• Individual entries may be listed in several horizontal "selection" lines.

• When a table is continued onto another page, a note to this effect has been added in red.

Body Part Definitions:

An exclusive Optum feature in the tables is the incorporation of the body part definitions provided in appendix E into the Medical and Surgical section (Ø) tables under their appropriate body part characters in the first column (character 4). This provides the user a direct reference to all anatomical descriptions, terms, and sites that could be coded to that particular body part value.

Paired body parts typically have values for the right and left side and in some cases a value for bilateral. These paired body parts often have the same list of inclusive body part definitions. When there are paired body parts with the same body part definitions, the first listed body part (usually the right side) contains the list of body part definitions while the second listed body part (usually the left side) contains a *See* instruction. This *See* instruction references the body part value that contains the body part definitions. In the table below, body part value P – Upper Eyelid, Left is followed by a *See* instruction that states *See N Upper Eyelid, Right*. All body part descriptions under value N also apply to body part value P.

Example:

Ø   Medical and Surgical
8   Eye
M   Reattachment   Definition: Putting back in or on all or a portion of a separated body part to its normal location or other suitable location
Explanation: Vascular circulation and nervous pathways may or may not be reestablished

Body Part Character 4	Approach Character 5	Device Character 6	Qualifier Character 7
N Upper Eyelid, Right Lateral canthus Levator palpebrae superioris muscle Orbicularis oculi muscle Superior tarsal plate **P Upper Eyelid, Left** *See N Upper Eyelid, Right* **Q Lower Eyelid, Right** Inferior tarsal plate Medial canthus **R Lower Eyelid, Left** *See Q Lower Eyelid, Right*	**X External**	**Z No Device**	**Z No Qualifier**

ICD-10-PCS Additional Features

Use of Official Sources

Color-coding, icons, and other annotations in this manual identify coding and reimbursement edits derived from the inpatient prospective payment system (IPPS) official tables and data files and from the MS-DRG Grouper software.

In most instances, FY 2024 data from the above sources were not available at the time this book was printed. In an effort to make available the most current source information, Optum has provided a document identifying FY 2024 changes to edit designations for ICD-10-PCS codes. Edit changes identified in this document may include:

- Sex
- Hospital-acquired condition
- Noncovered procedures
- Limited coverage procedures
- Valid operating room procedures
- DRG nonoperating room procedures
- Nonoperating room procedures
- New-technology add-on payment

This document can be accessed at the following:

> https://www.optumcoding.com/ProductUpdates/
> Title: "2024 ICD-10-PCS Edit Changes"
> Password: 24PCS

Table Notations

Many tables in ICD-10-PCS contain color or symbol annotations that may aid in code selection, provide clinical or coding information, or alert the coder to reimbursement issues affected by the PCS code assignment. These annotations may be displayed on or next to a character 4, character 6, or character 7 value. Please note that some values may have more than one annotation; this is true most often with the character 4 value.

Refer to the color/symbol legend at the bottom of each page in the tables section for an abridged description of each color and symbol.

Annotation Box

An annotation box has been appended to all tables that contain color-coding or symbol annotations. The color bar or symbol attached to a character value is provided in the box, as well as a list of the valid PCS code(s) to which that edit applies. The box may also list conditional criteria that must be met to satisfy the edit.

For example, see Table 00F. Four character 4 body part values have a gray color bar. In the annotation box below the table, the gray color bar is defined as "Non-OR," or a nonoperating room procedure edit. Following the Non-OR annotation are the PCS codes that are considered nonoperating room procedures from that row of Table 00F.

Bracketed Code Notation

The use of bracketed codes is an efficient convention to provide all valid character value alternatives for a specific set of circumstances. The character values in the brackets correspond to the valid values for the character in the position the bracket appears.

Examples:

In the annotation box for Table 00F the Noncovered Procedure edit (NC) applies to codes represented in the bracketed code 00F[3,4,5,6]XZZ.

> 00F[3,4,5,6]XZZ   Fragmentation in (Central Nervous System and Cranial Nerves), External Approach

The valid fourth character values (body part) that may be selected for this specific circumstance are as follows:

3	Epidural Space, Intracranial
4	Subdural Space, Intracranial
5	Subarachnoid Space, Intracranial
6	Cerebral Ventricle

The fragmentation of matter in the spinal canal, Body Part value U, is not included in the noncovered procedure code edit.

Color-Coding/Symbols

New and Revised Text

Changes within the ICD-10-PCS tables, since the last published edition of this manual, are highlighted in two ways:

- **Red font** identifies new or revised text effective April 1, 2023.
- **Green font** identifies new or revised text effective October 1, 2023.

Medicare Code Edits

Medicare administrative contractors (MACs) and many payers use Medicare code edits to check the coding accuracy on claims. The coding edits provided in this manual include only those directly related to ICD-10-PCS codes used for acute care hospital inpatient admissions.

Sex Edit Symbols

The sex edit symbols below are used to detect inconsistencies between the patient's sex and the procedure. The symbols below most often appear to the right of the body part (character 4) value but may also be found to the right of the qualifier (character 7) value:

♂ Male procedure only

♀ Female procedure only

QA Questionable Obstetric Admission

An inpatient admission is considered questionable when a vaginal or cesarean delivery code is assigned without a corresponding secondary diagnosis code describing the outcome of delivery. Both a delivery (ICD-10-PCS) code and an outcome-of-delivery (ICD-10-CM) code must be present to avoid errors in MS-DRG assignment. This symbol is found only in the Obstetrics Section, appearing to the right of the body part (character 4) value.

NC Noncovered Procedure

Medicare does not cover all procedures. However, some noncovered procedures, due to the presence of certain diagnoses, are reimbursed.

ICD-10-PCS Additional Features

Limited Coverage

For certain procedures whose medical complexity and serious nature incur extraordinary associated costs, Medicare limits coverage to a portion of the cost. The limited coverage edit indicates the type of limited coverage.

ICD-10 MS-DRG Definitions Manual Edits

An MS-DRG is assigned based on specific patient attributes, such as principal diagnosis, secondary diagnoses, procedures, and discharge status. The attributes (edits) provided in this manual include only those directly related to ICD-10-PCS codes used for acute care hospital inpatient admissions.

Non-Operating Room Procedures Not Affecting MS-DRG Assignment

In the Medical and Surgical section (ØØ1-ØYW) and the Obstetric section (1Ø2-1ØY) tables **only,** ICD-10-PCS procedures codes that DO NOT affect MS-DRG assignment are identified by a gray color bar over the body part (character 4) value and are considered non-operating room (non-OR) procedures.

Note: The majority of the ICD-10-PCS codes in the Medical and Surgical-Related, Ancillary and New Technology section tables are non-operating room procedures that do not typically affect MS-DRG assignment. Only the Valid Operating Room and DRG Non-Operating Room procedures are highlighted in these sections, *see* Non-Operating Room Procedures Affecting MS-DRG Assignment and Valid OR Procedure description below.

Non-Operating Room Procedures Affecting MS-DRG Assignment

Some ICD-10-PCS procedure codes, although considered non-operating room procedures, may still affect MS-DRG assignment. In all sections of the ICD-10-PCS book, these procedures are identified by a **purple color bar** over the body part (character 4) value.

Valid OR Procedure

In the Medical and Surgical-Related (2WØ-9WB), Ancillary (BØØ-HZ9) and New Technology (X2A-XYØ) section tables **only**, any codes that are considered a valid operating room procedure are identified with a **blue color bar** over the body part (character 4) value and will affect MS-DRG assignment. All codes without a color bar (blue or purple) are considered non-operating room procedures.

Hospital-Acquired Condition Related Procedures

Procedures associated with hospital-acquired conditions (HAC) are identified with the **yellow color bar** over the body part (character 4) value. Appendix K provides each specific HAC category and its associated ICD-10-CM and ICD-10-PCS codes.

Combination Only

Some ICD-10-PCS procedure codes that describe non-operating room procedures can group to a specific MS-DRG but only when used in combination with certain other ICD-10-PCS procedure codes. Such codes are designated by a **red color bar** over the body part (character 4) value.

Combination Member

A combination member, which can be either a valid operating room procedure or a non-operating room procedure, is an ICD-10-PCS procedure code that can influence MS-DRG assignment either on its own or in combination with other specific ICD-10-PCS procedure codes. Combination member codes are

designated by a plus sign (⊞) to the right of the body part (character 4) value.

Note: In the few instances when a code is both a combination member and a non-operating room procedure affecting the MS-DRG assignment, the body part (character 4) value will have a purple color bar and the combination member icon.

See Appendix L for Procedure Combinations

Under certain circumstances, more than one procedure code is needed in order to group to a specific MS-DRG. When codes within a table have been identified as a Combination Only (**red color bar**) or Combination Member (⊞) code, there is also a footnote instructing the coder to *see Appendix L*. Appendix L contains tables that identify the other procedure codes needed in the combination and the title and number of the MS-DRG to which the combination will group.

Other Table Notations

AHA Coding Clinic:

Official citations from AHA's *Coding Clinic for ICD-10-CM/PCS* have been provided at the beginning of each section, when applicable. Each specific citation is listed below a header identifying the table to which that particular *Coding Clinic* citation applies. The citations appear in purple type with the year, quarter, and page of the reference as well as the title of the question as it appears in that *Coding Clinic's* table of contents. *Coding Clinic* citations included in this edition have been updated through second quarter 2023.

New Technology Add-on Payment

This symbol identifies procedure codes that involve new technologies or medical services that have qualified for a new technology add-on payment (NTAP). CMS provides incremental payment, in addition to the DRG payment, for technologies that have received the NTAP designation. This symbol appears to the right of the sixth character value.

Note: Only specific brand or trade named devices, substances, or technologies receive NTAP approval. The sixth character value in the PCS table provides a generalized description that may be applicable to several brand or trade names. Unless otherwise specified in the annotation box, refer to appendix H or I to determine the specific brand or trade name of the device, substance, or technology that is applicable to the new technology add-on payment. New technology add-on payments are not exclusive to the New Technology (X) section.

Appendixes

The resources described below have been included as appendixes for *ICD-10-PCS The Complete Official Code Set*. These resources further instruct the coder on the appropriate application of the ICD-10-PCS code set.

Appendix A: Components of the Medical and Surgical Approach Definitions

This resource further defines the approach characters used in the Medical and Surgical (Ø) section. Complementing the detailed definition of the approach, additional information includes whether or not instrumentation is a part of the approach, the typical access location, the method used to initiate the approach, related procedural examples, and illustrations all of which will help the user determine the appropriate approach value.

Appendix B: Root Operation Definitions

This resource is a compilation of all root operations found in the Medical and Surgical-related sections (Ø-9) of this PCS manual. It provides a definition and in some cases a more detailed explanation of the root operation, to better reflect the purpose or objective. Examples of related procedure(s) may also be provided.

Appendix C: Comparison of Medical and Surgical Root Operations

The Medical and Surgical (Ø) section root operations are divided into groups that share similar attributes. These groups, and the root operations in each group, are listed in this resource along with information identifying the target of the root operation, the action used to perform the root operation, any clarification or further explanation on the objective of the root operation, and procedure examples.

Appendix D: Body Part Key

When an anatomical term or description is provided in the documentation but does not have a specific body part character within a table, the user can reference this resource to search for the anatomical description or site noted in the documentation to determine if there is a specific PCS body part character (character 4) to which the anatomical description or site could be coded.

Appendix E: Body Part Definitions

This resource is the reverse look-up of the Body Part Key. Each table in the Medical and Surgical section (Ø) of the PCS manual contains anatomical terms linked to a body part character or value, for example, in Table ØBB the Body Part (character 4) of 1 is Trachea. The body part Trachea may have anatomical structures or descriptions that may be used in procedure documentation instead of the term trachea. The Body Part Definitions list other anatomical structures or synonyms that are included in specific ICD-10-PCS body part values. According to the body part definitions, in the example above, cricoid cartilage is included in the Trachea (character 1) body part.

Appendix F: Device Classification

This resource provides an explanation of how a device is defined in the ICD-10-PCS classification along with two tables. The first table groups devices used in the ICD-10-PCS tables into general categories, including a definition of each device type and related examples. The second table provides definitions of transplant and grafting tissue types and associated terminology that may be found in the documentation.

Appendix G: Device Key and Aggregation Table

The Device Key helps users code the appropriate PCS sixth character for device. Devices are listed alphabetically by brand name or commonly used medical terminology and are translated to the appropriate PCS language or value. The key also reflects the body system where the device is located. For example, a SAPIEN valve used for transaortic valve replacement translates to Zooplastic Tissue in Heart and Great Vessels.

The following symbol **NT** has been placed next to those devices that have received an NTAP (new technology add-on payment) designation. When the code for this device is applied to an inpatient encounter, CMS provides incremental payment in addition to the DRG payment.

The Aggregation Table crosswalks specific device character value definitions for specific root operations in a specific body system to the more general device character value to be used when the root operation covers a wide range of body parts and the device character represents an entire family of devices.

Appendix H: Device Definitions

This resource is a reverse look-up to the Device Key. The user may reference this resource to see all the specific devices that may be grouped to a particular device character (character 6).

Example:
The operative report states, "An internal fixation device was used to repair a fractured femur. Kirschner wire, bone screws and neutralization plate all used and left in the bone at the end of the procedure. "

Although PCS requires all devices left in the body to be coded and the operative report lists three different devices, a check in the device definitions shows that all of these devices are included in the PCS value "Internal Fixation Device" and require only one code.

The following symbol **NT** has been placed next to those devices that have received an NTAP (new technology add-on payment) designation. When the code for this device is applied to an inpatient encounter, CMS provides incremental payment in addition to the DRG payment.

Appendix I: Substance Key/Substance Definitions

The Substance Key lists substances by trade name or synonym and relates them to a PCS character in the Administration (3) or New Technology (X) section in the Substance (sixth character) or Qualifier (seventh character) column.

The Substance Definitions table is the reverse look-up of the substance key, relating all substance categories, the sixth- or seventh character values, to all trade name or synonyms that may be classified to that particular character.

The following symbol **NT** has been placed next to those substances/technologies that have received an NTAP (new technology add-on payment) designation. When the code for this substance/technology is applied to an inpatient encounter, CMS provides incremental payment in addition to the DRG payment.

Appendix J: Sections B-H Character Definitions

In each ancillary section (B-H) the characters in a particular column may have different meanings depending on which section the user is working from. This resource provides the values for the characters in these sections as well as a definition of the character value.

Appendix K: Hospital Acquired Conditions

Hospital acquired conditions (HACs) are conditions that are considered reasonably preventable when occurring during the hospital admission and may prevent a case from grouping to a higher-paying MS-DRG. In certain instances the HACs are conditional, requiring a specific ICD-10-CM diagnosis code in combination with a specific ICD-10-PCS procedure code. This resource identifies these conditional HACs, listing the diagnosis and procedure codes that, in combination, may trigger a HAC edit. All codes, ICD-10-CM and ICD-10-PCS, are listed with their full descriptions.

Appendix L: Procedure Combination Tables

The procedure combination tables provided in this resource illustrate certain procedure combinations that must occur in order to assign a specific MS-DRG.

Appendix M: Coding Exercises and Answers

This resource provides the coding exercises with answers, and in some cases a brief explanation as to the reason that particular code was used.

ICD-10-PCS Official Guidelines for Coding and Reporting 2024

Narrative changes appear in **bold** text.

The Centers for Medicare and Medicaid Services (CMS) and the National Center for Health Statistics (NCHS), two departments within the U.S. Federal Government's Department of Health and Human Services (DHHS) provide the following guidelines for coding and reporting using the International Classification of Diseases, 10th Revision, Procedure Coding System (ICD-10-PCS). These guidelines should be used as a companion document to the official version of the ICD-10-PCS as published on the CMS website. The ICD-10-PCS is a procedure classification published by the United States for classifying procedures performed in hospital inpatient health care settings.

These guidelines have been approved by the four organizations that make up the Cooperating Parties for the ICD-10-PCS: the American Hospital Association (AHA), the American Health Information Management Association (AHIMA), CMS, and NCHS.

These guidelines are a set of rules that have been developed to accompany and complement the official conventions and instructions provided within the ICD-10-PCS itself. They are intended to provide direction that is applicable in most circumstances. However, there may be unique circumstances where exceptions are applied. The instructions and conventions of the classification take precedence over guidelines. These guidelines are based on the coding and sequencing instructions in the Tables, Index and Definitions of ICD-10-PCS, but provide additional instruction. Adherence to these guidelines when assigning ICD-10-PCS procedure codes is required under the Health Insurance Portability and Accountability Act (HIPAA). The procedure codes have been adopted under HIPAA for hospital inpatient healthcare settings. A joint effort between the healthcare provider and the coder is essential to achieve complete and accurate documentation, code assignment, and reporting of diagnoses and procedures. These guidelines have been developed to assist both the healthcare provider and the coder in identifying those procedures that are to be reported. The importance of consistent, complete documentation in the medical record cannot be overemphasized. Without such documentation accurate coding cannot be achieved.

Conventions

A1. ICD-10-PCS codes are composed of seven characters. Each character is an axis of classification that specifies information about the procedure performed. Within a defined code range, a character specifies the same type of information in that axis of classification.

> *Example:*
> The fifth axis of classification specifies the approach in sections Ø through 4 and 7 through 9 of the system.

A2. One of 34 possible values can be assigned to each axis of classification in the seven-character code: they are the numbers Ø through 9 and the alphabet (except I and O because they are easily confused with the numbers 1 and Ø). The number of unique values used in an axis of classification differs as needed.

> *Example:*
> Where the fifth axis of classification specifies the approach, seven different approach values are currently used to specify the approach.

A3. The valid values for an axis of classification can be added to as needed.

> *Example:*
> If a significantly distinct type of device is used in a new procedure, a new device value can be added to the system.

A4. As with words in their context, the meaning of any single value is a combination of its axis of classification and any preceding values on which it may be dependent.

> *Example:*
> The meaning of a body part value in the Medical and Surgical section is always dependent on the body system value. The body part value Ø in the Central Nervous body system specifies Brain and the body part value Ø in the Peripheral Nervous body system specifies Cervical Plexus.

A5. As the system is expanded to become increasingly detailed, over time more values will depend on preceding values for their meaning.

> *Example:*
> In the Lower Joints body system, the device value 3 in the root operation Insertion specifies Infusion Device and the device value 3 in the root operation Replacement specifies Ceramic Synthetic Substitute.

A6. The purpose of the alphabetic index is to locate the appropriate table that contains all information necessary to construct a procedure code. The PCS Tables should always be consulted to find the most appropriate valid code.

A7. It is not required to consult the index first before proceeding to the tables to complete the code. A valid code may be chosen directly from the tables.

A8. All seven characters must be specified to be a valid code. If the documentation is incomplete for coding purposes, the physician should be queried for the necessary information.

A9. Within a PCS table, valid codes include all combinations of choices in characters 4 through 7 contained in the same row of the table. In the example below, ØJHT3VZ is a valid code, and ØJHW3VZ is *not* a valid code.

Section:	Ø	**Medical and Surgical**
Body System:	J	**Subcutaneous Tissue and Fascia**
Operation:	H	**Insertion** Putting in a nonbiological appliance that monitors, assists, performs, or prevents a physiological function but does not physically take the place of a body part

Body Part	Approach	Device	Qualifier
S Subcutaneous Tissue and Fascia, Head and Neck V Subcutaneous Tissue and Fascia, Upper Extremity W Subcutaneous Tissue and Fascia, Lower Extremity	Ø Open 3 Percutaneous	1 Radioactive Element 3 Infusion Device Y Other Device	Z No Qualifier
T Subcutaneous Tissue and Fascia, Trunk	Ø Open 3 Percutaneous	1 Radioactive Element 3 Infusion Device V Infusion Pump Y Other Device	Z No Qualifier

A10. "And," when used in a code description, means "and/or," except when used to describe a combination of multiple body parts for which separate values exist for each body part (e.g., Skin and Subcutaneous Tissue used as a qualifier, where there are separate body part values for "Skin" and "Subcutaneous Tissue").

Example:
Lower Arm and Wrist Muscle means lower arm and/or wrist muscle.

A11. Many of the terms used to construct PCS codes are defined within the system. It is the coder's responsibility to determine what the documentation in the medical record equates to in the PCS definitions. The physician is not expected to use the terms used in PCS code descriptions, nor is the coder required to query the physician when the correlation between the documentation and the defined PCS terms is clear.

Example:
When the physician documents "partial resection" the coder can independently correlate "partial resection" to the root operation Excision without querying the physician for clarification.

Medical and Surgical Section Guidelines (section Ø)

B2. Body System

General guidelines

B2.1a. The procedure codes in Anatomical Regions, General, Anatomical Regions, Upper Extremities and Anatomical Regions, Lower Extremities can be used when the procedure is performed on an anatomical region rather than a specific body part, or on the rare occasion when no information is available to support assignment of a code to a specific body part.

Examples:
Chest tube drainage of the pleural cavity is coded to the root operation Drainage found in the body system Anatomical Regions, General.

Suture repair of the abdominal wall is coded to the root operation Repair in the body system Anatomical Regions, General.

Amputation of the foot is coded to the root operation Detachment in the body system Anatomical Regions, Lower Extremities.

B2.1b. Where the general body part values "upper" and "lower" are provided as an option in the Upper Arteries, Lower Arteries, Upper Veins, Lower Veins, Muscles and Tendons body systems, "upper" or "lower" specifies body parts located above or below the diaphragm respectively.

Example:
Vein body parts above the diaphragm are found in the Upper Veins body system; vein body parts below the diaphragm are found in the Lower Veins body system.

B3. Root Operation

General guidelines

B3.1a. In order to determine the appropriate root operation, the full definition of the root operation as contained in the PCS Tables must be applied.

B3.1b. Components of a procedure specified in the root operation definition or explanation as integral to that root operation are not coded separately. Procedural steps necessary to reach the operative site and close the operative site, including anastomosis of a tubular body part, are also not coded separately.

Examples:
Resection of a joint as part of a joint replacement procedure is included in the root operation definition of Replacement and is not coded separately.

Laparotomy performed to reach the site of an open liver biopsy is not coded separately.

In a resection of sigmoid colon with anastomosis of descending colon to rectum, the anastomosis is not coded separately.

Multiple procedures

B3.2. During the same operative episode, multiple procedures are coded if:

a. The same root operation is performed on different body parts as defined by distinct values of the body part character.

Examples:
Diagnostic excision of liver and pancreas are coded separately.

Excision of lesion in the ascending colon and excision of lesion in the transverse colon are coded separately.

b. The same root operation is repeated in multiple body parts, and those body parts are separate and distinct body parts classified to a single ICD-10-PCS body part value.

Examples:
Excision of the sartorius muscle and excision of the gracilis muscle are both included in the upper leg muscle body part value, and multiple procedures are coded.

Extraction of multiple toenails are coded separately.

c. Multiple root operations with distinct objectives are performed on the same body part.

Example:
Destruction of sigmoid lesion and bypass of sigmoid colon are coded separately.

d. The intended root operation is attempted using one approach but is converted to a different approach.

Example:
Laparoscopic cholecystectomy converted to an open cholecystectomy is coded as percutaneous endoscopic Inspection and open Resection.

Discontinued or incomplete procedures

B3.3. If the intended procedure is discontinued or otherwise not completed, code the procedure to the root operation performed. If a procedure is discontinued before any other root operation is performed, code the root operation Inspection of the body part or anatomical region inspected.

Example:
A planned aortic valve replacement procedure is discontinued after the initial thoracotomy and before any incision is made in the heart muscle, when the patient becomes hemodynamically unstable. This procedure is coded as an open Inspection of the mediastinum.

Biopsy procedures

B3.4a. Biopsy procedures are coded using the root operations Excision, Extraction, or Drainage and the qualifier Diagnostic.

Examples:
Fine needle aspiration biopsy of fluid in the lung is coded to the root operation Drainage with the qualifier Diagnostic.

Biopsy of bone marrow is coded to the root operation Extraction with the qualifier Diagnostic.

Lymph node sampling for biopsy is coded to the root operation Excision with the qualifier Diagnostic.

Biopsy followed by more definitive treatment

B3.4b. If a diagnostic Excision, Extraction, or Drainage procedure (biopsy) is followed by a more definitive procedure, such as Destruction, Excision or Resection at the same procedure site, both the biopsy and the more definitive treatment are coded.

> *Example:*
> Biopsy of breast followed by partial mastectomy at the same procedure site, both the biopsy and the partial mastectomy procedure are coded.

Overlapping body layers

B3.5. If root operations such as Excision, Extraction, Repair or Inspection are performed on overlapping layers of the musculoskeletal system, the body part specifying the deepest layer is coded.

> *Example:*
> Excisional debridement that includes skin and subcutaneous tissue and muscle is coded to the muscle body part.

Bypass procedures

B3.6a. Bypass procedures are coded by identifying the body part bypassed "from" and the body part bypassed "to." The fourth character body part specifies the body part bypassed from, and the qualifier specifies the body part bypassed to.

> *Example:*
> Bypass from stomach to jejunum, stomach is the body part and jejunum is the qualifier.

B3.6b. Coronary artery bypass procedures are coded differently than other bypass procedures as described in the previous guideline. Rather than identifying the body part bypassed from, the body part identifies the number of coronary arteries bypassed to, and the qualifier specifies the vessel bypassed from.

> *Example:*
> Aortocoronary artery bypass of the left anterior descending coronary artery and the obtuse marginal coronary artery is classified in the body part axis of classification as two coronary arteries, and the qualifier specifies the aorta as the body part bypassed from.

B3.6c. If multiple coronary arteries are bypassed, a separate procedure is coded for each coronary artery that uses a different device and/or qualifier.

> *Example:*
> Aortocoronary artery bypass and internal mammary coronary artery bypass are coded separately.

Control vs. more specific root operations

B3.7. The root operation Control is defined as, "Stopping, or attempting to stop, postprocedural or other acute bleeding." Control is the root operation coded when the procedure performed to achieve hemostasis, beyond what would be considered integral to a procedure, utilizes techniques (e.g. cautery, application of substances or pressure, suturing or ligation or clipping of bleeding points at the site) that are not described by a more specific root operation definition, such as Bypass, Detachment, Excision, Extraction, Reposition, Replacement, or Resection. If a more specific root operation definition applies to the procedure performed, then the more specific root operation is coded instead of Control.

> *Example:*
> Silver nitrate cautery to treat acute nasal bleeding is coded to the root operation Control.

> *Example:*
> Liquid embolization of the right internal iliac artery to treat acute hematoma by stopping blood flow is coded to the root operation Occlusion.

> *Example:*
> Suctioning of residual blood to achieve hemostasis during a transbronchial cryobiopsy is considered integral to the cryobiopsy procedure and is not coded separately.

Excision vs. Resection

B3.8. PCS contains specific body parts for anatomical subdivisions of a body part, such as lobes of the lungs or liver and regions of the intestine. Resection of the specific body part is coded whenever all of the body part is cut out or off, rather than coding Excision of a less specific body part.

> *Example:*
> Left upper lung lobectomy is coded to Resection of Upper Lung Lobe, Left rather than Excision of Lung, Left.

Excision for graft

B3.9. If an autograft is obtained from a different procedure site in order to complete the objective of the procedure, a separate procedure is coded, except when the seventh character qualifier value in the ICD-10-PCS table fully specifies the site from which the autograft was obtained.

> *Examples:*
> Coronary bypass with excision of saphenous vein graft, excision of saphenous vein is coded separately.
>
> Replacement of breast with autologous deep inferior epigastric artery perforator (DIEP) flap, excision of the DIEP flap is not coded separately. The seventh character qualifier value Deep Inferior Epigastric Artery Perforator Flap in the Replacement table fully specifies the site of the autograft harvest.

Fusion procedures of the spine

B3.10a. The body part coded for a spinal vertebral joint(s) rendered immobile by a spinal fusion procedure is classified by the level of the spine (e.g. thoracic). There are distinct body part values for a single vertebral joint and for multiple vertebral joints at each spinal level.

> *Example:*
> Body part values specify Lumbar Vertebral Joint, Lumbar Vertebral Joints, 2 or More and Lumbosacral Vertebral Joint.

B3.10b. If multiple vertebral joints are fused, a separate procedure is coded for each vertebral joint that uses a different device and/or qualifier.

> *Example:*
> Fusion of lumbar vertebral joint, posterior approach, anterior column and fusion of lumbar vertebral joint, posterior approach, posterior column are coded separately.

B3.10c. Combinations of devices and materials are often used on a vertebral joint to render the joint immobile. When combinations of devices are used on the same vertebral joint, the device value coded for the procedure is as follows:

- If an interbody fusion device is used to render the joint immobile (containing bone graft or bone graft substitute), the procedure is coded with the device value Interbody Fusion Device

- If bone graft is the *only* device used to render the joint immobile, the procedure is coded with the device value Nonautologous Tissue Substitute or Autologous Tissue Substitute

- If a mixture of autologous and nonautologous bone graft (with or without biological or synthetic extenders or binders) is used to render the joint immobile, code the procedure with the device value Autologous Tissue Substitute

Examples:
Fusion of a vertebral joint using a cage style interbody fusion device containing morsellized bone graft is coded to the device Interbody Fusion Device.

Fusion of a vertebral joint using a bone dowel interbody fusion device made of cadaver bone and packed with a mixture of local morsellized bone and demineralized bone matrix is coded to the device Interbody Fusion Device.

Fusion of a vertebral joint using both autologous bone graft and bone bank bone graft is coded to the device Autologous Tissue Substitute.

Inspection procedures

B3.11a. Inspection of a body part(s) performed in order to achieve the objective of a procedure is not coded separately.

Example:
Fiberoptic bronchoscopy performed for irrigation of bronchus, only the irrigation procedure is coded.

B3.11b. If multiple tubular body parts are inspected, the most distal body part (the body part furthest from the starting point of the inspection) is coded. If multiple non-tubular body parts in a region are inspected, the body part that specifies the entire area inspected is coded.

Examples:
Cystoureteroscopy with inspection of bladder and ureters is coded to the ureter body part value.

Exploratory laparotomy with general inspection of abdominal contents is coded to the peritoneal cavity body part value.

B3.11c. When both an Inspection procedure and another procedure are performed on the same body part during the same episode, if the Inspection procedure is performed using a different approach than the other procedure, the Inspection procedure is coded separately.

Example:
Endoscopic Inspection of the duodenum is coded separately when open Excision of the duodenum is performed during the same procedural episode.

Occlusion vs. Restriction for vessel embolization procedures

B3.12. If the objective of an embolization procedure is to completely close a vessel, the root operation Occlusion is coded. If the objective of an embolization procedure is to narrow the lumen of a vessel, the root operation Restriction is coded.

Examples:
Tumor embolization is coded to the root operation Occlusion, because the objective of the procedure is to cut off the blood supply to the vessel.

Embolization of a cerebral aneurysm is coded to the root operation Restriction, because the objective of the procedure is not to close off the vessel entirely, but to narrow the lumen of the vessel at the site of the aneurysm where it is abnormally wide.

Release procedures

B3.13. In the root operation Release, the body part value coded is the body part being freed and not the tissue being manipulated or cut to free the body part.

Example:
Lysis of intestinal adhesions is coded to the specific intestine body part value.

Release vs. Division

B3.14. If the sole objective of the procedure is freeing a body part without cutting the body part, the root operation is Release. If the sole objective of the procedure is separating or transecting a body part, the root operation is Division.

Examples:
Freeing a nerve root from surrounding scar tissue to relieve pain is coded to the root operation Release.

Severing a nerve root to relieve pain is coded to the root operation Division.

Reposition for fracture treatment

B3.15. Reduction of a displaced fracture is coded to the root operation Reposition and the application of a cast or splint in conjunction with the Reposition procedure is not coded separately. Treatment of a nondisplaced fracture is coded to the procedure performed.

Examples:
Casting of a nondisplaced fracture is coded to the root operation Immobilization in the Placement section.

Putting a pin in a nondisplaced fracture is coded to the root operation Insertion.

Transplantation vs. Administration

B3.16. Putting in a mature and functioning living body part taken from another individual or animal is coded to the root operation Transplantation. Putting in autologous or nonautologous cells is coded to the Administration section.

Example:
Putting in autologous or nonautologous bone marrow, pancreatic islet cells or stem cells is coded to the Administration section.

Transfer procedures using multiple tissue layers

B3.17. The root operation Transfer contains qualifiers that can be used to specify when a transfer flap is composed of more than one tissue layer, such as a musculocutaneous flap. For procedures involving transfer of multiple tissue layers including skin, subcutaneous tissue, fascia or muscle, the procedure is coded to the body part value that describes the deepest tissue layer in the flap, and the qualifier can be used to describe the other tissue layer(s) in the transfer flap.

Example:
A musculocutaneous flap transfer is coded to the appropriate body part value in the body system Muscles, and the qualifier is used to describe the additional tissue layer(s) in the transfer flap.

Excision/Resection followed by replacement

B3.18. If an excision or resection of a body part is followed by a replacement procedure, code both procedures to identify each distinct objective, except when the excision or resection is considered integral and preparatory for the replacement procedure.

Examples:
Mastectomy followed by reconstruction, both resection and replacement of the breast are coded to fully capture the distinct objectives of the procedures performed.

Maxillectomy with obturator reconstruction, both excision and replacement of the maxilla are coded to fully capture the distinct objectives of the procedures performed.

Excisional debridement of tendon with skin graft, both the excision of the tendon and the replacement of the skin with a graft are coded to fully capture the distinct objectives of the procedures performed.

Esophagectomy followed by reconstruction with colonic interposition, both the resection and the transfer of the large intestine to function as the esophagus are coded to fully capture the distinct objectives of the procedures performed.

Examples:
Resection of a joint as part of a joint replacement procedure is considered integral and preparatory for the replacement of the joint and the resection is not coded separately.

Resection of a valve as part of a valve replacement procedure is considered integral and preparatory for the valve replacement and the resection is not coded separately.

Detachment procedures of extremities

B3.19. The root operation Detachment contains qualifiers that can be used to specify the level where the extremity was amputated. These qualifiers are dependent on the body part value in the "upper extremities" and "lower extremities" body systems. For procedures involving the detachment of all or part of the upper or lower extremities, the procedure is coded to the body part value that describes the site of the detachment.

Example:
An amputation at the proximal portion of the shaft of the tibia and fibula is coded to the Lower leg body part value in the body system Anatomical Regions, Lower Extremities, and the qualifier High is used to specify the level where the extremity was detached.

The following definitions were developed for the Detachment qualifiers

Body Part	Qualifier	Definition
Upper arm and upper leg	1	High: Amputation at the proximal portion of the shaft of the humerus or femur
	2	Mid: Amputation at the middle portion of the shaft of the humerus or femur
	3	Low: Amputation at the distal portion of the shaft of the humerus or femur
Lower arm and lower leg	1	High: Amputation at the proximal portion of the shaft of the radius/ulna or tibia/fibula
	2	Mid: Amputation at the middle portion of the shaft of the radius/ulna or tibia/fibula
	3	Low: Amputation at the distal portion of the shaft of the radius/ulna or tibia/fibula
Hand and Foot	Ø	Complete*
	4	Complete 1st Ray
	5	Complete 2nd Ray
	6	Complete 3rd Ray
	7	Complete 4th Ray
	8	Complete 5th Ray
	9	Partial 1st Ray
	B	Partial 2nd Ray
	C	Partial 3rd Ray
	D	Partial 4th Ray
	F	Partial 5th Ray

Body Part	Qualifier	Definition
Thumb, finger, or toe	Ø	Complete: Amputation at the metacarpophalangeal/metatarsal-phalangeal joint
	1	High: Amputation anywhere along the proximal phalanx
	2	Mid: Amputation through the proximal interphalangeal joint or anywhere along the middle phalanx
	3	Low: Amputation through the distal interphalangeal joint or anywhere along the distal phalanx

*When coding amputation of Hand and Foot, the following definitions are followed:

- Complete: Amputation through the carpometacarpal joint of the hand, or through the tarsal-metatarsal joint of the foot.
- Partial: Amputation anywhere along the shaft or head of the metacarpal bone of the hand, or of the metatarsal bone of the foot.

B4. Body Part

General guidelines

B4.1a. If a procedure is performed on a portion of a body part that does not have a separate body part value, code the body part value corresponding to the whole body part.

Example:
A procedure performed on the alveolar process of the mandible is coded to the mandible body part.

B4.1b. If the prefix "peri" is combined with a body part to identify the site of the procedure, and the site of the procedure is not further specified, then the procedure is coded to the body part named. This guideline applies only when a more specific body part value is not available.

Examples:
A procedure site identified as perirenal is coded to the kidney body part when the site of the procedure is not further specified.

A procedure site described in the documentation as peri-urethral, and the documentation also indicates that it is the vulvar tissue and not the urethral tissue that is the site of the procedure, then the procedure is coded to the vulva body part.

A procedure site documented as involving the periosteum is coded to the corresponding bone body part.

B4.1c. If a single vascular procedure is performed on a continuous section of an arterial or venous body part, code the body part value corresponding to the anatomically most proximal (closest to the heart) portion of the arterial or venous body part.

Example:
A procedure performed on a continuous section of artery from the femoral artery to the external iliac artery with the point of entry at the femoral artery is coded to the external iliac body part.

A procedure performed on a continuous section of artery from the femoral artery to the external iliac artery with the point of entry at the external iliac artery is also coded to the external iliac artery body part.

Branches of body parts

B4.2. Where a specific branch of a body part does not have its own body part value in PCS, the body part is typically coded to the closest proximal branch that has a specific body part value. In the cardiovascular body systems, if a general body part is available in the correct root operation table, and coding to a proximal branch would require assigning a code in a different body system, the procedure is coded using the general body part value.

> *Examples:*
> A procedure performed on the mandibular branch of the trigeminal nerve is coded to the trigeminal nerve body part value.
>
> Occlusion of the bronchial artery is coded to the body part value Upper Artery in the body system Upper Arteries, and not to the body part value Thoracic Aorta, Descending in the body system Heart and Great Vessels.

Bilateral body part values

B4.3. Bilateral body part values are available for a limited number of body parts. If the identical procedure is performed on contralateral body parts, and a bilateral body part value exists for that body part, a single procedure is coded using the bilateral body part value. If no bilateral body part value exists, each procedure is coded separately using the appropriate body part value.

> *Examples:*
> The identical procedure performed on both fallopian tubes is coded once using the body part value Fallopian Tube, Bilateral.
>
> The identical procedure performed on both knee joints is coded twice using the body part values Knee Joint, Right and Knee Joint, Left.

Coronary arteries

B4.4. The coronary arteries are classified as a single body part that is further specified by number of arteries treated. One procedure code specifying multiple arteries is used when the same procedure is performed, including the same device and qualifier values.

> *Examples:*
> Angioplasty of two distinct coronary arteries with placement of two stents is coded as Dilation of Coronary Artery, Two Arteries with Two Intraluminal Devices.
>
> Angioplasty of two distinct coronary arteries, one with stent placed and one without, is coded separately as Dilation of Coronary Artery, One Artery with Intraluminal Device, and Dilation of Coronary Artery, One Artery with no device.

Tendons, ligaments, bursae and fascia near a joint

B4.5. Procedures performed on tendons, ligaments, bursae and fascia supporting a joint are coded to the body part in the respective body system that is the focus of the procedure. Procedures performed on joint structures themselves are coded to the body part in the joint body systems.

> *Examples:*
> Repair of the anterior cruciate ligament of the knee is coded to the knee bursa and ligament body part in the bursae and ligaments body system.
>
> Knee arthroscopy with shaving of articular cartilage is coded to the knee joint body part in the Lower Joints body system.

Skin, subcutaneous tissue and fascia overlying a joint

B4.6. If a procedure is performed on the skin, subcutaneous tissue or fascia overlying a joint, the procedure is coded to the following body part:

- Shoulder is coded to Upper Arm
- Elbow is coded to Lower Arm
- Wrist is coded to Lower Arm
- Hip is coded to Upper Leg
- Knee is coded to Lower Leg
- Ankle is coded to Foot

Fingers and toes

B4.7. If a body system does not contain a separate body part value for fingers, procedures performed on the fingers are coded to the body part value for the hand. If a body system does not contain a separate body part value for toes, procedures performed on the toes are coded to the body part value for the foot.

> *Example:*
> Excision of finger muscle is coded to one of the hand muscle body part values in the Muscles body system.

Upper and lower intestinal tract

B4.8. In the Gastrointestinal body system, the general body part values Upper Intestinal Tract and Lower Intestinal Tract are provided as an option for the root operations such as Change, Insertion, Inspection, Removal and Revision. Upper Intestinal Tract includes the portion of the gastrointestinal tract from the esophagus down to and including the duodenum, and Lower Intestinal Tract includes the portion of the gastrointestinal tract from the jejunum down to and including the rectum and anus.

> *Example:*
> In the root operation Change table, change of a device in the jejunum is coded using the body part Lower Intestinal Tract.

B5. Approach

Open approach with percutaneous endoscopic assistance

B5.2a. Procedures performed using the open approach with percutaneous endoscopic assistance are coded to the approach Open.

> *Example:*
> Laparoscopic-assisted sigmoidectomy is coded to the approach Open.

*Percutaneous endoscopic approach with **hand-assistance or** extension of incision*

B5.2b. Procedures performed using the percutaneous endoscopic approach, **with hand-assistance, or with an** incision or extension of an incision to assist in the removal of all or a portion of a body part, or to anastomose a tubular body part **with or without the temporary exteriorization of a body structure,** are coded to the approach value Percutaneous Endoscopic.

> *Examples:*
> **Hand-assisted laparoscopic sigmoid colon resection with exteriorization of a segment of the colon for removal of specimen with return of colon back into abdominal cavity is coded to the approach value percutaneous endoscopic.**
>
> Laparoscopic sigmoid colectomy with extension of stapling port for removal of specimen and direct anastomosis is coded to the approach value percutaneous endoscopic.
>
> Laparoscopic nephrectomy with midline incision for removing the resected kidney is coded to the approach value percutaneous endoscopic.
>
> Robotic-assisted laparoscopic prostatectomy with extension of incision for removal of the resected prostate is coded to the approach value percutaneous endoscopic.

External approach

B5.3a. Procedures performed within an orifice on structures that are visible without the aid of any instrumentation are coded to the approach External.

> *Example:*
> Resection of tonsils is coded to the approach External.

B5.3b. Procedures performed indirectly by the application of external force through the intervening body layers are coded to the approach External.

> *Example:*
> Closed reduction of fracture is coded to the approach External.

Percutaneous procedure via device

B5.4. Procedures performed percutaneously via a device placed for the procedure are coded to the approach Percutaneous.

> *Example:*
> Fragmentation of kidney stone performed via percutaneous nephrostomy is coded to the approach Percutaneous.

B6. Device

General guidelines

B6.1a. A device is coded only if a device remains after the procedure is completed. If no device remains, the device value No Device is coded. In limited root operations, the classification provides the qualifier values Temporary and Intraoperative, for specific procedures involving clinically significant devices, where the purpose of the device is to be utilized for a brief duration during the procedure or current inpatient stay. If a device that is intended to remain after the procedure is completed requires removal before the end of the operative episode in which it was inserted, both the insertion and removal of the device should be coded.

B6.1b. Materials such as sutures, ligatures, radiological markers and temporary post-operative wound drains are considered integral to the performance of a procedure and are not coded as devices.

B6.1c. Procedures performed on a device only and not on a body part are specified in the root operations Change, Irrigation, Removal and Revision, and are coded to the procedure performed.

> *Example:*
> Irrigation of percutaneous nephrostomy tube is coded to the root operation Irrigation of indwelling device in the Administration section.

Drainage device

B6.2. A separate procedure to put in a drainage device is coded to the root operation Drainage with the device value Drainage Device.

Obstetric Section Guidelines (section 1)

C. Obstetrics Section

Products of conception

C1. Procedures performed on the products of conception are coded to the Obstetrics section. Procedures performed on the pregnant female other than the products of conception are coded to the appropriate root operation in the Medical and Surgical section.

> *Examples:*
> Amniocentesis is coded to the products of conception body part in the Obstetrics section.
>
> Repair of obstetric urethral laceration is coded to the urethra body part in the Medical and Surgical section.

Procedures following delivery or abortion

C2. Procedures performed following a delivery or abortion for curettage of the endometrium or evacuation of retained products of conception are all coded in the Obstetrics section, to the root operation Extraction and the body part Products of Conception, Retained.

Diagnostic or therapeutic dilation and curettage performed during times other than the postpartum or post-abortion period are all coded in the Medical and Surgical section, to the root operation Extraction and the body part Endometrium.

Radiation Therapy Section Guidelines (section D)

D. Radiation Therapy Section

Brachytherapy

D1.a. Brachytherapy is coded to the modality Brachytherapy in the Radiation Therapy section. When a radioactive brachytherapy source is left in the body at the end of the procedure, it is coded separately to the root operation Insertion with the device value Radioactive Element.

> *Example:*
> Brachytherapy with implantation of a low dose rate brachytherapy source left in the body at the end of the procedure is coded to the applicable treatment site in section D, Radiation Therapy, with the modality Brachytherapy, the modality qualifier value Low Dose Rate, and the applicable isotope value and qualifier value. The implantation of the brachytherapy source is coded separately to the device value Radioactive Element in the appropriate Insertion table of the Medical and Surgical section. The Radiation Therapy section code identifies the specific modality and isotope of the brachytherapy, and the root operation Insertion code identifies the implantation of the brachytherapy source that remains in the body at the end of the procedure.

> *Exception:*
> Implantation of Cesium-131 brachytherapy seeds embedded in a collagen matrix to the treatment site after resection of brain tumor is coded to the root operation Insertion with the device value Radioactive Element, Cesium-131 Collagen Implant. The procedure is coded to the root operation Insertion only, because the device value identifies both the implantation of the radioactive element and a specific brachytherapy isotope that is not included in the Radiation Therapy section tables.

D1.b. A separate procedure to place a temporary applicator for delivering the brachytherapy is coded to the root operation Insertion and the device value Other Device.

> *Examples:*
> Intrauterine brachytherapy applicator placed as a separate procedure from the brachytherapy procedure is coded to Insertion of Other Device, and the brachytherapy is coded separately using the modality Brachytherapy in the Radiation Therapy section.
>
> Intrauterine brachytherapy applicator placed concomitantly with delivery of the brachytherapy dose is coded with a single code using the modality Brachytherapy in the Radiation Therapy section.

New Technology Section Guidelines (section X)

E. New Technology Section

General guidelines

E1.a. Section X codes fully represent the specific procedure described in the code title, and do not require additional codes from other sections of ICD-10-PCS. When section X contains a code title which fully describes a specific new technology procedure, and it is the only procedure performed, only the section X code is reported for the procedure. There is no need to report an additional code in another section of ICD-10-PCS.

> *Example:*
> XWØ43A6 Introduction of Cefiderocol Anti-infective into Central Vein, Percutaneous Approach, New Technology Group 6, can be coded to indicate that Cefiderocol Anti-infective was administered via a central vein. A separate code from table 3EØ in the Administration section of ICD-10-PCS is not coded in addition to this code.

E1.b. When multiple procedures are performed, New Technology section X codes are coded following the multiple procedures guideline.

> *Examples:*
> Dual filter cerebral embolic filtration used during transcatheter aortic valve replacement (TAVR), X2A5312 Cerebral Embolic Filtration, Dual Filter in Innominate Artery and Left Common Carotid Artery, Percutaneous Approach, New Technology Group 2, is coded for the cerebral embolic filtration, along with an ICD-10-PCS code for the TAVR procedure.

> An extracorporeal flow reversal circuit for embolic neuroprotection placed during a transcarotid arterial revascularization procedure, a code from table X2A, Assistance of the Cardiovascular System is coded for the use of the extracorporeal flow reversal circuit, along with an ICD-10-PCS code for the transcarotid arterial revascularization procedure.

F. Selection of Principal Procedure

The following instructions should be applied in the selection of principal procedure and clarification on the importance of the relation to the principal diagnosis when more than one procedure is performed:

1. Procedure performed for definitive treatment of both principal diagnosis and secondary diagnosis

   a. Sequence procedure performed for definitive treatment most related to principal diagnosis as principal procedure.

2. Procedure performed for definitive treatment and diagnostic procedures performed for both principal diagnosis and secondary diagnosis.

   a. Sequence procedure performed for definitive treatment most related to principal diagnosis as principal procedure

3. A diagnostic procedure was performed for the principal diagnosis and a procedure is performed for definitive treatment of a secondary diagnosis.

   a. Sequence diagnostic procedure as principal procedure, since the procedure most related to the principal diagnosis takes precedence.

4. No procedures performed that are related to principal diagnosis; procedures performed for definitive treatment and diagnostic procedures were performed for secondary diagnosis

   a. Sequence procedure performed for definitive treatment of secondary diagnosis as principal procedure, since there are no procedures (definitive or nondefinitive treatment) related to principal diagnosis.

# #

3f (Aortic) Bioprosthesis valve *use* Zooplastic Tissue in Heart and Great Vessels

A

Abdominal aortic plexus *use* Abdominal Sympathetic Nerve
Abdominal cavity *use* Peritoneal Cavity
Abdominal esophagus *use* Esophagus, Lower
Abdominohysterectomy *see* Resection, Uterus 0UT9
Abdominoplasty
　see Alteration, Abdominal Wall 0W0F
　see Repair, Abdominal Wall 0WQF
　see Supplement, Abdominal Wall 0WUF
Abductor hallucis muscle
　use Foot Muscle, Left
　use Foot Muscle, Right
ABECMA® *use* Idecabtagene Vicleucel Immunotherapy
AbioCor® Total Replacement Heart *use* Synthetic Substitute
Ablation
　see Control bleeding in
　see Destruction
Abortion
　Abortifacient 10A07ZX
　Laminaria 10A07ZW
　Products of Conception 10A0
　Vacuum 10A07Z6
Abrasion *see* Extraction
Absolute Pro Vascular (OTW) Self-Expanding Stent System *use* Intraluminal Device
Accelerate PhenoTest™ BC XXE5XN6
Accessory cephalic vein
　use Cephalic Vein, Left
　use Cephalic Vein, Right
Accessory obturator nerve *use* Lumbar Plexus
Accessory phrenic nerve *use* Phrenic Nerve
Accessory spleen *use* Spleen
Acculink (RX) Carotid Stent System *use* Intraluminal Device
Acellular Hydrated Dermis *use* Nonautologous Tissue Substitute
Acetabular cup *use* Liner in Lower Joints
Acetabulectomy
　see Excision, Lower Bones 0QB
　see Resection, Lower Bones 0QT
Acetabulofemoral joint
　use Hip Joint, Left
　use Hip Joint, Right
Acetabuloplasty
　see Repair, Lower Bones 0QQ
　see Replacement, Lower Bones 0QR
　see Supplement, Lower Bones 0QU
Achilles tendon
　use Lower Leg Tendon, Left
　use Lower Leg Tendon, Right
Achillorrhaphy *see* Repair, Tendons 0LQ
Achillotenotomy, achillotomy
　see Division, Tendons 0L8
　see Drainage, Tendons 0L9
Acoustic Pulse Thrombolysis *see* Fragmentation, Artery
Acromioclavicular ligament
　use Shoulder Bursa and Ligament, Left
　use Shoulder Bursa and Ligament, Right
Acromion (process)
　use Scapula, Left
　use Scapula, Right
Acromionectomy
　see Excision, Upper Joints 0RB
　see Resection, Upper Joints 0RT
Acromioplasty
　see Repair, Upper Joints 0RQ
　see Replacement, Upper Joints 0RR
　see Supplement, Upper Joints 0RU
ACTEMRA® *use* Tocilizumab
Activa PC neurostimulator *use* Stimulator Generator, Multiple Array in 0JH
Activa RC neurostimulator *use* Stimulator Generator, Multiple Array Rechargeable in 0JH
Activa SC neurostimulator *use* Stimulator Generator, Single Array in 0JH
Activities of Daily Living Assessment F02

Activities of Daily Living Treatment F08
ACUITY™ Steerable Lead
　use Cardiac Lead, Defibrillator in 02H
　use Cardiac Lead, Pacemaker in 02H
Acupuncture
　Breast
　　Anesthesia 8E0H300
　　No Qualifier 8E0H30Z
　Integumentary System
　　Anesthesia 8E0H300
　　No Qualifier 8E0H30Z
Adductor brevis muscle
　use Upper Leg Muscle, Left
　use Upper Leg Muscle, Right
Adductor hallucis muscle
　use Foot Muscle, Left
　use Foot Muscle, Right
Adductor longus muscle
　use Upper Leg Muscle, Left
　use Upper Leg Muscle, Right
Adductor magnus muscle
　use Upper Leg Muscle, Left
　use Upper Leg Muscle, Right
Adenohypophysis *use* Pituitary Gland
Adenoidectomy
　see Excision, Adenoids 0CBQ
　see Resection, Adenoids 0CTQ
Adenoidotomy *see* Drainage, Adenoids 0C9Q
Adhesiolysis *see* Release
Administration
　Blood products *see* Transfusion
　Other substance *see* Introduction of substance in or on
Adrenalectomy
　see Excision, Endocrine System 0GB
　see Resection, Endocrine System 0GT
Adrenalorrhaphy *see* Repair, Endocrine System 0GQ
Adrenalotomy *see* Drainage, Endocrine System 0G9
Advancement
　see Reposition
　see Transfer
Advisa (MRI) *use* Pacemaker, Dual Chamber in 0JH
afami-cel *use* Afamitresgene Autoleucel Immunotherapy
Afamitresgene Autoleucel Immunotherapy XW0
AFX® Endovascular AAA System *use* Intraluminal Device
Aidoc Briefcase for PE (pulmonary embolism) XXE3X27
AIGISRx Antibacterial Envelope *use* Anti-Infective Envelope
Alar ligament of axis *use* Head and Neck Bursa and Ligament
Alfapump® system *use* Other Device
Alfieri Stitch Valvuloplasty *see* Restriction, Valve, Mitral 02VG
Alimentation *see* Introduction of substance in or on
ALPPS (Associating liver partition and portal vein ligation)
　see Division, Hepatobiliary System and Pancreas 0F8
　see Resection, Hepatobiliary System and Pancreas 0FT
Alteration
　Abdominal Wall 0W0F
　Ankle Region
　　Left 0Y0L
　　Right 0Y0K
　Arm
　　Lower
　　　Left 0X0F
　　　Right 0X0D
　　Upper
　　　Left 0X09
　　　Right 0X08
　Axilla
　　Left 0X05
　　Right 0X04
　Back
　　Lower 0W0L
　　Upper 0W0K
　Breast
　　Bilateral 0H0V
　　Left 0H0U
　　Right 0H0T
　Buttock
　　Left 0Y01

Alteration — *continued*
　Buttock — *continued*
　　Right 0Y00
　Chest Wall 0W08
　Ear
　　Bilateral 0902
　　Left 0901
　　Right 0900
　Elbow Region
　　Left 0X0C
　　Right 0X0B
　Extremity
　　Lower
　　　Left 0Y0B
　　　Right 0Y09
　　Upper
　　　Left 0X07
　　　Right 0X06
　Eyelid
　　Lower
　　　Left 080R
　　　Right 080Q
　　Upper
　　　Left 080P
　　　Right 080N
　Face 0W02
　Head 0W00
　Jaw
　　Lower 0W05
　　Upper 0W04
　Knee Region
　　Left 0Y0G
　　Right 0Y0F
　Leg
　　Lower
　　　Left 0Y0J
　　　Right 0Y0H
　　Upper
　　　Left 0Y0D
　　　Right 0Y0C
　Lip
　　Lower 0C01X
　　Upper 0C00X
　Nasal Mucosa and Soft Tissue 090K
　Neck 0W06
　Perineum
　　Female 0W0N
　　Male 0W0M
　Shoulder Region
　　Left 0X03
　　Right 0X02
　Subcutaneous Tissue and Fascia
　　Abdomen 0J08
　　Back 0J07
　　Buttock 0J09
　　Chest 0J06
　　Face 0J01
　　Lower Arm
　　　Left 0J0H
　　　Right 0J0G
　　Lower Leg
　　　Left 0J0P
　　　Right 0J0N
　　Neck
　　　Left 0J05
　　　Right 0J04
　　Upper Arm
　　　Left 0J0F
　　　Right 0J0D
　　Upper Leg
　　　Left 0J0M
　　　Right 0J0L
　Wrist Region
　　Left 0X0H
　　Right 0X0G
Alveolar process of mandible
　use Mandible, Left
　use Mandible, Right
Alveolar process of maxilla *use* Maxilla
Alveolectomy
　see Excision, Head and Facial Bones 0NB
　see Resection, Head and Facial Bones 0NT
Alveoloplasty
　see Repair, Head and Facial Bones 0NQ
　see Replacement, Head and Facial Bones 0NR
　see Supplement, Head and Facial Bones 0NU
Alveolotomy
　see Division, Head and Facial Bones 0N8

Alveolotomy — *continued*
  see Drainage, Head and Facial Bones ØN9
Ambulatory cardiac monitoring 4A12X45
Amivantamab Monoclonal Antibody XWØ
Amniocentesis *see* Drainage, Products of Conception 1Ø9Ø
Amnioinfusion *see* Introduction of substance in or on, Products of Conception 3EØE
Amnioscopy 1ØJØ8ZZ
Amniotomy *see* Drainage, Products of Conception 1Ø9Ø
AMPLATZER® Muscular VSD Occluder *use* Synthetic Substitute
Amputation *see* Detachment
AMS 800® Urinary Control System *use* Artificial Sphincter in Urinary System
Anacaulase-bcdb XWØ
Anal orifice *use* Anus
Analog radiography *see* Plain Radiography
Analog radiology *see* Plain Radiography
Anastomosis *see* Bypass
Anatomical snuffbox
  use Lower Arm and Wrist Muscle, Left
  use Lower Arm and Wrist Muscle, Right
Andexanet Alfa, Factor Xa Inhibitor Reversal Agent
  use Coagulation Factor Xa, Inactivated
Andexxa *use* Coagulation Factor Xa, Inactivated
AneuRx® AAA Advantage® *use* Intraluminal Device
Angiectomy
  see Excision, Heart and Great Vessels Ø2B
  see Excision, Lower Arteries Ø4B
  see Excision, Lower Veins Ø6B
  see Excision, Upper Arteries Ø3B
  see Excision, Upper Veins Ø5B
Angiocardiography
  Combined right and left heart *see* Fluoroscopy, Heart, Right and Left B216
  Left Heart *see* Fluoroscopy, Heart, Left B215
  Right Heart *see* Fluoroscopy, Heart, Right B214
  SPY system intravascular fluorescence *see* Monitoring, Physiological Systems 4A1
Angiography
  see Computerized Tomography (CT Scan), Artery
  see Fluoroscopy, Artery
  see Magnetic Resonance Imaging (MRI), Artery
  see Plain Radiography, Artery
Angioplasty
  see Dilation, Heart and Great Vessels Ø27
  see Dilation, Lower Arteries Ø47
  see Dilation, Upper Arteries Ø37
  see Repair, Heart and Great Vessels Ø2Q
  see Repair, Lower Arteries Ø4Q
  see Repair, Upper Arteries Ø3Q
  see Replacement, Heart and Great Vessels Ø2R
  see Replacement, Lower Arteries Ø4R
  see Replacement, Upper Arteries Ø3R
  see Supplement, Heart and Great Vessels Ø2U
  see Supplement, Lower Arteries Ø4U
  see Supplement, Upper Arteries Ø3U
Angiorrhaphy
  see Repair, Heart and Great Vessels Ø2Q
  see Repair, Lower Arteries Ø4Q
  see Repair, Upper Arteries Ø3Q
Angioscopy Ø2JY4ZZ, Ø3JY4ZZ, Ø4JY4ZZ
Angiotensin II *use* Vasopressor
Angiotripsy
  see Occlusion, Lower Arteries Ø4L
  see Occlusion, Upper Arteries Ø3L
Angular artery *use* Face Artery
Angular vein
  use Face Vein, Left
  use Face Vein, Right
Ankle Truss System™ (ATS) *use* Internal Fixation Device, Open-truss Design in New Technology
Annular ligament
  use Elbow Bursa and Ligament, Left
  use Elbow Bursa and Ligament, Right
Annuloplasty
  see Repair, Heart and Great Vessels Ø2Q
  see Supplement, Heart and Great Vessels Ø2U
Annuloplasty ring *use* Synthetic Substitute
Anoplasty
  see Repair, Anus ØDQQ
  see Supplement, Anus ØDUQ
Anorectal junction *use* Rectum
Anoscopy ØDJD8ZZ
Ansa cervicalis *use* Cervical Plexus

Antabuse therapy HZ93ZZZ
Antebrachial fascia
  use Subcutaneous Tissue and Fascia, Left Lower Arm
  use Subcutaneous Tissue and Fascia, Right Lower Arm
Anterior cerebral artery *use* Intracranial Artery
Anterior cerebral vein *use* Intracranial Vein
Anterior choroidal artery *use* Intracranial Artery
Anterior circumflex humeral artery
  use Axillary Artery, Left
  use Axillary Artery, Right
Anterior communicating artery *use* Intracranial Artery
Anterior cruciate ligament (ACL)
  use Knee Bursa and Ligament, Left
  use Knee Bursa and Ligament, Right
Anterior crural nerve *use* Femoral Nerve
Anterior facial vein
  use Face Vein, Left
  use Face Vein, Right
Anterior intercostal artery
  use Internal Mammary Artery, Left
  use Internal Mammary Artery, Right
Anterior interosseous nerve *use* Median Nerve
Anterior lateral malleolar artery
  use Anterior Tibial Artery, Left
  use Anterior Tibial Artery, Right
Anterior lingual gland *use* Minor Salivary Gland
Anterior (pectoral) lymph node
  use Lymphatic, Left Axillary
  use Lymphatic, Right Axillary
Anterior medial malleolar artery
  use Anterior Tibial Artery, Left
  use Anterior Tibial Artery, Right
Anterior spinal artery
  use Vertebral Artery, Left
  use Vertebral Artery, Right
Anterior tibial recurrent artery
  use Anterior Tibial Artery, Left
  use Anterior Tibial Artery, Right
Anterior ulnar recurrent artery
  use Ulnar Artery, Left
  use Ulnar Artery, Right
Anterior vagal trunk *use* Vagus Nerve
Anterior vertebral muscle
  use Neck Muscle, Left
  use Neck Muscle, Right
Antibacterial Envelope (TYRX) (AIGISRx) *use* Anti-Infective Envelope
Antibiotic-eluting Bone Void Filler XWØVØP7
Antigen-free air conditioning *see* Atmospheric Control, Physiological Systems 6AØ
Antihelix
  use External Ear, Bilateral
  use External Ear, Left
  use External Ear, Right
Antimicrobial envelope *use* Anti-Infective Envelope
Anti-SARS-CoV-2 hyperimmune globulin *use* Hyperimmune Globulin
Antitragus
  use External Ear, Bilateral
  use External Ear, Left
  use External Ear, Right
Antrostomy *see* Drainage, Ear, Nose, Sinus Ø99
Antrotomy *see* Drainage, Ear, Nose, Sinus Ø99
Antrum of Highmore
  use Maxillary Sinus, Left
  use Maxillary Sinus, Right
Aortic annulus *use* Aortic Valve
Aortic arch *use* Thoracic Aorta, Ascending/Arch
Aortic intercostal artery *use* Upper Artery
Aortix™ System *use* Short-term External Heart Assist System in Heart and Great Vessels
Aortography
  see Fluoroscopy, Lower Arteries B41
  see Fluoroscopy, Upper Arteries B31
  see Plain Radiography, Lower Arteries B4Ø
  see Plain Radiography, Upper Arteries B3Ø
Aortoplasty
  see Repair, Aorta, Abdominal Ø4QØ
  see Repair, Aorta, Thoracic, Ascending/Arch Ø2QX
  see Repair, Aorta, Thoracic, Descending Ø2QW
  see Replacement, Aorta, Abdominal Ø4RØ
  see Replacement, Aorta, Thoracic, Ascending/Arch Ø2RX

Aortoplasty — *continued*
  see Replacement, Aorta, Thoracic, Descending Ø2RW
  see Supplement, Aorta, Abdominal Ø4UØ
  see Supplement, Aorta, Thoracic, Ascending/Arch Ø2UX
  see Supplement, Aorta, Thoracic, Descending Ø2UW
Apalutamide Antineoplastic XWØDXJ5
Apical (subclavicular) lymph node
  use Lymphatic, Left Axillary
  use Lymphatic, Right Axillary
ApiFix® Minimally Invasive Deformity Correction (MID-C) System *use* Posterior (Dynamic) Distraction Device in New Technology
Apneustic center *use* Pons
Appendectomy
  see Excision, Appendix ØDBJ
  see Resection, Appendix ØDTJ
Appendiceal orifice *use* Appendix
Appendicolysis *see* Release, Appendix ØDNJ
Appendicotomy *see* Drainage, Appendix ØD9J
Application *see* Introduction of substance in or on
aprevo™ *use* Interbody Fusion Device, Custom-Made Anatomically Designed in New Technology
Aquablation therapy, prostate ØV5Ø8ZZ
Aquapheresis 6A55ØZ3
Aqueduct of Sylvius *use* Cerebral Ventricle
Aqueous humour
  use Anterior Chamber, Left
  use Anterior Chamber, Right
Arachnoid mater, intracranial *use* Cerebral Meninges
Arachnoid mater, spinal *use* Spinal Meninges
Arcuate artery
  use Foot Artery, Left
  use Foot Artery, Right
Areola
  use Nipple, Left
  use Nipple, Right
AROM (artificial rupture of membranes) 1Ø9Ø7ZC
Arterial canal (duct) *use* Pulmonary Artery, Left
Arterial pulse tracing *see* Measurement, Arterial 4AØ3
Arteriectomy
  see Excision, Heart and Great Vessels Ø2B
  see Excision, Lower Arteries Ø4B
  see Excision, Upper Arteries Ø3B
Arteriography
  see Fluoroscopy, Heart B21
  see Fluoroscopy, Lower Arteries B41
  see Fluoroscopy, Upper Arteries B31
  see Plain Radiography, Heart B2Ø
  see Plain Radiography, Lower Arteries B4Ø
  see Plain Radiography, Upper Arteries B3Ø
Arterioplasty
  see Repair, Heart and Great Vessels Ø2Q
  see Repair, Lower Arteries Ø4Q
  see Repair, Upper Arteries Ø3Q
  see Replacement, Heart and Great Vessels Ø2R
  see Replacement, Lower Arteries Ø4R
  see Replacement, Upper Arteries Ø3R
  see Supplement, Heart and Great Vessels Ø2U
  see Supplement, Lower Arteries Ø4U
  see Supplement, Upper Arteries Ø3U
Arteriorrhaphy
  see Repair, Heart and Great Vessels Ø2Q
  see Repair, Lower Arteries Ø4Q
  see Repair, Upper Arteries Ø3Q
Arterioscopy
  see Inspection, Artery, Lower Ø4JY
  see Inspection, Artery, Upper Ø3JY
  see Inspection, Great Vessel Ø2JY
Arteriovenous Fistula, Extraluminal Support Device, Supplement X2U
Arthrectomy
  see Excision, Lower Joints ØSB
  see Excision, Upper Joints ØRB
  see Resection, Lower Joints ØST
  see Resection, Upper Joints ØRT
Arthrocentesis
  see Drainage, Lower Joints ØS9
  see Drainage, Upper Joints ØR9
Arthrodesis
  see Fusion, Lower Joints ØSG
  see Fusion, Upper Joints ØRG
Arthrography
  see Plain Radiography, Non-Axial Lower Bones BQØ

▽ **Subterms under main terms may continue to next column or page**

Arthrography — *continued*
  see Plain Radiography, Non-Axial Upper Bones BPØ
  see Plain Radiography, Skull and Facial Bones BNØ
Arthrolysis
  see Release, Lower Joints ØSN
  see Release, Upper Joints ØRN
Arthropexy
  see Repair, Lower Joints ØSQ
  see Repair, Upper Joints ØRQ
  see Reposition, Lower Joints ØSS
  see Reposition, Upper Joints ØRS
Arthroplasty
  see Repair, Lower Joints ØSQ
  see Repair, Upper Joints ØRQ
  see Replacement, Lower Joints ØSR
  see Replacement, Upper Joints ØRR
  see Supplement, Lower Joints ØSU
  see Supplement, Upper Joints ØRU
Arthroplasty, radial head
  see Replacement, Radius, Left ØPRJ
  see Replacement, Radius, Right ØPRH
Arthroscopy
  see Inspection, Lower Joints ØSJ
  see Inspection, Upper Joints ØRJ
Arthrotomy
  see Drainage, Lower Joints ØS9
  see Drainage, Upper Joints ØR9
Articulating Spacer (Antibiotic) *use* Articulating
  Spacer in Lower Joints
Artificial anal sphincter (AAS) *use* Artificial Sphincter
  in Gastrointestinal System
Artificial bowel sphincter (neosphincter) *use* Artifi-
  cial Sphincter in Gastrointestinal System
Artificial Sphincter
  Insertion of device in
    Anus ØDHQ
    Bladder ØTHB
    Bladder Neck ØTHC
    Urethra ØTHD
  Removal of device from
    Anus ØDPQ
    Bladder ØTPB
    Urethra ØTPD
  Revision of device in
    Anus ØDWQ
    Bladder ØTWB
    Urethra ØTWD
Artificial urinary sphincter (AUS) *use* Artificial
  Sphincter in Urinary System
Aryepiglottic fold *use* Larynx
Arytenoid cartilage *use* Larynx
Arytenoid muscle
  use Neck Muscle, Left
  use Neck Muscle, Right
Arytenoidectomy *see* Excision, Larynx ØCBS
Arytenoidopexy *see* Repair, Larynx ØCQS
Ascenda Intrathecal Catheter *use* Infusion Device
Ascending aorta *use* Thoracic Aorta, Ascending/Arch
Ascending palatine artery *use* Face Artery
Ascending pharyngeal artery
  use External Carotid Artery, Left
  use External Carotid Artery, Right
aScope™ Duodeno *see* New Technology, Hepatobiliary
  System and Pancreas XFJ
Aspiration, fine needle
  Fluid or gas *see* Drainage
  Tissue biopsy
    see Excision
    see Extraction
Assessment
  Activities of daily living *see* Activities of Daily Living
    Assessment, Rehabilitation FØ2
  Hearing *see* Hearing Assessment, Diagnostic Audi-
    ology F13
  Hearing aid *see* Hearing Aid Assessment, Diagnos-
    tic Audiology F14
  Intravascular perfusion, using indocyanine green
    (ICG) dye *see* Monitoring, Physiological Sys-
    tems 4A1
  Motor function *see* Motor Function Assessment,
    Rehabilitation FØ1
  Nerve function *see* Motor Function Assessment,
    Rehabilitation FØ1
  Speech *see* Speech Assessment, Rehabilitation FØØ
  Vestibular *see* Vestibular Assessment, Diagnostic
    Audiology F15

Assessment — *continued*
  Vocational *see* Activities of Daily Living Treatment,
    Rehabilitation FØ8
Assistance
  Cardiac
    Continuous
      Output
        Balloon Pump 5AØ221Ø
        Impeller Pump 5AØ221D
        Other Pump 5AØ2216
        Pulsatile Compression 5AØ2215
      Oxygenation, Supersaturated 5AØ222C
    Intermittent
      Balloon Pump 5AØ211Ø
      Impeller Pump 5AØ211D
      Other Pump 5AØ2116
      Pulsatile Compression 5AØ2115
  Circulatory
    Continuous, Oxygenation, Hyperbaric
      5AØ5221
    Intermittent, Oxygenation, Hyperbaric
      5AØ5121
  Respiratory
    24-96 Consecutive Hours
      Continuous Negative Airway Pressure
        5AØ9459
      Continuous Positive Airway Pressure
        5AØ9457
      High Nasal Flow/Velocity 5AØ945A
      Intermittent Negative Airway Pressure
        5AØ945B
      Intermittent Positive Airway Pressure
        5AØ9458
      No Qualifier 5AØ945Z
    8-24 Consecutive Hours, Ventilation, Intubat-
      ed Prone Positioning 5AØ9C5K
    Continuous, Filtration 5AØ92ØZ
    Greater than 24 Consecutive Hours, Ventila-
      tion, Intubated Prone Positioning
      5AØ9D5K
    Greater than 96 Consecutive Hours
      Continuous Negative Airway Pressure
        5AØ9559
      Continuous Positive Airway Pressure
        5AØ9557
      High Nasal Flow/Velocity 5AØ955A
      Intermittent Negative Airway Pressure
        5AØ955B
      Intermittent Positive Airway Pressure
        5AØ9558
      No Qualifier 5AØ955Z
    Less than 24 Consecutive Hours
      Continuous Negative Airway Pressure
        5AØ9359
      Continuous Positive Airway Pressure
        5AØ9357
      High Nasal Flow/Velocity 5AØ935A
      Intermittent Negative Airway Pressure
        5AØ935B
      Intermittent Positive Airway Pressure
        5AØ9358
      No Qualifier 5AØ935Z
    Less than 8 Consecutive Hours, Ventilation,
      Intubated Prone Positioning 5AØ9B5K
**Associating liver partition and portal vein ligation
  (ALPPS)**
  see Division, Hepatobiliary System and Pancreas
    ØF8
  see Resection, Hepatobiliary System and Pancreas
    ØFT
Assurant (Cobalt) stent *use* Intraluminal Device
Atezolizumab Antineoplastic XWØ
Atherectomy
  see Extirpation, Heart and Great Vessels Ø2C
  see Extirpation, Lower Arteries Ø4C
  see Extirpation, Upper Arteries Ø3C
Atlantoaxial joint *use* Cervical Vertebral Joint
Atmospheric Control 6AØZ
AtriClip LAA Exclusion System *use* Extraluminal De-
  vice
Atrioseptoplasty
  see Repair, Heart and Great Vessels Ø2Q
  see Replacement, Heart and Great Vessels Ø2R
  see Supplement, Heart and Great Vessels Ø2U
Atrioventricular node *use* Conduction Mechanism
Atrium dextrum cordis *use* Atrium, Right
Atrium pulmonale *use* Atrium, Left
Attain Ability® lead Ø2H

Attain Ability® lead — *continued*
  use Cardiac Lead, Defibrillator in Ø2H
  use Cardiac Lead, Pacemaker in Ø2H
Attain Starfix® (OTW) lead
  use Cardiac Lead, Defibrillator in Ø2H
  use Cardiac Lead, Pacemaker in Ø2H
Audiology, diagnostic
  see Hearing Aid Assessment, Diagnostic Audiology
    F14
  see Hearing Assessment, Diagnostic Audiology
    F13
  see Vestibular Assessment, Diagnostic Audiology
    F15
Audiometry *see* Hearing Assessment, Diagnostic Audiology F13
Auditory tube
  use Eustachian Tube, Left
  use Eustachian Tube, Right
Auerbach's (myenteric) plexus *use* Abdominal Sympathetic Nerve
Auricle
  use External Ear, Bilateral
  use External Ear, Left
  use External Ear, Right
Auricularis muscle *use* Head Muscle
Autograft *use* Autologous Tissue Substitute
AutoLITT® System *see* Destruction
Autologous artery graft
  use Autologous Arterial Tissue in Heart and Great
    Vessels
  use Autologous Arterial Tissue in Lower Arteries
  use Autologous Arterial Tissue in Lower Veins
  use Autologous Arterial Tissue in Upper Arteries
  use Autologous Arterial Tissue in Upper Veins
Autologous vein graft
  use Autologous Venous Tissue in Heart and Great
    Vessels
  use Autologous Venous Tissue in Lower Arteries
  use Autologous Venous Tissue in Lower Veins
  use Autologous Venous Tissue in Upper Arteries
  use Autologous Venous Tissue in Upper Veins
Automated Chest Compression (ACC) 5A1221J
AutoPulse® Resuscitation System 5A1221J
Autotransfusion *see* Transfusion
Autotransplant
  Adrenal tissue *see* Reposition, Endocrine System
    ØGS
  Kidney *see* Reposition, Urinary System ØTS
  Pancreatic tissue *see* Reposition, Pancreas ØFSG
  Parathyroid tissue *see* Reposition, Endocrine Sys-
    tem ØGS
  Thyroid tissue *see* Reposition, Endocrine System
    ØGS
  Tooth *see* Reattachment, Mouth and Throat ØCM
Aveir™ AR, as dual chamber *use* Intracardiac Pace-
  maker, Dual-Chamber in New Technology
Aveir™ DR, dual chamber *use* Intracardiac Pacemaker,
  Dual-Chamber in New Technology
Aveir™ VR, as single chamber *use* Intracardiac Pace-
  maker in Heart and Great Vessels
Avulsion *see* Extraction
AVYCAZ® (ceftazidime-avibactam) *use* Other Anti-
  infective
Axial Lumbar Interbody Fusion System *use* Inter-
  body Fusion Device in Lower Joints
AxiaLIF® System *use* Interbody Fusion Device in Lower
  Joints
Axicabtagene Ciloleucel *use* Axicabtagene Ciloleucel
  Immunotherapy
Axicabtagene Ciloleucel Immunotherapy XWØ
Axillary fascia
  use Subcutaneous Tissue and Fascia, Left Upper
    Arm
  use Subcutaneous Tissue and Fascia, Right Upper
    Arm
Axillary nerve *use* Brachial Plexus
AZEDRA® *use* Iobenguane I-131 Antineoplastic

B

BAK/C® Interbody Cervical Fusion System *use* Inter-
  body Fusion Device in Upper Joints
BAL (bronchial alveolar lavage), diagnostic *see*
  Drainage, Respiratory System ØB9
Balanoplasty
  see Repair, Penis ØVQS

Balanoplasty — *continued*
see Supplement, Penis ØVUS
Balloon atrial septostomy (BAS) Ø2163Z7
Balloon Pump
Continuous, Output 5AØ221Ø
Intermittent, Output 5AØ211Ø
Bamlanivimab Monoclonal Antibody XWØ
Bandage, Elastic *see* Compression
Banding
see Occlusion
see Restriction
Banding, esophageal varices *see* Occlusion, Vein, Esophageal Ø6L3
Banding, laparoscopic (adjustable) gastric
Initial procedure ØDV64CZ
Surgical correction *see* Revision of device in, Stomach ØDW6
Bard® Composix® Kugel® patch *use* Synthetic Substitute
Bard® Composix® (E/X) (LP) mesh *use* Synthetic Substitute
Bard® Dulex™ mesh *use* Synthetic Substitute
Bard® Ventralex™ hernia patch *use* Synthetic Substitute
Baricitinib XWØ
Barium swallow *see* Fluoroscopy, Gastrointestinal System BD1
Baroreflex Activation Therapy® (BAT®)
use Stimulator Generator in Subcutaneous Tissue and Fascia
use Stimulator Lead in Upper Arteries
Barricaid® Annular Closure Device (ACD) *use* Synthetic Substitute
Bartholin's (greater vestibular) gland *use* Vestibular Gland
Basal (internal) cerebral vein *use* Intracranial Vein
Basal metabolic rate (BMR) *see* Measurement, Physiological Systems 4AØZ
Basal nuclei *use* Basal Ganglia
Base of Tongue *use* Pharynx
Basilar artery *use* Intracranial Artery
Basis pontis *use* Pons
Beam Radiation
Abdomen DWØ3
Intraoperative DWØ33ZØ
Adrenal Gland DGØ2
Intraoperative DGØ23ZØ
Bile Ducts DFØ2
Intraoperative DFØ23ZØ
Bladder DTØ2
Intraoperative DTØ23ZØ
Bone
Intraoperative DPØC3ZØ
Other DPØC
Bone Marrow D7ØØ
Intraoperative D7ØØ3ZØ
Brain DØØØ
Intraoperative DØØØ3ZØ
Brain Stem DØØ1
Intraoperative DØØ13ZØ
Breast
Left DMØØ
Intraoperative DMØØ3ZØ
Right DMØ1
Intraoperative DMØ13ZØ
Bronchus DBØ1
Intraoperative DBØ13ZØ
Cervix DUØ1
Intraoperative DUØ13ZØ
Chest DWØ2
Intraoperative DWØ23ZØ
Chest Wall DBØ7
Intraoperative DBØ73ZØ
Colon DDØ5
Intraoperative DDØ53ZØ
Diaphragm DBØ8
Intraoperative DBØ83ZØ
Duodenum DDØ2
Intraoperative DDØ23ZØ
Ear D9ØØ
Intraoperative D9ØØ3ZØ
Esophagus DDØØ
Intraoperative DDØØ3ZØ
Eye D8ØØ
Intraoperative D8ØØ3ZØ
Femur DPØ9
Intraoperative DPØ93ZØ
Fibula DPØB

Beam Radiation — *continued*
Fibula — *continued*
Intraoperative DPØB3ZØ
Gallbladder DFØ1
Intraoperative DFØ13ZØ
Gland
Adrenal DGØ2
Intraoperative DGØ23ZØ
Parathyroid DGØ4
Intraoperative DGØ43ZØ
Pituitary DGØØ
Intraoperative DGØØ3ZØ
Thyroid DGØ5
Intraoperative DGØ53ZØ
Glands
Intraoperative D9Ø63ZØ
Salivary D9Ø6
Head and Neck DWØ1
Intraoperative DWØ13ZØ
Hemibody DWØ4
Intraoperative DWØ43ZØ
Humerus DPØ6
Intraoperative DPØ63ZØ
Hypopharynx D9Ø3
Intraoperative D9Ø33ZØ
Ileum DDØ4
Intraoperative DDØ43ZØ
Jejunum DDØ3
Intraoperative DDØ33ZØ
Kidney DTØØ
Intraoperative DTØØ3ZØ
Larynx D9ØB
Intraoperative D9ØB3ZØ
Liver DFØØ
Intraoperative DFØØ3ZØ
Lung DBØ2
Intraoperative DBØ23ZØ
Lymphatics
Abdomen D7Ø6
Intraoperative D7Ø63ZØ
Axillary D7Ø4
Intraoperative D7Ø43ZØ
Inguinal D7Ø8
Intraoperative D7Ø83ZØ
Neck D7Ø3
Intraoperative D7Ø33ZØ
Pelvis D7Ø7
Intraoperative D7Ø73ZØ
Thorax D7Ø5
Intraoperative D7Ø53ZØ
Mandible DPØ3
Intraoperative DPØ33ZØ
Maxilla DPØ2
Intraoperative DPØ23ZØ
Mediastinum DBØ6
Intraoperative DBØ63ZØ
Mouth D9Ø4
Intraoperative D9Ø43ZØ
Nasopharynx D9ØD
Intraoperative D9ØD3ZØ
Neck and Head DWØ1
Intraoperative DWØ13ZØ
Nerve
Intraoperative DØØ73ZØ
Peripheral DØØ7
Nose D9Ø1
Intraoperative D9Ø13ZØ
Oropharynx D9ØF
Intraoperative D9ØF3ZØ
Ovary DUØØ
Intraoperative DUØØ3ZØ
Palate
Hard D9Ø8
Intraoperative D9Ø83ZØ
Soft D9Ø9
Intraoperative D9Ø93ZØ
Pancreas DFØ3
Intraoperative DFØ33ZØ
Parathyroid Gland DGØ4
Intraoperative DGØ43ZØ
Pelvic Bones DPØ8
Intraoperative DPØ83ZØ
Pelvic Region DWØ6
Intraoperative DWØ63ZØ
Pineal Body DGØ1
Intraoperative DGØ13ZØ
Pituitary Gland DGØØ
Intraoperative DGØØ3ZØ
Pleura DBØ5

Beam Radiation — *continued*
Pleura — *continued*
Intraoperative DBØ53ZØ
Prostate DVØØ
Intraoperative DVØØ3ZØ
Radius DPØ7
Intraoperative DPØ73ZØ
Rectum DDØ7
Intraoperative DDØ73ZØ
Rib DPØ5
Intraoperative DPØ53ZØ
Sinuses D9Ø7
Intraoperative D9Ø73ZØ
Skin
Abdomen DHØ8
Intraoperative DHØ83ZØ
Arm DHØ4
Intraoperative DHØ43ZØ
Back DHØ7
Intraoperative DHØ73ZØ
Buttock DHØ9
Intraoperative DHØ93ZØ
Chest DHØ6
Intraoperative DHØ63ZØ
Face DHØ2
Intraoperative DHØ23ZØ
Leg DHØB
Intraoperative DHØB3ZØ
Neck DHØ3
Intraoperative DHØ33ZØ
Skull DPØØ
Intraoperative DPØØ3ZØ
Spinal Cord DØØ6
Intraoperative DØØ63ZØ
Spleen D7Ø2
Intraoperative D7Ø23ZØ
Sternum DPØ4
Intraoperative DPØ43ZØ
Stomach DDØ1
Intraoperative DDØ13ZØ
Testis DVØ1
Intraoperative DVØ13ZØ
Thymus D7Ø1
Intraoperative D7Ø13ZØ
Thyroid Gland DGØ5
Intraoperative DGØ53ZØ
Tibia DPØB
Intraoperative DPØB3ZØ
Tongue D9Ø5
Intraoperative D9Ø53ZØ
Trachea DBØØ
Intraoperative DBØØ3ZØ
Ulna DPØ7
Intraoperative DPØ73ZØ
Ureter DTØ1
Intraoperative DTØ13ZØ
Urethra DTØ3
Intraoperative DTØ33ZØ
Uterus DUØ2
Intraoperative DUØ23ZØ
Whole Body DWØ5
Intraoperative DWØ53ZØ
Bedside swallow FØØZJWZ
Berlin Heart Ventricular Assist Device *use* Implantable Heart Assist System in Heart and Great Vessels
Betibeglogene Autotemcel XW1
beti-cel *use* Betibeglogene Autotemcel
Bezlotoxumab infusion *see* Introduction with qualifier Other Therapeutic Monoclonal Antibody
Biceps brachii muscle
use Upper Arm Muscle, Left
use Upper Arm Muscle, Right
Biceps femoris muscle
use Upper Leg Muscle, Left
use Upper Leg Muscle, Right
Bicipital aponeurosis
use Subcutaneous Tissue and Fascia, Left Lower Arm
use Subcutaneous Tissue and Fascia, Right Lower Arm
Bicuspid valve *use* Mitral Valve
Bili light therapy *see* Phototherapy, Skin 6A6Ø
Bioactive embolization coil(s) *use* Intraluminal Device, Bioactive in Upper Arteries
Bioengineered Allogeneic Construct, Skin XHRPXF7
Biofeedback GZC9ZZZ
BioFire® FilmArray® Pneumonia Panel XXEBXQ6

Subterms under main terms may continue to next column or page

Biopsy
see Drainage with qualifier Diagnostic
see Excision with qualifier Diagnostic
see Extraction with qualifier Diagnostic
BiPAP see Assistance, Respiratory 5A09
Bisection see Division
Biventricular external heart assist system use Short-term External Heart Assist System in Heart and Great Vessels
Blepharectomy
see Excision, Eye 08B
see Resection, Eye 08T
Blepharoplasty
see Repair, Eye 08Q
see Replacement, Eye 08R
see Reposition, Eye 08S
see Supplement, Eye 08U
Blepharorrhaphy see Repair, Eye 08Q
Blepharotomy see Drainage, Eye 089
Blinatumomab use Other Antineoplastic
BLINCYTO® (blinatumomab) use Other Antineoplastic
Block, Nerve, anesthetic injection 3E0T3BZ
Blood glucose monitoring system use Monitoring Device
Blood pressure see Measurement, Arterial 4A03
BMR (basal metabolic rate) see Measurement, Physiological Systems 4A0Z
Body of femur
use Femoral Shaft, Left
use Femoral Shaft, Right
Body of fibula
use Fibula, Left
use Fibula, Right
Bone anchored hearing device
use Hearing Device, Bone Conduction in 09H
use Hearing Device in Head and Facial Bones
Bone bank bone graft use Nonautologous Tissue Substitute
Bone Growth Stimulator
Insertion of device in
Bone
Facial 0NHW
Lower 0QHY
Nasal 0NHB
Upper 0PHY
Skull 0NH0
Removal of device from
Bone
Facial 0NPW
Lower 0QPY
Nasal 0NPB
Upper 0PPY
Skull 0NP0
Revision of device in
Bone
Facial 0NWW
Lower 0QWY
Nasal 0NWB
Upper 0PWY
Skull 0NW0
Bone marrow transplant see Transfusion, Circulatory 302
Bone morphogenetic protein 2 (BMP 2) use Recombinant Bone Morphogenetic Protein
Bone screw (interlocking) (lag) (pedicle) (recessed)
use Internal Fixation Device in Head and Facial Bones
use Internal Fixation Device in Lower Bones
use Internal Fixation Device in Upper Bones
Bony labyrinth
use Inner Ear, Left
use Inner Ear, Right
Bony orbit
use Orbit, Left
use Orbit, Right
Bony vestibule
use Inner Ear, Left
use Inner Ear, Right
Botallo's duct use Pulmonary Artery, Left
Bovine pericardial valve use Zooplastic Tissue in Heart and Great Vessels
Bovine pericardium graft use Zooplastic Tissue in Heart and Great Vessels
BP (blood pressure) see Measurement, Arterial 4A03
Brachial (lateral) lymph node
use Lymphatic, Left Axillary
use Lymphatic, Right Axillary

Brachialis muscle
use Upper Arm Muscle, Left
use Upper Arm Muscle, Right
Brachiocephalic artery use Innominate Artery
Brachiocephalic trunk use Innominate Artery
Brachiocephalic vein
use Innominate Vein, Left
use Innominate Vein, Right
Brachioradialis muscle
use Lower Arm and Wrist Muscle, Left
use Lower Arm and Wrist Muscle, Right
Brachytherapy
Abdomen DW13
Adrenal Gland DG12
Back
Lower DW1LBB
Upper DW1KBB
Bile Ducts DF12
Bladder DT12
Bone Marrow D710
Brain D010
Brain Stem D011
Breast
Left DM10
Right DM11
Bronchus DB11
Cervix DU11
Chest DW12
Chest Wall DB17
Colon DD15
Cranial Cavity DW10BB
Diaphragm DB18
Duodenum DD12
Ear D910
Esophagus DD10
Extremity
Lower DW1YBB
Upper DW1XBB
Eye D810
Gallbladder DF11
Gastrointestinal Tract DW1PBB
Genitourinary Tract DW1RBB
Gland
Adrenal DG12
Parathyroid DG14
Pituitary DG10
Thyroid DG15
Glands, Salivary D916
Head and Neck DW11
Hypopharynx D913
Ileum DD14
Jejunum DD13
Kidney DT10
Larynx D91B
Liver DF10
Lung DB12
Lymphatics
Abdomen D716
Axillary D714
Inguinal D718
Neck D713
Pelvis D717
Thorax D715
Mediastinum DB16
Mouth D914
Nasopharynx D91D
Neck and Head DW11
Nerve, Peripheral D017
Nose D911
Oropharynx D91F
Ovary DU10
Palate
Hard D918
Soft D919
Pancreas DF13
Parathyroid Gland DG14
Pelvic Region DW16
Pineal Body DG11
Pituitary Gland DG10
Pleura DB15
Prostate DV10
Rectum DD17
Respiratory Tract DW1QBB
Sinuses D917
Spinal Cord D016
Spleen D712
Stomach DD11
Testis DV11

Brachytherapy — continued
Thymus D711
Thyroid Gland DG15
Tongue D915
Trachea DB10
Ureter DT11
Urethra DT13
Uterus DU12
Brachytherapy, CivaSheet®
see Brachytherapy with qualifier Unidirectional Source
see Insertion with device Radioactive Element
Brachytherapy seeds use Radioactive Element
Brain Electrical Activity
Computer-aided Detection and Notification XX20X89
Computer-aided Semiologic Analysis XXE0X48
Breast procedures, skin only use Skin, Chest
Brexanolone XW0
Brexucabtagene Autoleucel use Brexucabtagene Autoleucel Immunotherapy
Brexucabtagene Autoleucel Immunotherapy XW0
Breyanzi® use Lisocabtagene Maraleucel Immunotherapy
Broad Consortium Microbiota-based Live Biotherapeutic Suspension XW0H7X8
Broad ligament use Uterine Supporting Structure
Bromelain-enriched Proteolytic Enzyme use Anacaulase-bcdb
Bronchial artery use Upper Artery
Bronchography
see Fluoroscopy, Respiratory System BB1
see Plain Radiography, Respiratory System BB0
Bronchoplasty
see Repair, Respiratory System 0BQ
see Supplement, Respiratory System 0BU
Bronchorrhaphy see Repair, Respiratory System 0BQ
Bronchoscopy 0BJ08ZZ
Bronchotomy see Drainage, Respiratory System 0B9
Bronchus Intermedius use Main Bronchus, Right
BRYAN® Cervical Disc System use Synthetic Substitute
Buccal gland use Buccal Mucosa
Buccinator lymph node use Lymphatic, Head
Buccinator muscle use Facial Muscle
Buckling, scleral with implant see Supplement, Eye 08U
Bulbospongiosus muscle use Perineum Muscle
Bulbourethral (Cowper's) gland use Urethra
Bundle of His use Conduction Mechanism
Bundle of Kent use Conduction Mechanism
Bunionectomy see Excision, Lower Bones 0QB
Bursectomy
see Excision, Bursae and Ligaments 0MB
see Resection, Bursae and Ligaments 0MT
Bursocentesis see Drainage, Bursae and Ligaments 0M9
Bursography
see Plain Radiography, Non-Axial Lower Bones BQ0
see Plain Radiography, Non-Axial Upper Bones BP0
Bursotomy
see Division, Bursae and Ligaments 0M8
see Drainage, Bursae and Ligaments 0M9
BVS 5000 Ventricular Assist Device use Short-term External Heart Assist System in Heart and Great Vessels
Bypass
Anterior Chamber
Left 08133
Right 08123
Aorta
Abdominal 0410
Thoracic
Ascending/Arch 021X
Descending 021W
Artery
Anterior Tibial
Left 041Q
Right 041P
Axillary
Left 03160
Right 03150
Brachial
Left 0318
Right 0317
Common Carotid
Left 031J0
Right 031H0

Bypass — *continued*
  Artery — *continued*
    Common Iliac
      Left 041D
      Right 041C
    Coronary
      Four or More Arteries 0213
      One Artery 0210
      Three Arteries 0212
      Two Arteries 0211
    External Carotid
      Left 031N0
      Right 031M0
    External Iliac
      Left 041J
      Right 041H
    Femoral
      Left 041L
      Right 041K
    Foot
      Left 041W
      Right 041V
    Hepatic 0413
    Innominate 03120
    Internal Carotid
      Left 031L0
      Right 031K0
    Internal Iliac
      Left 041F
      Right 041E
    Intracranial 031G0
    Peroneal
      Left 041U
      Right 041T
    Popliteal
      Left 041N
      Right 041M
    Posterior Tibial
      Left 041S
      Right 041R
    Pulmonary
      Left 021R
      Right 021Q
    Pulmonary Trunk 021P
    Radial
      Left 031C
      Right 031B
    Splenic 0414
    Subclavian
      Left 03140
      Right 03130
    Temporal
      Left 031T0
      Right 031S0
    Ulnar
      Left 031A
      Right 0319
  Atrium
    Left 0217
    Right 0216
  Bladder 0T1B
  Cavity, Cranial 0W110J
  Cecum 0D1H
  Cerebral Ventricle 0016
  Colon
    Ascending 0D1K
    Descending 0D1M
    Sigmoid 0D1N
    Transverse 0D1L
  Conduit through Femoral Vein to Popliteal Artery X2K
  Conduit through Femoral Vein to Superficial Femoral Artery X2K
  Duct
    Common Bile 0F19
    Cystic 0F18
    Hepatic
      Common 0F17
      Left 0F16
      Right 0F15
    Lacrimal
      Left 081Y
      Right 081X
    Pancreatic 0F1D
      Accessory 0F1F
  Duodenum 0D19
  Ear
    Left 091E0
    Right 091D0

Bypass — *continued*
  Esophagus 0D15
    Lower 0D13
    Middle 0D12
    Upper 0D11
  Fallopian Tube
    Left 0U16
    Right 0U15
  Gallbladder 0F14
  Ileum 0D1B
  Intestine
    Large 0D1E
    Small 0D18
  Jejunum 0D1A
  Kidney Pelvis
    Left 0T14
    Right 0T13
  Pancreas 0F1G
  Pelvic Cavity 0W1J
  Peritoneal Cavity 0W1G
  Pleural Cavity
    Left 0W1B
    Right 0W19
  Spinal Canal 001U
  Stomach 0D16
  Trachea 0B11
  Ureter
    Left 0T17
    Right 0T16
  Ureters, Bilateral 0T18
  Vas Deferens
    Bilateral 0V1Q
    Left 0V1P
    Right 0V1N
  Vein
    Axillary
      Left 0518
      Right 0517
    Azygos 0510
    Basilic
      Left 051C
      Right 051B
    Brachial
      Left 051A
      Right 0519
    Cephalic
      Left 051F
      Right 051D
    Colic 0617
    Common Iliac
      Left 061D
      Right 061C
    Esophageal 0613
    External Iliac
      Left 061G
      Right 061F
    External Jugular
      Left 051Q
      Right 051P
    Face
      Left 051V
      Right 051T
    Femoral
      Left 061N
      Right 061M
    Foot
      Left 061V
      Right 061T
    Gastric 0612
    Hand
      Left 051H
      Right 051G
    Hemiazygos 0511
    Hepatic 0614
    Hypogastric
      Left 061J
      Right 061H
    Inferior Mesenteric 0616
    Innominate
      Left 0514
      Right 0513
    Internal Jugular
      Left 051N
      Right 051M
    Intracranial 051L
    Portal 0618
    Renal
      Left 061B
      Right 0619

Bypass — *continued*
  Vein — *continued*
    Saphenous
      Left 061Q
      Right 061P
    Splenic 0611
    Subclavian
      Left 0516
      Right 0515
    Superior Mesenteric 0615
    Vertebral
      Left 051S
      Right 051R
    Vena Cava
      Inferior 0610
      Superior 021V
    Ventricle
      Left 021L
      Right 021K
Bypass, cardiopulmonary 5A1221Z

C

Caesarean section *see* Extraction, Products of Conception 10D0
Calcaneocuboid joint
  use Tarsal Joint, Left
  use Tarsal Joint, Right
Calcaneocuboid ligament
  use Foot Bursa and Ligament, Left
  use Foot Bursa and Ligament, Right
Calcaneofibular ligament
  use Ankle Bursa and Ligament, Left
  use Ankle Bursa and Ligament, Right
Calcaneus
  use Tarsal, Left
  use Tarsal, Right
Cannulation
  see Bypass
  see Dilation
  see Drainage
  see Irrigation
Canthorrhaphy *see* Repair, Eye 08Q
Canthotomy *see* Release, Eye 08N
Canturio™ te (Tibial Extension) *use* Tibial Extension with Motion Sensors in New Technology
Capitate bone
  use Carpal, Left
  use Carpal, Right
Caplacizumab XW0
Capsulectomy, lens *see* Excision, Eye 08B
Capsulorrhaphy, joint
  see Repair, Lower Joints 0SQ
  see Repair, Upper Joints 0RQ
Caption Guidance system X2JAX47
Cardia *use* Esophagogastric Junction
Cardiac contractility modulation lead *use* Cardiac Lead in Heart and Great Vessels
Cardiac event recorder *use* Monitoring Device
Cardiac Lead
  Defibrillator
    Atrium
      Left 02H7
      Right 02H6
    Pericardium 02HN
    Vein, Coronary 02H4
    Ventricle
      Left 02HL
      Right 02HK
  Insertion of device in
    Atrium
      Left 02H7
      Right 02H6
    Pericardium 02HN
    Vein, Coronary 02H4
    Ventricle
      Left 02HL
      Right 02HK
  Pacemaker
    Atrium
      Left 02H7
      Right 02H6
    Pericardium 02HN
    Vein, Coronary 02H4
    Ventricle
      Left 02HL
      Right 02HK

Cardiac Lead — *continued*
  Removal of device from, Heart Ø2PA
  Revision of device in, Heart Ø2WA
Cardiac plexus *use* Thoracic Sympathetic Nerve
Cardiac Resynchronization Defibrillator Pulse Generator
  Abdomen ØJH8
  Chest ØJH6
Cardiac Resynchronization Pacemaker Pulse Generator
  Abdomen ØJH8
  Chest ØJH6
Cardiac resynchronization therapy (CRT) lead
  use Cardiac Lead, Defibrillator in Ø2H
  use Cardiac Lead, Pacemaker in Ø2H
Cardiac Rhythm Related Device
  Insertion of device in
    Abdomen ØJH8
    Chest ØJH6
  Removal of device from, Subcutaneous Tissue and Fascia, Trunk ØJPT
  Revision of device in, Subcutaneous Tissue and Fascia, Trunk ØJWT
Cardiocentesis *see* Drainage, Pericardial Cavity ØW9D
Cardioesophageal junction *use* Esophagogastric Junction
Cardiolysis *see* Release, Heart and Great Vessels Ø2N
CardioMEMS® pressure sensor *use* Monitoring Device, Pressure Sensor in Ø2H
Cardiomyotomy *see* Division, Esophagogastric Junction ØD84
Cardioplegia *see* Introduction of substance in or on, Heart 3EØ8
Cardiorrhaphy *see* Repair, Heart and Great Vessels Ø2Q
Cardioversion 5A22Ø4Z
Caregiver Training FØFZ
Carmat total artificial heart (TAH) *use* Biologic with Synthetic Substitute, Autoregulated Electrohydraulic in Ø2R
Caroticotympanic artery
  use Internal Carotid Artery, Left
  use Internal Carotid Artery, Right
Carotid glomus
  use Carotid Bodies, Bilateral
  use Carotid Body, Left
  use Carotid Body, Right
Carotid sinus
  use Internal Carotid Artery, Left
  use Internal Carotid Artery, Right
Carotid (artery) sinus (baroreceptor) lead *use* Stimulator Lead in Upper Arteries
Carotid sinus nerve *use* Glossopharyngeal Nerve
Carotid WALLSTENT® Monorail® Endoprosthesis *use* Intraluminal Device
Carpectomy
  see Excision, Upper Bones ØPB
  see Resection, Upper Bones ØPT
Carpometacarpal ligament
  use Hand Bursa and Ligament, Left
  use Hand Bursa and Ligament, Right
CARVYKTI™ *use* Ciltacabtagene Autoleucel
Casirivimab (REGN1Ø933) and Imdevimab (REGN1Ø987) *use* REGN-COV2 Monoclonal Antibody
Casting *see* Immobilization
CAT scan *see* Computerized Tomography (CT Scan)
Catheterization
  see Dilation
  see Drainage
  see Insertion of device in
  see Irrigation
  Heart *see* Measurement, Cardiac 4AØ2
  Umbilical vein, for infusion Ø6HØ33T
Cauda equina *use* Lumbar Spinal Cord
Cauterization
  see Destruction
  see Repair
Cavernous plexus *use* Head and Neck Sympathetic Nerve
Cavoatrial junction *use* Superior Vena Cava
CBMA (Concentrated Bone Marrow Aspirate) *use* Other Substance
CBMA (Concentrated Bone Marrow Aspirate) injection *see* Introduction of substance in or on, Muscle 3EØ2
CD24Fc Immunomodulator XWØ

Cecectomy
  see Excision, Cecum ØDBH
  see Resection, Cecum ØDTH
Cecocolostomy
  see Bypass, Gastrointestinal System ØD1
  see Drainage, Gastrointestinal System ØD9
Cecopexy
  see Repair, Cecum ØDQH
  see Reposition, Cecum ØDSH
Cecoplication *see* Restriction, Cecum ØDVH
Cecorrhaphy *see* Repair, Cecum ØDQH
Cecostomy
  see Bypass, Cecum ØD1H
  see Drainage, Cecum ØD9H
Cecotomy *see* Drainage, Cecum ØD9H
Cefiderocol Anti-infective XWØ
Ceftazidime-avibactam *use* Other Anti-infective
Ceftolozane/Tazobactam Anti-infective XWØ
Celiac ganglion *use* Abdominal Sympathetic Nerve
Celiac lymph node *use* Lymphatic, Aortic
Celiac (solar) plexus *use* Abdominal Sympathetic Nerve
Celiac trunk *use* Celiac Artery
Central axillary lymph node
  use Lymphatic, Left Axillary
  use Lymphatic, Right Axillary
Central venous pressure *see* Measurement, Venous 4AØ4
Centrimag® Blood Pump *use* Short-term External Heart Assist System in Heart and Great Vessels
Cephalogram BNØØZZZ
CERAMENT® G *use* Antibiotic-eluting Bone Void Filler
Ceramic on ceramic bearing surface *use* Synthetic Substitute, Ceramic in ØSR
Cerclage *see* Restriction
Cerebral aqueduct (Sylvius) *use* Cerebral Ventricle
Cerebral Embolic Filtration
  Dual Filter X2A5312
  Extracorporeal Flow Reversal Circuit X2A
  Single Deflection Filter X2A6325
Cerebrum *use* Brain
Ceribell® Monitor XX2ØX89
Cervical esophagus *use* Esophagus, Upper
Cervical facet joint
  use Cervical Vertebral Joint
  use Cervical Vertebral Joint, 2 or more
Cervical ganglion *use* Head and Neck Sympathetic Nerve
Cervical interspinous ligament *use* Head and Neck Bursa and Ligament
Cervical intertransverse ligament *use* Head and Neck Bursa and Ligament
Cervical Ligamentum Flavum *use* Head and Neck Bursa and Ligament
Cervical Lymph Node
  use Lymphatic, Left Neck
  use Lymphatic, Right Neck
Cervicectomy
  see Excision, Cervix ØUBC
  see Resection, Cervix ØUTC
Cervicothoracic facet joint *use* Cervicothoracic Vertebral Joint
Cesarean section *see* Extraction, Products of Conception 1ØDØ
Cesium-131 Collagen Implant *use* Radioactive Element, Cesium-131 Collagen Implant in ØØH
Change Device in
  Abdominal Wall ØW2FX
  Back
    Lower ØW2LX
    Upper ØW2KX
  Bladder ØT2BX
  Bone
    Facial ØN2WX
    Lower ØQ2YX
    Nasal ØN2BX
    Upper ØP2YX
  Bone Marrow Ø72TX
  Brain ØØ2ØX
  Breast
    Left ØH2UX
    Right ØH2TX
  Bursa and Ligament
    Lower ØM2YX
    Upper ØM2XX
  Cavity, Cranial ØW21X
  Chest Wall ØW28X

Change Device in — *continued*
  Cisterna Chyli Ø72LX
  Diaphragm ØB2TX
  Duct
    Hepatobiliary ØF2BX
    Pancreatic ØF2DX
  Ear
    Left Ø92JX
    Right Ø92HX
  Epididymis and Spermatic Cord ØV2MX
  Extremity
    Lower
      Left ØY2BX
      Right ØY29X
    Upper
      Left ØX27X
      Right ØX26X
  Eye
    Left Ø821X
    Right Ø82ØX
  Face ØW22X
  Fallopian Tube ØU28X
  Gallbladder ØF24X
  Gland
    Adrenal ØG25X
    Endocrine ØG2SX
    Pituitary ØG2ØX
    Salivary ØC2AX
  Head ØW2ØX
  Intestinal Tract
    Lower Intestinal Tract ØD2DXUZ
    Upper Intestinal Tract ØD2ØXUZ
  Jaw
    Lower ØW25X
    Upper ØW24X
  Joint
    Lower ØS2YX
    Upper ØR2YX
  Kidney ØT25X
  Larynx ØC2SX
  Liver ØF2ØX
  Lung
    Left ØB2LX
    Right ØB2KX
  Lymphatic Ø72NX
    Thoracic Duct Ø72KX
  Mediastinum ØW2CX
  Mesentery ØD2VX
  Mouth and Throat ØC2YX
  Muscle
    Lower ØK2YX
    Upper ØK2XX
  Nasal Mucosa and Soft Tissue Ø92KX
  Neck ØW26X
  Nerve
    Cranial ØØ2EX
    Peripheral Ø12YX
  Omentum ØD2UX
  Ovary ØU23X
  Pancreas ØF2GX
  Parathyroid Gland ØG2RX
  Pelvic Cavity ØW2JX
  Penis ØV2SX
  Pericardial Cavity ØW2DX
  Perineum
    Female ØW2NX
    Male ØW2MX
  Peritoneal Cavity ØW2GX
  Peritoneum ØD2WX
  Pineal Body ØG21X
  Pleura ØB2QX
  Pleural Cavity
    Left ØW2BX
    Right ØW29X
  Products of Conception 1Ø2Ø7
  Prostate and Seminal Vesicles ØV24X
  Retroperitoneum ØW2HX
  Scrotum and Tunica Vaginalis ØV28X
  Sinus Ø92YX
  Skin ØH2PX
  Skull ØN2ØX
  Spinal Canal ØØ2UX
  Spleen Ø72PX
  Subcutaneous Tissue and Fascia
    Head and Neck ØJ2SX
    Lower Extremity ØJ2WX
    Trunk ØJ2TX
    Upper Extremity ØJ2VX

Index

Change Device in — Colpopexy

Change Device in — *continued*
    Tendon
        Lower ØL2YX
        Upper ØL2XX
    Testis ØV2DX
    Thymus Ø72MX
    Thyroid Gland ØG2KX
    Trachea ØB21
    Tracheobronchial Tree ØB2ØX
    Ureter ØT29X
    Urethra ØT2DX
    Uterus and Cervix ØU2DXHZ
    Vagina and Cul-de-sac ØU2HXGZ
    Vas Deferens ØV2RX
    Vulva ØU2MX
Change Device in or on
    Abdominal Wall 2WØ3X
    Anorectal 2YØ3X5Z
    Arm
        Lower
            Left 2WØDX
            Right 2WØCX
        Upper
            Left 2WØBX
            Right 2WØAX
    Back 2WØ5X
    Chest Wall 2WØ4X
    Ear 2YØ2X5Z
    Extremity
        Lower
            Left 2WØMX
            Right 2WØLX
        Upper
            Left 2WØ9X
            Right 2WØ8X
    Face 2WØ1X
    Finger
        Left 2WØKX
        Right 2WØJX
    Foot
        Left 2WØTX
        Right 2WØSX
    Genital Tract, Female 2YØ4X5Z
    Hand
        Left 2WØFX
        Right 2WØEX
    Head 2WØØX
    Inguinal Region
        Left 2WØ7X
        Right 2WØ6X
    Leg
        Lower
            Left 2WØRX
            Right 2WØQX
        Upper
            Left 2WØPX
            Right 2WØNX
    Mouth and Pharynx 2YØØX5Z
    Nasal 2YØ1X5Z
    Neck 2WØ2X
    Thumb
        Left 2WØHX
        Right 2WØGX
    Toe
        Left 2WØVX
        Right 2WØUX
    Urethra 2YØ5X5Z
Chemoembolization *see* Introduction of substance in or on
Chemosurgery, Skin 3EØØXTZ
Chemothalamectomy *see* Destruction, Thalamus ØØ59
Chemotherapy, Infusion for Cancer *see* Introduction of substance in or on
Chest compression (CPR), external
    Manual 5A12Ø12
    Mechanical 5A1221J
Chest x-ray *see* Plain Radiography, Chest BWØ3
Chin *use* Subcutaneous Tissue and Fascia, Face
Chiropractic Manipulation
    Abdomen 9WB9X
    Cervical 9WB1X
    Extremities
        Lower 9WB6X
        Upper 9WB7X
    Head 9WBØX
    Lumbar 9WB3X
    Pelvis 9WB5X
    Rib Cage 9WB8X

Chiropractic Manipulation — *continued*
    Sacrum 9WB4X
    Thoracic 9WB2X
Choana *use* Nasopharynx
Cholangiogram
    see Fluoroscopy, Hepatobiliary System and Pancreas BF1
    see Plain Radiography, Hepatobiliary System and Pancreas BFØ
Cholecystectomy
    see Excision, Gallbladder ØFB4
    see Resection, Gallbladder ØFT4
Cholecystojejunostomy
    see Bypass, Hepatobiliary System and Pancreas ØF1
    see Drainage, Hepatobiliary System and Pancreas ØF9
Cholecystopexy
    see Repair, Gallbladder ØFQ4
    see Reposition, Gallbladder ØFS4
Cholecystoscopy ØFJ44ZZ
Cholecystostomy
    see Bypass, Gallbladder ØF14
    see Drainage, Gallbladder ØF94
Cholecystotomy *see* Drainage, Gallbladder ØF94
Choledochectomy
    see Excision, Hepatobiliary System and Pancreas ØFB
    see Resection, Hepatobiliary System and Pancreas ØFT
Choledocholithotomy *see* Extirpation, Duct, Common Bile ØFC9
Choledochoplasty
    see Repair, Hepatobiliary System and Pancreas ØFQ
    see Replacement, Hepatobiliary System and Pancreas ØFR
    see Supplement, Hepatobiliary System and Pancreas ØFU
Choledochoscopy ØFJB8ZZ
Choledochotomy *see* Drainage, Hepatobiliary System and Pancreas ØF9
Cholelithotomy *see* Extirpation, Hepatobiliary System and Pancreas ØFC
Chondrectomy
    see Excision, Lower Joints ØSB
    see Excision, Upper Joints ØRB
    Knee *see* Excision, Lower Joints ØSB
    Semilunar cartilage *see* Excision, Lower Joints ØSB
Chondroglossus muscle *use* Tongue, Palate, Pharynx Muscle
Chorda tympani *use* Facial Nerve
Chordotomy *see* Division, Central Nervous System and Cranial Nerves ØØ8
Choroid plexus *use* Cerebral Ventricle
Choroidectomy
    see Excision, Eye Ø8B
    see Resection, Eye Ø8T
Ciliary body
    use Eye, Left
    use Eye, Right
Ciliary ganglion *use* Head and Neck Sympathetic Nerve
Ciltacabtagene Autoleucel XWØ
cilta-cel *use* Ciltacabtagene Autoleucel
Circle of Willis *use* Intracranial Artery
Circumcision ØVTTXZZ
Circumflex iliac artery
    use Femoral Artery, Left
    use Femoral Artery, Right
CivaSheet® *use* Radioactive Element
CivaSheet® Brachytherapy
    see Brachytherapy with qualifier Unidirectional Source
    see Insertion with device Radioactive Element
Clamp and rod internal fixation system (CRIF)
    use Internal Fixation Device in Lower Bones
    use Internal Fixation Device in Upper Bones
Clamping *see* Occlusion
Claustrum *use* Basal Ganglia
Claviculectomy
    see Excision, Upper Bones ØPB
    see Resection, Upper Bones ØPT
Claviculotomy
    see Division, Upper Bones ØP8
    see Drainage, Upper Bones ØP9
Clipping, aneurysm
    see Occlusion using Extraluminal Device
    see Restriction using Extraluminal Device

Clitorectomy, clitoridectomy
    see Excision, Clitoris ØUBJ
    see Resection, Clitoris ØUTJ
Clolar *use* Clofarabine
Closure
    see Occlusion
    see Repair
Clysis *see* Introduction of substance in or on
Coagulation *see* Destruction
Coagulation Factor Xa, Inactivated XWØ
Coagulation Factor Xa, (Recombinant) Inactivated
    use Coagulation Factor Xa, Inactivated
COALESCE® radiolucent interbody fusion device
    use Interbody Fusion Device in Lower Joints
    use Interbody Fusion Device in Upper Joints
CoAxia NeuroFlo catheter *use* Intraluminal Device
Cobalt/chromium head and polyethylene socket
    use Synthetic Substitute, Metal on Polyethylene in ØSR
Cobalt/chromium head and socket *use* Synthetic Substitute, Metal in ØSR
Coccygeal body *use* Coccygeal Glomus
Coccygeus muscle
    use Trunk Muscle, Left
    use Trunk Muscle, Right
Cochlea
    use Inner Ear, Left
    use Inner Ear, Right
Cochlear implant (CI), multiple channel (electrode)
    use Hearing Device, Multiple Channel Cochlear Prosthesis in Ø9H
Cochlear implant (CI), single channel (electrode)
    use Hearing Device, Single Channel Cochlear Prosthesis in Ø9H
Cochlear Implant Treatment FØBZØ
Cochlear nerve *use* Acoustic Nerve
COGNIS® CRT-D *use* Cardiac Resynchronization Defibrillator Pulse Generator in ØJH
COHERE® radiolucent interbody fusion device
    use Interbody Fusion Device in Lower Joints
    use Interbody Fusion Device in Upper Joints
Colectomy
    see Excision, Gastrointestinal System ØDB
    see Resection, Gastrointestinal System ØDT
Collapse *see* Occlusion
Collection from
    Breast, Breast Milk 8EØHX62
    Indwelling Device
        Circulatory System
            Blood 8CØ2X6K
            Other Fluid 8CØ2X6L
        Nervous System
            Cerebrospinal Fluid 8CØ1X6J
            Other Fluid 8CØ1X6L
    Integumentary System, Breast Milk 8EØHX62
    Reproductive System, Male, Sperm 8EØVX63
Colocentesis *see* Drainage, Gastrointestinal System ØD9
Colofixation
    see Repair, Gastrointestinal System ØDQ
    see Reposition, Gastrointestinal System ØDS
Cololysis *see* Release, Gastrointestinal System ØDN
Colonic Z-Stent® *use* Intraluminal Device
Colonoscopy ØDJD8ZZ
Colopexy
    see Repair, Gastrointestinal System ØDQ
    see Reposition, Gastrointestinal System ØDS
Coloplication *see* Restriction, Gastrointestinal System ØDV
Coloproctectomy
    see Excision, Gastrointestinal System ØDB
    see Resection, Gastrointestinal System ØDT
Coloproctostomy
    see Bypass, Gastrointestinal System ØD1
    see Drainage, Gastrointestinal System ØD9
Colopuncture *see* Drainage, Gastrointestinal System ØD9
Colorrhaphy *see* Repair, Gastrointestinal System ØDQ
Colostomy
    see Bypass, Gastrointestinal System ØD1
    see Drainage, Gastrointestinal System ØD9
Colpectomy
    see Excision, Vagina ØUBG
    see Resection, Vagina ØUTG
Colpocentesis *see* Drainage, Vagina ØU9G
Colpopexy
    see Repair, Vagina ØUQG

Colpopexy — *continued*
  see Reposition, Vagina ØUSG
Colpoplasty
  see Repair, Vagina ØUQG
  see Supplement, Vagina ØUUG
Colporrhaphy *see* Repair, Vagina ØUQG
Colposcopy ØUJH8ZZ
Columella *use* Nasal Mucosa and Soft Tissue
COMIRNATY®
  use COVID-19 Vaccine
  use COVID-19 Vaccine Booster
  use COVID-19 Vaccine Dose 1
  use COVID-19 Vaccine Dose 2
  use COVID-19 Vaccine Dose 3
Common digital vein
  use Foot Vein, Left
  use Foot Vein, Right
Common facial vein
  use Face Vein, Left
  use Face Vein, Right
Common fibular nerve *use* Peroneal Nerve
Common hepatic artery *use* Hepatic Artery
Common iliac (subaortic) lymph node *use* Lymphatic, Pelvis
Common interosseous artery
  use Ulnar Artery, Left
  use Ulnar Artery, Right
Common peroneal nerve *use* Peroneal Nerve
Complete (SE) stent *use* Intraluminal Device
Compression
  see Restriction
  Abdominal Wall 2W13X
  Arm
    Lower
      Left 2W1DX
      Right 2W1CX
    Upper
      Left 2W1BX
      Right 2W1AX
  Back 2W15X
  Chest Wall 2W14X
  Extremity
    Lower
      Left 2W1MX
      Right 2W1LX
    Upper
      Left 2W19X
      Right 2W18X
  Face 2W11X
  Finger
    Left 2W1KX
    Right 2W1JX
  Foot
    Left 2W1TX
    Right 2W1SX
  Hand
    Left 2W1FX
    Right 2W1EX
  Head 2W10X
  Inguinal Region
    Left 2W17X
    Right 2W16X
  Leg
    Lower
      Left 2W1RX
      Right 2W1QX
    Upper
      Left 2W1PX
      Right 2W1NX
  Neck 2W12X
  Thumb
    Left 2W1HX
    Right 2W1GX
  Toe
    Left 2W1VX
    Right 2W1UX
Computer Assisted Procedure
  Extremity
    Lower
      No Qualifier 8EØYXBZ
      With Computerized Tomography
        8EØYXBG
      With Fluoroscopy 8EØYXBF
      With Magnetic Resonance Imaging
        8EØYXBH
    Upper
      No Qualifier 8EØXXBZ

Computer Assisted Procedure — *continued*
  Extremity — *continued*
    Upper — *continued*
      With Computerized Tomography
        8EØXXBG
      With Fluoroscopy 8EØXXBF
      With Magnetic Resonance Imaging
        8EØXXBH
  Head and Neck Region
    No Qualifier 8EØ9XBZ
    With Computerized Tomography 8EØ9XBG
    With Fluoroscopy 8EØ9XBF
    With Magnetic Resonance Imaging 8EØ9XBH
  Trunk Region
    No Qualifier 8EØWXBZ
    With Computerized Tomography 8EØWXBG
    With Fluoroscopy 8EØWXBF
    With Magnetic Resonance Imaging 8EØWXBH
Computer-aided Assessment
  Cardiac Output XXE2X19
  Intracranial Vascular Activity XXEØX07
Computer-aided Guidance, Transthoracic Echocardiography X2JAX47
Computer-aided Mechanical Aspiration X2C
Computer-aided Triage and Notification, Pulmonary Artery Flow XXE3X27
Computer-aided Valve Modeling and Notification, Coronary Artery Flow XXE3X68
Computer-assisted Intermittent Aspiration *see* New Technology, Cardiovascular System X2C
Computer-assisted Transcranial Magnetic Stimulation XØZØX18
Computerized Tomography (CT Scan)
  Abdomen BW2Ø
    Chest and Pelvis BW25
  Abdomen and Chest BW24
  Abdomen and Pelvis BW21
  Airway, Trachea BB2F
  Ankle
    Left BQ2H
    Right BQ2G
  Aorta
    Abdominal B42Ø
      Intravascular Optical Coherence
        B42ØZ2Z
    Thoracic B32Ø
      Intravascular Optical Coherence
        B32ØZ2Z
  Arm
    Left BP2F
    Right BP2E
  Artery
    Celiac B421
      Intravascular Optical Coherence
        B421Z2Z
    Common Carotid
      Bilateral B325
      Intravascular Optical Coherence
        B325Z2Z
    Coronary
      Bypass Graft
        Intravascular Optical Coherence
          B223Z2Z
        Multiple B223
      Multiple B221
        Intravascular Optical Coherence
          B221Z2Z
    Internal Carotid
      Bilateral B328
      Intravascular Optical Coherence
        B328Z2Z
    Intracranial B32R
      Intravascular Optical Coherence
        B32RZ2Z
    Lower Extremity
      Bilateral B42H
        Intravascular Optical Coherence
          B42HZ2Z
      Left B42G
        Intravascular Optical Coherence
          B42GZ2Z
      Right B42F
        Intravascular Optical Coherence
          B42FZ2Z
    Pelvic B42C
      Intravascular Optical Coherence
        B42CZ2Z

Computerized Tomography (CT Scan) — *continued*
  Artery — *continued*
    Pulmonary
      Left B32T
        Intravascular Optical Coherence
          B32TZ2Z
      Right B32S
        Intravascular Optical Coherence
          B32SZ2Z
    Renal
      Bilateral B428
        Intravascular Optical Coherence
          B428Z2Z
      Transplant B42M
        Intravascular Optical Coherence
          B42MZ2Z
    Superior Mesenteric B424
      Intravascular Optical Coherence
        B424Z2Z
    Vertebral
      Bilateral B32G
      Intravascular Optical Coherence
        B32GZ2Z
  Bladder BT2Ø
  Bone
    Facial BN25
    Temporal BN2F
  Brain BØ2Ø
  Calcaneus
    Left BQ2K
    Right BQ2J
  Cerebral Ventricle BØ28
  Chest, Abdomen and Pelvis BW25
  Chest and Abdomen BW24
  Cisterna BØ27
  Clavicle
    Left BP25
    Right BP24
  Coccyx BR2F
  Colon BD24
  Ear B92Ø
  Elbow
    Left BP2H
    Right BP2G
  Extremity
    Lower
      Left BQ2S
      Right BQ2R
    Upper
      Bilateral BP2V
      Left BP2U
      Right BP2T
  Eye
    Bilateral B827
    Left B826
    Right B825
  Femur
    Left BQ24
    Right BQ23
  Fibula
    Left BQ2C
    Right BQ2B
  Finger
    Left BP2S
    Right BP2R
  Foot
    Left BQ2M
    Right BQ2L
  Forearm
    Left BP2K
    Right BP2J
  Gland
    Adrenal, Bilateral BG22
    Parathyroid BG23
    Parotid, Bilateral B926
    Salivary, Bilateral B92D
    Submandibular, Bilateral B929
    Thyroid BG24
  Hand
    Left BP2P
    Right BP2N
  Hands and Wrists, Bilateral BP2Q
  Head BW28
  Head and Neck BW29
  Heart
    Intravascular Optical Coherence B226Z2Z
    Right and Left B226
  Hepatobiliary System, All BF2C

Computerized Tomography (CT Scan) — *continued*
- Hip
  - Left BQ21
  - Right BQ2Ø
- Humerus
  - Left BP2B
  - Right BP2A
- Intracranial Sinus B522
  - Intravascular Optical Coherence B522Z2Z
- Joint
  - Acromioclavicular, Bilateral BP23
  - Finger
    - Left BP2DZZZ
    - Right BP2CZZZ
  - Foot
    - Left BQ2Y
    - Right BQ2X
  - Hand
    - Left BP2DZZZ
    - Right BP2CZZZ
  - Sacroiliac BR2D
  - Sternoclavicular
    - Bilateral BP22
    - Left BP21
    - Right BP2Ø
  - Temporomandibular, Bilateral BN29
  - Toe
    - Left BQ2Y
    - Right BQ2X
- Kidney
  - Bilateral BT23
  - Left BT22
  - Right BT21
  - Transplant BT29
- Knee
  - Left BQ28
  - Right BQ27
- Larynx B92J
- Leg
  - Left BQ2F
  - Right BQ2D
- Liver BF25
- Liver and Spleen BF26
- Lung, Bilateral BB24
- Mandible BN26
- Nasopharynx B92F
- Neck BW2F
- Neck and Head BW29
- Orbit, Bilateral BN23
- Oropharynx B92F
- Pancreas BF27
- Patella
  - Left BQ2W
  - Right BQ2V
- Pelvic Region BW2G
- Pelvis BR2C
  - Chest and Abdomen BW25
- Pelvis and Abdomen BW21
- Pituitary Gland BØ29
- Prostate BV23
- Ribs
  - Left BP2Y
  - Right BP2X
- Sacrum BR2F
- Scapula
  - Left BP27
  - Right BP26
- Sella Turcica BØ29
- Shoulder
  - Left BP29
  - Right BP28
- Sinus
  - Intracranial B522
    - Intravascular Optical Coherence B522Z2Z
  - Paranasal B922
- Skull BN2Ø
- Spinal Cord BØ2B
- Spine
  - Cervical BR2Ø
  - Lumbar BR29
  - Thoracic BR27
- Spleen and Liver BF26
- Thorax BP2W
- Tibia
  - Left BQ2C
  - Right BQ2B
- Toe
  - Left BQ2Q

Computerized Tomography (CT Scan) — *continued*
- Toe — *continued*
  - Right BQ2P
- Trachea BB2F
- Tracheobronchial Tree
  - Bilateral BB29
  - Left BB28
  - Right BB27
- Vein
  - Pelvic (Iliac)
    - Left B52G
      - Intravascular Optical Coherence B52GZ2Z
    - Right B52F
      - Intravascular Optical Coherence B52FZ2Z
  - Pelvic (Iliac) Bilateral B52H
    - Intravascular Optical Coherence B52HZ2Z
  - Portal B52T
    - Intravascular Optical Coherence B52TZ2Z
  - Pulmonary
    - Bilateral B52S
      - Intravascular Optical Coherence B52SZ2Z
    - Left B52R
      - Intravascular Optical Coherence B52RZ2Z
    - Right B52Q
      - Intravascular Optical Coherence B52QZ2Z
  - Renal
    - Bilateral B52L
      - Intravascular Optical Coherence B52LZ2Z
    - Left B52K
      - Intravascular Optical Coherence B52KZ2Z
    - Right B52J
      - Intravascular Optical Coherence B52JZ2Z
  - Spanchnic B52T
    - Intravascular Optical Coherence B52TZ2Z
- Vena Cava
  - Inferior B529
    - Intravascular Optical Coherence B529Z2Z
  - Superior B528
    - Intravascular Optical Coherence B528Z2Z
- Ventricle, Cerebral BØ28
- Wrist
  - Left BP2M
  - Right BP2L

Concerto II CRT-D *use* Cardiac Resynchronization Defibrillator Pulse Generator in ØJH

Conduit through Femoral Vein to Popliteal Artery, Bypass X2K

Conduit through Femoral Vein to Superficial Femoral Artery, Bypass X2K

Conduit to Short-term External Heart Assist System, Insertion X2H

Condylectomy
- *see* Excision, Head and Facial Bones ØNB
- *see* Excision, Lower Bones ØQB
- *see* Excision, Upper Bones ØPB

Condyloid process
- *use* Mandible, Left
- *use* Mandible, Right

Condylotomy
- *see* Division, Head and Facial Bones ØN8
- *see* Division, Lower Bones ØQ8
- *see* Division, Upper Bones ØP8
- *see* Drainage, Head and Facial Bones ØN9
- *see* Drainage, Lower Bones ØQ9
- *see* Drainage, Upper Bones ØP9

Condylysis
- *see* Release, Head and Facial Bones ØNN
- *see* Release, Lower Bones ØQN
- *see* Release, Upper Bones ØPN

Conization, cervix *see* Excision, Cervix ØUBC

Conjunctivoplasty
- *see* Repair, Eye Ø8Q
- *see* Replacement, Eye Ø8R

CONSERVE® PLUS Total Resurfacing Hip System *use* Resurfacing Device in Lower Joints

Construction
- Auricle, ear *see* Replacement, Ear, Nose, Sinus Ø9R
- Ileal conduit *see* Bypass, Urinary System ØT1

Consulta CRT-D *use* Cardiac Resynchronization Defibrillator Pulse Generator in ØJH

Consulta CRT-P *use* Cardiac Resynchronization Pacemaker Pulse Generator in ØJH

Contact Radiation
- Abdomen DWY37ZZ
- Adrenal Gland DGY27ZZ
- Bile Ducts DFY27ZZ
- Bladder DTY27ZZ
- Bone, Other DPYC7ZZ
- Brain DØY07ZZ
- Brain Stem DØY17ZZ
- Breast
  - Left DMY07ZZ
  - Right DMY17ZZ
- Bronchus DBY17ZZ
- Cervix DUY17ZZ
- Chest DWY27ZZ
- Chest Wall DBY77ZZ
- Colon DDY57ZZ
- Diaphragm DBY87ZZ
- Duodenum DDY27ZZ
- Ear D9Y07ZZ
- Esophagus DDY07ZZ
- Eye D8Y07ZZ
- Femur DPY97ZZ
- Fibula DPYB7ZZ
- Gallbladder DFY17ZZ
- Gland
  - Adrenal DGY27ZZ
  - Parathyroid DGY47ZZ
  - Pituitary DGY07ZZ
  - Thyroid DGY57ZZ
- Glands, Salivary D9Y67ZZ
- Head and Neck DWY17ZZ
- Hemibody DWY47ZZ
- Humerus DPY67ZZ
- Hypopharynx D9Y37ZZ
- Ileum DDY47ZZ
- Jejunum DDY37ZZ
- Kidney DTY07ZZ
- Larynx D9YB7ZZ
- Liver DFY07ZZ
- Lung DBY27ZZ
- Mandible DPY37ZZ
- Maxilla DPY27ZZ
- Mediastinum DBY67ZZ
- Mouth D9Y47ZZ
- Nasopharynx D9YD7ZZ
- Neck and Head DWY17ZZ
- Nerve, Peripheral DØY77ZZ
- Nose D9Y17ZZ
- Oropharynx D9YF7ZZ
- Ovary DUY07ZZ
- Palate
  - Hard D9Y87ZZ
  - Soft D9Y97ZZ
- Pancreas DFY37ZZ
- Parathyroid Gland DGY47ZZ
- Pelvic Bones DPY87ZZ
- Pelvic Region DWY67ZZ
- Pineal Body DGY17ZZ
- Pituitary Gland DGY07ZZ
- Pleura DBY57ZZ
- Prostate DVY07ZZ
- Radius DPY77ZZ
- Rectum DDY77ZZ
- Rib DPY57ZZ
- Sinuses D9Y77ZZ
- Skin
  - Abdomen DHY87ZZ
  - Arm DHY47ZZ
  - Back DHY77ZZ
  - Buttock DHY97ZZ
  - Chest DHY67ZZ
  - Face DHY27ZZ
  - Leg DHYB7ZZ
  - Neck DHY37ZZ
- Skull DPY07ZZ
- Spinal Cord DØY67ZZ
- Sternum DPY47ZZ
- Stomach DDY17ZZ
- Testis DVY17ZZ
- Thyroid Gland DGY57ZZ
- Tibia DPYB7ZZ
- Tongue D9Y57ZZ

▽ **Subterms under main terms may continue to next column or page**

Contact Radiation — *continued*
　Trachea DBY07ZZ
　Ulna DPY77ZZ
　Ureter DTY17ZZ
　Urethra DTY37ZZ
　Uterus DUY27ZZ
　Whole Body DWY57ZZ
ContaCT software (Measurement of intracranial arterial flow) 4A03X5D
CONTAK RENEWAL® 3 RF (HE) CRT-D *use* Cardiac Resynchronization Defibrillator Pulse Generator in 0JH
Contegra Pulmonary Valved Conduit *use* Zooplastic Tissue in Heart and Great Vessels
CONTEPO™ *use* Fosfomycin Anti-Infective
Continent ileostomy *see* Bypass, Ileum 0D1B
Continuous Glucose Monitoring (CGM) device *use* Monitoring Device
Continuous Negative Airway Pressure
　24-96 Consecutive Hours, Ventilation 5A09459
　Greater than 96 Consecutive Hours, Ventilation 5A09559
　Less than 24 Consecutive Hours, Ventilation 5A09359
Continuous Positive Airway Pressure
　24-96 Consecutive Hours, Ventilation 5A09457
　Greater than 96 Consecutive Hours, Ventilation 5A09557
　Less than 24 Consecutive Hours, Ventilation 5A09357
Continuous renal replacement therapy (CRRT) 5A1D90Z
Contraceptive Device
　Change device in, Uterus and Cervix 0U2DXHZ
　Insertion of device in
　　Cervix 0UHC
　　Subcutaneous Tissue and Fascia
　　　Abdomen 0JH8
　　　Chest 0JH6
　　　Lower Arm
　　　　Left 0JHH
　　　　Right 0JHG
　　　Lower Leg
　　　　Left 0JHP
　　　　Right 0JHN
　　　Upper Arm
　　　　Left 0JHF
　　　　Right 0JHD
　　　Upper Leg
　　　　Left 0JHM
　　　　Right 0JHL
　　Uterus 0UH9
　Removal of device from
　　Subcutaneous Tissue and Fascia
　　　Lower Extremity 0JPW
　　　Trunk 0JPT
　　　Upper Extremity 0JPV
　　Uterus and Cervix 0UPD
　Revision of device in
　　Subcutaneous Tissue and Fascia
　　　Lower Extremity 0JWW
　　　Trunk 0JWT
　　　Upper Extremity 0JWV
　　Uterus and Cervix 0UWD
Contractility Modulation Device
　Abdomen 0JH8
　Chest 0JH6
Control bleeding in
　Abdominal Wall 0W3F
　Ankle Region
　　Left 0Y3L
　　Right 0Y3K
　Arm
　　Lower
　　　Left 0X3F
　　　Right 0X3D
　　Upper
　　　Left 0X39
　　　Right 0X38
　Axilla
　　Left 0X35
　　Right 0X34
　Back
　　Lower 0W3L
　　Upper 0W3K
　Buttock
　　Left 0Y31
　　Right 0Y30

Control bleeding in — *continued*
　Cavity, Cranial 0W31
　Chest Wall 0W38
　Elbow Region
　　Left 0X3C
　　Right 0X3B
　Extremity
　　Lower
　　　Left 0Y3B
　　　Right 0Y39
　　Upper
　　　Left 0X37
　　　Right 0X36
　Face 0W32
　Femoral Region
　　Left 0Y38
　　Right 0Y37
　Foot
　　Left 0Y3N
　　Right 0Y3M
　Gastrointestinal Tract 0W3P
　Genitourinary Tract 0W3R
　Hand
　　Left 0X3K
　　Right 0X3J
　Head 0W30
　Inguinal Region
　　Left 0Y36
　　Right 0Y35
　Jaw
　　Lower 0W35
　　Upper 0W34
　Knee Region
　　Left 0Y3G
　　Right 0Y3F
　Leg
　　Lower
　　　Left 0Y3J
　　　Right 0Y3H
　　Upper
　　　Left 0Y3D
　　　Right 0Y3C
　Mediastinum 0W3C
　Nasal Mucosa and Soft Tissue 093K
　Neck 0W36
　Oral Cavity and Throat 0W33
　Pelvic Cavity 0W3J
　Pericardial Cavity 0W3D
　Perineum
　　Female 0W3N
　　Male 0W3M
　Peritoneal Cavity 0W3G
　Pleural Cavity
　　Left 0W3B
　　Right 0W39
　Respiratory Tract 0W3Q
　Retroperitoneum 0W3H
　Shoulder Region
　　Left 0X33
　　Right 0X32
　Wrist Region
　　Left 0X3H
　　Right 0X3G
Control bleeding using Tourniquet, External *see* Compression, Anatomical Regions 2W1
Control, Epistaxis *see* Control bleeding in, Nasal Mucosa and Soft Tissue 093K
Conus arteriosus *use* Ventricle, Right
Conus medullaris *use* Lumbar Spinal Cord
Convalescent Plasma (Nonautologous) *see* New Technology, Anatomical Regions XW1
Conversion
　Cardiac rhythm 5A2204Z
　Gastrostomy to jejunostomy feeding device *see* Insertion of device in, Jejunum 0DHA
Cook Biodesign® Fistula Plug(s) *use* Nonautologous Tissue Substitute
Cook Biodesign® Hernia Graft(s) *use* Nonautologous Tissue Substitute
Cook Biodesign® Layered Graft(s) *use* Nonautologous Tissue Substitute
Cook Zenaprom™ Layered Graft(s) *use* Nonautologous Tissue Substitute
Cook Zenith AAA Endovascular Graft *use* Intraluminal Device
Cook Zenith® Fenestrated AAA Endovascular Graft
　use Intraluminal Device, Branched or Fenestrated, One or Two Arteries in 04V

Cook Zenith® Fenestrated AAA Endovascular Graft — *continued*
　use Intraluminal Device, Branched or Fenestrated, Three or More Arteries in 04V
Coracoacromial ligament
　use Shoulder Bursa and Ligament, Left
　use Shoulder Bursa and Ligament, Right
Coracobrachialis muscle
　use Upper Arm Muscle, Left
　use Upper Arm Muscle, Right
Coracoclavicular ligament
　use Shoulder Bursa and Ligament, Left
　use Shoulder Bursa and Ligament, Right
Coracohumeral ligament
　use Shoulder Bursa and Ligament, Left
　use Shoulder Bursa and Ligament, Right
Coracoid process
　use Scapula, Left
　use Scapula, Right
Cordotomy *see* Division, Central Nervous System and Cranial Nerves 008
Core needle biopsy *see* Biopsy
CoreValve transcatheter aortic valve *use* Zooplastic Tissue in Heart and Great Vessels
Cormet Hip Resurfacing System *use* Resurfacing Device in Lower Joints
Corniculate cartilage *use* Larynx
CoRoent® XL *use* Interbody Fusion Device in Lower Joints
Coronary arteriography
　see Fluoroscopy, Heart B21
　see Plain Radiography, Heart B20
Corox (OTW) Bipolar Lead
　use Cardiac Lead, Defibrillator in 02H
　use Cardiac Lead, Pacemaker in 02H
Corpus callosum *use* Brain
Corpus cavernosum *use* Penis
Corpus spongiosum *use* Penis
Corpus striatum *use* Basal Ganglia
Corrugator supercilii muscle *use* Facial Muscle
Cortical strip neurostimulator lead *use* Neurostimulator Lead in Central Nervous System and Cranial Nerves
Corvia IASD® *use* Synthetic Substitute
COSELA™ *use* Trilaciclib
Costatectomy
　see Excision, Upper Bones 0PB
　see Resection, Upper Bones 0PT
Costectomy
　see Excision, Upper Bones 0PB
　see Resection, Upper Bones 0PT
Costocervical trunk
　use Subclavian Artery, Left
　use Subclavian Artery, Right
Costochondrectomy
　see Excision, Upper Bones 0PB
　see Resection, Upper Bones 0PT
Costoclavicular ligament
　use Shoulder Bursa and Ligament, Left
　use Shoulder Bursa and Ligament, Right
Costosternoplasty
　see Repair, Upper Bones 0PQ
　see Replacement, Upper Bones 0PR
　see Supplement, Upper Bones 0PU
Costotomy
　see Division, Upper Bones 0P8
　see Drainage, Upper Bones 0P9
Costotransverse joint *use* Thoracic Vertebral Joint
Costotransverse ligament *use* Rib(s) Bursa and Ligament
Costovertebral joint *use* Thoracic Vertebral Joint
Costoxiphoid ligament *use* Sternum Bursa and Ligament
Counseling
　Family, for substance abuse, Other Family Counseling HZ63ZZZ
　Group
　　12-Step HZ43ZZZ
　　Behavioral HZ41ZZZ
　　Cognitive HZ40ZZZ
　　Cognitive-Behavioral HZ42ZZZ
　　Confrontational HZ48ZZZ
　　Continuing Care HZ49ZZZ
　　Infectious Disease
　　　Post-Test HZ4CZZZ
　　　Pre-Test HZ4CZZZ
　　Interpersonal HZ44ZZZ

Counseling — *continued*
  Group — *continued*
    Motivational Enhancement HZ47ZZZ
    Psychoeducation HZ46ZZZ
    Spiritual HZ4BZZZ
    Vocational HZ45ZZZ
  Individual
    12-Step HZ33ZZZ
    Behavioral HZ31ZZZ
    Cognitive HZ30ZZZ
    Cognitive-Behavioral HZ32ZZZ
    Confrontational HZ38ZZZ
    Continuing Care HZ39ZZZ
    Infectious Disease
      Post-Test HZ3CZZZ
      Pre-Test HZ3CZZZ
    Interpersonal HZ34ZZZ
    Motivational Enhancement HZ37ZZZ
    Psychoeducation HZ36ZZZ
    Spiritual HZ3BZZZ
    Vocational HZ35ZZZ
  Mental Health Services
    Educational GZ60ZZZ
    Other Counseling GZ63ZZZ
    Vocational GZ61ZZZ
Countershock, cardiac 5A2204Z
COVID-19 Vaccine XW0
COVID-19 Vaccine Booster XW0
COVID-19 Vaccine Dose 1 XW0
COVID-19 Vaccine Dose 2 XW0
COVID-19 Vaccine Dose 3 XW0
Cowper's (bulbourethral) gland *use* Urethra
CPAP (continuous positive airway pressure) *see* Assistance, Respiratory 5A09
Craniectomy
  see Excision, Head and Facial Bones 0NB
  see Resection, Head and Facial Bones 0NT
Cranioplasty
  see Repair, Head and Facial Bones 0NQ
  see Replacement, Head and Facial Bones 0NR
  see Supplement, Head and Facial Bones 0NU
Craniotomy
  see Division, Head and Facial Bones 0N8
  see Drainage, Central Nervous System and Cranial Nerves 009
  see Drainage, Head and Facial Bones 0N9
Creation
  Perineum
    Female 0W4N0
    Male 0W4M0
  Valve
    Aortic 024F0
    Mitral 024G0
    Tricuspid 024J0
Cremaster muscle *use* Perineum Muscle
CRESEMBA® (isavuconazonium sulfate) *use* Other Anti-infective
Cribriform plate
  use Ethmoid Bone, Left
  use Ethmoid Bone, Right
Cricoid cartilage *use* Trachea
Cricoidectomy *see* Excision, Larynx 0CBS
Cricothyroid artery
  use Thyroid Artery, Left
  use Thyroid Artery, Right
Cricothyroid muscle
  use Neck Muscle, Left
  use Neck Muscle, Right
Crisis Intervention GZ2ZZZZ
CRRT (Continuous renal replacement therapy) 5A1D90Z
Crural fascia
  use Subcutaneous Tissue and Fascia, Left Upper Leg
  use Subcutaneous Tissue and Fascia, Right Upper Leg
Crushing, nerve
  Cranial *see* Destruction, Central Nervous System and Cranial Nerves 005
  Peripheral *see* Destruction, Peripheral Nervous System 015
Cryoablation *see* Destruction
Cryotherapy *see* Destruction
Cryptorchidectomy
  see Excision, Male Reproductive System 0VB
  see Resection, Male Reproductive System 0VT

Cryptorchiectomy
  see Excision, Male Reproductive System 0VB
  see Resection, Male Reproductive System 0VT
Cryptotomy
  see Division, Gastrointestinal System 0D8
  see Drainage, Gastrointestinal System 0D9
CT scan *see* Computerized Tomography (CT Scan)
CT sialogram *see* Computerized Tomography (CT Scan), Ear, Nose, Mouth and Throat B92
CTX001™ *use* Exagamglogene Autotemcel
Cubital lymph node
  use Lymphatic, Left Upper Extremity
  use Lymphatic, Right Upper Extremity
Cubital nerve *use* Ulnar Nerve
Cuboid bone
  use Tarsal, Left
  use Tarsal, Right
Cuboideonavicular joint
  use Tarsal Joint, Left
  use Tarsal Joint, Right
Culdocentesis *see* Drainage, Cul-de-sac 0U9F
Culdoplasty
  see Repair, Cul-de-sac 0UQF
  see Supplement, Cul-de-sac 0UUF
Culdoscopy 0UJH8ZZ
Culdotomy *see* Drainage, Cul-de-sac 0U9F
Culmen *use* Cerebellum
Cultured epidermal cell autograft *use* Autologous Tissue Substitute
Cuneiform cartilage *use* Larynx
Cuneonavicular joint
  use Joint, Tarsal, Left
  use Joint, Tarsal, Right
Cuneonavicular ligament
  use Foot Bursa and Ligament, Left
  use Foot Bursa and Ligament, Right
Curettage
  see Excision
  see Extraction
Cutaneous (transverse) cervical nerve *use* Cervical Plexus
CVP (central venous pressure) *see* Measurement, Venous 4A04
Cyclodiathermy *see* Destruction, Eye 085
Cyclophotocoagulation *see* Destruction, Eye 085
CYPHER® Stent *use* Intraluminal Device, Drug-eluting in Heart and Great Vessels
Cystectomy
  see Excision, Bladder 0TBB
  see Resection, Bladder 0TTB
Cystocele repair *see* Repair, Subcutaneous Tissue and Fascia, Pelvic Region 0JQC
Cystography
  see Fluoroscopy, Urinary System BT1
  see Plain Radiography, Urinary System BT0
Cystolithotomy *see* Extirpation, Bladder 0TCB
Cystopexy
  see Repair, Bladder 0TQB
  see Reposition, Bladder 0TSB
Cystoplasty
  see Repair, Bladder 0TQB
  see Replacement, Bladder 0TRB
  see Supplement, Bladder 0TUB
Cystorrhaphy *see* Repair, Bladder 0TQB
Cystoscopy 0TJB8ZZ
Cystostomy *see* Bypass, Bladder 0T1B
Cystostomy Tube *use* Drainage Device
Cystotomy *see* Drainage, Bladder 0T9B
Cystourethrography
  see Fluoroscopy, Urinary System BT1
  see Plain Radiography, Urinary System BT0
Cystourethroplasty
  see Repair, Urinary System 0TQ
  see Replacement, Urinary System 0TR
  see Supplement, Urinary System 0TU
CYTALUX® (Pafolacianine), in Fluorescence Guided Procedure *see* Fluorescence Guided Procedure
Cytarabine and Daunorubicin Liposome Antineoplastic XW0

D

Daratumumab and Hyaluronidase-fihj XW01318
Darzalex Faspro® *use* Daratumumab and Hyaluronidase-fihj

DBS lead *use* Neurostimulator Lead in Central Nervous System and Cranial Nerves
DeBakey Left Ventricular Assist Device *use* Implantable Heart Assist System in Heart and Great Vessels
Debridement
  Excisional *see* Excision
  Non-excisional *see* Extraction
Decompression, Circulatory 6A15
Decortication, lung
  see Extirpation, Respiratory System 0BC
  see Release, Respiratory System 0BN
Deep brain neurostimulator lead *use* Neurostimulator Lead in Central Nervous System and Cranial Nerves
Deep cervical fascia
  use Subcutaneous Tissue and Fascia, Left Neck
  use Subcutaneous Tissue and Fascia, Right Neck
Deep cervical vein
  use Vertebral Vein, Left
  use Vertebral Vein, Right
Deep circumflex iliac artery
  use External Iliac Artery, Left
  use External Iliac Artery, Right
Deep facial vein
  use Face Vein, Left
  use Face Vein, Right
Deep femoral artery
  use Femoral Artery, Left
  use Femoral Artery, Right
Deep femoral (profunda femoris) vein
  use Femoral Vein, Left
  use Femoral Vein, Right
Deep Inferior Epigastric Artery Perforator Flap
  Replacement
    Bilateral 0HRV077
    Left 0HRU077
    Right 0HRT077
  Transfer
    Left 0KXG
    Right 0KXF
Deep palmar arch
  use Hand Artery, Left
  use Hand Artery, Right
Deep transverse perineal muscle *use* Perineum Muscle
DefenCath™ *use* Taurolidine Anti-infective and Heparin Anticoagulant
Deferential artery
  use Internal Iliac Artery, Left
  use Internal Iliac Artery, Right
Defibrillator Generator
  Abdomen 0JH8
  Chest 0JH6
Defibrillator Lead
  Insertion of device in, Mediastinum 0WHC
  Removal of device from, Mediastinum 0WPC
  Revision of device in, Mediastinum 0WWC
Defibtech Automated Chest Compression (ACC) device 5A1221J
Defitelio *use* Other Substance
Defitelio® infusion *see* Introduction of substance in or on, Physiological Systems and Anatomical Regions 3E0
Delivery
  Cesarean *see* Extraction, Products of Conception 10D0
  Forceps *see* Extraction, Products of Conception 10D0
  Manually assisted 10E0XZZ
  Products of Conception 10E0XZZ
  Vacuum assisted *see* Extraction, Products of Conception 10D0
Delta frame external fixator
  use External Fixation Device, Hybrid in 0PH
  use External Fixation Device, Hybrid in 0PS
  use External Fixation Device, Hybrid in 0QH
  use External Fixation Device, Hybrid in 0QS
Delta III Reverse shoulder prosthesis *use* Synthetic Substitute, Reverse Ball and Socket in 0RR
Deltoid fascia
  use Subcutaneous Tissue and Fascia, Left Upper Arm
  use Subcutaneous Tissue and Fascia, Right Upper Arm
Deltoid ligament
  use Ankle Bursa and Ligament, Left

Deltoid ligament — *continued*
  use Ankle Bursa and Ligament, Right
Deltoid muscle
  use Shoulder Muscle, Left
  use Shoulder Muscle, Right
Deltopectoral (infraclavicular) lymph node
  use Lymphatic, Left Upper Extremity
  use Lymphatic, Right Upper Extremity
Denervation
  Cranial nerve *see* Destruction, Central Nervous
    System and Cranial Nerves 005
  Peripheral nerve *see* Destruction, Peripheral Nervous System 015
Dens *use* Cervical Vertebra
Densitometry
  Plain Radiography
    Femur
      Left BQ04ZZ1
      Right BQ03ZZ1
    Hip
      Left BQ01ZZ1
      Right BQ00ZZ1
    Spine
      Cervical BR00ZZ1
      Lumbar BR09ZZ1
      Thoracic BR07ZZ1
      Whole BR0GZZ1
  Ultrasonography
    Elbow
      Left BP4HZZ1
      Right BP4GZZ1
    Hand
      Left BP4PZZ1
      Right BP4NZZ1
    Shoulder
      Left BP49ZZ1
      Right BP48ZZ1
    Wrist
      Left BP4MZZ1
      Right BP4LZZ1
Denticulate (dentate) ligament *use* Spinal Meninges
Depressor anguli oris muscle *use* Facial Muscle
Depressor labii inferioris muscle *use* Facial Muscle
Depressor septi nasi muscle *use* Facial Muscle
Depressor supercilii muscle *use* Facial Muscle
Dermabrasion *see* Extraction, Skin and Breast 0HD
Dermis *use* Skin
Descending genicular artery
  use Femoral Artery, Left
  use Femoral Artery, Right
Destruction
  Acetabulum
    Left 0Q55
    Right 0Q54
  Adenoids 0C5Q
  Ampulla of Vater 0F5C
  Anal Sphincter 0D5R
  Anterior Chamber
    Left 08533ZZ
    Right 08523ZZ
  Anus 0D5Q
  Aorta
    Abdominal
    Thoracic
      Ascending/Arch 025X
      Descending 025W
  Aortic Body 0G5D
  Appendix 0D5J
  Artery
    Anterior Tibial
      Left 045Q
      Right 045P
    Axillary
      Left 0356
      Right 0355
    Brachial
      Left 0358
      Right 0357
    Celiac 0451
    Colic
      Left 0457
      Middle 0458
      Right 0456
    Common Carotid
      Left 035J
      Right 035H
    Common Iliac
      Left 045D

Destruction — *continued*
  Artery — *continued*
    Common Iliac — *continued*
      Right 045C
    External Carotid
      Left 035N
      Right 035M
    External Iliac
      Left 045J
      Right 045H
    Face 035R
    Femoral
      Left 045L
      Right 045K
    Foot
      Left 045W
      Right 045V
    Gastric 0452
    Hand
      Left 035F
      Right 035D
    Hepatic 0453
    Inferior Mesenteric 045B
    Innominate 0352
    Internal Carotid
      Left 035L
      Right 035K
    Internal Iliac
      Left 045F
      Right 045E
    Internal Mammary
      Left 0351
      Right 0350
    Intracranial 035G
    Lower 045Y
    Peroneal
      Left 045U
      Right 045T
    Popliteal
      Left 045N
      Right 045M
    Posterior Tibial
      Left 045S
      Right 045R
    Pulmonary
      Left 025R
      Right 025Q
    Pulmonary Trunk 025P
    Radial
      Left 035C
      Right 035B
    Renal
      Left 045A
      Right 0459
    Splenic 0454
    Subclavian
      Left 0354
      Right 0353
    Superior Mesenteric 0455
    Temporal
      Left 035T
      Right 035S
    Thyroid
      Left 035V
      Right 035U
    Ulnar
      Left 035A
      Right 0359
    Upper 035Y
    Vertebral
      Left 035Q
      Right 035P
  Atrium
    Left 0257
    Right 0256
  Auditory Ossicle
    Left 095A
    Right 0959
  Basal Ganglia 0058
  Bladder 0T5B
  Bladder Neck 0T5C
  Bone
    Ethmoid
      Left 0N5G
      Right 0N5F
    Frontal 0N51
    Hyoid 0N5X
    Lacrimal
      Left 0N5J

Destruction — *continued*
  Bone — *continued*
    Lacrimal — *continued*
      Right 0N5H
    Nasal 0N5B
    Occipital 0N57
    Palatine
      Left 0N5L
      Right 0N5K
    Parietal
      Left 0N54
      Right 0N53
    Pelvic
      Left 0Q53
      Right 0Q52
    Sphenoid 0N5C
    Temporal
      Left 0N56
      Right 0N55
    Zygomatic
      Left 0N5N
      Right 0N5M
  Brain 0050
  Breast
    Bilateral 0H5V
    Left 0H5U
    Right 0H5T
  Bronchus
    Lingula 0B59
    Lower Lobe
      Left 0B5B
      Right 0B56
    Main
      Left 0B57
      Right 0B53
    Middle Lobe, Right 0B55
    Upper Lobe
      Left 0B58
      Right 0B54
  Buccal Mucosa 0C54
  Bursa and Ligament
    Abdomen
      Left 0M5J
      Right 0M5H
    Ankle
      Left 0M5R
      Right 0M5Q
    Elbow
      Left 0M54
      Right 0M53
    Foot
      Left 0M5T
      Right 0M5S
    Hand
      Left 0M58
      Right 0M57
    Head and Neck 0M50
    Hip
      Left 0M5M
      Right 0M5L
    Knee
      Left 0M5P
      Right 0M5N
    Lower Extremity
      Left 0M5W
      Right 0M5V
    Perineum 0M5K
    Rib(s) 0M5G
    Shoulder
      Left 0M52
      Right 0M51
    Spine
      Lower 0M5D
      Upper 0M5C
    Sternum 0M5F
    Upper Extremity
      Left 0M5B
      Right 0M59
    Wrist
      Left 0M56
      Right 0M55
  Carina 0B52
  Carotid Bodies, Bilateral 0G58
  Carotid Body
    Left 0G56
    Right 0G57
  Carpal
    Left 0P5N
    Right 0P5M

Destruction — *continued*
Cecum 0D5H
Cerebellum 005C
Cerebral Hemisphere 0057
Cerebral Meninges 0051
Cerebral Ventricle 0056
Cervix 0U5C
Chordae Tendineae 0259
Choroid
    Left 085B
    Right 085A
Cisterna Chyli 075L
Clavicle
    Left 0P5B
    Right 0P59
Clitoris 0U5J
Coccygeal Glomus 0G5B
Coccyx 0Q5S
Colon
    Ascending 0D5K
    Descending 0D5M
    Sigmoid 0D5N
    Transverse 0D5L
Conduction Mechanism 0258
Conjunctiva
    Left 085TXZZ
    Right 085SXZZ
Cord
    Bilateral 0V5H
    Left 0V5G
    Right 0V5F
Cornea
    Left 0859XZZ
    Right 0858XZZ
Cul-de-sac 0U5F
Diaphragm 0B5T
Disc
    Cervical Vertebral 0R53
    Cervicothoracic Vertebral 0R55
    Lumbar Vertebral 0S52
    Lumbosacral 0S54
    Thoracic Vertebral 0R59
    Thoracolumbar Vertebral 0R5B
Duct
    Common Bile 0F59
    Cystic 0F58
    Hepatic
        Common 0F57
        Left 0F56
        Right 0F55
    Lacrimal
        Left 085Y
        Right 085X
    Pancreatic 0F5D
        Accessory 0F5F
    Parotid
        Left 0C5C
        Right 0C5B
Duodenum 0D59
Dura Mater 0052
Ear
    External
        Left 0951
        Right 0950
    External Auditory Canal
        Left 0954
        Right 0953
    Inner
        Left 095E
        Right 095D
    Middle
        Left 0956
        Right 0955
Endometrium 0U5B
Epididymis
    Bilateral 0V5L
    Left 0V5K
    Right 0V5J
Epiglottis 0C5R
Esophagogastric Junction 0D54
Esophagus 0D55
    Lower 0D53
    Middle 0D52
    Upper 0D51
Eustachian Tube
    Left 095G
    Right 095F
Eye
    Left 0851XZZ

Destruction — *continued*
Eye — *continued*
    Right 0850XZZ
Eyelid
    Lower
        Left 085R
        Right 085Q
    Upper
        Left 085P
        Right 085N
Fallopian Tube
    Left 0U56
    Right 0U55
Fallopian Tubes, Bilateral 0U57
Femoral Shaft
    Left 0Q59
    Right 0Q58
Femur
    Lower
        Left 0Q5C
        Right 0Q5B
    Upper
        Left 0Q57
        Right 0Q56
Fibula
    Left 0Q5K
    Right 0Q5J
Finger Nail 0H5QXZZ
Gallbladder 0F54
Gingiva
    Lower 0C56
    Upper 0C55
Gland
    Adrenal
        Bilateral 0G54
        Left 0G52
        Right 0G53
    Lacrimal
        Left 085W
        Right 085V
    Minor Salivary 0C5J
    Parotid
        Left 0C59
        Right 0C58
    Pituitary 0G50
    Sublingual
        Left 0C5F
        Right 0C5D
    Submaxillary
        Left 0C5H
        Right 0C5G
    Vestibular 0U5L
Glenoid Cavity
    Left 0P58
    Right 0P57
Glomus Jugulare 0G5C
Humeral Head
    Left 0P5D
    Right 0P5C
Humeral Shaft
    Left 0P5G
    Right 0P5F
Hymen 0U5K
Hypothalamus 005A
Ileocecal Valve 0D5C
Ileum 0D5B
Intestine
    Large 0D5E
        Left 0D5G
        Right 0D5F
    Small 0D58
Iris
    Left 085D3ZZ
    Right 085C3ZZ
Jejunum 0D5A
Joint
    Acromioclavicular
        Left 0R5H
        Right 0R5G
    Ankle
        Left 0S5G
        Right 0S5F
    Carpal
        Left 0R5R
        Right 0R5Q
    Carpometacarpal
        Left 0R5T
        Right 0R5S
    Cervical Vertebral 0R51

Destruction — *continued*
Joint — *continued*
    Cervicothoracic Vertebral 0R54
    Coccygeal 0S56
    Elbow
        Left 0R5M
        Right 0R5L
    Finger Phalangeal
        Left 0R5X
        Right 0R5W
    Hip
        Left 0S5B
        Right 0S59
    Knee
        Left 0S5D
        Right 0S5C
    Lumbar Vertebral 0S50
    Lumbosacral 0S53
    Metacarpophalangeal
        Left 0R5V
        Right 0R5U
    Metatarsal-Phalangeal
        Left 0S5N
        Right 0S5M
    Occipital-cervical 0R50
    Sacrococcygeal 0S55
    Sacroiliac
        Left 0S58
        Right 0S57
    Shoulder
        Left 0R5K
        Right 0R5J
    Sternoclavicular
        Left 0R5F
        Right 0R5E
    Tarsal
        Left 0S5J
        Right 0S5H
    Tarsometatarsal
        Left 0S5L
        Right 0S5K
    Temporomandibular
        Left 0R5D
        Right 0R5C
    Thoracic Vertebral 0R56
    Thoracolumbar Vertebral 0R5A
    Toe Phalangeal
        Left 0S5Q
        Right 0S5P
    Wrist
        Left 0R5P
        Right 0R5N
Kidney
    Left 0T51
    Right 0T50
Kidney Pelvis
    Left 0T54
    Right 0T53
Larynx 0C5S
Lens
    Left 085K3ZZ
    Right 085J3ZZ
Lip
    Lower 0C51
    Upper 0C50
Liver 0F50
    Left Lobe 0F52
    Right Lobe 0F51
    Ultrasound-guided Cavitation XF5
Lung
    Bilateral 0B5M
    Left 0B5L
    Lower Lobe
        Left 0B5J
        Right 0B5F
    Middle Lobe, Right 0B5D
    Right 0B5K
    Upper Lobe
        Left 0B5G
        Right 0B5C
Lung Lingula 0B5H
Lymphatic
    Aortic 075D
    Axillary
        Left 0756
        Right 0755
    Head 0750
    Inguinal
        Left 075J

▼ Subterms under main terms may continue to next column or page

Destruction — *continued*
  Lymphatic — *continued*
    Inguinal — *continued*
      Right Ø75H
    Internal Mammary
      Left Ø759
      Right Ø758
    Lower Extremity
      Left Ø75G
      Right Ø75F
    Mesenteric Ø75B
    Neck
      Left Ø752
      Right Ø751
    Pelvis Ø75C
    Thoracic Duct Ø75K
    Thorax Ø757
    Upper Extremity
      Left Ø754
      Right Ø753
  Mandible
    Left ØN5V
    Right ØN5T
  Maxilla ØN5R
  Medulla Oblongata ØØ5D
  Mesentery ØD5V
  Metacarpal
    Left ØP5Q
    Right ØP5P
  Metatarsal
    Left ØQ5P
    Right ØQ5N
  Muscle
    Abdomen
      Left ØK5L
      Right ØK5K
    Extraocular
      Left Ø85M
      Right Ø85L
    Facial ØK51
    Foot
      Left ØK5W
      Right ØK5V
    Hand
      Left ØK5D
      Right ØK5C
    Head ØK5Ø
    Hip
      Left ØK5P
      Right ØK5N
    Lower Arm and Wrist
      Left ØK5B
      Right ØK59
    Lower Leg
      Left ØK5T
      Right ØK5S
    Neck
      Left ØK53
      Right ØK52
    Papillary Ø25D
    Perineum ØK5M
    Shoulder
      Left ØK56
      Right ØK55
    Thorax
      Left ØK5J
      Right ØK5H
    Tongue, Palate, Pharynx ØK54
    Trunk
      Left ØK5G
      Right ØK5F
    Upper Arm
      Left ØK58
      Right ØK57
    Upper Leg
      Left ØK5R
      Right ØK5Q
  Nasal Mucosa and Soft Tissue Ø95K
  Nasopharynx Ø95N
  Nerve
    Abdominal Sympathetic Ø15M
    Abducens ØØ5L
    Accessory ØØ5R
    Acoustic ØØ5N
    Brachial Plexus Ø153
    Cervical Ø151
    Cervical Plexus Ø15Ø
    Facial ØØ5M
    Femoral Ø15D

Destruction — *continued*
  Nerve — *continued*
    Glossopharyngeal ØØ5P
    Head and Neck Sympathetic Ø15K
    Hypoglossal ØØ5S
    Lumbar Ø15B
    Lumbar Plexus Ø159
    Lumbar Sympathetic Ø15N
    Lumbosacral Plexus Ø15A
    Median Ø155
    Oculomotor ØØ5H
    Olfactory ØØ5F
    Optic ØØ5G
    Peroneal Ø15H
    Phrenic Ø152
    Pudendal Ø15C
    Radial Ø156
    Sacral Ø15R
    Sacral Plexus Ø15Q
    Sacral Sympathetic Ø15P
    Sciatic Ø15F
    Thoracic Ø158
    Thoracic Sympathetic Ø15L
    Tibial Ø15G
    Trigeminal ØØ5K
    Trochlear ØØ5J
    Ulnar Ø154
    Vagus ØØ5Q
  Nipple
    Left ØH5X
    Right ØH5W
  Omentum ØD5U
  Orbit
    Left ØN5Q
    Right ØN5P
  Ovary
    Bilateral ØU52
    Left ØU51
    Right ØU50
  Palate
    Hard ØC52
    Soft ØC53
  Pancreas ØF5G
  Para-aortic Body ØG59
  Paraganglion Extremity ØG5F
  Parathyroid Gland ØG5R
    Inferior
      Left ØG5P
      Right ØG5N
    Multiple ØG5Q
    Superior
      Left ØG5M
      Right ØG5L
  Patella
    Left ØQ5F
    Right ØQ5D
  Penis ØV5S
  Pericardium Ø25N
  Peritoneum ØD5W
  Phalanx
    Finger
      Left ØP5V
      Right ØP5T
    Thumb
      Left ØP5S
      Right ØP5R
    Toe
      Left ØQ5R
      Right ØQ5Q
  Pharynx ØC5M
  Pineal Body ØG51
  Pleura
    Left ØB5P
    Right ØB5N
  Pons ØØ5B
  Prepuce ØV5T
  Prostate ØV50
  Radius
    Left ØP5J
    Right ØP5H
  Rectum ØD5P
  Renal Sympathetic Nerve(s), Ultrasound Ablation
    X051329
  Retina
    Left Ø85F3ZZ
    Right Ø85E3ZZ
  Retinal Vessel
    Left Ø85H3ZZ
    Right Ø85G3ZZ

Destruction — *continued*
  Ribs
    1 to 2 ØP51
    3 or More ØP52
  Sacrum ØQ51
  Scapula
    Left ØP56
    Right ØP55
  Sclera
    Left Ø857XZZ
    Right Ø856XZZ
  Scrotum ØV55
  Septum
    Atrial Ø255
    Nasal Ø95M
    Ventricular Ø25M
  Sinus
    Accessory Ø95P
    Ethmoid
      Left Ø95V
      Right Ø95U
    Frontal
      Left Ø95T
      Right Ø95S
    Mastoid
      Left Ø95C
      Right Ø95B
    Maxillary
      Left Ø95R
      Right Ø95Q
    Sphenoid
      Left Ø95X
      Right Ø95W
  Skin
    Abdomen ØH57XZ
    Back ØH56XZ
    Buttock ØH58XZ
    Chest ØH55XZ
    Ear
      Left ØH53XZ
      Right ØH52XZ
    Face ØH51XZ
    Foot
      Left ØH5NXZ
      Right ØH5MXZ
    Hand
      Left ØH5GXZ
      Right ØH5FXZ
    Inguinal ØH5AXZ
    Lower Arm
      Left ØH5EXZ
      Right ØH5DXZ
    Lower Leg
      Left ØH5LXZ
      Right ØH5KXZ
    Neck ØH54XZ
    Perineum ØH59XZ
    Scalp ØH5ØXZ
    Upper Arm
      Left ØH5CXZ
      Right ØH5BXZ
    Upper Leg
      Left ØH5JXZ
      Right ØH5HXZ
  Skull ØN5Ø
  Spinal Cord
    Cervical ØØ5W
    Lumbar ØØ5Y
    Thoracic ØØ5X
  Spinal Meninges ØØ5T
  Spleen Ø75P
  Sternum ØP5Ø
  Stomach ØD56
    Pylorus ØD57
  Subcutaneous Tissue and Fascia
    Abdomen ØJ58
    Back ØJ57
    Buttock ØJ59
    Chest ØJ56
    Face ØJ51
    Foot
      Left ØJ5R
      Right ØJ5Q
    Hand
      Left ØJ5K
      Right ØJ5J
    Lower Arm
      Left ØJ5H
      Right ØJ5G

Destruction — *continued*
  Subcutaneous Tissue and Fascia — *continued*
    Lower Leg
      Left ØJ5P
      Right ØJ5N
    Neck
      Left ØJ55
      Right ØJ54
    Pelvic Region ØJ5C
    Perineum ØJ5B
    Scalp ØJ5Ø
    Upper Arm
      Left ØJ5F
      Right ØJ5D
    Upper Leg
      Left ØJ5M
      Right ØJ5L
  Tarsal
    Left ØQ5M
    Right ØQ5L
  Tendon
    Abdomen
      Left ØL5G
      Right ØL5F
    Ankle
      Left ØL5T
      Right ØL5S
    Foot
      Left ØL5W
      Right ØL5V
    Hand
      Left ØL58
      Right ØL57
    Head and Neck ØL5Ø
    Hip
      Left ØL5K
      Right ØL5J
    Knee
      Left ØL5R
      Right ØL5Q
    Lower Arm and Wrist
      Left ØL56
      Right ØL55
    Lower Leg
      Left ØL5P
      Right ØL5N
    Perineum ØL5H
    Shoulder
      Left ØL52
      Right ØL51
    Thorax
      Left ØL5D
      Right ØL5C
    Trunk
      Left ØL5B
      Right ØL59
    Upper Arm
      Left ØL54
      Right ØL53
    Upper Leg
      Left ØL5M
      Right ØL5L
  Testis
    Bilateral ØV5C
    Left ØV5B
    Right ØV59
  Thalamus ØØ59
  Thymus Ø75M
  Thyroid Gland ØG5K
    Left Lobe ØG5G
    Right Lobe ØG5H
  Tibia
    Left ØQ5H
    Right ØQ5G
  Toe Nail ØH5RXZZ
  Tongue ØC57
  Tonsils ØC5P
  Tooth
    Lower ØC5X
    Upper ØC5W
  Trachea ØB51
  Tunica Vaginalis
    Left ØV57
    Right ØV56
  Turbinate, Nasal Ø95L
  Tympanic Membrane
    Left Ø958
    Right Ø957

Destruction — *continued*
  Ulna
    Left ØP5L
    Right ØP5K
  Ureter
    Left ØT57
    Right ØT56
  Urethra ØT5D
  Uterine Supporting Structure ØU54
  Uterus ØU59
  Uvula ØC5N
  Vagina ØU5G
  Valve
    Aortic Ø25F
    Mitral Ø25G
    Pulmonary Ø25H
    Tricuspid Ø25J
  Vas Deferens
    Bilateral ØV5Q
    Left ØV5P
    Right ØV5N
  Vein
    Axillary
      Left Ø558
      Right Ø557
    Azygos Ø55Ø
    Basilic
      Left Ø55C
      Right Ø55B
    Brachial
      Left Ø55A
      Right Ø559
    Cephalic
      Left Ø55F
      Right Ø55D
    Colic Ø657
    Common Iliac
      Left Ø65D
      Right Ø65C
    Coronary Ø254
    Esophageal Ø653
    External Iliac
      Left Ø65G
      Right Ø65F
    External Jugular
      Left Ø55Q
      Right Ø55P
    Face
      Left Ø55V
      Right Ø55T
    Femoral
      Left Ø65N
      Right Ø65M
    Foot
      Left Ø65V
      Right Ø65T
    Gastric Ø652
    Hand
      Left Ø55H
      Right Ø55G
    Hemiazygos Ø551
    Hepatic Ø654
    Hypogastric
      Left Ø65J
      Right Ø65H
    Inferior Mesenteric Ø656
    Innominate
      Left Ø554
      Right Ø553
    Internal Jugular
      Left Ø55N
      Right Ø55M
    Intracranial Ø55L
    Lower Ø65Y
    Portal Ø658
    Pulmonary
      Left Ø25T
      Right Ø25S
    Renal
      Left Ø65B
      Right Ø659
    Saphenous
      Left Ø65Q
      Right Ø65P
    Splenic Ø651
    Subclavian
      Left Ø556
      Right Ø555
    Superior Mesenteric Ø655

Destruction — *continued*
  Vein — *continued*
    Upper Ø55Y
    Vertebral
      Left Ø55S
      Right Ø55R
  Vena Cava
    Inferior Ø65Ø
    Superior Ø25V
  Ventricle
    Left Ø25L
    Right Ø25K
  Vertebra
    Cervical ØP53
    Lumbar ØQ5Ø
    Thoracic ØP54
  Vesicle
    Bilateral ØV53
    Left ØV52
    Right ØV51
  Vitreous
    Left Ø8553ZZ
    Right Ø8543ZZ
  Vocal Cord
    Left ØC5V
    Right ØC5T
  Vulva ØU5M

Detachment
  Arm
    Lower
      Left ØX6FØZ
      Right ØX6DØZ
    Upper
      Left ØX69ØZ
      Right ØX68ØZ
  Elbow Region
    Left ØX6CØZZ
    Right ØX6BØZZ
  Femoral Region
    Left ØY68ØZZ
    Right ØY67ØZZ
  Finger
    Index
      Left ØX6PØZ
      Right ØX6NØZ
    Little
      Left ØX6WØZ
      Right ØX6VØZ
    Middle
      Left ØX6RØZ
      Right ØX6QØZ
    Ring
      Left ØX6TØZ
      Right ØX6SØZ
  Foot
    Left ØY6NØZ
    Right ØY6MØZ
  Forequarter
    Left ØX61ØZZ
    Right ØX6ØØZZ
  Hand
    Left ØX6KØZ
    Right ØX6JØZ
  Hindquarter
    Bilateral ØY64ØZZ
    Left ØY63ØZZ
    Right ØY62ØZZ
  Knee Region
    Left ØY6GØZZ
    Right ØY6FØZZ
  Leg
    Lower
      Left ØY6JØZ
      Right ØY6HØZ
    Upper
      Left ØY6DØZ
      Right ØY6CØZ
  Shoulder Region
    Left ØX63ØZZ
    Right ØX62ØZZ
  Thumb
    Left ØX6MØZ
    Right ØX6LØZ
  Toe
    1st
      Left ØY6QØZ
      Right ØY6PØZ
    2nd
      Left ØY6SØZ

Subterms under main terms may continue to next column or page

Detachment — *continued*
  Toe — *continued*
    2nd — *continued*
      Right 0Y6R0Z
    3rd
      Left 0Y6U0Z
      Right 0Y6T0Z
    4th
      Left 0Y6W0Z
      Right 0Y6V0Z
    5th
      Left 0Y6Y0Z
      Right 0Y6X0Z
Determination, Mental status GZ14ZZZ
Detorsion
  see Release
  see Reposition
DETOUR® System
  use Conduit through Femoral Vein to Popliteal
    Artery in New Technology
  use Conduit through Femoral Vein to Superficial
    Femoral Artery in New Technology
Detoxification Services, for substance abuse
  HZ2ZZZZ
Device Fitting F0DZ
Diagnostic Audiology *see* Audiology, Diagnostic
Diagnostic imaging *see* Imaging, Diagnostic
Diagnostic radiology *see* Imaging, Diagnostic
Dialysis
  Hemodialysis *see* Performance, Urinary 5A1D
  Peritoneal 3E1M39Z
Diaphragma sellae *use* Dura Mater
Diaphragmatic pacemaker generator *use* Stimulator
  Generator in Subcutaneous Tissue and Fascia
Diaphragmatic Pacemaker Lead
  Insertion of device in, Diaphragm 0BHT
  Removal of device from, Diaphragm 0BPT
  Revision of device in, Diaphragm 0BWT
Digital radiography, plain *see* Plain Radiography
Dilation
  Ampulla of Vater 0F7C
  Anus 0D7Q
  Aorta
    Abdominal
    Thoracic
      Ascending/Arch 027X
      Descending 027W
  Artery
    Anterior Tibial
      Left 047Q
        Sustained Release Drug-eluting
          Intraluminal Device
          X27Q385
        Four or More X27Q3C5
        Three X27Q3B5
        Two X27Q395
      Right 047P
        Sustained Release Drug-eluting
          Intraluminal Device
          X27P385
        Four or More X27P3C5
        Three X27P3B5
        Two X27P395
    Axillary
      Left 0376
      Right 0375
    Brachial
      Left 0378
      Right 0377
    Celiac 0471
    Colic
      Left 0477
      Middle 0478
      Right 0476
    Common Carotid
      Left 037J
      Right 037H
    Common Iliac
      Left 047D
      Right 047C
    Coronary
      Four or More Arteries 0273
      One Artery 0270
      Three Arteries 0272
      Two Arteries 0271
    External Carotid
      Left 037N
      Right 037M

Dilation — *continued*
  Artery — *continued*
    External Iliac
      Left 047J
      Right 047H
    Face 037R
    Femoral
      Left 047L
        Sustained Release Drug-eluting
          Intraluminal Device
          X27J385
        Four or More X27J3C5
        Three X27J3B5
        Two X27J395
      Right 047K
        Sustained Release Drug-eluting
          Intraluminal Device
          X27H385
        Four or More X27H3C5
        Three X27H3B5
        Two X27H395
    Foot
      Left 047W
      Right 047V
    Gastric 0472
    Hand
      Left 037F
      Right 037D
    Hepatic 0473
    Inferior Mesenteric 047B
    Innominate 0372
    Internal Carotid
      Left 037L
      Right 037K
    Internal Iliac
      Left 047F
      Right 047E
    Internal Mammary
      Left 0371
      Right 0370
    Intracranial 037G
    Lower 047Y
    Peroneal
      Left 047U
        Sustained Release Drug-eluting
          Intraluminal Device
          X27U385
        Four or More X27U3C5
        Three X27U3B5
        Two X27U395
      Right 047T
        Sustained Release Drug-eluting
          Intraluminal Device
          X27T385
        Four or More X27T3C5
        Three X27T3B5
        Two X27T395
    Popliteal
      Left 047N
      Left Distal
        Sustained Release Drug-eluting
          Intraluminal Device
          X27N385
        Four or More X27N3C5
        Three X27N3B5
        Two X27N395
      Left Proximal
        Sustained Release Drug-eluting
          Intraluminal Device
          X27L385
        Four or More X27L3C5
        Three X27L3B5
        Two X27L395
      Right 047M
      Right Distal
        Sustained Release Drug-eluting
          Intraluminal Device
          X27M385
        Four or More X27M3C5
        Three X27M3B5
        Two X27M395
      Right Proximal
        Sustained Release Drug-eluting
          Intraluminal Device
          X27K385
        Four or More X27K3C5
        Three X27K3B5
        Two X27K395

Dilation — *continued*
  Artery — *continued*
    Posterior Tibial
      Left 047S
        Sustained Release Drug-eluting
          Intraluminal Device
          X27S385
        Four or More X27S3C5
        Three X27S3B5
        Two X27S395
      Right 047R
        Sustained Release Drug-eluting
          Intraluminal Device
          X27R385
        Four or More X27R3C5
        Three X27R3B5
        Two X27R395
    Pulmonary
      Left 027R
      Right 027Q
    Pulmonary Trunk 027P
    Radial
      Left 037C
      Right 037B
    Renal
      Left 047A
      Right 0479
    Splenic 0474
    Subclavian
      Left 0374
      Right 0373
    Superior Mesenteric 0475
    Temporal
      Left 037T
      Right 037S
    Thyroid
      Left 037V
      Right 037U
    Ulnar
      Left 037A
      Right 0379
    Upper 037Y
    Vertebral
      Left 037Q
      Right 037P
  Bladder 0T7B
  Bladder Neck 0T7C
  Bronchus
    Lingula 0B79
    Lower Lobe
      Left 0B7B
      Right 0B76
    Main
      Left 0B77
      Right 0B73
    Middle Lobe, Right 0B75
    Upper Lobe
      Left 0B78
      Right 0B74
  Carina 0B72
  Cecum 0D7H
  Cerebral Ventricle 0076
  Cervix 0U7C
  Colon
    Ascending 0D7K
    Descending 0D7M
    Sigmoid 0D7N
    Transverse 0D7L
  Duct
    Common Bile 0F79
    Cystic 0F78
    Hepatic
      Common 0F77
      Left 0F76
      Right 0F75
    Lacrimal
      Left 087Y
      Right 087X
    Pancreatic 0F7D
      Accessory 0F7F
    Parotid
      Left 0C7C
      Right 0C7B
  Duodenum 0D79
  Esophagogastric Junction 0D74
  Esophagus 0D75
    Lower 0D73
    Middle 0D72
    Upper 0D71

Index

Detachment — Dilation

Dilation — *continued*
- Eustachian Tube
  - Left Ø97G
  - Right Ø97F
- Fallopian Tube
  - Left ØU76
  - Right ØU75
- Fallopian Tubes, Bilateral ØU77
- Hymen ØU7K
- Ileocecal Valve ØD7C
- Ileum ØD7B
- Intestine
  - Large ØD7E
    - Left ØD7G
    - Right ØD7F
  - Small ØD78
- Jejunum ØD7A
- Kidney Pelvis
  - Left ØT74
  - Right ØT73
- Larynx ØC7S
- Pharynx ØC7M
- Rectum ØD7P
- Stomach ØD76
  - Pylorus ØD77
- Trachea ØB71
- Ureter
  - Left ØT77
  - Right ØT76
- Ureters, Bilateral ØT78
- Urethra ØT7D
- Uterus ØU79
- Vagina ØU7G
- Valve
  - Aortic Ø27F
  - Mitral Ø27G
  - Pulmonary Ø27H
  - Tricuspid Ø27J
- Vas Deferens
  - Bilateral ØV7Q
  - Left ØV7P
  - Right ØV7N
- Vein
  - Axillary
    - Left Ø578
    - Right Ø577
  - Azygos Ø57Ø
  - Basilic
    - Left Ø57C
    - Right Ø57B
  - Brachial
    - Left Ø57A
    - Right Ø579
  - Cephalic
    - Left Ø57F
    - Right Ø57D
  - Colic Ø677
  - Common Iliac
    - Left Ø67D
    - Right Ø67C
  - Esophageal Ø673
  - External Iliac
    - Left Ø67G
    - Right Ø67F
  - External Jugular
    - Left Ø57Q
    - Right Ø57P
  - Face
    - Left Ø57V
    - Right Ø57T
  - Femoral
    - Left Ø67N
    - Right Ø67M
  - Foot
    - Left Ø67V
    - Right Ø67T
  - Gastric Ø672
  - Hand
    - Left Ø57H
    - Right Ø57G
  - Hemiazygos Ø571
  - Hepatic Ø674
  - Hypogastric
    - Left Ø67J
    - Right Ø67H
  - Inferior Mesenteric Ø676
  - Innominate
    - Left Ø574
    - Right Ø573

Dilation — *continued*
- Vein — *continued*
  - Internal Jugular
    - Left Ø57N
    - Right Ø57M
  - Intracranial Ø57L
  - Lower Ø67Y
  - Portal Ø678
  - Pulmonary
    - Left Ø27T
    - Right Ø27S
  - Renal
    - Left Ø67B
    - Right Ø679
  - Saphenous
    - Left Ø67Q
    - Right Ø67P
  - Splenic Ø671
  - Subclavian
    - Left Ø576
    - Right Ø575
  - Superior Mesenteric Ø675
  - Upper Ø57Y
  - Vertebral
    - Left Ø57S
    - Right Ø57R
  - Vena Cava
    - Inferior Ø67Ø
    - Superior Ø27V
  - Ventricle
    - Left Ø27L
    - Right Ø27K

Direct Lateral Interbody Fusion (DLIF) device *use* Interbody Fusion Device in Lower Joints

Disarticulation *see* Detachment

Discectomy, diskectomy
- *see* Excision, Lower Joints ØSB
- *see* Excision, Upper Joints ØRB
- *see* Resection, Lower Joints ØST
- *see* Resection, Upper Joints ØRT

Discography
- *see* Fluoroscopy, Axial Skeleton, Except Skull and Facial Bones BR1
- *see* Plain Radiography, Axial Skeleton, Except Skull and Facial Bones BRØ

Dismembered pyeloplasty *see* Repair, Kidney Pelvis

Distal humerus
- *use* Humeral Shaft, Left
- *use* Humeral Shaft, Right

Distal humerus, involving joint
- *use* Elbow Joint, Left
- *use* Elbow Joint, Right

Distal radioulnar joint
- *use* Wrist Joint, Left
- *use* Wrist Joint, Right

Diversion *see* Bypass

Diverticulectomy *see* Excision, Gastrointestinal System ØDB

Division
- Acetabulum
  - Left ØQ85
  - Right ØQ84
- Anal Sphincter ØD8R
- Basal Ganglia ØØ88
- Bladder Neck ØT8C
- Bone
  - Ethmoid
    - Left ØN8G
    - Right ØN8F
  - Frontal ØN81
  - Hyoid ØN8X
  - Lacrimal
    - Left ØN8J
    - Right ØN8H
  - Nasal ØN8B
  - Occipital ØN87
  - Palatine
    - Left ØN8L
    - Right ØN8K
  - Parietal
    - Left ØN84
    - Right ØN83
  - Pelvic
    - Left ØQ83
    - Right ØQ82
  - Sphenoid ØN8C
  - Temporal
    - Left ØN86

Division — *continued*
- Bone — *continued*
  - Temporal — *continued*
    - Right ØN85
  - Zygomatic
    - Left ØN8N
    - Right ØN8M
- Brain ØØ8Ø
- Bursa and Ligament
  - Abdomen
    - Left ØM8J
    - Right ØM8H
  - Ankle
    - Left ØM8R
    - Right ØM8Q
  - Elbow
    - Left ØM84
    - Right ØM83
  - Foot
    - Left ØM8T
    - Right ØM8S
  - Hand
    - Left ØM88
    - Right ØM87
  - Head and Neck ØM8Ø
  - Hip
    - Left ØM8M
    - Right ØM8L
  - Knee
    - Left ØM8P
    - Right ØM8N
  - Lower Extremity
    - Left ØM8W
    - Right ØM8V
  - Perineum ØM8K
  - Rib(s) ØM8G
  - Shoulder
    - Left ØM82
    - Right ØM81
  - Spine
    - Lower ØM8D
    - Upper ØM8C
  - Sternum ØM8F
  - Upper Extremity
    - Left ØM8B
    - Right ØM89
  - Wrist
    - Left ØM86
    - Right ØM85
- Carpal
  - Left ØP8N
  - Right ØP8M
- Cerebral Hemisphere ØØ87
- Chordae Tendineae Ø289
- Clavicle
  - Left ØP8B
  - Right ØP89
- Coccyx ØQ8S
- Conduction Mechanism Ø288
- Esophagogastric Junction ØD84
- Femoral Shaft
  - Left ØQ89
  - Right ØQ88
- Femur
  - Lower
    - Left ØQ8C
    - Right ØQ8B
  - Upper
    - Left ØQ87
    - Right ØQ86
- Fibula
  - Left ØQ8K
  - Right ØQ8J
- Gland, Pituitary ØG8Ø
- Glenoid Cavity
  - Left ØP88
  - Right ØP87
- Humeral Head
  - Left ØP8D
  - Right ØP8C
- Humeral Shaft
  - Left ØP8G
  - Right ØP8F
- Hymen ØU8K
- Kidneys, Bilateral ØT82
- Liver ØF8Ø
  - Left Lobe ØF82
  - Right Lobe ØF81

Division — continued	Division — continued	Division — continued
Mandible	Orbit	Subcutaneous Tissue and Fascia — continued
Left ØN8V	Left ØN8Q	Lower Leg
Right ØN8T	Right ØN8P	Left ØJ8P
Maxilla ØN8R	Ovary	Right ØJ8N
Metacarpal	Bilateral ØU82	Neck
Left ØP8Q	Left ØU81	Left ØJ85
Right ØP8P	Right ØU80	Right ØJ84
Metatarsal	Pancreas ØF8G	Pelvic Region ØJ8C
Left ØQ8P	Patella	Perineum ØJ8B
Right ØQ8N	Left ØQ8F	Scalp ØJ80
Muscle	Right ØQ8D	Trunk ØJ8T
Abdomen	Perineum, Female ØW8NXZZ	Upper Arm
Left ØK8L	Phalanx	Left ØJ8F
Right ØK8K	Finger	Right ØJ8D
Facial ØK81	Left ØP8V	Upper Extremity ØJ8V
Foot	Right ØP8T	Upper Leg
Left ØK8W	Thumb	Left ØJ8M
Right ØK8V	Left ØP8S	Right ØJ8L
Hand	Right ØP8R	Tarsal
Left ØK8D	Toe	Left ØQ8M
Right ØK8C	Left ØQ8R	Right ØQ8L
Head ØK80	Right ØQ8Q	Tendon
Hip	Radius	Abdomen
Left ØK8P	Left ØP8J	Left ØL8G
Right ØK8N	Right ØP8H	Right ØL8F
Lower Arm and Wrist	Ribs	Ankle
Left ØK8B	1 to 2 ØP81	Left ØL8T
Right ØK89	3 or More ØP82	Right ØL8S
Lower Leg	Sacrum ØQ81	Foot
Left ØK8T	Scapula	Left ØL8W
Right ØK8S	Left ØP86	Right ØL8V
Neck	Right ØP85	Hand
Left ØK83	Skin	Left ØL88
Right ØK82	Abdomen ØH87XZZ	Right ØL87
Papillary Ø28D	Back ØH86XZZ	Head and Neck ØL80
Perineum ØK8M	Buttock ØH88XZZ	Hip
Shoulder	Chest ØH85XZZ	Left ØL8K
Left ØK86	Ear	Right ØL8J
Right ØK85	Left ØH83XZZ	Knee
Thorax	Right ØH82XZZ	Left ØL8R
Left ØK8J	Face ØH81XZZ	Right ØL8Q
Right ØK8H	Foot	Lower Arm and Wrist
Tongue, Palate, Pharynx ØK84	Left ØH8NXZZ	Left ØL86
Trunk	Right ØH8MXZZ	Right ØL85
Left ØK8G	Hand	Lower Leg
Right ØK8F	Left ØH8GXZZ	Left ØL8P
Upper Arm	Right ØH8FXZZ	Right ØL8N
Left ØK88	Inguinal ØH8AXZZ	Perineum ØL8H
Right ØK87	Lower Arm	Shoulder
Upper Leg	Left ØH8EXZZ	Left ØL82
Left ØK8R	Right ØH8DXZZ	Right ØL81
Right ØK8Q	Lower Leg	Thorax
Nerve	Left ØH8LXZZ	Left ØL8D
Abdominal Sympathetic Ø18M	Right ØH8KXZZ	Right ØL8C
Abducens ØØ8L	Neck ØH84XZZ	Trunk
Accessory ØØ8R	Perineum ØH89XZZ	Left ØL8B
Acoustic ØØ8N	Scalp ØH80XZZ	Right ØL89
Brachial Plexus Ø183	Upper Arm	Upper Arm
Cervical Ø181	Left ØH8CXZZ	Left ØL84
Cervical Plexus Ø180	Right ØH8BXZZ	Right ØL83
Facial ØØ8M	Upper Leg	Upper Leg
Femoral Ø18D	Left ØH8JXZZ	Left ØL8M
Glossopharyngeal ØØ8P	Right ØH8HXZZ	Right ØL8L
Head and Neck Sympathetic Ø18K	Skull ØN80	Thyroid Gland Isthmus ØG8J
Hypoglossal ØØ8S	Spinal Cord	Tibia
Lumbar Ø18B	Cervical ØØ8W	Left ØQ8H
Lumbar Plexus Ø189	Lumbar ØØ8Y	Right ØQ8G
Lumbar Sympathetic Ø18N	Thoracic ØØ8X	Turbinate, Nasal Ø98L
Lumbosacral Plexus Ø18A	Sternum ØP80	Ulna
Median Ø185	Stomach, Pylorus ØD87	Left ØP8L
Oculomotor ØØ8H	Subcutaneous Tissue and Fascia	Right ØP8K
Olfactory ØØ8F	Abdomen ØJ88	Uterine Supporting Structure ØU84
Optic ØØ8G	Back ØJ87	Vertebra
Peroneal Ø18H	Buttock ØJ89	Cervical ØP83
Phrenic Ø182	Chest ØJ86	Lumbar ØQ80
Pudendal Ø18C	Face ØJ81	Thoracic ØP84
Radial Ø186	Foot	**Doppler study** *see* Ultrasonography
Sacral Ø18R	Left ØJ8R	**Dorsal digital nerve** *use* Radial Nerve
Sacral Plexus Ø18Q	Right ØJ8Q	**Dorsal metacarpal vein**
Sacral Sympathetic Ø18P	Hand	*use* Hand Vein, Left
Sciatic Ø18F	Left ØJ8K	*use* Hand Vein, Right
Thoracic Ø188	Right ØJ8J	**Dorsal metatarsal artery**
Thoracic Sympathetic Ø18L	Head and Neck ØJ8S	*use* Foot Artery, Left
Tibial Ø18G	Lower Arm	*use* Foot Artery, Right
Trigeminal ØØ8K	Left ØJ8H	**Dorsal metatarsal vein**
Trochlear ØØ8J	Right ØJ8G	*use* Foot Vein, Left
Ulnar Ø184	Lower Extremity ØJ8W	*use* Foot Vein, Right
Vagus ØØ8Q		

Dorsal root ganglion
    use Cervical Spinal Cord
    use Lumbar Spinal Cord
    use Spinal Cord
    use Thoracic Spinal Cord
Dorsal scapular artery
    use Subclavian Artery, Left
    use Subclavian Artery, Right
Dorsal scapular nerve *use* Brachial Plexus
Dorsal venous arch
    use Foot Vein, Left
    use Foot Vein, Right
Dorsalis pedis artery
    use Anterior Tibial Artery, Left
    use Anterior Tibial Artery, Right
DownStream® System 5A0512C, 5A0522C
Drainage
Abdominal Wall 0W9F
Acetabulum
    Left 0Q95
    Right 0Q94
Adenoids 0C9Q
Ampulla of Vater 0F9C
Anal Sphincter 0D9R
Ankle Region
    Left 0Y9L
    Right 0Y9K
Anterior Chamber
    Left 0893
    Right 0892
Anus 0D9Q
Aorta, Abdominal 0490
Aortic Body 0G9D
Appendix 0D9J
Arm
    Lower
        Left 0X9F
        Right 0X9D
    Upper
        Left 0X99
        Right 0X98
Artery
    Anterior Tibial
        Left 049Q
        Right 049P
    Axillary
        Left 0396
        Right 0395
    Brachial
        Left 0398
        Right 0397
    Celiac 0491
    Colic
        Left 0497
        Middle 0498
        Right 0496
    Common Carotid
        Left 039J
        Right 039H
    Common Iliac
        Left 049D
        Right 049C
    External Carotid
        Left 039N
        Right 039M
    External Iliac
        Left 049J
        Right 049H
    Face 039R
    Femoral
        Left 049L
        Right 049K
    Foot
        Left 049W
        Right 049V
    Gastric 0492
    Hand
        Left 039F
        Right 039D
    Hepatic 0493
    Inferior Mesenteric 049B
    Innominate 0392
    Internal Carotid
        Left 039L
        Right 039K
    Internal Iliac
        Left 049F
        Right 049E

Drainage — *continued*
    Artery — *continued*
        Internal Mammary
            Left 0391
            Right 0390
        Intracranial 039G
        Lower 049Y
        Peroneal
            Left 049U
            Right 049T
        Popliteal
            Left 049N
            Right 049M
        Posterior Tibial
            Left 049S
            Right 049R
        Radial
            Left 039C
            Right 039B
        Renal
            Left 049A
            Right 0499
        Splenic 0494
        Subclavian
            Left 0394
            Right 0393
        Superior Mesenteric 0495
        Temporal
            Left 039T
            Right 039S
        Thyroid
            Left 039V
            Right 039U
        Ulnar
            Left 039A
            Right 0399
        Upper 039Y
        Vertebral
            Left 039Q
            Right 039P
    Auditory Ossicle
        Left 099A
        Right 0999
    Axilla
        Left 0X95
        Right 0X94
    Back
        Lower 0W9L
        Upper 0W9K
    Basal Ganglia 0098
    Bladder 0T9B
    Bladder Neck 0T9C
    Bone
        Ethmoid
            Left 0N9G
            Right 0N9F
        Frontal 0N91
        Hyoid 0N9X
        Lacrimal
            Left 0N9J
            Right 0N9H
        Nasal 0N9B
        Occipital 0N97
        Palatine
            Left 0N9L
            Right 0N9K
        Parietal
            Left 0N94
            Right 0N93
        Pelvic
            Left 0Q93
            Right 0Q92
        Sphenoid 0N9C
        Temporal
            Left 0N96
            Right 0N95
        Zygomatic
            Left 0N9N
            Right 0N9M
    Bone Marrow 079T
    Brain 0090
    Breast
        Bilateral 0H9V
        Left 0H9U
        Right 0H9T
    Bronchus
        Lingula 0B99
        Lower Lobe
            Left 0B9B

Drainage — *continued*
    Bronchus — *continued*
        Lower Lobe — *continued*
            Right 0B96
        Main
            Left 0B97
            Right 0B93
        Middle Lobe, Right 0B95
        Upper Lobe
            Left 0B98
            Right 0B94
    Buccal Mucosa 0C94
    Bursa and Ligament
        Abdomen
            Left 0M9J
            Right 0M9H
        Ankle
            Left 0M9R
            Right 0M9Q
        Elbow
            Left 0M94
            Right 0M93
        Foot
            Left 0M9T
            Right 0M9S
        Hand
            Left 0M98
            Right 0M97
        Head and Neck 0M90
        Hip
            Left 0M9M
            Right 0M9L
        Knee
            Left 0M9P
            Right 0M9N
        Lower Extremity
            Left 0M9W
            Right 0M9V
        Perineum 0M9K
        Rib(s) 0M9G
        Shoulder
            Left 0M92
            Right 0M91
        Spine
            Lower 0M9D
            Upper 0M9C
        Sternum 0M9F
        Upper Extremity
            Left 0M9B
            Right 0M99
        Wrist
            Left 0M96
            Right 0M95
    Buttock
        Left 0Y91
        Right 0Y90
    Carina 0B92
    Carotid Bodies, Bilateral 0G98
    Carotid Body
        Left 0G96
        Right 0G97
    Carpal
        Left 0P9N
        Right 0P9M
    Cavity, Cranial 0W91
    Cecum 0D9H
    Cerebellum 009C
    Cerebral Hemisphere 0097
    Cerebral Meninges 0091
    Cerebral Ventricle 0096
    Cervix 0U9C
    Chest Wall 0W98
    Choroid
        Left 089B
        Right 089A
    Cisterna Chyli 079L
    Clavicle
        Left 0P9B
        Right 0P99
    Clitoris 0U9J
    Coccygeal Glomus 0G9B
    Coccyx 0Q9S
    Colon
        Ascending 0D9K
        Descending 0D9M
        Sigmoid 0D9N
        Transverse 0D9L
    Conjunctiva
        Left 089T

⧗ Subterms under main terms may continue to next column or page

Drainage — *continued*
  Conjunctiva — *continued*
    Right Ø89S
  Cord
    Bilateral ØV9H
    Left ØV9G
    Right ØV9F
  Cornea
    Left Ø899
    Right Ø898
  Cul-de-sac ØU9F
  Diaphragm ØB9T
  Disc
    Cervical Vertebral ØR93
    Cervicothoracic Vertebral ØR95
    Lumbar Vertebral ØS92
    Lumbosacral ØS94
    Thoracic Vertebral ØR99
    Thoracolumbar Vertebral ØR9B
  Duct
    Common Bile ØF99
    Cystic ØF98
    Hepatic
      Common ØF97
      Left ØF96
      Right ØF95
    Lacrimal
      Left Ø89Y
      Right Ø89X
    Pancreatic ØF9D
      Accessory ØF9F
    Parotid
      Left ØC9C
      Right ØC9B
  Duodenum ØD99
  Dura Mater ØØ92
  Ear
    External
      Left Ø991
      Right Ø99Ø
    External Auditory Canal
      Left Ø994
      Right Ø993
    Inner
      Left Ø99E
      Right Ø99D
    Middle
      Left Ø996
      Right Ø995
  Elbow Region
    Left ØX9C
    Right ØX9B
  Epididymis
    Bilateral ØV9L
    Left ØV9K
    Right ØV9J
  Epidural Space, Intracranial ØØ93
  Epiglottis ØC9R
  Esophagogastric Junction ØD94
  Esophagus ØD95
    Lower ØD93
    Middle ØD92
    Upper ØD91
  Eustachian Tube
    Left Ø99G
    Right Ø99F
  Extremity
    Lower
      Left ØY9B
      Right ØY99
    Upper
      Left ØX97
      Right ØX96
  Eye
    Left Ø891
    Right Ø89Ø
  Eyelid
    Lower
      Left Ø89R
      Right Ø89Q
    Upper
      Left Ø89P
      Right Ø89N
  Face ØW92
  Fallopian Tube
    Left ØU96
    Right ØU95
  Fallopian Tubes, Bilateral ØU97

Drainage — *continued*
  Femoral Region
    Left ØY98
    Right ØY97
  Femoral Shaft
    Left ØQ99
    Right ØQ98
  Femur
    Lower
      Left ØQ9C
      Right ØQ9B
    Upper
      Left ØQ97
      Right ØQ96
  Fibula
    Left ØQ9K
    Right ØQ9J
  Finger Nail ØH9Q
  Foot
    Left ØY9N
    Right ØY9M
  Gallbladder ØF94
  Gingiva
    Lower ØC96
    Upper ØC95
  Gland
    Adrenal
      Bilateral ØG94
      Left ØG92
      Right ØG93
    Lacrimal
      Left Ø89W
      Right Ø89V
    Minor Salivary ØC9J
    Parotid
      Left ØC99
      Right ØC98
    Pituitary ØG90
    Sublingual
      Left ØC9F
      Right ØC9D
    Submaxillary
      Left ØC9H
      Right ØC9G
    Vestibular ØU9L
  Glenoid Cavity
    Left ØP98
    Right ØP97
  Glomus Jugulare ØG9C
  Hand
    Left ØX9K
    Right ØX9J
  Head ØW90
  Humeral Head
    Left ØP9D
    Right ØP9C
  Humeral Shaft
    Left ØP9G
    Right ØP9F
  Hymen ØU9K
  Hypothalamus ØØ9A
  Ileocecal Valve ØD9C
  Ileum ØD9B
  Inguinal Region
    Left ØY96
    Right ØY95
  Intestine
    Large ØD9E
      Left ØD9G
      Right ØD9F
    Small ØD98
  Iris
    Left Ø89D
    Right Ø89C
  Jaw
    Lower ØW95
    Upper ØW94
  Jejunum ØD9A
  Joint
    Acromioclavicular
      Left ØR9H
      Right ØR9G
    Ankle
      Left ØS9G
      Right ØS9F
    Carpal
      Left ØR9R
      Right ØR9Q

Drainage — *continued*
  Joint — *continued*
    Carpometacarpal
      Left ØR9T
      Right ØR9S
    Cervical Vertebral ØR91
    Cervicothoracic Vertebral ØR94
    Coccygeal ØS96
    Elbow
      Left ØR9M
      Right ØR9L
    Finger Phalangeal
      Left ØR9X
      Right ØR9W
    Hip
      Left ØS9B
      Right ØS99
    Knee
      Left ØS9D
      Right ØS9C
    Lumbar Vertebral ØS90
    Lumbosacral ØS93
    Metacarpophalangeal
      Left ØR9V
      Right ØR9U
    Metatarsal-Phalangeal
      Left ØS9N
      Right ØS9M
    Occipital-cervical ØR90
    Sacrococcygeal ØS95
    Sacroiliac
      Left ØS98
      Right ØS97
    Shoulder
      Left ØR9K
      Right ØR9J
    Sternoclavicular
      Left ØR9F
      Right ØR9E
    Tarsal
      Left ØS9J
      Right ØS9H
    Tarsometatarsal
      Left ØS9L
      Right ØS9K
    Temporomandibular
      Left ØR9D
      Right ØR9C
    Thoracic Vertebral ØR96
    Thoracolumbar Vertebral ØR9A
    Toe Phalangeal
      Left ØS9Q
      Right ØS9P
    Wrist
      Left ØR9P
      Right ØR9N
  Kidney
    Left ØT91
    Right ØT90
  Kidney Pelvis
    Left ØT94
    Right ØT93
  Knee Region
    Left ØY9G
    Right ØY9F
  Larynx ØC9S
  Leg
    Lower
      Left ØY9J
      Right ØY9H
    Upper
      Left ØY9D
      Right ØY9C
  Lens
    Left Ø89K
    Right Ø89J
  Lip
    Lower ØC91
    Upper ØC90
  Liver ØF90
    Left Lobe ØF92
    Right Lobe ØF91
  Lung
    Bilateral ØB9M
    Left ØB9L
    Lower Lobe
      Left ØB9J
      Right ØB9F
    Middle Lobe, Right ØB9D

Drainage — *continued*
  Lung — *continued*
    Right 0B9K
    Upper Lobe
      Left 0B9G
      Right 0B9C
  Lung Lingula 0B9H
  Lymphatic
    Aortic 079D
    Axillary
      Left 0796
      Right 0795
    Head 0790
    Inguinal
      Left 079J
      Right 079H
    Internal Mammary
      Left 0799
      Right 0798
    Lower Extremity
      Left 079G
      Right 079F
    Mesenteric 079B
    Neck
      Left 0792
      Right 0791
    Pelvis 079C
    Thoracic Duct 079K
    Thorax 0797
    Upper Extremity
      Left 0794
      Right 0793
  Mandible
    Left 0N9V
    Right 0N9T
  Maxilla 0N9R
  Mediastinum 0W9C
  Medulla Oblongata 009D
  Mesentery 0D9V
  Metacarpal
    Left 0P9Q
    Right 0P9P
  Metatarsal
    Left 0Q9P
    Right 0Q9N
  Muscle
    Abdomen
      Left 0K9L
      Right 0K9K
    Extraocular
      Left 089M
      Right 089L
    Facial 0K91
    Foot
      Left 0K9W
      Right 0K9V
    Hand
      Left 0K9D
      Right 0K9C
    Head 0K90
    Hip
      Left 0K9P
      Right 0K9N
    Lower Arm and Wrist
      Left 0K9B
      Right 0K99
    Lower Leg
      Left 0K9T
      Right 0K9S
    Neck
      Left 0K93
      Right 0K92
    Perineum 0K9M
    Shoulder
      Left 0K96
      Right 0K95
    Thorax
      Left 0K9J
      Right 0K9H
    Tongue, Palate, Pharynx 0K94
    Trunk
      Left 0K9G
      Right 0K9F
    Upper Arm
      Left 0K98
      Right 0K97
    Upper Leg
      Left 0K9R
      Right 0K9Q

Drainage — *continued*
  Nasal Mucosa and Soft Tissue 099K
  Nasopharynx 099N
  Neck 0W96
  Nerve
    Abdominal Sympathetic 019M
    Abducens 009L
    Accessory 009R
    Acoustic 009N
    Brachial Plexus 0193
    Cervical 0191
    Cervical Plexus 0190
    Facial 009M
    Femoral 019D
    Glossopharyngeal 009P
    Head and Neck Sympathetic 019K
    Hypoglossal 009S
    Lumbar 019B
    Lumbar Plexus 0199
    Lumbar Sympathetic 019N
    Lumbosacral Plexus 019A
    Median 0195
    Oculomotor 009H
    Olfactory 009F
    Optic 009G
    Peroneal 019H
    Phrenic 0192
    Pudendal 019C
    Radial 0196
    Sacral 019R
    Sacral Plexus 019Q
    Sacral Sympathetic 019P
    Sciatic 019F
    Thoracic 0198
    Thoracic Sympathetic 019L
    Tibial 019G
    Trigeminal 009K
    Trochlear 009J
    Ulnar 0194
    Vagus 009Q
  Nipple
    Left 0H9X
    Right 0H9W
  Omentum 0D9U
  Oral Cavity and Throat 0W93
  Orbit
    Left 0N9Q
    Right 0N9P
  Ovary
    Bilateral 0U92
    Left 0U91
    Right 0U90
  Palate
    Hard 0C92
    Soft 0C93
  Pancreas 0F9G
  Para-aortic Body 0G99
  Paraganglion Extremity 0G9F
  Parathyroid Gland 0G9R
    Inferior
      Left 0G9P
      Right 0G9N
    Multiple 0G9Q
    Superior
      Left 0G9M
      Right 0G9L
  Patella
    Left 0Q9F
    Right 0Q9D
  Pelvic Cavity 0W9J
  Penis 0V9S
  Pericardial Cavity 0W9D
  Perineum
    Female 0W9N
    Male 0W9M
  Peritoneal Cavity 0W9G
  Peritoneum 0D9W
  Phalanx
    Finger
      Left 0P9V
      Right 0P9T
    Thumb
      Left 0P9S
      Right 0P9R
    Toe
      Left 0Q9R
      Right 0Q9Q
  Pharynx 0C9M
  Pineal Body 0G91

Drainage — *continued*
  Pleura
    Left 0B9P
    Right 0B9N
  Pleural Cavity
    Left 0W9B
    Right 0W99
  Pons 009B
  Prepuce 0V9T
  Products of Conception
    Amniotic Fluid
      Diagnostic 1090
      Therapeutic 1090
    Fetal Blood 1090
    Fetal Cerebrospinal Fluid 1090
    Fetal Fluid, Other 1090
    Fluid, Other 1090
  Prostate 0V90
  Radius
    Left 0P9J
    Right 0P9H
  Rectum 0D9P
  Retina
    Left 089F
    Right 089E
  Retinal Vessel
    Left 089H
    Right 089G
  Retroperitoneum 0W9H
  Ribs
    1 to 2 0P91
    3 or More 0P92
  Sacrum 0Q91
  Scapula
    Left 0P96
    Right 0P95
  Sclera
    Left 0897
    Right 0896
  Scrotum 0V95
  Septum, Nasal 099M
  Shoulder Region
    Left 0X93
    Right 0X92
  Sinus
    Accessory 099P
    Ethmoid
      Left 099V
      Right 099U
    Frontal
      Left 099T
      Right 099S
    Mastoid
      Left 099C
      Right 099B
    Maxillary
      Left 099R
      Right 099Q
    Sphenoid
      Left 099X
      Right 099W
  Skin
    Abdomen 0H97
    Back 0H96
    Buttock 0H98
    Chest 0H95
    Ear
      Left 0H93
      Right 0H92
    Face 0H91
    Foot
      Left 0H9N
      Right 0H9M
    Hand
      Left 0H9G
      Right 0H9F
    Inguinal 0H9A
    Lower Arm
      Left 0H9E
      Right 0H9D
    Lower Leg
      Left 0H9L
      Right 0H9K
    Neck 0H94
    Perineum 0H99
    Scalp 0H90
    Upper Arm
      Left 0H9C
      Right 0H9B

Drainage — *continued*
  Skin — *continued*
    Upper Leg
      Left ØH9J
      Right ØH9H
  Skull ØN9Ø
  Spinal Canal ØØ9U
  Spinal Cord
    Cervical ØØ9W
    Lumbar ØØ9Y
    Thoracic ØØ9X
  Spinal Meninges ØØ9T
  Spleen Ø79P
  Sternum ØP9Ø
  Stomach ØD96
    Pylorus ØD97
  Subarachnoid Space, Intracranial ØØ95
  Subcutaneous Tissue and Fascia
    Abdomen ØJ98
    Back ØJ97
    Buttock ØJ99
    Chest ØJ96
    Face ØJ91
    Foot
      Left ØJ9R
      Right ØJ9Q
    Hand
      Left ØJ9K
      Right ØJ9J
    Lower Arm
      Left ØJ9H
      Right ØJ9G
    Lower Leg
      Left ØJ9P
      Right ØJ9N
    Neck
      Left ØJ95
      Right ØJ94
    Pelvic Region ØJ9C
    Perineum ØJ9B
    Scalp ØJ9Ø
    Upper Arm
      Left ØJ9F
      Right ØJ9D
    Upper Leg
      Left ØJ9M
      Right ØJ9L
  Subdural Space, Intracranial ØØ94
  Tarsal
    Left ØQ9M
    Right ØQ9L
  Tendon
    Abdomen
      Left ØL9G
      Right ØL9F
    Ankle
      Left ØL9T
      Right ØL9S
    Foot
      Left ØL9W
      Right ØL9V
    Hand
      Left ØL98
      Right ØL97
    Head and Neck ØL9Ø
    Hip
      Left ØL9K
      Right ØL9J
    Knee
      Left ØL9R
      Right ØL9Q
    Lower Arm and Wrist
      Left ØL96
      Right ØL95
    Lower Leg
      Left ØL9P
      Right ØL9N
    Perineum ØL9H
    Shoulder
      Left ØL92
      Right ØL91
    Thorax
      Left ØL9D
      Right ØL9C
    Trunk
      Left ØL9B
      Right ØL99
    Upper Arm
      Left ØL94

Drainage — *continued*
  Tendon — *continued*
    Upper Arm — *continued*
      Right ØL93
    Upper Leg
      Left ØL9M
      Right ØL9L
  Testis
    Bilateral ØV9C
    Left ØV9B
    Right ØV99
  Thalamus ØØ99
  Thymus Ø79M
  Thyroid Gland ØG9K
    Left Lobe ØG9G
    Right Lobe ØG9H
  Tibia
    Left ØQ9H
    Right ØQ9G
  Toe Nail ØH9R
  Tongue ØC97
  Tonsils ØC9P
  Tooth
    Lower ØC9X
    Upper ØC9W
  Trachea ØB91
  Tunica Vaginalis
    Left ØV97
    Right ØV96
  Turbinate, Nasal Ø99L
  Tympanic Membrane
    Left Ø998
    Right Ø997
  Ulna
    Left ØP9L
    Right ØP9K
  Ureter
    Left ØT97
    Right ØT96
  Ureters, Bilateral ØT98
  Urethra ØT9D
  Uterine Supporting Structure ØU94
  Uterus ØU99
  Uvula ØC9N
  Vagina ØU9G
  Vas Deferens
    Bilateral ØV9Q
    Left ØV9P
    Right ØV9N
  Vein
    Axillary
      Left Ø598
      Right Ø597
    Azygos Ø59Ø
    Basilic
      Left Ø59C
      Right Ø59B
    Brachial
      Left Ø59A
      Right Ø599
    Cephalic
      Left Ø59F
      Right Ø59D
    Colic Ø697
    Common Iliac
      Left Ø69D
      Right Ø69C
    Esophageal Ø693
    External Iliac
      Left Ø69G
      Right Ø69F
    External Jugular
      Left Ø59Q
      Right Ø59P
    Face
      Left Ø59V
      Right Ø59T
    Femoral
      Left Ø69N
      Right Ø69M
    Foot
      Left Ø69V
      Right Ø69T
    Gastric Ø692
    Hand
      Left Ø59H
      Right Ø59G
    Hemiazygos Ø591
    Hepatic Ø694

Drainage — *continued*
  Vein — *continued*
    Hypogastric
      Left Ø69J
      Right Ø69H
    Inferior Mesenteric Ø696
    Innominate
      Left Ø594
      Right Ø593
    Internal Jugular
      Left Ø59N
      Right Ø59M
    Intracranial Ø59L
    Lower Ø69Y
    Portal Ø698
    Renal
      Left Ø69B
      Right Ø699
    Saphenous
      Left Ø69Q
      Right Ø69P
    Splenic Ø691
    Subclavian
      Left Ø596
      Right Ø595
    Superior Mesenteric Ø695
    Upper Ø59Y
    Vertebral
      Left Ø59S
      Right Ø59R
  Vena Cava, Inferior Ø69Ø
  Vertebra
    Cervical ØP93
    Lumbar ØQ9Ø
    Thoracic ØP94
  Vesicle
    Bilateral ØV93
    Left ØV92
    Right ØV91
  Vitreous
    Left Ø895
    Right Ø894
  Vocal Cord
    Left ØC9V
    Right ØC9T
  Vulva ØU9M
  Wrist Region
    Left ØX9H
    Right ØX9G

Dressing
  Abdominal Wall 2W23X4Z
  Arm
    Lower
      Left 2W2DX4Z
      Right 2W2CX4Z
    Upper
      Left 2W2BX4Z
      Right 2W2AX4Z
  Back 2W25X4Z
  Chest Wall 2W24X4Z
  Extremity
    Lower
      Left 2W2MX4Z
      Right 2W2LX4Z
    Upper
      Left 2W29X4Z
      Right 2W28X4Z
  Face 2W21X4Z
  Finger
    Left 2W2KX4Z
    Right 2W2JX4Z
  Foot
    Left 2W2TX4Z
    Right 2W2SX4Z
  Hand
    Left 2W2FX4Z
    Right 2W2EX4Z
  Head 2W2ØX4Z
  Inguinal Region
    Left 2W27X4Z
    Right 2W26X4Z
  Leg
    Lower
      Left 2W2RX4Z
      Right 2W2QX4Z
    Upper
      Left 2W2PX4Z
      Right 2W2NX4Z
  Neck 2W22X4Z

Dressing — *continued*
 Thumb
  Left 2W2HX4Z
  Right 2W2GX4Z
 Toe
  Left 2W2VX4Z
  Right 2W2UX4Z
Driver stent (RX) (OTW) *use* Intraluminal Device
Drotrecogin alfa, infusion *see* Introduction of Recombinant Human-activated Protein C
Duct of Santorini *use* Pancreatic Duct, Accessory
Duct of Wirsung *use* Pancreatic Duct
Ductogram, mammary *see* Plain Radiography, Skin, Subcutaneous Tissue and Breast BHØ
Ductography, mammary *see* Plain Radiography, Skin, Subcutaneous Tissue and Breast BHØ
Ductus deferens
 use Vas Deferens
 use Vas Deferens, Bilateral
 use Vas Deferens, Left
 use Vas Deferens, Right
Duodenal ampulla *use* Ampulla of Vater
Duodenectomy
 see Excision, Duodenum ØDB9
 see Resection, Duodenum ØDT9
Duodenocholedochotomy *see* Drainage, Gallbladder ØF94
Duodenocystostomy
 see Bypass, Gallbladder ØF14
 see Drainage, Gallbladder ØF94
Duodenoenterostomy
 see Bypass, Gastrointestinal System ØD1
 see Drainage, Gastrointestinal System ØD9
Duodenojejunal flexure *use* Jejunum
Duodenolysis *see* Release, Duodenum ØDN9
Duodenorrhaphy *see* Repair, Duodenum ØDQ9
Duodenoscopy, single-use (aScope™ Duodeno) (EXALT™ Model D) *see* New Technology, Hepatobiliary System and Pancreas XFJ
Duodenostomy
 see Bypass, Duodenum ØD19
 see Drainage, Duodenum ØD99
Duodenotomy *see* Drainage, Duodenum ØD99
Dura mater, intracranial *use* Dura Mater
Dura mater, spinal *use* Spinal Meninges
DuraGraft® Endothelial Damage Inhibitor *use* Endothelial Damage Inhibitor
DuraHeart Left Ventricular Assist System *use* Implantable Heart Assist System in Heart and Great Vessels
Dural venous sinus *use* Intracranial Vein
Durata® Defibrillation Lead *use* Cardiac Lead, Defibrillator in Ø2H
Durvalumab Antineoplastic XWØ
DynaClip® (Forte)
 use Internal Fixation Device, Sustained Compression in ØRG
 use Internal Fixation Device, Sustained Compression in ØSG
DynaNail® (Helix)(Hybrid) (Mini)
 use Internal Fixation Device, Sustained Compression in ØRG
 use Internal Fixation Device, Sustained Compression in ØSG
Dynesys® Dynamic Stabilization System
 use Spinal Stabilization Device, Pedicle-Based in ØRH
 use Spinal Stabilization Device, Pedicle-Based in ØSH

E

Earlobe
 use Ear, External, Bilateral
 use Ear, External, Left
 use Ear, External, Right
ECCO2R (Extracorporeal Carbon Dioxide Removal) 5AØ92ØZ
Echocardiogram *see* Ultrasonography, Heart B24
EchoGo Heart Failure 1.Ø software XXE2X19
Echography *see* Ultrasonography
EchoTip® Insight™ Portosystemic Pressure Gradient Measurement System 4AØ44B2
ECMO *see* Performance, Circulatory 5A15
ECMO, intraoperative *see* Performance, Circulatory 5A15A

Eculizumab XWØ
EDWARDS INTUITY Elite valve system (rapid deployment technique) *see* Replacement, Valve, Aortic Ø2RF
EEG (electroencephalogram) *see* Measurement, Central Nervous 4AØØ
EGD (esophagogastroduodenoscopy) ØDJØ8ZZ
Eighth cranial nerve *use* Acoustic Nerve
Ejaculatory duct
 use Vas Deferens
 use Vas Deferens, Bilateral
 use Vas Deferens, Left
 use Vas Deferens, Right
EKG (electrocardiogram) *see* Measurement, Cardiac 4AØ2
EKOS™ EkoSonic® Endovascular System *see* Fragmentation, Artery
Eladocagene exuparvovec XWØQ316
Electrical bone growth stimulator (EBGS)
 use Bone Growth Stimulator in Head and Facial Bones
 use Bone Growth Stimulator in Lower Bones
 use Bone Growth Stimulator in Upper Bones
Electrical muscle stimulation (EMS) lead *use* Stimulator Lead in Muscles
Electrocautery
 Destruction *see* Destruction
 Repair *see* Repair
Electroconvulsive Therapy
 Bilateral-Multiple Seizure GZB3ZZZ
 Bilateral-Single Seizure GZB2ZZZ
 Electroconvulsive Therapy, Other GZB4ZZZ
 Unilateral-Multiple Seizure GZB1ZZZ
 Unilateral-Single Seizure GZBØZZZ
Electroencephalogram (EEG) *see* Measurement, Central Nervous 4AØØ
Electromagnetic Therapy
 Central Nervous 6A22
 Urinary 6A21
Electronic muscle stimulator lead *use* Stimulator Lead in Muscles
Electrophysiologic stimulation (EPS) *see* Measurement, Cardiac 4AØ2
Electroshock therapy *see* Electroconvulsive Therapy
Elevation, bone fragments, skull *see* Reposition, Head and Facial Bones ØNS
Eleventh cranial nerve *use* Accessory Nerve
Ellipsys® vascular access system *see* New Technology, Cardiovascular System X2K
E-Luminexx™(Biliary) (Vascular) Stent *use* Intraluminal Device
Eluvia™ Drug-Eluting Vascular Stent System
 use Intraluminal Device, Sustained Release Drug-eluting in New Technology
 use Intraluminal Device, Sustained Release Drug-eluting, Two in New Technology
 use Intraluminal Device, Sustained Release Drug-eluting, Three in New Technology
 use Intraluminal Device, Sustained Release Drug-eluting, Four or More in New Technology
ELZONRIS™ *use* Tagraxofusp-erzs Antineoplastic
Embolectomy *see* Extirpation
Embolization
 see Occlusion
 see Restriction
Embolization coil(s) *use* Intraluminal Device
EMG (electromyogram) *see* Measurement, Musculoskeletal 4AØF
Encephalon *use* Brain
Endarterectomy
 see Extirpation, Lower Arteries Ø4C
 see Extirpation, Upper Arteries Ø3C
Endeavor® (III) (IV) (Sprint) Zotarolimus-eluting Coronary Stent System *use* Intraluminal Device, Drug-eluting in Heart and Great Vessels
EndoAVF procedure, using magnetic-guided radiofrequency *see* Bypass, Upper Arteries Ø31
EndoAVF procedure, using thermal resistance energy *see* New Technology, Cardiovascular System X2K
Endologix AFX® Endovascular AAA System *use* Intraluminal Device
EndoSure® sensor *use* Monitoring Device, Pressure Sensor in Ø2H
ENDOTAK RELIANCE® (G) Defibrillation Lead *use* Cardiac Lead, Defibrillator in Ø2H

Endothelial damage inhibitor, applied to vein graft XYØVX83
Endotracheal tube (cuffed) (double-lumen) *use* Intraluminal Device, Endotracheal Airway in Respiratory System
Endovascular fistula creation, using magnetic-guided radiofrequency *see* Bypass, Upper Arteries Ø31
Endovascular fistula creation, using thermal resistance energy *see* New Technology, Cardiovascular System X2K
Endurant® Endovascular Stent Graft *use* Intraluminal Device
Endurant® II AAA Stent Graft System *use* Intraluminal Device
Engineered Allogeneic Thymus Tissue XWØ20D8
Engineered Chimeric Antigen Receptor T-cell Immunotherapy
 Allogeneic XWØ
 Autologous XWØ
Enlargement
 see Dilation
 see Repair
EnRhythm *use* Pacemaker, Dual Chamber in ØJH
ENROUTE® Transcarotid Neuroprotection System *see* New Technology, Cardiovascular System X2A
ENSPRYNG™ *use* Satralizumab-mwge
Enterorrhaphy *see* Repair, Gastrointestinal System ØDQ
Enterra gastric neurostimulator *use* Stimulator Generator, Multiple Array in ØJH
Enucleation
 Eyeball *see* Resection, Eye Ø8T
 Eyeball with prosthetic implant *see* Replacement, Eye Ø8R
Epcoritamab Monoclonal Antibody XWØ13S9
Ependyma *use* Cerebral Ventricle
Epicel® cultured epidermal autograft *use* Autologous Tissue Substitute
Epic™ Stented Tissue Valve (aortic) *use* Zooplastic Tissue in Heart and Great Vessels
Epidermis *use* Skin
Epididymectomy
 see Excision, Male Reproductive System ØVB
 see Resection, Male Reproductive System ØVT
Epididymoplasty
 see Repair, Male Reproductive System ØVQ
 see Supplement, Male Reproductive System ØVU
Epididymorrhaphy *see* Repair, Male Reproductive System ØVQ
Epididymotomy *see* Drainage, Male Reproductive System ØV9
Epidural space, spinal *use* Spinal Canal
Epiphysiodesis
 see Insertion of device in, Lower Bones ØQH
 see Insertion of device in, Upper Bones ØPH
 see Repair, Lower Bones ØQQ
 see Repair, Upper Bones ØPQ
Epiploic foramen *use* Peritoneum
Epiretinal Visual Prosthesis
 Left Ø8H1Ø5Z
 Right Ø8HØØ5Z
Episiorrhaphy *see* Repair, Perineum, Female ØWQN
Episiotomy *see* Division, Perineum, Female ØW8N
Epithalamus *use* Thalamus
Epitrochlear lymph node
 use Lymphatic, Left Upper Extremity
 use Lymphatic, Right Upper Extremity
EPS (electrophysiologic stimulation) *see* Measurement, Cardiac 4AØ2
Eptifibatide, infusion *see* Introduction of Platelet Inhibitor
ERCP (endoscopic retrograde cholangiopancreatography) *see* Fluoroscopy, Hepatobiliary System and Pancreas BF1
Erdafitinib Antineoplastic XWØDXL5
Erector spinae muscle
 use Trunk Muscle, Left
 use Trunk Muscle, Right
ERLEADA™ *use* Apalutamide Antineoplastic
Esketamine Hydrochloride XWØ97M5
Esophageal artery *use* Upper Artery
Esophageal obturator airway (EOA) *use* Intraluminal Device, Airway in Gastrointestinal System
Esophageal plexus *use* Thoracic Sympathetic Nerve
Esophagectomy
 see Excision, Gastrointestinal System ØDB

▽ Subterms under main terms may continue to next column or page

Esophagectomy — *continued*
  see Resection, Gastrointestinal System ØDT
Esophagocoloplasty
  see Repair, Gastrointestinal System ØDQ
  see Supplement, Gastrointestinal System ØDU
Esophagoenterostomy
  see Bypass, Gastrointestinal System ØD1
  see Drainage, Gastrointestinal System ØD9
Esophagoesophagostomy
  see Bypass, Gastrointestinal System ØD1
  see Drainage, Gastrointestinal System ØD9
Esophagogastrectomy
  see Excision, Gastrointestinal System ØDB
  see Resection, Gastrointestinal System ØDT
Esophagogastroduodenoscopy (EGD) ØDJØ8ZZ
Esophagogastroplasty
  see Repair, Gastrointestinal System ØDQ
  see Supplement, Gastrointestinal System ØDU
Esophagogastroscopy ØDJ68ZZ
Esophagogastrostomy
  see Bypass, Gastrointestinal System ØD1
  see Drainage, Gastrointestinal System ØD9
Esophagojejunoplasty *see* Supplement, Gastrointestinal System ØDU
Esophagojejunostomy
  see Bypass, Gastrointestinal System ØD1
  see Drainage, Gastrointestinal System ØD9
Esophagomyotomy *see* Division, Esophagogastric Junction ØD84
Esophagoplasty
  see Repair, Gastrointestinal System ØDQ
  see Replacement, Esophagus ØDR5
  see Supplement, Gastrointestinal System ØDU
Esophagoplication *see* Restriction, Gastrointestinal System ØDV
Esophagorrhaphy *see* Repair, Gastrointestinal System ØDQ
Esophagoscopy ØDJØ8ZZ
Esophagotomy *see* Drainage, Gastrointestinal System ØD9
Esteem® implantable hearing system *use* Hearing Device in Ear, Nose, Sinus
ESWL (extracorporeal shock wave lithotripsy) *see* Fragmentation
Etesevimab Monoclonal Antibody XWØ
Ethmoidal air cell
  use Ethmoid Sinus, Left
  use Ethmoid Sinus, Right
Ethmoidectomy
  see Excision, Ear, Nose, Sinus Ø9B
  see Excision, Head and Facial Bones ØNB
  see Resection, Ear, Nose, Sinus Ø9T
  see Resection, Head and Facial Bones ØNT
Ethmoidotomy *see* Drainage, Ear, Nose, Sinus Ø99
EV ICD System (Extravascular implantable defibrillator lead) *use* Defibrillator Lead in Anatomical Regions, General
Evacuation
  Hematoma *see* Extirpation
  Other Fluid *see* Drainage
Evera (XT) (S) (DR/VR) *use* Defibrillator Generator in ØJH
Everolimus-eluting coronary stent *use* Intraluminal Device, Drug-eluting in Heart and Great Vessels
Evisceration
  Eyeball *see* Resection, Eye Ø8T
  Eyeball with prosthetic implant *see* Replacement, Eye Ø8R
EVUSHELD™ *use* Tixagevimab and Cilgavimab Monoclonal Antibody
Exagamglogene Autotemcel XW1
EXALT™ Model D Single-Use Duodenoscope *see* New Technology, Hepatobiliary System and Pancreas XFJ
Examination *see* Inspection
Exchange *see* Change device in
Excision
  Abdominal Wall ØWBF
  Acetabulum
    Left ØQB5
    Right ØQB4
  Adenoids ØCBQ
  Ampulla of Vater ØFBC
  Anal Sphincter ØDBR
  Ankle Region
    Left ØYBL
    Right ØYBK

Excision — *continued*
  Anus ØDBQ
  Aorta
    Abdominal
    Thoracic
      Ascending/Arch Ø2BX
      Descending Ø2BW
  Aortic Body ØGBD
  Appendix ØDBJ
  Arm
    Lower
      Left ØXBF
      Right ØXBD
    Upper
      Left ØXB9
      Right ØXB8
  Artery
    Anterior Tibial
      Left Ø4BQ
      Right Ø4BP
    Axillary
      Left Ø3B6
      Right Ø3B5
    Brachial
      Left Ø3B8
      Right Ø3B7
    Celiac Ø4B1
    Colic
      Left Ø4B7
      Middle Ø4B8
      Right Ø4B6
    Common Carotid
      Left Ø3BJ
      Right Ø3BH
    Common Iliac
      Left Ø4BD
      Right Ø4BC
    External Carotid
      Left Ø3BN
      Right Ø3BM
    External Iliac
      Left Ø4BJ
      Right Ø4BH
    Face Ø3BR
    Femoral
      Left Ø4BL
      Right Ø4BK
    Foot
      Left Ø4BW
      Right Ø4BV
    Gastric Ø4B2
    Hand
      Left Ø3BF
      Right Ø3BD
    Hepatic Ø4B3
    Inferior Mesenteric Ø4BB
    Innominate Ø3B2
    Internal Carotid
      Left Ø3BL
      Right Ø3BK
    Internal Iliac
      Left Ø4BF
      Right Ø4BE
    Internal Mammary
      Left Ø3B1
      Right Ø3BØ
    Intracranial Ø3BG
    Lower Ø4BY
    Peroneal
      Left Ø4BU
      Right Ø4BT
    Popliteal
      Left Ø4BN
      Right Ø4BM
    Posterior Tibial
      Left Ø4BS
      Right Ø4BR
    Pulmonary
      Left Ø2BR
      Right Ø2BQ
    Pulmonary Trunk Ø2BP
    Radial
      Left Ø3BC
      Right Ø3BB
    Renal
      Left Ø4BA
      Right Ø4B9
    Splenic Ø4B4

Excision — *continued*
  Artery — *continued*
    Subclavian
      Left Ø3B4
      Right Ø3B3
    Superior Mesenteric Ø4B5
    Temporal
      Left Ø3BT
      Right Ø3BS
    Thyroid
      Left Ø3BV
      Right Ø3BU
    Ulnar
      Left Ø3BA
      Right Ø3B9
    Upper Ø3BY
    Vertebral
      Left Ø3BQ
      Right Ø3BP
  Atrium
    Left Ø2B7
    Right Ø2B6
  Auditory Ossicle
    Left Ø9BA
    Right Ø9B9
  Axilla
    Left ØXB5
    Right ØXB4
  Back
    Lower ØWBL
    Upper ØWBK
  Basal Ganglia ØØB8
  Bladder ØTBB
  Bladder Neck ØTBC
  Bone
    Ethmoid
      Left ØNBG
      Right ØNBF
    Frontal ØNB1
    Hyoid ØNBX
    Lacrimal
      Left ØNBJ
      Right ØNBH
    Nasal ØNBB
    Occipital ØNB7
    Palatine
      Left ØNBL
      Right ØNBK
    Parietal
      Left ØNB4
      Right ØNB3
    Pelvic
      Left ØQB3
      Right ØQB2
    Sphenoid ØNBC
    Temporal
      Left ØNB6
      Right ØNB5
    Zygomatic
      Left ØNBN
      Right ØNBM
  Brain ØØBØ
  Breast
    Bilateral ØHBV
    Left ØHBU
    Right ØHBT
    Supernumerary ØHBY
  Bronchus
    Lingula ØBB9
    Lower Lobe
      Left ØBB8
      Right ØBB6
    Main
      Left ØBB7
      Right ØBB3
    Middle Lobe, Right ØBB5
    Upper Lobe
      Left ØBB8
      Right ØBB4
  Buccal Mucosa ØCB4
  Bursa and Ligament
    Abdomen
      Left ØMBJ
      Right ØMBH
    Ankle
      Left ØMBR
      Right ØMBQ
    Elbow
      Left ØMB4

Excision — *continued*
  Bursa and Ligament — *continued*
    Elbow — *continued*
      Right ØMB3
    Foot
      Left ØMBT
      Right ØMBS
    Hand
      Left ØMB8
      Right ØMB7
    Head and Neck ØMBØ
    Hip
      Left ØMBM
      Right ØMBL
    Knee
      Left ØMBP
      Right ØMBN
    Lower Extremity
      Left ØMBW
      Right ØMBV
    Perineum ØMBK
    Rib(s) ØMBG
    Shoulder
      Left ØMB2
      Right ØMB1
    Spine
      Lower ØMBD
      Upper ØMBC
    Sternum ØMBF
    Upper Extremity
      Left ØMBB
      Right ØMB9
    Wrist
      Left ØMB6
      Right ØMB5
  Buttock
    Left ØYB1
    Right ØYBØ
  Carina ØBB2
  Carotid Bodies, Bilateral ØGB8
  Carotid Body
    Left ØGB6
    Right ØGB7
  Carpal
    Left ØPBN
    Right ØPBM
  Cecum ØDBH
  Cerebellum ØØBC
  Cerebral Hemisphere ØØB7
  Cerebral Meninges ØØB1
  Cerebral Ventricle ØØB6
  Cervix ØUBC
  Chest Wall ØWB8
  Chordae Tendineae Ø2B9
  Choroid
    Left Ø8BB
    Right Ø8BA
  Cisterna Chyli Ø7BL
  Clavicle
    Left ØPBB
    Right ØPB9
  Clitoris ØUBJ
  Coccygeal Glomus ØGBB
  Coccyx ØQBS
  Colon
    Ascending ØDBK
    Descending ØDBM
    Sigmoid ØDBN
    Transverse ØDBL
  Conduction Mechanism Ø2B8
  Conjunctiva
    Left Ø8BTXZ
    Right Ø8BSXZ
  Cord
    Bilateral ØVBH
    Left ØVBG
    Right ØVBF
  Cornea
    Left Ø8B9XZ
    Right Ø8B8XZ
  Cul-de-sac ØUBF
  Diaphragm ØBBT
  Disc
    Cervical Vertebral ØRB3
    Cervicothoracic Vertebral ØRB5
    Lumbar Vertebral ØSB2
    Lumbosacral ØSB4
    Thoracic Vertebral ØRB9
    Thoracolumbar Vertebral ØRBB

Excision — *continued*
  Duct
    Common Bile ØFB9
    Cystic ØFB8
    Hepatic
      Common ØFB7
      Left ØFB6
      Right ØFB5
    Lacrimal
      Left Ø8BY
      Right Ø8BX
    Pancreatic ØFBD
      Accessory ØFBF
    Parotid
      Left ØCBC
      Right ØCBB
  Duodenum ØDB9
  Dura Mater ØØB2
  Ear
    External
      Left Ø9B1
      Right Ø9BØ
    External Auditory Canal
      Left Ø9B4
      Right Ø9B3
    Inner
      Left Ø9BE
      Right Ø9BD
    Middle
      Left Ø9B6
      Right Ø9B5
  Elbow Region
    Left ØXBC
    Right ØXBB
  Epididymis
    Bilateral ØVBL
    Left ØVBK
    Right ØVBJ
  Epiglottis ØCBR
  Esophagogastric Junction ØDB4
  Esophagus ØDB5
    Lower ØDB3
    Middle ØDB2
    Upper ØDB1
  Eustachian Tube
    Left Ø9BG
    Right Ø9BF
  Extremity
    Lower
      Left ØYBB
      Right ØYB9
    Upper
      Left ØXB7
      Right ØXB6
  Eye
    Left Ø8B1
    Right Ø8BØ
  Eyelid
    Lower
      Left Ø8BR
      Right Ø8BQ
    Upper
      Left Ø8BP
      Right Ø8BN
  Face ØWB2
  Fallopian Tube
    Left ØUB6
    Right ØUB5
  Fallopian Tubes, Bilateral ØUB7
  Femoral Region
    Left ØYB8
    Right ØYB7
  Femoral Shaft
    Left ØQB9
    Right ØQB8
  Femur
    Lower
      Left ØQBC
      Right ØQBB
    Upper
      Left ØQB7
      Right ØQB6
  Fibula
    Left ØQBK
    Right ØQBJ
  Finger Nail ØHBQXZ
  Floor of mouth *see* Excision, Oral Cavity and Throat
    ØWB3

Excision — *continued*
  Foot
    Left ØYBN
    Right ØYBM
  Gallbladder ØFB4
  Gingiva
    Lower ØCB6
    Upper ØCB5
  Gland
    Adrenal
      Bilateral ØGB4
      Left ØGB2
      Right ØGB3
    Lacrimal
      Left Ø8BW
      Right Ø8BV
    Minor Salivary ØCBJ
    Parotid
      Left ØCB9
      Right ØCB8
    Pituitary ØGBØ
    Sublingual
      Left ØCBF
      Right ØCBD
    Submaxillary
      Left ØCBH
      Right ØCBG
    Vestibular ØUBL
  Glenoid Cavity
    Left ØPB8
    Right ØPB7
  Glomus Jugulare ØGBC
  Hand
    Left ØXBK
    Right ØXBJ
  Head ØWBØ
  Humeral Head
    Left ØPBD
    Right ØPBC
  Humeral Shaft
    Left ØPBG
    Right ØPBF
  Hymen ØUBK
  Hypothalamus ØØBA
  Ileocecal Valve ØDBC
  Ileum ØDBB
  Inguinal Region
    Left ØYB6
    Right ØYB5
  Intestine
    Large ØDBE
      Left ØDBG
      Right ØDBF
    Small ØDB8
  Iris
    Left Ø8BD3Z
    Right Ø8BC3Z
  Jaw
    Lower ØWB5
    Upper ØWB4
  Jejunum ØDBA
  Joint
    Acromioclavicular
      Left ØRBH
      Right ØRBG
    Ankle
      Left ØSBG
      Right ØSBF
    Carpal
      Left ØRBR
      Right ØRBQ
    Carpometacarpal
      Left ØRBT
      Right ØRBS
    Cervical Vertebral ØRB1
    Cervicothoracic Vertebral ØRB4
    Coccygeal ØSB6
    Elbow
      Left ØRBM
      Right ØRBL
    Finger Phalangeal
      Left ØRBX
      Right ØRBW
    Hip
      Left ØSBB
      Right ØSB9
    Knee
      Left ØSBD
      Right ØSBC

Excision — *continued*
  Joint — *continued*
    Lumbar Vertebral ØSBØ
    Lumbosacral ØSB3
    Metacarpophalangeal
      Left ØRBV
      Right ØRBU
    Metatarsal-Phalangeal
      Left ØSBN
      Right ØSBM
    Occipital-cervical ØRBØ
    Sacrococcygeal ØSB5
    Sacroiliac
      Left ØSB8
      Right ØSB7
    Shoulder
      Left ØRBK
      Right ØRBJ
    Sternoclavicular
      Left ØRBF
      Right ØRBE
    Tarsal
      Left ØSBJ
      Right ØSBH
    Tarsometatarsal
      Left ØSBL
      Right ØSBK
    Temporomandibular
      Left ØRBD
      Right ØRBC
    Thoracic Vertebral ØRB6
    Thoracolumbar Vertebral ØRBA
    Toe Phalangeal
      Left ØSBQ
      Right ØSBP
    Wrist
      Left ØRBP
      Right ØRBN
  Kidney
    Left ØTB1
    Right ØTBØ
  Kidney Pelvis
    Left ØTB4
    Right ØTB3
  Knee Region
    Left ØYBG
    Right ØYBF
  Larynx ØCBS
  Leg
    Lower
      Left ØYBJ
      Right ØYBH
    Upper
      Left ØYBD
      Right ØYBC
  Lens
    Left Ø8BK3Z
    Right Ø8BJ3Z
  Lip
    Lower ØCB1
    Upper ØCBØ
  Liver ØFBØ
    Left Lobe ØFB2
    Right Lobe ØFB1
  Lung
    Bilateral ØBBM
    Left ØBBL
    Lower Lobe
      Left ØBBJ
      Right ØBBF
    Middle Lobe, Right ØBBD
    Right ØBBK
    Upper Lobe
      Left ØBBG
      Right ØBBC
  Lung Lingula ØBBH
  Lymphatic
    Aortic Ø7BD
    Axillary
      Left Ø7B6
      Right Ø7B5
    Head Ø7BØ
    Inguinal
      Left Ø7BJ
      Right Ø7BH
    Internal Mammary
      Left Ø7B9
      Right Ø7B8

Excision — *continued*
  Lymphatic — *continued*
    Lower Extremity
      Left Ø7BG
      Right Ø7BF
    Mesenteric Ø7BB
    Neck
      Left Ø7B2
      Right Ø7B1
    Pelvis Ø7BC
    Thoracic Duct Ø7BK
    Thorax Ø7B7
    Upper Extremity
      Left Ø7B4
      Right Ø7B3
  Mandible
    Left ØNBV
    Right ØNBT
  Maxilla ØNBR
  Mediastinum ØWBC
  Medulla Oblongata ØØBD
  Mesentery ØDBV
  Metacarpal
    Left ØPBQ
    Right ØPBP
  Metatarsal
    Left ØQBP
    Right ØQBN
  Muscle
    Abdomen
      Left ØKBL
      Right ØKBK
    Extraocular
      Left Ø8BM
      Right Ø8BL
    Facial ØKB1
    Foot
      Left ØKBW
      Right ØKBV
    Hand
      Left ØKBD
      Right ØKBC
    Head ØKBØ
    Hip
      Left ØKBP
      Right ØKBN
    Lower Arm and Wrist
      Left ØKBB
      Right ØKB9
    Lower Leg
      Left ØKBT
      Right ØKBS
    Neck
      Left ØKB3
      Right ØKB2
    Papillary Ø2BD
    Perineum ØKBM
    Shoulder
      Left ØKB6
      Right ØKB5
    Thorax
      Left ØKBJ
      Right ØKBH
    Tongue, Palate, Pharynx ØKB4
    Trunk
      Left ØKBG
      Right ØKBF
    Upper Arm
      Left ØKB8
      Right ØKB7
    Upper Leg
      Left ØKBR
      Right ØKBQ
  Nasal Mucosa and Soft Tissue Ø9BK
  Nasopharynx Ø9BN
  Neck ØWB6
  Nerve
    Abdominal Sympathetic Ø1BM
    Abducens ØØBL
    Accessory ØØBR
    Acoustic ØØBN
    Brachial Plexus Ø1B3
    Cervical Ø1B1
    Cervical Plexus Ø1BØ
    Facial ØØBM
    Femoral Ø1BD
    Glossopharyngeal ØØBP
    Head and Neck Sympathetic Ø1BK
    Hypoglossal ØØBS

Excision — *continued*
  Nerve — *continued*
    Lumbar Ø1BB
    Lumbar Plexus Ø1B9
    Lumbar Sympathetic Ø1BN
    Lumbosacral Plexus Ø1BA
    Median Ø1B5
    Oculomotor ØØBH
    Olfactory ØØBF
    Optic ØØBG
    Peroneal Ø1BH
    Phrenic Ø1B2
    Pudendal Ø1BC
    Radial Ø1B6
    Sacral Ø1BR
    Sacral Plexus Ø1BQ
    Sacral Sympathetic Ø1BP
    Sciatic Ø1BF
    Thoracic Ø1B8
    Thoracic Sympathetic Ø1BL
    Tibial Ø1BG
    Trigeminal ØØBK
    Trochlear ØØBJ
    Ulnar Ø1B4
    Vagus ØØBQ
  Nipple
    Left ØHBX
    Right ØHBW
  Omentum ØDBU
  Oral Cavity and Throat ØWB3
  Orbit
    Left ØNBQ
    Right ØNBP
  Ovary
    Bilateral ØUB2
    Left ØUB1
    Right ØUBØ
  Palate
    Hard ØCB2
    Soft ØCB3
  Pancreas ØFBG
  Para-aortic Body ØGB9
  Paraganglion Extremity ØGBF
  Parathyroid Gland ØGBR
    Inferior
      Left ØGBP
      Right ØGBN
    Multiple ØGBQ
    Superior
      Left ØGBM
      Right ØGBL
  Patella
    Left ØQBF
    Right ØQBD
  Penis ØVBS
  Pericardium Ø2BN
  Perineum
    Female ØWBN
    Male ØWBM
  Peritoneum ØDBW
  Phalanx
    Finger
      Left ØPBV
      Right ØPBT
    Thumb
      Left ØPBS
      Right ØPBR
    Toe
      Left ØQBR
      Right ØQBQ
  Pharynx ØCBM
  Pineal Body ØGB1
  Pleura
    Left ØBBP
    Right ØBBN
  Pons ØØBB
  Prepuce ØVBT
  Prostate ØVBØ
  Radius
    Left ØPBJ
    Right ØPBH
  Rectum ØDBP
  Retina
    Left Ø8BF3Z
    Right Ø8BE3Z
  Retroperitoneum ØWBH
  Ribs
    1 to 2 ØPB1
    3 or More ØPB2

Excision — *continued*

Sacrum 0QB1
Scapula
  Left 0PB6
  Right 0PB5
Sclera
  Left 08B7XZ
  Right 08B6XZ
Scrotum 0VB5
Septum
  Atrial 02B5
  Nasal 09BM
  Ventricular 02BM
Shoulder Region
  Left 0XB3
  Right 0XB2
Sinus
  Accessory 09BP
  Ethmoid
    Left 09BV
    Right 09BU
  Frontal
    Left 09BT
    Right 09BS
  Mastoid
    Left 09BC
    Right 09BB
  Maxillary
    Left 09BR
    Right 09BQ
  Sphenoid
    Left 09BX
    Right 09BW
Skin
  Abdomen 0HB7XZ
  Back 0HB6XZ
  Buttock 0HB8XZ
  Chest 0HB5XZ
  Ear
    Left 0HB3XZ
    Right 0HB2XZ
  Face 0HB1XZ
  Foot
    Left 0HBNXZ
    Right 0HBMXZ
  Hand
    Left 0HBGXZ
    Right 0HBFXZ
  Inguinal 0HBAXZ
  Lower Arm
    Left 0HBEXZ
    Right 0HBDXZ
  Lower Leg
    Left 0HBLXZ
    Right 0HBKXZ
  Neck 0HB4XZ
  Perineum 0HB9XZ
  Scalp 0HB0XZ
  Upper Arm
    Left 0HBCXZ
    Right 0HBBXZ
  Upper Leg
    Left 0HBJXZ
    Right 0HBHXZ
Skull 0NB0
Spinal Cord
  Cervical 00BW
  Lumbar 00BY
  Thoracic 00BX
Spinal Meninges 00BT
Spleen 07BP
Sternum 0PB0
Stomach 0DB6
  Pylorus 0DB7
Subcutaneous Tissue and Fascia
  Abdomen 0JB8
  Back 0JB7
  Buttock 0JB9
  Chest 0JB6
  Face 0JB1
  Foot
    Left 0JBR
    Right 0JBQ
  Hand
    Left 0JBK
    Right 0JBJ
  Lower Arm
    Left 0JBH
    Right 0JBG

Excision — *continued*

Subcutaneous Tissue and Fascia — *continued*
  Lower Leg
    Left 0JBP
    Right 0JBN
  Neck
    Left 0JB5
    Right 0JB4
  Pelvic Region 0JBC
  Perineum 0JBB
  Scalp 0JB0
  Upper Arm
    Left 0JBF
    Right 0JBD
  Upper Leg
    Left 0JBM
    Right 0JBL
Tarsal
  Left 0QBM
  Right 0QBL
Tendon
  Abdomen
    Left 0LBG
    Right 0LBF
  Ankle
    Left 0LBT
    Right 0LBS
  Foot
    Left 0LBW
    Right 0LBV
  Hand
    Left 0LB8
    Right 0LB7
  Head and Neck 0LB0
  Hip
    Left 0LBK
    Right 0LBJ
  Knee
    Left 0LBR
    Right 0LBQ
  Lower Arm and Wrist
    Left 0LB6
    Right 0LB5
  Lower Leg
    Left 0LBP
    Right 0LBN
  Perineum 0LBH
  Shoulder
    Left 0LB2
    Right 0LB1
  Thorax
    Left 0LBD
    Right 0LBC
  Trunk
    Left 0LBB
    Right 0LB9
  Upper Arm
    Left 0LB4
    Right 0LB3
  Upper Leg
    Left 0LBM
    Right 0LBL
Testis
  Bilateral 0VBC
  Left 0VBB
  Right 0VB9
Thalamus 00B9
Thymus 07BM
Thyroid Gland
  Left Lobe 0GBG
  Right Lobe 0GBH
Thyroid Gland Isthmus 0GBJ
Tibia
  Left 0QBH
  Right 0QBG
Toe Nail 0HBRXZ
Tongue 0CB7
Tonsils 0CBP
Tooth
  Lower 0CBX
  Upper 0CBW
Trachea 0BB1
Tunica Vaginalis
  Left 0VB7
  Right 0VB6
Turbinate, Nasal 09BL
Tympanic Membrane
  Left 09B8
  Right 09B7

Excision — *continued*

Ulna
  Left 0PBL
  Right 0PBK
Ureter
  Left 0TB7
  Right 0TB6
Urethra 0TBD
Uterine Supporting Structure 0UB4
Uterus 0UB9
Uvula 0CBN
Vagina 0UBG
Valve
  Aortic 02BF
  Mitral 02BG
  Pulmonary 02BH
  Tricuspid 02BJ
Vas Deferens
  Bilateral 0VBQ
  Left 0VBP
  Right 0VBN
Vein
  Axillary
    Left 05B8
    Right 05B7
  Azygos 05B0
  Basilic
    Left 05BC
    Right 05BB
  Brachial
    Left 05BA
    Right 05B9
  Cephalic
    Left 05BF
    Right 05BD
  Colic 06B7
  Common Iliac
    Left 06BD
    Right 06BC
  Coronary 02B4
  Esophageal 06B3
  External Iliac
    Left 06BG
    Right 06BF
  External Jugular
    Left 05BQ
    Right 05BP
  Face
    Left 05BV
    Right 05BT
  Femoral
    Left 06BN
    Right 06BM
  Foot
    Left 06BV
    Right 06BT
  Gastric 06B2
  Hand
    Left 05BH
    Right 05BG
  Hemiazygos 05B1
  Hepatic 06B4
  Hypogastric
    Left 06BJ
    Right 06BH
  Inferior Mesenteric 06B6
  Innominate
    Left 05B4
    Right 05B3
  Internal Jugular
    Left 05BN
    Right 05BM
  Intracranial 05BL
  Lower 06BY
  Portal 06B8
  Pulmonary
    Left 02BT
    Right 02BS
  Renal
    Left 06BB
    Right 06B9
  Saphenous
    Left 06BQ
    Right 06BP
  Splenic 06B1
  Subclavian
    Left 05B6
    Right 05B5
  Superior Mesenteric 06B5

▼ **Subterms under main terms may continue to next column or page**

Excision — *continued*
  Vein — *continued*
    Upper 05BY
    Vertebral
      Left 05BS
      Right 05BR
  Vena Cava
    Inferior 06B0
    Superior 02BV
  Ventricle
    Left 02BL
    Right 02BK
  Vertebra
    Cervical 0PB3
    Lumbar 0QB0
    Thoracic 0PB4
  Vesicle
    Bilateral 0VB3
    Left 0VB2
    Right 0VB1
  Vitreous
    Left 08B53Z
    Right 08B43Z
  Vocal Cord
    Left 0CBV
    Right 0CBT
  Vulva 0UBM
  Wrist Region
    Left 0XBH
    Right 0XBG
EXCLUDER® AAA Endoprosthesis
  use Intraluminal Device
  use Intraluminal Device, Branched or Fenestrated, One or Two Arteries in 04V
  use Intraluminal Device, Branched or Fenestrated, Three or More Arteries in 04V
EXCLUDER® IBE Endoprosthesis *use* Intraluminal Device, Branched or Fenestrated, One or Two Arteries in 04V
Exclusion, Left atrial appendage (LAA) *see* Occlusion, Atrium, Left 02L7
Exercise, rehabilitation *see* Motor Treatment, Rehabilitation F07
Exploration *see* Inspection
Express® Biliary SD Monorail® Premounted Stent System *use* Intraluminal Device
Express® (LD) Premounted Stent System *use* Intraluminal Device
Express® SD Renal Monorail® Premounted Stent System *use* Intraluminal Device
Ex-PRESS™ mini glaucoma shunt *use* Synthetic Substitute
Extensor carpi radialis muscle
  use Lower Arm and Wrist Muscle, Left
  use Lower Arm and Wrist Muscle, Right
Extensor carpi ulnaris muscle
  use Lower Arm and Wrist Muscle, Left
  use Lower Arm and Wrist Muscle, Right
Extensor digitorum brevis muscle
  use Foot Muscle, Left
  use Foot Muscle, Right
Extensor digitorum longus muscle
  use Lower Leg Muscle, Left
  use Lower Leg Muscle, Right
Extensor hallucis brevis muscle
  use Foot Muscle, Left
  use Foot Muscle, Right
Extensor hallucis longus muscle
  use Lower Leg Muscle, Left
  use Lower Leg Muscle, Right
External anal sphincter *use* Anal Sphincter
External auditory meatus
  use External Auditory Canal, Left
  use External Auditory Canal, Right
External fixator
  use External Fixation Device in Head and Facial Bones
  use External Fixation Device in Lower Bones
  use External Fixation Device in Lower Joints
  use External Fixation Device in Upper Bones
  use External Fixation Device in Upper Joints
External maxillary artery *use* Face Artery
External naris *use* Nasal Mucosa and Soft Tissue
External oblique aponeurosis *use* Subcutaneous Tissue and Fascia, Trunk
External oblique muscle
  use Abdomen Muscle, Left

External oblique muscle — *continued*
  use Abdomen Muscle, Right
External popliteal nerve *use* Peroneal Nerve
External pudendal artery
  use Femoral Artery, Left
  use Femoral Artery, Right
External pudendal vein
  use Saphenous Vein, Left
  use Saphenous Vein, Right
External urethral sphincter *use* Urethra
Extirpation
  Acetabulum
    Left 0QC5
    Right 0QC4
  Adenoids 0CCQ
  Ampulla of Vater 0FCC
  Anal Sphincter 0DCR
  Anterior Chamber
    Left 08C3
    Right 08C2
  Anus 0DCQ
  Aorta
    Abdominal 04C0
    Thoracic
      Ascending/Arch 02CX
      Descending 02CW
  Aortic Body 0GCD
  Appendix 0DCJ
  Artery
    Anterior Tibial
      Left 04CQ
      Right 04CP
    Axillary
      Left 03C6
      Right 03C5
    Brachial
      Left 03C8
      Right 03C7
    Celiac 04C1
    Colic
      Left 04C7
      Middle 04C8
      Right 04C6
    Common Carotid
      Left 03CJ
      Right 03CH
    Common Iliac
      Left 04CD
      Right 04CC
    Coronary
      Four or More Arteries 02C3
      One Artery 02C0
      Three Arteries 02C2
      Two Arteries 02C1
    External Carotid
      Left 03CN
      Right 03CM
    External Iliac
      Left 04CJ
      Right 04CH
    Face 03CR
    Femoral
      Left 04CL
      Right 04CK
    Foot
      Left 04CW
      Right 04CV
    Gastric 04C2
    Hand
      Left 03CF
      Right 03CD
    Hepatic 04C3
    Inferior Mesenteric 04CB
    Innominate 03C2
    Internal Carotid
      Left 03CL
      Right 03CK
    Internal Iliac
      Left 04CF
      Right 04CE
    Internal Mammary
      Left 03C1
      Right 03C0
    Intracranial 03CG
    Lower 04CY
    Peroneal
      Left 04CU
      Right 04CT

Extirpation — *continued*
  Artery — *continued*
    Popliteal
      Left 04CN
      Right 04CM
    Posterior Tibial
      Left 04CS
      Right 04CR
    Pulmonary
      Left 02CR
      Right 02CQ
    Pulmonary Trunk 02CP
    Radial
      Left 03CC
      Right 03CB
    Renal
      Left 04CA
      Right 04C9
    Splenic 04C4
    Subclavian
      Left 03C4
      Right 03C3
    Superior Mesenteric 04C5
    Temporal
      Left 03CT
      Right 03CS
    Thyroid
      Left 03CV
      Right 03CU
    Ulnar
      Left 03CA
      Right 03C9
    Upper 03CY
    Vertebral
      Left 03CQ
      Right 03CP
  Atrium
    Left 02C7
    Right 02C6
  Auditory Ossicle
    Left 09CA
    Right 09C9
  Basal Ganglia 00C8
  Bladder 0TCB
  Bladder Neck 0TCC
  Bone
    Ethmoid
      Left 0NCG
      Right 0NCF
    Frontal 0NC1
    Hyoid 0NCX
    Lacrimal
      Left 0NCJ
      Right 0NCH
    Nasal 0NCB
    Occipital 0NC7
    Palatine
      Left 0NCL
      Right 0NCK
    Parietal
      Left 0NC4
      Right 0NC3
    Pelvic
      Left 0QC3
      Right 0QC2
    Sphenoid 0NCC
    Temporal
      Left 0NC6
      Right 0NC5
    Zygomatic
      Left 0NCN
      Right 0NCM
  Brain 00C0
  Breast
    Bilateral 0HCV
    Left 0HCU
    Right 0HCT
  Bronchus
    Lingula 0BC9
    Lower Lobe
      Left 0BCB
      Right 0BC6
    Main
      Left 0BC7
      Right 0BC3
    Middle Lobe, Right 0BC5
    Upper Lobe
      Left 0BC8
      Right 0BC4

Extirpation — *continued*
  Buccal Mucosa ØCC4
  Bursa and Ligament
    Abdomen
      Left ØMCJ
      Right ØMCH
    Ankle
      Left ØMCR
      Right ØMCQ
    Elbow
      Left ØMC4
      Right ØMC3
    Foot
      Left ØMCT
      Right ØMCS
    Hand
      Left ØMC8
      Right ØMC7
    Head and Neck ØMCØ
    Hip
      Left ØMCM
      Right ØMCL
    Knee
      Left ØMCP
      Right ØMCN
    Lower Extremity
      Left ØMCW
      Right ØMCV
    Perineum ØMCK
    Rib(s) ØMCG
    Shoulder
      Left ØMC2
      Right ØMC1
    Spine
      Lower ØMCD
      Upper ØMCC
    Sternum ØMCF
    Upper Extremity
      Left ØMCB
      Right ØMC9
    Wrist
      Left ØMC6
      Right ØMC5
  Carina ØBC2
  Carotid Bodies, Bilateral ØGC8
  Carotid Body
    Left ØGC6
    Right ØGC7
  Carpal
    Left ØPCN
    Right ØPCM
  Cavity, Cranial ØWC1
  Cecum ØDCH
  Cerebellum ØØCC
  Cerebral Hemisphere ØØC7
  Cerebral Meninges ØØC1
  Cerebral Ventricle ØØC6
  Cervix ØUCC
  Chordae Tendineae Ø2C9
  Choroid
    Left Ø8CB
    Right Ø8CA
  Cisterna Chyli Ø7CL
  Clavicle
    Left ØPCB
    Right ØPC9
  Clitoris ØUCJ
  Coccygeal Glomus ØGCB
  Coccyx ØQCS
  Colon
    Ascending ØDCK
    Descending ØDCM
    Sigmoid ØDCN
    Transverse ØDCL
  Computer-aided Mechanical Aspiration X2C
  Conduction Mechanism Ø2C8
  Conjunctiva
    Left Ø8CTXZZ
    Right Ø8CSXZZ
  Cord
    Bilateral ØVCH
    Left ØVCG
    Right ØVCF
  Cornea
    Left Ø8C9XZZ
    Right Ø8C8XZZ
  Cul-de-sac ØUCF
  Diaphragm ØBCT

Extirpation — *continued*
  Disc
    Cervical Vertebral ØRC3
    Cervicothoracic Vertebral ØRC5
    Lumbar Vertebral ØSC2
    Lumbosacral ØSC4
    Thoracic Vertebral ØRC9
    Thoracolumbar Vertebral ØRCB
  Duct
    Common Bile ØFC9
    Cystic ØFC8
    Hepatic
      Common ØFC7
      Left ØFC6
      Right ØFC5
    Lacrimal
      Left Ø8CY
      Right Ø8CX
    Pancreatic ØFCD
      Accessory ØFCF
    Parotid
      Left ØCCC
      Right ØCCB
  Duodenum ØDC9
  Dura Mater ØØC2
  Ear
    External
      Left Ø9C1
      Right Ø9CØ
    External Auditory Canal
      Left Ø9C4
      Right Ø9C3
    Inner
      Left Ø9CE
      Right Ø9CD
    Middle
      Left Ø9C6
      Right Ø9C5
  Endometrium ØUCB
  Epididymis
    Bilateral ØVCL
    Left ØVCK
    Right ØVCJ
  Epidural Space, Intracranial ØØC3
  Epiglottis ØCCR
  Esophagogastric Junction ØDC4
  Esophagus ØDC5
    Lower ØDC3
    Middle ØDC2
    Upper ØDC1
  Eustachian Tube
    Left Ø9CG
    Right Ø9CF
  Eye
    Left Ø8C1XZZ
    Right Ø8CØXZZ
  Eyelid
    Lower
      Left Ø8CR
      Right Ø8CQ
    Upper
      Left Ø8CP
      Right Ø8CN
  Fallopian Tube
    Left ØUC6
    Right ØUC5
  Fallopian Tubes, Bilateral ØUC7
  Femoral Shaft
    Left ØQC9
    Right ØQC8
  Femur
    Lower
      Left ØQCC
      Right ØQCB
    Upper
      Left ØQC7
      Right ØQC6
  Fibula
    Left ØQCK
    Right ØQCJ
  Finger Nail ØHCQXZZ
  Gallbladder ØFC4
  Gastrointestinal Tract ØWCP
  Genitourinary Tract ØWCR
  Gingiva
    Lower ØCC6
    Upper ØCC5

Extirpation — *continued*
  Gland
    Adrenal
      Bilateral ØGC4
      Left ØGC2
      Right ØGC3
    Lacrimal
      Left Ø8CW
      Right Ø8CV
    Minor Salivary ØCCJ
    Parotid
      Left ØCC9
      Right ØCC8
    Pituitary ØGCØ
    Sublingual
      Left ØCCF
      Right ØCCD
    Submaxillary
      Left ØCCH
      Right ØCCG
    Vestibular ØUCL
  Glenoid Cavity
    Left ØPC8
    Right ØPC7
  Glomus Jugulare ØGCC
  Humeral Head
    Left ØPCD
    Right ØPCC
  Humeral Shaft
    Left ØPCG
    Right ØPCF
  Hymen ØUCK
  Hypothalamus ØØCA
  Ileocecal Valve ØDCC
  Ileum ØDCB
  Intestine
    Large ØDCE
      Left ØDCG
      Right ØDCF
    Small ØDC8
  Iris
    Left Ø8CD
    Right Ø8CC
  Jaw
    Lower ØWC5
    Upper ØWC4
  Jejunum ØDCA
  Joint
    Acromioclavicular
      Left ØRCH
      Right ØRCG
    Ankle
      Left ØSCG
      Right ØSCF
    Carpal
      Left ØRCR
      Right ØRCQ
    Carpometacarpal
      Left ØRCT
      Right ØRCS
    Cervical Vertebral ØRC1
    Cervicothoracic Vertebral ØRC4
    Coccygeal ØSC6
    Elbow
      Left ØRCM
      Right ØRCL
    Finger Phalangeal
      Left ØRCX
      Right ØRCW
    Hip
      Left ØSCB
      Right ØSC9
    Knee
      Left ØSCD
      Right ØSCC
    Lumbar Vertebral ØSCØ
    Lumbosacral ØSC3
    Metacarpophalangeal
      Left ØRCV
      Right ØRCU
    Metatarsal-Phalangeal
      Left ØSCN
      Right ØSCM
    Occipital-cervical ØRCØ
    Sacrococcygeal ØSC5
    Sacroiliac
      Left ØSC8
      Right ØSC7

Subterms under main terms may continue to next column or page

Extirpation — *continued*
- Joint — *continued*
  - Shoulder
    - Left ØRCK
    - Right ØRCJ
  - Sternoclavicular
    - Left ØRCF
    - Right ØRCE
  - Tarsal
    - Left ØSCJ
    - Right ØSCH
  - Tarsometatarsal
    - Left ØSCL
    - Right ØSCK
  - Temporomandibular
    - Left ØRCD
    - Right ØRCC
  - Thoracic Vertebral ØRC6
  - Thoracolumbar Vertebral ØRCA
  - Toe Phalangeal
    - Left ØSCQ
    - Right ØSCP
  - Wrist
    - Left ØRCP
    - Right ØRCN
- Kidney
  - Left ØTC1
  - Right ØTCØ
- Kidney Pelvis
  - Left ØTC4
  - Right ØTC3
- Larynx ØCCS
- Lens
  - Left Ø8CK
  - Right Ø8CJ
- Lip
  - Lower ØCC1
  - Upper ØCCØ
- Liver ØFCØ
  - Left Lobe ØFC2
  - Right Lobe ØFC1
- Lung
  - Bilateral ØBCM
  - Left ØBCL
  - Lower Lobe
    - Left ØBCJ
    - Right ØBCF
  - Middle Lobe, Right ØBCD
  - Right ØBCK
  - Upper Lobe
    - Left ØBCG
    - Right ØBCC
- Lung Lingula ØBCH
- Lymphatic
  - Aortic Ø7CD
  - Axillary
    - Left Ø7C6
    - Right Ø7C5
  - Head Ø7CØ
  - Inguinal
    - Left Ø7CJ
    - Right Ø7CH
  - Internal Mammary
    - Left Ø7C9
    - Right Ø7C8
  - Lower Extremity
    - Left Ø7CG
    - Right Ø7CF
  - Mesenteric Ø7CB
  - Neck
    - Left Ø7C2
    - Right Ø7C1
  - Pelvis Ø7CC
  - Thoracic Duct Ø7CK
  - Thorax Ø7C7
  - Upper Extremity
    - Left Ø7C4
    - Right Ø7C3
- Mandible
  - Left ØNCV
  - Right ØNCT
- Maxilla ØNCR
- Mediastinum ØWCC
- Medulla Oblongata ØØCD
- Mesentery ØDCV
- Metacarpal
  - Left ØPCQ
  - Right ØPCP

Extirpation — *continued*
- Metatarsal
  - Left ØQCP
  - Right ØQCN
- Muscle
  - Abdomen
    - Left ØKCL
    - Right ØKCK
  - Extraocular
    - Left Ø8CM
    - Right Ø8CL
  - Facial ØKC1
  - Foot
    - Left ØKCW
    - Right ØKCV
  - Hand
    - Left ØKCD
    - Right ØKCC
  - Head ØKCØ
  - Hip
    - Left ØKCP
    - Right ØKCN
  - Lower Arm and Wrist
    - Left ØKCB
    - Right ØKC9
  - Lower Leg
    - Left ØKCT
    - Right ØKCS
  - Neck
    - Left ØKC3
    - Right ØKC2
  - Papillary Ø2CD
  - Perineum ØKCM
  - Shoulder
    - Left ØKC6
    - Right ØKC5
  - Thorax
    - Left ØKCJ
    - Right ØKCH
  - Tongue, Palate, Pharynx ØKC4
  - Trunk
    - Left ØKCG
    - Right ØKCF
  - Upper Arm
    - Left ØKC8
    - Right ØKC7
  - Upper Leg
    - Left ØKCR
    - Right ØKCQ
- Nasal Mucosa and Soft Tissue Ø9CK
- Nasopharynx Ø9CN
- Nerve
  - Abdominal Sympathetic Ø1CM
  - Abducens ØØCL
  - Accessory ØØCR
  - Acoustic ØØCN
  - Brachial Plexus Ø1C3
  - Cervical Ø1C1
  - Cervical Plexus Ø1CØ
  - Facial ØØCM
  - Femoral Ø1CD
  - Glossopharyngeal ØØCP
  - Head and Neck Sympathetic Ø1CK
  - Hypoglossal ØØCS
  - Lumbar Ø1CB
  - Lumbar Plexus Ø1C9
  - Lumbar Sympathetic Ø1CN
  - Lumbosacral Plexus Ø1CA
  - Median Ø1C5
  - Oculomotor ØØCH
  - Olfactory ØØCF
  - Optic ØØCG
  - Peroneal Ø1CH
  - Phrenic Ø1C2
  - Pudendal Ø1CC
  - Radial Ø1C6
  - Sacral Ø1CR
  - Sacral Plexus Ø1CQ
  - Sacral Sympathetic Ø1CP
  - Sciatic Ø1CF
  - Thoracic Ø1C8
  - Thoracic Sympathetic Ø1CL
  - Tibial Ø1CG
  - Trigeminal ØØCK
  - Trochlear ØØCJ
  - Ulnar Ø1C4
  - Vagus ØØCQ
- Nipple
  - Left ØHCX

Extirpation — *continued*
- Nipple — *continued*
  - Right ØHCW
- Omentum ØDCU
- Oral Cavity and Throat ØWC3
- Orbit
  - Left ØNCQ
  - Right ØNCP
- Orbital Atherectomy *see* Extirpation, Heart and Great Vessels Ø2C
- Ovary
  - Bilateral ØUC2
  - Left ØUC1
  - Right ØUCØ
- Palate
  - Hard ØCC2
  - Soft ØCC3
- Pancreas ØFCG
- Para-aortic Body ØGC9
- Paraganglion Extremity ØGCF
- Parathyroid Gland ØGCR
  - Inferior
    - Left ØGCP
    - Right ØGCN
  - Multiple ØGCQ
  - Superior
    - Left ØGCM
    - Right ØGCL
- Patella
  - Left ØQCF
  - Right ØQCD
- Pelvic Cavity ØWCJ
- Penis ØVCS
- Pericardial Cavity ØWCD
- Pericardium Ø2CN
- Peritoneal Cavity ØWCG
- Peritoneum ØDCW
- Phalanx
  - Finger
    - Left ØPCV
    - Right ØPCT
  - Thumb
    - Left ØPCS
    - Right ØPCR
  - Toe
    - Left ØQCR
    - Right ØQCQ
- Pharynx ØCCM
- Pineal Body ØGC1
- Pleura
  - Left ØBCP
  - Right ØBCN
- Pleural Cavity
  - Left ØWCB
  - Right ØWC9
- Pons ØØCB
- Prepuce ØVCT
- Prostate ØVCØ
- Radius
  - Left ØPCJ
  - Right ØPCH
- Rectum ØDCP
- Respiratory Tract ØWCQ
- Retina
  - Left Ø8CF
  - Right Ø8CE
- Retinal Vessel
  - Left Ø8CH
  - Right Ø8CG
- Retroperitoneum ØWCH
- Ribs
  - 1 to 2 ØPC1
  - 3 or More ØPC2
- Sacrum ØQC1
- Scapula
  - Left ØPC6
  - Right ØPC5
- Sclera
  - Left Ø8C7XZZ
  - Right Ø8C6XZZ
- Scrotum ØVC5
- Septum
  - Atrial Ø2C5
  - Nasal Ø9CM
  - Ventricular Ø2CM
- Sinus
  - Accessory Ø9CP
  - Ethmoid
    - Left Ø9CV

Extirpation — *continued*
Sinus — *continued*
  Ethmoid — *continued*
    Right 09CU
  Frontal
    Left 09CT
    Right 09CS
  Mastoid
    Left 09CC
    Right 09CB
  Maxillary
    Left 09CR
    Right 09CQ
  Sphenoid
    Left 09CX
    Right 09CW
Skin
  Abdomen 0HC7XZZ
  Back 0HC6XZZ
  Buttock 0HC8XZZ
  Chest 0HC5XZZ
  Ear
    Left 0HC3XZZ
    Right 0HC2XZZ
  Face 0HC1XZZ
  Foot
    Left 0HCNXZZ
    Right 0HCMXZZ
  Hand
    Left 0HCGXZZ
    Right 0HCFXZZ
  Inguinal 0HCAXZZ
  Lower Arm
    Left 0HCEXZZ
    Right 0HCDXZZ
  Lower Leg
    Left 0HCLXZZ
    Right 0HCKXZZ
  Neck 0HC4XZZ
  Perineum 0HC9XZZ
  Scalp 0HC0XZZ
  Upper Arm
    Left 0HCCXZZ
    Right 0HCBXZZ
  Upper Leg
    Left 0HCJXZZ
    Right 0HCHXZZ
Spinal Canal 00CU
Spinal Cord
  Cervical 00CW
  Lumbar 00CY
  Thoracic 00CX
Spinal Meninges 00CT
Spleen 07CP
Sternum 0PC0
Stomach 0DC6
  Pylorus 0DC7
Subarachnoid Space, Intracranial 00C5
Subcutaneous Tissue and Fascia
  Abdomen 0JC8
  Back 0JC7
  Buttock 0JC9
  Chest 0JC6
  Face 0JC1
  Foot
    Left 0JCR
    Right 0JCQ
  Hand
    Left 0JCK
    Right 0JCJ
  Lower Arm
    Left 0JCH
    Right 0JCG
  Lower Leg
    Left 0JCP
    Right 0JCN
  Neck
    Left 0JC5
    Right 0JC4
  Pelvic Region 0JCC
  Perineum 0JCB
  Scalp 0JC0
  Upper Arm
    Left 0JCF
    Right 0JCD
  Upper Leg
    Left 0JCM
    Right 0JCL
Subdural Space, Intracranial 00C4

Extirpation — *continued*
Tarsal
  Left 0QCM
  Right 0QCL
Tendon
  Abdomen
    Left 0LCG
    Right 0LCF
  Ankle
    Left 0LCT
    Right 0LCS
  Foot
    Left 0LCW
    Right 0LCV
  Hand
    Left 0LC8
    Right 0LC7
  Head and Neck 0LC0
  Hip
    Left 0LCK
    Right 0LCJ
  Knee
    Left 0LCR
    Right 0LCQ
  Lower Arm and Wrist
    Left 0LC6
    Right 0LC5
  Lower Leg
    Left 0LCP
    Right 0LCN
  Perineum 0LCH
  Shoulder
    Left 0LC2
    Right 0LC1
  Thorax
    Left 0LCD
    Right 0LCC
  Trunk
    Left 0LCB
    Right 0LC9
  Upper Arm
    Left 0LC4
    Right 0LC3
  Upper Leg
    Left 0LCM
    Right 0LCL
Testis
  Bilateral 0VCC
  Left 0VCB
  Right 0VC9
Thalamus 00C9
Thymus 07CM
Thyroid Gland 0GCK
  Left Lobe 0GCG
  Right Lobe 0GCH
Tibia
  Left 0QCH
  Right 0QCG
Toe Nail 0HCRXZZ
Tongue 0CC7
Tonsils 0CCP
Tooth
  Lower 0CCX
  Upper 0CCW
Trachea 0BC1
Tunica Vaginalis
  Left 0VC7
  Right 0VC6
Turbinate, Nasal 09CL
Tympanic Membrane
  Left 09C8
  Right 09C7
Ulna
  Left 0PCL
  Right 0PCK
Ureter
  Left 0TC7
  Right 0TC6
Urethra 0TCD
Uterine Supporting Structure 0UC4
Uterus 0UC9
Uvula 0CCN
Vagina 0UCG
Valve
  Aortic 02CF
  Mitral 02CG
  Pulmonary 02CH
  Tricuspid 02CJ

Extirpation — *continued*
Vas Deferens
  Bilateral 0VCQ
  Left 0VCP
  Right 0VCN
Vein
  Axillary
    Left 05C8
    Right 05C7
  Azygos 05C0
  Basilic
    Left 05CC
    Right 05CB
  Brachial
    Left 05CA
    Right 05C9
  Cephalic
    Left 05CF
    Right 05CD
  Colic 06C7
  Common Iliac
    Left 06CD
    Right 06CC
  Coronary 02C4
  Esophageal 06C3
  External Iliac
    Left 06CG
    Right 06CF
  External Jugular
    Left 05CQ
    Right 05CP
  Face
    Left 05CV
    Right 05CT
  Femoral
    Left 06CN
    Right 06CM
  Foot
    Left 06CV
    Right 06CT
  Gastric 06C2
  Hand
    Left 05CH
    Right 05CG
  Hemiazygos 05C1
  Hepatic 06C4
  Hypogastric
    Left 06CJ
    Right 06CH
  Inferior Mesenteric 06C6
  Innominate
    Left 05C4
    Right 05C3
  Internal Jugular
    Left 05CN
    Right 05CM
  Intracranial 05CL
  Lower 06CY
  Portal 06C8
  Pulmonary
    Left 02CT
    Right 02CS
  Renal
    Left 06CB
    Right 06C9
  Saphenous
    Left 06CQ
    Right 06CP
  Splenic 06C1
  Subclavian
    Left 05C6
    Right 05C5
  Superior Mesenteric 06C5
  Upper 05CY
  Vertebral
    Left 05CS
    Right 05CR
Vena Cava
  Inferior 06C0
  Superior 02CV
Ventricle
  Left 02CL
  Right 02CK
Vertebra
  Cervical 0PC3
  Lumbar 0QC0
  Thoracic 0PC4
Vesicle
  Bilateral 0VC3

Extirpation — continued
  Vesicle — continued
    Left 0VC2
    Right 0VC1
  Vitreous
    Left 08C5
    Right 08C4
  Vocal Cord
    Left 0CCV
    Right 0CCT
  Vulva 0UCM
Extracorporeal Carbon Dioxide Removal (ECCO2R)
  5A0920Z
Extracorporeal shock wave lithotripsy see Fragmentation
Extracranial-intracranial bypass (EC-IC) see Bypass, Upper Arteries 031
Extraction
  Acetabulum
    Left 0QD50ZZ
    Right 0QD40ZZ
  Ampulla of Vater 0FDC
  Anus 0DDQ
  Appendix 0DDJ
  Auditory Ossicle
    Left 09DA0ZZ
    Right 09D90ZZ
  Bone
    Ethmoid
      Left 0NDG0ZZ
      Right 0NDF0ZZ
    Frontal 0ND10ZZ
    Hyoid 0NDX0ZZ
    Lacrimal
      Left 0NDJ0ZZ
      Right 0NDH0ZZ
    Nasal 0NDB0ZZ
    Occipital 0ND70ZZ
    Palatine
      Left 0NDL0ZZ
      Right 0NDK0ZZ
    Parietal
      Left 0ND40ZZ
      Right 0ND30ZZ
    Pelvic
      Left 0QD30ZZ
      Right 0QD20ZZ
    Sphenoid 0NDC0ZZ
    Temporal
      Left 0ND60ZZ
      Right 0ND50ZZ
    Zygomatic
      Left 0NDN0ZZ
      Right 0NDM0ZZ
  Bone Marrow 07DT
    Iliac 07DR
    Sternum 07DQ
    Vertebral 07DS
  Brain 00D0
  Breast
    Bilateral 0HDV0ZZ
    Left 0HDU0ZZ
    Right 0HDT0ZZ
    Supernumerary 0HDY0ZZ
  Bronchus
    Lingula 0BD9
    Lower Lobe
      Left 0BDB
      Right 0BD6
    Main
      Left 0BD7
      Right 0BD3
    Middle Lobe, Right 0BD5
    Upper Lobe
      Left 0BD8
      Right 0BD4
  Bursa and Ligament
    Abdomen
      Left 0MDJ
      Right 0MDH
    Ankle
      Left 0MDR
      Right 0MDQ
    Elbow
      Left 0MD4
      Right 0MD3
    Foot
      Left 0MDT
      Right 0MDS

Extraction — continued
  Bursa and Ligament — continued
    Hand
      Left 0MD8
      Right 0MD7
    Head and Neck 0MD0
    Hip
      Left 0MDM
      Right 0MDL
    Knee
      Left 0MDP
      Right 0MDN
    Lower Extremity
      Left 0MDW
      Right 0MDV
    Perineum 0MDK
    Rib(s) 0MDG
    Shoulder
      Left 0MD2
      Right 0MD1
    Spine
      Lower 0MDD
      Upper 0MDC
    Sternum 0MDF
    Upper Extremity
      Left 0MDB
      Right 0MD9
    Wrist
      Left 0MD6
      Right 0MD5
  Carina 0BD2
  Carpal
    Left 0PDN0ZZ
    Right 0PDM0ZZ
  Cecum 0DDH
  Cerebellum 00DC
  Cerebral Hemisphere 00D7
  Cerebral Meninges 00D1
  Cisterna Chyli 07DL
  Clavicle
    Left 0PDB0ZZ
    Right 0PD90ZZ
  Coccyx 0QDS0ZZ
  Colon
    Ascending 0DDK
    Descending 0DDM
    Sigmoid 0DDN
    Transverse 0DDL
  Cornea
    Left 08D9XZ
    Right 08D8XZ
  Duct
    Common Bile 0FD9
    Cystic 0FD8
    Hepatic
      Common 0FD7
      Left 0FD6
      Right 0FD5
    Pancreatic 0FDD
      Accessory 0FDF
  Duodenum 0DD9
  Dura Mater 00D2
  Endometrium 0UDB
  Esophagogastric Junction 0DD4
  Esophagus 0DD5
    Lower 0DD3
    Middle 0DD2
    Upper 0DD1
  Femoral Shaft
    Left 0QD90ZZ
    Right 0QD80ZZ
  Femur
    Lower
      Left 0QDC0ZZ
      Right 0QDB0ZZ
    Upper
      Left 0QD70ZZ
      Right 0QD60ZZ
  Fibula
    Left 0QDK0ZZ
    Right 0QDJ0ZZ
  Finger Nail 0HDQXZZ
  Gallbladder 0FD4
  Glenoid Cavity
    Left 0PD80ZZ
    Right 0PD70ZZ
  Hair 0HDSXZZ
  Humeral Head
    Left 0PDD0ZZ

Extraction — continued
  Humeral Head — continued
    Right 0PDC0ZZ
  Humeral Shaft
    Left 0PDG0ZZ
    Right 0PDF0ZZ
  Ileocecal Valve 0DDC
  Ileum 0DDB
  Intestine
    Large 0DDE
      Left 0DDG
      Right 0DDF
    Small 0DD8
  Jejunum 0DDA
  Kidney
    Left 0TD1
    Right 0TD0
  Lens
    Left 08DK3ZZ
    Right 08DJ3ZZ
  Liver 0FD0
    Left Lobe 0FD2
    Right Lobe 0FD1
  Lung
    Bilateral 0BDM
    Left 0BDL
    Lower Lobe
      Left 0BDJ
      Right 0BDF
    Middle Lobe, Right 0BDD
    Right 0BDK
    Upper Lobe
      Left 0BDG
      Right 0BDC
  Lung Lingula 0BDH
  Lymphatic
    Aortic 07DD
    Axillary
      Left 07D6
      Right 07D5
    Head 07D0
    Inguinal
      Left 07DJ
      Right 07DH
    Internal Mammary
      Left 07D9
      Right 07D8
    Lower Extremity
      Left 07DG
      Right 07DF
    Mesenteric 07DB
    Neck
      Left 07D2
      Right 07D1
    Pelvis 07DC
    Thoracic Duct 07DK
    Thorax 07D7
    Upper Extremity
      Left 07D4
      Right 07D3
  Mandible
    Left 0NDV0ZZ
    Right 0NDT0ZZ
  Maxilla 0NDR0ZZ
  Metacarpal
    Left 0PDQ0ZZ
    Right 0PDP0ZZ
  Metatarsal
    Left 0QDP0ZZ
    Right 0QDN0ZZ
  Muscle
    Abdomen
      Left 0KDL0ZZ
      Right 0KDK0ZZ
    Facial 0KD10ZZ
    Foot
      Left 0KDW0ZZ
      Right 0KDV0ZZ
    Hand
      Left 0KDD0ZZ
      Right 0KDC0ZZ
    Head 0KD00ZZ
    Hip
      Left 0KDP0ZZ
      Right 0KDN0ZZ
    Lower Arm and Wrist
      Left 0KDB0ZZ
      Right 0KD90ZZ

Extraction — *continued*
  Muscle — *continued*
    Lower Leg
      Left 0KDT0ZZ
      Right 0KDS0ZZ
    Neck
      Left 0KD30ZZ
      Right 0KD20ZZ
    Perineum 0KDM0ZZ
    Shoulder
      Left 0KD60ZZ
      Right 0KD50ZZ
    Thorax
      Left 0KDJ0ZZ
      Right 0KDH0ZZ
    Tongue, Palate, Pharynx 0KD40ZZ
    Trunk
      Left 0KDG0ZZ
      Right 0KDF0ZZ
    Upper Arm
      Left 0KD80ZZ
      Right 0KD70ZZ
    Upper Leg
      Left 0KDR0ZZ
      Right 0KDQ0ZZ
  Nerve
    Abdominal Sympathetic 01DM
    Abducens 00DL
    Accessory 00DR
    Acoustic 00DN
    Brachial Plexus 01D3
    Cervical 01D1
    Cervical Plexus 01D0
    Facial 00DM
    Femoral 01DD
    Glossopharyngeal 00DP
    Head and Neck Sympathetic 01DK
    Hypoglossal 00DS
    Lumbar 01DB
    Lumbar Plexus 01D9
    Lumbar Sympathetic 01DN
    Lumbosacral Plexus 01DA
    Median 01D5
    Oculomotor 00DH
    Olfactory 00DF
    Optic 00DG
    Peroneal 01DH
    Phrenic 01D2
    Pudendal 01DC
    Radial 01D6
    Sacral 01DR
    Sacral Plexus 01DQ
    Sacral Sympathetic 01DP
    Sciatic 01DF
    Thoracic 01D8
    Thoracic Sympathetic 01DL
    Tibial 01DG
    Trigeminal 00DK
    Trochlear 00DJ
    Ulnar 01D4
    Vagus 00DQ
  Orbit
    Left 0NDQ0ZZ
    Right 0NDP0ZZ
  Ova 0UDN
  Pancreas 0FDG
  Patella
    Left 0QDF0ZZ
    Right 0QDD0ZZ
  Phalanx
    Finger
      Left 0PDV0ZZ
      Right 0PDT0ZZ
    Thumb
      Left 0PDS0ZZ
      Right 0PDR0ZZ
    Toe
      Left 0QDR0ZZ
      Right 0QDQ0ZZ
  Pleura
    Left 0BDP
    Right 0BDN
  Products of Conception
    Ectopic 10D2
    Extraperitoneal 10D00Z2
    High 10D00Z0
    High Forceps 10D07Z5
    Internal Version 10D07Z7
    Low 10D00Z1

Extraction — *continued*
  Products of Conception — *continued*
    Low Forceps 10D07Z3
    Mid Forceps 10D07Z4
    Other 10D07Z8
    Retained 10D1
    Vacuum 10D07Z6
  Radius
    Left 0PDJ0ZZ
    Right 0PDH0ZZ
  Rectum 0DDP
  Ribs
    1 to 2 0PD10ZZ
    3 or More 0PD20ZZ
  Sacrum 0QD10ZZ
  Scapula
    Left 0PD60ZZ
    Right 0PD50ZZ
  Septum, Nasal 09DM
  Sinus
    Accessory 09DP
    Ethmoid
      Left 09DV
      Right 09DU
    Frontal
      Left 09DT
      Right 09DS
    Mastoid
      Left 09DC
      Right 09DB
    Maxillary
      Left 09DR
      Right 09DQ
    Sphenoid
      Left 09DX
      Right 09DW
  Skin
    Abdomen 0HD7XZZ
    Back 0HD6XZZ
    Buttock 0HD8XZZ
    Chest 0HD5XZZ
    Ear
      Left 0HD3XZZ
      Right 0HD2XZZ
    Face 0HD1XZZ
    Foot
      Left 0HDNXZZ
      Right 0HDMXZZ
    Hand
      Left 0HDGXZZ
      Right 0HDFXZZ
    Inguinal 0HDAXZZ
    Lower Arm
      Left 0HDEXZZ
      Right 0HDDXZZ
    Lower Leg
      Left 0HDLXZZ
      Right 0HDKXZZ
    Neck 0HD4XZZ
    Perineum 0HD9XZZ
    Scalp 0HD0XZZ
    Upper Arm
      Left 0HDCXZZ
      Right 0HDBXZZ
    Upper Leg
      Left 0HDJXZZ
      Right 0HDHXZZ
  Skull 0ND00ZZ
  Spinal Meninges 00DT
  Spleen 07DP
  Sternum 0PD00ZZ
  Stomach 0DD6
    Pylorus 0DD7
  Subcutaneous Tissue and Fascia
    Abdomen 0JD8
    Back 0JD7
    Buttock 0JD9
    Chest 0JD6
    Face 0JD1
    Foot
      Left 0JDR
      Right 0JDQ
    Hand
      Left 0JDK
      Right 0JDJ
    Lower Arm
      Left 0JDH
      Right 0JDG

Extraction — *continued*
  Subcutaneous Tissue and Fascia — *continued*
    Lower Leg
      Left 0JDP
      Right 0JDN
    Neck
      Left 0JD5
      Right 0JD4
    Pelvic Region 0JDC
    Perineum 0JDB
    Scalp 0JD0
    Upper Arm
      Left 0JDF
      Right 0JDD
    Upper Leg
      Left 0JDM
      Right 0JDL
  Tarsal
    Left 0QDM0ZZ
    Right 0QDL0ZZ
  Tendon
    Abdomen
      Left 0LDG0ZZ
      Right 0LDF0ZZ
    Ankle
      Left 0LDT0ZZ
      Right 0LDS0ZZ
    Foot
      Left 0LDW0ZZ
      Right 0LDV0ZZ
    Hand
      Left 0LD80ZZ
      Right 0LD70ZZ
    Head and Neck 0LD00ZZ
    Hip
      Left 0LDK0ZZ
      Right 0LDJ0ZZ
    Knee
      Left 0LDR0ZZ
      Right 0LDQ0ZZ
    Lower Arm and Wrist
      Left 0LD60ZZ
      Right 0LD50ZZ
    Lower Leg
      Left 0LDP0ZZ
      Right 0LDN0ZZ
    Perineum 0LDH0ZZ
    Shoulder
      Left 0LD20ZZ
      Right 0LD10ZZ
    Thorax
      Left 0LDD0ZZ
      Right 0LDC0ZZ
    Trunk
      Left 0LDB0ZZ
      Right 0LD90ZZ
    Upper Arm
      Left 0LD40ZZ
      Right 0LD30ZZ
    Upper Leg
      Left 0LDM0ZZ
      Right 0DLL0ZZ
  Thymus 07DM
  Tibia
    Left 0QDH0ZZ
    Right 0QDG0ZZ
  Toe Nail 0HDRXZZ
  Tooth
    Lower 0CDXXZ
    Upper 0CDWXZ
  Trachea 0BD1
  Turbinate, Nasal 09DL
  Tympanic Membrane
    Left 09D8
    Right 09D7
  Ulna
    Left 0PDL0ZZ
    Right 0PDK0ZZ
  Vein
    Basilic
      Left 05DC
      Right 05DB
    Brachial
      Left 05DA
      Right 05D9
    Cephalic
      Left 05DF
      Right 05DD

▽ **Subterms under main terms may continue to next column or page**

Extraction — *continued*
  Vein — *continued*
    Femoral
      Left Ø6DN
      Right Ø6DM
    Foot
      Left Ø6DV
      Right Ø6DT
    Hand
      Left Ø5DH
      Right Ø5DG
    Lower Ø6DY
    Saphenous
      Left Ø6DQ
      Right Ø6DP
    Upper Ø5DY
  Vertebra
    Cervical ØPD3ØZZ
    Lumbar ØQDØØZZ
    Thoracic ØPD4ØZZ
  Vocal Cord
    Left ØCDV
    Right ØCDT
Extradural space, intracranial *use* Epidural Space, Intracranial
Extradural space, spinal *use* Spinal Canal
EXtreme Lateral Interbody Fusion (XLIF) device *use* Interbody Fusion Device in Lower Joints

F

Face lift *see* Alteration, Face ØWØ2
Facet replacement spinal stabilization device
  use Spinal Stabilization Device, Facet Replacement in ØRH
  use Spinal Stabilization Device, Facet Replacement in ØSH
Facial artery *use* Face Artery
Factor Xa Inhibitor Reversal Agent, Andexanet Alfa *use* Coagulation Factor Xa, Inactivated
False vocal cord *use* Larynx
Falx cerebri *use* Dura Mater
Fascia lata
  use Subcutaneous Tissue and Fascia, Left Upper Leg
  use Subcutaneous Tissue and Fascia, Right Upper Leg
Fasciaplasty, fascioplasty
  see Repair, Subcutaneous Tissue and Fascia ØJQ
  see Replacement, Subcutaneous Tissue and Fascia ØJR
Fasciectomy *see* Excision, Subcutaneous Tissue and Fascia ØJB
Fasciorrhaphy *see* Repair, Subcutaneous Tissue and Fascia ØJQ
Fasciotomy
  see Division, Subcutaneous Tissue and Fascia ØJ8
  see Drainage, Subcutaneous Tissue and Fascia ØJ9
  see Release
Feeding Device
  Change device in
    Lower Intestinal Tract ØD2DXUZ
    Upper Intestinal Tract ØD2ØXUZ
  Insertion of device in
    Duodenum ØDH9
    Esophagus ØDH5
    Ileum ØDHB
    Intestine, Small ØDH8
    Jejunum ØDHA
    Stomach ØDH6
  Removal of device from
    Esophagus ØDP5
    Intestinal Tract
      Lower Intestinal Tract ØDPD
      Upper Intestinal Tract ØDPØ
    Stomach ØDP6
  Revision of device in
    Intestinal Tract
      Lower Intestinal Tract ØDWD
      Upper Intestinal Tract ØDWØ
    Stomach ØDW6
    Upper Intestinal Tract ØDWØ
Femoral head
  use Upper Femur, Left
  use Upper Femur, Right
Femoral lymph node
  use Lymphatic, Left Lower Extremity

Femoral lymph node — *continued*
  use Lymphatic, Right Lower Extremity
Femoropatellar joint
  use Knee Joint, Left
  use Knee Joint, Left, Tibial Surface
  use Knee Joint, Right
  use Knee Joint, Right, Femoral Surface
Femorotibial joint
  use Knee Joint, Left
  use Knee Joint, Left, Tibial Surface
  use Knee Joint, Right
  use Knee Joint, Right, Tibial Surface
FETROJA® *use* Cefiderocol Anti-infective
FGS (fluorescence-guided surgery) *see* Fluorescence Guided Procedure
Fibular artery
  use Peroneal Artery, Left
  use Peroneal Artery, Right
Fibular sesamoid
  use Metatarsal, Left
  use Metatarsal, Right
Fibularis brevis muscle
  use Lower Leg Muscle, Left
  use Lower Leg Muscle, Right
Fibularis longus muscle
  use Lower Leg Muscle, Left
  use Lower Leg Muscle, Right
Fifth cranial nerve *use* Trigeminal Nerve
Filum terminale *use* Spinal Meninges
Fimbriectomy
  see Excision, Female Reproductive System ØUB
  see Resection, Female Reproductive System ØUT
Fine needle aspiration
  Fluid or gas *see* Drainage
  Tissue biopsy
    see Excision
    see Extraction
First cranial nerve *use* Olfactory Nerve
First intercostal nerve *use* Brachial Plexus
Fistulization
  see Bypass
  see Drainage
  see Repair
Fitting
  Arch bars, for fracture reduction *see* Reposition, Mouth and Throat ØCS
  Arch bars, for immobilization *see* Immobilization, Face 2W31
  Artificial limb *see* Device Fitting, Rehabilitation FØD
  Hearing aid *see* Device Fitting, Rehabilitation FØD
  Ocular prosthesis FØDZ8UZ
  Prosthesis, limb *see* Device Fitting, Rehabilitation FØD
  Prosthesis, ocular FØDZ8UZ
Fixation, bone
  External, with fracture reduction *see* Reposition
  External, without fracture reduction *see* Insertion
  Internal, with fracture reduction *see* Reposition
  Internal, without fracture reduction *see* Insertion
FLAIR® Endovascular Stent Graft *use* Intraluminal Device
Flexible Composite Mesh *use* Synthetic Substitute
Flexor carpi radialis muscle
  use Lower Arm and Wrist Muscle, Left
  use Lower Arm and Wrist Muscle, Right
Flexor carpi ulnaris muscle
  use Lower Arm and Wrist Muscle, Left
  use Lower Arm and Wrist Muscle, Right
Flexor digitorum brevis muscle
  use Foot Muscle, Left
  use Foot Muscle, Right
Flexor digitorum longus muscle
  use Lower Leg Muscle, Left
  use Lower Leg Muscle, Right
Flexor hallucis brevis muscle
  use Foot Muscle, Left
  use Foot Muscle, Right
Flexor hallucis longus muscle
  use Lower Leg Muscle, Left
  use Lower Leg Muscle, Right
Flexor pollicis longus muscle
  use Lower Arm and Wrist Muscle, Left
  use Lower Arm and Wrist Muscle, Right

Flourish® Pediatric Esophageal Atresia Device *use* Magnetic Lengthening Device in Gastrointestinal System
Flow Diverter embolization device *use* Intraluminal Device, Flow Diverter in Ø3V
FlowSense Noninvasive Thermal Sensor 4BØØXWØ
Fluorescence Guided Procedure
  Extremity
    Lower 8EØY
    Upper 8EØX
  Head and Neck Region 8EØ9
    Aminolevulinic Acid 8EØ9ØEM
    No Qualifier 8EØ9ØEZ
  Reproductive System, Female, Pafolacianine (CYTALUX®) EØU
  Trunk Region
    No Qualifier 8EØW
    Pafolacianine (CYTALUX®) 8EØW
Fluorescent Pyrazine, Kidney XT25XE5
Fluoroscopy
  Abdomen and Pelvis BW11
  Airway, Upper BB1DZZZ
  Ankle
    Left BQ1H
    Right BQ1G
  Aorta
    Abdominal B41Ø
      Laser, Intraoperative B41Ø
    Thoracic B31Ø
      Laser, Intraoperative B31Ø
    Thoraco-Abdominal B31P
      Laser, Intraoperative B31P
  Aorta and Bilateral Lower Extremity Arteries B41D
    Laser, Intraoperative B41D
  Arm
    Left BP1FZZZ
    Right BP1EZZZ
  Artery
    Brachiocephalic-Subclavian
      Laser, Intraoperative B311
      Right B311
    Bronchial B31L
      Laser, Intraoperative B31L
    Bypass Graft, Other B21F
    Cervico-Cerebral Arch B31Q
      Laser, Intraoperative B31Q
    Common Carotid
      Bilateral B315
        Laser, Intraoperative B315
      Left B314
        Laser, Intraoperative B314
      Right B313
        Laser, Intraoperative B313
    Coronary
      Bypass Graft
        Multiple B213
          Laser, Intraoperative B213
        Single B212
          Laser, Intraoperative B212
      Multiple B211
        Laser, Intraoperative B211
      Single B21Ø
        Laser, Intraoperative B21Ø
    External Carotid
      Bilateral B31C
        Laser, Intraoperative B31C
      Left B31B
        Laser, Intraoperative B31B
      Right B319
        Laser, Intraoperative B319
    Hepatic B412
      Laser, Intraoperative B412
    Inferior Mesenteric B415
      Laser, Intraoperative B415
    Intercostal B31L
      Laser, Intraoperative B31L
    Internal Carotid
      Bilateral B318
        Laser, Intraoperative B318
      Left B317
        Laser, Intraoperative B317
      Right B316
        Laser, Intraoperative B316
    Internal Mammary Bypass Graft
      Left B218
      Right B217
    Intra-Abdominal
      Laser, Intraoperative B41B
      Other B41B

Fluoroscopy — *continued*
  Artery — *continued*
    Intracranial B31R
      Laser, Intraoperative B31R
    Lower
      Laser, Intraoperative B41J
      Other B41J
    Lower Extremity
      Bilateral and Aorta B41D
        Laser, Intraoperative B41D
      Left B41G
        Laser, Intraoperative B41G
      Right B41F
        Laser, Intraoperative B41F
    Lumbar B419
      Laser, Intraoperative B419
    Pelvic B41C
      Laser, Intraoperative B41C
    Pulmonary
      Left B31T
        Laser, Intraoperative B31T
      Right B31S
        Laser, Intraoperative B31S
    Pulmonary Trunk B31U
      Laser, Intraoperative B31U
    Renal
      Bilateral B418
        Laser, Intraoperative B418
      Left B417
        Laser, Intraoperative B417
      Right B416
        Laser, Intraoperative B416
    Spinal B31M
      Laser, Intraoperative B31M
    Splenic B413
      Laser, Intraoperative B413
    Subclavian
      Laser, Intraoperative B312
      Left B312
    Superior Mesenteric B414
      Laser, Intraoperative B414
    Upper
      Laser, Intraoperative B31N
      Other B31N
    Upper Extremity
      Bilateral B31K
        Laser, Intraoperative B31K
      Left B31J
        Laser, Intraoperative B31J
      Right B31H
        Laser, Intraoperative B31H
    Vertebral
      Bilateral B31G
        Laser, Intraoperative B31G
      Left B31F
        Laser, Intraoperative B31F
      Right B31D
        Laser, Intraoperative B31D
  Bile Duct BF1Ø
    Pancreatic Duct and Gallbladder BF14
  Bile Duct and Gallbladder BF13
  Biliary Duct BF11
  Bladder BT1Ø
    Kidney and Ureter BT14
      Left BT1F
      Right BT1D
  Bladder and Urethra BT1B
  Bowel, Small BD1
  Calcaneus
    Left BQ1KZZZ
    Right BQ1JZZZ
  Clavicle
    Left BP15ZZZ
    Right BP14ZZZ
  Coccyx BR1F
  Colon BD14
  Corpora Cavernosa BV1Ø
  Dialysis Fistula B51W
  Dialysis Shunt B51W
  Diaphragm BB16ZZZ
  Disc
    Cervical BR11
    Lumbar BR13
    Thoracic BR12
  Duodenum BD19
  Elbow
    Left BP1H
    Right BP1G
  Epiglottis B91G

Fluoroscopy — *continued*
  Esophagus BD11
  Extremity
    Lower BW1C
    Upper BW1J
  Facet Joint
    Cervical BR14
    Lumbar BR16
    Thoracic BR15
  Fallopian Tube
    Bilateral BU12
    Left BU11
    Right BU1Ø
  Fallopian Tube and Uterus BU18
  Femur
    Left BQ14ZZZ
    Right BQ13ZZZ
  Finger
    Left BP1SZZZ
    Right BP1RZZZ
  Foot
    Left BQ1MZZZ
    Right BQ1LZZZ
  Forearm
    Left BP1KZZZ
    Right BP1JZZZ
  Gallbladder BF12
    Bile Duct and Pancreatic Duct BF14
  Gallbladder and Bile Duct BF13
  Gastrointestinal, Upper BD1
  Hand
    Left BP1PZZZ
    Right BP1NZZZ
  Head and Neck BW19
  Heart
    Left B215
    Right B214
    Right and Left B216
  Hip
    Left BQ11
    Right BQ1Ø
  Humerus
    Left BP1BZZZ
    Right BP1AZZZ
  Ileal Diversion Loop BT1C
  Ileal Loop, Ureters and Kidney BT1G
  Intracranial Sinus B512
  Joint
    Acromioclavicular, Bilateral BP13ZZZ
    Finger
      Left BP1D
      Right BP1C
    Foot
      Left BQ1Y
      Right BQ1X
    Hand
      Left BP1D
      Right BP1C
    Lumbosacral BR1B
    Sacroiliac BR1D
    Sternoclavicular
      Bilateral BP12ZZZ
      Left BP11ZZZ
      Right BP1ØZZZ
    Temporomandibular
      Bilateral BN19
      Left BN18
      Right BN17
    Thoracolumbar BR18
    Toe
      Left BQ1Y
      Right BQ1X
  Kidney
    Bilateral BT13
    Ileal Loop and Ureter BT1G
    Left BT12
    Right BT11
    Ureter and Bladder BT14
      Left BT1F
      Right BT1D
  Knee
    Left BQ18
    Right BQ17
  Larynx B91J
  Leg
    Left BQ1FZZZ
    Right BQ1DZZZ
  Liver BF15

Fluoroscopy — *continued*
  Lung
    Bilateral BB14ZZZ
    Left BB13ZZZ
    Right BB12ZZZ
  Mediastinum BB1CZZZ
  Mouth BD1B
  Neck and Head BW19
  Oropharynx BD1B
  Pancreatic Duct BF1
    Gallbladder and Bile Buct BF14
  Patella
    Left BQ1WZZZ
    Right BQ1VZZZ
  Pelvis BR1C
  Pelvis and Abdomen BW11
  Pharynix B91G
  Ribs
    Left BP1YZZZ
    Right BP1XZZZ
  Sacrum BR1F
  Scapula
    Left BP17ZZZ
    Right BP16ZZZ
  Shoulder
    Left BP19
    Right BP18
  Sinus, Intracranial B512
  Spinal Cord BØ1B
  Spine
    Cervical BR1Ø
    Lumbar BR19
    Thoracic BR17
    Whole BR1G
  Sternum BR1H
  Stomach BD12
  Toe
    Left BQ1QZZZ
    Right BQ1PZZZ
  Tracheobronchial Tree
    Bilateral BB19YZZ
    Left BB18YZZ
    Right BB17YZZ
  Ureter
    Ileal Loop and Kidney BT1G
    Kidney and Bladder BT14
      Left BT1F
      Right BT1D
    Left BT17
    Right BT16
  Urethra BT15
  Urethra and Bladder BT1B
  Uterus BU16
  Uterus and Fallopian Tube BU18
  Vagina BU19
  Vasa Vasorum BV18
  Vein
    Cerebellar B511
    Cerebral B511
    Epidural B51Ø
    Jugular
      Bilateral B515
      Left B514
      Right B513
    Lower Extremity
      Bilateral B51D
      Left B51C
      Right B51B
    Other B51V
    Pelvic (Iliac)
      Left B51G
      Right B51F
    Pelvic (Iliac) Bilateral B51H
    Portal B51T
    Pulmonary
      Bilateral B51S
      Left B51R
      Right B51Q
    Renal
      Bilateral B51L
      Left B51K
      Right B51J
    Spanchnic B51T
    Subclavian
      Left B517
      Right B516
    Upper Extremity
      Bilateral B51P
      Left B51N

Fluoroscopy — *continued*
  Vein — *continued*
    Upper Extremity — *continued*
      Right B51M
    Vena Cava
      Inferior B519
      Superior B518
    Wrist
      Left BP1M
      Right BP1L
Fluoroscopy, laser intraoperative
  see Fluoroscopy, Heart B21
  see Fluoroscopy, Lower Arteries B41
  see Fluoroscopy, Upper Arteries B31
Flushing *see* Irrigation
Foley catheter *use* Drainage Device
Fontan completion procedure Stage II *see* Bypass, Vena Cava, Inferior 0610
Foramen magnum *use* Occipital Bone
Foramen of Monro (intraventricular) *use* Cerebral Ventricle
Foreskin *use* Prepuce
Formula™ Balloon-Expandable Renal Stent System *use* Intraluminal Device
Fosfomycin Anti-infective XW0
Fosfomycin injection *use* Fosfomycin Anti-infective
Fossa of Rosenmuller *use* Nasopharynx
Fostamatinib XW0
Fourth cranial nerve *use* Trochlear Nerve
Fourth ventricle *use* Cerebral Ventricle
Fovea
  use Retina, Left
  use Retina, Right
Fragmentation
  Ampulla of Vater 0FFC
  Anus 0DFQ
  Appendix 0DFJ
  Artery
    Anterior Tibial
      Left 04FQ3Z
      Right 04FP3Z
    Axillary
      Left 03F63Z
      Right 03F53Z
    Brachial
      Left 03F83Z
      Right 03F73Z
    Common Iliac
      Left 04FD3Z
      Right 04FC3Z
    Coronary
      Four or More Arteries 02F33ZZ
      One Artery 02F03ZZ
      Three Arteries 02F23ZZ
      Two Arteries 02F13ZZ
    External Iliac
      Left 04FJ3Z
      Right 04FH3Z
    Femoral
      Left 04FL3Z
      Right 04FK3Z
    Innominate 03F23Z
    Internal Iliac
      Left 04FF3Z
      Right 04FE3Z
    Intracranial 03FG3Z
    Lower 04FY3Z
    Peroneal
      Left 04FU3Z
      Right 04FT3Z
    Popliteal
      Left 04FN3Z
      Right 04FM3Z
    Posterior Tibial
      Left 04FS3Z
      Right 04FR3Z
    Pulmonary
      Left 02FR3Z
      Right 02FQ3Z
    Pulmonary Trunk 02FP3Z
    Radial
      Left 03FC3Z
      Right 03FB3Z
    Subclavian
      Left 03F43Z
      Right 03F33Z
    Ulnar
      Left 03FA3Z

Fragmentation — *continued*
  Artery — *continued*
    Ulnar — *continued*
      Right 03F93Z
    Upper 03FY3Z
  Bladder 0TFB
  Bladder Neck 0TFC
  Bronchus
    Lingula 0BF9
    Lower Lobe
      Left 0BFB
      Right 0BF6
    Main
      Left 0BF7
      Right 0BF3
    Middle Lobe, Right 0BF5
    Upper Lobe
      Left 0BF8
      Right 0BF4
  Carina 0BF2
  Cavity, Cranial 0WF1
  Cecum 0DFH
  Cerebral Ventricle 00F6
  Colon
    Ascending 0DFK
    Descending 0DFM
    Sigmoid 0DFN
    Transverse 0DFL
  Duct
    Common Bile 0FF9
    Cystic 0FF8
    Hepatic
      Common 0FF7
      Left 0FF6
      Right 0FF5
    Pancreatic 0FFD
      Accessory 0FFF
    Parotid
      Left 0CFC
      Right 0CFB
  Duodenum 0DF9
  Epidural Space, Intracranial 00F3
  Esophagus 0DF5
  Fallopian Tube
    Left 0UF6
    Right 0UF5
  Fallopian Tubes, Bilateral 0UF7
  Gallbladder 0FF4
  Gastrointestinal Tract 0WFP
  Genitourinary Tract 0WFR
  Ileum 0DFB
  Intestine
    Large 0DFE
      Left 0DFG
      Right 0DFF
    Small 0DF8
  Jejunum 0DFA
  Kidney Pelvis
    Left 0TF4
    Right 0TF3
  Mediastinum 0WFC
  Oral Cavity and Throat 0WF3
  Pelvic Cavity 0WFJ
  Pericardial Cavity 0WFD
  Pericardium 02FN
  Peritoneal Cavity 0WFG
  Pleural Cavity
    Left 0WFB
    Right 0WF9
  Rectum 0DFP
  Respiratory Tract 0WFQ
  Spinal Canal 00FU
  Stomach 0DF6
  Subarachnoid Space, Intracranial 00F5
  Subdural Space, Intracranial 00F4
  Trachea 0BF1
  Ureter
    Left 0TF7
    Right 0TF6
  Urethra 0TFD
  Uterus 0UF9
  Vein
    Axillary
      Left 05F83Z
      Right 05F73Z
    Basilic
      Left 05FC3Z
      Right 05FB3Z

Fragmentation — *continued*
  Vein — *continued*
    Brachial
      Left 05FA3Z
      Right 05F93Z
    Cephalic
      Left 05FF3Z
      Right 05FD3Z
    Common Iliac
      Left 06FD3Z
      Right 06FC3Z
    External Iliac
      Left 06FG3Z
      Right 06FF3Z
    Femoral
      Left 06FN3Z
      Right 06FM3Z
    Hypogastric
      Left 06FJ3Z
      Right 06FH3Z
    Innominate
      Left 05F43Z
      Right 05F33Z
    Lower 06FY3Z
    Pulmonary
      Left 02FT3Z
      Right 02FS3Z
    Saphenous
      Left 06FQ3Z
      Right 06FP3Z
    Subclavian
      Left 05F63Z
      Right 05F53Z
    Upper 05FY3Z
  Vitreous
    Left 08F5
    Right 08F4
Fragmentation, Ultrasonic *see* Fragmentation, Artery
Freestyle (Stentless) Aortic Root Bioprosthesis *use* Zooplastic Tissue in Heart and Great Vessels
Frenectomy
  see Excision, Mouth and Throat 0CB
  see Resection, Mouth and Throat 0CT
Frenoplasty, frenuloplasty
  see Repair, Mouth and Throat 0CQ
  see Replacement, Mouth and Throat 0CR
  see Supplement, Mouth and Throat 0CU
Frenotomy
  see Drainage, Mouth and Throat 0C9
  see Release, Mouth and Throat 0CN
Frenulotomy
  see Drainage, Mouth and Throat 0C9
  see Release, Mouth and Throat 0CN
Frenulum labii inferioris *use* Lower Lip
Frenulum labii superioris *use* Upper Lip
Frenulum linguae *use* Tongue
Frenulumectomy
  see Excision, Mouth and Throat 0CB
  see Resection, Mouth and Throat 0CT
Frontal lobe *use* Cerebral Hemisphere
Frontal vein
  use Face Vein, Left
  use Face Vein, Right
Frozen elephant trunk (FET) technique, aortic arch replacement
  see New Technology, Cardiovascular System X2R
  see Replacement, Heart and Great Vessels 02R
Frozen elephant trunk (FET) technique, thoracic aorta restriction
  see New Technology, Cardiovascular System X2V
  see Restriction, Heart and Great Vessels 02V
FUJIFILM EP-7000X System for Oxygen Saturation Endoscopic Imaging (OXEI) *see* New Technology, Gastrointestinal System XD2
Fulguration *see* Destruction
Fundoplication, gastroesophageal *see* Restriction, Esophagogastric Junction 0DV4
Fundus uteri *use* Uterus
Fusion
  Acromioclavicular
    Left 0RGH
    Right 0RGG
  Ankle
    Left 0SGG
      Open-truss Design Internal Fixation Device XRGK0B9
    Right 0SGF

Index

Fusion — Greater trochanter

Fusion — *continued*
Ankle — *continued*
Right — *continued*
Open-truss Design Internal Fixation Device XRGJØB9
Carpal
Left ØRGR
Right ØRGQ
Carpometacarpal
Left ØRGT
Right ØRGS
Cervical Vertebral ØRG1
2 or more ØRG2
Cervicothoracic Vertebral ØRG4
Coccygeal ØSG6
Elbow
Left ØRGM
Right ØRGL
Finger Phalangeal
Left ØRGX
Right ØRGW
Hip
Left ØSGB
Right ØSG9
Knee
Left ØSGD
Right ØSGC
Lumbar Vertebral ØSGØ
2 or more ØSG1
Interbody Fusion Device, Custom-Made Anatomically Designed XRGC
Interbody Fusion Device, Custom-Made Anatomically Designed XRGB
Lumbosacral ØSG3
Interbody Fusion Device, Custom-Made Anatomically Designed XRGD
Metacarpophalangeal
Left ØRGV
Right ØRGU
Metatarsal-Phalangeal
Left ØSGN
Right ØSGM
Occipital-cervical ØRGØ
Sacrococcygeal ØSG5
Sacroiliac
Internal Fixation Device with Tulip Connector XRG
Left ØSG8
Right ØSG7
Shoulder
Left ØRGK
Right ØRGJ
Sternoclavicular
Left ØRGF
Right ØRGE
Tarsal
Left ØSGJ
Open-truss Design Internal Fixation Device XRGMØB9
Right ØSGH
Open-truss Design Internal Fixation Device XRGLØB9
Tarsometatarsal
Left ØSGL
Right ØSGK
Temporomandibular
Left ØRGD
Right ØRGC
Thoracic Vertebral ØRG6
2 to 7 ØRG7
8 or more ØRG8
Thoracolumbar Vertebral ØRGA
Interbody Fusion Device, Custom-Made Anatomically Designed XRGA
Toe Phalangeal
Left ØSGQ
Right ØSGP
Wrist
Left ØRGP
Right ØRGN
Fusion screw (compression) (lag) (locking)
use Internal Fixation Device in Lower Joints
use Internal Fixation Device in Upper Joints

G

Gait training *see* Motor Treatment, Rehabilitation FØ7

Galea aponeurotica *use* Subcutaneous Tissue and Fascia, Scalp
Gammaglobulin *use* Globulin
GammaTile™ *use* Radioactive Element, Cesium-131 Collagen Implant in ØØH
GAMUNEX-C, for COVID-19 treatment *use* High-Dose Intravenous Immune Globulin
Ganglion impar (ganglion of Walther) *use* Sacral Sympathetic Nerve
Ganglionectomy
Destruction of lesion *see* Destruction
Excision of lesion *see* Excision
Gasserian ganglion *use* Trigeminal Nerve
Gastrectomy
Partial *see* Excision, Stomach ØDB6
Total *see* Resection, Stomach ØDT6
Vertical (sleeve) *see* Excision, Stomach ØDB6
Gastric electrical stimulation (GES) lead *use* Stimulator Lead in Gastrointestinal System
Gastric lymph node *use* Lymphatic, Aortic
Gastric pacemaker lead *use* Stimulator Lead in Gastrointestinal System
Gastric plexus *use* Abdominal Sympathetic Nerve
Gastrocnemius muscle
use Lower Leg Muscle, Left
use Lower Leg Muscle, Right
Gastrocolic ligament *use* Omentum
Gastrocolic omentum *use* Omentum
Gastrocolostomy
see Bypass, Gastrointestinal System ØD1
see Drainage, Gastrointestinal System ØD9
Gastroduodenal artery *use* Hepatic Artery
Gastroduodenectomy
see Excision, Gastrointestinal System ØDB
see Resection, Gastrointestinal System ØDT
Gastroduodenoscopy ØDJØ8ZZ
Gastroenteroplasty
see Repair, Gastrointestinal System ØDQ
see Supplement, Gastrointestinal System ØDU
Gastroenterostomy
see Bypass, Gastrointestinal System ØD1
see Drainage, Gastrointestinal System ØD9
Gastroesophageal (GE) junction *use* Esophagogastric Junction
Gastrogastrostomy
see Bypass, Stomach ØD16
see Drainage, Stomach ØD96
Gastrohepatic omentum *use* Omentum
Gastrojejunostomy
see Bypass, Stomach ØD16
see Drainage, Stomach ØD96
Gastrolysis *see* Release, Stomach ØDN6
Gastropexy
see Repair, Stomach ØDQ6
see Reposition, Stomach ØDS6
Gastrophrenic ligament *use* Omentum
Gastroplasty
see Repair, Stomach ØDQ6
see Supplement, Stomach ØDU6
Gastroplication *see* Restriction, Stomach ØDV6
Gastropylorectomy *see* Excision, Gastrointestinal System ØDB
Gastrorrhaphy *see* Repair, Stomach ØDQ6
Gastroscopy ØDJ68ZZ
Gastrosplenic ligament *use* Omentum
Gastrostomy
see Bypass, Stomach ØD16
see Drainage, Stomach ØD96
Gastrotomy *see* Drainage, Stomach ØD96
Gemellus muscle
use Hip Muscle, Left
use Hip Muscle, Right
Geniculate ganglion *use* Facial Nerve
Geniculate nucleus *use* Thalamus
Genioglossus muscle *use* Tongue, Palate, Pharynx Muscle
Genioplasty *see* Alteration, Jaw, Lower ØW05
Genitofemoral nerve *use* Lumbar Plexus
GIAPREZA™ *use* Vasopressor
Gilteritinib Antineoplastic XWØDXV5
Gingivectomy *see* Excision, Mouth and Throat ØCB
Gingivoplasty
see Repair, Mouth and Throat ØCQ
see Replacement, Mouth and Throat ØCR
see Supplement, Mouth and Throat ØCU
Glans penis *use* Prepuce

Glenohumeral joint
use Shoulder Joint, Left
use Shoulder Joint, Right
Glenohumeral ligament
use Shoulder Bursa and Ligament, Left
use Shoulder Bursa and Ligament, Right
Glenoid fossa (of scapula)
use Glenoid Cavity, Left
use Glenoid Cavity, Right
Glenoid ligament (labrum)
use Shoulder Joint, Left
use Shoulder Joint, Right
Globus pallidus *use* Basal Ganglia
Glofitamab Antineoplastic XWØ
Glomectomy
see Excision, Endocrine System ØGB
see Resection, Endocrine System ØGT
Glossectomy
see Excision, Tongue ØCB7
see Resection, Tongue ØCT7
Glossoepiglottic fold *use* Epiglottis
Glossopexy
see Repair, Tongue ØCQ7
see Reposition, Tongue ØCS7
Glossoplasty
see Repair, Tongue ØCQ7
see Replacement, Tongue ØCR7
see Supplement, Tongue ØCU7
Glossorrhaphy *see* Repair, Tongue ØCQ7
Glossotomy *see* Drainage, Tongue ØC97
Glottis *use* Larynx
Gluteal Artery Perforator Flap
Replacement
Bilateral ØHRVØ79
Left ØHRUØ79
Right ØHRTØ79
Transfer
Left ØKXG
Right ØKXF
Gluteal lymph node *use* Lymphatic, Pelvis
Gluteal vein
use Hypogastric Vein, Left
use Hypogastric Vein, Right
Gluteus maximus muscle
use Hip Muscle, Left
use Hip Muscle, Right
Gluteus medius muscle
use Hip Muscle, Left
use Hip Muscle, Right
Gluteus minimus muscle
use Hip Muscle, Left
use Hip Muscle, Right
GORE EXCLUDER® AAA Endoprosthesis
use Intraluminal Device
use Intraluminal Device, Branched or Fenestrated, One or Two Arteries in Ø4V
use Intraluminal Device, Branched or Fenestrated, Three or More Arteries in Ø4V
GORE EXCLUDER® IBE Endoprosthesis *use* Intraluminal Device, Branched or Fenestrated, One or Two Arteries in Ø4V
GORE TAG® Thoracic Endoprosthesis *use* Intraluminal Device
GORE® DUALMESH® *use* Synthetic Substitute
Gracilis muscle
use Upper Leg Muscle, Left
use Upper Leg Muscle, Right
Graft
see Replacement
see Supplement
Great auricular nerve *use* Cervical Plexus
Great cerebral vein *use* Intracranial Vein
Great(er) saphenous vein
use Saphenous Vein, Left
use Saphenous Vein, Right
Greater alar cartilage *use* Nasal Mucosa and Soft Tissue
Greater occipital nerve *use* Cervical Nerve
Greater Omentum *use* Omentum
Greater splanchnic nerve *use* Thoracic Sympathetic Nerve
Greater superficial petrosal nerve *use* Facial Nerve
Greater trochanter
use Upper Femur, Left
use Upper Femur, Right

Greater tuberosity
use Humeral Head, Left
use Humeral Head, Right
Greater vestibular (Bartholin's) gland use Vestibular Gland
Greater wing use Sphenoid Bone
GS-5734 use Remdesivir Anti-infective
Guedel airway use Intraluminal Device, Airway in Mouth and Throat
Guidance, catheter placement
EKG see Measurement, Physiological Systems 4A0
Fluoroscopy see Fluoroscopy, Veins B51
Ultrasound see Ultrasonography, Veins B54

H

Hallux
use 1st Toe, Left
use 1st Toe, Right
Hamate bone
use Carpal, Left
use Carpal, Right
Hancock Bioprosthesis (aortic) (mitral) valve use Zooplastic Tissue in Heart and Great Vessels
Hancock Bioprosthetic Valved Conduit use Zooplastic Tissue in Heart and Great Vessels
Harmony™ transcatheter pulmonary valve (TPV) placement 02RH38M
Harvesting, Stem Cells see Pheresis, Circulatory 6A55
hdIVIG (high-dose intravenous immunoglobulin), for COVID-19 treatment use High-Dose Intravenous Immune Globulin
Head of fibula
use Fibula, Left
use Fibula, Right
Hearing Aid Assessment F14Z
Hearing Assessment F13Z
Hearing Device
Bone Conduction
Left 09HE
Right 09HD
Insertion of device in
Left 0NH6
Right 0NH5
Multiple Channel Cochlear Prosthesis
Left 09HE
Right 09HD
Removal of device from, Skull 0NP0
Revision of device in, Skull 0NW0
Single Channel Cochlear Prosthesis
Left 09HE
Right 09HD
Hearing Treatment F09Z
Heart Assist System
Implantable
Insertion of device in, Heart 02HA
Removal of device from, Heart 02PA
Revision of device in, Heart 02WA
Short-term External
Insertion of device in
Aorta, Thoracic, Descending 02HW3RZ
Heart 02HA
Removal of device from
Aorta, Thoracic, Descending 02PW3RZ
Heart 02PA
Revision of device in
Aorta, Thoracic, Descending 02WW3RZ
Heart 02WA
HeartMate 3™ LVAS use Implantable Heart Assist System in Heart and Great Vessels
HeartMate II® Left Ventricular Assist Device (LVAD) use Implantable Heart Assist System in Heart and Great Vessels
HeartMate XVE® Left Ventricular Assist Device (LVAD) use Implantable Heart Assist System in Heart and Great Vessels
HeartMate® implantable heart assist system see Insertion of device in, Heart 02HA
Helix
use Ear, External, Bilateral
use Ear, External, Left
use Ear, External, Right
Hematopoietic cell transplant (HCT) see Transfusion, Circulatory 302
Hemicolectomy see Resection, Gastrointestinal System 0DT
Hemicystectomy see Excision, Urinary System 0TB

Hemigastrectomy see Excision, Gastrointestinal System 0DB
Hemiglossectomy see Excision, Mouth and Throat 0CB
Hemilaminectomy
see Excision, Lower Bones 0QB
see Excision, Upper Bones 0PB
Hemilaminotomy
see Drainage, Lower Bones 0Q9
see Drainage, Upper Bones 0P9
see Excision, Lower Bones 0QB
see Excision, Upper Bones 0PB
see Release, Central Nervous System and Cranial Nerves 00N
see Release, Lower Bones 0QN
see Release, Peripheral Nervous System 01N
see Release, Upper Bones 0PN
Hemilaryngectomy see Excision, Larynx 0CBS
Hemimandibulectomy see Excision, Head and Facial Bones 0NB
Hemimaxillectomy see Excision, Head and Facial Bones 0NB
Hemipylorectomy see Excision, Gastrointestinal System 0DB
Hemispherectomy
see Excision, Central Nervous System and Cranial Nerves 00B
see Resection, Central Nervous System and Cranial Nerves 00T
Hemithyroidectomy
see Excision, Endocrine System 0GB
see Resection, Endocrine System 0GT
Hemodialysis see Performance, Urinary 5A1D
Hemolung® Respiratory Assist System (RAS) 5A0920Z
Hemospray® Endoscopic Hemostat use Mineral-based Topical Hemostatic Agent
Hepatectomy
see Excision, Hepatobiliary System and Pancreas 0FB
see Resection, Hepatobiliary System and Pancreas 0FT
Hepatic artery proper use Hepatic Artery
Hepatic flexure use Transverse Colon
Hepatic lymph node use Lymphatic, Aortic
Hepatic plexus use Abdominal Sympathetic Nerve
Hepatic portal vein use Portal Vein
Hepaticoduodenostomy
see Bypass, Hepatobiliary System and Pancreas 0F1
see Drainage, Hepatobiliary System and Pancreas 0F9
Hepaticotomy see Drainage, Hepatobiliary System and Pancreas 0F9
Hepatocholedochostomy see Drainage, Duct, Common Bile 0F99
Hepatogastric ligament use Omentum
Hepatopancreatic ampulla use Ampulla of Vater
Hepatopexy
see Repair, Hepatobiliary System and Pancreas 0FQ
see Reposition, Hepatobiliary System and Pancreas 0FS
Hepatorrhaphy see Repair, Hepatobiliary System and Pancreas 0FQ
Hepatotomy see Drainage, Hepatobiliary System and Pancreas 0F9
HEPZATO™ KIT (melphalan hydrochloride Hepatic Delivery System) use Melphalan Hydrochloride Antineoplastic
Herculink (RX) Elite Renal Stent System use Intraluminal Device
Herniorrhaphy
see Repair, Anatomical Regions, General 0WQ
see Repair, Anatomical Regions, Lower Extremities 0YQ
With synthetic substitute
see Supplement, Anatomical Regions, General 0WU
see Supplement, Anatomical Regions, Lower Extremities 0YU
HIG (hyperimmune globulin), for COVID-19 treatment use Hyperimmune Globulin
High-Dose Intravenous Immune Globulin, for COVID-19 treatment XW1
High-dose intravenous immunoglobulin (hdIVIG), for COVID-19 treatment use High-Dose Intravenous Immune Globulin
Hip (joint) liner use Liner in Lower Joints

HIPEC (hyperthermic intraperitoneal chemotherapy) 3E0M30Y
HistoSonics® System see New Technology, Hepatobiliary System and Pancreas XF5
Histotripsy, liver see New Technology, Hepatobiliary System and Pancreas XF5
hIVIG (hyperimmune intravenous immunoglobulin), for COVID-19 treatment use Hyperimmune Globulin
Holter Monitoring 4A12X45
Holter valve ventricular shunt use Synthetic Substitute
Human angiotensin II, synthetic use Vasopressor
Humeroradial joint
use Elbow Joint, Left
use Elbow Joint, Right
Humeroulnar joint
use Elbow Joint, Left
use Elbow Joint, Right
Humerus, distal
use Humeral Shaft, Left
use Humeral Shaft, Right
Hydrocelectomy see Excision, Male Reproductive System 0VB
Hydrotherapy
Assisted exercise in pool see Motor Treatment, Rehabilitation F07
Whirlpool see Activities of Daily Living Treatment, Rehabilitation F08
Hymenectomy
see Excision, Hymen 0UBK
see Resection, Hymen 0UTK
Hymenoplasty
see Repair, Hymen 0UQK
see Supplement, Hymen 0UUK
Hymenorrhaphy see Repair, Hymen 0UQK
Hymenotomy
see Division, Hymen 0U8K
see Drainage, Hymen 0U9K
Hyoglossus muscle use Tongue, Palate, Pharynx Muscle
Hyoid artery
use Thyroid Artery, Left
use Thyroid Artery, Right
Hyperalimentation see Introduction of substance in or on
Hyperbaric oxygenation
Decompression sickness treatment see Decompression, Circulatory 6A15
Other treatment see Assistance, Circulatory 5A05
Hyperimmune globulin use Globulin
Hyperimmune Globulin, for COVID-19 treatment XW1
Hyperimmune intravenous immunoglobulin (hIVIG), for COVID-19 treatment use Hyperimmune Globulin
Hyperthermia
Radiation Therapy
Abdomen DWY38ZZ
Adrenal Gland DGY28ZZ
Bile Ducts DFY28ZZ
Bladder DTY28ZZ
Bone Marrow D7Y08ZZ
Bone, Other DPYC8ZZ
Brain D0Y08ZZ
Brain Stem D0Y18ZZ
Breast
Left DMY08ZZ
Right DMY18ZZ
Bronchus DBY18ZZ
Cervix DUY18ZZ
Chest DWY28ZZ
Chest Wall DBY78ZZ
Colon DDY58ZZ
Diaphragm DBY88ZZ
Duodenum DDY28ZZ
Ear D9Y08ZZ
Esophagus DDY08ZZ
Eye D8Y08ZZ
Femur DPY98ZZ
Fibula DPYB8ZZ
Gallbladder DFY18ZZ
Gland
Adrenal DGY28ZZ
Parathyroid DGY48ZZ
Pituitary DGY08ZZ
Thyroid DGY58ZZ

Hyperthermia — *continued*
  Radiation Therapy — *continued*
    Glands, Salivary D9Y68ZZ
    Head and Neck DWY18ZZ
    Hemibody DWY48ZZ
    Humerus DPY68ZZ
    Hypopharynx D9Y38ZZ
    Ileum DDY48ZZ
    Jejunum DDY38ZZ
    Kidney DTY08ZZ
    Larynx D9YB8ZZ
    Liver DFY08ZZ
    Lung DBY28ZZ
    Lymphatics
      Abdomen D7Y68ZZ
      Axillary D7Y48ZZ
      Inguinal D7Y88ZZ
      Neck D7Y38ZZ
      Pelvis D7Y78ZZ
      Thorax D7Y58ZZ
    Mandible DPY38ZZ
    Maxilla DPY28ZZ
    Mediastinum DBY68ZZ
    Mouth D9Y48ZZ
    Nasopharynx D9YD8ZZ
    Neck and Head DWY18ZZ
    Nerve, Peripheral D0Y78ZZ
    Nose D9Y18ZZ
    Oropharynx D9YF8ZZ
    Ovary DUY08ZZ
    Palate
      Hard D9Y88ZZ
      Soft D9Y98ZZ
    Pancreas DFY38ZZ
    Parathyroid Gland DGY48ZZ
    Pelvic Bones DPY88ZZ
    Pelvic Region DWY68ZZ
    Pineal Body DGY18ZZ
    Pituitary Gland DGY08ZZ
    Pleura DBY58ZZ
    Prostate DVY08ZZ
    Radius DPY78ZZ
    Rectum DDY78ZZ
    Rib DPY58ZZ
    Sinuses D9Y78ZZ
    Skin
      Abdomen DHY88ZZ
      Arm DHY48ZZ
      Back DHY78ZZ
      Buttock DHY98ZZ
      Chest DHY68ZZ
      Face DHY28ZZ
      Leg DHYB8ZZ
      Neck DHY38ZZ
    Skull DPY08ZZ
    Spinal Cord D0Y68ZZ
    Spleen D7Y28ZZ
    Sternum DPY48ZZ
    Stomach DDY18ZZ
    Testis DVY18ZZ
    Thymus D7Y18ZZ
    Thyroid Gland DGY58ZZ
    Tibia DPYB8ZZ
    Tongue D9Y58ZZ
    Trachea DBY08ZZ
    Ulna DPY78ZZ
    Ureter DTY18ZZ
    Urethra DTY38ZZ·
    Uterus DUY28ZZ
    Whole Body DWY58ZZ
  Whole Body 6A3Z
Hyperthermic Intraperitoneal Chemotherapy (HIPEC) 3E0M30Y
Hypnosis GZFZZZZ
Hypogastric artery
  use Internal Iliac Artery, Left
  use Internal Iliac Artery, Right
Hypopharynx *use* Pharynx
Hypophysectomy
  see Excision, Gland, Pituitary 0GB0
  see Resection, Gland, Pituitary 0GT0
Hypophysis *use* Pituitary Gland
Hypothalamotomy *see* Destruction, Thalamus 0059
Hypothenar muscle
  use Hand Muscle, Left
  use Hand Muscle, Right
Hypothermia, Whole Body 6A4Z

Hysterectomy
  Supracervical *see* Resection, Uterus 0UT9
  Total *see* Resection, Uterus 0UT9
Hysterolysis *see* Release, Uterus 0UN9
Hysteropexy
  see Repair, Uterus 0UQ9
  see Reposition, Uterus 0US9
Hysteroplasty *see* Repair, Uterus 0UQ9
Hysterorrhaphy *see* Repair, Uterus 0UQ9
Hysteroscopy 0UJD8ZZ
Hysterotomy *see* Drainage, Uterus 0U99
Hysterotrachelectomy
  see Resection, Cervix 0UTC
  see Resection, Uterus 0UT9
Hysterotracheloplasty *see* Repair, Uterus 0UQ9
Hysterotrachelorrhaphy *see* Repair, Uterus 0UQ9

I

IABP (Intra-aortic balloon pump) *see* Assistance, Cardiac 5A02
IAEMT (Intraoperative anesthetic effect monitoring and titration) *see* Monitoring, Central Nervous 4A10
IASD® (InterAtrial Shunt Device), Corvia *use* Synthetic Substitute
Idarucizumab, Pradaxa® (dabigatran) reversal agent *use* Other Therapeutic Substance
Idecabtagene Vicleucel *use* Idecabtagene Vicleucel Immunotherapy
Idecabtagene Vicleucel Immunotherapy XW0
Ide-cel *use* Idecabtagene Vicleucel Immunotherapy
iFuse Bedrock™ Granite Implant System *use* Internal Fixation Device with Tulip Connector in New Technology
IGIV-C, for COVID-19 treatment *use* Hyperimmune Globulin
IHD (Intermittent hemodialysis) 5A1D70Z
Ileal artery *use* Superior Mesenteric Artery
Ileectomy
  see Excision, Ileum 0DBB
  see Resection, Ileum 0DTB
Ileocolic artery *use* Superior Mesenteric Artery
Ileocolic vein *use* Colic Vein
Ileopexy
  see Repair, Ileum 0DQB
  see Reposition, Ileum 0DSB
Ileorrhaphy *see* Repair, Ileum 0DQB
Ileoscopy 0DJD8ZZ
Ileostomy
  see Bypass, Ileum 0D1B
  see Drainage, Ileum 0D9B
Ileotomy *see* Drainage, Ileum 0D9B
Ileoureterostomy *see* Bypass, Urinary System 0T1
Iliac crest
  use Pelvic Bone, Left
  use Pelvic Bone, Right
Iliac fascia
  use Subcutaneous Tissue and Fascia, Left Upper Leg
  use Subcutaneous Tissue and Fascia, Right Upper Leg
Iliac lymph node *use* Lymphatic, Pelvis
Iliacus muscle
  use Hip Muscle, Left
  use Hip Muscle, Right
Iliofemoral ligament
  use Hip Bursa and Ligament, Left
  use Hip Bursa and Ligament, Right
Iliohypogastric nerve *use* Lumbar Plexus
Ilioinguinal nerve *use* Lumbar Plexus
Iliolumbar artery
  use Internal Iliac Artery, Left
  use Internal Iliac Artery, Right
Iliolumbar ligament *use* Lower Spine Bursa and Ligament
Iliotibial tract (band)
  use Subcutaneous Tissue and Fascia, Left Upper Leg
  use Subcutaneous Tissue and Fascia, Right Upper Leg
Ilium
  use Pelvic Bone, Left
  use Pelvic Bone, Right
Ilizarov external fixator
  use External Fixation Device, Ring in 0PH

Ilizarov external fixator — *continued*
  use External Fixation Device, Ring in 0PS
  use External Fixation Device, Ring in 0QH
  use External Fixation Device, Ring in 0QS
Ilizarov-Vecklich device
  use External Fixation Device, Limb Lengthening in 0PH
  use External Fixation Device, Limb Lengthening in 0QH
Imaging, diagnostic
  see Computerized Tomography (CT Scan)
  see Fluoroscopy
  see Magnetic Resonance Imaging (MRI)
  see Plain Radiography
  see Ultrasonography
Imdevimab (REGN10987) and Casirivimab (REGN10933) *use* REGN-COV2 Monoclonal Antibody
IMFINZI® *use* Durvalumab Antineoplastic
Imipenem-cilastatin-relebactam Anti-infective XW0
IMI/REL *use* Imipenem-cilastatin-relebactam Anti-infective
Immobilization
  Abdominal Wall 2W33X
  Arm
    Lower
      Left 2W3DX
      Right 2W3CX
    Upper
      Left 2W3BX
      Right 2W3AX
  Back 2W35X
  Chest Wall 2W34X
  Extremity
    Lower
      Left 2W3MX
      Right 2W3LX
    Upper
      Left 2W39X
      Right 2W38X
  Face 2W31X
  Finger
    Left 2W3KX
    Right 2W3JX
  Foot
    Left 2W3TX
    Right 2W3SX
  Hand
    Left 2W3FX
    Right 2W3EX
  Head 2W30X
  Inguinal Region
    Left 2W37X
    Right 2W36X
  Leg
    Lower
      Left 2W3RX
      Right 2W3QX
    Upper
      Left 2W3PX
      Right 2W3NX
  Neck 2W32X
  Thumb
    Left 2W3HX
    Right 2W3GX
  Toe
    Left 2W3VX
    Right 2W3UX
Immunization *see* Introduction of Serum, Toxoid, and Vaccine
Immunoglobulin *use* Globulin
Immunotherapy *see* Introduction of Immunotherapeutic Substance
Immunotherapy, antineoplastic
  Interferon *see* Introduction of Low-dose Interleukin
  Interleukin-2, high-dose *see* Introduction of High-dose Interleukin-2
  Interleukin-2, low-dose *see* Introduction of Low-dose Interleukin-2
  Monoclonal antibody *see* Introduction of Monoclonal Antibody
  Proleukin, high-dose *see* Introduction of High-dose Interleukin-2
  Proleukin, low-dose *see* Introduction of Low-dose Interleukin-2

Impella® 5.5 with SmartAssist® System *use* Conduit to Short-term External Heart Assist System in New Technology

Impella® heart pump *use* Short-term External Heart Assist System in Heart and Great Vessels

Impeller Pump
Continuous, Output 5A0221D
Intermittent, Output 5A0211D

Implantable cardioverter-defibrillator (ICD) *use* Defibrillator Generator in ØJH

Implantable drug infusion pump (anti-spasmodic) (chemotherapy) (pain) *use* Infusion Device, Pump in Subcutaneous Tissue and Fascia

Implantable glucose monitoring device *use* Monitoring Device

Implantable hemodynamic monitor (IHM) *use* Monitoring Device, Hemodynamic in ØJH

Implantable hemodynamic monitoring system (IHMS) *use* Monitoring Device, Hemodynamic in ØJH

Implantable Miniature Telescope™ (IMT) *use* Synthetic Substitute, Intraocular Telescope in Ø8R

Implantation
see Insertion
see Replacement

Implanted (venous)(access) port *use* Vascular Access Device, Totally Implantable in Subcutaneous Tissue and Fascia

IMV (intermittent mandatory ventilation) *see* Assistance, Respiratory 5AØ9

In Vitro Fertilization 8EØZXY1

Incision, abscess *see* Drainage

Incudectomy
see Excision, Ear, Nose, Sinus Ø9B
see Resection, Ear, Nose, Sinus Ø9T

Incudopexy
see Repair, Ear, Nose, Sinus Ø9Q
see Reposition, Ear, Nose, Sinus Ø9S

Incus
use Auditory Ossicle, Left
use Auditory Ossicle, Right

Induction of labor
Artificial rupture of membranes *see* Drainage, Pregnancy 1Ø9
Oxytocin *see* Introduction of Hormone

InDura, intrathecal catheter (1P) (spinal) *use* Infusion Device

Inebilizumab-cdon XWØ

Inferior cardiac nerve *use* Thoracic Sympathetic Nerve

Inferior cerebellar vein *use* Intracranial Vein

Inferior cerebral vein *use* Intracranial Vein

Inferior epigastric artery
use External Iliac Artery, Left
use External Iliac Artery, Right

Inferior epigastric lymph node *use* Lymphatic, Pelvis

Inferior genicular artery
use Popliteal Artery, Left
use Popliteal Artery, Right

Inferior gluteal artery
use Internal Iliac Artery, Left
use Internal Iliac Artery, Right

Inferior gluteal nerve *use* Sacral Plexus

Inferior hypogastric plexus *use* Abdominal Sympathetic Nerve

Inferior labial artery *use* Face Artery

Inferior longitudinal muscle *use* Tongue, Palate, Pharynx Muscle

Inferior mesenteric ganglion *use* Abdominal Sympathetic Nerve

Inferior mesenteric lymph node *use* Lymphatic, Mesenteric

Inferior mesenteric plexus *use* Abdominal Sympathetic Nerve

Inferior oblique muscle
use Extraocular Muscle, Left
use Extraocular Muscle, Right

Inferior pancreaticoduodenal artery *use* Superior Mesenteric Artery

Inferior phrenic artery *use* Abdominal Aorta

Inferior rectus muscle
use Extraocular Muscle, Left
use Extraocular Muscle, Right

Inferior suprarenal artery
use Renal Artery, Left
use Renal Artery, Right

Inferior tarsal plate
use Lower Eyelid, Left

Inferior tarsal plate — *continued*
use Lower Eyelid, Right

Inferior thyroid vein
use Innominate Vein, Left
use Innominate Vein, Right

Inferior tibiofibular joint
use Ankle Joint, Left
use Ankle Joint, Right

Inferior turbinate *use* Nasal Turbinate

Inferior ulnar collateral artery
use Brachial Artery, Left
use Brachial Artery, Right

Inferior vesical artery
use Internal Iliac Artery, Left
use Internal Iliac Artery, Right

Infraauricular lymph node *use* Lymphatic, Head

Infraclavicular (deltopectoral) lymph node
use Lymphatic, Left Upper Extremity
use Lymphatic, Right Upper Extremity

Infrahyoid muscle
use Neck Muscle, Left
use Neck Muscle, Right

Infraparotid lymph node *use* Lymphatic, Head

Infraspinatus fascia
use Subcutaneous Tissue and Fascia, Left Upper Arm
use Subcutaneous Tissue and Fascia, Right Upper Arm

Infraspinatus muscle
use Shoulder Muscle, Left
use Shoulder Muscle, Right

Infundibulopelvic ligament *use* Uterine Supporting Structure

Infusion *see* Introduction of substance in or on

Infusion Device, Pump
Insertion of device in
Abdomen ØJH8
Back ØJH7
Chest ØJH6
Lower Arm
Left ØJHH
Right ØJHG
Lower Leg
Left ØJHP
Right ØJHN
Trunk ØJHT
Upper Arm
Left ØJHF
Right ØJHD
Upper Leg
Left ØJHM
Right ØJHL
Removal of device from
Lower Extremity ØJPW
Trunk ØJPT
Upper Extremity ØJPV
Revision of device in
Lower Extremity ØJWW
Trunk ØJWT
Upper Extremity ØJWV

Infusion, glucarpidase
Central Vein 3E043GQ
Peripheral Vein 3E033GQ

Inguinal canal
use Inguinal Region, Bilateral
use Inguinal Region, Left
use Inguinal Region, Right

Inguinal triangle
use Inguinal Region, Bilateral
use Inguinal Region, Left
use Inguinal Region, Right

Injection *see* Introduction of substance in or on

Injection reservoir, port *use* Vascular Access Device, Totally Implantable in Subcutaneous Tissue and Fascia

Injection reservoir, pump *use* Infusion Device, Pump in Subcutaneous Tissue and Fascia

Insemination, artificial 3EØP7LZ

Insertion
Antimicrobial envelope *see* Introduction of Anti-infective
Aqueous drainage shunt
see Bypass, Eye Ø81
see Drainage, Eye Ø89
Bone, Pelvic, Internal Fixation Device with Tulip Connector XNH

Insertion — *continued*
Conduit to Short-term External Heart Assist System X2H
Intracardiac Pacemaker, Dual-Chamber X2H
Intraluminal Device, Bioprosthetic Valve X2H
Joint
Lumbar Vertebral, Posterior Spinal Motion Preservation Device XRHBØ18
Lumbosacral, Posterior Spinal Motion Preservation Device XRHDØ18
Neurostimulator Lead, Sphenopalatine Ganglion XØHK3Q8
Neurostimulator Lead with Paired Stimulation System XØHQ3R8
Products of Conception 1ØHØ
Spinal Stabilization Device
see Insertion of device in, Lower Joints ØSH
see Insertion of device in, Upper Joints ØRH
Tibial Extension with Motion Sensors XNH

Insertion of device in
Abdominal Wall ØWHF
Acetabulum
Left ØQH5
Right ØQH4
Anal Sphincter ØDHR
Ankle Region
Left ØYHL
Right ØYHK
Anus ØDHQ
Aorta
Abdominal Ø4HØ
Thoracic
Ascending/Arch Ø2HX
Descending Ø2HW
Arm
Lower
Left ØXHF
Right ØXHD
Upper
Left ØXH9
Right ØXH8
Artery
Anterior Tibial
Left Ø4HQ
Right Ø4HP
Axillary
Left Ø3H6
Right Ø3H5
Brachial
Left Ø3H8
Right Ø3H7
Celiac Ø4H1
Colic
Left Ø4H7
Middle Ø4H8
Right Ø4H6
Common Carotid
Left Ø3HJ
Right Ø3HH
Common Iliac
Left Ø4HD
Right Ø4HC
Coronary
Four or More Arteries Ø2H3
One Artery Ø2HØ
Three Arteries Ø2H2
Two Arteries Ø2H1
External Carotid
Left Ø3HN
Right Ø3HM
External Iliac
Left Ø4HJ
Right Ø4HH
Face Ø3HR
Femoral
Left Ø4HL
Right Ø4HK
Foot
Left Ø4HW
Right Ø4HV
Gastric Ø4H2
Hand
Left Ø3HF
Right Ø3HD
Hepatic Ø4H3
Inferior Mesenteric Ø4HB
Innominate Ø3H2
Internal Carotid
Left Ø3HL

Insertion of device in — *continued*
  Artery — *continued*
    Internal Carotid — *continued*
      Right 03HK
    Internal Iliac
      Left 04HF
      Right 04HE
    Internal Mammary
      Left 03H1
      Right 03H0
    Intracranial 03HG
    Lower 04HY
    Peroneal
      Left 04HU
      Right 04HT
    Popliteal
      Left 04HN
      Right 04HM
    Posterior Tibial
      Left 04HS
      Right 04HR
    Pulmonary
      Left 02HR
      Right 02HQ
    Pulmonary Trunk 02HP
    Radial
      Left 03HC
      Right 03HB
    Renal
      Left 04HA
      Right 04H9
    Splenic 04H4
    Subclavian
      Left 03H4
      Right 03H3
    Superior Mesenteric 04H5
    Temporal
      Left 03HT
      Right 03HS
    Thyroid
      Left 03HV
      Right 03HU
    Ulnar
      Left 03HA
      Right 03H9
    Upper 03HY
    Vertebral
      Left 03HQ
      Right 03HP
  Atrium
    Left 02H7
    Right 02H6
  Axilla
    Left 0XH5
    Right 0XH4
  Back
    Lower 0WHL
    Upper 0WHK
  Bladder 0THB
  Bladder Neck 0THC
  Bone
    Ethmoid
      Left 0NHG
      Right 0NHF
    Facial 0NHW
    Frontal 0NH1
    Hyoid 0NHX
    Lacrimal
      Left 0NHJ
      Right 0NHH
    Lower 0QHY
    Nasal 0NHB
    Occipital 0NH7
    Palatine
      Left 0NHL
      Right 0NHK
    Parietal
      Left 0NH4
      Right 0NH3
    Pelvic
      Left 0QH3
      Right 0QH2
    Sphenoid 0NHC
    Temporal
      Left 0NH6
      Right 0NH5
    Upper 0PHY
    Zygomatic
      Left 0NHN

Insertion of device in — *continued*
  Bone — *continued*
    Zygomatic — *continued*
      Right 0NHM
  Bone Marrow 07HT
  Brain 00H0
  Breast
    Bilateral 0HHV
    Left 0HHU
    Right 0HHT
  Bronchus
    Lingula 0BH9
    Lower Lobe
      Left 0BHB
      Right 0BH6
    Main
      Left 0BH7
      Right 0BH3
    Middle Lobe, Right 0BH5
    Upper Lobe
      Left 0BH8
      Right 0BH4
  Bursa and Ligament
    Lower 0MHY
    Upper 0MHX
  Buttock
    Left 0YH1
    Right 0YH0
  Carpal
    Left 0PHN
    Right 0PHM
  Cavity, Cranial 0WH1
  Cerebral Ventricle 00H6
  Cervix 0UHC
  Chest Wall 0WH8
  Cisterna Chyli 07HL
  Clavicle
    Left 0PHB
    Right 0PH9
  Coccyx 0QHS
  Cul-de-sac 0UHF
  Diaphragm 0BHT
  Disc
    Cervical Vertebral 0RH3
    Cervicothoracic Vertebral 0RH5
    Lumbar Vertebral 0SH2
    Lumbosacral 0SH4
    Thoracic Vertebral 0RH9
    Thoracolumbar Vertebral 0RHB
  Duct
    Hepatobiliary 0FHB
    Pancreatic 0FHD
  Duodenum 0DH9
  Ear
    Inner
      Left 09HE
      Right 09HD
    Left 09HJ
    Right 09HH
  Elbow Region
    Left 0XHC
    Right 0XHB
  Epididymis and Spermatic Cord 0VHM
  Esophagus 0DH5
    Lower, Magnetic Lengthening Device 0DH37JZ
    Middle, Magnetic Lengthening Device 0DH27JZ
    Upper, Magnetic Lengthening Device 0DH17JZ
  Extremity
    Lower
      Left 0YHB
      Right 0YH9
    Upper
      Left 0XH7
      Right 0XH6
  Eye
    Left 08H1
    Right 08H0
  Face 0WH2
  Fallopian Tube 0UH8
  Femoral Region
    Left 0YH8
    Right 0YH7
  Femoral Shaft
    Left 0QH9
    Right 0QH8

Insertion of device in — *continued*
  Femur
    Lower
      Left 0QHC
      Right 0QHB
    Upper
      Left 0QH7
      Right 0QH6
  Fibula
    Left 0QHK
    Right 0QHJ
  Foot
    Left 0YHN
    Right 0YHM
  Gallbladder 0FH4
  Gastrointestinal Tract 0WHP
  Genitourinary Tract 0WHR
  Gland
    Endocrine 0GHS
    Salivary 0CHA
  Glenoid Cavity
    Left 0PH8
    Right 0PH7
  Hand
    Left 0XHK
    Right 0XHJ
  Head 0WH0
  Heart 02HA
  Humeral Head
    Left 0PHD
    Right 0PHC
  Humeral Shaft
    Left 0PHG
    Right 0PHF
  Ileum 0DHB
  Inguinal Region
    Left 0YH6
    Right 0YH5
  Intestinal Tract
    Lower Intestinal Tract 0DHD
    Upper Intestinal Tract 0DH0
  Intestine
    Large 0DHE
    Small 0DH8
  Jaw
    Lower 0WH5
    Upper 0WH4
  Jejunum 0DHA
  Joint
    Acromioclavicular
      Left 0RHH
      Right 0RHG
    Ankle
      Left 0SHG
      Right 0SHF
    Carpal
      Left 0RHR
      Right 0RHQ
    Carpometacarpal
      Left 0RHT
      Right 0RHS
    Cervical Vertebral 0RH1
    Cervicothoracic Vertebral 0RH4
    Coccygeal 0SH6
    Elbow
      Left 0RHM
      Right 0RHL
    Finger Phalangeal
      Left 0RHX
      Right 0RHW
    Hip
      Left 0SHB
      Right 0SH9
    Knee
      Left 0SHD
      Right 0SHC
    Lumbar Vertebral 0SH0
    Lumbosacral 0SH3
    Metacarpophalangeal
      Left 0RHV
      Right 0RHU
    Metatarsal-Phalangeal
      Left 0SHN
      Right 0SHM
    Occipital-cervical 0RH0
    Sacrococcygeal 0SH5
    Sacroiliac
      Left 0SH8
      Right 0SH7

Insertion of device in — continued

Joint — continued
Shoulder
　Left ØRHK
　Right ØRHJ
Sternoclavicular
　Left ØRHF
　Right ØRHE
Tarsal
　Left ØSHJ
　Right ØSHH
Tarsometatarsal
　Left ØSHL
　Right ØSHK
Temporomandibular
　Left ØRHD
　Right ØRHC
Thoracic Vertebral ØRH6
Thoracolumbar Vertebral ØRHA
Toe Phalangeal
　Left ØSHQ
　Right ØSHP
Wrist
　Left ØRHP
　Right ØRHN
Kidney ØTH5
Knee Region
　Left ØYHG
　Right ØYHF
Larynx ØCHS
Leg
　Lower
　　Left ØYHJ
　　Right ØYHH
　Upper
　　Left ØYHD
　　Right ØYHC
Liver ØFHØ
　Left Lobe ØFH2
　Right Lobe ØFH1
Lung
　Left ØBHL
　Right ØBHK
Lymphatic Ø7HN
　Thoracic Duct Ø7HK
Mandible
　Left ØNHV
　Right ØNHT
Maxilla ØNHR
Mediastinum ØWHC
Metacarpal
　Left ØPHQ
　Right ØPHP
Metatarsal
　Left ØQHP
　Right ØQHN
Mouth and Throat ØCHY
Muscle
　Lower ØKHY
　Upper ØKHX
Nasal Mucosa and Soft Tissue Ø9HK
Nasopharynx Ø9HN
Neck ØWH6
Nerve
　Cranial ØØHE
　Peripheral Ø1HY
Nipple
　Left ØHHX
　Right ØHHW
Oral Cavity and Throat ØWH3
Orbit
　Left ØNHQ
　Right ØNHP
Ovary ØUH3
Pancreas ØFHG
Patella
　Left ØQHF
　Right ØQHD
Pelvic Cavity ØWHJ
Penis ØVHS
Pericardial Cavity ØWHD
Pericardium Ø2HN
Perineum
　Female ØWHN
　Male ØWHM
Peritoneal Cavity ØWHG
Phalanx
　Finger
　　Left ØPHV

Insertion of device in — continued

Phalanx — continued
Finger — continued
　　Right ØPHT
　Thumb
　　Left ØPHS
　　Right ØPHR
　Toe
　　Left ØQHR
　　Right ØQHQ
Pleura ØBHQ
Pleural Cavity
　Left ØWHB
　Right ØWH9
Prostate ØVHØ
Prostate and Seminal Vesicles ØVH4
Radius
　Left ØPHJ
　Right ØPHH
Rectum ØDHP
Respiratory Tract ØWHQ
Retroperitoneum ØWHH
Ribs
　1 to 2 ØPH1
　3 or More ØPH2
Sacrum ØQH1
Scapula
　Left ØPH6
　Right ØPH5
Scrotum and Tunica Vaginalis ØVH8
Shoulder Region
　Left ØXH3
　Right ØXH2
Sinus Ø9HY
Skin ØHHPXYZ
Skull ØNHØ
Spinal Canal ØØHU
Spinal Cord ØØHV
Spleen Ø7HP
Sternum ØPHØ
Stomach ØDH6
Subcutaneous Tissue and Fascia
　Abdomen ØJH8
　Back ØJH7
　Buttock ØJH9
　Chest ØJH6
　Face ØJH1
　Foot
　　Left ØJHR
　　Right ØJHQ
　Hand
　　Left ØJHK
　　Right ØJHJ
　Head and Neck ØJHS
　Lower Arm
　　Left ØJHH
　　Right ØJHG
　Lower Extremity ØJHW
　Lower Leg
　　Left ØJHP
　　Right ØJHN
　Neck
　　Left ØJH5
　　Right ØJH4
　Pelvic Region ØJHC
　Perineum ØJHB
　Scalp ØJHØ
　Trunk ØJHT
　Upper Arm
　　Left ØJHF
　　Right ØJHD
　Upper Extremity ØJHV
　Upper Leg
　　Left ØJHM
　　Right ØJHL
Tarsal
　Left ØQHM
　Right ØQHL
Tendon
　Lower ØLHY
　Upper ØLHX
Testis ØVHD
Thymus Ø7HM
Tibia
　Left ØQHH
　Right ØQHG
Tongue ØCH7
Trachea ØBH1
Tracheobronchial Tree ØBHØ

Insertion of device in — continued

Ulna
Left ØPHL
Right ØPHK
Ureter ØTH9
Urethra ØTHD
Uterus ØUH9
Uterus and Cervix ØUHD
Vagina ØUHG
Vagina and Cul-de-sac ØUHH
Vas Deferens ØVHR
Vein
　Axillary
　　Left Ø5H8
　　Right Ø5H7
　Azygos Ø5HØ
　Basilic
　　Left Ø5HC
　　Right Ø5HB
　Brachial
　　Left Ø5HA
　　Right Ø5H9
　Cephalic
　　Left Ø5HF
　　Right Ø5HD
　Colic Ø6H7
　Common Iliac
　　Left Ø6HD
　　Right Ø6HC
　Coronary Ø2H4
　Esophageal Ø6H3
　External Iliac
　　Left Ø6HG
　　Right Ø6HF
　External Jugular
　　Left Ø5HQ
　　Right Ø5HP
　Face
　　Left Ø5HV
　　Right Ø5HT
　Femoral
　　Left Ø6HN
　　Right Ø6HM
　Foot
　　Left Ø6HV
　　Right Ø6HT
　Gastric Ø6H2
　Hand
　　Left Ø5HH
　　Right Ø5HG
　Hemiazygos Ø5H1
　Hepatic Ø6H4
　Hypogastric
　　Left Ø6HJ
　　Right Ø6HH
　Inferior Mesenteric Ø6H6
　Innominate
　　Left Ø5H4
　　Right Ø5H3
　Internal Jugular
　　Left Ø5HN
　　Right Ø5HM
　Intracranial Ø5HL
　Lower Ø6HY
　Portal Ø6H8
　Pulmonary
　　Left Ø2HT
　　Right Ø2HS
　Renal
　　Left Ø6HB
　　Right Ø6H9
　Saphenous
　　Left Ø6HQ
　　Right Ø6HP
　Splenic Ø6H1
　Subclavian
　　Left Ø5H6
　　Right Ø5H5
　Superior Mesenteric Ø6H5
　Upper Ø5HY
　Vertebral
　　Left Ø5HS
　　Right Ø5HR
Vena Cava
　Inferior Ø6HØ
　Superior Ø2HV
Ventricle
　Left Ø2HL
　Right Ø2HK

Subterms under main terms may continue to next column or page

Index

Insertion of device in — Inspection

Inspection — *continued*
  Tympanic Membrane
    Left Ø9J8
    Right Ø9J7
  Ureter ØTJ9
  Urethra ØTJD
  Uterus and Cervix ØUJD
  Vagina and Cul-de-sac ØUJH
  Vas Deferens ØVJR
  Vein
    Lower Ø6JY
    Upper Ø5JY
  Vulva ØUJM
  Wrist Region
    Left ØXJH
    Right ØXJG
Instillation *see* Introduction of substance in or on
Insufflation *see* Introduction of substance in or on
Intellis™ neurostimulator *use* Stimulator Generator, Multiple Array Rechargeable in ØJH
Interatrial septum *use* Atrial Septum
InterAtrial Shunt Device IASD®, Corvia *use* Synthetic Substitute
Interbody fusion (spine) cage
  use Interbody Fusion Device in Lower Joints
  use Interbody Fusion Device in Upper Joints
Interbody Fusion Device, Custom-Made Anatomically Designed
  Lumbar Vertebral XRGB
    2 or more XRGC
  Lumbosacral XRGD
  Thoracolumbar Vertebral XRGA
Intercarpal joint
  use Carpal Joint, Left
  use Carpal Joint, Right
Intercarpal ligament
  use Hand Bursa and Ligament, Left
  use Hand Bursa and Ligament, Right
INTERCEPT Blood System for Plasma Pathogen Reduced Cryoprecipitated Fibrinogen Complex *use* Pathogen Reduced Cryoprecipitated Fibrinogen Complex
INTERCEPT Fibrinogen Complex *use* Pathogen Reduced Cryoprecipitated Fibrinogen Complex
Interclavicular ligament
  use Shoulder Bursa and Ligament, Left
  use Shoulder Bursa and Ligament, Right
Intercostal lymph node *use* Lymphatic, Thorax
Intercostal muscle
  use Thorax Muscle, Left
  use Thorax Muscle, Right
Intercostal nerve *use* Thoracic Nerve
Intercostobrachial nerve *use* Thoracic Nerve
Intercuneiform joint
  use Tarsal Joint, Left
  use Tarsal Joint, Right
Intercuneiform ligament
  use Foot Bursa and Ligament, Left
  use Foot Bursa and Ligament, Right
Intermediate bronchus *use* Main Bronchus, Right
Intermediate cuneiform bone
  use Tarsal, Left
  use Tarsal, Right
Intermittent Coronary Sinus Occlusion X2A7358
Intermittent hemodialysis (IHD) 5A1D70Z
Intermittent mandatory ventilation *see* Assistance, Respiratory 5AØ9
Intermittent Negative Airway Pressure
  24-96 Consecutive Hours, Ventilation 5AØ945B
  Greater than 96 Consecutive Hours, Ventilation 5AØ955B
  Less than 24 Consecutive Hours, Ventilation 5AØ935B
Intermittent Positive Airway Pressure
  24-96 Consecutive Hours, Ventilation 5AØ9458
  Greater than 96 Consecutive Hours, Ventilation 5AØ9558
  Less than 24 Consecutive Hours, Ventilation 5AØ9358
Intermittent positive pressure breathing *see* Assistance, Respiratory 5AØ9
Internal anal sphincter *use* Anal Sphincter
Internal carotid artery, intracranial portion *use* Intracranial Artery
Internal carotid plexus *use* Head and Neck Sympathetic Nerve
Internal (basal) cerebral vein *use* Intracranial Vein

Internal Fixation Device with Tulip Connector
  Fusion, Joint, Sacroiliac XRG
  Insertion, Bone, Pelvic XNH
Internal iliac vein
  use Hypogastric Vein, Left
  use Hypogastric Vein, Right
Internal maxillary artery
  use External Carotid Artery, Left
  use External Carotid Artery, Right
Internal naris *use* Nasal Mucosa and Soft Tissue
Internal oblique muscle
  use Abdomen Muscle, Left
  use Abdomen Muscle, Right
Internal pudendal artery
  use Internal Iliac Artery, Left
  use Internal Iliac Artery, Right
Internal pudendal vein
  use Hypogastric Vein, Left
  use Hypogastric Vein, Right
Internal thoracic artery
  use Internal Mammary Artery, Left
  use Internal Mammary Artery, Right
  use Subclavian Artery, Left
  use Subclavian Artery, Right
Internal urethral sphincter *use* Urethra
Interphalangeal (IP) joint
  use Finger Phalangeal Joint, Left
  use Finger Phalangeal Joint, Right
  use Toe Phalangeal Joint, Left
  use Toe Phalangeal Joint, Right
Interphalangeal ligament
  use Foot Bursa and Ligament, Left
  use Foot Bursa and Ligament, Right
  use Hand Bursa and Ligament, Left
  use Hand Bursa and Ligament, Right
Interrogation, cardiac rhythm related device
  Interrogation only *see* Measurement, Cardiac 4BØ2
  With cardiac function testing *see* Measurement, Cardiac 4AØ2
Interruption *see* Occlusion
Interspinalis muscle
  use Trunk Muscle, Left
  use Trunk Muscle, Right
Interspinous ligament, cervical *use* Head and Neck Bursa and Ligament
Interspinous ligament, lumbar *use* Lower Spine Bursa and Ligament
Interspinous ligament, thoracic *use* Upper Spine Bursa and Ligament
Interspinous process spinal stabilization device
  use Spinal Stabilization Device, Interspinous Process in ØRH
  use Spinal Stabilization Device, Interspinous Process in ØSH
InterStim® Therapy lead *use* Neurostimulator Lead in Peripheral Nervous System
InterStim™ II Therapy neurostimulator *use* Stimulator Generator, Single Array in ØJH
InterStim™ Micro Therapy neurostimulator *use* Stimulator Generator, Single Array Rechargeable in ØJH
Intertransversarius muscle
  use Trunk Muscle, Left
  use Trunk Muscle, Right
Intertransverse ligament, cervical *use* Head and Neck Bursa and Ligament
Intertransverse ligament, lumbar *use* Lower Spine Bursa and Ligament
Intertransverse ligament, thoracic *use* Upper Spine Bursa and Ligament
Interventricular foramen (Monro) *use* Cerebral Ventricle
Interventricular septum *use* Ventricular Septum
Intestinal lymphatic trunk *use* Cisterna Chyli
Intracardiac Pacemaker, Dual-Chamber, Insertion X2H
Intracranial Arterial Flow, Whole Blood mRNA XXE5XT7
Intraluminal Device
  Airway
    Esophagus ØDH5
    Mouth and Throat ØCHY
    Nasopharynx Ø9HN
  Bioactive
    Occlusion
      Common Carotid
        Left Ø3LJ

Intraluminal Device — *continued*
  Bioactive — *continued*
    Occlusion — *continued*
      Common Carotid — *continued*
        Right Ø3LH
      External Carotid
        Left Ø3LN
        Right Ø3LM
      Internal Carotid
        Left Ø3LL
        Right Ø3LK
      Intracranial Ø3LG
      Vertebral
        Left Ø3LQ
        Right Ø3LP
    Restriction
      Common Carotid
        Left Ø3VJ
        Right Ø3VH
      External Carotid
        Left Ø3VN
        Right Ø3VM
      Internal Carotid
        Left Ø3VL
        Right Ø3VK
      Intracranial Ø3VG
      Vertebral
        Left Ø3VQ
        Right Ø3VP
  Bioprosthetic Valve, Insertion X2H
  Endobronchial Valve
    Lingula ØBH9
    Lower Lobe
      Left ØBHB
      Right ØBH6
    Main
      Left ØBH7
      Right ØBH3
    Middle Lobe, Right ØBH5
    Upper Lobe
      Left ØBH8
      Right ØBH4
  Endotracheal Airway
    Change device in, Trachea ØB21XEZ
    Insertion of device in, Trachea ØBH1
  Pessary
    Change device in, Vagina and Cul-de-sac ØU2HXGZ
    Insertion of device in
      Cul-de-sac ØUHF
      Vagina ØUHG
Intramedullary (IM) rod (nail)
  use Internal Fixation Device, Intramedullary in Lower Bones
  use Internal Fixation Device, Intramedullary in Upper Bones
Intramedullary skeletal kinetic distractor (ISKD)
  use Internal Fixation Device, Intramedullary in Lower Bones
  use Internal Fixation Device, Intramedullary in Upper Bones
Intraocular Telescope
  Left Ø8RK3ØZ
  Right Ø8RJ3ØZ
Intraoperative Radiation Therapy (IORT)
  Anus DDY8CZZ
  Bile Ducts DFY2CZZ
  Bladder DTY2CZZ
  Brain DØYØCZZ
  Brain Stem DØY1CZZ
  Cervix DUY1CZZ
  Colon DDY5CZZ
  Duodenum DDY2CZZ
  Gallbladder DFY1CZZ
  Ileum DDY4CZZ
  Jejunum DDY3CZZ
  Kidney DTYØCZZ
  Larynx D9YBCZZ
  Liver DFYØCZZ
  Mouth D9Y4CZZ
  Nasopharynx D9YDCZZ
  Nerve, Peripheral DØY7CZZ
  Ovary DUYØCZZ
  Pancreas DFY3CZZ
  Pharynx D9YCCZZ
  Prostate DVYØCZZ
  Rectum DDY7CZZ
  Spinal Cord DØY6CZZ

Introduction of substance in or on — *continued*	Introduction of substance in or on — *continued*	Introduction of substance in or on — *continued*

Mouth — *continued*
- Electrolytic Substance 3E0D
- Hypnotics 3E0D
- Nutritional Substance 3E0D
- Radioactive Substance 3E0D
- Sedatives 3E0D
- Serum 3E0D
- Toxoid 3E0D
- Vaccine 3E0D
- Water Balance Substance 3E0D

Mucous Membrane 3E00XGC
- Analgesics 3E00XNZ
- Anesthetic Agent 3E00XBZ
- Anti-infective 3E00X2
- Anti-inflammatory 3E00X3Z
- Antineoplastic 3E00X0
- Destructive Agent 3E00XTZ
- Diagnostic Substance, Other 3E00XKZ
- Hypnotics 3E00XNZ
- Pigment 3E00XMZ
- Sedatives 3E00XNZ
- Serum 3E00X4Z
- Toxoid 3E00X4Z
- Vaccine 3E00X4Z

Muscle 3E023GC
- Analgesics 3E023NZ
- Anesthetic Agent 3E023BZ
- Anti-infective 3E0232
- Anti-inflammatory 3E0233Z
- Antineoplastic 3E0230
- Destructive Agent 3E023TZ
- Diagnostic Substance, Other 3E023KZ
- Electrolytic Substance 3E0237Z
- Hypnotics 3E023NZ
- Nutritional Substance 3E0236Z
- Radioactive Substance 3E023HZ
- Sedatives 3E023NZ
- Serum 3E0234Z
- Toxoid 3E0234Z
- Vaccine 3E0234Z
- Water Balance Substance 3E0237Z

Nerve
- Cranial 3E0X3GC
  - Anesthetic Agent 3E0X3BZ
  - Anti-inflammatory 3E0X33Z
  - Destructive Agent 3E0X3TZ
- Peripheral 3E0T3GC
  - Anesthetic Agent 3E0T3BZ
  - Anti-inflammatory 3E0T33Z
  - Destructive Agent 3E0T3TZ
- Plexus 3E0T3GC
  - Anesthetic Agent 3E0T3BZ
  - Anti-inflammatory 3E0T33Z
  - Destructive Agent 3E0T3TZ

Nose 3E09
- Analgesics 3E09
- Anesthetic Agent 3E09
- Anti-infective 3E09
- Anti-inflammatory 3E09
- Antineoplastic 3E09
- Destructive Agent 3E09
- Diagnostic Substance, Other 3E09
- Hypnotics 3E09
- Radioactive Substance 3E09
- Sedatives 3E09
- Serum 3E09
- Toxoid 3E09
- Vaccine 3E09

Pancreatic Tract 3E0J
- Analgesics 3E0J
- Anesthetic Agent 3E0J
- Anti-infective 3E0J
- Anti-inflammatory 3E0J
- Antineoplastic 3E0J
- Destructive Agent 3E0J
- Diagnostic Substance, Other 3E0J
- Electrolytic Substance 3E0J
- Gas 3E0J
- Hypnotics 3E0J
- Islet Cells, Pancreatic 3E0J
- Nutritional Substance 3E0J
- Radioactive Substance 3E0J
- Sedatives 3E0J
- Water Balance Substance 3E0J

Pericardial Cavity 3E0Y
- Analgesics 3E0Y3NZ
- Anesthetic Agent 3E0Y3BZ
- Anti-infective 3E0Y32

Pericardial Cavity — *continued*
- Anti-inflammatory 3E0Y33Z
- Antineoplastic 3E0Y
- Destructive Agent 3E0Y3TZ
- Diagnostic Substance, Other 3E0Y3KZ
- Electrolytic Substance 3E0Y37Z
- Gas 3E0Y
- Hypnotics 3E0Y3NZ
- Nutritional Substance 3E0Y36Z
- Radioactive Substance 3E0Y3HZ
- Sedatives 3E0Y3NZ
- Water Balance Substance 3E0Y37Z

Peritoneal Cavity 3E0M
- Adhesion Barrier 3E0M
- Analgesics 3E0M3NZ
- Anesthetic Agent 3E0M3BZ
- Anti-infective 3E0M32
- Anti-inflammatory 3E0M33Z
- Antineoplastic 3E0M
- Destructive Agent 3E0M3TZ
- Diagnostic Substance, Other 3E0M3KZ
- Electrolytic Substance 3E0M37Z
- Gas 3E0M
- Hypnotics 3E0M3NZ
- Nutritional Substance 3E0M36Z
- Radioactive Substance 3E0M3HZ
- Sedatives 3E0M3NZ
- Water Balance Substance 3E0M37Z

Pharynx 3E0D
- Analgesics 3E0D
- Anesthetic Agent 3E0D
- Antiarrhythmic 3E0D
- Anti-infective 3E0D
- Anti-inflammatory 3E0D
- Antineoplastic 3E0D
- Destructive Agent 3E0D
- Diagnostic Substance, Other 3E0D
- Electrolytic Substance 3E0D
- Hypnotics 3E0D
- Nutritional Substance 3E0D
- Radioactive Substance 3E0D
- Sedatives 3E0D
- Serum 3E0D
- Toxoid 3E0D
- Vaccine 3E0D
- Water Balance Substance 3E0D

Pleural Cavity 3E0L
- Adhesion Barrier 3E0L
- Analgesics 3E0L3NZ
- Anesthetic Agent 3E0L3BZ
- Anti-infective 3E0L32
- Anti-inflammatory 3E0L33Z
- Antineoplastic 3E0L
- Destructive Agent 3E0L3TZ
- Diagnostic Substance, Other 3E0L3KZ
- Electrolytic Substance 3E0L37Z
- Gas 3E0L
- Hypnotics 3E0L3NZ
- Nutritional Substance 3E0L36Z
- Radioactive Substance 3E0L3HZ
- Sedatives 3E0L3NZ
- Water Balance Substance 3E0L37Z

Products of Conception 3E0E
- Analgesics 3E0E
- Anesthetic Agent 3E0E
- Anti-infective 3E0E
- Anti-inflammatory 3E0E
- Antineoplastic 3E0E
- Destructive Agent 3E0E
- Diagnostic Substance, Other 3E0E
- Electrolytic Substance 3E0E
- Gas 3E0E
- Hypnotics 3E0E
- Nutritional Substance 3E0E
- Radioactive Substance 3E0E
- Sedatives 3E0E
- Water Balance Substance 3E0E

Reproductive
- Female 3E0P
  - Adhesion Barrier 3E0P
  - Analgesics 3E0P
  - Anesthetic Agent 3E0P
  - Anti-infective 3E0P
  - Anti-inflammatory 3E0P
  - Antineoplastic 3E0P
  - Destructive Agent 3E0P
  - Diagnostic Substance, Other 3E0P
  - Electrolytic Substance 3E0P

Reproductive — *continued*
- Female — *continued*
  - Gas 3E0P
  - Hormone 3E0P
  - Hypnotics 3E0P
  - Nutritional Substance 3E0P
  - Ovum, Fertilized 3E0P
  - Radioactive Substance 3E0P
  - Sedatives 3E0P
  - Sperm 3E0P
  - Water Balance Substance 3E0P
- Male 3E0N
  - Analgesics 3E0N
  - Anesthetic Agent 3E0N
  - Anti-infective 3E0N
  - Anti-inflammatory 3E0N
  - Antineoplastic 3E0N
  - Destructive Agent 3E0N
  - Diagnostic Substance, Other 3E0N
  - Electrolytic Substance 3E0N
  - Gas 3E0N
  - Hypnotics 3E0N
  - Nutritional Substance 3E0N
  - Radioactive Substance 3E0N
  - Sedatives 3E0N
  - Water Balance Substance 3E0N

Respiratory Tract 3E0F
- Analgesics 3E0F
- Anesthetic Agent 3E0F
- Anti-infective 3E0F
- Anti-inflammatory 3E0F
- Antineoplastic 3E0F
- Destructive Agent 3E0F
- Diagnostic Substance, Other 3E0F
- Electrolytic Substance 3E0F
- Gas 3E0F
- Hypnotics 3E0F
- Nutritional Substance 3E0F
- Radioactive Substance 3E0F
- Sedatives 3E0F
- Water Balance Substance 3E0F

Skin 3E00XGC
- Analgesics 3E00XNZ
- Anesthetic Agent 3E00XBZ
- Anti-infective 3E00X2
- Anti-inflammatory 3E00X3Z
- Antineoplastic 3E00X0
- Destructive Agent 3E00XTZ
- Diagnostic Substance, Other 3E00XKZ
- Hypnotics 3E00XNZ
- Pigment 3E00XMZ
- Sedatives 3E00XNZ
- Serum 3E00X4Z
- Toxoid 3E00X4Z
- Vaccine 3E00X4Z

Spinal Canal 3E0R3GC
- Analgesics 3E0R3NZ
- Anesthetic Agent 3E0R3BZ
- Anti-infective 3E0R32
- Anti-inflammatory 3E0R33Z
- Antineoplastic 3E0R30
- Destructive Agent 3E0R3TZ
- Diagnostic Substance, Other 3E0R3KZ
- Electrolytic Substance 3E0R37Z
- Gas 3E0R
- Hypnotics 3E0R3NZ
- Nutritional Substance 3E0R36Z
- Radioactive Substance 3E0R3HZ
- Sedatives 3E0R3NZ
- Stem Cells
  - Embryonic 3E0R
  - Somatic 3E0R
- Water Balance Substance 3E0R37Z

Subcutaneous Tissue 3E013GC
- Analgesics 3E013NZ
- Anesthetic Agent 3E013BZ
- Anti-infective 3E01
- Anti-inflammatory 3E0133Z
- Antineoplastic 3E0130
- Destructive Agent 3E013TZ
- Diagnostic Substance, Other 3E013KZ
- Electrolytic Substance 3E0137Z
- Hormone 3E013V
- Hypnotics 3E013NZ
- Nutritional Substance 3E0136Z
- Radioactive Substance 3E013HZ
- Sedatives 3E013NZ
- Serum 3E0134Z

Introduction of substance in or on — *continued*
　Subcutaneous Tissue — *continued*
　　Toxoid 3E0134Z
　　Vaccine 3E0134Z
　　Water Balance Substance 3E0137Z
　Vein
　　Central 3E04
　　　Analgesics 3E04
　　　Anesthetic, Intracirculatory 3E04
　　　Antiarrhythmic 3E04
　　　Anti-infective 3E04
　　　Anti-inflammatory 3E04
　　　Antineoplastic 3E04
　　　Destructive Agent 3E04
　　　Diagnostic Substance, Other 3E04
　　　Electrolytic Substance 3E04
　　　Hormone 3E04
　　　Hypnotics 3E04
　　　Immunotherapeutic 3E04
　　　Nutritional Substance 3E04
　　　Platelet Inhibitor 3E04
　　　Radioactive Substance 3E04
　　　Sedatives 3E04
　　　Serum 3E04
　　　Thrombolytic 3E04
　　　Toxoid 3E04
　　　Vaccine 3E04
　　　Vasopressor 3E04
　　　Water Balance Substance 3E04
　　Peripheral 3E03
　　　Analgesics 3E03
　　　Anesthetic, Intracirculatory 3E03
　　　Antiarrhythmic 3E03
　　　Anti-infective 3E03
　　　Anti-inflammatory 3E03
　　　Antineoplastic 3E03
　　　Destructive Agent 3E03
　　　Diagnostic Substance, Other 3E03
　　　Electrolytic Substance 3E03
　　　Hormone 3E03
　　　Hypnotics 3E03
　　　Immunotherapeutic 3E03
　　　Islet Cells, Pancreatic 3E03
　　　Nutritional Substance 3E03
　　　Platelet Inhibitor 3E03
　　　Radioactive Substance 3E03
　　　Sedatives 3E03
　　　Serum 3E03
　　　Thrombolytic 3E03
　　　Toxoid 3E03
　　　Vaccine 3E03
　　　Vasopressor 3E03
　　　Water Balance Substance 3E03
Intubated prone positioning *see* Assistance, Respiratory 5A09
Intubation
　Airway
　　see Insertion of device in, Esophagus 0DH5
　　see Insertion of device in, Mouth and Throat 0CHY
　　see Insertion of device in, Trachea 0BH1
　Drainage device *see* Drainage
　Feeding Device *see* Insertion of device in, Gastrointestinal System 0DH
INTUITY Elite valve system, EDWARDS (rapid deployment technique) *see* Replacement, Valve, Aortic 02RF
Iobenguane I-131 Antineoplastic XW0
Iobenguane I-131, High Specific Activity (HSA) *use* Iobenguane I-131 Antineoplastic
IPPB (intermittent positive pressure breathing) *see* Assistance, Respiratory 5A09
IRE (Irreversible Electroporation) *see* Destruction, Hepatobiliary System and Pancreas 0F5
Iridectomy
　see Excision, Eye 08B
　see Resection, Eye 08T
Iridoplasty
　see Repair, Eye 08Q
　see Replacement, Eye 08R
　see Supplement, Eye 08U
Iridotomy *see* Drainage, Eye 089
Irreversible Electroporation (IRE) *see* Destruction, Hepatobiliary System and Pancreas 0F5
Irrigation
　Biliary Tract, Irrigating Substance 3E1J
　Brain, Irrigating Substance 3E1Q38Z
　Cranial Cavity, Irrigating Substance 3E1Q38Z

Irrigation — *continued*
　Ear, Irrigating Substance 3E1B
　Epidural Space, Irrigating Substance 3E1S38Z
　Eye, Irrigating Substance 3E1C
　Gastrointestinal Tract
　　Lower, Irrigating Substance 3E1H
　　Upper, Irrigating Substance 3E1G
　Genitourinary Tract, Irrigating Substance 3E1K
　Irrigating Substance 3C1ZX8Z
　Joint, Irrigating Substance 3E1U
　Mucous Membrane, Irrigating Substance 3E10
　Nose, Irrigating Substance 3E19
　Pancreatic Tract, Irrigating Substance 3E1J
　Pericardial Cavity, Irrigating Substance 3E1Y38Z
　Peritoneal Cavity
　　Dialysate 3E1M39Z
　　Irrigating Substance 3E1M
　Pleural Cavity, Irrigating Substance 3E1L38Z
　Reproductive
　　Female, Irrigating Substance 3E1P
　　Male, Irrigating Substance 3E1N
　Respiratory Tract, Irrigating Substance 3E1F
　Skin, Irrigating Substance 3E10
　Spinal Canal, Irrigating Substance 3E1R38Z
Isavuconazole (isavuconazonium sulfate) *use* Other Anti-infective
Ischemic Stroke System (ISS500) *use* Neurostimulator Lead in New Technology
Ischiatic nerve *use* Sciatic Nerve
Ischiocavernosus muscle *use* Perineum Muscle
Ischiofemoral ligament
　use Hip Bursa and Ligament, Left
　use Hip Bursa and Ligament, Right
Ischium
　use Pelvic Bone, Left
　use Pelvic Bone, Right
ISC-REST kit
　ISCDx XXE5XT7
　QIAGEN Access Anti-SARS-CoV-2 Total Test XXE5XV7
　QIAstat-Dx Respiratory SARS-CoV-2 Panel XXE97U7
Isolation 8E0ZXY6
Isotope Administration, Other Radiation, Whole Body DWY5G
ISS500 (Ischemic Stroke System) *use* Neurostimulator Lead in New Technology
Itrel (3) (4) neurostimulator *use* Stimulator Generator, Single Array in 0JH

J

Jakafi® *use* Ruxolitinib
Jejunal artery *use* Superior Mesenteric Artery
Jejunectomy
　see Excision, Jejunum 0DBA
　see Resection, Jejunum 0DTA
Jejunocolostomy
　see Bypass, Gastrointestinal System 0D1
　see Drainage, Gastrointestinal System 0D9
Jejunopexy
　see Repair, Jejunum 0DQA
　see Reposition, Jejunum 0DSA
Jejunostomy
　see Bypass, Jejunum 0D1A
　see Drainage, Jejunum 0D9A
Jejunotomy *see* Drainage, Jejunum 0D9A
Joint fixation plate
　use Internal Fixation Device in Lower Joints
　use Internal Fixation Device in Upper Joints
Joint liner (insert) *use* Liner in Lower Joints
Joint spacer (antibiotic)
　use Spacer in Lower Joints
　use Spacer in Upper Joints
Jugular body *use* Glomus Jugulare
Jugular lymph node
　use Lymphatic, Left Neck
　use Lymphatic, Right Neck

K

Kappa *use* Pacemaker, Dual Chamber in 0JH
Kcentra *use* 4-Factor Prothrombin Complex Concentrate
Keratectomy, kerectomy
　see Excision, Eye 08B
　see Resection, Eye 08T

Keratocentesis *see* Drainage, Eye 089
Keratoplasty
　see Repair, Eye 08Q
　see Replacement, Eye 08R
　see Supplement, Eye 08U
Keratotomy
　see Drainage, Eye 089
　see Repair, Eye 08Q
KEVZARA® *use* Sarilumab
Keystone Heart TriGuard 3™ CEPD (cerebral embolic protection device) X2A6325
Kirschner wire (K-wire)
　use Internal Fixation Device in Head and Facial Bones
　use Internal Fixation Device in Lower Bones
　use Internal Fixation Device in Lower Joints
　use Internal Fixation Device in Upper Bones
　use Internal Fixation Device in Upper Joints
Knee (implant) insert *use* Liner in Lower Joints
KUB x-ray *see* Plain Radiography, Kidney, Ureter and Bladder BT04
Kuntscher nail
　use Internal Fixation Device, Intramedullary in Lower Bones
　use Internal Fixation Device, Intramedullary in Upper Bones
KYMRIAH® *use* Tisagenlecleucel Immunotherapy

L

Labia majora *use* Vulva
Labia minora *use* Vulva
Labial gland
　use Lower Lip
　use Upper Lip
Labiectomy
　see Excision, Female Reproductive System 0UB
　see Resection, Female Reproductive System 0UT
Lacrimal canaliculus
　use Lacrimal Duct, Left
　use Lacrimal Duct, Right
Lacrimal punctum
　use Lacrimal Duct, Left
　use Lacrimal Duct, Right
Lacrimal sac
　use Lacrimal Duct, Left
　use Lacrimal Duct, Right
LAGB (laparoscopic adjustable gastric banding)
　Initial procedure 0DV64CZ
　Surgical correction *see* Revision of device in, Stomach 0DW6
Laminectomy
　see Excision, Lower Bones 0QB
　see Excision, Upper Bones 0PB
　see Release, Central Nervous System and Cranial Nerves 00N
　see Release, Peripheral Nervous System 01N
Laminotomy
　see Drainage, Lower Bones 0Q9
　see Drainage, Upper Bones 0P9
　see Excision, Lower Bones 0QB
　see Excision, Upper Bones 0PB
　see Release, Central Nervous System and Cranial Nerves 00N
　see Release, Lower Bones 0QN
　see Release, Peripheral Nervous System 01N
　see Release, Upper Bones 0PN
Laparoscopic-assisted transanal pull-through
　see Excision, Gastrointestinal System 0DB
　see Resection, Gastrointestinal System 0DT
Laparoscopy *see* Inspection
Laparotomy
　Drainage *see* Drainage, Peritoneal Cavity 0W9G
　Exploratory *see* Inspection, Peritoneal Cavity 0WJG
LAP-BAND® adjustable gastric banding system *use* Extraluminal Device
Laryngectomy
　see Excision, Larynx 0CBS
　see Resection, Larynx 0CTS
Laryngocentesis *see* Drainage, Larynx 0C9S
Laryngogram *see* Fluoroscopy, Larynx B91J
Laryngopexy *see* Repair, Larynx 0CQS
Laryngopharynx *use* Pharynx
Laryngoplasty
　see Repair, Larynx 0CQS
　see Replacement, Larynx 0CRS

Laryngoplasty — *continued*
　see Supplement, Larynx ØCUS
Laryngorrhaphy *see* Repair, Larynx ØCQS
Laryngoscopy ØCJS8ZZ
Laryngotomy *see* Drainage, Larynx ØC9S
Laser Interstitial Thermal Therapy
　Ampulla of Vater ØF5C
　Anus ØD5Q
　Aortic Body ØG5D
　Appendix ØD5J
　Brain ØØ5Ø
　Breast
　　Bilateral ØH5V
　　Left ØH5U
　　Right ØH5T
　Carotid Bodies, Bilateral ØG58
　Carotid Body
　　Left ØG56
　　Right ØG57
　Cecum ØD5H
　Coccygeal Glomus ØG5B
　Colon
　　Ascending ØD5K
　　Descending ØD5M
　　Sigmoid ØD5N
　　Transverse ØD5L
　Duct
　　Common Bile ØF59
　　Cystic ØF58
　　Hepatic
　　　Common ØF57
　　　Left ØF56
　　　Right ØF55
　　Pancreatic ØF5D
　　　Accessory ØF5F
　Duodenum ØD59
　Esophagogastric Junction ØD54
　Esophagus ØD55
　　Lower ØD53
　　Middle ØD52
　　Upper ØD51
　Gallbladder ØF54
　Gland
　　Adrenal
　　　Bilateral ØG54
　　　Left ØG52
　　　Right ØG53
　　Pituitary ØG5Ø
　Glomus Jugulare ØG5C
　Ileocecal Valve ØD5C
　Ileum ØD5B
　Intestine
　　Large ØD5E
　　　Left ØD5G
　　　Right ØD5F
　　Small ØD58
　Jejunum ØD5A
　Liver ØF5Ø
　　Left Lobe ØF52
　　Right Lobe ØF51
　Lung
　　Bilateral ØB5M
　　Left ØB5L
　　Lower Lobe
　　　Left ØB5J
　　　Right ØB5F
　　Middle Lobe, Right ØB5D
　　Right ØB5K
　　Upper Lobe
　　　Left ØB5G
　　　Right ØB5C
　Lung Lingula ØB5H
　Pancreas ØF5G
　Para-aortic Body ØG59
　Paraganglion Extremity ØG5F
　Parathyroid Gland ØG5R
　　Inferior
　　　Left ØG5P
　　　Right ØG5N
　　Multiple ØG5Q
　　Superior
　　　Left ØG5M
　　　Right ØG5L
　Pineal Body ØG51
　Prostate ØV5Ø
　Rectum ØD5P
　Sacrum ØQ51
　Spinal Cord
　　Cervical ØØ5W

Laser Interstitial Thermal Therapy — *continued*
　Spinal Cord — *continued*
　　Lumbar ØØ5Y
　　Thoracic ØØ5X
　Stomach ØD56
　　Pylorus ØD57
　Thyroid Gland ØG5K
　　Left Lobe ØG5G
　　Right Lobe ØG5H
　Vertebra
　　Cervical ØP53
　　Lumbar ØQ5Ø
　　Thoracic ØP54
Lateral canthus
　use Upper Eyelid, Left
　use Upper Eyelid, Right
Lateral collateral ligament (LCL)
　use Knee Bursa and Ligament, Left
　use Knee Bursa and Ligament, Right
Lateral condyle of femur
　use Lower Femur, Left
　use Lower Femur, Right
Lateral condyle of tibia
　use Tibia, Left
　use Tibia, Right
Lateral cuneiform bone
　use Tarsal, Left
　use Tarsal, Right
Lateral epicondyle of femur
　use Lower Femur, Left
　use Lower Femur, Right
Lateral epicondyle of humerus
　use Humeral Shaft, Left
　use Humeral Shaft, Right
Lateral femoral cutaneous nerve *use* Lumbar Plexus
Lateral (brachial) lymph node
　use Lymphatic, Left Axillary
　use Lymphatic, Right Axillary
Lateral malleolus
　use Fibula, Left
　use Fibula, Right
Lateral meniscus
　use Knee Joint, Left
　use Knee Joint, Right
Lateral nasal cartilage *use* Nasal Mucosa and Soft
　　Tissue
Lateral plantar artery
　use Foot Artery, Left
　use Foot Artery, Right
Lateral plantar nerve *use* Tibial Nerve
Lateral rectus muscle
　use Extraocular Muscle, Left
　use Extraocular Muscle, Right
Lateral sacral artery
　use Internal Iliac Artery, Left
　use Internal Iliac Artery, Right
Lateral sacral vein
　use Hypogastric Vein, Left
　use Hypogastric Vein, Right
Lateral sural cutaneous nerve *use* Peroneal Nerve
Lateral tarsal artery
　use Foot Artery, Left
　use Foot Artery, Right
Lateral temporomandibular ligament *use* Head and
　　Neck Bursa and Ligament
Lateral thoracic artery
　use Axillary Artery, Left
　use Axillary Artery, Right
Latissimus dorsi muscle
　use Trunk Muscle, Left
　use Trunk Muscle, Right
Latissimus Dorsi Myocutaneous Flap
　Replacement
　　Bilateral ØHRVØ75
　　Left ØHRUØ75
　　Right ØHRTØ75
　Transfer
　　Left ØKXG
　　Right ØKXF
Lavage
　see Irrigation
　Bronchial alveolar, diagnostic *see* Drainage, Respira-
　　tory System ØB9
Least splanchnic nerve *use* Thoracic Sympathetic
　　Nerve
Lefamulin Anti-infective XWØ
Left ascending lumbar vein *use* Hemiazygos Vein

Left atrioventricular valve *use* Mitral Valve
Left auricular appendix *use* Atrium, Left
Left colic vein *use* Colic Vein
Left coronary sulcus *use* Heart, Left
Left gastric artery *use* Gastric Artery
Left gastroepiploic artery *use* Splenic Artery
Left gastroepiploic vein *use* Splenic Vein
Left inferior phrenic vein *use* Renal Vein, Left
Left inferior pulmonary vein *use* Pulmonary Vein,
　　Left
Left jugular trunk *use* Thoracic Duct
Left lateral ventricle *use* Cerebral Ventricle
Left ovarian vein *use* Renal Vein, Left
Left second lumbar vein *use* Renal Vein, Left
Left subclavian trunk *use* Thoracic Duct
Left subcostal vein *use* Hemiazygos Vein
Left superior pulmonary vein *use* Pulmonary Vein,
　　Left
Left suprarenal vein *use* Renal Vein, Left
Left testicular vein *use* Renal Vein, Left
Lengthening
　Bone, with device *see* Insertion of Limb Lengthen-
　　ing Device
　Muscle, by incision *see* Division, Muscles ØK8
　Tendon, by incision *see* Division, Tendons ØL8
Leptomeninges, intracranial *use* Cerebral Meninges
Leptomeninges, spinal *use* Spinal Meninges
Leronlimab Monoclonal Antibody XWØ13K6
Lesser alar cartilage *use* Nasal Mucosa and Soft Tissue
Lesser occipital nerve *use* Cervical Plexus
Lesser Omentum *use* Omentum
Lesser saphenous vein
　use Saphenous Vein, Left
　use Saphenous Vein, Right
Lesser splanchnic nerve *use* Thoracic Sympathetic
　　Nerve
Lesser trochanter
　use Upper Femur, Left
　use Upper Femur, Right
Lesser tuberosity
　use Humeral Head, Left
　use Humeral Head, Right
Lesser wing *use* Sphenoid Bone
Leukopheresis, therapeutic *see* Pheresis, Circulatory
　　6A55
Levator anguli oris muscle *use* Facial Muscle
Levator ani muscle *use* Perineum Muscle
Levator labii superioris alaeque nasi muscle *use*
　　Facial Muscle
Levator labii superioris muscle *use* Facial Muscle
Levator palpebrae superioris muscle
　use Upper Eyelid, Left
　use Upper Eyelid, Right
Levator scapulae muscle
　use Neck Muscle, Left
　use Neck Muscle, Right
Levator veli palatini muscle *use* Tongue, Palate,
　　Pharynx Muscle
Levatores costarum muscle
　use Thorax Muscle, Left
　use Thorax Muscle, Right
**Lifeline ARM Automated Chest Compression (ACC)
　　device** 5A1221J
LifeStent® (Flexstar) (XL) Vascular Stent System
　use Intraluminal Device
Lifileucel *use* Lifileucel Immunotherapy
Lifileucel Immunotherapy XWØ
Ligament of head of fibula
　use Knee Bursa and Ligament, Left
　use Knee Bursa and Ligament, Right
Ligament of the lateral malleolus
　use Ankle Bursa and Ligament, Left
　use Ankle Bursa and Ligament, Right
Ligamentum flavum, cervical *use* Head and Neck
　　Bursa and Ligament
Ligamentum flavum, lumbar *use* Lower Spine Bursa
　　and Ligament
Ligamentum flavum, thoracic *use* Upper Spine Bursa
　　and Ligament
LigaPASS 2.Ø™ PJK Prevention System *use* Posterior
　　Vertebral Tether in New Technology
Ligation *see* Occlusion
Ligation, hemorrhoid *see* Occlusion, Lower Veins,
　　Hemorrhoidal Plexus
Light Therapy GZJZZZZ

▽ Subterms under main terms may continue to next column or page

Liner
Removal of device from
Hip
Left ØSPBØ9Z
Right ØSP9Ø9Z
Knee
Left ØSPDØ9Z
Right ØSPCØ9Z
Revision of device in
Hip
Left ØSWBØ9Z
Right ØSW9Ø9Z
Knee
Left ØSWDØ9Z
Right ØSWCØ9Z
Supplement
Hip
Left ØSUBØ9Z
Acetabular Surface ØSUEØ9Z
Femoral Surface ØSUSØ9Z
Right ØSU9Ø9Z
Acetabular Surface ØSUAØ9Z
Femoral Surface ØSURØ9Z
Knee
Left ØSUDØ9
Femoral Surface ØSUUØ9Z
Tibial Surface ØSUWØ9Z
Right ØSUCØ9
Femoral Surface ØSUTØ9Z
Tibial Surface ØSUVØ9Z
Lingual artery
use External Carotid Artery, Left
use External Carotid Artery, Right
Lingual tonsil *use* Pharynx
Lingulectomy, lung
see Excision, Lung Lingula ØBBH
see Resection, Lung Lingula ØBTH
Lisocabtagene Maraleucel *use* Lisocabtagene Maraleucel Immunotherapy
Lisocabtagene Maraleucel Immunotherapy XWØ
Lithoplasty *see* Fragmentation
Lithotripsy
see Fragmentation
With removal of fragments *see* Extirpation
LITT (laser interstitial thermal therapy)
see Destruction
see Laser Interstitial Thermal Therapy
LIVIAN™ CRT-D *use* Cardiac Resynchronization Defibrillator Pulse Generator in ØJH
LIVTENCITY™ *use* Maribavir Anti-infective
Lobectomy
see Excision, Central Nervous System and Cranial Nerves ØØB
see Excision, Endocrine System ØGB
see Excision, Hepatobiliary System and Pancreas ØFB
see Excision, Respiratory System ØBB
see Resection, Endocrine System ØGT
see Resection, Hepatobiliary System and Pancreas ØFT
see Resection, Respiratory System ØBT
Lobotomy *see* Division, Brain ØØ8Ø
Localization
see Imaging
see Map
Locus ceruleus *use* Pons
Long thoracic nerve *use* Brachial Plexus
Longeviti ClearFit® Cranial Implant *use* Synthetic Substitute, Ultrasound Penetrable in New Technology
Longeviti ClearFit® OTS Cranial Implant *use* Synthetic Substitute, Ultrasound Penetrable in New Technology
Loop ileostomy *see* Bypass, Ileum ØD1B
Loop recorder, implantable *use* Monitoring Device
Lovotibeglogene Autotemcel XW1
Lower GI series *see* Fluoroscopy, Colon BD14
Lower Respiratory Fluid Nucleic Acid-base Microbial Detection XXEBXQ6
LTX Regional Anticoagulant *use* Nafamostat Anticoagulant
LUCAS® Chest Compression System 5A1221J
Lumbar artery *use* Abdominal Aorta
Lumbar facet joint *use* Lumbar Vertebral Joint
Lumbar ganglion *use* Lumbar Sympathetic Nerve
Lumbar lymph node *use* Lymphatic, Aortic
Lumbar lymphatic trunk *use* Cisterna Chyli

Lumbar splanchnic nerve *use* Lumbar Sympathetic Nerve
Lumbosacral facet joint *use* Lumbosacral Joint
Lumbosacral trunk *use* Lumbar Nerve
Lumpectomy *see* Excision
Lunate bone
use Carpal, Left
use Carpal, Right
Lunotriquetral ligament
use Hand Bursa and Ligament, Left
use Hand Bursa and Ligament, Right
LUNSUMIO™ *use* Mosunetuzumab Antineoplastic
Lurbinectedin XWØ
Lymphadenectomy
see Excision, Lymphatic and Hemic Systems Ø7B
see Resection, Lymphatic and Hemic Systems Ø7T
Lymphadenotomy *see* Drainage, Lymphatic and Hemic Systems Ø79
Lymphangiectomy
see Excision, Lymphatic and Hemic Systems Ø7B
see Resection, Lymphatic and Hemic Systems Ø7T
Lymphangiogram *see* Plain Radiography, Lymphatic System B7Ø
Lymphangioplasty
see Repair, Lymphatic and Hemic Systems Ø7Q
see Supplement, Lymphatic and Hemic Systems Ø7U
Lymphangiorrhaphy *see* Repair, Lymphatic and Hemic Systems Ø7Q
Lymphangiotomy *see* Drainage, Lymphatic and Hemic Systems Ø79
Lysis *see* Release

M

Macula XXE5XR7
use Retina, Left
use Retina, Right
MAGEC® Spinal Bracing and Distraction System *use* Magnetically Controlled Growth Rod(s) in New Technology
Magnet extraction, ocular foreign body *see* Extirpation, Eye Ø8C
Magnetic Resonance Imaging (MRI)
Abdomen BW3Ø
Ankle
Left BQ3H
Right BQ3G
Aorta
Abdominal B43Ø
Thoracic B33Ø
Arm
Left BP3F
Right BP3E
Artery
Celiac B431
Cervico-Cerebral Arch B33Q
Common Carotid, Bilateral B335
Coronary
Bypass Graft, Multiple B233
Multiple B231
Internal Carotid, Bilateral B338
Intracranial B33R
Lower Extremity
Bilateral B43H
Left B43G
Right B43F
Pelvic B43C
Renal, Bilateral B438
Spinal B33M
Superior Mesenteric B434
Upper Extremity
Bilateral B33K
Left B33J
Right B33H
Vertebral, Bilateral B33G
Bladder BT3Ø
Brachial Plexus BW3P
Brain BØ3Ø
Breast
Bilateral BH32
Left BH31
Right BH3Ø
Calcaneus
Left BQ3K
Right BQ3J
Chest BW33Y

Magnetic Resonance Imaging (MRI) — *continued*
Coccyx BR3F
Connective Tissue
Lower Extremity BL31
Upper Extremity BL3Ø
Corpora Cavernosa BV3Ø
Disc
Cervical BR31
Lumbar BR33
Thoracic BR32
Ear B93Ø
Elbow
Left BP3H
Right BP3G
Eye
Bilateral B837
Left B836
Right B835
Femur
Left BQ34
Right BQ33
Fetal Abdomen BY33
Fetal Extremity BY35
Fetal Head BY3Ø
Fetal Heart BY31
Fetal Spine BY34
Fetal Thorax BY32
Fetus, Whole BY36
Foot
Left BQ3M
Right BQ3L
Forearm
Left BP3K
Right BP3J
Gland
Adrenal, Bilateral BG32
Parathyroid BG33
Parotid, Bilateral B936
Salivary, Bilateral B93D
Submandibular, Bilateral B939
Thyroid BG34
Head BW38
Heart, Right and Left B236
Hip
Left BQ31
Right BQ3Ø
Intracranial Sinus B532
Joint
Finger
Left BP3D
Right BP3C
Hand
Left BP3D
Right BP3C
Temporomandibular, Bilateral BN39
Kidney
Bilateral BT33
Left BT32
Right BT31
Transplant BT39
Knee
Left BQ38
Right BQ37
Larynx B93J
Leg
Left BQ3F
Right BQ3D
Liver BF35
Liver and Spleen BF36
Lung Apices BB3G
Lung, Bilateral, Hyperpolarized Xenon 129 (Xe-129) BB34Z3Z
Nasopharynx B93F
Neck BW3F
Nerve
Acoustic BØ3C
Brachial Plexus BW3P
Oropharynx B93F
Ovary
Bilateral BU35
Left BU34
Right BU33
Ovary and Uterus BU3C
Pancreas BF37
Patella
Left BQ3W
Right BQ3V
Pelvic Region BW3G
Pelvis BR3C

Magnetic Resonance Imaging (MRI) — *continued*
Pituitary Gland B039
Plexus, Brachial BW3P
Prostate BV33
Retroperitoneum BW3H
Sacrum BR3F
Scrotum BV34
Sella Turcica B039
Shoulder
Left BP39
Right BP38
Sinus
Intracranial B532
Paranasal B932
Spinal Cord B03B
Spine
Cervical BR30
Lumbar BR39
Thoracic BR37
Spleen and Liver BF36
Subcutaneous Tissue
Abdomen BH3H
Extremity
Lower BH3J
Upper BH3F
Head BH3D
Neck BH3D
Pelvis BH3H
Thorax BH3G
Tendon
Lower Extremity BL33
Upper Extremity BL32
Testicle
Bilateral BV37
Left BV36
Right BV35
Toe
Left BQ3Q
Right BQ3P
Uterus BU36
Pregnant BU3B
Uterus and Ovary BU3C
Vagina BU39
Vein
Cerebellar B531
Cerebral B531
Jugular, Bilateral B535
Lower Extremity
Bilateral B53D
Left B53C
Right B53B
Other B53V
Pelvic (Iliac) Bilateral B53H
Portal B53T
Pulmonary, Bilateral B53S
Renal, Bilateral B53L
Spanchnic B53T
Upper Extremity
Bilateral B53P
Left B53N
Right B53M
Vena Cava
Inferior B539
Superior B538
Wrist
Left BP3M
Right BP3L
Magnetically Controlled Growth Rod(s)
Cervical XNS3
Lumbar XNS0
Thoracic XNS4
Magnetic-guided radiofrequency endovascular fistula
Radial Artery, Left 031C3ZF
Radial Artery, Right 031B3ZF
Ulnar Artery, Left 031A3ZF
Ulnar Artery, Right 03193ZF
Magnus Neuromodulation System (MNS) X0Z0X18
Malleotomy *see* Drainage, Ear, Nose, Sinus 099
Malleus
use Auditory Ossicle, Left
use Auditory Ossicle, Right
Mammaplasty, mammoplasty
see Alteration, Skin and Breast 0H0
see Repair, Skin and Breast 0HQ
see Replacement, Skin and Breast 0HR
see Supplement, Skin and Breast 0HU

Mammary duct
use Breast, Bilateral
use Breast, Left
use Breast, Right
Mammary gland
use Breast, Bilateral
use Breast, Left
use Breast, Right
Mammectomy
see Excision, Skin and Breast 0HB
see Resection, Skin and Breast 0HT
Mammillary body *use* Hypothalamus
Mammography *see* Plain Radiography, Skin, Subcutaneous Tissue and Breast BH0
Mammotomy *see* Drainage, Skin and Breast 0H9
Mandibular nerve *use* Trigeminal Nerve
Mandibular notch
use Mandible, Left
use Mandible, Right
Mandibulectomy
see Excision, Head and Facial Bones 0NB
see Resection, Head and Facial Bones 0NT
Manipulation
Adhesions *see* Release
Chiropractic *see* Chiropractic Manipulation
Manual removal, retained placenta *see* Extraction, Products of Conception, Retained 10D1
Manubrium *use* Sternum
Map
Basal Ganglia 00K8
Brain 00K0
Cerebellum 00KC
Cerebral Hemisphere 00K7
Conduction Mechanism 02K8
Hypothalamus 00KA
Medulla Oblongata 00KD
Pons 00KB
Thalamus 00K9
Mapping
Doppler ultrasound *see* Ultrasonography
Electrocardiogram only *see* Measurement, Cardiac 4A02
Maribavir Anti-infective XW0
Mark IV Breathing Pacemaker System *use* Stimulator Generator in Subcutaneous Tissue and Fascia
MarrowStim™ PAD Kit for CBMA (Concentrated Bone Marrow Aspirate) *use* Other Substance
MarrowStim™ PAD Kit, for injection of concentrated bone marrow aspirate *see* Introduction of substance in or on, Muscle 3E02
Marsupialization
see Drainage
see Excision
Massage, cardiac
External 5A12012
Open 02QA0ZZ
Masseter muscle *use* Head Muscle
Masseteric fascia *use* Subcutaneous Tissue and Fascia, Face
Mastectomy
see Excision, Skin and Breast 0HB
see Resection, Skin and Breast 0HT
Mastoid air cells
use Mastoid Sinus, Left
use Mastoid Sinus, Right
Mastoid (postauricular) lymph node
use Lymphatic, Left Neck
use Lymphatic, Right Neck
Mastoid process
use Temporal Bone, Left
use Temporal Bone, Right
Mastoidectomy
see Excision, Ear, Nose, Sinus 09B
see Resection, Ear, Nose, Sinus 09T
Mastoidotomy *see* Drainage, Ear, Nose, Sinus 099
Mastopexy
see Repair, Skin and Breast 0HQ
see Reposition, Skin and Breast 0HS
Mastorrhaphy *see* Repair, Skin and Breast 0HQ
Mastotomy *see* Drainage, Skin and Breast 0H9
Maxillary artery
use External Carotid Artery, Left
use External Carotid Artery, Right
Maxillary nerve *use* Trigeminal Nerve
Maximo II DR (VR) *use* Defibrillator Generator in 0JH
Maximo II DR CRT-D *use* Cardiac Resynchronization Defibrillator Pulse Generator in 0JH

Measurement
Arterial
Flow
Coronary 4A03
Intracranial 4A03X5D
Peripheral 4A03
Pulmonary 4A03
Pressure
Coronary 4A03
Peripheral 4A03
Pulmonary 4A03
Thoracic, Other 4A03
Pulse
Coronary 4A03
Peripheral 4A03
Pulmonary 4A03
Saturation, Peripheral 4A03
Sound, Peripheral 4A03
Biliary
Flow 4A0C
Pressure 4A0C
Cardiac
Action Currents 4A02
Defibrillator 4B02XTZ
Electrical Activity 4A02
Guidance 4A02X4A
No Qualifier 4A02X4Z
Output 4A02
Pacemaker 4B02XSZ
Rate 4A02
Rhythm 4A02
Sampling and Pressure
Bilateral 4A02
Left Heart 4A02
Right Heart 4A02
Sound 4A02
Total Activity, Stress 4A02XM4
Central Nervous
Cerebrospinal Fluid Shunt, Wireless Sensor 4B00XW0
Conductivity 4A00
Electrical Activity 4A00
Pressure 4A000BZ
Intracranial 4A00
Saturation, Intracranial 4A00
Stimulator 4B00XVZ
Temperature, Intracranial 4A00
Circulatory, Volume 4A05XLZ
Gastrointestinal
Motility 4A0B
Pressure 4A0B
Secretion 4A0B
Lower Respiratory Fluid Nucleic Acid-base Microbial Detection XXEBXQ6
Lymphatic
Flow 4A06
Pressure 4A06
Metabolism 4A0Z
Musculoskeletal
Contractility 4A0F
Pressure 4A0F3BE
Stimulator 4B0FXVZ
Olfactory, Acuity 4A08X0Z
Peripheral Nervous
Conductivity
Motor 4A01
Sensory 4A01
Electrical Activity 4A01
Stimulator 4B01XVZ
Positive Blood Culture Fluorescence Hybridization for Organism Identification, Concentration and Susceptibility XXE5XN6
Products of Conception
Cardiac
Electrical Activity 4A0H
Rate 4A0H
Rhythm 4A0H
Sound 4A0H
Nervous
Conductivity 4A0J
Electrical Activity 4A0J
Pressure 4A0J
Respiratory
Capacity 4A09
Flow 4A09
Pacemaker 4B09XSZ
Rate 4A09
Resistance 4A09
Total Activity 4A09

🔻 Subterms under main terms may continue to next column or page

Measurement — *continued*
  Respiratory — *continued*
    Volume 4A09
  Sleep 4A0ZXQZ
  Temperature 4A0Z
  Urinary
    Contractility 4A0D
    Flow 4A0D
    Pressure 4A0D
    Resistance 4A0D
    Volume 4A0D
  Venous
    Flow
      Central 4A04
      Peripheral 4A04
      Portal 4A04
      Pulmonary 4A04
    Pressure
      Central 4A04
      Peripheral 4A04
      Portal 4A04
      Pulmonary 4A04
    Pulse
      Central 4A04
      Peripheral 4A04
      Portal 4A04
      Pulmonary 4A04
    Saturation, Peripheral 4A04
  Visual
    Acuity 4A07X0Z
    Mobility 4A07X7Z
    Pressure 4A07XBZ
  Whole Blood Nucleic Acid-base Microbial Detection XXE5XM5

Meatoplasty, urethra *see* Repair, Urethra 0TQD
Meatotomy *see* Drainage, Urinary System 0T9
Mechanical chest compression (mCPR) 5A1221J
Mechanical Initial Specimen Diversion Technique Using Active Negative Pressure (blood collection) XXE5XR7
Mechanical ventilation *see* Performance, Respiratory 5A19
Medial canthus
  use Lower Eyelid, Left
  use Lower Eyelid, Right
Medial collateral ligament (MCL)
  use Knee Bursa and Ligament, Left
  use Knee Bursa and Ligament, Right
Medial condyle of femur
  use Lower Femur, Left
  use Lower Femur, Right
Medial condyle of tibia
  use Tibia, Left
  use Tibia, Right
Medial cuneiform bone
  use Tarsal, Left
  use Tarsal, Right
Medial epicondyle of femur
  use Lower Femur, Left
  use Lower Femur, Right
Medial epicondyle of humerus
  use Humeral Shaft, Left
  use Humeral Shaft, Right
Medial malleolus
  use Tibia, Left
  use Tibia, Right
Medial meniscus
  use Knee Joint, Left
  use Knee Joint, Right
Medial plantar artery
  use Foot Artery, Left
  use Foot Artery, Right
Medial plantar nerve *use* Tibial Nerve
Medial popliteal nerve *use* Tibial Nerve
Medial rectus muscle
  use Extraocular Muscle, Left
  use Extraocular Muscle, Right
Medial sural cutaneous nerve *use* Tibial Nerve
Median antebrachial vein
  use Basilic Vein, Left
  use Basilic Vein, Right
Median cubital vein
  use Basilic Vein, Left
  use Basilic Vein, Right
Median sacral artery *use* Abdominal Aorta
Mediastinal cavity *use* Mediastinum
Mediastinal lymph node *use* Lymphatic, Thorax

Mediastinal space *use* Mediastinum
Mediastinoscopy 0WJC4ZZ
Medication Management GZ3ZZZZ
  for substance abuse
    Antabuse HZ83ZZZ
    Bupropion HZ87ZZZ
    Clonidine HZ86ZZZ
    Levo-alpha-acetyl-methadol (LAAM) HZ82ZZZ
    Methadone Maintenance HZ81ZZZ
    Naloxone HZ85ZZZ
    Naltrexone HZ84ZZZ
    Nicotine Replacement HZ80ZZZ
    Other Replacement Medication HZ89ZZZ
    Psychiatric Medication HZ88ZZZ
Meditation 8E0ZXY5
Medtronic Endurant® II AAA stent graft system *use* Intraluminal Device
Meissner's (submucous) plexus *use* Abdominal Sympathetic Nerve
Melody® transcatheter pulmonary valve *use* Zooplastic Tissue in Heart and Great Vessels
Melphalan Hydrochloride Antineoplastic XW053T9
Membranous urethra *use* Urethra
Meningeorrhaphy
  see Repair, Cerebral Meninges 00Q1
  see Repair, Spinal Meninges 00QT
Meniscectomy, knee
  see Excision, Joint, Knee, Left 0SBD
  see Excision, Joint, Knee, Right 0SBC
Mental foramen
  use Mandible, Left
  use Mandible, Right
Mentalis muscle *use* Facial Muscle
Mentoplasty *see* Alteration, Jaw, Lower 0W05
Meropenem-vaborbactam Anti-infective XW0
Mesenterectomy *see* Excision, Mesentery 0DBV
Mesenteriorrhaphy, mesenterorrhaphy *see* Repair, Mesentery 0DQV
Mesenteriplication *see* Repair, Mesentery 0DQV
Mesoappendix *use* Mesentery
Mesocolon *use* Mesentery
Metacarpal ligament
  use Hand Bursa and Ligament, Left
  use Hand Bursa and Ligament, Right
Metacarpophalangeal ligament
  use Hand Bursa and Ligament, Left
  use Hand Bursa and Ligament, Right
Metal on metal bearing surface *use* Synthetic Substitute, Metal in 0SR
Metatarsal Ligament
  use Foot Bursa and Ligament, Left
  use Foot Bursa and Ligament, Right
Metatarsectomy
  see Excision, Lower Bones 0QB
  see Resection, Lower Bones 0QT
Metatarsophalangeal (MTP) joint
  use Metatarsal-Phalangeal Joint, Left
  use Metatarsal-Phalangeal Joint, Right
Metatarsophalangeal Ligament
  use Foot Bursa and Ligament, Left
  use Foot Bursa and Ligament, Right
Metathalamus *use* Thalamus
Micro-Driver stent (RX) (OTW) *use* Intraluminal Device
MicroMed HeartAssist *use* Implantable Heart Assist System in Heart and Great Vessels
Micrus CERECYTE Microcoil *use* Intraluminal Device, Bioactive in Upper Arteries
Midcarpal joint
  use Carpal Joint, Left
  use Carpal Joint, Right
Middle cardiac nerve *use* Thoracic Sympathetic Nerve
Middle cerebral artery *use* Intracranial Artery
Middle cerebral vein *use* Intracranial Vein
Middle colic vein *use* Colic Vein
Middle genicular artery
  use Popliteal Artery, Left
  use Popliteal Artery, Right
Middle hemorrhoidal vein
  use Hypogastric Vein, Left
  use Hypogastric Vein, Right
Middle meningeal artery, intracranial portion *use* Intracranial Artery
Middle rectal artery
  use Internal Iliac Artery, Left
  use Internal Iliac Artery, Right
Middle suprarenal artery *use* Abdominal Aorta

Middle temporal artery
  use Temporal Artery, Left
  use Temporal Artery, Right
Middle turbinate *use* Nasal Turbinate
Mineral-based Topical Hemostatic Agent XW0
MIRODERM™ Biologic Wound Matrix *use* Nonautologous Tissue Substitute
MIRODERM™ skin graft *see* Replacement, Skin and Breast 0HR
MitraClip valve repair system *use* Synthetic Substitute
Mitral annulus *use* Mitral Valve
Mitroflow® Aortic Pericardial Heart Valve *use* Zooplastic Tissue in Heart and Great Vessels
MNS (Magnus Neuromodulation System) X0Z0X18
Mobilization, adhesions *see* Release
Molar gland *use* Buccal Mucosa
MolecuLight i:X® wound imaging *see* Other Imaging, Anatomical Regions BW5
Monitoring
  Arterial
    Flow
      Coronary 4A13
      Peripheral 4A13
      Pulmonary 4A13
    Pressure
      Coronary 4A13
      Peripheral 4A13
      Pulmonary 4A13
    Pulse
      Coronary 4A13
      Peripheral 4A13
      Pulmonary 4A13
    Saturation, Peripheral 4A13
    Sound, Peripheral 4A13
  Brain Electrical Activity, Computer-aided Detection and Notification XX20X89
  Cardiac
    Electrical Activity 4A12
      Ambulatory 4A12X45
      No Qualifier 4A12X4Z
    Output 4A12
    Rate 4A12
    Rhythm 4A12
    Sound 4A12
    Total Activity, Stress 4A12XM4
    Vascular Perfusion, Indocyanine Green Dye 4A12XSH
  Central Nervous
    Conductivity 4A10
    Electrical Activity
      Intraoperative 4A10
      No Qualifier 4A10
    Pressure 4A100BZ
      Intracranial 4A10
    Saturation, Intracranial 4A10
    Temperature, Intracranial 4A10
  Gastrointestinal
    Motility 4A1B
    Pressure 4A1B
    Secretion 4A1B
    Vascular Perfusion, Indocyanine Green Dye 4A1BXSH
  Kidney, Fluorescent Pyrazine XT25XE5
  Lymphatic
    Flow
      Indocyanine Green Dye 4A16
      No Qualifier 4A16
    Pressure 4A16
  Muscle Compartment Pressure, Micro-Electro-Mechanical System XX2F3W9
  Oxygen Saturation Endoscopic Imaging (OXEI) XD2
  Peripheral Nervous
    Conductivity
      Motor 4A11
      Sensory 4A11
    Electrical Activity
      Intraoperative 4A11
      No Qualifier 4A11
  Products of Conception
    Cardiac
      Electrical Activity 4A1H
      Rate 4A1H
      Rhythm 4A1H
      Sound 4A1H
    Nervous
      Conductivity 4A1J
      Electrical Activity 4A1J

▽ Subterms under main terms may continue to next column or page

Monitoring — *continued*
    Products of Conception — *continued*
        Nervous — *continued*
            Pressure 4A1J
        Respiratory
            Capacity 4A19
            Flow 4A19
            Rate 4A19
            Resistance 4A19
            Volume 4A19
        Skin and Breast, Vascular Perfusion, Indocyanine
            Green Dye 4A1GXSH
        Sleep 4A1ZXQZ
        Temperature 4A1Z
        Urinary
            Contractility 4A1D
            Flow 4A1D
            Pressure 4A1D
            Resistance 4A1D
            Volume 4A1D
        Venous
            Flow
                Central 4A14
                Peripheral 4A14
                Portal 4A14
                Pulmonary 4A14
            Pressure
                Central 4A14
                Peripheral 4A14
                Portal 4A14
                Pulmonary 4A14
            Pulse
                Central 4A14
                Peripheral 4A14
                Portal 4A14
                Pulmonary 4A14
            Saturation
                Central 4A14
                Portal 4A14
                Pulmonary 4A14
Monitoring Device, Hemodynamic
    Abdomen ØJH8
    Chest ØJH6
Mosaic Bioprosthesis (aortic) (mitral) valve *use*
    Zooplastic Tissue in Heart and Great Vessels
Mosunetuzumab Antineoplastic XWØ
Motor Function Assessment FØ1
Motor Treatment FØ7
MR Angiography
    see Magnetic Resonance Imaging (MRI), Heart B23
    see Magnetic Resonance Imaging (MRI), Lower
        Arteries B43
    see Magnetic Resonance Imaging (MRI), Upper
        Arteries B33
MULTI-LINK (VISION) (MINI-VISION) (ULTRA)
    Coronary Stent System *use* Intraluminal Device
Multiple sleep latency test 4AØZXQZ
Muscle Compartment Pressure, Micro-Electro-
    Mechanical System XX2F3W9
Musculocutaneous nerve *use* Brachial Plexus
Musculopexy
    see Repair, Muscles ØKQ
    see Reposition, Muscles ØKS
Musculophrenic artery
    use Internal Mammary Artery, Left
    use Internal Mammary Artery, Right
Musculoplasty
    see Repair, Muscles ØKQ
    see Supplement, Muscles ØKU
Musculorrhaphy *see* Repair, Muscles ØKQ
Musculospiral nerve *use* Radial Nerve
MYØ1 Continuous Compartmental Pressure Moni-
    tor XX2F3W9
Myectomy
    see Excision, Muscles ØKB
    see Resection, Muscles ØKT
Myelencephalon *use* Medulla Oblongata
Myelogram
    CT *see* Computerized Tomography (CT Scan),
        Central Nervous System BØ2
    MRI *see* Magnetic Resonance Imaging (MRI), Cen-
        tral Nervous System BØ3
Myenteric (Auerbach's) plexus *use* Abdominal Sym-
    pathetic Nerve
Myocardial Bridge Release *see* Release, Artery,
    Coronary
Myomectomy *see* Excision, Female Reproductive Sys-
    tem ØUB

Myometrium *use* Uterus
Myopexy
    see Repair, Muscles ØKQ
    see Reposition, Muscles ØKS
Myoplasty
    see Repair, Muscles ØKQ
    see Supplement, Muscles ØKU
Myorrhaphy *see* Repair, Muscles ØKQ
Myoscopy *see* Inspection, Muscles ØKJ
Myotomy
    see Division, Muscles ØK8
    see Drainage, Muscles ØK9
Myringectomy
    see Excision, Ear, Nose, Sinus Ø9B
    see Resection, Ear, Nose, Sinus Ø9T
Myringoplasty
    see Repair, Ear, Nose, Sinus Ø9Q
    see Replacement, Ear, Nose, Sinus Ø9R
    see Supplement, Ear, Nose, Sinus Ø9U
Myringostomy *see* Drainage, Ear, Nose, Sinus Ø99
Myringotomy *see* Drainage, Ear, Nose, Sinus Ø99

N

NA-1 (Nerinitide) *use* Nerinitide
Nafamostat Anticoagulant XYØYX37
Nail bed
    use Finger Nail
    use Toe Nail
Nail plate
    use Finger Nail
    use Toe Nail
nanoLOCK™ interbody fusion device
    use Interbody Fusion Device in Lower Joints
    use Interbody Fusion Device in Upper Joints
Narcosynthesis GZGZZZZ
Narsoplimab Monoclonal Antibody XWØ
Nasal cavity *use* Nasal Mucosa and Soft Tissue
Nasal concha *use* Nasal Turbinate
Nasalis muscle *use* Facial Muscle
Nasolacrimal duct
    use Lacrimal Duct, Left
    use Lacrimal Duct, Right
Nasopharyngeal airway (NPA) *use* Intraluminal De-
    vice, Airway in Ear, Nose, Sinus
Navicular bone
    use Tarsal, Left
    use Tarsal, Right
Near Infrared Spectroscopy, Circulatory System
    8EØ2
Neck of femur
    use Upper Femur, Left
    use Upper Femur, Right
Neck of humerus (anatomical) (surgical)
    use Humeral Head, Left
    use Humeral Head, Right
Nelli® Seizure Monitoring System XXEØX48
Neovasc Reducer™ *use* Reduction Device in New
    Technology
Nephrectomy
    see Excision, Urinary System ØTB
    see Resection, Urinary System ØTT
Nephrolithotomy *see* Extirpation, Urinary System ØTC
Nephrolysis *see* Release, Urinary System ØTN
Nephropexy
    see Repair, Urinary System ØTQ
    see Reposition, Urinary System ØTS
Nephroplasty
    see Repair, Urinary System ØTQ
    see Supplement, Urinary System ØTU
Nephropyeloureterostomy
    see Bypass, Urinary System ØT1
    see Drainage, Urinary System ØT9
Nephrorrhaphy *see* Repair, Urinary System ØTQ
Nephroscopy, transurethral ØTJ58ZZ
Nephrostomy
    see Bypass, Urinary System ØT1
    see Drainage, Urinary System ØT9
Nephrotomography
    see Fluoroscopy, Urinary System BT1
    see Plain Radiography, Urinary System BTØ
Nephrotomy
    see Division, Urinary System ØT8
    see Drainage, Urinary System ØT9
Nerinitide XWØ

Nerve conduction study
    see Measurement, Central Nervous 4AØØ
    see Measurement, Peripheral Nervous 4AØ1
Nerve Function Assessment FØ1
Nerve to the stapedius *use* Facial Nerve
Nesiritide *use* Human B-Type Natriuretic Peptide
Neurectomy
    see Excision, Central Nervous System and Cranial
        Nerves ØØB
    see Excision, Peripheral Nervous System Ø1B
Neurexeresis
    see Extraction, Central Nervous System and Cranial
        Nerves ØØD
    see Extraction, Peripheral Nervous System Ø1D
NeuroBlate™ System *see* Destruction
Neurohypophysis *use* Pituitary Gland
Neurolysis
    see Release, Central Nervous System and Cranial
        Nerves ØØN
    see Release, Peripheral Nervous System Ø1N
Neuromuscular electrical stimulation (NEMS) lead
    use Stimulator Lead in Muscles
Neurophysiologic monitoring *see* Monitoring, Central
    Nervous 4A1Ø
Neuroplasty
    see Repair, Central Nervous System and Cranial
        Nerves ØØQ
    see Repair, Peripheral Nervous System Ø1Q
    see Supplement, Central Nervous System and
        Cranial Nerves ØØU
    see Supplement, Peripheral Nervous System Ø1U
Neurorrhaphy
    see Repair, Central Nervous System and Cranial
        Nerves ØØQ
    see Repair, Peripheral Nervous System Ø1Q
Neurostimulator Generator
    Insertion of device in, Skull ØNHØØNZ
    Removal of device from, Skull ØNPØØNZ
    Revision of device in, Skull ØNWØØNZ
Neurostimulator generator, multiple channel *use*
    Stimulator Generator, Multiple Array in ØJH
Neurostimulator generator, multiple channel
    rechargeable *use* Stimulator Generator, Multiple
    Array Rechargeable in ØJH
Neurostimulator generator, single channel *use*
    Stimulator Generator, Single Array in ØJH
Neurostimulator generator, single channel
    rechargeable *use* Stimulator Generator, Single
    Array Rechargeable in ØJH
Neurostimulator Lead
    Insertion of device in
        Brain ØØHØ
        Cerebral Ventricle ØØH6
        Nerve
            Cranial ØØHE
            Peripheral Ø1HY
        Spinal Canal ØØHU
        Spinal Cord ØØHV
        Vein
            Azygos Ø5HØ
            Innominate
                Left Ø5H4
                Right Ø5H3
    Removal of device from
        Brain ØØPØ
        Cerebral Ventricle ØØP6
        Nerve
            Cranial ØØPE
            Peripheral Ø1PY
        Spinal Canal ØØPU
        Spinal Cord ØØPV
        Vein
            Azygos Ø5PØ
            Innominate
                Left Ø5P4
                Right Ø5P3
    Revision of device in
        Brain ØØWØ
        Cerebral Ventricle ØØW6
        Nerve
            Cranial ØØWE
            Peripheral Ø1WY
        Spinal Canal ØØWU
        Spinal Cord ØØWV
        Vein
            Azygos Ø5WØ
            Innominate
                Left Ø5W4

Neurostimulator Lead — *continued*
  Revision of device in — *continued*
    Vein — *continued*
      Innominate — *continued*
        Right 05W3
    Sphenopalatine Ganglion, Insertion X0HK3Q8
Neurostimulator Lead in Oropharynx XWHD7Q7
Neurostimulator Lead with Paired Stimulation System, Insertion X0HQ3R8
Neurotomy
  see Division, Central Nervous System and Cranial Nerves 008
  see Division, Peripheral Nervous System 018
Neurotripsy
  see Destruction, Central Nervous System and Cranial Nerves 005
  see Destruction, Peripheral Nervous System 015
Neutralization plate
  use Internal Fixation Device in Head and Facial Bones
  use Internal Fixation Device in Lower Bones
  use Internal Fixation Device in Upper Bones
New Technology
  Afamitresgene Autoleucel Immunotherapy XW0
  Amivantamab Monoclonal Antibody XW0
  Anacaulase-bcdb XW0
  Antibiotic-eluting Bone Void Filler XW0V0P7
  Aorta
    Thoracic Arch using Branched Synthetic Substitute with Intraluminal Device X2RX0N7
    Thoracic Descending using Branched Synthetic Substitute with Intraluminal Device X2VW0N7
  Apalutamide Antineoplastic XW0DXJ5
  Atezolizumab Antineoplastic XW0
  Axicabtagene Ciloleucel Immunotherapy XW0
  Bamlanivimab Monoclonal Antibody XW0
  Baricitinib XW0
  Betibeglogene Autotemcel XW1
  Bioengineered Allogeneic Construct, Skin XHRPXF7
  Brain Electrical Activity
    Computer-aided Detection and Notification XX20X89
    Computer-aided Semiologic Analysis XXE0X48
  Brexanolone XW0
  Brexucabtagene Autoleucel Immunotherapy XW0
  Broad Consortium Microbiota-based Live Biotherapeutic Suspension XW0H7X8
  Bypass
    Conduit through Femoral Vein to Popliteal Artery X2K
    Conduit through Femoral Vein to Superficial Femoral Artery X2K
  Caplacizumab XW0
  CD24Fc Immunomodulator XW0
  Cefiderocol Anti-infective XW0
  Ceftolozane/Tazobactam Anti-infective XW0
  Cerebral Embolic Filtration
    Dual Filter X2A5312
    Extracorporeal Flow Reversal Circuit X2A
    Single Deflection Filter X2A6325
  Ciltacabtagene Autoleucel XW0
  Coagulation Factor Xa, Inactivated XW0
  Computer-aided Assessment
    Cardiac Output XXE2X19
    Intracranial Vascular Activity XXE0X07
  Computer-aided Guidance, Transthoracic Echocardiography X2JAX47
  Computer-aided Mechanical Aspiration X2C
  Computer-aided Triage and Notification, Pulmonary Artery Flow XXE3X27
  Computer-aided Valve Modeling and Notification, Coronary Artery Flow XXE3X68
  Computer-assisted Transcranial Magnetic Stimulation X0Z0X18
  Coronary Sinus, Reduction Device X2V73Q7
  COVID-19 Vaccine XW0
  COVID-19 Vaccine Booster XW0
  COVID-19 Vaccine Dose 1 XW0
  COVID-19 Vaccine Dose 2 XW0
  COVID-19 Vaccine Dose 3 XW0
  Cytarabine and Daunorubicin Liposome Antineoplastic XW0
  Daratumumab and Hyaluronidase-fihj XW01318
  Destruction
    Liver, Ultrasound-guided Cavitation XF5

New Technology — *continued*
  Destruction — *continued*
    Renal Sympathetic Nerve(s), Ultrasound Ablation X051329
  Dilation
    Anterior Tibial
      Left
        Sustained Release Drug-eluting Intraluminal Device X27Q385
        Four or More X27Q3C5
        Three X27Q3B5
        Two X27Q395
      Right
        Sustained Release Drug-eluting Intraluminal Device X27P385
        Four or More X27P3C5
        Three X27P3B5
        Two X27P395
    Femoral
      Left
        Sustained Release Drug-eluting Intraluminal Device X27J385
        Four or More X27J3C5
        Three X27J3B5
        Two X27J395
      Right
        Sustained Release Drug-eluting Intraluminal Device X27H385
        Four or More X27H3C5
        Three X27H3B5
        Two X27H395
    Peroneal
      Left
        Sustained Release Drug-eluting Intraluminal Device X27U385
        Four or More X27U3C5
        Three X27U3B5
        Two X27U395
      Right
        Sustained Release Drug-eluting Intraluminal Device X27T385
        Four or More X27T3C5
        Three X27T3B5
        Two X27T395
    Popliteal
      Left Distal
        Sustained Release Drug-eluting Intraluminal Device X27N385
        Four or More X27N3C5
        Three X27N3B5
        Two X27N395
      Left Proximal
        Sustained Release Drug-eluting Intraluminal Device X27L385
        Four or More X27L3C5
        Three X27L3B5
        Two X27L395
      Right Distal
        Sustained Release Drug-eluting Intraluminal Device X27M385
        Four or More X27M3C5
        Three X27M3B5
        Two X27M395
      Right Proximal
        Sustained Release Drug-eluting Intraluminal Device X27K385
        Four or More X27K3C5
        Three X27K3B5
        Two X27K395
    Posterior Tibial
      Left
        Sustained Release Drug-eluting Intraluminal Device X27S385
        Four or More X27S3C5
        Three X27S3B5
        Two X27S395

New Technology — *continued*
  Dilation — *continued*
    Posterior Tibial — *continued*
      Right
        Sustained Release Drug-eluting Intraluminal Device X27R385
        Four or More X27R3C5
        Three X27R3B5
        Two X27R395
  Durvalumab Antineoplastic XW0
  Eculizumab XW0
  Eladocagene exuparvovec XW0Q316
  Elranatamab Antineoplastic XW013L9
  Endothelial Damage Inhibitor XY0VX83
  Engineered Allogeneic Thymus Tissue XW020D8
  Engineered Chimeric Antigen Receptor T-cell Immunotherapy
    Allogeneic XW0
    Autologous XW0
  Epcoritamab Monoclonal Antibody XW013S9
  Erdafitinib Antineoplastic XW0DXL5
  Esketamine Hydrochloride XW097M5
  Etesevimab Monoclonal Antibody XW0
  Exagamglogene Autotemcel XW1
  Fosfomycin Anti-infective XW0
  Fostamatinib XW0
  Fusion
    Ankle
      Left, Open-truss Design Internal Fixation Device XRGK0B9
      Right, Open-truss Design Internal Fixation Device XRGJ0B9
    Lumbar Vertebral
      2 or more, Interbody Fusion Device, Custom-Made Anatomically Designed XRGC
      Interbody Fusion Device, Custom-Made Anatomically Designed XRGB
      Lumbosacral, Interbody Fusion Device, Custom-Made Anatomically Designed XRGD
      Sacroiliac, Internal Fixation Device with Tulip Connector XRG
    Tarsal
      Left, Open-truss Design Internal Fixation Device XRGM0B9
      Right, Open-truss Design Internal Fixation Device XRGL0B9
    Thoracolumbar Vertebral, Interbody Fusion Device, Custom-Made Anatomically Designed XRGA
  Gilteritinib Antineoplastic XW0DXV5
  Glofitamab Antineoplastic XW0
  High-Dose Intravenous Immune Globulin, for COVID-19 treatment XW1
  Hyperimmune Globulin, for COVID-19 treatment XW1
  Idecabtagene Vicleucel Immunotherapy XW0
  Imipenem-cilastatin-relebactam Anti-infective XW0
  Inebilizumab-cdon XW0
  Insertion
    Bone, Pelvic, Internal Fixation Device with Tulip Connector XNH
    Conduit to Short-term External Heart Assist System X2H
    Intracardiac Pacemaker, Dual-Chamber X2H
    Intraluminal Device, Bioprosthetic Valve X2H
    Joint
      Lumbar Vertebral, Posterior Spinal Motion Preservation Device XRHB018
      Lumbosacral, Posterior Spinal Motion Preservation Device XRHD018
    Neurostimulator Lead, Sphenopalatine Ganglion X0HK3Q8
    Neurostimulator Lead with Paired Stimulation System X0HQ3R8
    Tibial Extension with Motion Sensors XNH
  Intermittent Coronary Sinus Occlusion X2A7358
  Intracranial Arterial Flow, Whole Blood mRNA XXE5XT7
  Iobenguane I-131 Antineoplastic XW0
  Kidney, Fluorescent Pyrazine XT25XE5
  Lefamulin Anti-infective XW0
  Leronlimab Monoclonal Antibody XW013K6
  Lifileucel Immunotherapy XW0
  Lisocabtagene Maraleucel Immunotherapy XW0

New Technology — *continued*
  Lovotibeglogene Autotemcel XW1
  Lower Respiratory Fluid Nucleic Acid-base Microbial Detection XXEBXQ6
  Lurbinectedin XWØ
  Maribavir Anti-infective XWØ
  Mechanical Initial Specimen Diversion Technique Using Active Negative Pressure (blood collection) XXE5XR7
  Melphalan Hydrochloride Antineoplastic XWØ53T9
  Meropenem-vaborbactam Anti-infective XWØ
  Mineral-based Topical Hemostatic Agent XWØ
  Mosunetuzumab Antineoplastic XWØ
  Muscle Compartment Pressure, Micro-Electro-Mechanical System XX2F3W9
  Nafamostat Anticoagulant XYØYX37
  Narsoplimab Monoclonal Antibody XWØ
  Nerinitide XWØ
  Neurostimulator Lead in Oropharynx XWHD7Q7
  Omadacycline Anti-infective XWØ
  Omidubicel XW1
  Other New Technology Monoclonal Antibody XWØ
  Other New Technology Therapeutic Substance XWØ
  Other Positive Blood/Isolated Colonies Bimodal Phenotypic Susceptibility Technology XXE5XY9
  OTL-103 XW1
  OTL-200 XW1
  Oxygen Saturation Endoscopic Imaging (OXEI) XD2
  Plasma, Convalescent (Nonautologous) XW1
  Positive Blood Culture Fluorescence Hybridization for Organism Identification, Concentration and Susceptibility XXE5XN6
  Posoleucel XWØ
  Quantitative Flow Ratio Analysis, Coronary Artery Flow XXE3X58
  Quizartinib Antineoplastic XWØDXJ9
  Radial artery arteriovenous fistula, using Thermal Resistance Energy X2K
  REGN-COV2 Monoclonal Antibody XWØ
  Remdesivir Anti-infective XWØ
  Replacement
    Lateral Meniscus Synthetic Substitute XRR
    Medial Meniscus Synthetic Substitute XRR
  Reposition
    Cervical, Magnetically Controlled Growth Rod(s) XNS3
    Lumbar
      Magnetically Controlled Growth Rod(s) XNSØ
      Posterior (Dynamic) Distraction Device XNSØ
    Thoracic
      Magnetically Controlled Growth Rod(s) XNS4
      Posterior (Dynamic) Distraction Device XNS4
  Rezafungin XWØ
  Ruxolitinib XWØDXT5
  Sabizabulin XWØ
  Sarilumab XWØ
  SARS-CoV-2 Antibody Detection, Serum/Plasma Nanoparticle Fluorescence XXE5XV7
  SARS-CoV-2 Polymerase Chain Reaction, Nasopharyngeal Fluid XXE97U7
  Satralizumab-mwge XWØ1397
  SER-109 XWØDXN9
  Single-use Duodenoscope XFJ
  Single-use Oversleeve with Intraoperative Colonic Irrigation XDPH8K7
  Spesolimab Monoclonal Antibody XWØ
  Sulbactam-Durlobactam XWØ
  Supplement
    Arteriovenous Fistula, Extraluminal Support Device X2U
    Bursa and Ligament, Spine, Posterior Vertebral Tether XKU
    Coronary Artery/Arteries, Vein Graft Extraluminal Support Device(s) X2U4079
    Vertebra
      Lumbar, Mechanically Expandable (Paired) Synthetic Substitute XNUØ356
      Thoracic, Mechanically Expandable (Paired) Synthetic Substitute XNU4356
  Tabelecleucel Immunotherapy XWØ
  Tagraxofusp-erzs Antineoplastic XWØ

New Technology — *continued*
  Talar Prosthesis Synthetic Substitute XNR
  Taurolidine Anti-infective and Heparin Anticoagulant XYØYX28
  Teclistamab Antineoplastic XWØ1348
  Terlipressin XWØ
  Tisagenlecleucel Immunotherapy XWØ
  Tixagevimab and Cilgavimab Monoclonal Antibody XWØ23X7
  Tocilizumab XWØ
  Treosulfan XWØ
  Trilaciclib XWØ
  Ultrasound Penetrable Synthetic Substitute, Skull XNR80D9
  Uridine Triacetate XWØDX82
  Venetoclax Antineoplastic XWØDXR5
  Whole Blood Nucleic Acid-base Microbial Detection XXE5XM5
  Whole Blood Reverse Transcription and Quantitative Real-time Polymerase Chain Reaction XXE5X38
NexoBrid™ *use* Anacaulase-bcdb
Ninth cranial nerve *use* Glossopharyngeal Nerve
NIRS (Near Infrared Spectroscopy) *see* Physiological Systems and Anatomical Regions 8EØ
Nitinol framed polymer mesh *use* Synthetic Substitute
Niyad™ *use* Nafamostat Anticoagulant
Nonimaging Nuclear Medicine Assay
  Bladder, Kidneys and Ureters CT63
  Blood C763
  Kidneys, Ureters and Bladder CT63
  Lymphatics and Hematologic System C76YYZZ
  Ureters, Kidneys and Bladder CT63
  Urinary System CT6YYZZ
Nonimaging Nuclear Medicine Probe
  Abdomen CW50
  Abdomen and Chest CW54
  Abdomen and Pelvis CW51
  Brain C050
  Central Nervous System C05YYZZ
  Chest CW53
  Chest and Abdomen CW54
  Chest and Neck CW56
  Extremity
    Lower CP5PZZZ
    Upper CP5NZZZ
  Head and Neck CW5B
  Heart C25YYZZ
    Right and Left C256
  Lymphatics
    Head C75J
    Head and Neck C755
    Lower Extremity C75P
    Neck C75K
    Pelvic C75D
    Trunk C75M
    Upper Chest C75L
    Upper Extremity C75N
  Lymphatics and Hematologic System C75YYZZ
  Musculoskeletal System, Other CP5YYZZ
  Neck and Chest CW56
  Neck and Head CW5B
  Pelvic Region CW5J
  Pelvis and Abdomen CW51
  Spine CP55ZZZ
Nonimaging Nuclear Medicine Uptake
  Endocrine System CG4YYZZ
  Gland, Thyroid CG42
Non-tunneled central venous catheter *use* Infusion Device
Nostril *use* Nasal Mucosa and Soft Tissue
Novacor Left Ventricular Assist Device *use* Implantable Heart Assist System in Heart and Great Vessels
Novation® Ceramic AHS® (Articulation Hip System) *use* Synthetic Substitute, Ceramic in ØSR
Nuclear medicine
  see Nonimaging Nuclear Medicine Assay
  see Nonimaging Nuclear Medicine Probe
  see Nonimaging Nuclear Medicine Uptake
  see Planar Nuclear Medicine Imaging
  see Positron Emission Tomographic (PET) Imaging
  see Systemic Nuclear Medicine Therapy
  see Tomographic (Tomo) Nuclear Medicine Imaging
Nuclear scintigraphy *see* Nuclear Medicine

NUsurface® Meniscus Implant
  use Synthetic Substitute, Lateral Meniscus in New Technology
  use Synthetic Substitute, Medial Meniscus in New Technology
Nutrition, concentrated substances
  Enteral infusion 3EØG36Z
  Parenteral (peripheral) infusion *see* Introduction of Nutritional Substance
NUZYRA™ *use* Omadacycline Anti-infective

O

Obliteration *see* Destruction
Obturator artery
  use Internal Iliac Artery, Left
  use Internal Iliac Artery, Right
Obturator lymph node *use* Lymphatic, Pelvis
Obturator muscle
  use Hip Muscle, Left
  use Hip Muscle, Right
Obturator nerve *use* Lumbar Plexus
Obturator vein
  use Hypogastric Vein, Left
  use Hypogastric Vein, Right
Obtuse margin *use* Heart, Left
Occipital artery
  use External Carotid Artery, Left
  use External Carotid Artery, Right
Occipital lobe *use* Cerebral Hemisphere
Occipital lymph node
  use Lymphatic, Left Neck
  use Lymphatic, Right Neck
Occipitofrontalis muscle *use* Facial Muscle
Occlusion
  Ampulla of Vater ØFLC
  Anus ØDLQ
  Aorta
    Abdominal 04LØ
    Thoracic, Descending 02LW
  Artery
    Anterior Tibial
      Left 04LQ
      Right 04LP
    Axillary
      Left 03L6
      Right 03L5
    Brachial
      Left 03L8
      Right 03L7
    Celiac 04L1
    Colic
      Left 04L7
      Middle 04L8
      Right 04L6
    Common Carotid
      Left 03LJ
      Right 03LH
    Common Iliac
      Left 04LD
      Right 04LC
    External Carotid
      Left 03LN
      Right 03LM
    External Iliac
      Left 04LJ
      Right 04LH
    Face 03LR
    Femoral
      Left 04LL
      Right 04LK
    Foot
      Left 04LW
      Right 04LV
    Gastric 04L2
    Hand
      Left 03LF
      Right 03LD
    Hepatic 04L3
    Inferior Mesenteric 04LB
    Innominate 03L2
    Internal Carotid
      Left 03LL
      Right 03LK
    Internal Iliac
      Left 04LF
      Right 04LE

Occlusion — *continued*
  Artery — *continued*
    Internal Mammary
      Left 03L1
      Right 03L0
    Intracranial 03LG
    Lower 04LY
    Peroneal
      Left 04LU
      Right 04LT
    Popliteal
      Left 04LN
      Right 04LM
    Posterior Tibial
      Left 04LS
      Right 04LR
    Pulmonary
      Left 02LR
      Right 02LQ
    Pulmonary Trunk 02LP
    Radial
      Left 03LC
      Right 03LB
    Renal
      Left 04LA
      Right 04L9
    Splenic 04L4
    Subclavian
      Left 03L4
      Right 03L3
    Superior Mesenteric 04L5
    Temporal
      Left 03LT
      Right 03LS
    Thyroid
      Left 03LV
      Right 03LU
    Ulnar
      Left 03LA
      Right 03L9
    Upper 03LY
    Vertebral
      Left 03LQ
      Right 03LP
  Atrium, Left 02L7
  Bladder 0TLB
  Bladder Neck 0TLC
  Bronchus
    Lingula 0BL9
    Lower Lobe
      Left 0BLB
      Right 0BL6
    Main
      Left 0BL7
      Right 0BL3
    Middle Lobe, Right 0BL5
    Upper Lobe
      Left 0BL8
      Right 0BL4
  Carina 0BL2
  Cecum 0DLH
  Cisterna Chyli 07LL
  Colon
    Ascending 0DLK
    Descending 0DLM
    Sigmoid 0DLN
    Transverse 0DLL
  Cord
    Bilateral 0VLH
    Left 0VLG
    Right 0VLF
  Cul-de-sac 0ULF
  Duct
    Common Bile 0FL9
    Cystic 0FL8
    Hepatic
      Common 0FL7
      Left 0FL6
      Right 0FL5
    Lacrimal
      Left 08LY
      Right 08LX
    Pancreatic 0FLD
      Accessory 0FLF
    Parotid
      Left 0CLC
      Right 0CLB
  Duodenum 0DL9
  Esophagogastric Junction 0DL4

Occlusion — *continued*
  Esophagus 0DL5
    Lower 0DL3
    Middle 0DL2
    Upper 0DL1
  Fallopian Tube
    Left 0UL6
    Right 0UL5
  Fallopian Tubes, Bilateral 0UL7
  Ileocecal Valve 0DLC
  Ileum 0DLB
  Intestine
    Large 0DLE
      Left 0DLG
      Right 0DLF
    Small 0DL8
  Jejunum 0DLA
  Kidney Pelvis
    Left 0TL4
    Right 0TL3
  Left atrial appendage (LAA) *see* Occlusion, Atrium,
    Left 02L7
  Lymphatic
    Aortic 07LD
    Axillary
      Left 07L6
      Right 07L5
    Head 07L0
    Inguinal
      Left 07LJ
      Right 07LH
    Internal Mammary
      Left 07L9
      Right 07L8
    Lower Extremity
      Left 07LG
      Right 07LF
    Mesenteric 07LB
    Neck
      Left 07L2
      Right 07L1
    Pelvis 07LC
    Thoracic Duct 07LK
    Thorax 07L7
    Upper Extremity
      Left 07L4
      Right 07L3
  Rectum 0DLP
  Stomach 0DL6
    Pylorus 0DL7
  Trachea 0BL1
  Ureter
    Left 0TL7
    Right 0TL6
  Urethra 0TLD
  Vagina 0ULG
  Valve, Pulmonary 02LH
  Vas Deferens
    Bilateral 0VLQ
    Left 0VLP
    Right 0VLN
  Vein
    Axillary
      Left 05L8
      Right 05L7
    Azygos 05L0
    Basilic
      Left 05LC
      Right 05LB
    Brachial
      Left 05LA
      Right 05L9
    Cephalic
      Left 05LF
      Right 05LD
    Colic 06L7
    Common Iliac
      Left 06LD
      Right 06LC
    Esophageal 06L3
    External Iliac
      Left 06LG
      Right 06LF
    External Jugular
      Left 05LQ
      Right 05LP
    Face
      Left 05LV
      Right 05LT

Occlusion — *continued*
  Vein — *continued*
    Femoral
      Left 06LN
      Right 06LM
    Foot
      Left 06LV
      Right 06LT
    Gastric 06L2
    Hand
      Left 05LH
      Right 05LG
    Hemiazygos 05L1
    Hepatic 06L4
    Hypogastric
      Left 06LJ
      Right 06LH
    Inferior Mesenteric 06L6
    Innominate
      Left 05L4
      Right 05L3
    Internal Jugular
      Left 05LN
      Right 05LM
    Intracranial 05LL
    Lower 06LY
    Portal 06L8
    Pulmonary
      Left 02LT
      Right 02LS
    Renal
      Left 06LB
      Right 06L9
    Saphenous
      Left 06LQ
      Right 06LP
    Splenic 06L1
    Subclavian
      Left 05L6
      Right 05L5
    Superior Mesenteric 06L5
    Upper 05LY
    Vertebral
      Left 05LS
      Right 05LR
  Vena Cava
    Inferior 06L0
    Superior 02LV
Occlusion, REBOA (resuscitative endovascular balloon occlusion of the aorta)
  02LW3DJ
  04L03DJ
Occupational therapy *see* Activities of Daily Living Treatment, Rehabilitation F08
Octagam 10%, for COVID-19 treatment *use* High-Dose Intravenous Immune Globulin
Odentectomy
  see Excision, Mouth and Throat 0CB
  see Resection, Mouth and Throat 0CT
Odontoid process *use* Cervical Vertebra
Olecranon bursa
  use Elbow Bursa and Ligament, Left
  use Elbow Bursa and Ligament, Right
Olecranon process
  use Ulna, Left
  use Ulna, Right
Olfactory bulb *use* Olfactory Nerve
Olumiant® *use* Baricitinib
Omadacycline Anti-infective XW0
Omentectomy, omentumectomy
  see Excision, Gastrointestinal System 0DB
  see Resection, Gastrointestinal System 0DT
Omentofixation *see* Repair, Gastrointestinal System 0DQ
Omentoplasty
  see Repair, Gastrointestinal System 0DQ
  see Replacement, Gastrointestinal System 0DR
  see Supplement, Gastrointestinal System 0DU
Omentorrhaphy *see* Repair, Gastrointestinal System 0DQ
Omentotomy *see* Drainage, Gastrointestinal System 0D9
Omidubicel XW1
Omnilink Elite Vascular Balloon Expandable Stent System *use* Intraluminal Device
Onychectomy
  see Excision, Skin and Breast 0HB
  see Resection, Skin and Breast 0HT

Onychoplasty
  see Repair, Skin and Breast ØHQ
  see Replacement, Skin and Breast ØHR
Onychotomy *see* Drainage, Skin and Breast ØH9
Oophorectomy
  see Excision, Female Reproductive System ØUB
  see Resection, Female Reproductive System ØUT
Oophoropexy
  see Repair, Female Reproductive System ØUQ
  see Reposition, Female Reproductive System ØUS
Oophoroplasty
  see Repair, Female Reproductive System ØUQ
  see Supplement, Female Reproductive System ØUU
Oophororrhaphy *see* Repair, Female Reproductive
  System ØUQ
Oophorostomy *see* Drainage, Female Reproductive
  System ØU9
Oophorotomy
  see Division, Female Reproductive System ØU8
  see Drainage, Female Reproductive System ØU9
Oophorrhaphy *see* Repair, Female Reproductive Sys-
  tem ØUQ
Open Pivot Aortic Valve Graft (AVG) *use* Synthetic
  Substitute
Open Pivot (mechanical) Valve *use* Synthetic Substi-
  tute
Open-truss Design Internal Fixation Device
  Ankle
    Left XRGKØB9
    Right XRGJØB9
  Tarsal
    Left XRGMØB9
    Right XRGLØB9
Ophthalmic artery *use* Intracranial Artery
Ophthalmic nerve *use* Trigeminal Nerve
Ophthalmic vein *use* Intracranial Vein
Opponensplasty
  Tendon replacement *see* Replacement, Tendons
    ØLR
  Tendon transfer *see* Transfer, Tendons ØLX
Optic chiasma *use* Optic Nerve
Optic disc
  use Retina, Left
  use Retina, Right
Optic foramen *use* Sphenoid Bone
Optical coherence tomography, intravascular *see*
  Computerized Tomography (CT Scan)
Optimizer™ III implantable pulse generator *use*
  Contractility Modulation Device in ØJH
Orbicularis oculi muscle
  use Upper Eyelid, Left
  use Upper Eyelid, Right
Orbicularis oris muscle *use* Facial Muscle
Orbital Atherectomy *see* Extirpation, Heart and Great
  Vessels Ø2C
Orbital fascia *use* Subcutaneous Tissue and Fascia,
  Face
Orbital portion of ethmoid bone
  use Orbit, Left
  use Orbit, Right
Orbital portion of frontal bone
  use Orbit, Left
  use Orbit, Right
Orbital portion of lacrimal bone
  use Orbit, Left
  use Orbit, Right
Orbital portion of maxilla
  use Orbit, Left
  use Orbit, Right
Orbital portion of palatine bone
  use Orbit, Left
  use Orbit, Right
Orbital portion of sphenoid bone
  use Orbit, Left
  use Orbit, Right
Orbital portion of zygomatic bone
  use Orbit, Left
  use Orbit, Right
Orchectomy, orchidectomy, orchiectomy
  see Excision, Male Reproductive System ØVB
  see Resection, Male Reproductive System ØVT
Orchidoplasty, orchioplasty
  see Repair, Male Reproductive System ØVQ
  see Replacement, Male Reproductive System ØVR
  see Supplement, Male Reproductive System ØVU
Orchidorrhaphy, orchiorrhaphy *see* Repair, Male
  Reproductive System ØVQ

Orchidotomy, orchiotomy, orchotomy *see* Drainage,
  Male Reproductive System ØV9
Orchiopexy
  see Repair, Male Reproductive System ØVQ
  see Reposition, Male Reproductive System ØVS
Oropharyngeal airway (OPA) *use* Intraluminal Device,
  Airway in Mouth and Throat
Oropharynx *use* Pharynx
Ossiculectomy
  see Excision, Ear, Nose, Sinus Ø9B
  see Resection, Ear, Nose, Sinus Ø9T
Ossiculotomy *see* Drainage, Ear, Nose, Sinus Ø99
Ostectomy
  see Excision, Head and Facial Bones ØNB
  see Excision, Lower Bones ØQB
  see Excision, Upper Bones ØPB
  see Resection, Head and Facial Bones ØNT
  see Resection, Lower Bones ØQT
  see Resection, Upper Bones ØPT
Osteoclasis
  see Division, Head and Facial Bones ØN8
  see Division, Lower Bones ØQ8
  see Division, Upper Bones ØP8
Osteolysis
  see Release, Head and Facial Bones ØNN
  see Release, Lower Bones ØQN
  see Release, Upper Bones ØPN
Osteopathic Treatment
  Abdomen 7WØ9X
  Cervical 7WØ1X
  Extremity
    Lower 7WØ6X
    Upper 7WØ7X
  Head 7WØØX
  Lumbar 7WØ3X
  Pelvis 7WØ5X
  Rib Cage 7WØ8X
  Sacrum 7WØ4X
  Thoracic 7WØ2X
Osteopexy
  see Repair, Head and Facial Bones ØNQ
  see Repair, Lower Bones ØQQ
  see Repair, Upper Bones ØPQ
  see Reposition, Head and Facial Bones ØNS
  see Reposition, Lower Bones ØQS
  see Reposition, Upper Bones ØPS
Osteoplasty
  see Repair, Head and Facial Bones ØNQ
  see Repair, Lower Bones ØQQ
  see Repair, Upper Bones ØPQ
  see Replacement, Head and Facial Bones ØNR
  see Replacement, Lower Bones ØQR
  see Replacement, Upper Bones ØPR
  see Supplement, Head and Facial Bones ØNU
  see Supplement, Lower Bones ØQU
  see Supplement, Upper Bones ØPU
Osteorrhaphy
  see Repair, Head and Facial Bones ØNQ
  see Repair, Lower Bones ØQQ
  see Repair, Upper Bones ØPQ
Osteotomy, ostotomy
  see Division, Head and Facial Bones ØN8
  see Division, Lower Bones ØQ8
  see Division, Upper Bones ØP8
  see Drainage, Head and Facial Bones ØN9
  see Drainage, Lower Bones ØQ9
  see Drainage, Upper Bones ØP9
Other Imaging
  Bile Duct and Gallbladder, Indocyanine Green Dye,
    Intraoperative BF532ØØ
  Bile Duct, Indocyanine Green Dye, Intraoperative
    BF5Ø2ØØ
  Extremity
    Lower BW5CZ1Z
    Upper BW5JZ1Z
  Gallbladder and Bile Duct, Indocyanine Green Dye,
    Intraoperative BF532ØØ
  Gallbladder, Indocyanine Green Dye, Intraoperative
    BF52ØØ
  Head and Neck BW59Z1Z
  Hepatobiliary System, All, Indocyanine Green Dye,
    Intraoperative BF5C2ØØ
  Liver and Spleen, Indocyanine Green Dye, Intraop-
    erative BF56200
  Liver, Indocyanine Green Dye, Intraoperative
    BF55200
  Neck and Head BW59Z1Z

Other Imaging — *continued*
  Pancreas, Indocyanine Green Dye, Intraoperative
    BF572ØØ
  Spleen and Liver, Indocyanine Green Dye, Intraop-
    erative BF56200
  Trunk BW52Z1Z
Other New Technology Monoclonal Antibody XWØ
Other New Technology Therapeutic Substance
  XWØ
Other Positive Blood/Isolated Colonies Bimodal
  Phenotypic Susceptibility Technology
  XXE5XY9
Otic ganglion *use* Head and Neck Sympathetic Nerve
OTL-101 *use* Hematopoietic Stem/Progenitor Cells,
  Genetically Modified
OTL-103 XW1
OTL-200 XW1
Otoplasty
  see Repair, Ear, Nose, Sinus Ø9Q
  see Replacement, Ear, Nose, Sinus Ø9R
  see Supplement, Ear, Nose, Sinus Ø9U
Otoscopy *see* Inspection, Ear, Nose, Sinus Ø9J
Oval window
  use Middle Ear, Left
  use Middle Ear, Right
Ovarian artery *use* Abdominal Aorta
Ovarian ligament *use* Uterine Supporting Structure
Ovariectomy
  see Excision, Female Reproductive System ØUB
  see Resection, Female Reproductive System ØUT
Ovariocentesis *see* Drainage, Female Reproductive
  System ØU9
Ovariopexy
  see Repair, Female Reproductive System ØUQ
  see Reposition, Female Reproductive System ØUS
Ovariotomy
  see Division, Female Reproductive System ØU8
  see Drainage, Female Reproductive System ØU9
Ovatio™ CRT-D *use* Cardiac Resynchronization Defibril-
  lator Pulse Generator in ØJH
Oversewing
  Gastrointestinal ulcer *see* Repair, Gastrointestinal
    System ØDQ
  Pleural bleb *see* Repair, Respiratory System ØBQ
Oviduct
  use Fallopian Tube, Left
  use Fallopian Tube, Right
Oximetry, Fetal pulse 1ØHØ73Z
OXINIUM *use* Synthetic Substitute, Oxidized Zirconium
  on Polyethylene in ØSR
Oxygen Saturation Endoscopic Imaging (OXEI) XD2
Oxygenation
  Extracorporeal membrane (ECMO) *see* Perfor-
    mance, Circulatory 5A15
  Hyperbaric *see* Assistance, Circulatory 5AØ5
  Supersaturated *see* Assistance, Cardiac 5AØ2

P

Pacemaker
  Dual Chamber
    Abdomen ØJH8
    Chest ØJH6
  Intracardiac
    Insertion of device in
      Atrium
        Left Ø2H7
        Right Ø2H6
      Vein, Coronary Ø2H4
      Ventricle
        Left Ø2HL
        Right Ø2HK
    Removal of device from, Heart Ø2PA
    Revision of device in, Heart Ø2WA
  Single Chamber
    Abdomen ØJH8
    Chest ØJH6
  Single Chamber Rate Responsive
    Abdomen ØJH8
    Chest ØJH6
Packing
  Abdominal Wall 2W43X5Z
  Anorectal 2Y43X5Z
  Arm
    Lower
      Left 2W4DX5Z
      Right 2W4CX5Z

Packing — continued
  Arm — continued
    Upper
      Left 2W4BX5Z
      Right 2W4AX5Z
  Back 2W45X5Z
  Chest Wall 2W44X5Z
  Ear 2Y42X5Z
  Extremity
    Lower
      Left 2W4MX5Z
      Right 2W4LX5Z
    Upper
      Left 2W49X5Z
      Right 2W48X5Z
  Face 2W41X5Z
  Finger
    Left 2W4KX5Z
    Right 2W4JX5Z
  Foot
    Left 2W4TX5Z
    Right 2W4SX5Z
  Genital Tract, Female 2Y44X5Z
  Hand
    Left 2W4FX5Z
    Right 2W4EX5Z
  Head 2W40X5Z
  Inguinal Region
    Left 2W47X5Z
    Right 2W46X5Z
  Leg
    Lower
      Left 2W4RX5Z
      Right 2W4QX5Z
    Upper
      Left 2W4PX5Z
      Right 2W4NX5Z
  Mouth and Pharynx 2Y40X5Z
  Nasal 2Y41X5Z
  Neck 2W42X5Z
  Thumb
    Left 2W4HX5Z
    Right 2W4GX5Z
  Toe
    Left 2W4VX5Z
    Right 2W4UX5Z
  Urethra 2Y45X5Z
Paclitaxel-eluting coronary stent use Intraluminal Device, Drug-eluting in Heart and Great Vessels
Paclitaxel-eluting peripheral stent
  use Intraluminal Device, Drug-eluting in Lower Arteries
  use Intraluminal Device, Drug-eluting in Upper Arteries
Palatine gland use Buccal Mucosa
Palatine tonsil use Tonsils
Palatine uvula use Uvula
Palatoglossal muscle use Tongue, Palate, Pharynx Muscle
Palatopharyngeal muscle use Tongue, Palate, Pharynx Muscle
Palatoplasty
  see Repair, Mouth and Throat ØCQ
  see Replacement, Mouth and Throat ØCR
  see Supplement, Mouth and Throat ØCU
Palatorrhaphy see Repair, Mouth and Throat ØCQ
Palmar cutaneous nerve
  use Median Nerve
  use Radial Nerve
Palmar (volar) digital vein
  use Hand Vein, Left
  use Hand Vein, Right
Palmar fascia (aponeurosis)
  use Subcutaneous Tissue and Fascia, Left Hand
  use Subcutaneous Tissue and Fascia, Right Hand
Palmar interosseous muscle
  use Hand Muscle, Left
  use Hand Muscle, Right
Palmar (volar) metacarpal vein
  use Hand Vein, Left
  use Hand Vein, Right
Palmar ulnocarpal ligament
  use Wrist Bursa and Ligament, Left
  use Wrist Bursa and Ligament, Right
Palmaris longus muscle
  use Lower Arm and Wrist Muscle, Left
  use Lower Arm and Wrist Muscle, Right

Pancreatectomy
  see Excision, Pancreas ØFBG
  see Resection, Pancreas ØFTG
Pancreatic artery use Splenic Artery
Pancreatic plexus use Abdominal Sympathetic Nerve
Pancreatic vein use Splenic Vein
Pancreaticoduodenostomy see Bypass, Hepatobiliary System and Pancreas ØF1
Pancreaticosplenic lymph node use Lymphatic, Aortic
Pancreatogram, endoscopic retrograde see Fluoroscopy, Pancreatic Duct BF18
Pancreatolithotomy see Extirpation, Pancreas ØFCG
Pancreatotomy
  see Division, Pancreas ØF8G
  see Drainage, Pancreas ØF9G
Panniculectomy
  see Excision, Skin, Abdomen ØHB7
  see Excision, Subcutaneous Tissue and Fascia, Abdomen ØJB8
Paraaortic lymph node use Lymphatic, Aortic
Paracentesis
  Eye see Drainage, Eye Ø89
  Peritoneal Cavity see Drainage, Peritoneal Cavity ØW9G
  Tympanum see Drainage, Ear, Nose, Sinus Ø99
Paradise™ Ultrasound Renal Denervation System XØ51329
Parapharyngeal space use Neck
Pararectal lymph node use Lymphatic, Mesenteric
Parasternal lymph node use Lymphatic, Thorax
Parathyroidectomy
  see Excision, Endocrine System ØGB
  see Resection, Endocrine System ØGT
Paratracheal lymph node use Lymphatic, Thorax
Paraurethral (Skene's) gland use Vestibular Gland
Parenteral nutrition, total see Introduction of Nutritional Substance
Parietal lobe use Cerebral Hemisphere
Parotid lymph node use Lymphatic, Head
Parotid plexus use Facial Nerve
Parotidectomy
  see Excision, Mouth and Throat ØCB
  see Resection, Mouth and Throat ØCT
Pars flaccida
  use Tympanic Membrane, Left
  use Tympanic Membrane, Right
Partial joint replacement
  Hip see Replacement, Lower Joints ØSR
  Knee see Replacement, Lower Joints ØSR
  Shoulder see Replacement, Upper Joints ØRR
Partially absorbable mesh use Synthetic Substitute
Patch, blood, spinal 3EØR3GC
Patellapexy
  see Repair, Lower Bones ØQQ
  see Reposition, Lower Bones ØQS
Patellaplasty
  see Repair, Lower Bones ØQQ
  see Replacement, Lower Bones ØQR
  see Supplement, Lower Bones ØQU
Patellar ligament
  use Knee Bursa and Ligament, Left
  use Knee Bursa and Ligament, Right
Patellar tendon
  use Knee Tendon, Left
  use Knee Tendon, Right
Patellectomy
  see Excision, Lower Bones ØQB
  see Resection, Lower Bones ØQT
Patellofemoral joint
  use Knee Joint, Left
  use Knee Joint, Left, Femoral Surface
  use Knee Joint, Right
  use Knee Joint, Right, Femoral Surface
pAVF (percutaneous arteriovenous fistula), using magnetic-guided radiofrequency see Bypass, Upper Arteries Ø31
pAVF (percutaneous arteriovenous fistula), using thermal resistance energy see New Technology, Cardiovascular System X2K
Pectineus muscle
  use Upper Leg Muscle, Left
  use Upper Leg Muscle, Right
Pectoral fascia use Subcutaneous Tissue and Fascia, Chest

Pectoral (anterior) lymph node
  use Lymphatic Left, Axillary
  use Lymphatic Right, Axillary
Pectoralis major muscle
  use Thorax Muscle, Left
  use Thorax Muscle, Right
Pectoralis minor muscle
  use Thorax Muscle, Left
  use Thorax Muscle, Right
Pedicle-based dynamic stabilization device
  use Spinal Stabilization Device, Pedicle-Based in ØSH
  use Spinal Stabilization Device, Pedicle-Based in ØRH
PEEP (positive end expiratory pressure) see Assistance, Respiratory 5AØ9
PEG (percutaneous endoscopic gastrostomy) ØDH63UZ
PEJ (percutaneous endoscopic jejunostomy) ØDHA3UZ
Pelvic splanchnic nerve
  use Abdominal Sympathetic Nerve
  use Sacral Sympathetic Nerve
Penectomy
  see Excision, Male Reproductive System ØVB
  see Resection, Male Reproductive System ØVT
Penile urethra use Urethra
Penumbra Indigo® Aspiration System see New Technology, Cardiovascular System X2C
PERCEPT™ PC neurostimulator use Stimulator Generator, Multiple Array in ØJH
Perceval sutureless valve (rapid deployment technique) see Replacement, Valve, Aortic Ø2RF
Percutaneous endoscopic gastrojejunostomy (PEG/J) tube use Feeding Device in Gastrointestinal System
Percutaneous endoscopic gastrostomy (PEG) tube use Feeding Device in Gastrointestinal System
Percutaneous nephrostomy catheter use Drainage Device
Percutaneous transluminal coronary angioplasty (PTCA) see Dilation, Heart and Great Vessels Ø27
Performance
  Biliary
    Multiple, Filtration 5A1C6ØZ
    Single, Filtration 5A1CØØZ
  Cardiac
    Continuous
      Output 5A1221Z
      Pacing 5A1223Z
    Intermittent, Pacing 5A1213Z
    Single, Output, Manual 5A12Ø12
  Circulatory
    Continuous
      Central Membrane 5A1522F
      Peripheral Veno-arterial Membrane 5A1522G
      Peripheral Veno-venous Membrane 5A1522H
    Intraoperative
      Central Membrane 5A15A2F
      Peripheral Veno-arterial Membrane 5A15A2G
      Peripheral Veno-venous Membrane 5A15A2H
  Respiratory
    24-96 Consecutive Hours, Ventilation 5A1945Z
    Greater than 96 Consecutive Hours, Ventilation 5A1955Z
    Less than 24 Consecutive Hours, Ventilation 5A1935Z
    Single, Ventilation, Nonmechanical 5A19Ø54
  Urinary
    Continuous, Greater than 18 hours per day, Filtration 5A1D9ØZ
    Intermittent, Less than 6 Hours Per Day, Filtration 5A1D7ØZ
    Prolonged Intermittent, 6-18 hours per day, Filtration 5A1D8ØZ
Perfusion see Introduction of substance in or on
Perfusion, donor organ
  Heart 6AB5ØBZ
  Kidney(s) 6ABTØBZ
  Liver 6ABFØBZ
  Lung(s) 6ABBØBZ
Perianal skin use Skin, Perineum

Pericardiectomy
- *see* Excision, Pericardium 02BN
- *see* Resection, Pericardium 02TN

Pericardiocentesis *see* Drainage, Pericardial Cavity 0W9D

Pericardiolysis *see* Release, Pericardium 02NN

Pericardiophrenic artery
- *use* Internal Mammary Artery, Left
- *use* Internal Mammary Artery, Right

Pericardioplasty
- *see* Repair, Pericardium 02QN
- *see* Replacement, Pericardium 02RN
- *see* Supplement, Pericardium 02UN

Pericardiorrhaphy *see* Repair, Pericardium 02QN

Pericardiostomy *see* Drainage, Pericardial Cavity 0W9D

Pericardiotomy *see* Drainage, Pericardial Cavity 0W9D

Perimetrium *use* Uterus

Peripheral Intravascular Lithotripsy (Peripheral IVL) *see* Fragmentation

Peripheral parenteral nutrition *see* Introduction of Nutritional Substance

Peripherally inserted central catheter (PICC) *use* Infusion Device

Peritoneal dialysis 3E1M39Z

Peritoneocentesis
- *see* Drainage, Peritoneal Cavity 0W9G
- *see* Drainage, Peritoneum 0D9W

Peritoneoplasty
- *see* Repair, Peritoneum 0DQW
- *see* Replacement, Peritoneum 0DRW
- *see* Supplement, Peritoneum 0DUW

Peritoneoscopy 0DJW4ZZ

Peritoneotomy *see* Drainage, Peritoneum 0D9W

Peritoneumectomy *see* Excision, Peritoneum 0DBW

Peroneus brevis muscle
- *use* Lower Leg Muscle, Left
- *use* Lower Leg Muscle, Right

Peroneus longus muscle
- *use* Lower Leg Muscle, Left
- *use* Lower Leg Muscle, Right

Pessary ring *use* Intraluminal Device, Pessary in Female Reproductive System

PET scan *see* Positron Emission Tomographic (PET) Imaging

Petrous part of temporal bone
- *use* Temporal Bone, Left
- *use* Temporal Bone, Right

Phacoemulsification, lens
- With IOL implant *see* Replacement, Eye 08R
- Without IOL implant *see* Extraction, Eye 08D

Phagenyx® System XWHD7Q7

Phalangectomy
- *see* Excision, Lower Bones 0QB
- *see* Excision, Upper Bones 0PB
- *see* Resection, Lower Bones 0QT
- *see* Resection, Upper Bones 0PT

Phallectomy
- *see* Excision, Penis 0VBS
- *see* Resection, Penis 0VTS

Phalloplasty
- *see* Repair, Penis 0VQS
- *see* Supplement, Penis 0VUS

Phallotomy *see* Drainage, Penis 0V9S

Pharmacotherapy, for substance abuse
- Antabuse HZ93ZZZ
- Bupropion HZ97ZZZ
- Clonidine HZ96ZZZ
- Levo-alpha-acetyl-methadol (LAAM) HZ92ZZZ
- Methadone Maintenance HZ91ZZZ
- Naloxone HZ95ZZZ
- Naltrexone HZ94ZZZ
- Nicotine Replacement HZ90ZZZ
- Psychiatric Medication HZ98ZZZ
- Replacement Medication, Other HZ99ZZZ

Pharyngeal constrictor muscle *use* Tongue, Palate, Pharynx Muscle

Pharyngeal plexus *use* Vagus Nerve

Pharyngeal recess *use* Nasopharynx

Pharyngeal tonsil *use* Adenoids

Pharyngogram *see* Fluoroscopy, Pharynix B91G

Pharyngoplasty
- *see* Repair, Mouth and Throat 0CQ
- *see* Replacement, Mouth and Throat 0CR
- *see* Supplement, Mouth and Throat 0CU

Pharyngorrhaphy *see* Repair, Mouth and Throat 0CQ

Pharyngotomy *see* Drainage, Mouth and Throat 0C9

Pharyngotympanic tube
- *use* Eustachian Tube, Left
- *use* Eustachian Tube, Right

Pheresis
- Erythrocytes 6A55
- Leukocytes 6A55
- Plasma 6A55
- Platelets 6A55
- Stem Cells
  - Cord Blood 6A55
  - Hematopoietic 6A55

Phlebectomy
- *see* Excision, Lower Veins 06B
- *see* Excision, Upper Veins 05B
- *see* Extraction, Lower Veins 06D
- *see* Extraction, Upper Veins 05D

Phlebography
- *see* Plain Radiography, Veins B50
- Impedance 4A04X51

Phleborrhaphy
- *see* Repair, Lower Veins 06Q
- *see* Repair, Upper Veins 05Q

Phlebotomy
- *see* Drainage, Lower Veins 069
- *see* Drainage, Upper Veins 059

Photocoagulation
- For Destruction *see* Destruction
- For Repair *see* Repair

Photopheresis, therapeutic *see* Phototherapy, Circulatory 6A65

Phototherapy
- Circulatory 6A65
- Skin 6A60
- Ultraviolet light *see* Ultraviolet Light Therapy, Physiological Systems 6A8

Phrenectomy, phrenoneurectomy *see* Excision, Nerve, Phrenic 01B2

Phrenemphraxis *see* Destruction, Nerve, Phrenic 0152

Phrenic nerve stimulator generator *use* Stimulator Generator in Subcutaneous Tissue and Fascia

Phrenic nerve stimulator lead *use* Diaphragmatic Pacemaker Lead in Respiratory System

Phreniclasis *see* Destruction, Nerve, Phrenic 0152

Phrenicoexeresis *see* Extraction, Nerve, Phrenic 01D2

Phrenicotomy *see* Division, Nerve, Phrenic 0182

Phrenicotripsy *see* Destruction, Nerve, Phrenic 0152

Phrenoplasty
- *see* Repair, Respiratory System 0BQ
- *see* Supplement, Respiratory System 0BU

Phrenotomy *see* Drainage, Respiratory System 0B9

Physiatry *see* Motor Treatment, Rehabilitation F07

Physical medicine *see* Motor Treatment, Rehabilitation F07

Physical therapy *see* Motor Treatment, Rehabilitation F07

PHYSIOMESH™ Flexible Composite Mesh *use* Synthetic Substitute

Pia mater, intracranial *use* Cerebral Meninges

Pia mater, spinal *use* Spinal Meninges

PiCSO® Impulse System X2A7358

Pinealectomy
- *see* Excision, Pineal Body 0GB1
- *see* Resection, Pineal Body 0GT1

Pinealoscopy 0GJ14ZZ

Pinealotomy *see* Drainage, Pineal Body 0G91

Pinna
- *use* External Ear, Bilateral
- *use* External Ear, Left
- *use* External Ear, Right

Pipeline™ (Flex) embolization device *use* Intraluminal Device, Flow Diverter in 03V

Piriform recess (sinus) *use* Pharynx

Piriformis muscle
- *use* Hip Muscle, Left
- *use* Hip Muscle, Right

PIRRT (Prolonged intermittent renal replacement therapy) 5A1D80Z

Pisiform bone
- *use* Carpal, Left
- *use* Carpal, Right

Pisohamate ligament
- *use* Hand Bursa and Ligament, Left
- *use* Hand Bursa and Ligament, Right

Pisometacarpal ligament
- *use* Hand Bursa and Ligament, Left
- *use* Hand Bursa and Ligament, Right

Pituitectomy
- *see* Excision, Gland, Pituitary 0GB0
- *see* Resection, Gland, Pituitary 0GT0

Plain film radiology *see* Plain Radiography

Plain Radiography
- Abdomen BW00ZZZ
- Abdomen and Pelvis BW01ZZZ
- Abdominal Lymphatic
  - Bilateral B701
  - Unilateral B700
- Airway, Upper BB0DZZZ
- Ankle
  - Left BQ0H
  - Right BQ0G
- Aorta
  - Abdominal B400
  - Thoracic B300
  - Thoraco-Abdominal B30P
- Aorta and Bilateral Lower Extremity Arteries B40D
- Arch
  - Bilateral BN0DZZZ
  - Left BN0CZZZ
  - Right BN0BZZZ
- Arm
  - Left BP0FZZZ
  - Right BP0EZZZ
- Artery
  - Brachiocephalic-Subclavian, Right B301
  - Bronchial B30L
  - Bypass Graft, Other B20F
  - Cervico-Cerebral Arch B30Q
  - Common Carotid
    - Bilateral B305
    - Left B304
    - Right B303
  - Coronary
    - Bypass Graft
      - Multiple B203
      - Single B202
    - Multiple B201
    - Single B200
  - External Carotid
    - Bilateral B30C
    - Left B30B
    - Right B309
  - Hepatic B402
  - Inferior Mesenteric B405
  - Intercostal B30L
  - Internal Carotid
    - Bilateral B308
    - Left B307
    - Right B306
  - Internal Mammary Bypass Graft
    - Left B208
    - Right B207
  - Intra-Abdominal, Other B40B
  - Intracranial B30R
  - Lower Extremity
    - Bilateral and Aorta B40D
    - Left B40G
    - Right B40F
  - Lower, Other B40J
  - Lumbar B409
  - Pelvic B40C
  - Pulmonary
    - Left B30T
    - Right B30S
  - Renal
    - Bilateral B408
    - Left B407
    - Right B406
    - Transplant B40M
  - Spinal B30M
  - Splenic B403
  - Subclavian, Left B302
  - Superior Mesenteric B404
  - Upper Extremity
    - Bilateral B30K
    - Left B30J
    - Right B30H
  - Upper, Other B30N
  - Vertebral
    - Bilateral B30G
    - Left B30F
    - Right B30D
- Bile Duct BF00
- Bile Duct and Gallbladder BF03
- Bladder BT00
  - Kidney and Ureter BT04

Subterms under main terms may continue to next column or page

Planar Nuclear Medicine Imaging — *continued*
　Abdomen and Pelvis CW11
　Anatomical Region, Other CW1ZZZZ
　Anatomical Regions, Multiple CW1YYZZ
　Bladder and Ureters CT1H
　Bladder, Kidneys and Ureters CT13
　Blood C713
　Bone Marrow C710
　Brain C010
　Breast CH1YYZZ
　　Bilateral CH12
　　Left CH11
　　Right CH10
　Bronchi and Lungs CB12
　Central Nervous System C01YYZZ
　Cerebrospinal Fluid C015
　Chest CW13
　Chest and Abdomen CW14
　Chest and Neck CW16
　Digestive System CD1YYZZ
　Ducts, Lacrimal, Bilateral C819
　Ear, Nose, Mouth and Throat C91YYZZ
　Endocrine System CG1YYZZ
　Extremity
　　Lower CW1D
　　　Bilateral CP1F
　　　Left CP1D
　　　Right CP1C
　　Upper CW1M
　　　Bilateral CP1B
　　　Left CP19
　　　Right CP18
　Eye C81YYZZ
　Gallbladder CF14
　Gastrointestinal Tract CD17
　　Upper CD15
　Gland
　　Adrenal, Bilateral CG14
　　Parathyroid CG11
　　Thyroid CG12
　Glands, Salivary, Bilateral C91B
　Head and Neck CW1B
　Heart C21YYZZ
　　Right and Left C216
　Hepatobiliary System, All CF1C
　Hepatobiliary System and Pancreas CF1YYZZ
　Kidneys, Ureters and Bladder CT13
　Liver CF15
　Liver and Spleen CF16
　Lungs and Bronchi CB12
　Lymphatics
　　Head C71J
　　Head and Neck C715
　　Lower Extremity C71P
　　Neck C71K
　　Pelvic C71D
　　Trunk C71M
　　Upper Chest C71L
　　Upper Extremity C71N
　Lymphatics and Hematologic System C71YYZZ
　Musculoskeletal System
　　All CP1Z
　　Other CP1YYZZ
　Myocardium C21G
　Neck and Chest CW16
　Neck and Head CW1B
　Pancreas and Hepatobiliary System CF1YYZZ
　Pelvic Region CW1J
　Pelvis CP16
　Pelvis and Abdomen CW11
　Pelvis and Spine CP17
　Reproductive System, Male CV1YYZZ
　Respiratory System CB1YYZZ
　Skin CH1YYZZ
　Skull CP11
　Spine CP15
　Spine and Pelvis CP17
　Spleen C712
　Spleen and Liver CF16
　Subcutaneous Tissue CH1YYZZ
　Testicles, Bilateral CV19
　Thorax CP14
　Ureters and Bladder CT1H
　Ureters, Kidneys and Bladder CT13
　Urinary System CT1YYZZ
　Veins C51YYZZ
　　Central C51R
　　Lower Extremity
　　　Bilateral C51D

Planar Nuclear Medicine Imaging — *continued*
　Veins — *continued*
　　Lower Extremity — *continued*
　　　Left C51C
　　　Right C51B
　　Upper Extremity
　　　Bilateral C51Q
　　　Left C51P
　　　Right C51N
　Whole Body CW1N
Plantar digital vein
　use Foot Vein, Left
　use Foot Vein, Right
Plantar fascia (aponeurosis)
　use Subcutaneous Tissue and Fascia, Left Foot
　use Subcutaneous Tissue and Fascia, Right Foot
Plantar metatarsal vein
　use Foot Vein, Left
　use Foot Vein, Right
Plantar venous arch
　use Foot Vein, Left
　use Foot Vein, Right
Plaque Radiation
　Abdomen DWY3FZZ
　Adrenal Gland DGY2FZZ
　Anus DDY8FZZ
　Bile Ducts DFY2FZZ
　Bladder DTY2FZZ
　Bone Marrow D7Y0FZZ
　Bone, Other DPYCFZZ
　Brain D0Y0FZZ
　Brain Stem D0Y1FZZ
　Breast
　　Left DMY0FZZ
　　Right DMY1FZZ
　Bronchus DBY1FZZ
　Cervix DUY1FZZ
　Chest DWY2FZZ
　Chest Wall DBY7FZZ
　Colon DDY5FZZ
　Diaphragm DBY8FZZ
　Duodenum DDY2FZZ
　Ear D9Y0FZZ
　Esophagus DDY0FZZ
　Eye D8Y0FZZ
　Femur DPY9FZZ
　Fibula DPYBFZZ
　Gallbladder DFY1FZZ
　Gland
　　Adrenal DGY2FZZ
　　Parathyroid DGY4FZZ
　　Pituitary DGY0FZZ
　　Thyroid DGY5FZZ
　Glands, Salivary D9Y6FZZ
　Head and Neck DWY1FZZ
　Hemibody DWY4FZZ
　Humerus DPY6FZZ
　Ileum DDY4FZZ
　Jejunum DDY3FZZ
　Kidney DTY0FZZ
　Larynx D9YBFZZ
　Liver DFY0FZZ
　Lung DBY2FZZ
　Lymphatics
　　Abdomen D7Y6FZZ
　　Axillary D7Y4FZZ
　　Inguinal D7Y8FZZ
　　Neck D7Y3FZZ
　　Pelvis D7Y7FZZ
　　Thorax D7Y5FZZ
　Mandible DPY3FZZ
　Maxilla DPY2FZZ
　Mediastinum DBY6FZZ
　Mouth D9Y4FZZ
　Nasopharynx D9YDFZZ
　Neck and Head DWY1FZZ
　Nerve, Peripheral D0Y7FZZ
　Nose D9Y1FZZ
　Ovary DUY0FZZ
　Palate
　　Hard D9Y8FZZ
　　Soft D9Y9FZZ
　Pancreas DFY3FZZ
　Parathyroid Gland DGY4FZZ
　Pelvic Bones DPY8FZZ
　Pelvic Region DWY6FZZ
　Pharynx D9YCFZZ
　Pineal Body DGY1FZZ

Plaque Radiation — *continued*
　Pituitary Gland DGY0FZZ
　Pleura DBY5FZZ
　Prostate DVY0FZZ
　Radius DPY7FZZ
　Rectum DDY7FZZ
　Rib DPY5FZZ
　Sinuses D9Y7FZZ
　Skin
　　Abdomen DHY8FZZ
　　Arm DHY4FZZ
　　Back DHY7FZZ
　　Buttock DHY9FZZ
　　Chest DHY6FZZ
　　Face DHY2FZZ
　　Foot DHYCFZZ
　　Hand DHY5FZZ
　　Leg DHYBFZZ
　　Neck DHY3FZZ
　Skull DPY0FZZ
　Spinal Cord D0Y6FZZ
　Spleen D7Y2FZZ
　Sternum DPY4FZZ
　Stomach DDY1FZZ
　Testis DVY1FZZ
　Thymus D7Y1FZZ
　Thyroid Gland DGY5FZZ
　Tibia DPYBFZZ
　Tongue D9Y5FZZ
　Trachea DBY0FZZ
　Ulna DPY7FZZ
　Ureter DTY1FZZ
　Urethra DTY3FZZ
　Uterus DUY2FZZ
　Whole Body DWY5FZZ
Plasma, Convalescent (Nonautologous) XW1
Plasmapheresis, therapeutic *see* Pheresis, Physiological Systems 6A5
Plateletpheresis, therapeutic *see* Pheresis, Physiological Systems 6A5
Platysma muscle
　use Neck Muscle, Left
　use Neck Muscle, Right
Plazomicin *use* Other Anti-infective
Pleurectomy
　see Excision, Respiratory System 0BB
　see Resection, Respiratory System 0BT
Pleurocentesis *see* Drainage, Anatomical Regions, General 0W9
Pleurodesis, pleurosclerosis
　Chemical injection *see* Introduction of Substance in or on, Pleural Cavity 3E0L
　Surgical *see* Destruction, Respiratory System 0B5
Pleurolysis *see* Release, Respiratory System 0BN
Pleuroscopy 0BJQ4ZZ
Pleurotomy *see* Drainage, Respiratory System 0B9
Plica semilunaris
　use Conjunctiva, Left
　use Conjunctiva, Right
Plication *see* Restriction
Pneumectomy
　see Excision, Respiratory System 0BB
　see Resection, Respiratory System 0BT
Pneumocentesis *see* Drainage, Respiratory System 0B9
Pneumogastric nerve *use* Vagus Nerve
Pneumolysis *see* Release, Respiratory System 0BN
Pneumonectomy *see* Resection, Respiratory System 0BT
Pneumonolysis *see* Release, Respiratory System 0BN
Pneumonopexy
　see Repair, Respiratory System 0BQ
　see Reposition, Respiratory System 0BS
Pneumonorrhaphy *see* Repair, Respiratory System 0BQ
Pneumonotomy *see* Drainage, Respiratory System 0B9
Pneumotaxic center *use* Pons
Pneumotomy *see* Drainage, Respiratory System 0B9
Pollicization *see* Transfer, Anatomical Regions, Upper Extremities 0XX
Polyclonal hyperimmune globulin *use* Globulin
Polyethylene socket *use* Synthetic Substitute, Polyethylene in 0SR
Polymethylmethacrylate (PMMA) *use* Synthetic Substitute
Polypectomy, gastrointestinal *see* Excision, Gastrointestinal System 0DB

Polypropylene mesh *use* Synthetic Substitute
Polysomnogram 4A1ZXQZ
Pontine tegmentum *use* Pons
Popliteal ligament
   use Knee Bursa and Ligament, Left
   use Knee Bursa and Ligament, Right
Popliteal lymph node
   use Lymphatic, Left Lower Extremity
   use Lymphatic, Right Lower Extremity
Popliteal vein
   use Femoral Vein, Left
   use Femoral Vein, Right
Popliteus muscle
   use Lower Leg Muscle, Left
   use Lower Leg Muscle, Right
Porcine (bioprosthetic) valve *use* Zooplastic Tissue
   in Heart and Great Vessels
Positive Blood Culture Fluorescence Hybridization
   for Organism Identification, Concentration
   and Susceptibility XXE5XN6
Positive end expiratory pressure *see* Performance,
   Respiratory 5A19
Positron Emission Tomographic (PET) Imaging
   Brain C030
   Bronchi and Lungs CB32
   Central Nervous System C03YYZZ
   Heart C23YYZZ
   Lungs and Bronchi CB32
   Myocardium C23G
   Respiratory System CB3YYZZ
   Whole Body CW3NYZZ
Positron emission tomography *see* Positron Emission
   Tomographic (PET) Imaging
Posoleucel XW0
Postauricular (mastoid) lymph node
   use Lymphatic, Left Neck
   use Lymphatic, Right Neck
Postcava *use* Inferior Vena Cava
Posterior auricular artery
   use External Carotid Artery, Left
   use External Carotid Artery, Right
Posterior auricular nerve *use* Facial Nerve
Posterior auricular vein
   use External Jugular Vein, Left
   use External Jugular Vein, Right
Posterior cerebral artery *use* Intracranial Artery
Posterior chamber
   use Eye, Left
   use Eye, Right
Posterior circumflex humeral artery
   use Axillary Artery, Left
   use Axillary Artery, Right
Posterior communicating artery *use* Intracranial
   Artery
Posterior cruciate ligament (PCL)
   use Knee Bursa and Ligament, Left
   use Knee Bursa and Ligament, Right
Posterior (Dynamic) Distraction Device
   Lumbar XNS0
   Thoracic XNS4
Posterior facial (retromandibular) vein
   use Face Vein, Left
   use Face Vein, Right
Posterior femoral cutaneous nerve *use* Sacral Plexus
Posterior inferior cerebellar artery (PICA) *use* In-
   tracranial Artery
Posterior interosseous nerve *use* Radial Nerve
Posterior labial nerve *use* Pudendal Nerve
Posterior (subscapular) lymph node
   use Lymphatic, Left Axillary
   use Lymphatic, Right Axillary
Posterior scrotal nerve *use* Pudendal Nerve
Posterior spinal artery
   use Vertebral Artery, Left
   use Vertebral Artery, Right
Posterior tibial recurrent artery
   use Anterior Tibial Artery, Left
   use Anterior Tibial Artery, Right
Posterior ulnar recurrent artery
   use Ulnar Artery, Left
   use Ulnar Artery, Right
Posterior vagal trunk *use* Vagus Nerve
PPN (peripheral parenteral nutrition) *see* Introduction of Nutritional Substance
Praxbind® (idarucizumab), Pradaxa® (dabigatran)
   reversal agent *use* Other Therapeutic Substance
Preauricular lymph node *use* Lymphatic, Head

Precava *use* Superior Vena Cava
PRECICE intramedullary limb lengthening system
   use Internal Fixation Device, Intramedullary Limb
     Lengthening in 0PH
   use Internal Fixation Device, Intramedullary Limb
     Lengthening in 0QH
Precision TAVI™ Coronary Obstruction Module
   XXE3X68
Prepatellar bursa
   use Knee Bursa and Ligament, Left
   use Knee Bursa and Ligament, Right
Preputiotomy *see* Drainage, Male Reproductive System
   0V9
Pressure support ventilation *see* Performance, Respiratory 5A19
PRESTIGE® Cervical Disc *use* Synthetic Substitute
Pretracheal fascia
   use Subcutaneous Tissue and Fascia, Left Neck
   use Subcutaneous Tissue and Fascia, Right Neck
Prevertebral fascia
   use Subcutaneous Tissue and Fascia, Left Neck
   use Subcutaneous Tissue and Fascia, Right Neck
PrimeAdvanced neurostimulator (SureScan) (MRI
   Safe) *use* Stimulator Generator, Multiple Array in
   0JH
Princeps pollicis artery
   use Hand Artery, Left
   use Hand Artery, Right
Probing, duct
   Diagnostic *see* Inspection
   Dilation *see* Dilation
PROCEED™ Ventral Patch *use* Synthetic Substitute
Procerus muscle *use* Facial Muscle
Proctectomy
   see Excision, Rectum 0DBP
   see Resection, Rectum 0DTP
Proctoclysis *see* Introduction of substance in or on,
   Gastrointestinal Tract, Lower 3E0H
Proctocolectomy
   see Excision, Gastrointestinal System 0DB
   see Resection, Gastrointestinal System 0DT
Proctocolpoplasty
   see Repair, Gastrointestinal System 0DQ
   see Supplement, Gastrointestinal System 0DU
Proctoperineoplasty
   see Repair, Gastrointestinal System 0DQ
   see Supplement, Gastrointestinal System 0DU
Proctoperineorrhaphy *see* Repair, Gastrointestinal
   System 0DQ
Proctopexy
   see Repair, Rectum 0DQP
   see Reposition, Rectum 0DSP
Proctoplasty
   see Repair, Rectum 0DQP
   see Supplement, Rectum 0DUP
Proctorrhaphy *see* Repair, Rectum 0DQP
Proctoscopy 0DJD8ZZ
Proctosigmoidectomy
   see Excision, Gastrointestinal System 0DB
   see Resection, Gastrointestinal System 0DT
Proctosigmoidoscopy 0DJD8ZZ
Proctostomy *see* Drainage, Rectum 0D9P
Proctotomy *see* Drainage, Rectum 0D9P
Prodisc-C *use* Synthetic Substitute
Prodisc-L *use* Synthetic Substitute
Production, atrial septal defect *see* Excision, Septum,
   Atrial 02B5
Profunda brachii
   use Brachial Artery, Left
   use Brachial Artery, Right
Profunda femoris (deep femoral) vein
   use Femoral Vein, Left
   use Femoral Vein, Right
PROLENE Polypropylene Hernia System (PHS) *use*
   Synthetic Substitute
Prolonged intermittent renal replacement therapy
   (PIRRT) 5A1D80Z
Pronator quadratus muscle
   use Lower Arm and Wrist Muscle, Left
   use Lower Arm and Wrist Muscle, Right
Pronator teres muscle
   use Lower Arm and Wrist Muscle, Left
   use Lower Arm and Wrist Muscle, Right
Prone positioning, intubated *see* Assistance, Respiratory 5A09

Prostatectomy
   see Excision, Prostate 0VB0
   see Resection, Prostate 0VT0
Prostatic artery
   use Internal Iliac Artery, Left
   use Internal Iliac Artery, Right
Prostatic urethra *use* Urethra
Prostatomy, prostatotomy *see* Drainage, Prostate
   0V90
Protecta XT CRT-D *use* Cardiac Resynchronization
   Defibrillator Pulse Generator in 0JH
Protecta XT DR (XT VR) *use* Defibrillator Generator in
   0JH
Protege® RX Carotid Stent System *use* Intraluminal
   Device
Proximal radioulnar joint
   use Elbow Joint, Left
   use Elbow Joint, Right
Psoas muscle
   use Hip Muscle, Left
   use Hip Muscle, Right
PSV (pressure support ventilation) *see* Performance,
   Respiratory 5A19
Psychoanalysis GZ54ZZZ
Psychological Tests
   Cognitive Status GZ14ZZZ
   Developmental GZ10ZZZ
   Intellectual and Psychoeducational GZ12ZZZ
   Neurobehavioral Status GZ14ZZZ
   Neuropsychological GZ13ZZZ
   Personality and Behavioral GZ11ZZZ
Psychotherapy
   Family, Mental Health Services GZ72ZZZ
   Group GZHZZZZ
     Mental Health Services GZHZZZZ
   Individual
     see Psychotherapy, Individual, Mental Health
       Services
     for substance abuse
       12-Step HZ53ZZZ
       Behavioral HZ51ZZZ
       Cognitive HZ50ZZZ
       Cognitive-Behavioral HZ52ZZZ
       Confrontational HZ58ZZZ
       Interactive HZ55ZZZ
       Interpersonal HZ54ZZZ
       Motivational Enhancement HZ57ZZZ
       Psychoanalysis HZ5BZZZ
       Psychodynamic HZ5CZZZ
       Psychoeducation HZ56ZZZ
       Psychophysiological HZ5DZZZ
       Supportive HZ59ZZZ
     Mental Health Services
       Behavioral GZ51ZZZ
       Cognitive GZ52ZZZ
       Cognitive-Behavioral GZ58ZZZ
       Interactive GZ50ZZZ
       Interpersonal GZ53ZZZ
       Psychoanalysis GZ54ZZZ
       Psychodynamic GZ55ZZZ
       Psychophysiological GZ59ZZZ
       Supportive GZ56ZZZ
PTCA (percutaneous transluminal coronary angio-
   plasty) *see* Dilation, Heart and Great Vessels 027
Pterygoid muscle *use* Head Muscle
Pterygoid process *use* Sphenoid Bone
Pterygopalatine (sphenopalatine) ganglion *use*
   Head and Neck Sympathetic Nerve
Pubis
   use Pelvic Bone, Left
   use Pelvic Bone, Right
Pubofemoral ligament
   use Hip Bursa and Ligament, Left
   use Hip Bursa and Ligament, Right
Pudendal nerve *use* Sacral Plexus
Pull-through, laparoscopic-assisted transanal
   see Excision, Gastrointestinal System 0DB
   see Resection, Gastrointestinal System 0DT
Pull-through, rectal *see* Resection, Rectum 0DTP
Pulmoaortic canal *use* Pulmonary Artery, Left
Pulmonary annulus *use* Pulmonary Valve
Pulmonary artery wedge monitoring *see* Monitor-
   ing, Arterial 4A13
Pulmonary plexus
   use Thoracic Sympathetic Nerve
   use Vagus Nerve
Pulmonic valve *use* Pulmonary Valve

Pulpectomy *see* Excision, Mouth and Throat ØCB
Pulverization *see* Fragmentation
Pulvinar *use* Thalamus
Pump reservoir *use* Infusion Device, Pump in Subcutaneous Tissue and Fascia
Punch biopsy *see* Excision with qualifier Diagnostic
Puncture *see* Drainage
Puncture, lumbar *see* Drainage, Spinal Canal ØØ9U
Pure-Vu® System XDPH8K7
Pyelography
   see Fluoroscopy, Urinary System BT1
   see Plain Radiography, Urinary System BTØ
Pyeloileostomy, urinary diversion *see* Bypass, Urinary System ØT1
Pyeloplasty
   see Repair, Urinary System ØTQ
   see Replacement, Urinary System ØTR
   see Supplement, Urinary System ØTU
Pyeloplasty, dismembered *see* Repair, Kidney Pelvis
Pyelorrhaphy *see* Repair, Urinary System ØTQ
Pyeloscopy ØTJ58ZZ
Pyelostomy
   see Bypass, Urinary System ØT1
   see Drainage, Urinary System ØT9
Pyelotomy *see* Drainage, Urinary System ØT9
Pylorectomy
   see Excision, Stomach, Pylorus ØDB7
   see Resection, Stomach, Pylorus ØDT7
Pyloric antrum *use* Stomach, Pylorus
Pyloric canal *use* Stomach, Pylorus
Pyloric sphincter *use* Stomach, Pylorus
Pylorodiosis *see* Dilation, Stomach, Pylorus ØD77
Pylorogastrectomy
   see Excision, Gastrointestinal System ØDB
   see Resection, Gastrointestinal System ØDT
Pyloroplasty
   see Repair, Stomach, Pylorus ØDQ7
   see Supplement, Stomach, Pylorus ØDU7
Pyloroscopy ØDJ68ZZ
Pylorotomy *see* Drainage, Stomach, Pylorus ØD97
Pyramidalis muscle
   use Abdomen Muscle, Left
   use Abdomen Muscle, Right

Q

QAngio XA® 3D XXE3X58
QFR® (Quantitative Flow Ratio) analysis of coronary angiography XXE3X58
Quadrangular cartilage *use* Nasal Septum
Quadrant resection of breast *see* Excision, Skin and Breast ØHB
Quadrate lobe *use* Liver
Quadratus femoris muscle
   use Hip Muscle, Left
   use Hip Muscle, Right
Quadratus lumborum muscle
   use Trunk Muscle, Left
   use Trunk Muscle, Right
Quadratus plantae muscle
   use Foot Muscle, Left
   use Foot Muscle, Right
Quadriceps (femoris)
   use Upper Leg Muscle, Left
   use Upper Leg Muscle, Right
Quantitative Flow Ratio Analysis, Coronary Artery Flow XXE3X58
Quarantine 8EØZXY6
Quizartinib Antineoplastic XWØDXJ9

R

Radial artery arteriovenous fistula, using Thermal Resistance Energy X2K
Radial collateral carpal ligament
   use Wrist Bursa and Ligament, Left
   use Wrist Bursa and Ligament, Right
Radial collateral ligament
   use Elbow Bursa and Ligament, Left
   use Elbow Bursa and Ligament, Right
Radial notch
   use Ulna, Left
   use Ulna, Right
Radial recurrent artery
   use Radial Artery, Left

Radial recurrent artery — *continued*
   use Radial Artery, Right
Radial vein
   use Brachial Vein, Left
   use Brachial Vein, Right
Radialis indicis
   use Hand Artery, Left
   use Hand Artery, Right
Radiation Therapy
   see Beam Radiation
   see Brachytherapy
   see Other Radiation
   see Stereotactic Radiosurgery
Radiation treatment *see* Radiation Therapy
Radiocarpal joint
   use Wrist Joint, Left
   use Wrist Joint, Right
Radiocarpal ligament
   use Wrist Bursa and Ligament, Left
   use Wrist Bursa and Ligament, Right
Radiography *see* Plain Radiography
Radiology, analog *see* Plain Radiography
Radiology, diagnostic *see* Imaging, Diagnostic
Radioulnar ligament
   use Wrist Bursa and Ligament, Left
   use Wrist Bursa and Ligament, Right
Range of motion testing *see* Motor Function Assessment, Rehabilitation FØ1
Rapid ASPECTS XXEØX07
REALIZE® Adjustable Gastric Band *use* Extraluminal Device
Reattachment
   Abdominal Wall ØWMFØZZ
   Ampulla of Vater ØFMC
   Ankle Region
     Left ØYMLØZZ
     Right ØYMKØZZ
   Arm
     Lower
       Left ØXMFØZZ
       Right ØXMDØZZ
     Upper
       Left ØXM9ØZZ
       Right ØXM8ØZZ
   Axilla
     Left ØXM5ØZZ
     Right ØXM4ØZZ
   Back
     Lower ØWMLØZZ
     Upper ØWMKØZZ
   Bladder ØTMB
   Bladder Neck ØTMC
   Breast
     Bilateral ØHMVXZZ
     Left ØHMUXZZ
     Right ØHMTXZZ
   Bronchus
     Lingula ØBM9ØZZ
     Lower Lobe
       Left ØBMBØZZ
       Right ØBM6ØZZ
     Main
       Left ØBM7ØZZ
       Right ØBM3ØZZ
     Middle Lobe, Right ØBM5ØZZ
     Upper Lobe
       Left ØBM8ØZZ
       Right ØBM4ØZZ
   Bursa and Ligament
     Abdomen
       Left ØMMJ
       Right ØMMH
     Ankle
       Left ØMMR
       Right ØMMQ
     Elbow
       Left ØMM4
       Right ØMM3
     Foot
       Left ØMMT
       Right ØMMS
     Hand
       Left ØMM8
       Right ØMM7
     Head and Neck ØMMØ
     Hip
       Left ØMMM
       Right ØMML

Reattachment — *continued*
   Bursa and Ligament — *continued*
     Knee
       Left ØMMP
       Right ØMMN
     Lower Extremity
       Left ØMMW
       Right ØMMV
     Perineum ØMMK
     Rib(s) ØMMG
     Shoulder
       Left ØMM2
       Right ØMM1
     Spine
       Lower ØMMD
       Upper ØMMC
     Sternum ØMMF
     Upper Extremity
       Left ØMMB
       Right ØMM9
     Wrist
       Left ØMM6
       Right ØMM5
   Buttock
     Left ØYM1ØZZ
     Right ØYMØØZZ
   Carina ØBM2ØZZ
   Cecum ØDMH
   Cervix ØUMC
   Chest Wall ØWM8ØZZ
   Clitoris ØUMJXZZ
   Colon
     Ascending ØDMK
     Descending ØDMM
     Sigmoid ØDMN
     Transverse ØDML
   Cord
     Bilateral ØVMH
     Left ØVMG
     Right ØVMF
   Cul-de-sac ØUMF
   Diaphragm ØBMTØZZ
   Duct
     Common Bile ØFM9
     Cystic ØFM8
     Hepatic
       Common ØFM7
       Left ØFM6
       Right ØFM5
     Pancreatic ØFMD
       Accessory ØFMF
   Duodenum ØDM9
   Ear
     Left Ø9M1XZZ
     Right Ø9MØXZZ
   Elbow Region
     Left ØXMCØZZ
     Right ØXMBØZZ
   Esophagus ØDM5
   Extremity
     Lower
       Left ØYMBØZZ
       Right ØYM9ØZZ
     Upper
       Left ØXM7ØZZ
       Right ØXM6ØZZ
   Eyelid
     Lower
       Left Ø8MRXZZ
       Right Ø8MQXZZ
     Upper
       Left Ø8MPXZZ
       Right Ø8MNXZZ
   Face ØWM2ØZZ
   Fallopian Tube
     Left ØUM6
     Right ØUM5
   Fallopian Tubes, Bilateral ØUM7
   Femoral Region
     Left ØYM8ØZZ
     Right ØYM7ØZZ
   Finger
     Index
       Left ØXMPØZZ
       Right ØXMNØZZ
     Little
       Left ØXMWØZZ
       Right ØXMVØZZ

Reattachment — *continued*
  Finger — *continued*
    Middle
      Left ØXMRØZZ
      Right ØXMQØZZ
    Ring
      Left ØXMTØZZ
      Right ØXMSØZZ
  Foot
    Left ØYMNØZZ
    Right ØYMMØZZ
  Forequarter
    Left ØXM1ØZZ
    Right ØXMØØZZ
  Gallbladder ØFM4
  Gland
    Left ØGM2
    Right ØGM3
  Hand
    Left ØXMKØZZ
    Right ØXMJØZZ
  Hindquarter
    Bilateral ØYM4ØZZ
    Left ØYM3ØZZ
    Right ØYM2ØZZ
  Hymen ØUMK
  Ileum ØDMB
  Inguinal Region
    Left ØYM6ØZZ
    Right ØYM5ØZZ
  Intestine
    Large ØDME
      Left ØDMG
      Right ØDMF
    Small ØDM8
  Jaw
    Lower ØWM5ØZZ
    Upper ØWM4ØZZ
  Jejunum ØDMA
  Kidney
    Left ØTM1
    Right ØTMØ
  Kidney Pelvis
    Left ØTM4
    Right ØTM3
  Kidneys, Bilateral ØTM2
  Knee Region
    Left ØYMGØZZ
    Right ØYMFØZZ
  Leg
    Lower
      Left ØYMJØZZ
      Right ØYMHØZZ
    Upper
      Left ØYMDØZZ
      Right ØYMCØZZ
  Lip
    Lower ØCM1ØZZ
    Upper ØCMØØZZ
  Liver ØFMØ
    Left Lobe ØFM2
    Right Lobe ØFM1
  Lung
    Left ØBMLØZZ
    Lower Lobe
      Left ØBMJØZZ
      Right ØBMFØZZ
    Middle Lobe, Right ØBMDØZZ
    Right ØBMKØZZ
    Upper Lobe
      Left ØBMGØZZ
      Right ØBMCØZZ
  Lung Lingula ØBMHØZZ
  Muscle
    Abdomen
      Left ØKML
      Right ØKMK
    Facial ØKM1
    Foot
      Left ØKMW
      Right ØKMV
    Hand
      Left ØKMD
      Right ØKMC
    Head ØKMØ
    Hip
      Left ØKMP
      Right ØKMN

Reattachment — *continued*
  Muscle — *continued*
    Lower Arm and Wrist
      Left ØKMB
      Right ØKM9
    Lower Leg
      Left ØKMT
      Right ØKMS
    Neck
      Left ØKM3
      Right ØKM2
    Perineum ØKMM
    Shoulder
      Left ØKM6
      Right ØKM5
    Thorax
      Left ØKMJ
      Right ØKMH
    Tongue, Palate, Pharynx ØKM4
    Trunk
      Left ØKMG
      Right ØKMF
    Upper Arm
      Left ØKM8
      Right ØKM7
    Upper Leg
      Left ØKMR
      Right ØKMQ
  Nasal Mucosa and Soft Tissue Ø9MKXZZ
  Neck ØWM6ØZZ
  Nipple
    Left ØHMXXZZ
    Right ØHMWXZZ
  Ovary
    Bilateral ØUM2
    Left ØUM1
    Right ØUMØ
  Palate, Soft ØCM3ØZZ
  Pancreas ØFMG
  Parathyroid Gland ØGMR
    Inferior
      Left ØGMP
      Right ØGMN
    Multiple ØGMQ
    Superior
      Left ØGMM
      Right ØGML
  Penis ØVMSXZZ
  Perineum
    Female ØWMNØZZ
    Male ØWMMØZZ
  Rectum ØDMP
  Scrotum ØVM5XZZ
  Shoulder Region
    Left ØXM3ØZZ
    Right ØXM2ØZZ
  Skin
    Abdomen ØHM7XZZ
    Back ØHM6XZZ
    Buttock ØHM8XZZ
    Chest ØHM5XZZ
    Ear
      Left ØHM3XZZ
      Right ØHM2XZZ
    Face ØHM1XZZ
    Foot
      Left ØHMNXZZ
      Right ØHMMXZZ
    Hand
      Left ØHMGXZZ
      Right ØHMFXZZ
    Inguinal ØHMAXZZ
    Lower Arm
      Left ØHMEXZZ
      Right ØHMDXZZ
    Lower Leg
      Left ØHMLXZZ
      Right ØHMKXZZ
    Neck ØHM4XZZ
    Perineum ØHM9XZZ
    Scalp ØHMØXZZ
    Upper Arm
      Left ØHMCXZZ
      Right ØHMBXZZ
    Upper Leg
      Left ØHMJXZZ
      Right ØHMHXZZ
  Stomach ØDM6

Reattachment — *continued*
  Tendon
    Abdomen
      Left ØLMG
      Right ØLMF
    Ankle
      Left ØLMT
      Right ØLMS
    Foot
      Left ØLMW
      Right ØLMV
    Hand
      Left ØLM8
      Right ØLM7
    Head and Neck ØLMØ
    Hip
      Left ØLMK
      Right ØLMJ
    Knee
      Left ØLMR
      Right ØLMQ
    Lower Arm and Wrist
      Left ØLM6
      Right ØLM5
    Lower Leg
      Left ØLMP
      Right ØLMN
    Perineum ØLMH
    Shoulder
      Left ØLM2
      Right ØLM1
    Thorax
      Left ØLMD
      Right ØLMC
    Trunk
      Left ØLMB
      Right ØLM9
    Upper Arm
      Left ØLM4
      Right ØLM3
    Upper Leg
      Left ØLMM
      Right ØLML
  Testis
    Bilateral ØVMC
    Left ØVMB
    Right ØVM9
  Thumb
    Left ØXMMØZZ
    Right ØXMLØZZ
  Thyroid Gland
    Left Lobe ØGMG
    Right Lobe ØGMH
  Toe
    1st
      Left ØYMQØZZ
      Right ØYMPØZZ
    2nd
      Left ØYMSØZZ
      Right ØYMRØZZ
    3rd
      Left ØYMUØZZ
      Right ØYMTØZZ
    4th
      Left ØYMWØZZ
      Right ØYMVØZZ
    5th
      Left ØYMYØZZ
      Right ØYMXØZZ
  Tongue ØCM7ØZZ
  Tooth
    Lower ØCMX
    Upper ØCMW
  Trachea ØBM1ØZZ
  Tunica Vaginalis
    Left ØVM7
    Right ØVM6
  Ureter
    Left ØTM7
    Right ØTM6
  Ureters, Bilateral ØTM8
  Urethra ØTMD
  Uterine Supporting Structure ØUM4
  Uterus ØUM9
  Uvula ØCMNØZZ
  Vagina ØUMG
  Vulva ØUMMXZZ
  Wrist Region
    Left ØXMHØZZ

Reattachment — *continued*
  Wrist Region — *continued*
    Right 0XMG0ZZ
REBOA (resuscitative endovascular balloon occlusion of the aorta)
  02LW3DJ
  04L03DJ
Rebound HRD® (Hernia Repair Device) *use* Synthetic Substitute
REBYOTA® *use* Broad Consortium Microbiota-based Live Biotherapeutic Suspension
RECELL® cell suspension autograft *see* Replacement, Skin and Breast 0HR
Recession
  see Repair
  see Reposition
Reclosure, disrupted abdominal wall 0WQFXZZ
Reconstruction
  see Repair
  see Replacement
  see Supplement
Rectectomy
  see Excision, Rectum 0DBP
  see Resection, Rectum 0DTP
Rectocele repair *see* Repair, Subcutaneous Tissue and Fascia, Pelvic Region 0JQC
Rectopexy
  see Repair, Gastrointestinal System 0DQ
  see Reposition, Gastrointestinal System 0DS
Rectoplasty
  see Repair, Gastrointestinal System 0DQ
  see Supplement, Gastrointestinal System 0DU
Rectorrhaphy *see* Repair, Gastrointestinal System 0DQ
Rectoscopy 0DJD8ZZ
Rectosigmoid junction *use* Sigmoid Colon
Rectosigmoidectomy
  see Excision, Gastrointestinal System 0DB
  see Resection, Gastrointestinal System 0DT
Rectostomy *see* Drainage, Rectum 0D9P
Rectotomy *see* Drainage, Rectum 0D9P
Rectus abdominis muscle
  use Abdomen Muscle, Left
  use Abdomen Muscle, Right
Rectus femoris muscle
  use Upper Leg Muscle, Left
  use Upper Leg Muscle, Right
Recurrent laryngeal nerve *use* Vagus Nerve
Reducer™ System *use* Reduction Device in New Technology
Reduction
  Dislocation *see* Reposition
  Fracture *see* Reposition
  Intussusception, intestinal *see* Reposition, Gastrointestinal System 0DS
  Mammoplasty *see* Excision, Skin and Breast 0HB
  Prolapse *see* Reposition
  Torsion *see* Reposition
  Volvulus, gastrointestinal *see* Reposition, Gastrointestinal System 0DS
Reduction Device, Coronary Sinus X2V73Q7
Refusion *see* Fusion
REGN-COV2 Monoclonal Antibody XW0
Rehabilitation
  see Activities of Daily Living Assessment, Rehabilitation F02
  see Activities of Daily Living Treatment, Rehabilitation F08
  see Caregiver Training, Rehabilitation F0F
  see Cochlear Implant Treatment, Rehabilitation F0B
  see Device Fitting, Rehabilitation F0D
  see Hearing Treatment, Rehabilitation F09
  see Motor Function Assessment, Rehabilitation F01
  see Motor Treatment, Rehabilitation F07
  see Speech Assessment, Rehabilitation F00
  see Speech Treatment, Rehabilitation F06
  see Vestibular Treatment, Rehabilitation F0C
Reimplantation
  see Reattachment
  see Reposition
  see Transfer
Reinforcement
  see Repair
  see Supplement
Relaxation, scar tissue *see* Release

Release
  Acetabulum
    Left 0QN5
    Right 0QN4
  Adenoids 0CNQ
  Ampulla of Vater 0FNC
  Anal Sphincter 0DNR
  Anterior Chamber
    Left 08N33ZZ
    Right 08N23ZZ
  Anus 0DNQ
  Aorta
    Abdominal 04N0
    Thoracic
      Ascending/Arch 02NX
      Descending 02NW
  Aortic Body 0GND
  Appendix 0DNJ
  Artery
    Anterior Tibial
      Left 04NQ
      Right 04NP
    Axillary
      Left 03N6
      Right 03N5
    Brachial
      Left 03N8
      Right 03N7
    Celiac 04N1
    Colic
      Left 04N7
      Middle 04N8
      Right 04N6
    Common Carotid
      Left 03NJ
      Right 03NH
    Common Iliac
      Left 04ND
      Right 04NC
    Coronary
      Four or More Arteries 02N3
      One Artery 02N0
      Three Arteries 02N2
      Two Arteries 02N1
    External Carotid
      Left 03NN
      Right 03NM
    External Iliac
      Left 04NJ
      Right 04NH
    Face 03NR
    Femoral
      Left 04NL
      Right 04NK
    Foot
      Left 04NW
      Right 04NV
    Gastric 04N2
    Hand
      Left 03NF
      Right 03ND
    Hepatic 04N3
    Inferior Mesenteric 04NB
    Innominate 03N2
    Internal Carotid
      Left 03NL
      Right 03NK
    Internal Iliac
      Left 04NF
      Right 04NE
    Internal Mammary
      Left 03N1
      Right 03N0
    Intracranial 03NG
    Lower 04NY
    Peroneal
      Left 04NU
      Right 04NT
    Popliteal
      Left 04NN
      Right 04NM
    Posterior Tibial
      Left 04NS
      Right 04NR
    Pulmonary
      Left 02NR
      Right 02NQ
    Pulmonary Trunk 02NP

Release — *continued*
  Artery — *continued*
    Radial
      Left 03NC
      Right 03NB
    Renal
      Left 04NA
      Right 04N9
    Splenic 04N4
    Subclavian
      Left 03N4
      Right 03N3
    Superior Mesenteric 04N5
    Temporal
      Left 03NT
      Right 03NS
    Thyroid
      Left 03NV
      Right 03NU
    Ulnar
      Left 03NA
      Right 03N9
    Upper 03NY
    Vertebral
      Left 03NQ
      Right 03NP
  Atrium
    Left 02N7
    Right 02N6
  Auditory Ossicle
    Left 09NA
    Right 09N9
  Basal Ganglia 00N8
  Bladder 0TNB
  Bladder Neck 0TNC
  Bone
    Ethmoid
      Left 0NNG
      Right 0NNF
    Frontal 0NN1
    Hyoid 0NNX
    Lacrimal
      Left 0NNJ
      Right 0NNH
    Nasal 0NNB
    Occipital 0NN7
    Palatine
      Left 0NNL
      Right 0NNK
    Parietal
      Left 0NN4
      Right 0NN3
    Pelvic
      Left 0QN3
      Right 0QN2
    Sphenoid 0NNC
    Temporal
      Left 0NN6
      Right 0NN5
    Zygomatic
      Left 0NNN
      Right 0NNM
  Brain 00N0
  Breast
    Bilateral 0HNV
    Left 0HNU
    Right 0HNT
  Bronchus
    Lingula 0BN9
    Lower Lobe
      Left 0BNB
      Right 0BN6
    Main
      Left 0BN7
      Right 0BN3
    Middle Lobe, Right 0BN5
    Upper Lobe
      Left 0BN8
      Right 0BN4
  Buccal Mucosa 0CN4
  Bursa and Ligament
    Abdomen
      Left 0MNJ
      Right 0MNH
    Ankle
      Left 0MNR
      Right 0MNQ
    Elbow
      Left 0MN4

▽ **Subterms under main terms may continue to next column or page**

Index

Release — Release

Release — continued
  Joint — continued
    Toe Phalangeal
      Left ØSNQ
      Right ØSNP
    Wrist
      Left ØRNP
      Right ØRNN
  Kidney
    Left ØTN1
    Right ØTNØ
  Kidney Pelvis
    Left ØTN4
    Right ØTN3
  Larynx ØCNS
  Lens
    Left Ø8NK3ZZ
    Right Ø8NJ3ZZ
  Lip
    Lower ØCN1
    Upper ØCNØ
  Liver ØFNØ
    Left Lobe ØFN2
    Right Lobe ØFN1
  Lung
    Bilateral ØBNM
    Left ØBNL
    Lower Lobe
      Left ØBNJ
      Right ØBNF
    Middle Lobe, Right ØBND
    Right ØBNK
    Upper Lobe
      Left ØBNG
      Right ØBNC
  Lung Lingula ØBNH
  Lymphatic
    Aortic Ø7ND
    Axillary
      Left Ø7N6
      Right Ø7N5
    Head Ø7NØ
    Inguinal
      Left Ø7NJ
      Right Ø7NH
    Internal Mammary
      Left Ø7N9
      Right Ø7N8
    Lower Extremity
      Left Ø7NG
      Right Ø7NF
    Mesenteric Ø7NB
    Neck
      Left Ø7N2
      Right Ø7N1
    Pelvis Ø7NC
    Thoracic Duct Ø7NK
    Thorax Ø7N7
    Upper Extremity
      Left Ø7N4
      Right Ø7N3
  Mandible
    Left ØNNV
    Right ØNNT
  Maxilla ØNNR
  Medulla Oblongata ØØND
  Mesentery ØDNV
  Metacarpal
    Left ØPNQ
    Right ØPNP
  Metatarsal
    Left ØQNP
    Right ØQNN
  Muscle
    Abdomen
      Left ØKNL
      Right ØKNK
    Extraocular
      Left Ø8NM
      Right Ø8NL
    Facial ØKN1
    Foot
      Left ØKNW
      Right ØKNV
    Hand
      Left ØKND
      Right ØKNC
    Head ØKNØ

Release — continued
  Muscle — continued
    Hip
      Left ØKNP
      Right ØKNN
    Lower Arm and Wrist
      Left ØKNB
      Right ØKN9
    Lower Leg
      Left ØKNT
      Right ØKNS
    Neck
      Left ØKN3
      Right ØKN2
    Papillary Ø2ND
    Perineum ØKNM
    Shoulder
      Left ØKN6
      Right ØKN5
    Thorax
      Left ØKNJ
      Right ØKNH
    Tongue, Palate, Pharynx ØKN4
    Trunk
      Left ØKNG
      Right ØKNF
    Upper Arm
      Left ØKN8
      Right ØKN7
    Upper Leg
      Left ØKNR
      Right ØKNQ
  Myocardial Bridge *see* Release, Artery, Coronary
  Nasal Mucosa and Soft Tissue Ø9NK
  Nasopharynx Ø9NN
  Nerve
    Abdominal Sympathetic Ø1NM
    Abducens ØØNL
    Accessory ØØNR
    Acoustic ØØNN
    Brachial Plexus Ø1N3
    Cervical Ø1N1
    Cervical Plexus Ø1NØ
    Facial ØØNM
    Femoral Ø1ND
    Glossopharyngeal ØØNP
    Head and Neck Sympathetic Ø1NK
    Hypoglossal ØØNS
    Lumbar Ø1NB
    Lumbar Plexus Ø1N9
    Lumbar Sympathetic Ø1NN
    Lumbosacral Plexus Ø1NA
    Median Ø1N5
    Oculomotor ØØNH
    Olfactory ØØNF
    Optic ØØNG
    Peroneal Ø1NH
    Phrenic Ø1N2
    Pudendal Ø1NC
    Radial Ø1N6
    Sacral Ø1NR
    Sacral Plexus Ø1NQ
    Sacral Sympathetic Ø1NP
    Sciatic Ø1NF
    Thoracic Ø1N8
    Thoracic Sympathetic Ø1NL
    Tibial Ø1NG
    Trigeminal ØØNK
    Trochlear ØØNJ
    Ulnar Ø1N4
    Vagus ØØNQ
  Nipple
    Left ØHNX
    Right ØHNW
  Omentum ØDNU
  Orbit
    Left ØNNQ
    Right ØNNP
  Ovary
    Bilateral ØUN2
    Left ØUN1
    Right ØUNØ
  Palate
    Hard ØCN2
    Soft ØCN3
  Pancreas ØFNG
  Para-aortic Body ØGN9
  Paraganglion Extremity ØGNF
  Parathyroid Gland ØGNR

Release — continued
  Parathyroid Gland — continued
    Inferior
      Left ØGNP
      Right ØGNN
    Multiple ØGNQ
    Superior
      Left ØGNM
      Right ØGNL
  Patella
    Left ØQNF
    Right ØQND
  Penis ØVNS
  Pericardium Ø2NN
  Peritoneum ØDNW
  Phalanx
    Finger
      Left ØPNV
      Right ØPNT
    Thumb
      Left ØPNS
      Right ØPNR
    Toe
      Left ØQNR
      Right ØQNQ
  Pharynx ØCNM
  Pineal Body ØGN1
  Pleura
    Left ØBNP
    Right ØBNN
  Pons ØØNB
  Prepuce ØVNT
  Prostate ØVNØ
  Radius
    Left ØPNJ
    Right ØPNH
  Rectum ØDNP
  Retina
    Left Ø8NF3ZZ
    Right Ø8NE3ZZ
  Retinal Vessel
    Left Ø8NH3ZZ
    Right Ø8NG3ZZ
  Ribs
    1 to 2 ØPN1
    3 or More ØPN2
  Sacrum ØQN1
  Scapula
    Left ØPN6
    Right ØPN5
  Sclera
    Left Ø8N7XZZ
    Right Ø8N6XZZ
  Scrotum ØVN5
  Septum
    Atrial Ø2N5
    Nasal Ø9NM
    Ventricular Ø2NM
  Sinus
    Accessory Ø9NP
    Ethmoid
      Left Ø9NV
      Right Ø9NU
    Frontal
      Left Ø9NT
      Right Ø9NS
    Mastoid
      Left Ø9NC
      Right Ø9NB
    Maxillary
      Left Ø9NR
      Right Ø9NQ
    Sphenoid
      Left Ø9NX
      Right Ø9NW
  Skin
    Abdomen ØHN7XZZ
    Back ØHN6XZZ
    Buttock ØHN8XZZ
    Chest ØHN5XZZ
    Ear
      Left ØHN3XZZ
      Right ØHN2XZZ
    Face ØHN1XZZ
    Foot
      Left ØHNNXZZ
      Right ØHNMXZZ
    Hand
      Left ØHNGXZZ

Release — *continued*
  Skin — *continued*
    Hand — *continued*
      Right 0HNFXZZ
      Inguinal 0HNAXZZ
     Lower Arm
      Left 0HNEXZZ
      Right 0HNDXZZ
     Lower Leg
      Left 0HNLXZZ
      Right 0HNKXZZ
     Neck 0HN4XZZ
     Perineum 0HN9XZZ
     Scalp 0HN0XZZ
     Upper Arm
      Left 0HNCXZZ
      Right 0HNBXZZ
     Upper Leg
      Left 0HNJXZZ
      Right 0HNHXZZ
  Spinal Cord
   Cervical 00NW
   Lumbar 00NY
   Thoracic 00NX
  Spinal Meninges 00NT
  Spleen 07NP
  Sternum 0PN0
  Stomach 0DN6
   Pylorus 0DN7
  Subcutaneous Tissue and Fascia
   Abdomen 0JN8
   Back 0JN7
   Buttock 0JN9
   Chest 0JN6
   Face 0JN1
   Foot
    Left 0JNR
    Right 0JNQ
   Hand
    Left 0JNK
    Right 0JNJ
   Lower Arm
    Left 0JNH
    Right 0JNG
   Lower Leg
    Left 0JNP
    Right 0JNN
   Neck
    Left 0JN5
    Right 0JN4
   Pelvic Region 0JNC
   Perineum 0JNB
   Scalp 0JN0
   Upper Arm
    Left 0JNF
    Right 0JND
   Upper Leg
    Left 0JNM
    Right 0JNL
  Tarsal
   Left 0QNM
   Right 0QNL
  Tendon
   Abdomen
    Left 0LNG
    Right 0LNF
   Ankle
    Left 0LNT
    Right 0LNS
   Foot
    Left 0LNW
    Right 0LNV
   Hand
    Left 0LN8
    Right 0LN7
   Head and Neck 0LN0
   Hip
    Left 0LNK
    Right 0LNJ
   Knee
    Left 0LNR
    Right 0LNQ
   Lower Arm and Wrist
    Left 0LN6
    Right 0LN5
   Lower Leg
    Left 0LNP
    Right 0LNN
   Perineum 0LNH

Release — *continued*
  Tendon — *continued*
   Shoulder
    Left 0LN2
    Right 0LN1
   Thorax
    Left 0LND
    Right 0LNC
   Trunk
    Left 0LNB
    Right 0LN9
   Upper Arm
    Left 0LN4
    Right 0LN3
   Upper Leg
    Left 0LNM
    Right 0LNL
  Testis
   Bilateral 0VNC
   Left 0VNB
   Right 0VN9
  Thalamus 00N9
  Thymus 07NM
  Thyroid Gland 0GNK
   Left Lobe 0GNG
   Right Lobe 0GNH
  Tibia
   Left 0QNH
   Right 0QNG
  Toe Nail 0HNRXZZ
  Tongue 0CN7
  Tonsils 0CNP
  Tooth
   Lower 0CNX
   Upper 0CNW
  Trachea 0BN1
  Tunica Vaginalis
   Left 0VN7
   Right 0VN6
  Turbinate, Nasal 09NL
  Tympanic Membrane
   Left 09N8
   Right 09N7
  Ulna
   Left 0PNL
   Right 0PNK
  Ureter
   Left 0TN7
   Right 0TN6
  Urethra 0TND
  Uterine Supporting Structure 0UN4
  Uterus 0UN9
  Uvula 0CNN
  Vagina 0UNG
  Valve
   Aortic 02NF
   Mitral 02NG
   Pulmonary 02NH
   Tricuspid 02NJ
  Vas Deferens
   Bilateral 0VNQ
   Left 0VNP
   Right 0VNN
  Vein
   Axillary
    Left 05N8
    Right 05N7
   Azygos 05N0
   Basilic
    Left 05NC
    Right 05NB
   Brachial
    Left 05NA
    Right 05N9
   Cephalic
    Left 05NF
    Right 05ND
   Colic 06N7
   Common Iliac
    Left 06ND
    Right 06NC
   Coronary 02N4
   Esophageal 06N3
   External Iliac
    Left 06NG
    Right 06NF
   External Jugular
    Left 05NQ
    Right 05NP

Release — *continued*
  Vein — *continued*
   Face
    Left 05NV
    Right 05NT
   Femoral
    Left 06NN
    Right 06NM
   Foot
    Left 06NV
    Right 06NT
   Gastric 06N2
   Hand
    Left 05NH
    Right 05NG
   Hemiazygos 05N1
   Hepatic 06N4
   Hypogastric
    Left 06NJ
    Right 06NH
   Inferior Mesenteric 06N6
   Innominate
    Left 05N4
    Right 05N3
   Internal Jugular
    Left 05NN
    Right 05NM
   Intracranial 05NL
   Lower 06NY
   Portal 06N8
   Pulmonary
    Left 02NT
    Right 02NS
   Renal
    Left 06NB
    Right 06N9
   Saphenous
    Left 06NQ
    Right 06NP
   Splenic 06N1
   Subclavian
    Left 05N6
    Right 05N5
   Superior Mesenteric 06N5
   Upper 05NY
   Vertebral
    Left 05NS
    Right 05NR
  Vena Cava
   Inferior 06N0
   Superior 02NV
  Ventricle
   Left 02NL
   Right 02NK
  Vertebra
   Cervical 0PN3
   Lumbar 0QN0
   Thoracic 0PN4
  Vesicle
   Bilateral 0VN3
   Left 0VN2
   Right 0VN1
  Vitreous
   Left 08N53ZZ
   Right 08N43ZZ
  Vocal Cord
   Left 0CNV
   Right 0CNT
  Vulva 0UNM
Relocation *see* Reposition
Remdesivir Anti-infective XW0
Removal
  Abdominal Wall 2W53X
  Anorectal 2Y53X5Z
  Arm
   Lower
    Left 2W5DX
    Right 2W5CX
   Upper
    Left 2W5BX
    Right 2W5AX
  Back 2W55X
  Chest Wall 2W54X
  Ear 2Y52X5Z
  Extremity
   Lower
    Left 2W5MX
    Right 2W5LX

Subterms under main terms may continue to next column or page

Removal — *continued*
  Extremity — *continued*
    Upper
      Left 2W59X
      Right 2W58X
  Face 2W51X
  Finger
    Left 2W5KX
    Right 2W5JX
  Foot
    Left 2W5TX
    Right 2W5SX
  Genital Tract, Female 2Y54X5Z
  Hand
    Left 2W5FX
    Right 2W5EX
  Head 2W50X
  Inguinal Region
    Left 2W57X
    Right 2W56X
  Leg
    Lower
      Left 2W5RX
      Right 2W5QX
    Upper
      Left 2W5PX
      Right 2W5NX
  Mouth and Pharynx 2Y50X5Z
  Nasal 2Y51X5Z
  Neck 2W52X
  Thumb
    Left 2W5HX
    Right 2W5GX
  Toe
    Left 2W5VX
    Right 2W5UX
  Urethra 2Y55X5Z

Removal of device from
  Abdominal Wall ØWPF
  Acetabulum
    Left ØQP5
    Right ØQP4
  Anal Sphincter ØDPR
  Anus ØDPQ
  Aorta, Thoracic, Descending Ø2PW3RZ
  Artery
    Lower Ø4PY
    Upper Ø3PY
  Back
    Lower ØWPL
    Upper ØWPK
  Bladder ØTPB
  Bone
    Facial ØNPW
    Lower ØQPY
    Nasal ØNPB
    Pelvic
      Left ØQP3
      Right ØQP2
    Upper ØPPY
  Bone Marrow Ø7PT
  Brain ØØPØ
  Breast
    Left ØHPU
    Right ØHPT
  Bursa and Ligament
    Lower ØMPY
    Upper ØMPX
  Carpal
    Left ØPPN
    Right ØPPM
  Cavity, Cranial ØWP1
  Cerebral Ventricle ØØP6
  Chest Wall ØWP8
  Cisterna Chyli Ø7PL
  Clavicle
    Left ØPPB
    Right ØPP9
  Coccyx ØQPS
  Diaphragm ØBPT
  Disc
    Cervical Vertebral ØRP3
    Cervicothoracic Vertebral ØRP5
    Lumbar Vertebral ØSP2
    Lumbosacral ØSP4
    Thoracic Vertebral ØRP9
    Thoracolumbar Vertebral ØRPB
  Duct
    Hepatobiliary ØFPB

Removal of device from — *continued*
  Duct — *continued*
    Pancreatic ØFPD
  Ear
    Inner
      Left Ø9PJ
      Right Ø9PD
    Left Ø9PJ
    Right Ø9PH
  Epididymis and Spermatic Cord ØVPM
  Esophagus ØDP5
  Extremity
    Lower
      Left ØYPB
      Right ØYP9
    Upper
      Left ØXP7
      Right ØXP6
  Eye
    Left Ø8P1
    Right Ø8PØ
  Face ØWP2
  Fallopian Tube ØUP8
  Femoral Shaft
    Left ØQP9
    Right ØQP8
  Femur
    Lower
      Left ØQPC
      Right ØQPB
    Upper
      Left ØQP7
      Right ØQP6
  Fibula
    Left ØQPK
    Right ØQPJ
  Finger Nail ØHPQX
  Gallbladder ØFP4
  Gastrointestinal Tract ØWPP
  Genitourinary Tract ØWPR
  Gland
    Adrenal ØGP5
    Endocrine ØGPS
    Pituitary ØGPØ
    Salivary ØCPA
  Glenoid Cavity
    Left ØPP8
    Right ØPP7
  Great Vessel Ø2PY
  Hair ØHPSX
  Head ØWPØ
  Heart Ø2PA
  Humeral Head
    Left ØPPD
    Right ØPPC
  Humeral Shaft
    Left ØPPG
    Right ØPPF
  Intestinal Tract
    Lower Intestinal Tract ØDPD
    Upper Intestinal Tract ØDPØ
  Jaw
    Lower ØWP5
    Upper ØWP4
  Joint
    Acromioclavicular
      Left ØRPH
      Right ØRPG
    Ankle
      Left ØSPG
      Right ØSPF
    Carpal
      Left ØRPR
      Right ØRPQ
    Carpometacarpal
      Left ØRPT
      Right ØRPS
    Cervical Vertebral ØRP1
    Cervicothoracic Vertebral ØRP4
    Coccygeal ØSP6
    Elbow
      Left ØRPM
      Right ØRPL
    Finger Phalangeal
      Left ØRPX
      Right ØRPW
    Hip
      Left ØSPB
        Acetabular Surface ØSPE

Removal of device from — *continued*
  Joint — *continued*
    Hip — *continued*
      Left — *continued*
        Femoral Surface ØSPS
      Right ØSP9
        Acetabular Surface ØSPA
        Femoral Surface ØSPR
    Knee
      Left ØSPD
        Femoral Surface ØSPU
        Tibial Surface ØSPW
      Right ØSPC
        Femoral Surface ØSPT
        Tibial Surface ØSPV
    Lumbar Vertebral ØSPØ
    Lumbosacral ØSP3
    Metacarpophalangeal
      Left ØRPV
      Right ØRPU
    Metatarsal-Phalangeal
      Left ØSPN
      Right ØSPM
    Occipital-cervical ØRPØ
    Sacrococcygeal ØSP5
    Sacroiliac
      Left ØSP8
      Right ØSP7
    Shoulder
      Left ØRPK
      Right ØRPJ
    Sternoclavicular
      Left ØRPF
      Right ØRPE
    Tarsal
      Left ØSPJ
      Right ØSPH
    Tarsometatarsal
      Left ØSPL
      Right ØSPK
    Temporomandibular
      Left ØRPD
      Right ØRPC
    Thoracic Vertebral ØRP6
    Thoracolumbar Vertebral ØRPA
    Toe Phalangeal
      Left ØSPQ
      Right ØSPP
    Wrist
      Left ØRPP
      Right ØRPN
  Kidney ØTP5
  Larynx ØCPS
  Lens
    Left Ø8PK3
    Right Ø8PJ3
  Liver ØFPØ
  Lung
    Left ØBPL
    Right ØBPK
  Lymphatic Ø7PN
    Thoracic Duct Ø7PK
  Mediastinum ØWPC
  Mesentery ØDPV
  Metacarpal
    Left ØPPQ
    Right ØPPP
  Metatarsal
    Left ØQPP
    Right ØQPN
  Mouth and Throat ØCPY
  Muscle
    Extraocular
      Left Ø8PM
      Right Ø8PL
    Lower ØKPY
    Upper ØKPX
  Nasal Mucosa and Soft Tissue Ø9PK
  Neck ØWP6
  Nerve
    Cranial ØØPE
    Peripheral Ø1PY
  Omentum ØDPU
  Ovary ØUP3
  Pancreas ØFPG
  Parathyroid Gland ØGPR
  Patella
    Left ØQPF
    Right ØQPD

Removal of device from — *continued*
Pelvic Cavity 0WPJ
Penis 0VPS
Pericardial Cavity 0WPD
Perineum
  Female 0WPN
  Male 0WPM
Peritoneal Cavity 0WPG
Peritoneum 0DPW
Phalanx
  Finger
    Left 0PPV
    Right 0PPT
  Thumb
    Left 0PPS
    Right 0PPR
  Toe
    Left 0QPR
    Right 0QPQ
Pineal Body 0GP1
Pleura 0BPQ
Pleural Cavity
  Left 0WPB
  Right 0WP9
Products of Conception 10P0
Prostate and Seminal Vesicles 0VP4
Radius
  Left 0PPJ
  Right 0PPH
Rectum 0DPP
Respiratory Tract 0WPQ
Retroperitoneum 0WPH
Ribs
  1 to 2 0PP1
  3 or More 0PP2
Sacrum 0QP1
Scapula
  Left 0PP6
  Right 0PP5
Scrotum and Tunica Vaginalis 0VP8
Sinus 09PY
Skin 0HPPX
Skull 0NP0
Spinal Canal 00PU
Spinal Cord 00PV
Spleen 07PP
Sternum 0PP0
Stomach 0DP6
Subcutaneous Tissue and Fascia
  Head and Neck 0JPS
  Lower Extremity 0JPW
  Trunk 0JPT
  Upper Extremity 0JPV
Tarsal
  Left 0QPM
  Right 0QPL
Tendon
  Lower 0LPY
  Upper 0LPX
Testis 0VPD
Thymus 07PM
Thyroid Gland 0GPK
Tibia
  Left 0QPH
  Right 0QPG
Toe Nail 0HPRX
Trachea 0BP1
Tracheobronchial Tree 0BP0
Tympanic Membrane
  Left 09P8
  Right 09P7
Ulna
  Left 0PPL
  Right 0PPK
Ureter 0TP9
Urethra 0TPD
Uterus and Cervix 0UPD
Vagina and Cul-de-sac 0UPH
Vas Deferens 0VPR
Vein
  Azygos 05P0
  Innominate
    Left 05P4
    Right 05P3
  Lower 06PY
  Upper 05PY
Vertebra
  Cervical 0PP3
  Lumbar 0QP0

Removal of device from — *continued*
Vertebra — *continued*
  Thoracic 0PP4
Vulva 0UPM
Renal calyx
use Kidney
use Kidney, Left
use Kidney, Right
use Kidneys, Bilateral
Renal capsule
use Kidney
use Kidney, Left
use Kidney, Right
use Kidneys, Bilateral
Renal cortex
use Kidney
use Kidney, Left
use Kidney, Right
use Kidneys, Bilateral
Renal dialysis *see* Performance, Urinary 5A1D
Renal nerve *use* Abdominal Sympathetic Nerve
Renal plexus *use* Abdominal Sympathetic Nerve
Renal segment
use Kidney
use Kidney, Left
use Kidney, Right
use Kidneys, Bilateral
Renal segmental artery
use Renal Artery, Left
use Renal Artery, Right
Reopening, operative site
  Control of bleeding *see* Control bleeding in
  Inspection only *see* Inspection
Repair
Abdominal Wall 0WQF
Acetabulum
  Left 0QQ5
  Right 0QQ4
Adenoids 0CQQ
Ampulla of Vater 0FQC
Anal Sphincter 0DQR
Ankle Region
  Left 0YQL
  Right 0YQK
Anterior Chamber
  Left 08Q33ZZ
  Right 08Q23ZZ
Anus 0DQQ
Aorta
  Abdominal 04Q0
  Thoracic
    Ascending/Arch 02QX
    Descending 02QW
Aortic Body 0GQD
Appendix 0DQJ
Arm
  Lower
    Left 0XQF
    Right 0XQD
  Upper
    Left 0XQ9
    Right 0XQ8
Artery
  Anterior Tibial
    Left 04QQ
    Right 04QP
  Axillary
    Left 03Q6
    Right 03Q5
  Brachial
    Left 03Q8
    Right 03Q7
  Celiac 04Q1
  Colic
    Left 04Q7
    Middle 04Q8
    Right 04Q6
  Common Carotid
    Left 03QJ
    Right 03QH
  Common Iliac
    Left 04QD
    Right 04QC
  Coronary
    Four or More Arteries 02Q3
    One Artery 02Q0
    Three Arteries 02Q2
    Two Arteries 02Q1

Repair — *continued*
Artery — *continued*
  External Carotid
    Left 03QN
    Right 03QM
  External Iliac
    Left 04QJ
    Right 04QH
  Face 03QR
  Femoral
    Left 04QL
    Right 04QK
  Foot
    Left 04QW
    Right 04QV
  Gastric 04Q2
  Hand
    Left 03QF
    Right 03QD
  Hepatic 04Q3
  Inferior Mesenteric 04QB
  Innominate 03Q2
  Internal Carotid
    Left 03QL
    Right 03QK
  Internal Iliac
    Left 04QF
    Right 04QE
  Internal Mammary
    Left 03Q1
    Right 03Q0
  Intracranial 03QG
  Lower 04QY
  Peroneal
    Left 04QU
    Right 04QT
  Popliteal
    Left 04QN
    Right 04QM
  Posterior Tibial
    Left 04QS
    Right 04QR
  Pulmonary
    Left 02QR
    Right 02QQ
  Pulmonary Trunk 02QP
  Radial
    Left 03QC
    Right 03QB
  Renal
    Left 04QA
    Right 04Q9
  Splenic 04Q4
  Subclavian
    Left 03Q4
    Right 03Q3
  Superior Mesenteric 04Q5
  Temporal
    Left 03QT
    Right 03QS
  Thyroid
    Left 03QV
    Right 03QU
  Ulnar
    Left 03QA
    Right 03Q9
  Upper 03QY
  Vertebral
    Left 03QQ
    Right 03QP
Atrium
  Left 02Q7
  Right 02Q6
Auditory Ossicle
  Left 09QA
  Right 09Q9
Axilla
  Left 0XQ5
  Right 0XQ4
Back
  Lower 0WQL
  Upper 0WQK
Basal Ganglia 00Q8
Bladder 0TQB
Bladder Neck 0TQC
Bone
  Ethmoid
    Left 0NQG
    Right 0NQF

Repair — continued

Bone — continued
Frontal ØNQ1
Hyoid ØNQX
Lacrimal
  Left ØNQJ
  Right ØNQH
Nasal ØNQB
Occipital ØNQ7
Palatine
  Left ØNQL
  Right ØNQK
Parietal
  Left ØNQ4
  Right ØNQ3
Pelvic
  Left ØQQ3
  Right ØQQ2
Sphenoid ØNQC
Temporal
  Left ØNQ6
  Right ØNQ5
Zygomatic
  Left ØNQN
  Right ØNQM
Brain ØØQØ
Breast
  Bilateral ØHQV
  Left ØHQU
  Right ØHQT
  Supernumerary ØHQY
Bronchus
  Lingula ØBQ9
  Lower Lobe
    Left ØBQB
    Right ØBQ6
  Main
    Left ØBQ7
    Right ØBQ3
  Middle Lobe, Right ØBQ5
  Upper Lobe
    Left ØBQ8
    Right ØBQ4
Buccal Mucosa ØCQ4
Bursa and Ligament
  Abdomen
    Left ØMQJ
    Right ØMQH
  Ankle
    Left ØMQR
    Right ØMQQ
  Elbow
    Left ØMQ4
    Right ØMQ3
  Foot
    Left ØMQT
    Right ØMQS
  Hand
    Left ØMQ8
    Right ØMQ7
  Head and Neck ØMQØ
  Hip
    Left ØMQM
    Right ØMQL
  Knee
    Left ØMQP
    Right ØMQN
  Lower Extremity
    Left ØMQW
    Right ØMQV
  Perineum ØMQK
  Rib(s) ØMQG
  Shoulder
    Left ØMQ2
    Right ØMQ1
  Spine
    Lower ØMQD
    Upper ØMQC
  Sternum ØMQF
  Upper Extremity
    Left ØMQB
    Right ØMQ9
  Wrist
    Left ØMQ6
    Right ØMQ5
Buttock
  Left ØYQ1
  Right ØYQØ
Carina ØBQ2

Repair — continued

Carotid Bodies, Bilateral ØGQ8
Carotid Body
  Left ØGQ6
  Right ØGQ7
Carpal
  Left ØPQN
  Right ØPQM
Cecum ØDQH
Cerebellum ØØQC
Cerebral Hemisphere ØØQ7
Cerebral Meninges ØØQ1
Cerebral Ventricle ØØQ6
Cervix ØUQC
Chest Wall ØWQ8
Chordae Tendineae Ø2Q9
Choroid
  Left Ø8QB
  Right Ø8QA
Cisterna Chyli Ø7QL
Clavicle
  Left ØPQB
  Right ØPQ9
Clitoris ØUQJ
Coccygeal Glomus ØGQB
Coccyx ØQQS
Colon
  Ascending ØDQK
  Descending ØDQM
  Sigmoid ØDQN
  Transverse ØDQL
Conduction Mechanism Ø2Q8
Conjunctiva
  Left Ø8QTXZZ
  Right Ø8QSXZZ
Cord
  Bilateral ØVQH
  Left ØVQG
  Right ØVQF
Cornea
  Left Ø8Q9XZZ
  Right Ø8Q8XZZ
Cul-de-sac ØUQF
Diaphragm ØBQT
Disc
  Cervical Vertebral ØRQ3
  Cervicothoracic Vertebral ØRQ5
  Lumbar Vertebral ØSQ2
  Lumbosacral ØSQ4
  Thoracic Vertebral ØRQ9
  Thoracolumbar Vertebral ØRQB
Duct
  Common Bile ØFQ9
  Cystic ØFQ8
  Hepatic
    Common ØFQ7
    Left ØFQ6
    Right ØFQ5
  Lacrimal
    Left Ø8QY
    Right Ø8QX
  Pancreatic ØFQD
    Accessory ØFQF
  Parotid
    Left ØCQC
    Right ØCQB
Duodenum ØDQ9
Dura Mater ØØQ2
Ear
  External
    Bilateral Ø9Q2
    Left Ø9Q1
    Right Ø9QØ
  External Auditory Canal
    Left Ø9Q4
    Right Ø9Q3
  Inner
    Left Ø9QE
    Right Ø9QD
  Middle
    Left Ø9Q6
    Right Ø9Q5
Elbow Region
  Left ØXQC
  Right ØXQB
Epididymis
  Bilateral ØVQL
  Left ØVQK
  Right ØVQJ

Repair — continued

Epiglottis ØCQR
Esophagogastric Junction ØDQ4
Esophagus ØDQ5
  Lower ØDQ3
  Middle ØDQ2
  Upper ØDQ1
Eustachian Tube
  Left Ø9QG
  Right Ø9QF
Extremity
  Lower
    Left ØYQB
    Right ØYQ9
  Upper
    Left ØXQ7
    Right ØXQ6
Eye
  Left Ø8Q1XZZ
  Right Ø8QØXZZ
Eyelid
  Lower
    Left Ø8QR
    Right Ø8QQ
  Upper
    Left Ø8QP
    Right Ø8QN
Face ØWQ2
Fallopian Tube
  Left ØUQ6
  Right ØUQ5
Fallopian Tubes, Bilateral ØUQ7
Femoral Region
  Bilateral ØYQE
  Left ØYQ8
  Right ØYQ7
Femoral Shaft
  Left ØQQ9
  Right ØQQ8
Femur
  Lower
    Left ØQQC
    Right ØQQB
  Upper
    Left ØQQ7
    Right ØQQ6
Fibula
  Left ØQQK
  Right ØQQJ
Finger
  Index
    Left ØXQP
    Right ØXQN
  Little
    Left ØXQW
    Right ØXQV
  Middle
    Left ØXQR
    Right ØXQQ
  Ring
    Left ØXQT
    Right ØXQS
Finger Nail ØHQQXZZ
Floor of mouth *see* Repair, Oral Cavity and Throat ØWQ3
Foot
  Left ØYQN
  Right ØYQM
Gallbladder ØFQ4
Gingiva
  Lower ØCQ6
  Upper ØCQ5
Gland
  Adrenal
    Bilateral ØGQ4
    Left ØGQ2
    Right ØGQ3
  Lacrimal
    Left Ø8QW
    Right Ø8QV
  Minor Salivary ØCQJ
  Parotid
    Left ØCQ9
    Right ØCQ8
  Pituitary ØGQØ
  Sublingual
    Left ØCQF
    Right ØCQD

Repair — *continued*
  Gland — *continued*
    Submaxillary
      Left 0CQH
      Right 0CQG
    Vestibular 0UQL
  Glenoid Cavity
    Left 0PQ8
    Right 0PQ7
  Glomus Jugulare 0GQC
  Hand
    Left 0XQK
    Right 0XQJ
  Head 0WQ0
  Heart 02QA
    Left 02QC
    Right 02QB
  Humeral Head
    Left 0PQD
    Right 0PQC
  Humeral Shaft
    Left 0PQG
    Right 0PQF
  Hymen 0UQK
  Hypothalamus 00QA
  Ileocecal Valve 0DQC
  Ileum 0DQB
  Inguinal Region
    Bilateral 0YQA
    Left 0YQ6
    Right 0YQ5
  Intestine
    Large 0DQE
      Left 0DQG
      Right 0DQF
    Small 0DQ8
  Iris
    Left 08QD3ZZ
    Right 08QC3ZZ
  Jaw
    Lower 0WQ5
    Upper 0WQ4
  Jejunum 0DQA
  Joint
    Acromioclavicular
      Left 0RQH
      Right 0RQG
    Ankle
      Left 0SQG
      Right 0SQF
    Carpal
      Left 0RQR
      Right 0RQQ
    Carpometacarpal
      Left 0RQT
      Right 0RQS
    Cervical Vertebral 0RQ1
    Cervicothoracic Vertebral 0RQ4
    Coccygeal 0SQ6
    Elbow
      Left 0RQM
      Right 0RQL
    Finger Phalangeal
      Left 0RQX
      Right 0RQW
    Hip
      Left 0SQB
      Right 0SQ9
    Knee
      Left 0SQD
      Right 0SQC
    Lumbar Vertebral 0SQ0
    Lumbosacral 0SQ3
    Metacarpophalangeal
      Left 0RQV
      Right 0RQU
    Metatarsal-Phalangeal
      Left 0SQN
      Right 0SQM
    Occipital-cervical 0RQ0
    Sacrococcygeal 0SQ5
    Sacroiliac
      Left 0SQ8
      Right 0SQ7
    Shoulder
      Left 0RQK
      Right 0RQJ
    Sternoclavicular
      Left 0RQF

Repair — *continued*
  Joint — *continued*
    Sternoclavicular — *continued*
      Right 0RQE
    Tarsal
      Left 0SQJ
      Right 0SQH
    Tarsometatarsal
      Left 0SQL
      Right 0SQK
    Temporomandibular
      Left 0RQD
      Right 0RQC
    Thoracic Vertebral 0RQ6
    Thoracolumbar Vertebral 0RQA
    Toe Phalangeal
      Left 0SQQ
      Right 0SQP
    Wrist
      Left 0RQP
      Right 0RQN
  Kidney
    Left 0TQ1
    Right 0TQ0
  Kidney Pelvis
    Left 0TQ4
    Right 0TQ3
  Knee Region
    Left 0YQG
    Right 0YQF
  Larynx 0CQS
  Leg
    Lower
      Left 0YQJ
      Right 0YQH
    Upper
      Left 0YQD
      Right 0YQC
  Lens
    Left 08QK3ZZ
    Right 08QJ3ZZ
  Lip
    Lower 0CQ1
    Upper 0CQ0
  Liver 0FQ0
    Left Lobe 0FQ2
    Right Lobe 0FQ1
  Lung
    Bilateral 0BQM
    Left 0BQL
    Lower Lobe
      Left 0BQJ
      Right 0BQF
    Middle Lobe, Right 0BQD
    Right 0BQK
    Upper Lobe
      Left 0BQG
      Right 0BQC
  Lung Lingula 0BQH
  Lymphatic
    Aortic 07QD
    Axillary
      Left 07Q6
      Right 07Q5
    Head 07Q0
    Inguinal
      Left 07QJ
      Right 07QH
    Internal Mammary
      Left 07Q9
      Right 07Q8
    Lower Extremity
      Left 07QG
      Right 07QF
    Mesenteric 07QB
    Neck
      Left 07Q2
      Right 07Q1
    Pelvis 07QC
    Thoracic Duct 07QK
    Thorax 07Q7
    Upper Extremity
      Left 07Q4
      Right 07Q3
  Mandible
    Left 0NQV
    Right 0NQT
  Maxilla 0NQR
  Mediastinum 0WQC

Repair — *continued*
  Medulla Oblongata 00QD
  Mesentery 0DQV
  Metacarpal
    Left 0PQQ
    Right 0PQP
  Metatarsal
    Left 0QQP
    Right 0QQN
  Muscle
    Abdomen
      Left 0KQL
      Right 0KQK
    Extraocular
      Left 08QM
      Right 08QL
    Facial 0KQ1
    Foot
      Left 0KQW
      Right 0KQV
    Hand
      Left 0KQD
      Right 0KQC
    Head 0KQ0
    Hip
      Left 0KQP
      Right 0KQN
    Lower Arm and Wrist
      Left 0KQB
      Right 0KQ9
    Lower Leg
      Left 0KQT
      Right 0KQS
    Neck
      Left 0KQ3
      Right 0KQ2
    Papillary 02QD
    Perineum 0KQM
    Shoulder
      Left 0KQ6
      Right 0KQ5
    Thorax
      Left 0KQJ
      Right 0KQH
    Tongue, Palate, Pharynx 0KQ4
    Trunk
      Left 0KQG
      Right 0KQF
    Upper Arm
      Left 0KQ8
      Right 0KQ7
    Upper Leg
      Left 0KQR
      Right 0KQQ
  Nasal Mucosa and Soft Tissue 09QK
  Nasopharynx 09QN
  Neck 0WQ6
  Nerve
    Abdominal Sympathetic 01QM
    Abducens 00QL
    Accessory 00QR
    Acoustic 00QN
    Brachial Plexus 01Q3
    Cervical 01Q1
    Cervical Plexus 01Q0
    Facial 00QM
    Femoral 01QD
    Glossopharyngeal 00QP
    Head and Neck Sympathetic 01QK
    Hypoglossal 00QS
    Lumbar 01Q8
    Lumbar Plexus 01Q9
    Lumbar Sympathetic 01QN
    Lumbosacral Plexus 01QA
    Median 01Q5
    Oculomotor 00QH
    Olfactory 00QF
    Optic 00QG
    Peroneal 01QH
    Phrenic 01Q2
    Pudendal 01QC
    Radial 01Q6
    Sacral 01QR
    Sacral Plexus 01QQ
    Sacral Sympathetic 01QP
    Sciatic 01QF
    Thoracic 01Q8
    Thoracic Sympathetic 01QL
    Tibial 01QG

Repair — continued
 Nerve — continued
  Trigeminal ØØQK
  Trochlear ØØQJ
  Ulnar Ø1Q4
  Vagus ØØQQ
 Nipple
  Left ØHQX
  Right ØHQW
 Omentum ØDQU
 Oral Cavity and Throat ØWQ3
 Orbit
  Left ØNQQ
  Right ØNQP
 Ovary
  Bilateral ØUQ2
  Left ØUQ1
  Right ØUQØ
 Palate
  Hard ØCQ2
  Soft ØCQ3
 Pancreas ØFQG
 Para-aortic Body ØGQ9
 Paraganglion Extremity ØGQF
 Parathyroid Gland ØGQR
  Inferior
   Left ØGQP
   Right ØGQN
  Multiple ØGQQ
  Superior
   Left ØGQM
   Right ØGQL
 Patella
  Left ØQQF
  Right ØQQD
 Penis ØVQS
 Pericardium Ø2QN
 Perineum
  Female ØWQN
  Male ØWQM
 Peritoneum ØDQW
 Phalanx
  Finger
   Left ØPQV
   Right ØPQT
  Thumb
   Left ØPQS
   Right ØPQR
  Toe
   Left ØQQR
   Right ØQQQ
 Pharynx ØCQM
 Pineal Body ØGQ1
 Pleura
  Left ØBQP
  Right ØBQN
 Pons ØØQB
 Prepuce ØVQT
 Products of Conception 1ØQØ
 Prostate ØVQØ
 Radius
  Left ØPQJ
  Right ØPQH
 Rectum ØDQP
 Retina
  Left Ø8QF3ZZ
  Right Ø8QE3ZZ
 Retinal Vessel
  Left Ø8QH3ZZ
  Right Ø8QG3ZZ
 Ribs
  1 to 2 ØPQ1
  3 or More ØPQ2
 Sacrum ØQQ1
 Scapula
  Left ØPQ6
  Right ØPQ5
 Sclera
  Left Ø8Q7XZZ
  Right Ø8Q6XZZ
 Scrotum ØVQ5
 Septum
  Atrial Ø2Q5
  Nasal Ø9QM
  Ventricular Ø2QM
 Shoulder Region
  Left ØXQ3
  Right ØXQ2

Repair — continued
 Sinus
  Accessory Ø9QP
  Ethmoid
   Left Ø9QV
   Right Ø9QU
  Frontal
   Left Ø9QT
   Right Ø9QS
  Mastoid
   Left Ø9QC
   Right Ø9QB
  Maxillary
   Left Ø9QR
   Right Ø9QQ
  Sphenoid
   Left Ø9QX
   Right Ø9QW
 Skin
  Abdomen ØHQ7XZZ
  Back ØHQ6XZZ
  Buttock ØHQ8XZZ
  Chest ØHQ5XZZ
  Ear
   Left ØHQ3XZZ
   Right ØHQ2XZZ
  Face ØHQ1XZZ
  Foot
   Left ØHQNXZZ
   Right ØHQMXZZ
  Hand
   Left ØHQGXZZ
   Right ØHQFXZZ
  Inguinal ØHQAXZZ
  Lower Arm
   Left ØHQEXZZ
   Right ØHQDXZZ
  Lower Leg
   Left ØHQLXZZ
   Right ØHQKXZZ
  Neck ØHQ4XZZ
  Perineum ØHQ9XZZ
  Scalp ØHQØXZZ
  Upper Arm
   Left ØHQCXZZ
   Right ØHQBXZZ
  Upper Leg
   Left ØHQJXZZ
   Right ØHQHXZZ
 Skull ØNQØ
 Spinal Cord
  Cervical ØØQW
  Lumbar ØØQY
  Thoracic ØØQX
 Spinal Meninges ØØQT
 Spleen Ø7QP
 Sternum ØPQØ
 Stomach ØDQ6
  Pylorus ØDQ7
 Subcutaneous Tissue and Fascia
  Abdomen ØJQ8
  Back ØJQ7
  Buttock ØJQ9
  Chest ØJQ6
  Face ØJQ1
  Foot
   Left ØJQR
   Right ØJQQ
  Hand
   Left ØJQK
   Right ØJQJ
  Lower Arm
   Left ØJQH
   Right ØJQG
  Lower Leg
   Left ØJQP
   Right ØJQN
  Neck
   Left ØJQ5
   Right ØJQ4
  Pelvic Region ØJQC
  Perineum ØJQB
  Scalp ØJQØ
  Upper Arm
   Left ØJQF
   Right ØJQD
  Upper Leg
   Left ØJQM
   Right ØJQL

Repair — continued
 Tarsal
  Left ØQQM
  Right ØQQL
 Tendon
  Abdomen
   Left ØLQG
   Right ØLQF
  Ankle
   Left ØLQT
   Right ØLQS
  Foot
   Left ØLQW
   Right ØLQV
  Hand
   Left ØLQ8
   Right ØLQ7
  Head and Neck ØLQØ
  Hip
   Left ØLQK
   Right ØLQJ
  Knee
   Left ØLQR
   Right ØLQQ
  Lower Arm and Wrist
   Left ØLQ6
   Right ØLQ5
  Lower Leg
   Left ØLQP
   Right ØLQN
  Perineum ØLQH
  Shoulder
   Left ØLQ2
   Right ØLQ1
  Thorax
   Left ØLQD
   Right ØLQC
  Trunk
   Left ØLQB
   Right ØLQ9
  Upper Arm
   Left ØLQ4
   Right ØLQ3
  Upper Leg
   Left ØLQM
   Right ØLQL
 Testis
  Bilateral ØVQC
  Left ØVQB
  Right ØVQ9
 Thalamus ØØQ9
 Thumb
  Left ØXQM
  Right ØXQL
 Thymus Ø7QM
 Thyroid Gland ØGQK
  Left Lobe ØGQG
  Right Lobe ØGQH
 Thyroid Gland Isthmus ØGQJ
 Tibia
  Left ØQQH
  Right ØQQG
 Toe
  1st
   Left ØYQQ
   Right ØYQP
  2nd
   Left ØYQS
   Right ØYQR
  3rd
   Left ØYQU
   Right ØYQT
  4th
   Left ØYQW
   Right ØYQV
  5th
   Left ØYQY
   Right ØYQX
 Toe Nail ØHQRXZZ
 Tongue ØCQ7
 Tonsils ØCQP
 Tooth
  Lower ØCQX
  Upper ØCQW
 Trachea ØBQ1
 Tunica Vaginalis
  Left ØVQ7
  Right ØVQ6
 Turbinate, Nasal Ø9QL

Index

Repair — Repair

Repair — *continued*
    Tympanic Membrane
        Left 09Q8
        Right 09Q7
    Ulna
        Left 0PQL
        Right 0PQK
    Ureter
        Left 0TQ7
        Right 0TQ6
    Urethra 0TQD
    Uterine Supporting Structure 0UQ4
    Uterus 0UQ9
    Uvula 0CQN
    Vagina 0UQG
    Valve
        Aortic 02QF
        Mitral 02QG
        Pulmonary 02QH
        Tricuspid 02QJ
    Vas Deferens
        Bilateral 0VQQ
        Left 0VQP
        Right 0VQN
    Vein
        Axillary
            Left 05Q8
            Right 05Q7
        Azygos 05Q0
        Basilic
            Left 05QC
            Right 05QB
        Brachial
            Left 05QA
            Right 05Q9
        Cephalic
            Left 05QF
            Right 05QD
        Colic 06Q7
        Common Iliac
            Left 06QD
            Right 06QC
        Coronary 02Q4
        Esophageal 06Q3
        External Iliac
            Left 06QG
            Right 06QF
        External Jugular
            Left 05QQ
            Right 05QP
        Face
            Left 05QV
            Right 05QT
        Femoral
            Left 06QN
            Right 06QM
        Foot
            Left 06QV
            Right 06QT
        Gastric 06Q2
        Hand
            Left 05QH
            Right 05QG
        Hemiazygos 05Q1
        Hepatic 06Q4
        Hypogastric
            Left 06QJ
            Right 06QH
        Inferior Mesenteric 06Q6
        Innominate
            Left 05Q4
            Right 05Q3
        Internal Jugular
            Left 05QN
            Right 05QM
        Intracranial 05QL
        Lower 06QY
        Portal 06Q8
        Pulmonary
            Left 02QT
            Right 02QS
        Renal
            Left 06QB
            Right 06Q9
        Saphenous
            Left 06QQ
            Right 06QP
        Splenic 06Q1

Repair — *continued*
    Vein — *continued*
        Subclavian
            Left 05Q6
            Right 05Q5
        Superior Mesenteric 06Q5
        Upper 05QY
        Vertebral
            Left 05QS
            Right 05QR
    Vena Cava
        Inferior 06Q0
        Superior 02QV
    Ventricle
        Left 02QL
        Right 02QK
    Vertebra
        Cervical 0PQ3
        Lumbar 0QQ0
        Thoracic 0PQ4
    Vesicle
        Bilateral 0VQ3
        Left 0VQ2
        Right 0VQ1
    Vitreous
        Left 08Q53ZZ
        Right 08Q43ZZ
    Vocal Cord
        Left 0CQV
        Right 0CQT
    Vulva 0UQM
    Wrist Region
        Left 0XQH
        Right 0XQG

Repair, obstetric laceration, periurethral 0UQMXZZ
Replacement
    Acetabulum
        Left 0QR5
        Right 0QR4
    Ampulla of Vater 0FRC
    Anal Sphincter 0DRR
    Aorta
        Abdominal 04R0
        Thoracic
            Ascending/Arch 02RX
            Descending 02RW
    Artery
        Anterior Tibial
            Left 04RQ
            Right 04RP
        Axillary
            Left 03R6
            Right 03R5
        Brachial
            Left 03R8
            Right 03R7
        Celiac 04R1
        Colic
            Left 04R7
            Middle 04R8
            Right 04R6
        Common Carotid
            Left 03RJ
            Right 03RH
        Common Iliac
            Left 04RD
            Right 04RC
        External Carotid
            Left 03RN
            Right 03RM
        External Iliac
            Left 04RJ
            Right 04RH
        Face 03RR
        Femoral
            Left 04RL
            Right 04RK
        Foot
            Left 04RW
            Right 04RV
        Gastric 04R2
        Hand
            Left 03RF
            Right 03RD
        Hepatic 04R3
        Inferior Mesenteric 04RB
        Innominate 03R2
        Internal Carotid
            Left 03RL

Replacement — *continued*
    Artery — *continued*
        Internal Carotid — *continued*
            Right 03RK
        Internal Iliac
            Left 04RF
            Right 04RE
        Internal Mammary
            Left 03R1
            Right 03R0
        Intracranial 03RG
        Lower 04RY
        Peroneal
            Left 04RU
            Right 04RT
        Popliteal
            Left 04RN
            Right 04RM
        Posterior Tibial
            Left 04RS
            Right 04RR
        Pulmonary
            Left 02RR
            Right 02RQ
        Pulmonary Trunk 02RP
        Radial
            Left 03RC
            Right 03RB
        Renal
            Left 04RA
            Right 04R9
        Splenic 04R4
        Subclavian
            Left 03R4
            Right 03R3
        Superior Mesenteric 04R5
        Temporal
            Left 03RT
            Right 03RS
        Thyroid
            Left 03RV
            Right 03RU
        Ulnar
            Left 03RA
            Right 03R9
        Upper 03RY
        Vertebral
            Left 03RQ
            Right 03RP
    Atrium
        Left 02R7
        Right 02R6
    Auditory Ossicle
        Left 09RA0
        Right 09R90
    Bladder 0TRB
    Bladder Neck 0TRC
    Bone
        Ethmoid
            Left 0NRG
            Right 0NRF
        Frontal 0NR1
        Hyoid 0NRX
        Lacrimal
            Left 0NRJ
            Right 0NRH
        Nasal 0NRB
        Occipital 0NR7
        Palatine
            Left 0NRL
            Right 0NRK
        Parietal
            Left 0NR4
            Right 0NR3
        Pelvic
            Left 0QR3
            Right 0QR2
        Sphenoid 0NRC
        Temporal
            Left 0NR6
            Right 0NR5
        Zygomatic
            Left 0NRN
            Right 0NRM
    Breast
        Bilateral 0HRV
        Left 0HRU
        Right 0HRT

Subterms under main terms may continue to next column or page

Replacement — *continued*
   Bronchus
      Lingula ØBR9
      Lower Lobe
         Left ØBRB
         Right ØBR6
      Main
         Left ØBR7
         Right ØBR3
      Middle Lobe, Right ØBR5
      Upper Lobe
         Left ØBR8
         Right ØBR4
   Buccal Mucosa ØCR4
   Bursa and Ligament
      Abdomen
         Left ØMRJ
         Right ØMRH
      Ankle
         Left ØMRR
         Right ØMRQ
      Elbow
         Left ØMR4
         Right ØMR3
      Foot
         Left ØMRT
         Right ØMRS
      Hand
         Left ØMR8
         Right ØMR7
      Head and Neck ØMRØ
      Hip
         Left ØMRM
         Right ØMRL
      Knee
         Left ØMRP
         Right ØMRN
      Lower Extremity
         Left ØMRW
         Right ØMRV
      Perineum ØMRK
      Rib(s) ØMRG
      Shoulder
         Left ØMR2
         Right ØMR1
      Spine
         Lower ØMRD
         Upper ØMRC
      Sternum ØMRF
      Upper Extremity
         Left ØMRB
         Right ØMR9
      Wrist
         Left ØMR6
         Right ØMR5
   Carina ØBR2
   Carpal
      Left ØPRN
      Right ØPRM
   Cerebral Meninges ØØR1
   Cerebral Ventricle ØØR6
   Chordae Tendineae Ø2R9
   Choroid
      Left Ø8RB
      Right Ø8RA
   Clavicle
      Left ØPRB
      Right ØPR9
   Coccyx ØQRS
   Conjunctiva
      Left Ø8RTX
      Right Ø8RSX
   Cornea
      Left Ø8R9
      Right Ø8R8
   Diaphragm ØBRT
   Disc
      Cervical Vertebral ØRR3Ø
      Cervicothoracic Vertebral ØRR5Ø
      Lumbar Vertebral ØSR2Ø
      Lumbosacral ØSR4Ø
      Thoracic Vertebral ØRR9Ø
      Thoracolumbar Vertebral ØRRBØ
   Duct
      Common Bile ØFR9
      Cystic ØFR8
      Hepatic
         Common ØFR7
         Left ØFR6

Replacement — *continued*
   Duct — *continued*
      Hepatic — *continued*
         Right ØFR5
      Lacrimal
         Left Ø8RY
         Right Ø8RX
      Pancreatic ØFRD
         Accessory ØFRF
      Parotid
         Left ØCRC
         Right ØCRB
   Dura Mater ØØR2
   Ear
      External
         Bilateral Ø9R2
         Left Ø9R1
         Right Ø9RØ
      Inner
         Left Ø9REØ
         Right Ø9RDØ
      Middle
         Left Ø9R6Ø
         Right Ø9R5Ø
   Epiglottis ØCRR
   Esophagus ØDR5
   Eye
      Left Ø8R1
      Right Ø8RØ
   Eyelid
      Lower
         Left Ø8RR
         Right Ø8RQ
      Upper
         Left Ø8RP
         Right Ø8RN
   Femoral Shaft
      Left ØQR9
      Right ØQR8
   Femur
      Lower
         Left ØQRC
         Right ØQRB
      Upper
         Left ØQR7
         Right ØQR6
   Fibula
      Left ØQRK
      Right ØQRJ
   Finger Nail ØHRQX
   Gingiva
      Lower ØCR6
      Upper ØCR5
   Glenoid Cavity
      Left ØPR8
      Right ØPR7
   Hair ØHRSX
   Heart Ø2RAØ
   Humeral Head
      Left ØPRD
      Right ØPRC
   Humeral Shaft
      Left ØPRG
      Right ØPRF
   Iris
      Left Ø8RD3
      Right Ø8RC3
   Joint
      Acromioclavicular
         Left ØRRHØ
         Right ØRRGØ
      Ankle
         Left ØSRG
         Right ØSRF
      Carpal
         Left ØRRRØ
         Right ØRRQØ
      Carpometacarpal
         Left ØRRTØ
         Right ØRRSØ
      Cervical Vertebral ØRR1Ø
      Cervicothoracic Vertebral ØRR4Ø
      Coccygeal ØSR6Ø
      Elbow
         Left ØRRMØ
         Right ØRRLØ
      Finger Phalangeal
         Left ØRRXØ
         Right ØRRWØ

Replacement — *continued*
   Joint — *continued*
      Hip
         Left ØSRB
            Acetabular Surface ØSRE
            Femoral Surface ØSRS
         Right ØSR9
            Acetabular Surface ØSRA
            Femoral Surface ØSRR
      Knee
         Left ØSRD
            Femoral Surface ØSRU
            Tibial Surface ØSRW
         Right ØSRC
            Femoral Surface ØSRT
            Tibial Surface ØSRV
      Lumbar Vertebral ØSRØØ
      Lumbosacral ØSR3Ø
      Metacarpophalangeal
         Left ØRRVØ
         Right ØRRUØ
      Metatarsal-Phalangeal
         Left ØSRNØ
         Right ØSRMØ
      Occipital-cervical ØRRØØ
      Sacrococcygeal ØSR5Ø
      Sacroiliac
         Left ØSR8Ø
         Right ØSR7Ø
      Shoulder
         Left ØRRK
         Right ØRRJ
      Sternoclavicular
         Left ØRRFØ
         Right ØRREØ
      Tarsal
         Left ØSRJØ
         Right ØSRHØ
      Tarsometatarsal
         Left ØSRLØ
         Right ØSRKØ
      Temporomandibular
         Left ØRRDØ
         Right ØRRCØ
      Thoracic Vertebral ØRR6Ø
      Thoracolumbar Vertebral ØRRAØ
      Toe Phalangeal
         Left ØSRQØ
         Right ØSRPØ
      Wrist
         Left ØRRPØ
         Right ØRRNØ
   Kidney Pelvis
      Left ØTR4
      Right ØTR3
   Larynx ØCRS
   Lens
      Left Ø8RK3ØZ
      Right Ø8RJ3ØZ
   Lip
      Lower ØCR1
      Upper ØCRØ
   Mandible
      Left ØNRV
      Right ØNRT
   Maxilla ØNRR
   Mesentery ØDRV
   Metacarpal
      Left ØPRQ
      Right ØPRP
   Metatarsal
      Left ØQRP
      Right ØQRN
   Muscle
      Abdomen
         Left ØKRL
         Right ØKRK
      Facial ØKR1
      Foot
         Left ØKRW
         Right ØKRV
      Hand
         Left ØKRD
         Right ØKRC
      Head ØKRØ
      Hip
         Left ØKRP
         Right ØKRN

Replacement — *continued*
  Muscle — *continued*
    Lower Arm and Wrist
      Left ØKRB
      Right ØKR9
    Lower Leg
      Left ØKRT
      Right ØKRS
    Neck
      Left ØKR3
      Right ØKR2
    Papillary Ø2RD
    Perineum ØKRM
    Shoulder
      Left ØKR6
      Right ØKR5
    Thorax
      Left ØKRJ
      Right ØKRH
    Tongue, Palate, Pharynx ØKR4
    Trunk
      Left ØKRG
      Right ØKRF
    Upper Arm
      Left ØKR8
      Right ØKR7
    Upper Leg
      Left ØKRR
      Right ØKRQ
  Nasal Mucosa and Soft Tissue Ø9RK
  Nasopharynx Ø9RN
  Nerve
    Abducens ØØRL
    Accessory ØØRR
    Acoustic ØØRN
    Cervical Ø1R1
    Facial ØØRM
    Femoral Ø1RD
    Glossopharyngeal ØØRP
    Hypoglossal ØØRS
    Lumbar Ø1RB
    Median Ø1R5
    Oculomotor ØØRH
    Olfactory ØØRF
    Optic ØØRG
    Peroneal Ø1RH
    Phrenic Ø1R2
    Pudendal Ø1RC
    Radial Ø1R6
    Sacral Ø1RR
    Sciatic Ø1RF
    Thoracic Ø1R8
    Tibial Ø1RG
    Trigeminal ØØRK
    Trochlear ØØRJ
    Ulnar Ø1R4
    Vagus ØØRQ
  Nipple
    Left ØHRX
    Right ØHRW
  Omentum ØDRU
  Orbit
    Left ØNRQ
    Right ØNRP
  Palate
    Hard ØCR2
    Soft ØCR3
  Patella
    Left ØQRF
    Right ØQRD
  Pericardium Ø2RN
  Peritoneum ØDRW
  Phalanx
    Finger
      Left ØPRV
      Right ØPRT
    Thumb
      Left ØPRS
      Right ØPRR
    Toe
      Left ØQRR
      Right ØQRQ
  Pharynx ØCRM
  Radius
    Left ØPRJ
    Right ØPRH
  Retinal Vessel
    Left Ø8RH3
    Right Ø8RG3

Replacement — *continued*
  Ribs
    1 to 2 ØPR1
    3 or More ØPR2
  Sacrum ØQR1
  Scapula
    Left ØPR6
    Right ØPR5
  Sclera
    Left Ø8R7X
    Right Ø8R6X
  Septum
    Atrial Ø2R5
    Nasal Ø9RM
    Ventricular Ø2RM
  Skin
    Abdomen ØHR7
    Back ØHR6
    Buttock ØHR8
    Chest ØHR5
    Ear
      Left ØHR3
      Right ØHR2
    Face ØHR1
    Foot
      Left ØHRN
      Right ØHRM
    Hand
      Left ØHRG
      Right ØHRF
    Inguinal ØHRA
    Lower Arm
      Left ØHRE
      Right ØHRD
    Lower Leg
      Left ØHRL
      Right ØHRK
    Neck ØHR4
    Perineum ØHR9
    Scalp ØHRØ
    Upper Arm
      Left ØHRC
      Right ØHRB
    Upper Leg
      Left ØHRJ
      Right ØHRH
  Skull ØNRØ
  Spinal Meninges ØØRT
  Sternum ØPRØ
  Subcutaneous Tissue and Fascia
    Abdomen ØJR8
    Back ØJR7
    Buttock ØJR9
    Chest ØJR6
    Face ØJR1
    Foot
      Left ØJRR
      Right ØJRQ
    Hand
      Left ØJRK
      Right ØJRJ
    Lower Arm
      Left ØJRH
      Right ØJRG
    Lower Leg
      Left ØJRP
      Right ØJRN
    Neck
      Left ØJR5
      Right ØJR4
    Pelvic Region ØJRC
    Perineum ØJRB
    Scalp ØJRØ
    Upper Arm
      Left ØJRF
      Right ØJRD
    Upper Leg
      Left ØJRM
      Right ØJRL
  Tarsal
    Left ØQRM
    Right ØQRL
  Tendon
    Abdomen
      Left ØLRG
      Right ØLRF
    Ankle
      Left ØLRT
      Right ØLRS

Replacement — *continued*
  Tendon — *continued*
    Foot
      Left ØLRW
      Right ØLRV
    Hand
      Left ØLR8
      Right ØLR7
    Head and Neck ØLRØ
    Hip
      Left ØLRK
      Right ØLRJ
    Knee
      Left ØLRR
      Right ØLRQ
    Lower Arm and Wrist
      Left ØLR6
      Right ØLR5
    Lower Leg
      Left ØLRP
      Right ØLRN
    Perineum ØLRH
    Shoulder
      Left ØLR2
      Right ØLR1
    Thorax
      Left ØLRD
      Right ØLRC
    Trunk
      Left ØLRB
      Right ØLR9
    Upper Arm
      Left ØLR4
      Right ØLR3
    Upper Leg
      Left ØLRM
      Right ØLRL
  Testis
    Bilateral ØVRCØJZ
    Left ØVRBØJZ
    Right ØVR9ØJZ
  Thumb
    Left ØXRM
    Right ØXRL
  Tibia
    Left ØQRH
    Right ØQRG
  Toe Nail ØHRRX
  Tongue ØCR7
  Tooth
    Lower ØCRX
    Upper ØCRW
  Trachea ØBR1
  Turbinate, Nasal Ø9RL
  Tympanic Membrane
    Left Ø9R8
    Right Ø9R7
  Ulna
    Left ØPRL
    Right ØPRK
  Ureter
    Left ØTR7
    Right ØTR6
  Urethra ØTRD
  Uvula ØCRN
  Valve
    Aortic Ø2RF
    Mitral Ø2RG
    Pulmonary Ø2RH
    Tricuspid Ø2RJ
  Vein
    Axillary
      Left Ø5R8
      Right Ø5R7
    Azygos Ø5RØ
    Basilic
      Left Ø5RC
      Right Ø5RB
    Brachial
      Left Ø5RA
      Right Ø5R9
    Cephalic
      Left Ø5RF
      Right Ø5RD
    Colic Ø6R7
    Common Iliac
      Left Ø6RD
      Right Ø6RC
    Esophageal Ø6R3

Replacement — *continued*
- Vein — *continued*
  - External Iliac
    - Left Ø6RG
    - Right Ø6RF
  - External Jugular
    - Left Ø5RQ
    - Right Ø5RP
  - Face
    - Left Ø5RV
    - Right Ø5RT
  - Femoral
    - Left Ø6RN
    - Right Ø6RM
  - Foot
    - Left Ø6RV
    - Right Ø6RT
  - Gastric Ø6R2
  - Hand
    - Left Ø5RH
    - Right Ø5RG
  - Hemiazygos Ø5R1
  - Hepatic Ø6R4
  - Hypogastric
    - Left Ø6RJ
    - Right Ø6RH
  - Inferior Mesenteric Ø6R6
  - Innominate
    - Left Ø5R4
    - Right Ø5R3
  - Internal Jugular
    - Left Ø5RN
    - Right Ø5RM
  - Intracranial Ø5RL
  - Lower Ø6RY
  - Portal Ø6R8
  - Pulmonary
    - Left Ø2RT
    - Right Ø2RS
  - Renal
    - Left Ø6RB
    - Right Ø6R9
  - Saphenous
    - Left Ø6RQ
    - Right Ø6RP
  - Splenic Ø6R1
  - Subclavian
    - Left Ø5R6
    - Right Ø5R5
  - Superior Mesenteric Ø6R5
  - Upper Ø5RY
  - Vertebral
    - Left Ø5RS
    - Right Ø5RR
- Vena Cava
  - Inferior Ø6RØ
  - Superior Ø2RV
- Ventricle
  - Left Ø2RL
  - Right Ø2RK
- Vertebra
  - Cervical ØPR3
  - Lumbar ØQRØ
  - Thoracic ØPR4
- Vitreous
  - Left Ø8R53
  - Right Ø8R43
- Vocal Cord
  - Left ØCRV
  - Right ØCRT

Replacement, hip
- Partial or total *see* Replacement, Lower Joints ØSR
- Resurfacing only *see* Supplement, Lower Joints ØSU

Replacement, knee
- Meniscus implant only *see* New Technology, Joints XRR
- Partial or total *see* Replacement, Lower Joints ØSR

Replantation *see* Reposition

Replantation, scalp *see* Reattachment, Skin, Scalp ØHMØ

Reposition
- Acetabulum
  - Left ØQS5
  - Right ØQS4
- Ampulla of Vater ØFSC
- Anus ØDSQ

Reposition — *continued*
- Aorta
  - Abdominal Ø4SØ
  - Thoracic
    - Ascending/Arch Ø2SXØZZ
    - Descending Ø2SWØZZ
- Artery
  - Anterior Tibial
    - Left Ø4SQ
    - Right Ø4SP
  - Axillary
    - Left Ø3S6
    - Right Ø3S5
  - Brachial
    - Left Ø3S8
    - Right Ø3S7
  - Celiac Ø4S1
  - Colic
    - Left Ø4S7
    - Middle Ø4S8
    - Right Ø4S6
  - Common Carotid
    - Left Ø3SJ
    - Right Ø3SH
  - Common Iliac
    - Left Ø4SD
    - Right Ø4SC
  - Coronary
    - One Artery Ø2SØØZZ
    - Two Arteries Ø2S1ØZZ
  - External Carotid
    - Left Ø3SN
    - Right Ø3SM
  - External Iliac
    - Left Ø4SJ
    - Right Ø4SH
  - Face Ø3SR
  - Femoral
    - Left Ø4SL
    - Right Ø4SK
  - Foot
    - Left Ø4SW
    - Right Ø4SV
  - Gastric Ø4S2
  - Hand
    - Left Ø3SF
    - Right Ø3SD
  - Hepatic Ø4S3
  - Inferior Mesenteric Ø4SB
  - Innominate Ø3S2
  - Internal Carotid
    - Left Ø3SL
    - Right Ø3SK
  - Internal Iliac
    - Left Ø4SF
    - Right Ø4SE
  - Internal Mammary
    - Left Ø3S1
    - Right Ø3SØ
  - Intracranial Ø3SG
  - Lower Ø4SY
  - Peroneal
    - Left Ø4SU
    - Right Ø4ST
  - Popliteal
    - Left Ø4SN
    - Right Ø4SM
  - Posterior Tibial
    - Left Ø4SS
    - Right Ø4SR
  - Pulmonary
    - Left Ø2SRØZZ
    - Right Ø2SQØZZ
  - Pulmonary Trunk Ø2SPØZZ
  - Radial
    - Left Ø3SC
    - Right Ø3SB
  - Renal
    - Left Ø4SA
    - Right Ø4S9
  - Splenic Ø4S4
  - Subclavian
    - Left Ø3S4
    - Right Ø3S3
  - Superior Mesenteric Ø4S5
  - Temporal
    - Left Ø3ST
    - Right Ø3SS

Reposition — *continued*
- Artery — *continued*
  - Thyroid
    - Left Ø3SV
    - Right Ø3SU
  - Ulnar
    - Left Ø3SA
    - Right Ø3S9
  - Upper Ø3SY
  - Vertebral
    - Left Ø3SQ
    - Right Ø3SP
- Auditory Ossicle
  - Left Ø9SA
  - Right Ø9S9
- Bladder ØTSB
- Bladder Neck ØTSC
- Bone
  - Ethmoid
    - Left ØNSG
    - Right ØNSF
  - Frontal ØNS1
  - Hyoid ØNSX
  - Lacrimal
    - Left ØNSJ
    - Right ØNSH
  - Nasal ØNSB
  - Occipital ØNS7
  - Palatine
    - Left ØNSL
    - Right ØNSK
  - Parietal
    - Left ØNS4
    - Right ØNS3
  - Pelvic
    - Left ØQS3
    - Right ØQS2
  - Sphenoid ØNSC
  - Temporal
    - Left ØNS6
    - Right ØNS5
  - Zygomatic
    - Left ØNSN
    - Right ØNSM
- Breast
  - Bilateral ØHSVØZZ
  - Left ØHSUØZZ
  - Right ØHSTØZZ
- Bronchus
  - Lingula ØBS9ØZZ
  - Lower Lobe
    - Left ØBSBØZZ
    - Right ØBS6ØZZ
  - Main
    - Left ØBS7ØZZ
    - Right ØBS3ØZZ
  - Middle Lobe, Right ØBS5ØZZ
  - Upper Lobe
    - Left ØBS8ØZZ
    - Right ØBS4ØZZ
- Bursa and Ligament
  - Abdomen
    - Left ØMSJ
    - Right ØMSH
  - Ankle
    - Left ØMSR
    - Right ØMSQ
  - Elbow
    - Left ØMS4
    - Right ØMS3
  - Foot
    - Left ØMST
    - Right ØMSS
  - Hand
    - Left ØMS8
    - Right ØMS7
  - Head and Neck ØMSØ
  - Hip
    - Left ØMSM
    - Right ØMSL
  - Knee
    - Left ØMSP
    - Right ØMSN
  - Lower Extremity
    - Left ØMSW
    - Right ØMSV
  - Perineum ØMSK
  - Rib(s) ØMSG

Reposition — *continued*
  Bursa and Ligament — *continued*
    Shoulder
      Left 0MS2
      Right 0MS1
    Spine
      Lower 0MSD
      Upper 0MSC
    Sternum 0MSF
    Upper Extremity
      Left 0MSB
      Right 0MS9
    Wrist
      Left 0MS6
      Right 0MS5
  Carina 0BS20ZZ
  Carpal
    Left 0PSN
    Right 0PSM
  Cecum 0DSH
  Cervix 0USC
  Clavicle
    Left 0PSB
    Right 0PS9
  Coccyx 0QSS
  Colon
    Ascending 0DSK
    Descending 0DSM
    Sigmoid 0DSN
    Transverse 0DSL
  Cord
    Bilateral 0VSH
    Left 0VSG
    Right 0VSF
  Cul-de-sac 0USF
  Diaphragm 0BST0ZZ
  Duct
    Common Bile 0FS9
    Cystic 0FS8
    Hepatic
      Common 0FS7
      Left 0FS6
      Right 0FS5
    Lacrimal
      Left 08SY
      Right 08SX
    Pancreatic 0FSD
      Accessory 0FSF
    Parotid
      Left 0CSC
      Right 0CSB
  Duodenum 0DS9
  Ear
    Bilateral 09S2
    Left 09S1
    Right 09S0
  Epiglottis 0CSR
  Esophagus 0DS5
  Eustachian Tube
    Left 09SG
    Right 09SF
  Eyelid
    Lower
      Left 08SR
      Right 08SQ
    Upper
      Left 08SP
      Right 08SN
  Fallopian Tube
    Left 0US6
    Right 0US5
  Fallopian Tubes, Bilateral 0US7
  Femoral Shaft
    Left 0QS9
    Right 0QS8
  Femur
    Lower
      Left 0QSC
      Right 0QSB
    Upper
      Left 0QS7
      Right 0QS6
  Fibula
    Left 0QSK
    Right 0QSJ
  Gallbladder 0FS4
  Gland
    Adrenal
      Left 0GS2

Reposition — *continued*
  Gland — *continued*
    Adrenal — *continued*
      Right 0GS3
    Lacrimal
      Left 08SW
      Right 08SV
  Glenoid Cavity
    Left 0PS8
    Right 0PS7
  Hair 0HSSXZZ
  Humeral Head
    Left 0PSD
    Right 0PSC
  Humeral Shaft
    Left 0PSG
    Right 0PSF
  Ileum 0DSB
  Intestine
    Large 0DSE
    Small 0DS8
  Iris
    Left 08SD3ZZ
    Right 08SC3ZZ
  Jejunum 0DSA
  Joint
    Acromioclavicular
      Left 0RSH
      Right 0RSG
    Ankle
      Left 0SSG
      Right 0SSF
    Carpal
      Left 0RSR
      Right 0RSQ
    Carpometacarpal
      Left 0RST
      Right 0RSS
    Cervical Vertebral 0RS1
    Cervicothoracic Vertebral 0RS4
    Coccygeal 0SS6
    Elbow
      Left 0RSM
      Right 0RSL
    Finger Phalangeal
      Left 0RSX
      Right 0RSW
    Hip
      Left 0SSB
      Right 0SS9
    Knee
      Left 0SSD
      Right 0SSC
    Lumbar Vertebral 0SS0
    Lumbosacral 0SS3
    Metacarpophalangeal
      Left 0RSV
      Right 0RSU
    Metatarsal-Phalangeal
      Left 0SSN
      Right 0SSM
    Occipital-cervical 0RS0
    Sacrococcygeal 0SS5
    Sacroiliac
      Left 0SS8
      Right 0SS7
    Shoulder
      Left 0RSK
      Right 0RSJ
    Sternoclavicular
      Left 0RSF
      Right 0RSE
    Tarsal
      Left 0SSJ
      Right 0SSH
    Tarsometatarsal
      Left 0SSL
      Right 0SSK
    Temporomandibular
      Left 0RSD
      Right 0RSC
    Thoracic Vertebral 0RS6
    Thoracolumbar Vertebral 0RSA
    Toe Phalangeal
      Left 0SSQ
      Right 0SSP
    Wrist
      Left 0RSP
      Right 0RSN

Reposition — *continued*
  Kidney
    Left 0TS1
    Right 0TS0
  Kidney Pelvis
    Left 0TS4
    Right 0TS3
  Kidneys, Bilateral 0TS2
  Larynx 0CSS
  Lens
    Left 08SK3ZZ
    Right 08SJ3ZZ
  Lip
    Lower 0CS1
    Upper 0CS0
  Liver 0FS0
  Lung
    Left 0BSL0ZZ
    Lower Lobe
      Left 0BSJ0ZZ
      Right 0BSF0ZZ
    Middle Lobe, Right 0BSD0ZZ
    Right 0BSK0ZZ
    Upper Lobe
      Left 0BSG0ZZ
      Right 0BSC0ZZ
  Lung Lingula 0BSH0ZZ
  Mandible
    Left 0NSV
    Right 0NST
  Maxilla 0NSR
  Metacarpal
    Left 0PSQ
    Right 0PSP
  Metatarsal
    Left 0QSP
    Right 0QSN
  Muscle
    Abdomen
      Left 0KSL
      Right 0KSK
    Extraocular
      Left 08SM
      Right 08SL
    Facial 0KS1
    Foot
      Left 0KSW
      Right 0KSV
    Hand
      Left 0KSD
      Right 0KSC
    Head 0KS0
    Hip
      Left 0KSP
      Right 0KSN
    Lower Arm and Wrist
      Left 0KSB
      Right 0KS9
    Lower Leg
      Left 0KST
      Right 0KSS
    Neck
      Left 0KS3
      Right 0KS2
    Perineum 0KSM
    Shoulder
      Left 0KS6
      Right 0KS5
    Thorax
      Left 0KSJ
      Right 0KSH
    Tongue, Palate, Pharynx 0KS4
    Trunk
      Left 0KSG
      Right 0KSF
    Upper Arm
      Left 0KS8
      Right 0KS7
    Upper Leg
      Left 0KSR
      Right 0KSQ
  Nasal Mucosa and Soft Tissue 09SK
  Nerve
    Abducens 00SL
    Accessory 00SR
    Acoustic 00SN
    Brachial Plexus 01S3
    Cervical 01S1
    Cervical Plexus 01S0

▽ **Subterms under main terms may continue to next column or page**

Resection — *continued*
Anus ØDTQ
Aortic Body ØGTD
Appendix ØDTJ
Auditory Ossicle
  Left Ø9TA
  Right Ø9T9
Bladder ØTTB
Bladder Neck ØTTC
Bone
  Ethmoid
    Left ØNTGØZZ
    Right ØNTFØZZ
  Frontal ØNT1ØZZ
  Hyoid ØNTXØZZ
  Lacrimal
    Left ØNTJØZZ
    Right ØNTHØZZ
  Nasal ØNTBØZZ
  Occipital ØNT7ØZZ
  Palatine
    Left ØNTLØZZ
    Right ØNTKØZZ
  Parietal
    Left ØNT4ØZZ
    Right ØNT3ØZZ
  Pelvic
    Left ØQT3ØZZ
    Right ØQT2ØZZ
  Sphenoid ØNTCØZZ
  Temporal
    Left ØNT6ØZZ
    Right ØNT5ØZZ
  Zygomatic
    Left ØNTNØZZ
    Right ØNTMØZZ
Breast
  Bilateral ØHTVØZZ
  Left ØHTUØZZ
  Right ØHTTØZZ
  Supernumerary ØHTYØZZ
Bronchus
  Lingula ØBT9
  Lower Lobe
    Left ØBTB
    Right ØBT6
  Main
    Left ØBT7
    Right ØBT3
  Middle Lobe, Right ØBT5
  Upper Lobe
    Left ØBT8
    Right ØBT4
Bursa and Ligament
  Abdomen
    Left ØMTJ
    Right ØMTH
  Ankle
    Left ØMTR
    Right ØMTQ
  Elbow
    Left ØMT4
    Right ØMT3
  Foot
    Left ØMTT
    Right ØMTS
  Hand
    Left ØMT8
    Right ØMT7
  Head and Neck ØMTØ
  Hip
    Left ØMTM
    Right ØMTL
  Knee
    Left ØMTP
    Right ØMTN
  Lower Extremity
    Left ØMTW
    Right ØMTV
  Perineum ØMTK
  Rib(s) ØMTG
  Shoulder
    Left ØMT2
    Right ØMT1
  Spine
    Lower ØMTD
    Upper ØMTC
  Sternum ØMTF

Resection — *continued*
Bursa and Ligament — *continued*
  Upper Extremity
    Left ØMTB
    Right ØMT9
  Wrist
    Left ØMT6
    Right ØMT5
Carina ØBT2
Carotid Bodies, Bilateral ØGT8
Carotid Body
  Left ØGT6
  Right ØGT7
Carpal
  Left ØPTNØZZ
  Right ØPTMØZZ
Cecum ØDTH
Cerebral Hemisphere ØØT7
Cervix ØUTC
Chordae Tendineae Ø2T9
Cisterna Chyli Ø7TL
Clavicle
  Left ØPTBØZZ
  Right ØPT9ØZZ
Clitoris ØUTJ
Coccygeal Glomus ØGTB
Coccyx ØQTSØZZ
Colon
  Ascending ØDTK
  Descending ØDTM
  Sigmoid ØDTN
  Transverse ØDTL
Conduction Mechanism Ø2T8
Cord
  Bilateral ØVTH
  Left ØVTG
  Right ØVTF
Cornea
  Left Ø8T9XZZ
  Right Ø8T8XZZ
Cul-de-sac ØUTF
Diaphragm ØBTT
Disc
  Cervical Vertebral ØRT3ØZZ
  Cervicothoracic Vertebral ØRT5ØZZ
  Lumbar Vertebral ØST2ØZZ
  Lumbosacral ØST4ØZZ
  Thoracic Vertebral ØRT9ØZZ
  Thoracolumbar Vertebral ØRTBØZZ
Duct
  Common Bile ØFT9
  Cystic ØFT8
  Hepatic
    Common ØFT7
    Left ØFT6
    Right ØFT5
  Lacrimal
    Left Ø8TY
    Right Ø8TX
  Pancreatic ØFTD
    Accessory ØFTF
  Parotid
    Left ØCTCØZZ
    Right ØCTBØZZ
Duodenum ØDT9
Ear
  External
    Left Ø9T1
    Right Ø9TØ
  Inner
    Left Ø9TE
    Right Ø9TD
  Middle
    Left Ø9T6
    Right Ø9T5
Epididymis
  Bilateral ØVTL
  Left ØVTK
  Right ØVTJ
Epiglottis ØCTR
Esophagogastric Junction ØDT4
Esophagus ØDT5
  Lower ØDT3
  Middle ØDT2
  Upper ØDT1
Eustachian Tube
  Left Ø9TG
  Right Ø9TF

Resection — *continued*
Eye
  Left Ø8T1XZZ
  Right Ø8TØXZZ
Eyelid
  Lower
    Left Ø8TR
    Right Ø8TQ
  Upper
    Left Ø8TP
    Right Ø8TN
Fallopian Tube
  Left ØUT6
  Right ØUT5
Fallopian Tubes, Bilateral ØUT7
Femoral Shaft
  Left ØQT9ØZZ
  Right ØQT8ØZZ
Femur
  Lower
    Left ØQTCØZZ
    Right ØQTBØZZ
  Upper
    Left ØQT7ØZZ
    Right ØQT6ØZZ
Fibula
  Left ØQTKØZZ
  Right ØQTJØZZ
Finger Nail ØHTQXZZ
Gallbladder ØFT4
Gland
  Adrenal
    Bilateral ØGT4
    Left ØGT2
    Right ØGT3
  Lacrimal
    Left Ø8TW
    Right Ø8TV
  Minor Salivary ØCTJØZZ
  Parotid
    Left ØCT9ØZZ
    Right ØCT8ØZZ
  Pituitary ØGTØ
  Sublingual
    Left ØCTFØZZ
    Right ØCTDØZZ
  Submaxillary
    Left ØCTHØZZ
    Right ØCTGØZZ
  Vestibular ØUTL
Glenoid Cavity
  Left ØPT8ØZZ
  Right ØPT7ØZZ
Glomus Jugulare ØGTC
Humeral Head
  Left ØPTDØZZ
  Right ØPTCØZZ
Humeral Shaft
  Left ØPTGØZZ
  Right ØPTFØZZ
Hymen ØUTK
Ileocecal Valve ØDTC
Ileum ØDTB
Intestine
  Large ØDTE
    Left ØDTG
    Right ØDTF
  Small ØDT8
Iris
  Left Ø8TD3ZZ
  Right Ø8TC3ZZ
Jejunum ØDTA
Joint
  Acromioclavicular
    Left ØRTHØZZ
    Right ØRTGØZZ
  Ankle
    Left ØSTGØZZ
    Right ØSTFØZZ
  Carpal
    Left ØRTRØZZ
    Right ØRTQØZZ
  Carpometacarpal
    Left ØRTTØZZ
    Right ØRTSØZZ
  Cervicothoracic Vertebral ØRT4ØZZ
  Coccygeal ØST6ØZZ
  Elbow
    Left ØRTMØZZ

▽ **Subterms under main terms may continue to next column or page**

Resection — continued
Joint — continued
Elbow — continued
Right ØRTLØZZ
Finger Phalangeal
Left ØRTXØZZ
Right ØRTWØZZ
Hip
Left ØSTBØZZ
Right ØST9ØZZ
Knee
Left ØSTDØZZ
Right ØSTCØZZ
Metacarpophalangeal
Left ØRTVØZZ
Right ØRTUØZZ
Metatarsal-Phalangeal
Left ØSTNØZZ
Right ØSTMØZZ
Sacrococcygeal ØST5ØZZ
Sacroiliac
Left ØST8ØZZ
Right ØST7ØZZ
Shoulder
Left ØRTKØZZ
Right ØRTJØZZ
Sternoclavicular
Left ØRTFØZZ
Right ØRTEØZZ
Tarsal
Left ØSTJØZZ
Right ØSTHØZZ
Tarsometatarsal
Left ØSTLØZZ
Right ØSTKØZZ
Temporomandibular
Left ØRTDØZZ
Right ØRTCØZZ
Toe Phalangeal
Left ØSTQØZZ
Right ØSTPØZZ
Wrist
Left ØRTPØZZ
Right ØRTNØZZ
Kidney
Left ØTT1
Right ØTTØ
Kidney Pelvis
Left ØTT4
Right ØTT3
Kidneys, Bilateral ØTT2
Larynx ØCTS
Lens
Left Ø8TK3ZZ
Right Ø8TJ3ZZ
Lip
Lower ØCT1
Upper ØCTØ
Liver ØFTØ
Left Lobe ØFT2
Right Lobe ØFT1
Lung
Bilateral ØBTM
Left ØBTL
Lower Lobe
Left ØBTJ
Right ØBTF
Middle Lobe, Right ØBTD
Right ØBTK
Upper Lobe
Left ØBTG
Right ØBTC
Lung Lingula ØBTH
Lymphatic
Aortic Ø7TD
Axillary
Left Ø7T6
Right Ø7T5
Head Ø7TØ
Inguinal
Left Ø7TJ
Right Ø7TH
Internal Mammary
Left Ø7T9
Right Ø7T8
Lower Extremity
Left Ø7TG
Right Ø7TF
Mesenteric Ø7TB

Resection — continued
Lymphatic — continued
Neck
Left Ø7T2
Right Ø7T1
Pelvis Ø7TC
Thoracic Duct Ø7TK
Thorax Ø7T7
Upper Extremity
Left Ø7T4
Right Ø7T3
Mandible
Left ØNTVØZZ
Right ØNTTØZZ
Maxilla ØNTRØZZ
Metacarpal
Left ØPTQØZZ
Right ØPTPØZZ
Metatarsal
Left ØQTPØZZ
Right ØQTNØZZ
Muscle
Abdomen
Left ØKTL
Right ØKTK
Extraocular
Left Ø8TM
Right Ø8TL
Facial ØKT1
Foot
Left ØKTW
Right ØKTV
Hand
Left ØKTD
Right ØKTC
Head ØKTØ
Hip
Left ØKTP
Right ØKTN
Lower Arm and Wrist
Left ØKTB
Right ØKT9
Lower Leg
Left ØKTT
Right ØKTS
Neck
Left ØKT3
Right ØKT2
Papillary Ø2TD
Perineum ØKTM
Shoulder
Left ØKT6
Right ØKT5
Thorax
Left ØKTJ
Right ØKTH
Tongue, Palate, Pharynx ØKT4
Trunk
Left ØKTG
Right ØKTF
Upper Arm
Left ØKT8
Right ØKT7
Upper Leg
Left ØKTR
Right ØKTQ
Nasal Mucosa and Soft Tissue Ø9TK
Nasopharynx Ø9TN
Nipple
Left ØHTXXZZ
Right ØHTWXZZ
Omentum ØDTU
Orbit
Left ØNTQØZZ
Right ØNTPØZZ
Ovary
Bilateral ØUT2
Left ØUT1
Right ØUTØ
Palate
Hard ØCT2
Soft ØCT3
Pancreas ØFTG
Para-aortic Body ØGT9
Paraganglion Extremity ØGTF
Parathyroid Gland ØGTR
Inferior
Left ØGTP
Right ØGTN

Resection — continued
Parathyroid Gland — continued
Multiple ØGTQ
Superior
Left ØGTM
Right ØGTL
Patella
Left ØQTFØZZ
Right ØQTDØZZ
Penis ØVTS
Pericardium Ø2TN
Phalanx
Finger
Left ØPTVØZZ
Right ØPTTØZZ
Thumb
Left ØPTSØZZ
Right ØPTRØZZ
Toe
Left ØQTRØZZ
Right ØQTQØZZ
Pharynx ØCTM
Pineal Body ØGT1
Prepuce ØVTT
Products of Conception, Ectopic 1ØT2
Prostate ØVTØ
Radius
Left ØPTJØZZ
Right ØPTHØZZ
Rectum ØDTP
Ribs
1 to 2 ØPT1ØZZ
3 or More ØPT2ØZZ
Scapula
Left ØPT6ØZZ
Right ØPT5ØZZ
Scrotum ØVT5
Septum
Atrial Ø2T5
Nasal Ø9TM
Ventricular Ø2TM
Sinus
Accessory Ø9TP
Ethmoid
Left Ø9TV
Right Ø9TU
Frontal
Left Ø9TT
Right Ø9TS
Mastoid
Left Ø9TC
Right Ø9TB
Maxillary
Left Ø9TR
Right Ø9TQ
Sphenoid
Left Ø9TX
Right Ø9TW
Spleen Ø7TP
Sternum ØPTØØZZ
Stomach ØDT6
Pylorus ØDT7
Tarsal
Left ØQTMØZZ
Right ØQTLØZZ
Tendon
Abdomen
Left ØLTG
Right ØLTF
Ankle
Left ØLTT
Right ØLTS
Foot
Left ØLTW
Right ØLTV
Hand
Left ØLT8
Right ØLT7
Head and Neck ØLTØ
Hip
Left ØLTK
Right ØLTJ
Knee
Left ØLTR
Right ØLTQ
Lower Arm and Wrist
Left ØLT6
Right ØLT5

⛟ Subterms under main terms may continue to next column or page

Resection — *continued*
 Tendon — *continued*
  Lower Leg
   Left ØLTP
   Right ØLTN
  Perineum ØLTH
  Shoulder
   Left ØLT2
   Right ØLT1
  Thorax
   Left ØLTD
   Right ØLTC
  Trunk
   Left ØLTB
   Right ØLT9
  Upper Arm
   Left ØLT4
   Right ØLT3
  Upper Leg
   Left ØLTM
   Right ØLTL
 Testis
  Bilateral ØVTC
  Left ØVTB
  Right ØVT9
 Thymus Ø7TM
 Thyroid Gland ØGTK
  Left Lobe ØGTG
  Right Lobe ØGTH
 Thyroid Gland Isthmus ØGTJ
 Tibia
  Left ØQTHØZZ
  Right ØQTGØZZ
 Toe Nail ØHTRXZZ
 Tongue ØCT7
 Tonsils ØCTP
 Tooth
  Lower ØCTXØZ
  Upper ØCTWØZ
 Trachea ØBT1
 Tunica Vaginalis
  Left ØVT7
  Right ØVT6
 Turbinate, Nasal Ø9TL
 Tympanic Membrane
  Left Ø9T8
  Right Ø9T7
 Ulna
  Left ØPTLØZZ
  Right ØPTKØZZ
 Ureter
  Left ØTT7
  Right ØTT6
 Urethra ØTTD
 Uterine Supporting Structure ØUT4
 Uterus ØUT9
 Uvula ØCTN
 Vagina ØUTG
 Valve, Pulmonary Ø2TH
 Vas Deferens
  Bilateral ØVTQ
  Left ØVTP
  Right ØVTN
 Vesicle
  Bilateral ØVT3
  Left ØVT2
  Right ØVT1
 Vitreous
  Left Ø8T53ZZ
  Right Ø8T43ZZ
 Vocal Cord
  Left ØCTV
  Right ØCTT
 Vulva ØUTM
Resection, Left ventricular outflow tract obstruction (LVOT) *see* Dilation, Ventricle, Left Ø27L
Resection, Subaortic membrane (Left ventricular outflow tract obstruction) *see* Dilation, Ventricle, Left Ø27L
Restoration, Cardiac, Single, Rhythm 5A22Ø4Z
RestoreAdvanced neurostimulator (SureScan) (MRI Safe) *use* Stimulator Generator, Multiple Array Rechargeable in ØJH
RestoreSensor neurostimulator (SureScan) (MRI Safe) *use* Stimulator Generator, Multiple Array Rechargeable in ØJH

RestoreUltra neurostimulator (SureScan) (MRI Safe) *use* Stimulator Generator, Multiple Array Rechargeable in ØJH
Restriction
 Ampulla of Vater ØFVC
 Anus ØDVQ
 Aorta
  Abdominal Ø4VØ
   Intraluminal Device, Branched or Fenestrated Ø4VØ
  Thoracic
   Ascending/Arch, Intraluminal Device, Branched or Fenestrated Ø2VX
   Descending, Intraluminal Device, Branched or Fenestrated Ø2VW
 Artery
  Anterior Tibial
   Left Ø4VQ
   Right Ø4VP
  Axillary
   Left Ø3V6
   Right Ø3V5
  Brachial
   Left Ø3V8
   Right Ø3V7
  Celiac Ø4V1
  Colic
   Left Ø4V7
   Middle Ø4V8
   Right Ø4V6
  Common Carotid
   Left Ø3VJ
   Right Ø3VH
  Common Iliac
   Left Ø4VD
   Right Ø4VC
  External Carotid
   Left Ø3VN
   Right Ø3VM
  External Iliac
   Left Ø4VJ
   Right Ø4VH
  Face Ø3VR
  Femoral
   Left Ø4VL
   Right Ø4VK
  Foot
   Left Ø4VW
   Right Ø4VV
  Gastric Ø4V2
  Hand
   Left Ø3VF
   Right Ø3VD
  Hepatic Ø4V3
  Inferior Mesenteric Ø4VB
  Innominate Ø3V2
  Internal Carotid
   Left Ø3VL
   Right Ø3VK
  Internal Iliac
   Left Ø4VF
   Right Ø4VE
  Internal Mammary
   Left Ø3V1
   Right Ø3VØ
  Intracranial Ø3VG
  Lower Ø4VY
  Peroneal
   Left Ø4VU
   Right Ø4VT
  Popliteal
   Left Ø4VN
   Right Ø4VM
  Posterior Tibial
   Left Ø4VS
   Right Ø4VR
  Pulmonary
   Left Ø2VR
   Right Ø2VQ
  Pulmonary Trunk Ø2VP
  Radial
   Left Ø3VC
   Right Ø3VB
  Renal
   Left Ø4VA
   Right Ø4V9
  Splenic Ø4V4
  Subclavian
   Left Ø3V4

Restriction — *continued*
 Artery — *continued*
  Subclavian — *continued*
   Right Ø3V3
  Superior Mesenteric Ø4V5
  Temporal
   Left Ø3VT
   Right Ø3VS
  Thyroid
   Left Ø3VV
   Right Ø3VU
  Ulnar
   Left Ø3VA
   Right Ø3V9
  Upper Ø3VY
  Vertebral
   Left Ø3VQ
   Right Ø3VP
 Bladder ØTVB
 Bladder Neck ØTVC
 Bronchus
  Lingula ØBV9
  Lower Lobe
   Left ØBVB
   Right ØBV6
  Main
   Left ØBV7
   Right ØBV3
  Middle Lobe, Right ØBV5
  Upper Lobe
   Left ØBV8
   Right ØBV4
 Carina ØBV2
 Cecum ØDVH
 Cervix ØUVC
 Cisterna Chyli Ø7VL
 Colon
  Ascending ØDVK
  Descending ØDVM
  Sigmoid ØDVN
  Transverse ØDVL
 Duct
  Common Bile ØFV9
  Cystic ØFV8
  Hepatic
   Common ØFV7
   Left ØFV6
   Right ØFV5
  Lacrimal
   Left Ø8VY
   Right Ø8VX
  Pancreatic ØFVD
   Accessory ØFVF
  Parotid
   Left ØCVC
   Right ØCVB
 Duodenum ØDV9
 Esophagogastric Junction ØDV4
 Esophagus ØDV5
  Lower ØDV3
  Middle ØDV2
  Upper ØDV1
 Heart Ø2VA
 Ileocecal Valve ØDVC
 Ileum ØDVB
 Intestine
  Large ØDVE
   Left ØDVG
   Right ØDVF
  Small ØDV8
 Jejunum ØDVA
 Kidney Pelvis
  Left ØTV4
  Right ØTV3
 Lymphatic
  Aortic Ø7VD
  Axillary
   Left Ø7V6
   Right Ø7V5
  Head Ø7VØ
  Inguinal
   Left Ø7VJ
   Right Ø7VH
  Internal Mammary
   Left Ø7V9
   Right Ø7V8
  Lower Extremity
   Left Ø7VG
   Right Ø7VF

▽ Subterms under main terms may continue to next column or page

Restriction — *continued*
  Lymphatic — *continued*
    Mesenteric 07VB
    Neck
      Left 07V2
      Right 07V1
    Pelvis 07VC
    Thoracic Duct 07VK
    Thorax 07V7
    Upper Extremity
      Left 07V4
      Right 07V3
  Rectum 0DVP
  Stomach 0DV6
    Pylorus 0DV7
  Trachea 0BV1
  Ureter
    Left 0TV7
    Right 0TV6
  Urethra 0TVD
  Valve, Mitral 02VG
  Vein
    Axillary
      Left 05V8
      Right 05V7
    Azygos 05V0
    Basilic
      Left 05VC
      Right 05VB
    Brachial
      Left 05VA
      Right 05V9
    Cephalic
      Left 05VF
      Right 05VD
    Colic 06V7
    Common Iliac
      Left 06VD
      Right 06VC
    Esophageal 06V3
    External Iliac
      Left 06VG
      Right 06VF
    External Jugular
      Left 05VQ
      Right 05VP
    Face
      Left 05VV
      Right 05VT
    Femoral
      Left 06VN
      Right 06VM
    Foot
      Left 06VV
      Right 06VT
    Gastric 06V2
    Hand
      Left 05VH
      Right 05VG
    Hemiazygos 05V1
    Hepatic 06V4
    Hypogastric
      Left 06VJ
      Right 06VH
    Inferior Mesenteric 06V6
    Innominate
      Left 05V4
      Right 05V3
    Internal Jugular
      Left 05VN
      Right 05VM
    Intracranial 05VL
    Lower 06VY
    Portal 06V8
    Pulmonary
      Left 02VT
      Right 02VS
    Renal
      Left 06VB
      Right 06V9
    Saphenous
      Left 06VQ
      Right 06VP
    Splenic 06V1
    Subclavian
      Left 05V6
      Right 05V5
    Superior Mesenteric 06V5
    Upper 05VY

Restriction — *continued*
  Vein — *continued*
    Vertebral
      Left 05VS
      Right 05VR
    Vena Cava
      Inferior 06V0
      Superior 02VV
    Ventricle, Left 02VL
Resurfacing Device
  Removal of device from
    Left 0SPB0BZ
    Right 0SP90BZ
  Revision of device in
    Left 0SWB0BZ
    Right 0SW90BZ
  Supplement
    Left 0SUB0BZ
      Acetabular Surface 0SUE0BZ
      Femoral Surface 0SUS0BZ
    Right 0SU90BZ
      Acetabular Surface 0SUA0BZ
      Femoral Surface 0SUR0BZ
Resuscitation
  Cardiopulmonary *see* Assistance, Cardiac 5A02
  Cardioversion 5A2204Z
  Defibrillation 5A2204Z
  Endotracheal intubation *see* Insertion of device in,
    Trachea 0BH1
  External chest compression, manual 5A12012
  External chest compression, mechanical 5A1221J
  Pulmonary 5A19054
Resuscitative endovascular balloon occlusion of
  the aorta (REBOA)
  02LW3DJ
  04L03DJ
Resuture, Heart valve prosthesis *see* Revision of
  device in, Heart and Great Vessels 02W
Retained placenta, manual removal *see* Extraction,
  Products of Conception, Retained 10D1
RETHYMIC® *use* Engineered Allogeneic Thymus Tissue
Retraining
  Cardiac *see* Motor Treatment, Rehabilitation F07
  Vocational *see* Activities of Daily Living Treatment,
    Rehabilitation F08
Retrogasserian rhizotomy *see* Division, Nerve,
  Trigeminal 008K
Retroperitoneal cavity *use* Retroperitoneum
Retroperitoneal lymph node *use* Lymphatic, Aortic
Retroperitoneal space *use* Retroperitoneum
Retropharyngeal lymph node
  use Lymphatic, Left Neck
  use Lymphatic, Right Neck
Retropharyngeal space *use* Neck
Retropubic space *use* Pelvic Cavity
Reveal (LINQ) (DX) (XT) *use* Monitoring Device
Reverse total shoulder replacement *see* Replace-
  ment, Upper Joints 0RR
Reverse® Shoulder Prosthesis *use* Synthetic Substi-
  tute, Reverse Ball and Socket in 0RR
Revision
  Correcting a portion of existing device *see* Revision
    of device in
  Removal of device without replacement *see* Re-
    moval of device from
  Replacement of existing device
    see Removal of device from
    see Root operation to place new device, e.g.,
      Insertion, Replacement, Supplement
Revision of device in
  Abdominal Wall 0WWF
  Acetabulum
    Left 0QW5
    Right 0QW4
  Anal Sphincter 0DWR
  Anus 0DWQ
  Aorta, Thoracic, Descending 02WW3RZ
  Artery
    Lower 04WY
    Upper 03WY
  Auditory Ossicle
    Left 09WA
    Right 09W9
  Back
    Lower 0WWL
    Upper 0WWK
  Bladder 0TWB

Revision of device in — *continued*
  Bone
    Facial 0NWW
    Lower 0QWY
    Nasal 0NWB
    Pelvic
      Left 0QW3
      Right 0QW2
    Upper 0PWY
  Bone Marrow 07WT
  Brain 00W0
  Breast
    Left 0HWU
    Right 0HWT
  Bursa and Ligament
    Lower 0MWY
    Upper 0MWX
  Carpal
    Left 0PWN
    Right 0PWM
  Cavity, Cranial 0WW1
  Cerebral Ventricle 00W6
  Chest Wall 0WW8
  Cisterna Chyli 07WL
  Clavicle
    Left 0PWB
    Right 0PW9
  Coccyx 0QWS
  Diaphragm 0BWT
  Disc
    Cervical Vertebral 0RW3
    Cervicothoracic Vertebral 0RW5
    Lumbar Vertebral 0SW2
    Lumbosacral 0SW4
    Thoracic Vertebral 0RW9
    Thoracolumbar Vertebral 0RWB
  Duct
    Hepatobiliary 0FWB
    Pancreatic 0FWD
  Ear
    Inner
      Left 09WE
      Right 09WD
    Left 09WJ
    Right 09WH
  Epididymis and Spermatic Cord 0VWM
  Esophagus 0DW5
  Extremity
    Lower
      Left 0YWB
      Right 0YW9
    Upper
      Left 0XW7
      Right 0XW6
  Eye
    Left 08W1
    Right 08W0
  Face 0WW2
  Fallopian Tube 0UW8
  Femoral Shaft
    Left 0QW9
    Right 0QW8
  Femur
    Lower
      Left 0QWC
      Right 0QWB
    Upper
      Left 0QW7
      Right 0QW6
  Fibula
    Left 0QWK
    Right 0QWJ
  Finger Nail 0HWQX
  Gallbladder 0FW4
  Gastrointestinal Tract 0WWP
  Genitourinary Tract 0WWR
  Gland
    Adrenal 0GW5
    Endocrine 0GWS
    Pituitary 0GW0
    Salivary 0CWA
  Glenoid Cavity
    Left 0PW8
    Right 0PW7
  Great Vessel 02WY
  Hair 0HWSX
  Head 0WW0
  Heart 02WA

Revision of device in — *continued*
Humeral Head
  Left ØPWD
  Right ØPWC
Humeral Shaft
  Left ØPWG
  Right ØPWF
Intestinal Tract
  Lower Intestinal Tract ØDWD
  Upper Intestinal Tract ØDWØ
Intestine
  Large ØDWE
  Small ØDW8
Jaw
  Lower ØWW5
  Upper ØWW4
Joint
  Acromioclavicular
    Left ØRWH
    Right ØRWG
  Ankle
    Left ØSWG
    Right ØSWF
  Carpal
    Left ØRWR
    Right ØRWQ
  Carpometacarpal
    Left ØRWT
    Right ØRWS
  Cervical Vertebral ØRW1
  Cervicothoracic Vertebral ØRW4
  Coccygeal ØSW6
  Elbow
    Left ØRWM
    Right ØRWL
  Finger Phalangeal
    Left ØRWX
    Right ØRWW
  Hip
    Left ØSWB
      Acetabular Surface ØSWE
      Femoral Surface ØSWS
    Right ØSW9
      Acetabular Surface ØSWA
      Femoral Surface ØSWR
  Knee
    Left ØSWD
      Femoral Surface ØSWU
      Tibial Surface ØSWW
    Right ØSWC
      Femoral Surface ØSWT
      Tibial Surface ØSWV
  Lumbar Vertebral ØSWØ
  Lumbosacral ØSW3
  Metacarpophalangeal
    Left ØRWV
    Right ØRWU
  Metatarsal-Phalangeal
    Left ØSWN
    Right ØSWM
  Occipital-cervical ØRWØ
  Sacrococcygeal ØSW5
  Sacroiliac
    Left ØSW8
    Right ØSW7
  Shoulder
    Left ØRWK
    Right ØRWJ
  Sternoclavicular
    Left ØRWF
    Right ØRWE
  Tarsal
    Left ØSWJ
    Right ØSWH
  Tarsometatarsal
    Left ØSWL
    Right ØSWK
  Temporomandibular
    Left ØRWD
    Right ØRWC
  Thoracic Vertebral ØRW6
  Thoracolumbar Vertebral ØRWA
  Toe Phalangeal
    Left ØSWQ
    Right ØSWP
  Wrist
    Left ØRWP
    Right ØRWN
Kidney ØTW5

Revision of device in — *continued*
Larynx ØCWS
Lens
  Left Ø8WK
  Right Ø8WJ
Liver ØFWØ
Lung
  Left ØBWL
  Right ØBWK
Lymphatic Ø7WN
  Thoracic Duct Ø7WK
Mediastinum ØWWC
Mesentery ØDWV
Metacarpal
  Left ØPWQ
  Right ØPWP
Metatarsal
  Left ØQWP
  Right ØQWN
Mouth and Throat ØCWY
Muscle
  Extraocular
    Left Ø8WM
    Right Ø8WL
  Lower ØKWY
  Upper ØKWX
Nasal Mucosa and Soft Tissue Ø9WK
Neck ØWW6
Nerve
  Cranial ØØWE
  Peripheral Ø1WY
Omentum ØDWU
Ovary ØUW3
Pancreas ØFWG
Parathyroid Gland ØGWR
Patella
  Left ØQWF
  Right ØQWD
Pelvic Cavity ØWWJ
Penis ØVWS
Pericardial Cavity ØWWD
Perineum
  Female ØWWN
  Male ØWWM
Peritoneal Cavity ØWWG
Peritoneum ØDWW
Phalanx
  Finger
    Left ØPWV
    Right ØPWT
  Thumb
    Left ØPWS
    Right ØPWR
  Toe
    Left ØQWR
    Right ØQWQ
Pineal Body ØGW1
Pleura ØBWQ
Pleural Cavity
  Left ØWWB
  Right ØWW9
Prostate and Seminal Vesicles ØVW4
Radius
  Left ØPWJ
  Right ØPWH
Respiratory Tract ØWWQ
Retroperitoneum ØWWH
Ribs
  1 to 2 ØPW1
  3 or More ØPW2
Sacrum ØQW1
Scapula
  Left ØPW6
  Right ØPW5
Scrotum and Tunica Vaginalis ØVW8
Septum
  Atrial Ø2W5
  Ventricular Ø2WM
Sinus Ø9WY
Skin ØHWPX
Skull ØNWØ
Spinal Canal ØØWU
Spinal Cord ØØWV
Spleen Ø7WP
Sternum ØPWØ
Stomach ØDW6
Subcutaneous Tissue and Fascia
  Head and Neck ØJWS
  Lower Extremity ØJWW

Revision of device in — *continued*
Subcutaneous Tissue and Fascia — *continued*
  Trunk ØJWT
  Upper Extremity ØJWV
Tarsal
  Left ØQWM
  Right ØQWL
Tendon
  Lower ØLWY
  Upper ØLWX
Testis ØVWD
Thymus Ø7WM
Thyroid Gland ØGWK
Tibia
  Left ØQWH
  Right ØQWG
Toe Nail ØHWRX
Trachea ØBW1
Tracheobronchial Tree ØBWØ
Tympanic Membrane
  Left Ø9W8
  Right Ø9W7
Ulna
  Left ØPWL
  Right ØPWK
Ureter ØTW9
Urethra ØTWD
Uterus and Cervix ØUWD
Vagina and Cul-de-sac ØUWH
Valve
  Aortic Ø2WF
  Mitral Ø2WG
  Pulmonary Ø2WH
  Tricuspid Ø2WJ
Vas Deferens ØVWR
Vein
  Azygos Ø5WØ
  Innominate
    Left Ø5W4
    Right Ø5W3
  Lower Ø6WY
  Upper Ø5WY
Vertebra
  Cervical ØPW3
  Lumbar ØQWØ
  Thoracic ØPW4
Vulva ØUWM
Revo MRI™ SureScan® pacemaker *use* Pacemaker, Dual Chamber in ØJH
Rezafungin XWØ
rhBMP-2 *use* Recombinant Bone Morphogenetic Protein
Rheos® System device *use* Stimulator Generator in Subcutaneous Tissue and Fascia
Rheos® System lead *use* Stimulator Lead in Upper Arteries
Rhinopharynx *use* Nasopharynx
Rhinoplasty
  see Alteration, Nasal Mucosa and Soft Tissue Ø9ØK
  see Repair, Nasal Mucosa and Soft Tissue Ø9QK
  see Replacement, Nasal Mucosa and Soft Tissue Ø9RK
  see Supplement, Nasal Mucosa and Soft Tissue Ø9UK
Rhinorrhaphy *see* Repair, Nasal Mucosa and Soft Tissue Ø9QK
Rhinoscopy Ø9JKXZZ
Rhizotomy
  see Division, Central Nervous System and Cranial Nerves ØØ8
  see Division, Peripheral Nervous System Ø18
Rhomboid major muscle
  use Trunk Muscle, Left
  use Trunk Muscle, Right
Rhomboid minor muscle
  use Trunk Muscle, Left
  use Trunk Muscle, Right
Rhythm electrocardiogram *see* Measurement, Cardiac 4AØ2
Rhytidectomy *see* Alteration, Face ØWØ2
Right ascending lumbar vein *use* Azygos Vein
Right atrioventricular valve *use* Tricuspid Valve
Right auricular appendix *use* Atrium, Right
Right colic vein *use* Colic Vein
Right coronary sulcus *use* Heart, Right
Right gastric artery *use* Gastric Artery
Right gastroepiploic vein *use* Superior Mesenteric Vein

Right inferior phrenic vein use Inferior Vena Cava
Right inferior pulmonary vein use Pulmonary Vein, Right
Right jugular trunk use Lymphatic, Right Neck
Right lateral ventricle use Cerebral Ventricle
Right lymphatic duct use Lymphatic, Right Neck
Right ovarian vein use Inferior Vena Cava
Right second lumbar vein use Inferior Vena Cava
Right subclavian trunk use Lymphatic, Right Neck
Right subcostal vein use Azygos Vein
Right superior pulmonary vein use Pulmonary Vein, Right
Right suprarenal vein use Inferior Vena Cava
Right testicular vein use Inferior Vena Cava
Rima glottidis use Larynx
Risorius muscle use Facial Muscle
RNS System lead use Neurostimulator Lead in Central Nervous System and Cranial Nerves
RNS system neurostimulator generator use Neurostimulator Generator in Head and Facial Bones
Robotic Assisted Procedure
  Extremity
    Lower 8E0Y
    Upper 8E0X
  Head and Neck Region 8E09
  Trunk Region 8E0W
Rotation of fetal head
  Forceps 10S07ZZ
  Manual 10S0XZZ
Round ligament of uterus use Uterine Supporting Structure
Round window
  use Inner Ear, Left
  use Inner Ear, Right
Roux-en-Y operation
  see Bypass, Gastrointestinal System 0D1
  see Bypass, Hepatobiliary System and Pancreas 0F1
Rupture
  Adhesions see Release
  Fluid collection see Drainage
Ruxolitinib XW0DXT5
RYBREVANT™ use Amivantamab Monoclonal Antibody

S

Sabizabulin XW0
Sacral ganglion use Sacral Sympathetic Nerve
Sacral lymph node use Lymphatic, Pelvis
Sacral nerve modulation (SNM) lead use Stimulator Lead in Urinary System
Sacral neuromodulation lead use Stimulator Lead in Urinary System
Sacral splanchnic nerve use Sacral Sympathetic Nerve
Sacrectomy see Excision, Lower Bones 0QB
Sacrococcygeal ligament use Lower Spine Bursa and Ligament
Sacrococcygeal symphysis use Sacrococcygeal Joint
Sacroiliac ligament use Lower Spine Bursa and Ligament
Sacrospinous ligament use Lower Spine Bursa and Ligament
Sacrotuberous ligament use Lower Spine Bursa and Ligament
Salpingectomy
  see Excision, Female Reproductive System 0UB
  see Resection, Female Reproductive System 0UT
Salpingolysis see Release, Female Reproductive System 0UN
Salpingopexy
  see Repair, Female Reproductive System 0UQ
  see Reposition, Female Reproductive System 0US
Salpingopharyngeus muscle use Tongue, Palate, Pharynx Muscle
Salpingoplasty
  see Repair, Female Reproductive System 0UQ
  see Supplement, Female Reproductive System 0UU
Salpingorrhaphy see Repair, Female Reproductive System 0UQ
Salpingoscopy 0UJ88ZZ
Salpingostomy see Drainage, Female Reproductive System 0U9
Salpingotomy see Drainage, Female Reproductive System 0U9
Salpinx
  use Fallopian Tube, Left

Salpinx — continued
  use Fallopian Tube, Right
Saphenous nerve use Femoral Nerve
SAPIEN transcatheter aortic valve use Zooplastic Tissue in Heart and Great Vessels
Sarilumab XW0
SARS-CoV-2 Antibody Detection, Serum/Plasma Nanoparticle Fluorescence XXE5XV7
SARS-CoV-2 Polymerase Chain Reaction, Nasopharyngeal Fluid XXE97U7
Sartorius muscle
  use Upper Leg Muscle, Left
  use Upper Leg Muscle, Right
Satralizumab-mwge XW01397
SAVAL below-the-knee (BTK) drug-eluting stent system
  use Intraluminal Device, Sustained Release Drug-eluting in New Technology
  use Intraluminal Device, Sustained Release Drug-eluting, Two in New Technology
  use Intraluminal Device, Sustained Release Drug-eluting, Three in New Technology
  use Intraluminal Device, Sustained Release Drug-eluting, Four or More in New Technology
Scalene muscle
  use Neck Muscle, Left
  use Neck Muscle, Right
Scan
  Computerized Tomography (CT) see Computerized Tomography (CT Scan)
  Radioisotope see Planar Nuclear Medicine Imaging
Scaphoid bone
  use Carpal, Left
  use Carpal, Right
Scapholunate ligament
  use Wrist Bursa and Ligament, Left
  use Wrist Bursa and Ligament, Right
Scaphotrapezium ligament
  use Hand Bursa and Ligament, Left
  use Hand Bursa and Ligament, Right
Scapulectomy
  see Excision, Upper Bones 0PB
  see Resection, Upper Bones 0PT
Scapulopexy
  see Repair, Upper Bones 0PQ
  see Reposition, Upper Bones 0PS
Scarpa's (vestibular) ganglion use Acoustic Nerve
Sclerectomy see Excision, Eye 08B
Sclerotherapy, mechanical see Destruction
Sclerotherapy, via injection of sclerosing agent see Introduction, Destructive Agent
Sclerotomy see Drainage, Eye 089
Scrotectomy
  see Excision, Male Reproductive System 0VB
  see Resection, Male Reproductive System 0VT
Scrotoplasty
  see Repair, Male Reproductive System 0VQ
  see Supplement, Male Reproductive System 0VU
Scrotorrhaphy see Repair, Male Reproductive System 0VQ
Scrototomy see Drainage, Male Reproductive System 0V9
Sebaceous gland use Skin
Second cranial nerve use Optic Nerve
Section, cesarean see Extraction, Pregnancy 10D
Secura (DR) (VR) use Defibrillator Generator in 0JH
Sella turcica use Sphenoid Bone
Selux Rapid AST Platform XXE5XY9
Semicircular canal
  use Inner Ear, Left
  use Inner Ear, Right
Semimembranosus muscle
  use Upper Leg Muscle, Left
  use Upper Leg Muscle, Right
Semitendinosus muscle
  use Upper Leg Muscle, Left
  use Upper Leg Muscle, Right
Sentinel™ Cerebral Protection System (CPS) X2A5312
Seprafilm use Adhesion Barrier
Septal cartilage use Nasal Septum
Septectomy
  see Excision, Ear, Nose, Sinus 09B
  see Excision, Heart and Great Vessels 02B
  see Resection, Ear, Nose, Sinus 09T
  see Resection, Heart and Great Vessels 02T

SeptiCyte® RAPID XXE5X38
Septoplasty
  see Repair, Ear, Nose, Sinus 09Q
  see Repair, Heart and Great Vessels 02Q
  see Replacement, Ear, Nose, Sinus 09R
  see Replacement, Heart and Great Vessels 02R
  see Reposition, Ear, Nose, Sinus 09S
  see Supplement, Ear, Nose, Sinus 09U
  see Supplement, Heart and Great Vessels 02U
Septostomy, balloon atrial 02163Z7
Septotomy see Drainage, Ear, Nose, Sinus 099
Sequestrectomy, bone see Extirpation
SER-109 XW0DXN9
Serratus anterior muscle
  use Thorax Muscle, Left
  use Thorax Muscle, Right
Serratus posterior muscle
  use Trunk Muscle, Left
  use Trunk Muscle, Right
Seventh cranial nerve use Facial Nerve
Shapshot_NIR 8E02XDZ
Sheffield hybrid external fixator
  use External Fixation Device, Hybrid in 0PH
  use External Fixation Device, Hybrid in 0PS
  use External Fixation Device, Hybrid in 0QH
  use External Fixation Device, Hybrid in 0QS
Sheffield ring external fixator
  use External Fixation Device, Ring in 0PH
  use External Fixation Device, Ring in 0PS
  use External Fixation Device, Ring in 0QH
  use External Fixation Device, Ring in 0QS
Shirodkar cervical cerclage 0UVC7ZZ
Shock Wave Therapy, Musculoskeletal 6A93
Shockwave Intravascular Lithotripsy (Shockwave IVL) see Fragmentation
Short gastric artery use Splenic Artery
Shortening
  see Excision
  see Repair
  see Reposition
Shunt creation see Bypass
Sialoadenectomy
  Complete see Resection, Mouth and Throat 0CT
  Partial see Excision, Mouth and Throat 0CB
Sialodochoplasty
  see Repair, Mouth and Throat 0CQ
  see Replacement, Mouth and Throat 0CR
  see Supplement, Mouth and Throat 0CU
Sialoectomy
  see Excision, Mouth and Throat 0CB
  see Resection, Mouth and Throat 0CT
Sialography see Plain Radiography, Ear, Nose, Mouth and Throat B90
Sialolithotomy see Extirpation, Mouth and Throat 0CC
S-ICD™ lead use Subcutaneous Defibrillator Lead in Subcutaneous Tissue and Fascia
Sigmoid artery use Inferior Mesenteric Artery
Sigmoid flexure use Sigmoid Colon
Sigmoid vein use Inferior Mesenteric Vein
Sigmoidectomy
  see Excision, Gastrointestinal System 0DB
  see Resection, Gastrointestinal System 0DT
Sigmoidorrhaphy see Repair, Gastrointestinal System 0DQ
Sigmoidoscopy 0DJD8ZZ
Sigmoidotomy see Drainage, Gastrointestinal System 0D9
Single lead pacemaker (atrium) (ventricle) use Pacemaker, Single Chamber in 0JH
Single lead rate responsive pacemaker (atrium) (ventricle) use Pacemaker, Single Chamber Rate Responsive in 0JH
Single-use Duodenoscope XFJ
Single-use Oversleeve with Intraoperative Colonic Irrigation XDPH8K7
Sinoatrial node use Conduction Mechanism
Sinogram
  Abdominal Wall see Fluoroscopy, Abdomen and Pelvis BW11
  Chest Wall see Plain Radiography, Chest BW03
  Retroperitoneum see Fluoroscopy, Abdomen and Pelvis BW11
Sinus venosus use Atrium, Right
Sinusectomy
  see Excision, Ear, Nose, Sinus 09B
  see Resection, Ear, Nose, Sinus 09T

Sinusoscopy Ø9JY4ZZ
Sinusotomy *see* Drainage, Ear, Nose, Sinus Ø99
Sirolimus-eluting coronary stent *use* Intraluminal Device, Drug-eluting in Heart and Great Vessels
Sixth cranial nerve *use* Abducens Nerve
Size reduction, breast *see* Excision, Skin and Breast ØHB
SJM Biocor® Stented Valve System *use* Zooplastic Tissue in Heart and Great Vessels
Skene's (paraurethral) gland *use* Vestibular Gland
Sling
    Fascial, orbicularis muscle (mouth) *see* Supplement, Muscle, Facial ØKU1
    Levator muscle, for urethral suspension *see* Reposition, Bladder Neck ØTSC
    Pubococcygeal, for urethral suspension *see* Reposition, Bladder Neck ØTSC
    Rectum *see* Reposition, Rectum ØDSP
Small bowel series *see* Fluoroscopy, Bowel, Small BD13
Small saphenous vein
    use Saphenous Vein, Left
    use Saphenous Vein, Right
Snapshot_NIR 8EØ2XDZ
Snaring, polyp, colon *see* Excision, Gastrointestinal System ØDB
Solar (celiac) plexus *use* Abdominal Sympathetic Nerve
Soleus muscle
    use Lower Leg Muscle, Left
    use Lower Leg Muscle, Right
Soliris® *use* Eculizumab
Space of Retzius *use* Pelvic Cavity
Spacer
    Insertion of device in
      Disc
        Lumbar Vertebral ØSH2
        Lumbosacral ØSH4
      Joint
        Acromioclavicular
          Left ØRHH
          Right ØRHG
        Ankle
          Left ØSHG
          Right ØSHF
        Carpal
          Left ØRHR
          Right ØRHQ
        Carpometacarpal
          Left ØRHT
          Right ØRHS
        Cervical Vertebral ØRH1
        Cervicothoracic Vertebral ØRH4
        Coccygeal ØSH6
        Elbow
          Left ØRHM
          Right ØRHL
        Finger Phalangeal
          Left ØRHX
          Right ØRHW
        Hip
          Left ØSHB
          Right ØSH9
        Knee
          Left ØSHD
          Right ØSHC
        Lumbar Vertebral ØSHØ
        Lumbosacral ØSH3
        Metacarpophalangeal
          Left ØRHV
          Right ØRHU
        Metatarsal-Phalangeal
          Left ØSHN
          Right ØSHM
        Occipital-cervical ØRHØ
        Sacrococcygeal ØSH5
        Sacroiliac
          Left ØSH8
          Right ØSH7
        Shoulder
          Left ØRHK
          Right ØRHJ
        Sternoclavicular
          Left ØRHF
          Right ØRHE
        Tarsal
          Left ØSHJ
          Right ØSHH

Spacer — *continued*
    Insertion of device in — *continued*
      Joint — *continued*
        Tarsometatarsal
          Left ØSHL
          Right ØSHK
        Temporomandibular
          Left ØRHD
          Right ØRHC
        Thoracic Vertebral ØRH6
        Thoracolumbar Vertebral ØRHA
        Toe Phalangeal
          Left ØSHQ
          Right ØSHP
        Wrist
          Left ØRHP
          Right ØRHN
    Removal of device from
      Acromioclavicular
        Left ØRPH
        Right ØRPG
      Ankle
        Left ØSPG
        Right ØSPF
      Carpal
        Left ØRPR
        Right ØRPQ
      Carpometacarpal
        Left ØRPT
        Right ØRPS
      Cervical Vertebral ØRP1
      Cervicothoracic Vertebral ØRP4
      Coccygeal ØSP6
      Elbow
        Left ØRPM
        Right ØRPL
      Finger Phalangeal
        Left ØRPX
        Right ØRPW
      Hip
        Left ØSPB
        Right ØSP9
      Knee
        Left ØSPD
        Right ØSPC
      Lumbar Vertebral ØSPØ
      Lumbosacral ØSP3
      Metacarpophalangeal
        Left ØRPV
        Right ØRPU
      Metatarsal-Phalangeal
        Left ØSPN
        Right ØSPM
      Occipital-cervical ØRPØ
      Sacrococcygeal ØSP5
      Sacroiliac
        Left ØSP8
        Right ØSP7
      Shoulder
        Left ØRPK
        Right ØRPJ
      Sternoclavicular
        Left ØRPF
        Right ØRPE
      Tarsal
        Left ØSPJ
        Right ØSPH
      Tarsometatarsal
        Left ØSPL
        Right ØSPK
      Temporomandibular
        Left ØRPD
        Right ØRPC
      Thoracic Vertebral ØRP6
      Thoracolumbar Vertebral ØRPA
      Toe Phalangeal
        Left ØSPQ
        Right ØSPP
      Wrist
        Left ØRPP
        Right ØRPN
    Revision of device in
      Acromioclavicular
        Left ØRWH
        Right ØRWG
      Ankle
        Left ØSWG
        Right ØSWF

Spacer — *continued*
    Revision of device in — *continued*
      Carpal
        Left ØRWR
        Right ØRWQ
      Carpometacarpal
        Left ØRWT
        Right ØRWS
      Cervical Vertebral ØRW1
      Cervicothoracic Vertebral ØRW4
      Coccygeal ØSW6
      Elbow
        Left ØRWM
        Right ØRWL
      Finger Phalangeal
        Left ØRWX
        Right ØRWW
      Hip
        Left ØSWB
        Right ØSW9
      Knee
        Left ØSWD
        Right ØSWC
      Lumbar Vertebral ØSWØ
      Lumbosacral ØSW3
      Metacarpophalangeal
        Left ØRWV
        Right ØRWU
      Metatarsal-Phalangeal
        Left ØSWN
        Right ØSWM
      Occipital-cervical ØRWØ
      Sacrococcygeal ØSW5
      Sacroiliac
        Left ØSW8
        Right ØSW7
      Shoulder
        Left ØRWK
        Right ØRWJ
      Sternoclavicular
        Left ØRWF
        Right ØRWE
      Tarsal
        Left ØSWJ
        Right ØSWH
      Tarsometatarsal
        Left ØSWL
        Right ØSWK
      Temporomandibular
        Left ØRWD
        Right ØRWC
      Thoracic Vertebral ØRW6
      Thoracolumbar Vertebral ØRWA
      Toe Phalangeal
        Left ØSWQ
        Right ØSWP
      Wrist
        Left ØRWP
        Right ØRWN
Spacer, Articulating (Antibiotic) *use* Articulating Spacer in Lower Joints
Spacer, Static (Antibiotic) *use* Spacer in Lower Joints
Spectroscopy
    Intravascular Near Infrared 8EØ23DZ
    Near Infrared *see* Physiological Systems and Anatomical Regions 8EØ
Speech Assessment FØØ
Speech therapy *see* Speech Treatment, Rehabilitation FØ6
Speech Treatment FØ6
Spesolimab Monoclonal Antibody XWØ
Sphenoidectomy
    see Excision, Ear, Nose, Sinus Ø9B
    see Excision, Head and Facial Bones ØNB
    see Resection, Ear, Nose, Sinus Ø9T
    see Resection, Head and Facial Bones ØNT
Sphenoidotomy *see* Drainage, Ear, Nose, Sinus Ø99
Sphenomandibular ligament *use* Head and Neck Bursa and Ligament
Sphenopalatine (pterygopalatine) ganglion *use* Head and Neck Sympathetic Nerve
Sphincterorrhaphy, anal *see* Repair, Anal Sphincter ØDQR
Sphincterotomy, anal
    see Division, Anal Sphincter ØD8R
    see Drainage, Anal Sphincter ØD9R
SPIKEVAX™
    use COVID-19 Vaccine

▽ **Subterms under main terms may continue to next column or page**

SPIKEVAX™ — *continued*
   use COVID-19 Vaccine Booster
   use COVID-19 Vaccine Dose 1
   use COVID-19 Vaccine Dose 2
   use COVID-19 Vaccine Dose 3
Spinal cord neurostimulator lead *use* Neurostimulator Lead in Central Nervous System and Cranial Nerves
Spinal growth rods, magnetically controlled *use* Magnetically Controlled Growth Rod(s) in New Technology
Spinal nerve, cervical *use* Cervical Nerve
Spinal nerve, lumbar *use* Lumbar Nerve
Spinal nerve, sacral *use* Sacral Nerve
Spinal nerve, thoracic *use* Thoracic Nerve
Spinal Stabilization Device
  Facet Replacement
    Cervical Vertebral ØRH1
    Cervicothoracic Vertebral ØRH4
    Lumbar Vertebral ØSHØ
    Lumbosacral ØSH3
    Occipital-cervical ØRHØ
    Thoracic Vertebral ØRH6
    Thoracolumbar Vertebral ØRHA
  Interspinous Process
    Cervical Vertebral ØRH1
    Cervicothoracic Vertebral ØRH4
    Lumbar Vertebral ØSHØ
    Lumbosacral ØSH3
    Occipital-cervical ØRHØ
    Thoracic Vertebral ØRH6
    Thoracolumbar Vertebral ØRHA
  Pedicle-Based
    Cervical Vertebral ØRH1
    Cervicothoracic Vertebral ØRH4
    Lumbar Vertebral ØSHØ
    Lumbosacral ØSH3
    Occipital-cervical ØRHØ
    Thoracic Vertebral ØRH6
    Thoracolumbar Vertebral ØRHA
SpineJack® system *use* Synthetic Substitute, Mechanically Expandable (Paired) in New Technology
Spinous process
   use Cervical Vertebra
   use Lumbar Vertebra
   use Thoracic Vertebra
Spiral ganglion *use* Acoustic Nerve
Spiration IBV™ Valve System *use* Intraluminal Device, Endobronchial Valve in Respiratory System
Splenectomy
   see Excision, Lymphatic and Hemic Systems Ø7B
   see Resection, Lymphatic and Hemic Systems Ø7T
Splenic flexure *use* Transverse Colon
Splenic plexus *use* Abdominal Sympathetic Nerve
Splenius capitis muscle *use* Head Muscle
Splenius cervicis muscle
   use Neck Muscle, Left
   use Neck Muscle, Right
Splenolysis *see* Release, Lymphatic and Hemic Systems Ø7N
Splenopexy
   see Repair, Lymphatic and Hemic Systems Ø7Q
   see Reposition, Lymphatic and Hemic Systems Ø7S
Splenoplasty *see* Repair, Lymphatic and Hemic Systems Ø7Q
Splenorrhaphy *see* Repair, Lymphatic and Hemic Systems Ø7Q
Splenotomy *see* Drainage, Lymphatic and Hemic Systems Ø79
Splinting, musculoskeletal *see* Immobilization, Anatomical Regions 2W3
SPRAVATO™ *use* Esketamine Hydrochloride
SPY PINPOINT fluorescence imaging system
   see Monitoring, Physiological Systems 4A1
   see Other Imaging, Hepatobiliary System and Pancreas BF5
SPY system intraoperative fluorescence cholangiography *see* Other Imaging, Hepatobiliary System and Pancreas BF5
SPY system intravascular fluorescence angiography *see* Monitoring, Physiological Systems 4A1
SSO2 (Supersaturated Oxygen) therapy, cardiac intra-arterial 5A0222C
Staged hepatectomy
   see Division, Hepatobiliary System and Pancreas ØF8

Staged hepatectomy — *continued*
   see Resection, Hepatobiliary System and Pancreas ØFT
Stapedectomy
   see Excision, Ear, Nose, Sinus Ø9B
   see Resection, Ear, Nose, Sinus Ø9T
Stapediolysis *see* Release, Ear, Nose, Sinus Ø9N
Stapedioplasty
   see Repair, Ear, Nose, Sinus Ø9Q
   see Replacement, Ear, Nose, Sinus Ø9R
   see Supplement, Ear, Nose, Sinus Ø9U
Stapedotomy *see* Drainage, Ear, Nose, Sinus Ø99
Stapes
   use Auditory Ossicle, Left
   use Auditory Ossicle, Right
Static Spacer (Antibiotic) *use* Spacer in Lower Joints
STELARA® *use* Other New Technology Therapeutic Substance
Stellate ganglion *use* Head and Neck Sympathetic Nerve
Stem cell transplant *see* Transfusion, Circulatory 3Ø2
Stensen's duct
   use Parotid Duct, Left
   use Parotid Duct, Right
Stent, intraluminal (cardiovascular) (gastrointestinal) (hepatobiliary) (urinary) *use* Intraluminal Device
Stent retriever thrombectomy *see* Extirpation, Upper Arteries Ø3C
Stented tissue valve *use* Zooplastic Tissue in Heart and Great Vessels
Stereotactic Radiosurgery
  Abdomen DW23
  Adrenal Gland DG22
  Bile Ducts DF22
  Bladder DT22
  Bone Marrow D72Ø
  Brain DØ2Ø
  Brain Stem DØ21
  Breast
    Left DM2Ø
    Right DM21
  Bronchus DB21
  Cervix DU21
  Chest DW22
  Chest Wall DB27
  Colon DD25
  Diaphragm DB28
  Duodenum DD22
  Ear D92Ø
  Esophagus DD2Ø
  Eye D82Ø
  Gallbladder DF21
  Gamma Beam
    Abdomen DW23JZZ
    Adrenal Gland DG22JZZ
    Bile Ducts DF22JZZ
    Bladder DT22JZZ
    Bone Marrow D72ØJZZ
    Brain DØ2ØJZZ
    Brain Stem DØ21JZZ
    Breast
      Left DM2ØJZZ
      Right DM21JZZ
    Bronchus DB21JZZ
    Cervix DU21JZZ
    Chest DW22JZZ
    Chest Wall DB27JZZ
    Colon DD25JZZ
    Diaphragm DB28JZZ
    Duodenum DD22JZZ
    Ear D92ØJZZ
    Esophagus DD2ØJZZ
    Eye D82ØJZZ
    Gallbladder DF21JZZ
    Gland
      Adrenal DG22JZZ
      Parathyroid DG24JZZ
      Pituitary DG2ØJZZ
      Thyroid DG25JZZ
    Glands, Salivary D926JZZ
    Head and Neck DW21JZZ
    Ileum DD24JZZ
    Jejunum DD23JZZ
    Kidney DT2ØJZZ
    Larynx D92BJZZ
    Liver DF2ØJZZ
    Lung DB22JZZ

Stereotactic Radiosurgery — *continued*
  Gamma Beam — *continued*
    Lymphatics
      Abdomen D726JZZ
      Axillary D724JZZ
      Inguinal D728JZZ
      Neck D723JZZ
      Pelvis D727JZZ
      Thorax D725JZZ
    Mediastinum DB26JZZ
    Mouth D924JZZ
    Nasopharynx D92DJZZ
    Neck and Head DW21JZZ
    Nerve, Peripheral DØ27JZZ
    Nose D921JZZ
    Ovary DU2ØJZZ
    Palate
      Hard D928JZZ
      Soft D929JZZ
    Pancreas DF23JZZ
    Parathyroid Gland DG24JZZ
    Pelvic Region DW26JZZ
    Pharynx D92CJZZ
    Pineal Body DG21JZZ
    Pituitary Gland DG2ØJZZ
    Pleura DB25JZZ
    Prostate DV2ØJZZ
    Rectum DD27JZZ
    Sinuses D927JZZ
    Spinal Cord DØ26JZZ
    Spleen D722JZZ
    Stomach DD21JZZ
    Testis DV21JZZ
    Thymus D721JZZ
    Thyroid Gland DG25JZZ
    Tongue D925JZZ
    Trachea DB2ØJZZ
    Ureter DT21JZZ
    Urethra DT23JZZ
    Uterus DU22JZZ
  Gland
    Adrenal DG22
    Parathyroid DG24
    Pituitary DG2Ø
    Thyroid DG25
  Glands, Salivary D926
  Head and Neck DW21
  Ileum DD24
  Jejunum DD23
  Kidney DT2Ø
  Larynx D92B
  Liver DF2Ø
  Lung DB22
  Lymphatics
    Abdomen D726
    Axillary D724
    Inguinal D728
    Neck D723
    Pelvis D727
    Thorax D725
  Mediastinum DB26
  Mouth D924
  Nasopharynx D92D
  Neck and Head DW21
  Nerve, Peripheral DØ27
  Nose D921
  Other Photon
    Abdomen DW23DZZ
    Adrenal Gland DG22DZZ
    Bile Ducts DF22DZZ
    Bladder DT22DZZ
    Bone Marrow D72ØDZZ
    Brain DØ2ØDZZ
    Brain Stem DØ21DZZ
    Breast
      Left DM2ØDZZ
      Right DM21DZZ
    Bronchus DB21DZZ
    Cervix DU21DZZ
    Chest DW22DZZ
    Chest Wall DB27DZZ
    Colon DD25DZZ
    Diaphragm DB28DZZ
    Duodenum DD22DZZ
    Ear D92ØDZZ
    Esophagus DD2ØDZZ
    Eye D82ØDZZ
    Gallbladder DF21DZZ

Stereotactic Radiosurgery — *continued*
  Other Photon — *continued*
    Gland
      Adrenal DG22DZZ
      Parathyroid DG24DZZ
      Pituitary DG20DZZ
      Thyroid DG25DZZ
    Glands, Salivary D926DZZ
    Head and Neck DW21DZZ
    Ileum DD24DZZ
    Jejunum DD23DZZ
    Kidney DT20DZZ
    Larynx D92BDZZ
    Liver DF20DZZ
    Lung DB22DZZ
    Lymphatics
      Abdomen D726DZZ
      Axillary D724DZZ
      Inguinal D728DZZ
      Neck D723DZZ
      Pelvis D727DZZ
      Thorax D725DZZ
    Mediastinum DB26DZZ
    Mouth D924DZZ
    Nasopharynx D92DDZZ
    Neck and Head DW21DZZ
    Nerve, Peripheral D027DZZ
    Nose D921DZZ
    Ovary DU20DZZ
    Palate
      Hard D928DZZ
      Soft D929DZZ
    Pancreas DF23DZZ
    Parathyroid Gland DG24DZZ
    Pelvic Region DW26DZZ
    Pharynx D92CDZZ
    Pineal Body DG21DZZ
    Pituitary Gland DG20DZZ
    Pleura DB25DZZ
    Prostate DV20DZZ
    Rectum DD27DZZ
    Sinuses D927DZZ
    Spinal Cord D026DZZ
    Spleen D722DZZ
    Stomach DD21DZZ
    Testis DV21DZZ
    Thymus D721DZZ
    Thyroid Gland DG25DZZ
    Tongue D925DZZ
    Trachea DB20DZZ
    Ureter DT21DZZ
    Urethra DT23DZZ
    Uterus DU22DZZ
  Ovary DU20
  Palate
    Hard D928
    Soft D929
  Pancreas DF23
  Parathyroid Gland DG24
  Particulate
    Abdomen DW23HZZ
    Adrenal Gland DG22HZZ
    Bile Ducts DF22HZZ
    Bladder DT22HZZ
    Bone Marrow D720HZZ
    Brain D020HZZ
    Brain Stem D021HZZ
    Breast
      Left DM20HZZ
      Right DM21HZZ
    Bronchus DB21HZZ
    Cervix DU21HZZ
    Chest DW22HZZ
    Chest Wall DB27HZZ
    Colon DD25HZZ
    Diaphragm DB28HZZ
    Duodenum DD22HZZ
    Ear D920HZZ
    Esophagus DD20HZZ
    Eye D820HZZ
    Gallbladder DF21HZZ
    Gland
      Adrenal DG22HZZ
      Parathyroid DG24HZZ
      Pituitary DG20HZZ
      Thyroid DG25HZZ
    Glands, Salivary D926HZZ
    Head and Neck DW21HZZ
    Ileum DD24HZZ

Stereotactic Radiosurgery — *continued*
  Particulate — *continued*
    Jejunum DD23HZZ
    Kidney DT20HZZ
    Larynx D92BHZZ
    Liver DF20HZZ
    Lung DB22HZZ
    Lymphatics
      Abdomen D726HZZ
      Axillary D724HZZ
      Inguinal D728HZZ
      Neck D723HZZ
      Pelvis D727HZZ
      Thorax D725HZZ
    Mediastinum DB26HZZ
    Mouth D924HZZ
    Nasopharynx D92DHZZ
    Neck and Head DW21HZZ
    Nerve, Peripheral D027HZZ
    Nose D921HZZ
    Ovary DU20HZZ
    Palate
      Hard D928HZZ
      Soft D929HZZ
    Pancreas DF23HZZ
    Parathyroid Gland DG24HZZ
    Pelvic Region DW26HZZ
    Pharynx D92CHZZ
    Pineal Body DG21HZZ
    Pituitary Gland DG20HZZ
    Pleura DB25HZZ
    Prostate DV20HZZ
    Rectum DD27HZZ
    Sinuses D927HZZ
    Spinal Cord D026HZZ
    Spleen D722HZZ
    Stomach DD21HZZ
    Testis DV21HZZ
    Thymus D721HZZ
    Thyroid Gland DG25HZZ
    Tongue D925HZZ
    Trachea DB20HZZ
    Ureter DT21HZZ
    Urethra DT23HZZ
    Uterus DU22HZZ
  Pelvic Region DW26
  Pharynx D92C
  Pineal Body DG21
  Pituitary Gland DG20
  Pleura DB25
  Prostate DV20
  Rectum DD27
  Sinuses D927
  Spinal Cord D026
  Spleen D722
  Stomach DD21
  Testis DV21
  Thymus D721
  Thyroid Gland DG25
  Tongue D925
  Trachea DB20
  Ureter DT21
  Urethra DT23
  Uterus DU22

Steripath® Micro™ Blood Collection System
  XXE5XR7

Sternoclavicular ligament
  use Shoulder Bursa and Ligament, Left
  use Shoulder Bursa and Ligament, Right

Sternocleidomastoid artery
  use Thyroid Artery, Left
  use Thyroid Artery, Right

Sternocleidomastoid muscle
  use Neck Muscle, Left
  use Neck Muscle, Right

Sternocostal ligament *use* Sternum Bursa and Ligament

Sternotomy
  see Division, Sternum 0P80
  see Drainage, Sternum 0P90

Stimulation, cardiac
  Cardioversion 5A2204Z
  Electrophysiologic testing *see* Measurement, Cardiac 4A02

Stimulator Generator
  Insertion of device in
    Abdomen 0JH8
    Back 0JH7

Stimulator Generator — *continued*
  Insertion of device in — *continued*
    Chest 0JH6
    Multiple Array
      Abdomen 0JH8
      Back 0JH7
      Chest 0JH6
    Multiple Array Rechargeable
      Abdomen 0JH8
      Back 0JH7
      Chest 0JH6
    Removal of device from, Subcutaneous Tissue and Fascia, Trunk 0JPT
    Revision of device in, Subcutaneous Tissue and Fascia, Trunk 0JWT
    Single Array
      Abdomen 0JH8
      Back 0JH7
      Chest 0JH6
    Single Array Rechargeable
      Abdomen 0JH8
      Back 0JH7
      Chest 0JH6

Stimulator Lead
  Insertion of device in
    Anal Sphincter 0DHR
    Artery
      Left 03HL
      Right 03HK
    Bladder 0THB
    Muscle
      Lower 0KHY
      Upper 0KHX
    Stomach 0DH6
    Ureter 0TH9
  Removal of device from
    Anal Sphincter 0DPR
    Artery, Upper 03PY
    Bladder 0TPB
    Muscle
      Lower 0KPY
      Upper 0KPX
    Stomach 0DP6
    Ureter 0TP9
  Revision of device in
    Anal Sphincter 0DWR
    Artery, Upper 03WY
    Bladder 0TWB
    Muscle
      Lower 0KWY
      Upper 0KWX
    Stomach 0DW6
    Ureter 0TW9

Stoma
  Excision
    Abdominal Wall 0WBFXZ2
    Neck 0WB6XZ2
  Repair
    Abdominal Wall 0WQFXZ2
    Neck 0WQ6XZ2

Stomatoplasty
  see Repair, Mouth and Throat 0CQ
  see Replacement, Mouth and Throat 0CR
  see Supplement, Mouth and Throat 0CU

Stomatorrhaphy *see* Repair, Mouth and Throat 0CQ

StrataGraft® *use* Bioengineered Allogeneic Construct

Stratos LV *use* Cardiac Resynchronization Pacemaker Pulse Generator in 0JH

Stress test 4A02XM4, 4A12XM4

Stripping *see* Extraction

Study
  Electrophysiologic stimulation, cardiac *see* Measurement, Cardiac 4A02
  Ocular motility 4A07X7Z
  Pulmonary airway flow measurement *see* Measurement, Respiratory 4A09
  Visual acuity 4A07X0Z

Styloglossus muscle *use* Tongue, Palate, Pharynx Muscle

Stylomandibular ligament *use* Head and Neck Bursa and Ligament

Stylopharyngeus muscle *use* Tongue, Palate, Pharynx Muscle

Subacromial bursa
  use Shoulder Bursa and Ligament, Left
  use Shoulder Bursa and Ligament, Right

Subaortic (common iliac) lymph node *use* Lymphatic, Pelvis

Subarachnoid space, spinal *use* Spinal Canal
Subclavicular (apical) lymph node
   use Lymphatic, Left Axillary
   use Lymphatic, Right Axillary
Subclavius muscle
   use Thorax Muscle, Left
   use Thorax Muscle, Right
Subclavius nerve *use* Brachial Plexus
Subcostal artery *use* Upper Artery
Subcostal muscle
   use Thorax Muscle, Left
   use Thorax Muscle, Right
Subcostal nerve *use* Thoracic Nerve
Subcutaneous Defibrillator Lead
   Insertion of device in, Subcutaneous Tissue and
      Fascia, Chest ØJH6
   Removal of device from, Subcutaneous Tissue and
      Fascia, Trunk ØJPT
   Revision of device in, Subcutaneous Tissue and
      Fascia, Trunk ØJWT
Subcutaneous injection reservoir, port *use* Vascular
   Access Device, Totally Implantable in Subcuta-
   neous Tissue and Fascia
Subcutaneous injection reservoir, pump *use* Infu-
   sion Device, Pump in Subcutaneous Tissue and
   Fascia
Subdermal progesterone implant *use* Contraceptive
   Device in Subcutaneous Tissue and Fascia
Subdural space, spinal *use* Spinal Canal
Submandibular ganglion
   use Facial Nerve
   use Head and Neck Sympathetic Nerve
Submandibular gland
   use Submaxillary Gland, Left
   use Submaxillary Gland, Right
Submandibular lymph node *use* Lymphatic, Head
Submandibular space *use* Subcutaneous Tissue and
   Fascia, Face
Submaxillary ganglion *use* Head and Neck Sympa-
   thetic Nerve
Submaxillary lymph node *use* Lymphatic, Head
Submental artery *use* Face Artery
Submental lymph node *use* Lymphatic, Head
Submucous (Meissner's) plexus *use* Abdominal
   Sympathetic Nerve
Suboccipital nerve *use* Cervical Nerve
Suboccipital venous plexus
   use Vertebral Vein, Left
   use Vertebral Vein, Right
Subparotid lymph node *use* Lymphatic, Head
Subscapular aponeurosis
   use Subcutaneous Tissue and Fascia, Left Upper
      Arm
   use Subcutaneous Tissue and Fascia, Right Upper
      Arm
Subscapular artery
   use Axillary Artery, Left
   use Axillary Artery, Right
Subscapular (posterior) lymph node
   use Lymphatic, Axillary, Left
   use Lymphatic, Axillary, Right
Subscapularis muscle
   use Shoulder Muscle, Left
   use Shoulder Muscle, Right
Substance Abuse Treatment
   Counseling
      Family, for substance abuse, Other Family
         Counseling HZ63ZZZ
      Group
         12-Step HZ43ZZZ
         Behavioral HZ41ZZZ
         Cognitive HZ40ZZZ
         Cognitive-Behavioral HZ42ZZZ
         Confrontational HZ48ZZZ
         Continuing Care HZ49ZZZ
         Infectious Disease
            Post-Test HZ4CZZZ
            Pre-Test HZ4CZZZ
         Interpersonal HZ44ZZZ
         Motivational Enhancement HZ47ZZZ
         Psychoeducation HZ46ZZZ
         Spiritual HZ4BZZZ
         Vocational HZ45ZZZ
      Individual
         12-Step HZ33ZZZ
         Behavioral HZ31ZZZ
         Cognitive HZ30ZZZ

Substance Abuse Treatment — *continued*
   Counseling — *continued*
      Individual — *continued*
         Cognitive-Behavioral HZ32ZZZ
         Confrontational HZ38ZZZ
         Continuing Care HZ39ZZZ
         Infectious Disease
            Post-Test HZ3CZZZ
            Pre-Test HZ3CZZZ
         Interpersonal HZ34ZZZ
         Motivational Enhancement HZ37ZZZ
         Psychoeducation HZ36ZZZ
         Spiritual HZ3BZZZ
         Vocational HZ35ZZZ
   Detoxification Services, for substance abuse
      HZ2ZZZZ
   Medication Management
      Antabuse HZ83ZZZ
      Bupropion HZ87ZZZ
      Clonidine HZ86ZZZ
      Levo-alpha-acetyl-methadol (LAAM)
         HZ82ZZZ
      Methadone Maintenance HZ81ZZZ
      Naloxone HZ85ZZZ
      Naltrexone HZ84ZZZ
      Nicotine Replacement HZ80ZZZ
      Other Replacement Medication HZ89ZZZ
      Psychiatric Medication HZ88ZZZ
   Pharmacotherapy
      Antabuse HZ93ZZZ
      Bupropion HZ97ZZZ
      Clonidine HZ96ZZZ
      Levo-alpha-acetyl-methadol (LAAM)
         HZ92ZZZ
      Methadone Maintenance HZ91ZZZ
      Naloxone HZ95ZZZ
      Naltrexone HZ94ZZZ
      Nicotine Replacement HZ90ZZZ
      Psychiatric Medication HZ98ZZZ
      Replacement Medication, Other HZ99ZZZ
   Psychotherapy
      12-Step HZ53ZZZ
      Behavioral HZ51ZZZ
      Cognitive HZ50ZZZ
      Cognitive-Behavioral HZ52ZZZ
      Confrontational HZ58ZZZ
      Interactive HZ55ZZZ
      Interpersonal HZ54ZZZ
      Motivational Enhancement HZ57ZZZ
      Psychoanalysis HZ5BZZZ
      Psychodynamic HZ5CZZZ
      Psychoeducation HZ56ZZZ
      Psychophysiological HZ5DZZZ
      Supportive HZ59ZZZ
Substantia nigra *use* Basal Ganglia
Subtalar (talocalcaneal) joint
   use Tarsal Joint, Left
   use Tarsal Joint, Right
Subtalar ligament
   use Foot Bursa and Ligament, Left
   use Foot Bursa and Ligament, Right
Subthalamic nucleus *use* Basal Ganglia
Suction curettage (D&C), nonobstetric *see* Extraction, Endometrium ØUDB
Suction curettage, obstetric post-delivery *see* Ex-
   traction, Products of Conception, Retained 1ØD1
Sulbactam-Durlobactam XWØ
SUL-DUR *use* Sulbactam-Durlobactam
Superficial circumflex iliac vein
   use Saphenous Vein, Left
   use Saphenous Vein, Right
Superficial epigastric artery
   use Femoral Artery, Left
   use Femoral Artery, Right
Superficial epigastric vein
   use Saphenous Vein, Left
   use Saphenous Vein, Right
Superficial Inferior Epigastric Artery Flap
   Replacement
      Bilateral ØHRVØ78
      Left ØHRUØ78
      Right ØHRTØ78
   Transfer
      Left ØKXG
      Right ØKXF
Superficial palmar arch
   use Hand Artery, Left
   use Hand Artery, Right

Superficial palmar venous arch
   use Hand Vein, Left
   use Hand Vein, Right
Superficial temporal artery
   use Temporal Artery, Left
   use Temporal Artery, Right
Superficial transverse perineal muscle *use* Perineum
   Muscle
Superior cardiac nerve *use* Thoracic Sympathetic
   Nerve
Superior cerebellar vein *use* Intracranial Vein
Superior cerebral vein *use* Intracranial Vein
Superior clunic (cluneal) nerve *use* Lumbar Nerve
Superior epigastric artery
   use Internal Mammary Artery, Left
   use Internal Mammary Artery, Right
Superior genicular artery
   use Popliteal Artery, Left
   use Popliteal Artery, Right
Superior gluteal artery
   use Internal Iliac Artery, Left
   use Internal Iliac Artery, Right
Superior gluteal nerve *use* Lumbar Plexus
Superior hypogastric plexus *use* Abdominal Sympa-
   thetic Nerve
Superior labial artery *use* Face Artery
Superior laryngeal artery
   use Thyroid Artery, Left
   use Thyroid Artery, Right
Superior laryngeal nerve *use* Vagus Nerve
Superior longitudinal muscle *use* Tongue, Palate,
   Pharynx Muscle
Superior mesenteric ganglion *use* Abdominal Sym-
   pathetic Nerve
Superior mesenteric lymph node *use* Lymphatic,
   Mesenteric
Superior mesenteric plexus *use* Abdominal Sympa-
   thetic Nerve
Superior oblique muscle
   use Extraocular Muscle, Left
   use Extraocular Muscle, Right
Superior olivary nucleus *use* Pons
Superior rectal artery *use* Inferior Mesenteric Artery
Superior rectal vein *use* Inferior Mesenteric Vein
Superior rectus muscle
   use Extraocular Muscle, Left
   use Extraocular Muscle, Right
Superior tarsal plate
   use Upper Eyelid, Left
   use Upper Eyelid, Right
Superior thoracic artery
   use Axillary Artery, Left
   use Axillary Artery, Right
Superior thyroid artery
   use External Carotid Artery, Left
   use External Carotid Artery, Right
   use Thyroid Artery, Left
   use Thyroid Artery, Right
Superior turbinate *use* Nasal Turbinate
Superior ulnar collateral artery
   use Brachial Artery, Left
   use Brachial Artery, Right
Superior vesical artery
   use Internal Iliac Artery, Left
   use Internal Iliac Artery, Right
Supersaturated Oxygen (SSO2) therapy, cardiac
   intra-arterial 5A0222C
Supplement
   Abdominal Wall ØWUF
   Acetabulum
      Left ØQU5
      Right ØQU4
   Ampulla of Vater ØFUC
   Anal Sphincter ØDUR
   Ankle Region
      Left ØYUL
      Right ØYUK
   Anus ØDUQ
   Aorta
      Abdominal Ø4UØ
      Thoracic
         Ascending/Arch Ø2UX
         Descending Ø2UW
   Arm
      Lower
         Left ØXUF
         Right ØXUD

Supplement — *continued*
  Arm — *continued*
    Upper
      Left ØXU9
      Right ØXU8
  Arteriovenous Fistula, Extraluminal Support Device
    X2U
  Artery
    Anterior Tibial
      Left 04UQ
      Right 04UP
    Axillary
      Left 03U6
      Right 03U5
    Brachial
      Left 03U8
      Right 03U7
    Celiac 04U1
    Colic
      Left 04U7
      Middle 04U8
      Right 04U6
    Common Carotid
      Left 03UJ
      Right 03UH
    Common Iliac
      Left 04UD
      Right 04UC
    Coronary
      Four or More Arteries 02U3
      One Artery 02UØ
      Three Arteries 02U2
      Two Arteries 02U1
    External Carotid
      Left 03UN
      Right 03UM
    External Iliac
      Left 04UJ
      Right 04UH
    Face 03UR
    Femoral
      Left 04UL
      Right 04UK
    Foot
      Left 04UW
      Right 04UV
    Gastric 04U2
    Hand
      Left 03UF
      Right 03UD
    Hepatic 04U3
    Inferior Mesenteric 04UB
    Innominate 03U2
    Internal Carotid
      Left 03UL
      Right 03UK
    Internal Iliac
      Left 04UF
      Right 04UE
    Internal Mammary
      Left 03U1
      Right 03UØ
    Intracranial 03UG
    Lower 04UY
    Peroneal
      Left 04UU
      Right 04UT
    Popliteal
      Left 04UN
      Right 04UM
    Posterior Tibial
      Left 04US
      Right 04UR
    Pulmonary
      Left 02UR
      Right 02UQ
    Pulmonary Trunk 02UP
    Radial
      Left 03UC
      Right 03UB
    Renal
      Left 04UA
      Right 04U9
    Splenic 04U4
    Subclavian
      Left 03U4
      Right 03U3
    Superior Mesenteric 04U5

Supplement — *continued*
  Artery — *continued*
    Temporal
      Left 03UT
      Right 03US
    Thyroid
      Left 03UV
      Right 03UU
    Ulnar
      Left 03UA
      Right 03U9
    Upper 03UY
    Vertebral
      Left 03UQ
      Right 03UP
  Atrium
    Left 02U7
    Right 02U6
  Auditory Ossicle
    Left 09UA
    Right 09U9
  Axilla
    Left ØXU5
    Right ØXU4
  Back
    Lower ØWUL
    Upper ØWUK
  Bladder ØTUB
  Bladder Neck ØTUC
  Bone
    Ethmoid
      Left ØNUG
      Right ØNUF
    Frontal ØNU1
    Hyoid ØNUX
    Lacrimal
      Left ØNUJ
      Right ØNUH
    Nasal ØNUB
    Occipital ØNU7
    Palatine
      Left ØNUL
      Right ØNUK
    Parietal
      Left ØNU4
      Right ØNU3
    Pelvic
      Left ØQU3
      Right ØQU2
    Sphenoid ØNUC
    Temporal
      Left ØNU6
      Right ØNU5
    Zygomatic
      Left ØNUN
      Right ØNUM
  Breast
    Bilateral ØHUV
    Left ØHUU
    Right ØHUT
  Bronchus
    Lingula ØBU9
    Lower Lobe
      Left ØBUB
      Right ØBU6
    Main
      Left ØBU7
      Right ØBU3
    Middle Lobe, Right ØBU5
    Upper Lobe
      Left ØBU8
      Right ØBU4
  Buccal Mucosa ØCU4
  Bursa and Ligament
    Abdomen
      Left ØMUJ
      Right ØMUH
    Ankle
      Left ØMUR
      Right ØMUQ
    Elbow
      Left ØMU4
      Right ØMU3
    Foot
      Left ØMUT
      Right ØMUS
    Hand
      Left ØMU8
      Right ØMU7

Supplement — *continued*
  Bursa and Ligament — *continued*
    Head and Neck ØMUØ
    Hip
      Left ØMUM
      Right ØMUL
    Knee
      Left ØMUP
      Right ØMUN
    Lower Extremity
      Left ØMUW
      Right ØMUV
    Perineum ØMUK
    Rib(s) ØMUG
    Shoulder
      Left ØMU2
      Right ØMU1
    Spine
      Lower ØMUD
      Posterior Vertebral Tether XKU
      Upper ØMUC
    Sternum ØMUF
    Upper Extremity
      Left ØMUB
      Right ØMU9
    Wrist
      Left ØMU6
      Right ØMU5
  Buttock
    Left ØYU1
    Right ØYUØ
  Carina ØBU2
  Carpal
    Left ØPUN
    Right ØPUM
  Cecum ØDUH
  Cerebral Meninges ØØU1
  Cerebral Ventricle ØØU6
  Chest Wall ØWU8
  Chordae Tendineae 02U9
  Cisterna Chyli 07UL
  Clavicle
    Left ØPUB
    Right ØPU9
  Clitoris ØUUJ
  Coccyx ØQUS
  Colon
    Ascending ØDUK
    Descending ØDUM
    Sigmoid ØDUN
    Transverse ØDUL
  Cord
    Bilateral ØVUH
    Left ØVUG
    Right ØVUF
  Cornea
    Left Ø8U9
    Right Ø8U8
  Coronary Artery/Arteries, Vein Graft Extraluminal
    Support Device(s) X2U4079
  Cul-de-sac ØUUF
  Diaphragm ØBUT
  Disc
    Cervical Vertebral ØRU3
    Cervicothoracic Vertebral ØRU5
    Lumbar Vertebral ØSU2
    Lumbosacral ØSU4
    Thoracic Vertebral ØRU9
    Thoracolumbar Vertebral ØRUB
  Duct
    Common Bile ØFU9
    Cystic ØFU8
    Hepatic
      Common ØFU7
      Left ØFU6
      Right ØFU5
    Lacrimal
      Left Ø8UY
      Right Ø8UX
    Pancreatic ØFUD
      Accessory ØFUF
  Duodenum ØDU9
  Dura Mater ØØU2
  Ear
    External
      Bilateral Ø9U2
      Left Ø9U1
      Right Ø9UØ

Supplement — *continued*
  Ear — *continued*
    Inner
      Left Ø9UE
      Right Ø9UD
    Middle
      Left Ø9U6
      Right Ø9U5
  Elbow Region
    Left ØXUC
    Right ØXUB
  Epididymis
    Bilateral ØVUL
    Left ØVUK
    Right ØVUJ
  Epiglottis ØCUR
  Esophagogastric Junction ØDU4
  Esophagus ØDU5
    Lower ØDU3
    Middle ØDU2
    Upper ØDU1
  Extremity
    Lower
      Left ØYUB
      Right ØYU9
    Upper
      Left ØXU7
      Right ØXU6
  Eye
    Left Ø8U1
    Right Ø8UØ
  Eyelid
    Lower
      Left Ø8UR
      Right Ø8UQ
    Upper
      Left Ø8UP
      Right Ø8UN
  Face ØWU2
  Fallopian Tube
    Left ØUU6
    Right ØUU5
  Fallopian Tubes, Bilateral ØUU7
  Femoral Region
    Bilateral ØYUE
    Left ØYU8
    Right ØYU7
  Femoral Shaft
    Left ØQU9
    Right ØQU8
  Femur
    Lower
      Left ØQUC
      Right ØQUB
    Upper
      Left ØQU7
      Right ØQU6
  Fibula
    Left ØQUK
    Right ØQUJ
  Finger
    Index
      Left ØXUP
      Right ØXUN
    Little
      Left ØXUW
      Right ØXUV
    Middle
      Left ØXUR
      Right ØXUQ
    Ring
      Left ØXUT
      Right ØXUS
  Foot
    Left ØYUN
    Right ØYUM
  Gingiva
    Lower ØCU6
    Upper ØCU5
  Glenoid Cavity
    Left ØPU8
    Right ØPU7
  Hand
    Left ØXUK
    Right ØXUJ
  Head ØWUØ
  Heart Ø2UA
  Humeral Head
    Left ØPUD

Supplement — *continued*
  Humeral Head — *continued*
    Right ØPUC
  Humeral Shaft
    Left ØPUG
    Right ØPUF
  Hymen ØUUK
  Ileocecal Valve ØDUC
  Ileum ØDUB
  Inguinal Region
    Bilateral ØYUA
    Left ØYU6
    Right ØYU5
  Intestine
    Large ØDUE
      Left ØDUG
      Right ØDUF
    Small ØDU8
  Iris
    Left Ø8UD
    Right Ø8UC
  Jaw
    Lower ØWU5
    Upper ØWU4
  Jejunum ØDUA
  Joint
    Acromioclavicular
      Left ØRUH
      Right ØRUG
    Ankle
      Left ØSUG
      Right ØSUF
    Carpal
      Left ØRUR
      Right ØRUQ
    Carpometacarpal
      Left ØRUT
      Right ØRUS
    Cervical Vertebral ØRU1
    Cervicothoracic Vertebral ØRU4
    Coccygeal ØSU6
    Elbow
      Left ØRUM
      Right ØRUL
    Finger Phalangeal
      Left ØRUX
      Right ØRUW
    Hip
      Left ØSUB
        Acetabular Surface ØSUE
        Femoral Surface ØSUS
      Right ØSU9
        Acetabular Surface ØSUA
        Femoral Surface ØSUR
    Knee
      Left ØSUD
        Femoral Surface ØSUUØ9Z
        Tibial Surface ØSUWØ9Z
      Right ØSUC
        Femoral Surface ØSUTØ9Z
        Tibial Surface ØSUVØ9Z
    Lumbar Vertebral ØSUØ
    Lumbosacral ØSU3
    Metacarpophalangeal
      Left ØRUV
      Right ØRUU
    Metatarsal-Phalangeal
      Left ØSUN
      Right ØSUM
    Occipital-cervical ØRUØ
    Sacrococcygeal ØSU5
    Sacroiliac
      Left ØSU8
      Right ØSU7
    Shoulder
      Left ØRUK
      Right ØRUJ
    Sternoclavicular
      Left ØRUF
      Right ØRUE
    Tarsal
      Left ØSUJ
      Right ØSUH
    Tarsometatarsal
      Left ØSUL
      Right ØSUK
    Temporomandibular
      Left ØRUD
      Right ØRUC

Supplement — *continued*
  Joint — *continued*
    Thoracic Vertebral ØRU6
    Thoracolumbar Vertebral ØRUA
    Toe Phalangeal
      Left ØSUQ
      Right ØSUP
    Wrist
      Left ØRUP
      Right ØRUN
  Kidney Pelvis
    Left ØTU4
    Right ØTU3
  Knee Region
    Left ØYUG
    Right ØYUF
  Larynx ØCUS
  Leg
    Lower
      Left ØYUJ
      Right ØYUH
    Upper
      Left ØYUD
      Right ØYUC
  Lip
    Lower ØCU1
    Upper ØCUØ
  Lymphatic
    Aortic Ø7UD
    Axillary
      Left Ø7U6
      Right Ø7U5
    Head Ø7UØ
    Inguinal
      Left Ø7UJ
      Right Ø7UH
    Internal Mammary
      Left Ø7U9
      Right Ø7U8
    Lower Extremity
      Left Ø7UG
      Right Ø7UF
    Mesenteric Ø7UB
    Neck
      Left Ø7U2
      Right Ø7U1
    Pelvis Ø7UC
    Thoracic Duct Ø7UK
    Thorax Ø7U7
    Upper Extremity
      Left Ø7U4
      Right Ø7U3
  Mandible
    Left ØNUV
    Right ØNUT
  Maxilla ØNUR
  Mediastinum ØWUC
  Mesentery ØDUV
  Metacarpal
    Left ØPUQ
    Right ØPUP
  Metatarsal
    Left ØQUP
    Right ØQUN
  Muscle
    Abdomen
      Left ØKUL
      Right ØKUK
    Extraocular
      Left Ø8UM
      Right Ø8UL
    Facial ØKU1
    Foot
      Left ØKUW
      Right ØKUV
    Hand
      Left ØKUD
      Right ØKUC
    Head ØKUØ
    Hip
      Left ØKUP
      Right ØKUN
    Lower Arm and Wrist
      Left ØKUB
      Right ØKU9
    Lower Leg
      Left ØKUT
      Right ØKUS

Supplement — *continued*
  Muscle — *continued*
    Neck
      Left 0KU3
      Right 0KU2
    Papillary 02UD
    Perineum 0KUM
    Shoulder
      Left 0KU6
      Right 0KU5
    Thorax
      Left 0KUJ
      Right 0KUH
    Tongue, Palate, Pharynx 0KU4
    Trunk
      Left 0KUG
      Right 0KUF
    Upper Arm
      Left 0KU8
      Right 0KU7
    Upper Leg
      Left 0KUR
      Right 0KUQ
  Nasal Mucosa and Soft Tissue 09UK
  Nasopharynx 09UN
  Neck 0WU6
  Nerve
    Abducens 00UL
    Accessory 00UR
    Acoustic 00UN
    Cervical 01U1
    Facial 00UM
    Femoral 01UD
    Glossopharyngeal 00UP
    Hypoglossal 00US
    Lumbar 01UB
    Median 01U5
    Oculomotor 00UH
    Olfactory 00UF
    Optic 00UG
    Peroneal 01UH
    Phrenic 01U2
    Pudendal 01UC
    Radial 01U6
    Sacral 01UR
    Sciatic 01UF
    Thoracic 01U8
    Tibial 01UG
    Trigeminal 00UK
    Trochlear 00UJ
    Ulnar 01U4
    Vagus 00UQ
  Nipple
    Left 0HUX
    Right 0HUW
  Omentum 0DUU
  Orbit
    Left 0NUQ
    Right 0NUP
  Palate
    Hard 0CU2
    Soft 0CU3
  Patella
    Left 0QUF
    Right 0QUD
  Penis 0VUS
  Pericardium 02UN
  Perineum
    Female 0WUN
    Male 0WUM
  Peritoneum 0DUW
  Phalanx
    Finger
      Left 0PUV
      Right 0PUT
    Thumb
      Left 0PUS
      Right 0PUR
    Toe
      Left 0QUR
      Right 0QUQ
  Pharynx 0CUM
  Prepuce 0VUT
  Radius
    Left 0PUJ
    Right 0PUH
  Rectum 0DUP
  Retina
    Left 08UF

Supplement — *continued*
  Retina — *continued*
    Right 08UE
  Retinal Vessel
    Left 08UH
    Right 08UG
  Ribs
    1 to 2 0PU1
    3 or More 0PU2
  Sacrum 0QU1
  Scapula
    Left 0PU6
    Right 0PU5
  Scrotum 0VU5
  Septum
    Atrial 02U5
    Nasal 09UM
    Ventricular 02UM
  Shoulder Region
    Left 0XU3
    Right 0XU2
  Sinus
    Accessory 09UP
    Ethmoid
      Left 09UV
      Right 09UU
    Frontal
      Left 09UT
      Right 09US
    Mastoid
      Left 09UC
      Right 09UB
    Maxillary
      Left 09UR
      Right 09UQ
    Sphenoid
      Left 09UX
      Right 09UW
  Skull 0NU0
  Spinal Meninges 00UT
  Sternum 0PU0
  Stomach 0DU6
    Pylorus 0DU7
  Subcutaneous Tissue and Fascia
    Abdomen 0JU8
    Back 0JU7
    Buttock 0JU9
    Chest 0JU6
    Face 0JU1
    Foot
      Left 0JUR
      Right 0JUQ
    Hand
      Left 0JUK
      Right 0JUJ
    Lower Arm
      Left 0JUH
      Right 0JUG
    Lower Leg
      Left 0JUP
      Right 0JUN
    Neck
      Left 0JU5
      Right 0JU4
    Pelvic Region 0JUC
    Perineum 0JUB
    Scalp 0JU0
    Upper Arm
      Left 0JUF
      Right 0JUD
    Upper Leg
      Left 0JUM
      Right 0JUL
  Tarsal
    Left 0QUM
    Right 0QUL
  Tendon
    Abdomen
      Left 0LUG
      Right 0LUF
    Ankle
      Left 0LUT
      Right 0LUS
    Foot
      Left 0LUW
      Right 0LUV
    Hand
      Left 0LU8
      Right 0LU7

Supplement — *continued*
  Tendon — *continued*
    Head and Neck 0LU0
    Hip
      Left 0LUK
      Right 0LUJ
    Knee
      Left 0LUR
      Right 0LUQ
    Lower Arm and Wrist
      Left 0LU6
      Right 0LU5
    Lower Leg
      Left 0LUP
      Right 0LUN
    Perineum 0LUH
    Shoulder
      Left 0LU2
      Right 0LU1
    Thorax
      Left 0LUD
      Right 0LUC
    Trunk
      Left 0LUB
      Right 0LU9
    Upper Arm
      Left 0LU4
      Right 0LU3
    Upper Leg
      Left 0LUM
      Right 0LUL
  Testis
    Bilateral 0VUC0
    Left 0VUB0
    Right 0VU90
  Thumb
    Left 0XUM
    Right 0XUL
  Tibia
    Left 0QUH
    Right 0QUG
  Toe
    1st
      Left 0YUQ
      Right 0YUP
    2nd
      Left 0YUS
      Right 0YUR
    3rd
      Left 0YUU
      Right 0YUT
    4th
      Left 0YUW
      Right 0YUV
    5th
      Left 0YUY
      Right 0YUX
  Tongue 0CU7
  Trachea 0BU1
  Tunica Vaginalis
    Left 0VU7
    Right 0VU6
  Turbinate, Nasal 09UL
  Tympanic Membrane
    Left 09U8
    Right 09U7
  Ulna
    Left 0PUL
    Right 0PUK
  Ureter
    Left 0TU7
    Right 0TU6
  Urethra 0TUD
  Uterine Supporting Structure 0UU4
  Uvula 0CUN
  Vagina 0UUG
  Valve
    Aortic 02UF
    Mitral 02UG
    Pulmonary 02UH
    Tricuspid 02UJ
  Vas Deferens
    Bilateral 0VUQ
    Left 0VUP
    Right 0VUN
  Vein
    Axillary
      Left 05U8
      Right 05U7

Subterms under main terms may continue to next column or page

Supplement — *continued*
　Vein — *continued*
　　Azygos Ø5UØ
　　Basilic
　　　Left Ø5UC
　　　Right Ø5UB
　　Brachial
　　　Left Ø5UA
　　　Right Ø5U9
　　Cephalic
　　　Left Ø5UF
　　　Right Ø5UD
　　Colic Ø6U7
　　Common Iliac
　　　Left Ø6UD
　　　Right Ø6UC
　　Esophageal Ø6U3
　　External Iliac
　　　Left Ø6UG
　　　Right Ø6UF
　　External Jugular
　　　Left Ø5UQ
　　　Right Ø5UP
　　Face
　　　Left Ø5UV
　　　Right Ø5UT
　　Femoral
　　　Left Ø6UN
　　　Right Ø6UM
　　Foot
　　　Left Ø6UV
　　　Right Ø6UT
　　Gastric Ø6U2
　　Hand
　　　Left Ø5UH
　　　Right Ø5UG
　　Hemiazygos Ø5U1
　　Hepatic Ø6U4
　　Hypogastric
　　　Left Ø6UJ
　　　Right Ø6UH
　　Inferior Mesenteric Ø6U6
　　Innominate
　　　Left Ø5U4
　　　Right Ø5U3
　　Internal Jugular
　　　Left Ø5UN
　　　Right Ø5UM
　　Intracranial Ø5UL
　　Lower Ø6UY
　　Portal Ø6U8
　　Pulmonary
　　　Left Ø2UT
　　　Right Ø2US
　　Renal
　　　Left Ø6UB
　　　Right Ø6U9
　　Saphenous
　　　Left Ø6UQ
　　　Right Ø6UP
　　Splenic Ø6U1
　　Subclavian
　　　Left Ø5U6
　　　Right Ø5U5
　　Superior Mesenteric Ø6U5
　　Upper Ø5UY
　　Vertebral
　　　Left Ø5US
　　　Right Ø5UR
　Vena Cava
　　Inferior Ø6UØ
　　Superior Ø2UV
　Ventricle
　　Left Ø2UL
　　Right Ø2UK
　Vertebra
　　Cervical ØPU3
　　Lumbar ØQUØ
　　　Mechanically Expandable (Paired) Synthetic Substitute XNUØ356
　　Thoracic ØPU4
　　　Mechanically Expandable (Paired) Synthetic Substitute XNU4356
　Vesicle
　　Bilateral ØVU3
　　Left ØVU2
　　Right ØVU1
　Vocal Cord
　　Left ØCUV

Supplement — *continued*
　Vocal Cord — *continued*
　　Right ØCUT
　Vulva ØUUM
　Wrist Region
　　Left ØXUH
　　Right ØXUG
Supraclavicular (Virchow's) lymph node
　use Lymphatic, Left Neck
　use Lymphatic, Right Neck
Supraclavicular nerve *use* Cervical Plexus
Suprahyoid lymph node *use* Lymphatic, Head
Suprahyoid muscle
　use Neck Muscle, Left
　use Neck Muscle, Right
Suprainguinal lymph node *use* Lymphatic, Pelvis
Supraorbital vein
　use Face Vein, Left
　use Face Vein, Right
Suprarenal gland
　use Adrenal Gland
　use Adrenal Gland, Bilateral
　use Adrenal Gland, Left
　use Adrenal Gland, Right
Suprarenal plexus *use* Abdominal Sympathetic Nerve
Suprascapular nerve *use* Brachial Plexus
Supraspinatus fascia
　use Subcutaneous Tissue and Fascia, Left Upper Arm
　use Subcutaneous Tissue and Fascia, Right Upper Arm
Supraspinatus muscle
　use Shoulder Muscle, Left
　use Shoulder Muscle, Right
Supraspinous ligament
　use Lower Spine Bursa and Ligament
　use Upper Spine Bursa and Ligament
Suprasternal notch *use* Sternum
Supratrochlear lymph node
　use Lymphatic, Left Upper Extremity
　use Lymphatic, Right Upper Extremity
Sural artery
　use Popliteal Artery, Left
　use Popliteal Artery, Right
Surpass Streamline™ Flow Diverter *use* Intraluminal Device, Flow Diverter in Ø3V
Suspension
　Bladder Neck *see* Reposition, Bladder Neck ØTSC
　Kidney *see* Reposition, Urinary System ØTS
　Urethra *see* Reposition, Urinary System ØTS
　Urethrovesical *see* Reposition, Bladder Neck ØTSC
　Uterus *see* Reposition, Uterus ØUS9
　Vagina *see* Reposition, Vagina ØUSG
Sustained Release Drug-eluting Intraluminal Device
　Dilation
　　Anterior Tibial
　　　Left X27Q385
　　　Right X27P385
　　Femoral
　　　Left X27J385
　　　Right X27H385
　　Peroneal
　　　Left X27U385
　　　Right X27T385
　　Popliteal
　　　Left Distal X27N385
　　　Left Proximal X27L385
　　　Right Distal X27M385
　　　Right Proximal X27K385
　　Posterior Tibial
　　　Left X27S385
　　　Right X27R385
　　Four or More
　　　Anterior Tibial
　　　　Left X27Q3C5
　　　　Right X27P3C5
　　　Femoral
　　　　Left X27J3C5
　　　　Right X27H3C5
　　　Peroneal
　　　　Left X27U3C5
　　　　Right X27T3C5
　　　Popliteal
　　　　Left Distal X27N3C5
　　　　Left Proximal X27L3C5
　　　　Right Distal X27M3C5

Sustained Release Drug-eluting Intraluminal Device — *continued*
　Four or More — *continued*
　　Popliteal — *continued*
　　　Right Proximal X27K3C5
　　Posterior Tibial
　　　Left X27S3C5
　　　Right X27R3C5
　Three
　　Anterior Tibial
　　　Left X27Q3B5
　　　Right X27P3B5
　　Femoral
　　　Left X27J3B5
　　　Right X27H3B5
　　Peroneal
　　　Left X27U3B5
　　　Right X27T3B5
　　Popliteal
　　　Left Distal X27N3B5
　　　Left Proximal X27L3B5
　　　Right Distal X27M3B5
　　　Right Proximal X27K3B5
　　Posterior Tibial
　　　Left X27S3B5
　　　Right X27R3B5
　Two
　　Anterior Tibial
　　　Left X27Q395
　　　Right X27P395
　　Femoral
　　　Left X27J395
　　　Right X27H395
　　Peroneal
　　　Left X27U395
　　　Right X27T395
　　Popliteal
　　　Left Distal X27N395
　　　Left Proximal X27L395
　　　Right Distal X27M395
　　　Right Proximal X27K395
　　Posterior Tibial
　　　Left X27S395
　　　Right X27R395
Suture
　Laceration repair *see* Repair
　Ligation *see* Occlusion
Suture Removal
　Extremity
　　Lower 8EØYXY8
　　Upper 8EØXXY8
　Head and Neck Region 8EØ9XY8
　Trunk Region 8EØWXY8
Sutureless valve, Perceval (rapid deployment technique) *see* Replacement, Valve, Aortic Ø2RF
Sweat gland *use* Skin
Sympathectomy *see* Excision, Peripheral Nervous System Ø1B
SynCardia (temporary) total artificial heart (TAH) *use* Synthetic Substitute, Pneumatic in Ø2R
SynCardia Total Artificial Heart *use* Synthetic Substitute
Synchra CRT-P *use* Cardiac Resynchronization Pacemaker Pulse Generator in ØJH
SynchroMed pump *use* Infusion Device, Pump in Subcutaneous Tissue and Fascia
Synechiotomy, iris *see* Release, Eye Ø8N
Synovectomy
　Lower joint *see* Excision, Lower Joints ØSB
　Upper joint *see* Excision, Upper Joints ØRB
Systemic Nuclear Medicine Therapy
　Abdomen CW7Ø
　Anatomical Regions, Multiple CW7YYZZ
　Chest CW73
　Thyroid CW7G
　Whole Body CW7N

T

tab-cel® *use* Tabelecleucel Immunotherapy
Tabelecleucel Immunotherapy XWØ
Tagraxofusp-erzs Antineoplastic XWØ
Takedown
　Arteriovenous shunt *see* Removal of device from, Upper Arteries Ø3P
　Arteriovenous shunt, with creation of new shunt *see* Bypass, Upper Arteries Ø31

▽ Subterms under main terms may continue to next column or page

Takedown — *continued*
 Stoma
  see Excision
  see Reposition
Talent® Converter *use* Intraluminal Device
Talent® Occluder *use* Intraluminal Device
Talent® Stent Graft (abdominal) (thoracic) *use* Intraluminal Device
Talocalcaneal (subtalar) joint
 use Tarsal Joint, Left
 use Tarsal Joint, Right
Talocalcaneal ligament
 use Foot Bursa and Ligament, Left
 use Foot Bursa and Ligament, Right
Talocalcaneonavicular joint
 use Tarsal Joint, Left
 use Tarsal Joint, Right
Talocalcaneonavicular ligament
 use Foot Bursa and Ligament, Left
 use Foot Bursa and Ligament, Right
Talocrural joint
 use Ankle Joint, Left
 use Joint, Ankle, Right
Talofibular ligament
 use Ankle Bursa and Ligament, Left
 use Ankle Bursa and Ligament, Right
Talus bone
 use Tarsal, Left
 use Tarsal, Right
TandemHeart® System *use* Short-term External Heart Assist System in Heart and Great Vessels
Tarsectomy
 see Excision, Lower Bones ØQB
 see Resection, Lower Bones ØQT
Tarsometatarsal ligament
 use Foot Bursa and Ligament, Left
 use Foot Bursa and Ligament, Right
Tarsorrhaphy *see* Repair, Eye Ø8Q
Tattooing
 Cornea 3EØCXMZ
 Skin *see* Introduction of substance in or on, Skin 3EØØ
Taurolidine Anti-infective and Heparin Anticoagulant XYØYX28
TAXUS® Liberte® Paclitaxel-eluting Coronary Stent System *use* Intraluminal Device, Drug-eluting in Heart and Great Vessels
TBNA (transbronchial needle aspiration)
 Fluid or gas *see* Drainage, Respiratory System ØB9
 Tissue biopsy *see* Extraction, Respiratory System ØBD
Tecartus™ *use* Brexucabtagene Autoleucel Immunotherapy
TECENTRIQ® *use* Atezolizumab Antineoplastic
Teclistamab Antineoplastic XWØ1348
Telemetry 4A12X4Z
 Ambulatory 4A12X45
Temperature gradient study 4AØZXKZ
Temporal lobe *use* Cerebral Hemisphere
Temporalis muscle *use* Head Muscle
Temporoparietalis muscle *use* Head Muscle
Tendolysis *see* Release, Tendons ØLN
Tendonectomy
 see Excision, Tendons ØLB
 see Resection, Tendons ØLT
Tendonoplasty, tenoplasty
 see Repair, Tendons ØLQ
 see Replacement, Tendons ØLR
 see Supplement, Tendons ØLU
Tendorrhaphy *see* Repair, Tendons ØLQ
Tendototomy
 see Division, Tendons ØL8
 see Drainage, Tendons ØL9
Tenectomy, tenonectomy
 see Excision, Tendons ØLB
 see Resection, Tendons ØLT
Tenolysis *see* Release, Tendons ØLN
Tenontorrhaphy *see* Repair, Tendons ØLQ
Tenontotomy
 see Division, Tendons ØL8
 see Drainage, Tendons ØL9
Tenorrhaphy *see* Repair, Tendons ØLQ
Tenosynovectomy
 see Excision, Tendons ØLB
 see Resection, Tendons ØLT

Tenotomy
 see Division, Tendons ØL8
 see Drainage, Tendons ØL9
Tensor fasciae latae muscle
 use Hip Muscle, Left
 use Hip Muscle, Right
Tensor veli palatini muscle *use* Tongue, Palate, Pharynx Muscle
Tenth cranial nerve *use* Vagus Nerve
Tentorium cerebelli *use* Dura Mater
Teres major muscle
 use Shoulder Muscle, Left
 use Shoulder Muscle, Right
Teres minor muscle
 use Shoulder Muscle, Left
 use Shoulder Muscle, Right
Terlipressin XWØ
TERLIVAZ® *use* Terlipressin
Termination of pregnancy
 Aspiration curettage 10A07ZZ
 Dilation and curettage 10A07ZZ
 Hysterotomy 10A00ZZ
 Intra-amniotic injection 10A03ZZ
 Laminaria 10A07ZW
 Vacuum 10A07Z6
Testectomy
 see Excision, Male Reproductive System ØVB
 see Resection, Male Reproductive System ØVT
Testicular artery *use* Abdominal Aorta
Testing
 Glaucoma 4A07XBZ
 Hearing *see* Hearing Assessment, Diagnostic Audiology F13
 Mental health *see* Psychological Tests
 Muscle function, electromyography (EMG) *see* Measurement, Musculoskeletal 4AØF
 Muscle function, manual *see* Motor Function Assessment, Rehabilitation FØ1
 Neurophysiologic monitoring, intra-operative *see* Monitoring, Physiological Systems 4A1
 Range of motion *see* Motor Function Assessment, Rehabilitation FØ1
 Vestibular function *see* Vestibular Assessment, Diagnostic Audiology F15
Thalamectomy *see* Excision, Thalamus ØØB9
Thalamotomy *see* Drainage, Thalamus ØØ99
Thenar muscle
 use Hand Muscle, Left
 use Hand Muscle, Right
Therapeutic Massage
 Musculoskeletal System 8EØKX1Z
 Reproductive System
  Prostate 8EØVX1C
  Rectum 8EØVX1D
Therapeutic occlusion coil(s) *use* Intraluminal Device
Thermography 4AØZXKZ
Thermotherapy, prostate *see* Destruction, Prostate ØV5Ø
Third cranial nerve *use* Oculomotor Nerve
Third occipital nerve *use* Cervical Nerve
Third ventricle *use* Cerebral Ventricle
Thoracectomy *see* Excision, Anatomical Regions, General ØWB
Thoracentesis *see* Drainage, Anatomical Regions, General ØW9
Thoracic aortic plexus *use* Thoracic Sympathetic Nerve
Thoracic esophagus *use* Esophagus, Middle
Thoracic facet joint *use* Thoracic Vertebral Joint
Thoracic ganglion *use* Thoracic Sympathetic Nerve
Thoracoacromial artery
 use Axillary Artery, Left
 use Axillary Artery, Right
Thoracocentesis *see* Drainage, Anatomical Regions, General ØW9
Thoracolumbar facet joint *use* Thoracolumbar Vertebral Joint
Thoracoplasty
 see Repair, Anatomical Regions, General ØWQ
 see Supplement, Anatomical Regions, General ØWU
Thoracostomy, for lung collapse *see* Drainage, Respiratory System ØB9
Thoracostomy tube *use* Drainage Device
Thoracotomy *see* Drainage, Anatomical Regions, General ØW9
Thoraflex™ Hybrid device *use* Branched Synthetic Substitute with Intraluminal Device in New Technology

Thoratec IVAD (Implantable Ventricular Assist Device) *use* Implantable Heart Assist System in Heart and Great Vessels
Thoratec Paracorporeal Ventricular Assist Device *use* Short-term External Heart Assist System in Heart and Great Vessels
Thrombectomy *see* Extirpation
Thrombolysis, Ultrasound assisted *see* Fragmentation, Artery
Thymectomy
 see Excision, Lymphatic and Hemic Systems Ø7B
 see Resection, Lymphatic and Hemic Systems Ø7T
Thymopexy
 see Repair, Lymphatic and Hemic Systems Ø7Q
 see Reposition, Lymphatic and Hemic Systems Ø7S
Thymus gland *use* Thymus
Thyroarytenoid muscle
 use Neck Muscle, Left
 use Neck Muscle, Right
Thyrocervical trunk
 use Thyroid Artery, Left
 use Thyroid Artery, Right
Thyroid cartilage *use* Larynx
Thyroidectomy
 see Excision, Endocrine System ØGB
 see Resection, Endocrine System ØGT
Thyroidorrhaphy *see* Repair, Endocrine System ØGQ
Thyroidoscopy ØGJK4ZZ
Thyroidotomy *see* Drainage, Endocrine System ØG9
Tibial Extension with Motion Sensors, Insertion XNH
Tibial insert *use* Liner in Lower Joints
Tibial sesamoid
 use Metatarsal, Left
 use Metatarsal, Right
Tibialis anterior muscle
 use Lower Leg Muscle, Left
 use Lower Leg Muscle, Right
Tibialis posterior muscle
 use Lower Leg Muscle, Left
 use Lower Leg Muscle, Right
Tibiofemoral joint
 use Knee Joint, Left
 use Knee Joint, Right
 use Knee Joint, Tibial Surface, Left
 use Knee Joint, Tibial Surface, Right
Tibioperoneal trunk
 use Popliteal Artery, Left
 use Popliteal Artery, Right
Tisagenlecleucel *use* Tisagenlecleucel Immunotherapy
Tisagenlecleucel Immunotherapy XWØ
Tissue bank graft *use* Nonautologous Tissue Substitute
Tissue expander (inflatable) (injectable)
 use Tissue Expander in Skin and Breast
 use Tissue Expander in Subcutaneous Tissue and Fascia
Tissue Expander
 Insertion of device in
  Breast
   Bilateral ØHHV
   Left ØHHU
   Right ØHHT
  Nipple
   Left ØHHX
   Right ØHHW
  Subcutaneous Tissue and Fascia
   Abdomen ØJH8
   Back ØJH7
   Buttock ØJH9
   Chest ØJH6
   Face ØJH1
   Foot
    Left ØJHR
    Right ØJHQ
   Hand
    Left ØJHK
    Right ØJHJ
   Lower Arm
    Left ØJHH
    Right ØJHG
   Lower Leg
    Left ØJHP
    Right ØJHN
   Neck
    Left ØJH5
    Right ØJH4
   Pelvic Region ØJHC

Tissue Expander — *continued*
  Insertion of device in — *continued*
    Subcutaneous Tissue and Fascia — *continued*
      Perineum ØJHB
      Scalp ØJHØ
      Upper Arm
        Left ØJHF
        Right ØJHD
      Upper Leg
        Left ØJHM
        Right ØJHL
  Removal of device from
    Breast
      Left ØHPU
      Right ØHPT
    Subcutaneous Tissue and Fascia
      Head and Neck ØJPS
      Lower Extremity ØJPW
      Trunk ØJPT
      Upper Extremity ØJPV
  Revision of device in
    Breast
      Left ØHWU
      Right ØHWT
    Subcutaneous Tissue and Fascia
      Head and Neck ØJWS
      Lower Extremity ØJWW
      Trunk ØJWT
      Upper Extremity ØJWV
Tissue Plasminogen Activator (tPA) (r-tPA) *use* Other Thrombolytic
Titan Endoskeleton™
  use Interbody Fusion Device in Lower Joints
  use Interbody Fusion Device in Upper Joints
Titanium Sternal Fixation System (TSFS)
  use Internal Fixation Device, Rigid Plate in ØPS
  use Internal Fixation Device, Rigid Plate in ØPH
Tixagevimab and Cilgavimab Monoclonal Antibody XW023X7
Tocilizumab XWØ
Tomographic (Tomo) Nuclear Medicine Imaging
  Abdomen CW2Ø
  Abdomen and Chest CW24
  Abdomen and Pelvis CW21
  Anatomical Regions, Multiple CW2YYZZ
  Bladder, Kidneys and Ureters CT23
  Brain CØ2Ø
  Breast CH2YYZZ
    Bilateral CH22
    Left CH21
    Right CH2Ø
  Bronchi and Lungs CB22
  Central Nervous System CØ2YYZZ
  Cerebrospinal Fluid CØ25
  Chest CW23
  Chest and Abdomen CW24
  Chest and Neck CW26
  Digestive System CD2YYZZ
  Endocrine System CG2YYZZ
  Extremity
    Lower CW2D
      Bilateral CP2F
      Left CP2D
      Right CP2C
    Upper CW2M
      Bilateral CP2B
      Left CP29
      Right CP28
  Gallbladder CF24
  Gastrointestinal Tract CD27
  Gland, Parathyroid CG21
  Head and Neck CW2B
  Heart C22YYZZ
    Right and Left C226
  Hepatobiliary System and Pancreas CF2YYZZ
  Kidneys, Ureters and Bladder CT23
  Liver CF25
  Liver and Spleen CF26
  Lungs and Bronchi CB22
  Lymphatics and Hematologic System C72YYZZ
  Musculoskeletal System, Other CP2YYZZ
  Myocardium C22G
  Neck and Chest CW26
  Neck and Head CW2B
  Pancreas and Hepatobiliary System CF2YYZZ
  Pelvic Region CW2J
  Pelvis CP26

Tomographic (Tomo) Nuclear Medicine Imaging — *continued*
  Pelvis and Abdomen CW21
  Pelvis and Spine CP27
  Respiratory System CB2YYZZ
  Skin CH2YYZZ
  Skull CP21
  Skull and Cervical Spine CP23
  Spine
    Cervical CP22
    Cervical and Skull CP23
    Lumbar CP2H
    Thoracic CP2G
    Thoracolumbar CP2J
  Spine and Pelvis CP27
  Spleen C722
  Spleen and Liver CF26
  Subcutaneous Tissue CH2YYZZ
  Thorax CP24
  Ureters, Kidneys and Bladder CT23
  Urinary System CT2YYZZ
Tomography, computerized *see* Computerized Tomography (CT Scan)
Tongue, base of *use* Pharynx
Tonometry 4AØ7XBZ
Tonsillectomy
  see Excision, Mouth and Throat ØCB
  see Resection, Mouth and Throat ØCT
Tonsillotomy *see* Drainage, Mouth and Throat ØC9
TOPS™ System *use* Posterior Spinal Motion Preservation Device in New Technology
Total Ankle Talar Replacement™ (TATR) *use* Synthetic Substitute, Talar Prosthesis in New Technology
Total Anomalous Pulmonary Venous Return (TAPVR) repair
  see Bypass, Atrium, Left Ø217
  see Bypass, Vena Cava, Superior Ø21V
Total artificial (replacement) heart *use* Synthetic Substitute
Total parenteral nutrition (TPN) *see* Introduction of Nutritional Substance
Tourniquet, External *see* Compression, Anatomical Regions 2W1
Trachectomy
  see Excision, Trachea ØBB1
  see Resection, Trachea ØBT1
Trachelectomy
  see Excision, Cervix ØUBC
  see Resection, Cervix ØUTC
Trachelopexy
  see Repair, Cervix ØUQC
  see Reposition, Cervix ØUSC
Tracheloplasty *see* Repair, Cervix ØUQC
Trachelorrhaphy *see* Repair, Cervix ØUQC
Trachelotomy *see* Drainage, Cervix ØU9C
Tracheobronchial lymph node *use* Lymphatic, Thorax
Tracheoesophageal fistulization ØB110D6
Tracheolysis *see* Release, Respiratory System ØBN
Tracheoplasty
  see Repair, Respiratory System ØBQ
  see Supplement, Respiratory System ØBU
Tracheorrhaphy *see* Repair, Respiratory System ØBQ
Tracheoscopy ØBJ18ZZ
Tracheostomy *see* Bypass, Respiratory System ØB1
Tracheostomy Device
  Bypass, Trachea ØB11
  Change device in, Trachea ØB21XFZ
  Removal of device from, Trachea ØBP1
  Revision of device in, Trachea ØBW1
Tracheostomy tube *use* Tracheostomy Device in Respiratory System
Tracheotomy *see* Drainage, Respiratory System ØB9
Traction
  Abdominal Wall 2W63X
  Arm
    Lower
      Left 2W6DX
      Right 2W6CX
    Upper
      Left 2W6BX
      Right 2W6AX
  Back 2W65X
  Chest Wall 2W64X
  Extremity
    Lower
      Left 2W6MX
      Right 2W6LX

Traction — *continued*
  Extremity — *continued*
    Upper
      Left 2W69X
      Right 2W68X
  Face 2W61X
  Finger
    Left 2W6KX
    Right 2W6JX
  Foot
    Left 2W6TX
    Right 2W6SX
  Hand
    Left 2W6FX
    Right 2W6EX
  Head 2W6ØX
  Inguinal Region
    Left 2W67X
    Right 2W66X
  Leg
    Lower
      Left 2W6RX
      Right 2W6QX
    Upper
      Left 2W6PX
      Right 2W6NX
  Neck 2W62X
  Thumb
    Left 2W6HX
    Right 2W6GX
  Toe
    Left 2W6VX
    Right 2W6UX
Tractotomy *see* Division, Central Nervous System and Cranial Nerves ØØ8
Tragus
  use External Ear, Bilateral
  use External Ear, Left
  use External Ear, Right
Training, caregiver *see* Caregiver Training
TRAM (transverse rectus abdominis myocutaneous) flap reconstruction
  Free *see* Replacement, Skin and Breast ØHR
  Pedicled *see* Transfer, Muscles ØKX
Transcatheter Pulmonary Valve (TPV) placement
  In conduit Ø2RH38L
  Native site Ø2RH38M
Transdermal Glomerular Filtration Rate (GFR) Measurement System XT25XE5
Transection *see* Division
Transfer
  Buccal Mucosa ØCX4
  Bursa and Ligament
    Abdomen
      Left ØMXJ
      Right ØMXH
    Ankle
      Left ØMXR
      Right ØMXQ
    Elbow
      Left ØMX4
      Right ØMX3
    Foot
      Left ØMXT
      Right ØMXS
    Hand
      Left ØMX8
      Right ØMX7
    Head and Neck ØMXØ
    Hip
      Left ØMXM
      Right ØMXL
    Knee
      Left ØMXP
      Right ØMXN
    Lower Extremity
      Left ØMXW
      Right ØMXV
    Perineum ØMXK
    Rib(s) ØMXG
    Shoulder
      Left ØMX2
      Right ØMX1
    Spine
      Lower ØMXD
      Upper ØMXC
    Sternum ØMXF

Transfer — continued
  Bursa and Ligament — continued
    Upper Extremity
      Left 0MXB
      Right 0MX9
    Wrist
      Left 0MX6
      Right 0MX5
  Finger
    Left 0XXP0ZM
    Right 0XXN0ZL
  Gingiva
    Lower 0CX6
    Upper 0CX5
  Intestine
    Large 0DXE
    Small 0DX8
  Lip
    Lower 0CX1
    Upper 0CX0
  Muscle
    Abdomen
      Left 0KXL
      Right 0KXK
    Extraocular
      Left 08XM
      Right 08XL
    Facial 0KX1
    Foot
      Left 0KXW
      Right 0KXV
    Hand
      Left 0KXD
      Right 0KXC
    Head 0KX0
    Hip
      Left 0KXP
      Right 0KXN
    Lower Arm and Wrist
      Left 0KXB
      Right 0KX9
    Lower Leg
      Left 0KXT
      Right 0KXS
    Neck
      Left 0KX3
      Right 0KX2
    Perineum 0KXM
    Shoulder
      Left 0KX6
      Right 0KX5
    Thorax
      Left 0KXJ
      Right 0KXH
    Tongue, Palate, Pharynx 0KX4
    Trunk
      Left 0KXG
      Right 0KXF
    Upper Arm
      Left 0KX8
      Right 0KX7
    Upper Leg
      Left 0KXR
      Right 0KXQ
  Nerve
    Abducens 00XL
    Accessory 00XR
    Acoustic 00XN
    Cervical 01X1
    Facial 00XM
    Femoral 01XD
    Glossopharyngeal 00XP
    Hypoglossal 00XS
    Lumbar 01XB
    Median 01X5
    Oculomotor 00XH
    Olfactory 00XF
    Optic 00XG
    Peroneal 01XH
    Phrenic 01X2
    Pudendal 01XC
    Radial 01X6
    Sciatic 01XF
    Thoracic 01X8
    Tibial 01XG
    Trigeminal 00XK
    Trochlear 00XJ
    Ulnar 01X4
    Vagus 00XQ

Transfer — continued
  Palate, Soft 0CX3
  Prepuce 0VXT
  Skin
    Abdomen 0HX7XZZ
    Back 0HX6XZZ
    Buttock 0HX8XZZ
    Chest 0HX5XZZ
    Ear
      Left 0HX3XZZ
      Right 0HX2XZZ
    Face 0HX1XZZ
    Foot
      Left 0HXNXZZ
      Right 0HXMXZZ
    Hand
      Left 0HXGXZZ
      Right 0HXFXZZ
    Inguinal 0HXAXZZ
    Lower Arm
      Left 0HXEXZZ
      Right 0HXDXZZ
    Lower Leg
      Left 0HXLXZZ
      Right 0HXKXZZ
    Neck 0HX4XZZ
    Perineum 0HX9XZZ
    Scalp 0HX0XZZ
    Upper Arm
      Left 0HXCXZZ
      Right 0HXBXZZ
    Upper Leg
      Left 0HXJXZZ
      Right 0HXHXZZ
  Stomach 0DX6
  Subcutaneous Tissue and Fascia
    Abdomen 0JX8
    Back 0JX7
    Buttock 0JX9
    Chest 0JX6
    Face 0JX1
    Foot
      Left 0JXR
      Right 0JXQ
    Hand
      Left 0JXK
      Right 0JXJ
    Lower Arm
      Left 0JXH
      Right 0JXG
    Lower Leg
      Left 0JXP
      Right 0JXN
    Neck
      Left 0JX5
      Right 0JX4
    Pelvic Region 0JXC
    Perineum 0JXB
    Scalp 0JX0
    Upper Arm
      Left 0JXF
      Right 0JXD
    Upper Leg
      Left 0JXM
      Right 0JXL
  Tendon
    Abdomen
      Left 0LXG
      Right 0LXF
    Ankle
      Left 0LXT
      Right 0LXS
    Foot
      Left 0LXW
      Right 0LXV
    Hand
      Left 0LX8
      Right 0LX7
    Head and Neck 0LX0
    Hip
      Left 0LXK
      Right 0LXJ
    Knee
      Left 0LXR
      Right 0LXQ
    Lower Arm and Wrist
      Left 0LX6
      Right 0LX5

Transfer — continued
  Tendon — continued
    Lower Leg
      Left 0LXP
      Right 0LXN
    Perineum 0LXH
    Shoulder
      Left 0LX2
      Right 0LX1
    Thorax
      Left 0LXD
      Right 0LXC
    Trunk
      Left 0LXB
      Right 0LX9
    Upper Arm
      Left 0LX4
      Right 0LX3
    Upper Leg
      Left 0LXM
      Right 0LXL
  Tongue 0CX7
Transfusion
  Bone Marrow
    Blood
      Platelets 302A3R
      Red Cells 302A3N
        Frozen 302A3P
      Whole 302A3H
    Plasma
      Fresh 302A3L
      Frozen 302A3K
    Serum Albumin 302A3J
  New Technology see New Technology, Anatomical
      Regions XW1
  Products of Conception
    Antihemophilic Factors 3027
    Blood
      Platelets 3027
      Red Cells 3027
        Frozen 3027
      White Cells 3027
      Whole 3027
    Factor IX 3027
    Fibrinogen 3027
    Globulin 3027
    Plasma
      Fresh 3027
      Frozen 3027
    Plasma Cryoprecipitate 3027
    Serum Albumin 3027
  Vein
    4-Factor Prothrombin Complex Concentrate
        30283B1
    Central
      Antihemophilic Factors 30243V
      Blood
        Platelets 30243R
        Red Cells 30243N
          Frozen 30243P
        White Cells 30243Q
        Whole 30243H
      Bone Marrow 30243G
      Factor IX 30243W
      Fibrinogen 30243T
      Globulin 30243S
      Hematopoietic Stem/Progenitor Cells
          (HSPC), Genetically Modified
          30243C0
      Pathogen Reduced Cryoprecipitated
          Fibrinogen Complex 30243D1
      Plasma
        Fresh 30243L
        Frozen 30243K
      Plasma Cryoprecipitate 30243M
      Serum Albumin 30243J
      Stem Cells
        Cord Blood 30243X
        Embryonic 30243AZ
        Hematopoietic 30243Y
        T-cell Depleted Hematopoietic
            30243U
    Peripheral
      Antihemophilic Factors 30233V
      Blood
        Platelets 30233R
        Red Cells 30233N
          Frozen 30233P
        White Cells 30233Q

Transfusion — *continued*
  Vein — *continued*
    Peripheral — *continued*
      Blood — *continued*
        Whole 30233H
      Bone Marrow 30233G
      Factor IX 30233W
      Fibrinogen 30233T
      Globulin 30233S
      Hematopoietic Stem/Progenitor Cells (HSPC), Genetically Modified 30233C0
      Pathogen Reduced Cryoprecipitated Fibrinogen Complex 30233D1
      Plasma
        Fresh 30233L
        Frozen 30233K
      Plasma Cryoprecipitate 30233M
      Serum Albumin 30233J
      Stem Cells
        Cord Blood 30233X
        Embryonic 30233AZ
        Hematopoietic 30233Y
        T-cell Depleted Hematopoietic 30233U
Transplant *see* Transplantation
Transplantation
  Bone marrow *see* Transfusion, Circulatory 302
  Esophagus ØDY50Z
  Face ØWY20Z
  Hand
    Left ØXYKØZ
    Right ØXYJØZ
  Heart Ø2YAØZ
  Hematopoietic cell *see* Transfusion, Circulatory 302
  Intestine
    Large ØDYEØZ
    Small ØDY8ØZ
  Kidney
    Left ØTY1ØZ
    Right ØTYØØZ
  Liver ØFYØØZ
  Lung
    Bilateral ØBYMØZ
    Left ØBYLØZ
    Lower Lobe
      Left ØBYJØZ
      Right ØBYFØZ
    Middle Lobe, Right ØBYDØZ
    Right ØBYKØZ
    Upper Lobe
      Left ØBYGØZ
      Right ØBYCØZ
  Lung Lingula ØBYHØZ
  Ovary
    Left ØUY1ØZ
    Right ØUYØØZ
  Pancreas ØFYGØZ
  Penis ØVYSØZ
  Products of Conception 10Y0
  Scrotum ØVY5ØZ
  Spleen Ø7YPØZ
  Stem cell *see* Transfusion, Circulatory 302
  Stomach ØDY6ØZ
  Thymus Ø7YMØZ
  Uterus ØUY9ØZ
Transposition
  see Bypass
  see Reposition
  see Transfer
Transversalis fascia *use* Subcutaneous Tissue and Fascia, Trunk
Transverse acetabular ligament
  use Hip Bursa and Ligament, Left
  use Hip Bursa and Ligament, Right
Transverse (cutaneous) cervical nerve *use* Cervical Plexus
Transverse facial artery
  use Temporal Artery, Left
  use Temporal Artery, Right
Transverse foramen *use* Cervical Vertebra
Transverse humeral ligament
  use Shoulder Bursa and Ligament, Left
  use Shoulder Bursa and Ligament, Right
Transverse ligament of atlas *use* Head and Neck Bursa and Ligament

Transverse process
  use Cervical Vertebra
  use Lumbar Vertebra
  use Thoracic Vertebra
Transverse Rectus Abdominis Myocutaneous Flap
  Replacement
    Bilateral ØHRVØ76
    Left ØHRUØ76
    Right ØHRTØ76
  Transfer
    Left ØKXL
    Right ØKXK
Transverse scapular ligament
  use Shoulder Bursa and Ligament, Left
  use Shoulder Bursa and Ligament, Right
Transverse thoracis muscle
  use Thorax Muscle, Left
  use Thorax Muscle, Right
Transversospinalis muscle
  use Trunk Muscle, Left
  use Trunk Muscle, Right
Transversus abdominis muscle
  use Abdomen Muscle, Left
  use Abdomen Muscle, Right
Trapezium bone
  use Carpal, Left
  use Carpal, Right
Trapezius muscle
  use Trunk Muscle, Left
  use Trunk Muscle, Right
Trapezoid bone
  use Carpal, Left
  use Carpal, Right
Treosulfan XWØ
Triceps brachii muscle
  use Upper Arm Muscle, Left
  use Upper Arm Muscle, Right
Tricuspid annulus *use* Tricuspid Valve
TricValve® Transcatheter Bicaval Valve System *use* Intraluminal Device, Bioprosthetic Valve in New Technology
Trifacial nerve *use* Trigeminal Nerve
Trifecta™ Valve (aortic) *use* Zooplastic Tissue in Heart and Great Vessels
Trigone of bladder *use* Bladder
TriGuard 3™ CEPD (cerebral embolic protection device) X2A6325
Trilaciclib XWØ
Trimming, excisional *see* Excision
Triquetral bone
  use Carpal, Left
  use Carpal, Right
Trochanteric bursa
  use Hip Bursa and Ligament, Left
  use Hip Bursa and Ligament, Right
TUMT (transurethral microwave thermotherapy of prostate) ØV5Ø7ZZ
TUNA (transurethral needle ablation of prostate) ØV5Ø7ZZ
Tunneled central venous catheter *use* Vascular Access Device, Tunneled in Subcutaneous Tissue and Fascia
Tunneled spinal (intrathecal) catheter *use* Infusion Device
Turbinectomy
  see Excision, Ear, Nose, Sinus Ø9B
  see Resection, Ear, Nose, Sinus Ø9T
Turbinoplasty
  see Repair, Ear, Nose, Sinus Ø9Q
  see Replacement, Ear, Nose, Sinus Ø9R
  see Supplement, Ear, Nose, Sinus Ø9U
Turbinotomy
  see Division, Ear, Nose, Sinus Ø98
  see Drainage, Ear, Nose, Sinus Ø99
TURP (transurethral resection of prostate) ØVBØ7ZZ
  see Excision, Prostate ØVBØ
  see Resection, Prostate ØVTØ
Twelfth cranial nerve *use* Hypoglossal Nerve
Two lead pacemaker *use* Pacemaker, Dual Chamber in ØJH
Tympanic cavity
  use Middle Ear, Left
  use Middle Ear, Right
Tympanic nerve *use* Glossopharyngeal Nerve
Tympanic part of temoporal bone
  use Temporal Bone, Left

Tympanic part of temporal bone — *continued*
  use Temporal Bone, Right
Tympanogram *see* Hearing Assessment, Diagnostic Audiology F13
Tympanoplasty
  see Repair, Ear, Nose, Sinus Ø9Q
  see Replacement, Ear, Nose, Sinus Ø9R
  see Supplement, Ear, Nose, Sinus Ø9U
Tympanosympathectomy *see* Excision, Nerve, Head and Neck Sympathetic Ø1BK
Tympanotomy *see* Drainage, Ear, Nose, Sinus Ø99
TYRX Antibacterial Envelope *use* Anti-Infective Envelope

U

Ulnar collateral carpal ligament
  use Wrist Bursa and Ligament, Left
  use Wrist Bursa and Ligament, Right
Ulnar collateral ligament
  use Elbow Bursa and Ligament, Left
  use Elbow Bursa and Ligament, Right
Ulnar notch
  use Radius, Left
  use Radius, Right
Ulnar vein
  use Brachial Vein, Left
  use Brachial Vein, Right
Ultrafiltration
  Hemodialysis *see* Performance, Urinary 5A1D
  Therapeutic plasmapheresis *see* Pheresis, Circulatory 6A55
Ultraflex™ Precision Colonic Stent System *use* Intraluminal Device
ULTRAPRO Hernia System (UHS) *use* Synthetic Substitute
ULTRAPRO Partially Absorbable Lightweight Mesh *use* Synthetic Substitute
ULTRAPRO Plug *use* Synthetic Substitute
Ultrasonic osteogenic stimulator
  use Bone Growth Stimulator in Head and Facial Bones
  use Bone Growth Stimulator in Lower Bones
  use Bone Growth Stimulator in Upper Bones
Ultrasonography
  Abdomen BW40ZZZ
  Abdomen and Pelvis BW41ZZZ
  Abdominal Wall BH49ZZZ
  Aorta
    Abdominal, Intravascular B440ZZ3
    Thoracic, Intravascular B340ZZ3
  Appendix BD48ZZZ
  Artery
    Brachiocephalic-Subclavian, Right, Intravascular B341ZZ3
    Celiac and Mesenteric, Intravascular B44KZZ3
    Common Carotid
      Bilateral, Intravascular B345ZZ3
      Left, Intravascular B344ZZ3
      Right, Intravascular B343ZZ3
    Coronary
      Multiple B241YZZ
        Intravascular B241ZZ3
        Transesophageal B241ZZ4
      Single B240YZZ
        Intravascular B240ZZ3
        Transesophageal B240ZZ4
    Femoral, Intravascular B44LZZ3
    Inferior Mesenteric, Intravascular B445ZZ3
    Internal Carotid
      Bilateral, Intravascular B348ZZ3
      Left, Intravascular B347ZZ3
      Right, Intravascular B346ZZ3
    Intra-Abdominal, Other, Intravascular B44BZZ3
    Intracranial, Intravascular B34RZZ3
    Lower Extremity
      Bilateral, Intravascular B44HZZ3
      Left, Intravascular B44GZZ3
      Right, Intravascular B44FZZ3
    Mesenteric and Celiac, Intravascular B44KZZ3
    Ophthalmic, Intravascular B34VZZ3
    Penile, Intravascular B44NZZ3
    Pulmonary
      Left, Intravascular B34TZZ3
      Right, Intravascular B34SZZ3

Ultrasonography — *continued*
Artery — *continued*
  Renal
    Bilateral, Intravascular B448ZZ3
    Left, Intravascular B447ZZ3
    Right, Intravascular B446ZZ3
  Subclavian, Left, Intravascular B342ZZ3
  Superior Mesenteric, Intravascular B444ZZ3
  Upper Extremity
    Bilateral, Intravascular B34KZZ3
    Left, Intravascular B34JZZ3
    Right, Intravascular B34HZZ3
Bile Duct BF40ZZZ
Bile Duct and Gallbladder BF43ZZZ
Bladder BT40ZZZ
  and Kidney BT4JZZZ
Brain B040ZZZ
Breast
  Bilateral BH42ZZZ
  Left BH41ZZZ
  Right BH40ZZZ
Chest Wall BH4BZZZ
Coccyx BR4FZZZ
Connective Tissue
  Lower Extremity BL41ZZZ
  Upper Extremity BL40ZZZ
Duodenum BD49ZZZ
Elbow
  Left, Densitometry BP4HZZ1
  Right, Densitometry BP4GZZ1
Esophagus BD41ZZZ
Extremity
  Lower BH48ZZZ
  Upper BH47ZZZ
Eye
  Bilateral B847ZZZ
  Left B846ZZZ
  Right B845ZZZ
Fallopian Tube
  Bilateral BU42
  Left BU41
  Right BU40
Fetal Umbilical Cord BY47ZZZ
Fetus
  First Trimester, Multiple Gestation BY4BZZZ
  Second Trimester, Multiple Gestation
    BY4DZZZ
  Single
    First Trimester BY49ZZZ
    Second Trimester BY4CZZZ
    Third Trimester BY4FZZZ
  Third Trimester, Multiple Gestation BY4GZZZ
Gallbladder BF42ZZZ
Gallbladder and Bile Duct BF43ZZZ
Gastrointestinal Tract BD47ZZZ
Gland
  Adrenal
    Bilateral BG42ZZZ
    Left BG41ZZZ
    Right BG40ZZZ
  Parathyroid BG43ZZZ
  Thyroid BG44ZZZ
Hand
  Left, Densitometry BP4PZZ1
  Right, Densitometry BP4NZZ1
Head and Neck BH4CZZZ
Heart
  Left B245YZZ
    Intravascular B245ZZ3
    Transesophageal B245ZZ4
  Pediatric B24DYZZ
    Intravascular B24DZZ3
    Transesophageal B24DZZ4
  Right B244YZZ
    Intravascular B244ZZ3
    Transesophageal B244ZZ4
  Right and Left B246YZZ
    Intravascular B246ZZ3
    Transesophageal B246ZZ4
Heart with Aorta B24BYZZ
  Intravascular B24BZZ3
  Transesophageal B24BZZ4
Hepatobiliary System, All BF4CZZZ
Hip
  Bilateral BQ42ZZZ
  Left BQ41ZZZ
  Right BQ40ZZZ
Kidney
  and Bladder BT4JZZZ

Ultrasonography — *continued*
Kidney — *continued*
  Bilateral BT43ZZZ
  Left BT42ZZZ
  Right BT41ZZZ
  Transplant BT49ZZZ
Knee
  Bilateral BQ49ZZZ
  Left BQ48ZZZ
  Right BQ47ZZZ
Liver BF45ZZZ
Liver and Spleen BF46ZZZ
Mediastinum BB4CZZZ
Neck BW4FZZZ
Ovary
  Bilateral BU45
  Left BU44
  Right BU43
Ovary and Uterus BU4C
Pancreas BF47ZZZ
Pelvic Region BW4GZZZ
Pelvis and Abdomen BW41ZZZ
Penis BV4BZZZ
Pericardium B24CYZZ
  Intravascular B24CZZ3
  Transesophageal B24CZZ4
Placenta BY48ZZZ
Pleura BB4BZZZ
Prostate and Seminal Vesicle BV49ZZZ
Rectum BD4CZZZ
Sacrum BR4FZZZ
Scrotum BV44ZZZ
Seminal Vesicle and Prostate BV49ZZZ
Shoulder
  Left, Densitometry BP49ZZ1
  Right, Densitometry BP48ZZ1
Spinal Cord B04BZZZ
Spine
  Cervical BR40ZZZ
  Lumbar BR49ZZZ
  Thoracic BR47ZZZ
Spleen and Liver BF46ZZZ
Stomach BD42ZZZ
Tendon
  Lower Extremity BL43ZZZ
  Upper Extremity BL42ZZZ
Ureter
  Bilateral BT48ZZZ
  Left BT47ZZZ
  Right BT46ZZZ
Urethra BT45ZZZ
Uterus BU46
Uterus and Ovary BU4C
Vein
  Jugular
    Left, Intravascular B544ZZ3
    Right, Intravascular B543ZZ3
  Lower Extremity
    Bilateral, Intravascular B54DZZ3
    Left, Intravascular B54CZZ3
    Right, Intravascular B54BZZ3
  Portal, Intravascular B54TZZ3
  Renal
    Bilateral, Intravascular B54LZZ3
    Left, Intravascular B54KZZ3
    Right, Intravascular B54JZZ3
  Spanchnic, Intravascular B54TZZ3
  Subclavian
    Left, Intravascular B547ZZ3
    Right, Intravascular B546ZZ3
  Upper Extremity
    Bilateral, Intravascular B54PZZ3
    Left, Intravascular B54NZZ3
    Right, Intravascular B54MZZ3
Vena Cava
  Inferior, Intravascular B549ZZ3
  Superior, Intravascular B548ZZ3
Wrist
  Left, Densitometry BP4MZZ1
  Right, Densitometry BP4LZZ1
Ultrasound Ablation, Destruction, Renal Sympathetic Nerve(s) X051329
Ultrasound bone healing system
  use Bone Growth Stimulator in Head and Facial Bones
  use Bone Growth Stimulator in Lower Bones
  use Bone Growth Stimulator in Upper Bones

Ultrasound Penetrable Synthetic Substitute, Skull XNR80D9
Ultrasound Therapy
  Heart 6A75
  No Qualifier 6A75
  Vessels
    Head and Neck 6A75
    Other 6A75
    Peripheral 6A75
Ultraviolet Light Therapy, Skin 6A80
Umbilical artery
  use Internal Iliac Artery, Left
  use Internal Iliac Artery, Right
  use Lower Artery
Uniplanar external fixator
  use External Fixation Device, Monoplanar in 0PH
  use External Fixation Device, Monoplanar in 0PS
  use External Fixation Device, Monoplanar in 0QH
  use External Fixation Device, Monoplanar in 0QS
UPLIZNA® *use* Inebilizumab-cdon
Upper GI series *see* Fluoroscopy, Gastrointestinal, Upper BD15
Ureteral orifice
  use Ureter
  use Ureter, Left
  use Ureter, Right
  use Ureters, Bilateral
Ureterectomy
  see Excision, Urinary System 0TB
  see Resection, Urinary System 0TT
Ureterocolostomy *see* Bypass, Urinary System 0T1
Ureterocystostomy *see* Bypass, Urinary System 0T1
Ureteroenterostomy *see* Bypass, Urinary System 0T1
Ureteroileostomy *see* Bypass, Urinary System 0T1
Ureterolithotomy *see* Extirpation, Urinary System 0TC
Ureterolysis *see* Release, Urinary System 0TN
Ureteroneocystostomy
  see Bypass, Urinary System 0T1
  see Reposition, Urinary System 0TS
Ureteropelvic junction (UPJ)
  use Kidney Pelvis, Left
  use Kidney Pelvis, Right
Ureteropexy
  see Repair, Urinary System 0TQ
  see Reposition, Urinary System 0TS
Ureteroplasty
  see Repair, Urinary System 0TQ
  see Replacement, Urinary System 0TR
  see Supplement, Urinary System 0TU
Ureteroplication *see* Restriction, Urinary System 0TV
Ureteropyelography *see* Fluoroscopy, Urinary System BT1
Ureterorrhaphy *see* Repair, Urinary System 0TQ
Ureteroscopy 0TJ98ZZ
Ureterostomy
  see Bypass, Urinary System 0T1
  see Drainage, Urinary System 0T9
Ureterotomy *see* Drainage, Urinary System 0T9
Ureteroureterostomy *see* Bypass, Urinary System 0T1
Ureterovesical orifice
  use Ureter
  use Ureter, Left
  use Ureter, Right
  use Ureters, Bilateral
Urethral catheterization, indwelling 0T9B70Z
Urethrectomy
  see Excision, Urethra 0TBD
  see Resection, Urethra 0TTD
Urethrolithotomy *see* Extirpation, Urethra 0TCD
Urethrolysis *see* Release, Urethra 0TND
Urethropexy
  see Repair, Urethra 0TQD
  see Reposition, Urethra 0TSD
Urethroplasty
  see Repair, Urethra 0TQD
  see Replacement, Urethra 0TRD
  see Supplement, Urethra 0TUD
Urethrorrhaphy *see* Repair, Urethra 0TQD
Urethroscopy 0TJD8ZZ
Urethrotomy *see* Drainage, Urethra 0T9D
Uridine Triacetate XW0DX82
Urinary incontinence stimulator lead *use* Stimulator Lead in Urinary System
Urography *see* Fluoroscopy, Urinary System BT1
Ustekinumab *use* Other New Technology Therapeutic Substance

Uterine Artery
use Internal Iliac Artery, Left
use Internal Iliac Artery, Right
Uterine artery embolization (UAE) see Occlusion,
Lower Arteries Ø4L
Uterine cornu use Uterus
Uterine tube
use Fallopian Tube, Left
use Fallopian Tube, Right
Uterine vein
use Hypogastric Vein, Left
use Hypogastric Vein, Right
Uvulectomy
see Excision, Uvula ØCBN
see Resection, Uvula ØCTN
Uvulorrhaphy see Repair, Uvula ØCQN
Uvulotomy see Drainage, Uvula ØC9N

V

Vabomere™ use Meropenem-vaborbactam Anti-infective
Vaccination see Introduction of Serum, Toxoid, and Vaccine
Vacuum extraction, obstetric 10D07Z6
Vaginal artery
use Internal Iliac Artery, Left
use Internal Iliac Artery, Right
Vaginal pessary use Intraluminal Device, Pessary in Female Reproductive System
Vaginal vein
use Hypogastric Vein, Left
use Hypogastric Vein, Right
Vaginectomy
see Excision, Vagina ØUBG
see Resection, Vagina ØUTG
Vaginofixation
see Repair, Vagina ØUQG
see Reposition, Vagina ØUSG
Vaginoplasty
see Repair, Vagina ØUQG
see Supplement, Vagina ØUUG
Vaginorrhaphy see Repair, Vagina ØUQG
Vaginoscopy ØUJH8ZZ
Vaginotomy see Drainage, Female Reproductive System ØU9
Vagotomy see Division, Nerve, Vagus ØØ8Q
Valiant Thoracic Stent Graft use Intraluminal Device
Valvotomy, valvulotomy
see Division, Heart and Great Vessels Ø28
see Release, Heart and Great Vessels Ø2N
Valvuloplasty
see Repair, Heart and Great Vessels Ø2Q
see Replacement, Heart and Great Vessels Ø2R
see Supplement, Heart and Great Vessels Ø2U
Valvuloplasty, Alfieri Stitch see Restriction, Valve, Mitral Ø2VG
Vanta™ PC neurostimulator use Stimulator Generator, Multiple Array in ØJH
Vascular Access Device
Totally Implantable
Insertion of device in
Abdomen ØJH8
Chest ØJH6
Lower Arm
Left ØJHH
Right ØJHG
Lower Leg
Left ØJHP
Right ØJHN
Upper Arm
Left ØJHF
Right ØJHD
Upper Leg
Left ØJHM
Right ØJHL
Removal of device from
Lower Extremity ØJPW
Trunk ØJPT
Upper Extremity ØJPV
Revision of device in
Lower Extremity ØJWW
Trunk ØJWT
Upper Extremity ØJWV

Vascular Access Device — continued
Tunneled
Insertion of device in
Abdomen ØJH8
Chest ØJH6
Lower Arm
Left ØJHH
Right ØJHG
Lower Leg
Left ØJHP
Right ØJHN
Upper Arm
Left ØJHF
Right ØJHD
Upper Leg
Left ØJHM
Right ØJHL
Removal of device from
Lower Extremity ØJPW
Trunk ØJPT
Upper Extremity ØJPV
Revision of device in
Lower Extremity ØJWW
Trunk ØJWT
Upper Extremity ØJWV
Vasectomy see Excision, Male Reproductive System ØVB
Vasography
see Fluoroscopy, Male Reproductive System BV1
see Plain Radiography, Male Reproductive System BVØ
Vasoligation see Occlusion, Male Reproductive System ØVL
Vasorrhaphy see Repair, Male Reproductive System ØVQ
Vasostomy see Bypass, Male Reproductive System ØV1
Vasotomy
Drainage see Drainage, Male Reproductive System ØV9
With ligation see Occlusion, Male Reproductive System ØVL
Vasovasostomy see Repair, Male Reproductive System ØVQ
VasQ™ External Support device use Synthetic Substitute, Extraluminal Support Device in New Technology
Vastus intermedius muscle
use Upper Leg Muscle, Left
use Upper Leg Muscle, Right
Vastus lateralis muscle
use Upper Leg Muscle, Left
use Upper Leg Muscle, Right
Vastus medialis muscle
use Upper Leg Muscle, Left
use Upper Leg Muscle, Right
VCG (vectorcardiogram) see Measurement, Cardiac 4A02
Vectra® Vascular Access Graft use Vascular Access Device, Tunneled in Subcutaneous Tissue and Fascia
Vein Graft Extraluminal Support Device(s), Supplement, Coronary Artery/Arteries X2U4079
Veklury use Remdesivir Anti-infective
Venclexta® use Venetoclax Antineoplastic
Venectomy
see Excision, Lower Veins Ø6B
see Excision, Upper Veins Ø5B
Venetoclax Antineoplastic XW0DXR5
Venography
see Fluoroscopy, Veins B51
see Plain Radiography, Veins B50
Venorrhaphy
see Repair, Lower Veins Ø6Q
see Repair, Upper Veins Ø5Q
Venotripsy
see Occlusion, Lower Veins Ø6L
see Occlusion, Upper Veins Ø5L
VenoValve® use Intraluminal Device, Bioprosthetic Valve in New Technology
Ventricular fold use Larynx
Ventriculoatriostomy see Bypass, Central Nervous System and Cranial Nerves ØØ1
Ventriculocisternostomy see Bypass, Central Nervous System and Cranial Nerves ØØ1
Ventriculogram, cardiac
Combined left and right heart see Fluoroscopy, Heart, Right and Left B216

Ventriculogram, cardiac — continued
Left ventricle see Fluoroscopy, Heart, Left B215
Right ventricle see Fluoroscopy, Heart, Right B214
Ventriculopuncture, through previously implanted catheter 8C01X6J
Ventriculoscopy 00J04ZZ
Ventriculostomy
External drainage see Drainage, Cerebral Ventricle 0096
Internal shunt see Bypass, Cerebral Ventricle 0016
Ventriculovenostomy see Bypass, Cerebral Ventricle 0016
Ventrio™ Hernia Patch use Synthetic Substitute
VEP (visual evoked potential) 4A07X0Z
Vermiform appendix use Appendix
Vermilion border
use Lower Lip
use Upper Lip
Versa use Pacemaker, Dual Chamber in ØJH
Version, obstetric
External 10S0XZZ
Internal 10S07ZZ
Vertebral arch
use Cervical Vertebra
use Lumbar Vertebra
use Thoracic Vertebra
Vertebral artery, intracranial portion use Intracranial Artery
Vertebral body
use Cervical Vertebra
use Lumbar Vertebra
use Thoracic Vertebra
Vertebral canal use Spinal Canal
Vertebral foramen
use Cervical Vertebra
use Lumbar Vertebra
use Thoracic Vertebra
Vertebral lamina
use Cervical Vertebra
use Lumbar Vertebra
use Thoracic Vertebra
Vertebral pedicle
use Cervical Vertebra
use Lumbar Vertebra
use Thoracic Vertebra
Vesical vein
use Hypogastric Vein, Left
use Hypogastric Vein, Right
Vesicotomy see Drainage, Urinary System ØT9
Vesiculectomy
see Excision, Male Reproductive System ØVB
see Resection, Male Reproductive System ØVT
Vesiculogram, seminal see Plain Radiography, Male Reproductive System BVØ
Vesiculotomy see Drainage, Male Reproductive System ØV9
Vestibular Assessment F15Z
Vestibular (Scarpa's) ganglion use Acoustic Nerve
Vestibular nerve use Acoustic Nerve
Vestibular Treatment FØC
Vestibulocochlear nerve use Acoustic Nerve
VEST™ Venous External Support device use Vein Graft Extraluminal Support Device(s) in New Technology
VH-IVUS (virtual histology intravascular ultrasound) see Ultrasonography, Heart B24
Virchow's (supraclavicular) lymph node
use Lymphatic, Left Neck
use Lymphatic, Right Neck
Virtuoso (II) (DR) (VR) use Defibrillator Generator in ØJH
Vistogard® use Uridine Triacetate
Visualase™ MRI-Guided Laser Ablation System see Destruction
Vitrectomy
see Excision, Eye Ø8B
see Resection, Eye Ø8T
Vitreous body
use Vitreous, Left
use Vitreous, Right
Viva (XT) (S) use Cardiac Resynchronization Defibrillator Pulse Generator in ØJH
Vivistim® Paired VNS System Lead use Neurostimulator Lead with Paired Stimulation System in New Technology

Vocal fold
use Vocal Cord, Left
use Vocal Cord, Right
Vocational
Assessment see Activities of Daily Living Assessment, Rehabilitation FØ2
Retraining see Activities of Daily Living Treatment, Rehabilitation FØ8
Volar (palmar) digital vein
use Hand Vein, Left
use Hand Vein, Right
Volar (palmar) metacarpal vein
use Hand Vein, Left
use Hand Vein, Right
Vomer bone use Nasal Septum
Vomer of nasal septum use Nasal Bone
Voraxaze use Glucarpidase
Vulvectomy
see Excision, Female Reproductive System ØUB
see Resection, Female Reproductive System ØUT
V-Wave Interatrial Shunt System use Synthetic Substitute
VYXEOS™ use Cytarabine and Daunorubicin Liposome Antineoplastic

W

WALLSTENT® Endoprosthesis use Intraluminal Device
Washing see Irrigation
WavelinQ EndoAVF system
Radial Artery, Left Ø31C3ZF
Radial Artery, Right Ø31B3ZF
Ulnar Artery, Left Ø31A3ZF
Ulnar Artery, Right Ø3193ZF
Wedge resection, pulmonary see Excision, Respiratory System ØBB
Whole Blood Nucleic Acid-base Microbial Detection XXE5XM5
Whole Blood Reverse Transcription and Quantitative Real-time Polymerase Chain Reaction XXE5X38

Window see Drainage
Wiring, dental 2W31X9Z

X

Xact Carotid Stent System use Intraluminal Device
XENLETA™ use Lefamulin Anti-infective
Xenograft use Zooplastic Tissue in Heart and Great Vessels
XENOVIEW™ BB34Z3Z
XIENCE Everolimus Eluting Coronary Stent System
use Intraluminal Device, Drug-eluting in Heart and Great Vessels
Xiphoid process use Sternum
XLIF® System use Interbody Fusion Device in Lower Joints
XOSPATA® use Gilteritinib Antineoplastic
X-ray see Plain Radiography
X-Spine Axle Cage
use Spinal Stabilization Device, Interspinous Process in ØRH
use Spinal Stabilization Device, Interspinous Process in ØSH
X-STOP® Spacer
use Spinal Stabilization Device, Interspinous Process in ØRH
use Spinal Stabilization Device, Interspinous Process in ØSH

Y

Yescarta® use Axicabtagene Ciloleucel Immunotherapy
Yoga Therapy 8EØZXY4

Z

Zenith AAA Endovascular Graft use Intraluminal Device

Zenith Flex® AAA Endovascular Graft use Intraluminal Device
Zenith TX2® TAA Endovascular Graft use Intraluminal Device
Zenith® Fenestrated AAA Endovascular Graft
use Intraluminal Device, Branched or Fenestrated, One or Two Arteries in Ø4V
use Intraluminal Device, Branched or Fenestrated, Three or More Arteries in Ø4V
Zenith® Renu™ AAA Ancillary Graft use Intraluminal Device
ZEPZELCA™ use Lurbinectedin
ZERBAXA® use Ceftolozane/Tazobactam Anti-infective
Zilver® PTX® (paclitaxel) Drug-Eluting Peripheral Stent
use Intraluminal Device, Drug-eluting in Lower Arteries
use Intraluminal Device, Drug-eluting in Upper Arteries
Zimmer® NexGen® LPS Mobile Bearing Knee use Synthetic Substitute
Zimmer® NexGen® LPS-Flex Mobile Knee use Synthetic Substitute
Zonule of Zinn
use Lens, Left
use Lens, Right
Zotarolimus-eluting Coronary Stent use Intraluminal Device, Drug-eluting in Heart and Great Vessels
Z-plasty, skin for scar contracture see Release, Skin and Breast ØHN
ZULRESSO™ use Brexanolone
Zygomatic process of frontal bone use Frontal Bone
Zygomatic process of temporal bone
use Temporal Bone, Left
use Temporal Bone, Right
Zygomaticus muscle use Facial Muscle
ZYNTEGLO® use Betibeglogene Autotemcel
Zyvox use Oxazolidinones

ICD-10-PCS Tables

Central Nervous System and Cranial Nerves ØØ1–ØØX

Character Meanings

This Character Meaning table is provided as a guide to assist the user in the identification of character members that may be found in this section of code tables. It **SHOULD NOT** be used to build a PCS code.

Operation–Character 3		Body Part–Character 4		Approach–Character 5		Device–Character 6		Qualifier–Character 7	
1	Bypass	Ø	Brain	Ø	Open	Ø	Drainage Device	Ø	Nasopharynx
2	Change	1	Cerebral Meninges	3	Percutaneous	1	Radioactive Element	1	Mastoid Sinus
5	Destruction	2	Dura Mater	4	Percutaneous Endoscopic	2	Monitoring Device	2	Atrium
7	Dilation	3	Epidural Space, Intracranial	X	External	3	Infusion Device	3	Blood Vessel OR Laser Interstitial Thermal Therapy
8	Division	4	Subdural Space, Intracranial			4	Radioactive Element, Cesium-131 Collagen Implant	4	Pleural Cavity
9	Drainage	5	Subarachnoid Space, Intracranial			7	Autologous Tissue Substitute	5	Intestine
B	Excision	6	Cerebral Ventricle			J	Synthetic Substitute	6	Peritoneal Cavity
C	Extirpation	7	Cerebral Hemisphere			K	Nonautologous Tissue Substitute	7	Urinary Tract
D	Extraction	8	Basal Ganglia			M	Neurostimulator Lead	8	Bone Marrow
F	Fragmentation	9	Thalamus			Y	Other Device	9	Fallopian Tube
H	Insertion	A	Hypothalamus			Z	No Device	A	Subgaleal Space
J	Inspection	B	Pons					B	Cerebral Cisterns
K	Map	C	Cerebellum					F	Olfactory Nerve
N	Release	D	Medulla Oblongata					G	Optic Nerve
P	Removal	E	Cranial Nerve					H	Oculomotor Nerve
Q	Repair	F	Olfactory Nerve					J	Trochlear Nerve
R	Replacement	G	Optic Nerve					K	Trigeminal Nerve
S	Reposition	H	Oculomotor Nerve					L	Abducens Nerve
T	Resection	J	Trochlear Nerve					M	Facial Nerve
U	Supplement	K	Trigeminal Nerve					N	Acoustic Nerve
W	Revision	L	Abducens Nerve					P	Glossopharyngeal Nerve
X	Transfer	M	Facial Nerve					Q	Vagus Nerve
		N	Acoustic Nerve					R	Accessory Nerve
		P	Glossopharyngeal Nerve					S	Hypoglossal Nerve
		Q	Vagus Nerve					X	Diagnostic
		R	Accessory Nerve					Z	No Qualifier
		S	Hypoglossal Nerve						
		T	Spinal Meninges						
		U	Spinal Canal						
		V	Spinal Cord						
		W	Cervical Spinal Cord						
		X	Thoracic Spinal Cord						
		Y	Lumbar Spinal Cord						

AHA Coding Clinic for table 001

2021, 2Q, 19	Electromagnetic stealth guided ventriculoperitoneal shunt insertion with endoscopy
2019, 4Q, 21-22	Cerebral ventricle bypass Qualifier
2018, 4Q, 86	Placement of lumboatrial shunt
2017, 4Q, 39-41	Dilation and bypass of cerebral ventricle
2015, 2Q, 9	Revision of ventriculoperitoneal (VP) shunt
2013, 2Q, 36	Insertion of ventriculoperitoneal shunt with laparoscopic assistance

AHA Coding Clinic for table 005

2022, 4Q, 53-54	Laser interstitial thermal therapy
2022, 1Q, 50	Percutaneous ganglion balloon compression
2021, 3Q, 16	Decompression of Chiari malformation by excision
2021, 2Q, 17	Dorsal root entry zone procedure

AHA Coding Clinic for table 007

2017, 4Q, 39-41	Dilation and bypass of cerebral ventricle

AHA Coding Clinic for table 009

2018, 4Q, 85	Externalization of lumboatrial shunt
2017, 1Q, 50	Failed lumbar puncture
2015, 3Q, 10	Open evacuation of subdural hematoma
2015, 3Q, 11	Percutaneous drainage of subdural hematoma
2015, 3Q, 12	Subdural evacuation portal system (SEPS) placement
2015, 3Q, 12	Placement of ventriculostomy catheter via burr hole
2015, 2Q, 30	Drainage of syrinx
2015, 1Q, 31	Intrathecal chemotherapy
2014, 1Q, 8	Diagnostic lumbar tap
2014, 1Q, 8	Lumbar drainage port aspiration

AHA Coding Clinic for table 00B

2021, 3Q, 16	Decompression of Chiari malformation by excision
2017, 3Q, 17	Resection of schwannoma and placement of DuraGen and Lorenz cranial plating system
2016, 2Q, 12	Resection of malignant neoplasm of inframtemporal fossa
2016, 2Q, 18	Amygdalohippocampectomy
2014, 4Q, 34	Resection of brain malignancy with implantation of chemotherapeutic wafer
2014, 3Q, 24	Repair of lipomyelomeningocele and tethered cord

AHA Coding Clinic for table 00C

2019, 3Q, 4	Evacuation of subdural hematoma and control of bleeding artery
2019, 2Q, 36	Evacuation of hematoma using NICO Brainpath® technology
2017, 4Q, 48	New and revised body part values - Extirpation spinal canal
2016, 2Q, 29	Decompressive craniectomy with cryopreservation and storage of bone flap
2015, 3Q, 10	Open evacuation of subdural hematoma
2015, 3Q, 11	Percutaneous drainage of subdural hematoma
2015, 3Q, 13	Evacuation of intracerebral hematoma

AHA Coding Clinic for table 00D

2022, 4Q, 54	Ultrasonic surgical aspiration of brain
2021, 4Q, 38-40	Ultrasonic surgical aspiration of brain
2015, 3Q, 13	Nonexcisional debridement of cranial wound with removal and replacement of hardware

AHA Coding Clinic for table 00H

2020, 4Q, 43-44	Insertion of radioactive element
2020, 2Q, 15	Ommaya reservoir with ventricular catheter placement
2020, 2Q, 16	Ommaya reservoir placement for cerebrospinal fluid infusion therapy
2017, 4Q, 30-31	Radiotherapeutic brain implant
2017, 3Q, 13	Implantation of bilateral neurostimulator electrodes
2014, 3Q, 19	End of life replacement of Baclofen pump

AHA Coding Clinic for table 00J

2021, 2Q, 19	Electromagnetic stealth guided ventriculoperitoneal shunt insertion with endoscopy
2019, 2Q, 36	Evacuation of hematoma using NICO Brainpath® technology
2017, 1Q, 50	Failed lumbar puncture

AHA Coding Clinic for table 00N

2019, 2Q, 19	Cervical spinal fusion, decompression and placement of interfacet stabilization device
2019, 1Q, 28	Decompressive laminectomy of both spinal cord and nerve roots
2018, 3Q, 30	Decompressive laminectomy (release of spinal cord versus release of spinal meninges)
2017, 3Q, 10	Repair of Chiari malformation
2017, 2Q, 23	Decompression of spinal cord and placement of instrumentation
2016, 2Q, 29	Decompressive craniectomy with cryopreservation and storage of bone flap
2015, 2Q, 20	Cervical laminoplasty
2015, 2Q, 21	Multiple decompressive cervical laminectomies
2015, 2Q, 34	Decompressive laminectomy
2014, 3Q, 24	Repair of lipomyelomeningocele and tethered cord

AHA Coding Clinic for table 00P

2014, 3Q, 19	End of life replacement of Baclofen pump

AHA Coding Clinic for table 00Q

2014, 3Q, 7	Hemi-cranioplasty for repair of cranial defect
2013, 3Q, 25	Fracture of frontal bone with repair and coagulation for hemostasis

AHA Coding Clinic for table 00S

2014, 4Q, 35	Reimplantation of buccal nerve

AHA Coding Clinic for table 00U

2021, 3Q, 16	Decompression of Chiari malformation by excision
2018, 1Q, 9	Craniectomy with DuraGaurd placement
2017, 4Q, 62	Added and revised device values - Nerve substitutes
2017, 3Q, 10	Repair of Chiari malformation
2017, 3Q, 17	Resection of schwannoma and placement of DuraGen and Lorenz cranial plating system
2015, 4Q, 39	Dural patch graft
2014, 3Q, 24	Repair of lipomyelomeningocele and tethered cord

AHA Coding Clinic for table 00W

2018, 4Q, 86	Placement of lumboatrial shunt

Brain

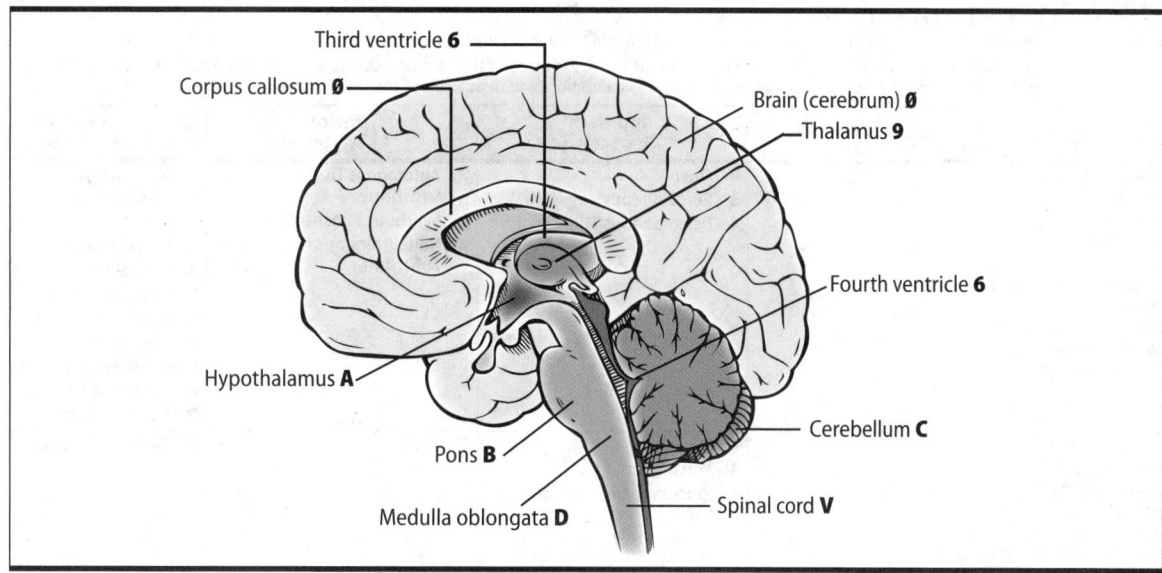

Third ventricle **6**

Corpus callosum **Ø**

Brain (cerebrum) **Ø**

Thalamus **9**

Fourth ventricle **6**

Hypothalamus **A**

Cerebellum **C**

Pons **B**

Spinal cord **V**

Medulla oblongata **D**

Cranial Nerves

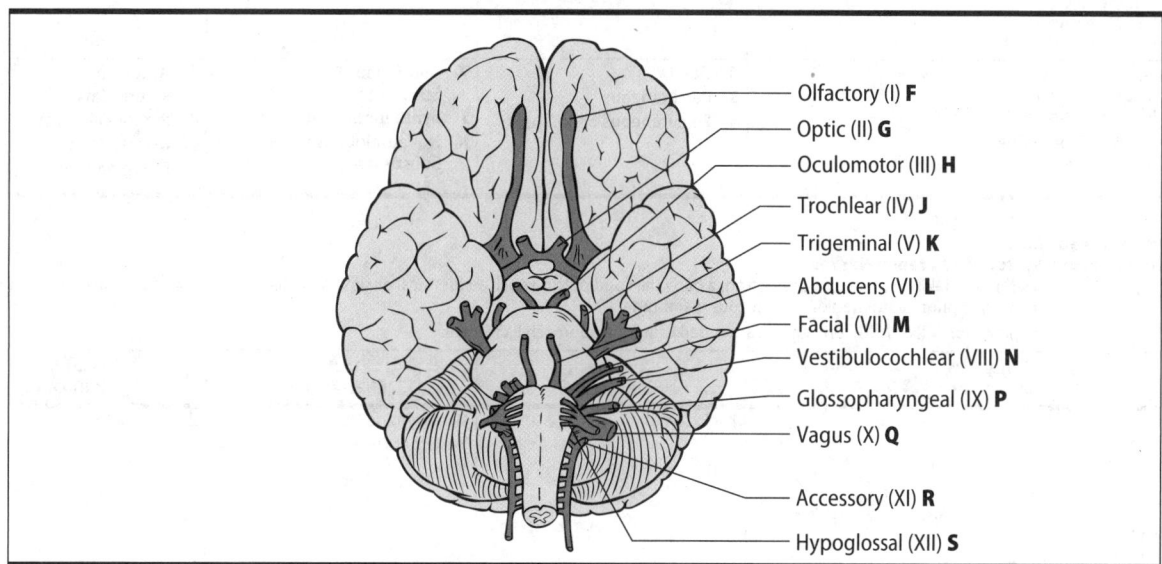

Olfactory (I) **F**

Optic (II) **G**

Oculomotor (III) **H**

Trochlear (IV) **J**

Trigeminal (V) **K**

Abducens (VI) **L**

Facial (VII) **M**

Vestibulocochlear (VIII) **N**

Glossopharyngeal (IX) **P**

Vagus (X) **Q**

Accessory (XI) **R**

Hypoglossal (XII) **S**

Ø   **Medical and Surgical**
Ø   **Central Nervous System and Cranial Nerves**
1   **Bypass**   Definition: Altering the route of passage of the contents of a tubular body part

Explanation: Rerouting contents of a body part to a downstream area of the normal route, to a similar route and body part, or to an abnormal route and dissimilar body part. Includes one or more anastomoses, with or without the use of a device.

Body Part Character 4	Approach Character 5	Device Character 6	Qualifier Character 7
6 **Cerebral Ventricle** Aqueduct of Sylvius Cerebral aqueduct (Sylvius) Choroid plexus Ependyma Foramen of Monro (intraventricular) Fourth ventricle Interventricular foramen (Monro) Left lateral ventricle Right lateral ventricle Third ventricle	**Ø** Open **3** Percutaneous **4** Percutaneous Endoscopic	**7** Autologous Tissue Substitute **J** Synthetic Substitute **K** Nonautologous Tissue Substitute	**Ø** Nasopharynx **1** Mastoid Sinus **2** Atrium **3** Blood Vessel **4** Pleural Cavity **5** Intestine **6** Peritoneal Cavity **7** Urinary Tract **8** Bone Marrow **A** Subgaleal Space **B** Cerebral Cisterns
6 **Cerebral Ventricle** Aqueduct of Sylvius Cerebral aqueduct (Sylvius) Choroid plexus Ependyma Foramen of Monro (intraventricular) Fourth ventricle Interventricular foramen (Monro) Left lateral ventricle Right lateral ventricle Third ventricle	**Ø** Open **3** Percutaneous **4** Percutaneous Endoscopic	**Z** No Device	**B** Cerebral Cisterns
U **Spinal Canal** Epidural space, spinal Extradural space, spinal Subarachnoid space, spinal Subdural space, spinal Vertebral canal	**Ø** Open **3** Percutaneous **4** Percutaneous Endoscopic	**7** Autologous Tissue Substitute **J** Synthetic Substitute **K** Nonautologous Tissue Substitute	**2** Atrium **4** Pleural Cavity **6** Peritoneal Cavity **7** Urinary Tract **9** Fallopian Tube

Ø   **Medical and Surgical**
Ø   **Central Nervous System and Cranial Nerves**
2   **Change**   Definition: Taking out or off a device from a body part and putting back an identical or similar device in or on the same body part without cutting or puncturing the skin or a mucous membrane

Explanation: All CHANGE procedures are coded using the approach EXTERNAL

Body Part Character 4	Approach Character 5	Device Character 6	Qualifier Character 7
Ø **Brain** Cerebrum Corpus callosum Encephalon **E** **Cranial Nerve** **U** **Spinal Canal** Epidural space, spinal Extradural space, spinal Subarachnoid space, spinal Subdural space, spinal Vertebral canal	**X** External	**Ø** Drainage Device **Y** Other Device	**Z** No Qualifier

Non-OR   All body part, approach, device, and qualifier values

---

Ø   **Medical and Surgical**
Ø   **Central Nervous System and Cranial Nerves**
5   **Destruction**   Definition: Physical eradication of all or a portion of a body part by the direct use of energy, force, or a destructive agent
                          Explanation: None of the body part is physically taken out

Body Part Character 4		Approach Character 5	Device Character 6	Qualifier Character 7
Ø **Brain** Cerebrum Corpus callosum Encephalon W **Cervical Spinal Cord** Dorsal root ganglion	X **Thoracic Spinal Cord** Dorsal root ganglion Y **Lumbar Spinal Cord** Cauda equina Conus medullaris Dorsal root ganglion	Ø Open 3 Percutaneous 4 Percutaneous Endoscopic	Z No Device	3 Laser Interstitial Thermal Therapy Z No Qualifier
1 **Cerebral Meninges** Arachnoid mater, intracranial Leptomeninges, intracranial Pia mater, intracranial 2 **Dura Mater** Diaphragma sellae Dura mater, intracranial Falx cerebri Tentorium cerebelli 6 **Cerebral Ventricle** Aqueduct of Sylvius Cerebral aqueduct (Sylvius) Choroid plexus Ependyma Foramen of Monro (intraventricular) Fourth ventricle Interventricular foramen (Monro) Left lateral ventricle Right lateral ventricle Third ventricle 7 **Cerebral Hemisphere** Frontal lobe Occipital lobe Parietal lobe Temporal lobe 8 **Basal Ganglia** Basal nuclei Claustrum Corpus striatum Globus pallidus Substantia nigra Subthalamic nucleus 9 **Thalamus** Epithalamus Geniculate nucleus Metathalamus Pulvinar A **Hypothalamus** Mammillary body B **Pons** Apneustic center Basis pontis Locus ceruleus Pneumotaxic center Pontine tegmentum Superior olivary nucleus C **Cerebellum** Culmen D **Medulla Oblongata** Myelencephalon F **Olfactory Nerve** First cranial nerve Olfactory bulb G **Optic Nerve** Optic chiasma Second cranial nerve	H **Oculomotor Nerve** Third cranial nerve J **Trochlear Nerve** Fourth cranial nerve K **Trigeminal Nerve** Fifth cranial nerve Gasserian ganglion Mandibular nerve Maxillary nerve Ophthalmic nerve Trifacial nerve L **Abducens Nerve** Sixth cranial nerve M **Facial Nerve** Chorda tympani Geniculate ganglion Greater superficial petrosal nerve Nerve to the stapedius Parotid plexus Posterior auricular nerve Seventh cranial nerve Submandibular ganglion N **Acoustic Nerve** Cochlear nerve Eighth cranial nerve Scarpa's (vestibular) ganglion Spiral ganglion Vestibular (Scarpa's) ganglion Vestibular nerve Vestibulocochlear nerve P **Glossopharyngeal Nerve** Carotid sinus nerve Ninth cranial nerve Tympanic nerve Q **Vagus Nerve** Anterior vagal trunk Pharyngeal plexus Pneumogastric nerve Posterior vagal trunk Pulmonary plexus Recurrent laryngeal nerve Superior laryngeal nerve Tenth cranial nerve R **Accessory Nerve** Eleventh cranial nerve S **Hypoglossal Nerve** Twelfth cranial nerve T **Spinal Meninges** Arachnoid mater, spinal Denticulate (dentate) ligament Dura mater, spinal Filum terminale Leptomeninges, spinal Pia mater, spinal	Ø Open 3 Percutaneous 4 Percutaneous Endoscopic	Z No Device	Z No Qualifier

Non-OR   ØØ5[F,G,H,J,K,L,M,N,P,Q,R,S][Ø,3,4]ZZ

Central Nervous System and Cranial Nerves

Ø   **Medical and Surgical**
Ø   **Central Nervous System and Cranial Nerves**
7   **Dilation**   Definition: Expanding an orifice or the lumen of a tubular body part

Explanation: The orifice can be a natural orifice or an artificially created orifice. Accomplished by stretching a tubular body part using intraluminal pressure or by cutting part of the orifice or wall of the tubular body part.

Body Part Character 4	Approach Character 5	Device Character 6	Qualifier Character 7
6 Cerebral Ventricle Aqueduct of Sylvius Cerebral aqueduct (Sylvius) Choroid plexus Ependyma Foramen of Monro (intraventricular) Fourth ventricle Interventricular foramen (Monro) Left lateral ventricle Right lateral ventricle Third ventricle	**Ø** Open **3** Percutaneous **4** Percutaneous Endoscopic	**Z** No Device	**Z** No Qualifier

Ø   **Medical and Surgical**
Ø   **Central Nervous System and Cranial Nerves**
8   **Division**   Definition: Cutting into a body part, without draining fluids and/or gases from the body part, in order to separate or transect a body part

Explanation: All or a portion of the body part is separated into two or more portions

Body Part Character 4	Approach Character 5	Device Character 6	Qualifier Character 7

Ø Brain
Cerebrum
Corpus callosum
Encephalon
7 Cerebral Hemisphere
Frontal lobe
Occipital lobe
Parietal lobe
Temporal lobe
8 Basal Ganglia
Basal nuclei
Claustrum
Corpus striatum
Globus pallidus
Substantia nigra
Subthalamic nucleus
F Olfactory Nerve
First cranial nerve
Olfactory bulb
G Optic Nerve
Optic chiasma
Second cranial nerve
H Oculomotor Nerve
Third cranial nerve
J Trochlear Nerve
Fourth cranial nerve
K Trigeminal Nerve
Fifth cranial nerve
Gasserian ganglion
Mandibular nerve
Maxillary nerve
Ophthalmic nerve
Trifacial nerve
L Abducens Nerve
Sixth cranial nerve
M Facial Nerve
Chorda tympani
Geniculate ganglion
Greater superficial petrosal
  nerve
Nerve to the stapedius
Parotid plexus
Posterior auricular nerve
Seventh cranial nerve
Submandibular ganglion
 	
N Acoustic Nerve
Cochlear nerve
Eighth cranial nerve
Scarpa's (vestibular)
  ganglion
Spiral ganglion
Vestibular (Scarpa's)
  ganglion
Vestibular nerve
Vestibulocochlear nerve
P Glossopharyngeal Nerve
Carotid sinus nerve
Ninth cranial nerve
Tympanic nerve
Q Vagus Nerve
Anterior vagal trunk
Pharyngeal plexus
Pneumogastric nerve
Posterior vagal trunk
Pulmonary plexus
Recurrent laryngeal nerve
Superior laryngeal nerve
Tenth cranial nerve
R Accessory Nerve
Eleventh cranial nerve
S Hypoglossal Nerve
Twelfth cranial nerve
W Cervical Spinal Cord
Dorsal root ganglion
X Thoracic Spinal Cord
Dorsal root ganglion
Y Lumbar Spinal Cord
Cauda equina
Conus medullaris
Dorsal root ganglion
	Ø Open
	3 Percutaneous
	4 Percutaneous Endoscopic
		Z No Device	**Z** No Qualifier

Non-OR Procedure   DRG Non-OR Procedure   Valid OR Procedure   HAC Associated Procedure   Combination Only   New/Revised April   New/Revised October

136   ICD-10-PCS 2024

007–008

Ø   **Medical and Surgical**
Ø   **Central Nervous System and Cranial Nerves**
9   **Drainage**   Definition: Taking or letting out fluids and/or gases from a body part
                       Explanation: The qualifier DIAGNOSTIC is used to identify drainage procedures that are biopsies

Body Part Character 4		Approach Character 5	Device Character 6	Qualifier Character 7

Ø Brain
  Cerebrum
  Corpus callosum
  Encephalon
1 Cerebral Meninges
  Arachnoid mater,
    intracranial
  Leptomeninges,
    intracranial
  Pia mater, intracranial
2 Dura Mater
  Diaphragma sellae
  Dura mater, intracranial
  Falx cerebri
  Tentorium cerebelli
**3 Epidural Space,
  Intracranial**
  Extradural space,
    intracranial
**4 Subdural Space,
  Intracranial**
**5 Subarachnoid Space,
  Intracranial**
6 Cerebral Ventricle
  Aqueduct of Sylvius
  Cerebral aqueduct
    (Sylvius)
  Choroid plexus
  Ependyma
  Foramen of Monro
    (intraventricular)
  Fourth ventricle
  Interventricular foramen
    (Monro)
  Left lateral ventricle
  Right lateral ventricle
  Third ventricle
7 Cerebral Hemisphere
  Frontal lobe
  Occipital lobe
  Parietal lobe
  Temporal lobe
8 Basal Ganglia
  Basal nuclei
  Claustrum
  Corpus striatum
  Globus pallidus
  Substantia nigra
  Subthalamic nucleus
9 Thalamus
  Epithalamus
  Geniculate nucleus
  Metathalamus
  Pulvinar
A Hypothalamus
  Mammillary body
B Pons
  Apneustic center
  Basis pontis
  Locus ceruleus
  Pneumotaxic center
  Pontine tegmentum
  Superior olivary nucleus
C Cerebellum
  Culmen
D Medulla Oblongata
  Myelencephalon
F Olfactory Nerve
  First cranial nerve
  Olfactory bulb
	G Optic Nerve
	  Optic chiasma
	  Second cranial nerve
	H Oculomotor Nerve
	  Third cranial nerve
	J Trochlear Nerve
	  Fourth cranial nerve
	K Trigeminal Nerve
	  Fifth cranial nerve
	  Gasserian ganglion
	  Mandibular nerve
	  Maxillary nerve
	  Ophthalmic nerve
	  Trifacial nerve
	L Abducens Nerve
	  Sixth cranial nerve
	M Facial Nerve
	  Chorda tympani
	  Geniculate ganglion
	  Greater superficial petrosal
	    nerve
	  Nerve to the stapedius
	  Parotid plexus
	  Posterior auricular nerve
	  Seventh cranial nerve
	  Submandibular ganglion
	N Acoustic Nerve
	  Cochlear nerve
	  Eighth cranial nerve
	  Scarpa's (vestibular) ganglion
	  Spiral ganglion
	  Vestibular (Scarpa's) ganglion
	  Vestibular nerve
	  Vestibulocochlear nerve
	P Glossopharyngeal Nerve
	  Carotid sinus nerve
	  Ninth cranial nerve
	  Tympanic nerve
	Q Vagus Nerve
	  Anterior vagal trunk
	  Pharyngeal plexus
	  Pneumogastric nerve
	  Posterior vagal trunk
	  Pulmonary plexus
	  Recurrent laryngeal nerve
	  Superior laryngeal nerve
	  Tenth cranial nerve
	R Accessory Nerve
	  Eleventh cranial nerve
	S Hypoglossal Nerve
	  Twelfth cranial nerve
	T Spinal Meninges
	  Arachnoid mater, spinal
	  Denticulate (dentate)
	    ligament
	  Dura mater, spinal
	  Filum terminale
	  Leptomeninges, spinal
	  Pia mater, spinal
	U Spinal Canal
	  Epidural space, spinal
	  Extradural space, spinal
	  Subarachnoid space, spinal
	  Subdural space, spinal
	  Vertebral canal
	W Cervical Spinal Cord
	  Dorsal root ganglion
	X Thoracic Spinal Cord
	  Dorsal root ganglion
	Y Lumbar Spinal Cord
	  Cauda equina
	  Conus medullaris
	  Dorsal root ganglion
		Ø Open
		3 Percutaneous
		4 Percutaneous Endoscopic
			Ø Drainage Device	**Z No Qualifier**

Non-OR   ØØ9[T,W,X,Y]3ØZ
Non-OR   ØØ9U[3,4]ØZ

ØØ9 Continued on next page

NC Noncovered Procedure   **LC** Limited Coverage   **QA** Questionable OB Admit   **NT** New Tech Add-on   ⊞ Combination Member   ♂ Male   ♀ Female

Central Nervous System and Cranial Nerves

Ø   **Medical and Surgical**   *009 Continued*
Ø   **Central Nervous System and Cranial Nerves**
9   **Drainage**   Definition: Taking or letting out fluids and/or gases from a body part
                     Explanation: The qualifier DIAGNOSTIC is used to identify drainage procedures that are biopsies

Body Part Character 4		Approach Character 5	Device Character 6	Qualifier Character 7

Ø **Brain**
  Cerebrum
  Corpus callosum
  Encephalon
1 **Cerebral Meninges**
  Arachnoid mater,
    intracranial
  Leptomeninges,
    intracranial
  Pia mater, intracranial
2 **Dura Mater**
  Diaphragma sellae
  Dura mater, intracranial
  Falx cerebri
  Tentorium cerebelli
3 **Epidural Space,
Intracranial**
  Extradural space,
    intracranial
4 **Subdural Space,
Intracranial**
5 **Subarachnoid Space,
Intracranial**
6 **Cerebral Ventricle**
  Aqueduct of Sylvius
  Cerebral aqueduct
    (Sylvius)
  Choroid plexus
  Ependyma
  Foramen of Monro
    (intraventricular)
  Fourth ventricle
  Interventricular foramen
    (Monro)
  Left lateral ventricle
  Right lateral ventricle
  Third ventricle
7 **Cerebral Hemisphere**
  Frontal lobe
  Occipital lobe
  Parietal lobe
  Temporal lobe
8 **Basal Ganglia**
  Basal nuclei
  Claustrum
  Corpus striatum
  Globus pallidus
  Substantia nigra
  Subthalamic nucleus
9 **Thalamus**
  Epithalamus
  Geniculate nucleus
  Metathalamus
  Pulvinar
A **Hypothalamus**
  Mammillary body
B **Pons**
  Apneustic center
  Basis pontis
  Locus ceruleus
  Pneumotaxic center
  Pontine tegmentum
  Superior olivary nucleus
C **Cerebellum**
  Culmen
D **Medulla Oblongata**
  Myelencephalon
F **Olfactory Nerve**
  First cranial nerve
  Olfactory bulb
	G **Optic Nerve**
	  Optic chiasma
	  Second cranial nerve
	H **Oculomotor Nerve**
	  Third cranial nerve
	J **Trochlear Nerve**
	  Fourth cranial nerve
	K **Trigeminal Nerve**
	  Fifth cranial nerve
	  Gasserian ganglion
	  Mandibular nerve
	  Maxillary nerve
	  Ophthalmic nerve
	  Trifacial nerve
	L **Abducens Nerve**
	  Sixth cranial nerve
	M **Facial Nerve**
	  Chorda tympani
	  Geniculate ganglion
	  Greater superficial petrosal
	    nerve
	  Nerve to the stapedius
	  Parotid plexus
	  Posterior auricular nerve
	  Seventh cranial nerve
	  Submandibular ganglion
	N **Acoustic Nerve**
	  Cochlear nerve
	  Eighth cranial nerve
	  Scarpa's (vestibular) ganglion
	  Spiral ganglion
	  Vestibular (Scarpa's) ganglion
	  Vestibular nerve
	  Vestibulocochlear nerve
	P **Glossopharyngeal Nerve**
	  Carotid sinus nerve
	  Ninth cranial nerve
	  Tympanic nerve
	Q **Vagus Nerve**
	  Anterior vagal trunk
	  Pharyngeal plexus
	  Pneumogastric nerve
	  Posterior vagal trunk
	  Pulmonary plexus
	  Recurrent laryngeal nerve
	  Superior laryngeal nerve
	  Tenth cranial nerve
	R **Accessory Nerve**
	  Eleventh cranial nerve
	S **Hypoglossal Nerve**
	  Twelfth cranial nerve
	T **Spinal Meninges**
	  Arachnoid mater, spinal
	  Denticulate (dentate)
	    ligament
	  Dura mater, spinal
	  Filum terminale
	  Leptomeninges, spinal
	  Pia mater, spinal
	U **Spinal Canal**
	  Epidural space, spinal
	  Extradural space, spinal
	  Subarachnoid space, spinal
	  Subdural space, spinal
	  Vertebral canal
	W **Cervical Spinal Cord**
	  Dorsal root ganglion
	X **Thoracic Spinal Cord**
	  Dorsal root ganglion
	Y **Lumbar Spinal Cord**
	  Cauda equina
	  Conus medullaris
	  Dorsal root ganglion
		Ø Open
		3 Percutaneous
		4 Percutaneous Endoscopic
			Z No Device	X Diagnostic
				Z No Qualifier

Non-OR	009[Ø,1,2,3,4,5,6,7,8,9,A,B,C,D,F,G,H,J,K,L,M,N,P,Q,R,S][3,4]ZX
Non-OR	009[T,W,X,Y]3Z[X,Z]
Non-OR	009U[3,4]Z[X,Z]

Non-OR Procedure   DRG Non-OR Procedure   Valid OR Procedure   HAC Associated Procedure   Combination Only   New/Revised April   New/Revised October

138   **ICD-10-PCS 2024**

Ø   **Medical and Surgical**
Ø   **Central Nervous System and Cranial Nerves**
B   **Excision**   Definition: Cutting out or off, without replacement, a portion of a body part
                     Explanation: The qualifier DIAGNOSTIC is used to identify excision procedures that are biopsies

Body Part Character 4		Approach Character 5	Device Character 6	Qualifier Character 7

Ø Brain
  Cerebrum
  Corpus callosum
  Encephalon
1 Cerebral Meninges
  Arachnoid mater,
    intracranial
  Leptomeninges,
    intracranial
  Pia mater, intracranial
2 Dura Mater
  Diaphragma sellae
  Dura mater, intracranial
  Falx cerebri
  Tentorium cerebelli
6 Cerebral Ventricle
  Aqueduct of Sylvius
  Cerebral aqueduct
    (Sylvius)
  Choroid plexus
  Ependyma
  Foramen of Monro
    (intraventricular)
  Fourth ventricle
  Interventricular foramen
    (Monro)
  Left lateral ventricle
  Right lateral ventricle
  Third ventricle
7 Cerebral Hemisphere
  Frontal lobe
  Occipital lobe
  Parietal lobe
  Temporal lobe
8 Basal Ganglia
  Basal nuclei
  Claustrum
  Corpus striatum
  Globus pallidus
  Substantia nigra
  Subthalamic nucleus
9 Thalamus
  Epithalamus
  Geniculate nucleus
  Metathalamus
  Pulvinar
A Hypothalamus
  Mammillary body
B Pons
  Apneustic center
  Basis pontis
  Locus ceruleus
  Pneumotaxic center
  Pontine tegmentum
  Superior olivary nucleus
C Cerebellum
  Culmen
D Medulla Oblongata
  Myelencephalon
F Olfactory Nerve
  First cranial nerve
  Olfactory bulb
G Optic Nerve
  Optic chiasma
  Second cranial nerve
	H Oculomotor Nerve
	  Third cranial nerve
	J Trochlear Nerve
	  Fourth cranial nerve
	K Trigeminal Nerve
	  Fifth cranial nerve
	  Gasserian ganglion
	  Mandibular nerve
	  Maxillary nerve
	  Ophthalmic nerve
	  Trifacial nerve
	L Abducens Nerve
	  Sixth cranial nerve
	M Facial Nerve
	  Chorda tympani
	  Geniculate ganglion
	  Greater superficial petrosal
	    nerve
	  Nerve to the stapedius
	  Parotid plexus
	  Posterior auricular nerve
	  Seventh cranial nerve
	  Submandibular ganglion
	N Acoustic Nerve
	  Cochlear nerve
	  Eighth cranial nerve
	  Scarpa's (vestibular)
	    ganglion
	  Spiral ganglion
	  Vestibular (Scarpa's)
	    ganglion
	  Vestibular nerve
	  Vestibulocochlear nerve
	P Glossopharyngeal Nerve
	  Carotid sinus nerve
	  Ninth cranial nerve
	  Tympanic nerve
	Q Vagus Nerve
	  Anterior vagal trunk
	  Pharyngeal plexus
	  Pneumogastric nerve
	  Posterior vagal trunk
	  Pulmonary plexus
	  Recurrent laryngeal nerve
	  Superior laryngeal nerve
	  Tenth cranial nerve
	R Accessory Nerve
	  Eleventh cranial nerve
	S Hypoglossal Nerve
	  Twelfth cranial nerve
	T Spinal Meninges
	  Arachnoid mater, spinal
	  Denticulate (dentate)
	    ligament
	  Dura mater, spinal
	  Filum terminale
	  Leptomeninges, spinal
	  Pia mater, spinal
	W Cervical Spinal Cord
	  Dorsal root ganglion
	X Thoracic Spinal Cord
	  Dorsal root ganglion
	Y Lumbar Spinal Cord
	  Cauda equina
	  Conus medullaris
	  Dorsal root ganglion
		Ø Open
		3 Percutaneous
		4 Percutaneous Endoscopic
			Z No Device	**X** Diagnostic
				Z No Qualifier

Non-OR   ØØB[F,G,H,J,K,L,M,N,P,Q,R,S][3,4]ZX

NC Noncovered Procedure   **LC** Limited Coverage   **QA** Questionable OB Admit   **NT** New Tech Add-on   ✚ Combination Member   ♂ Male   ♀ Female

ICD-10-PCS 2024   139

ØØB–ØØB

Ø   Medical and Surgical
Ø   Central Nervous System and Cranial Nerves
C   Extirpation   Definition: Taking or cutting out solid matter from a body part

           Explanation: The solid matter may be an abnormal byproduct of a biological function or a foreign body; it may be imbedded in a body part or in the lumen of a tubular body part. The solid matter may or may not have been previously broken into pieces.

Body Part Character 4	Approach Character 5	Device Character 6	Qualifier Character 7

Ø **Brain**
  Cerebrum
  Corpus callosum
  Encephalon
1 **Cerebral Meninges**
  Arachnoid mater,
    intracranial
  Leptomeninges,
    intracranial
  Pia mater, intracranial
2 **Dura Mater**
  Diaphragma sellae
  Dura mater, intracranial
  Falx cerebri
  Tentorium cerebelli
3 **Epidural Space,**
  Intracranial
  Extradural space,
    intracranial
4 **Subdural Space,**
  Intracranial
5 **Subarachnoid Space,**
  Intracranial
6 **Cerebral Ventricle**
  Aqueduct of Sylvius
  Cerebral aqueduct
    (Sylvius)
  Choroid plexus
  Ependyma
  Foramen of Monro
    (intraventricular)
  Fourth ventricle
  Interventricular foramen
    (Monro)
  Left lateral ventricle
  Right lateral ventricle
  Third ventricle
7 **Cerebral Hemisphere**
  Frontal lobe
  Occipital lobe
  Parietal lobe
  Temporal lobe
8 **Basal Ganglia**
  Basal nuclei
  Claustrum
  Corpus striatum
  Globus pallidus
  Substantia nigra
  Subthalamic nucleus
9 **Thalamus**
  Epithalamus
  Geniculate nucleus
  Metathalamus
  Pulvinar
A **Hypothalamus**
  Mammillary body
B **Pons**
  Apneustic center
  Basis pontis
  Locus ceruleus
  Pneumotaxic center
  Pontine tegmentum
  Superior olivary nucleus
C **Cerebellum**
  Culmen
D **Medulla Oblongata**
  Myelencephalon
F **Olfactory Nerve**
  First cranial nerve
  Olfactory bulb
	G **Optic Nerve**
	  Optic chiasma
	  Second cranial nerve
	H **Oculomotor Nerve**
	  Third cranial nerve
	J **Trochlear Nerve**
	  Fourth cranial nerve
	K **Trigeminal Nerve**
	  Fifth cranial nerve
	  Gasserian ganglion
	  Mandibular nerve
	  Maxillary nerve
	  Ophthalmic nerve
	  Trifacial nerve
	L **Abducens Nerve**
	  Sixth cranial nerve
	M **Facial Nerve**
	  Chorda tympani
	  Geniculate ganglion
	  Greater superficial petrosal
	    nerve
	  Nerve to the stapedius
	  Parotid plexus
	  Posterior auricular nerve
	  Seventh cranial nerve
	  Submandibular ganglion
	N **Acoustic Nerve**
	  Cochlear nerve
	  Eighth cranial nerve
	  Scarpa's (vestibular)
	    ganglion
	  Spiral ganglion
	  Vestibular (Scarpa's)
	    ganglion
	  Vestibular nerve
	  Vestibulocochlear nerve
	P **Glossopharyngeal Nerve**
	  Carotid sinus nerve
	  Ninth cranial nerve
	  Tympanic nerve
	Q **Vagus Nerve**
	  Anterior vagal trunk
	  Pharyngeal plexus
	  Pneumogastric nerve
	  Posterior vagal trunk
	  Pulmonary plexus
	  Recurrent laryngeal nerve
	  Superior laryngeal nerve
	  Tenth cranial nerve
	R **Accessory Nerve**
	  Eleventh cranial nerve
	S **Hypoglossal Nerve**
	  Twelfth cranial nerve
	T **Spinal Meninges**
	  Arachnoid mater, spinal
	  Denticulate (dentate)
	    ligament
	  Dura mater, spinal
	  Filum terminale
	  Leptomeninges, spinal
	  Pia mater, spinal
	U **Spinal Canal**
	W **Cervical Spinal Cord**
	  Dorsal root ganglion
	X **Thoracic Spinal Cord**
	  Dorsal root ganglion
	Y **Lumbar Spinal Cord**
	  Cauda equina
	  Conus medullaris
	  Dorsal root ganglion
		Ø Open
		3 Percutaneous
		4 Percutaneous Endoscopic
			Z No Device	Z No Qualifier

Non-OR Procedure   DRG Non-OR Procedure   Valid OR Procedure   HAC Associated Procedure   Combination Only   New/Revised April   New/Revised October

140   ICD-10-PCS 2024

Ø   **Medical and Surgical**
Ø   **Central Nervous System and Cranial Nerves**
D   **Extraction**   Definition: Pulling or stripping out or off all or a portion of a body part by the use of force
                         Explanation: The qualifier DIAGNOSTIC is used to identify extraction procedures that are biopsies

Body Part Character 4		Approach Character 5	Device Character 6	Qualifier Character 7

Ø Brain
  Cerebrum
  Corpus callosum
  Encephalon
1 Cerebral Meninges
  Arachnoid mater,
    intracranial
  Leptomeninges,
    intracranial
  Pia mater, intracranial
2 Dura Mater
  Diaphragma sellae
  Dura mater, intracranial
  Falx cerebri
  Tentorium cerebelli
7 Cerebral Hemisphere
  Frontal lobe
  Occipital lobe
  Parietal lobe
  Temporal lobe
C Cerebellum
  Culmen
F Olfactory Nerve
  First cranial nerve
  Olfactory bulb
G Optic Nerve
  Optic chiasma
  Second cranial nerve
H Oculomotor Nerve
  Third cranial nerve
J Trochlear Nerve
  Fourth cranial nerve
K Trigeminal Nerve
  Fifth cranial nerve
  Gasserian ganglion
  Mandibular nerve
  Maxillary nerve
  Ophthalmic nerve
  Trifacial nerve
L Abducens Nerve
  Sixth cranial nerve
	M Facial Nerve
	  Chorda tympani
	  Geniculate ganglion
	  Greater superficial petrosal
	    nerve
	  Nerve to the stapedius
	  Parotid plexus
	  Posterior auricular nerve
	  Seventh cranial nerve
	  Submandibular ganglion
	N Acoustic Nerve
	  Cochlear nerve
	  Eighth cranial nerve
	  Scarpa's (vestibular)
	    ganglion
	  Spiral ganglion
	  Vestibular (Scarpa's)
	    ganglion
	  Vestibular nerve
	  Vestibulocochlear nerve
	P Glossopharyngeal Nerve
	  Carotid sinus nerve
	  Ninth cranial nerve
	  Tympanic nerve
	Q Vagus Nerve
	  Anterior vagal trunk
	  Pharyngeal plexus
	  Pneumogastric nerve
	  Posterior vagal trunk
	  Pulmonary plexus
	  Recurrent laryngeal nerve
	  Superior laryngeal nerve
	  Tenth cranial nerve
	R Accessory Nerve
	  Eleventh cranial nerve
	S Hypoglossal Nerve
	  Twelfth cranial nerve
	T Spinal Meninges
	  Arachnoid mater, spinal
	  Denticulate (dentate)
	    ligament
	  Dura mater, spinal
	  Filum terminale
	  Leptomeninges, spinal
	  Pia mater, spinal
		Ø Open
		3 Percutaneous
		4 Percutaneous Endoscopic
			Z No Device	**Z No Qualifier**

Central Nervous System and Cranial Nerves *(left margin)*

Ø   **Medical and Surgical**
Ø   **Central Nervous System and Cranial Nerves**
F   **Fragmentation**   Definition: Breaking solid matter in a body part into pieces

Explanation: Physical force (e.g., manual, ultrasonic) applied directly or indirectly is used to break the solid matter into pieces. The solid matter may be an abnormal byproduct of a biological function or a foreign body. The pieces of solid matter are not taken out.

Body Part Character 4	Approach Character 5	Device Character 6	Qualifier Character 7

3 Epidural Space, Intracranial **NC**
  Extradural space, intracranial
4 Subdural Space, Intracranial **NC**
5 Subarachnoid Space, Intracranial **NC**
6 Cerebral Ventricle **NC**
  Aqueduct of Sylvius
  Cerebral aqueduct (Sylvius)
  Choroid plexus
  Ependyma
  Foramen of Monro (intraventricular)
  Fourth ventricle
  Interventricular foramen (Monro)
  Left lateral ventricle
  Right lateral ventricle
  Third ventricle
U Spinal Canal
  Epidural space, spinal
  Extradural space, spinal
  Subarachnoid space, spinal
  Subdural space, spinal
  Vertebral canal
	Ø Open
	3 Percutaneous
	4 Percutaneous Endoscopic
	X External
		Z No Device	Z No Qualifier

Non-OR   ØØF[3,4,5,6]XZZ
NC   ØØF[3,4,5,6]XZZ

Ø   **Medical and Surgical**
Ø   **Central Nervous System and Cranial Nerves**
H   **Insertion**   Definition: Putting in a nonbiological appliance that monitors, assists, performs, or prevents a physiological function but does not physically take the place of a body part

Explanation: None

Body Part Character 4	Approach Character 5	Device Character 6	Qualifier Character 7

Ø Brain ⊞
  Cerebrum
  Corpus callosum
  Encephalon
	Ø Open	1 Radioactive Element
		2 Monitoring Device
		3 Infusion Device
		4 Radioactive Element, Cesium-131 Collagen Implant
		M Neurostimulator Lead
		Y Other Device
			Z No Qualifier

Ø Brain ⊞
  Cerebrum
  Corpus callosum
  Encephalon
	3 Percutaneous
	4 Percutaneous Endoscopic
		1 Radioactive Element
		2 Monitoring Device
		3 Infusion Device
		M Neurostimulator Lead
		Y Other Device
			Z No Qualifier

6 Cerebral Ventricle ⊞
  Aqueduct of Sylvius
  Cerebral aqueduct (Sylvius)
  Choroid plexus
  Ependyma
  Foramen of Monro (intraventricular)
  Fourth ventricle Interventricular foramen (Monro)
  Left lateral ventricle
  Right lateral ventricle
  Third ventricle
E Cranial Nerve ⊞
U Spinal Canal ⊞
  Epidural space, spinal
  Extradural space, spinal
  Subarachnoid space, spinal
  Subdural space, spinal
  Vertebral canal
V Spinal Cord ⊞
  Dorsal root ganglion
	Ø Open
	3 Percutaneous
	4 Percutaneous Endoscopic
		1 Radioactive Element
		2 Monitoring Device
		3 Infusion Device
		M Neurostimulator Lead
		Y Other Device
			Z No Qualifier

DRG Non-OR   ØØHØØ4Z
Non-OR   ØØH[E,U,V]32Z
Non-OR   ØØH[E,U][3,4]YZ
Non-OR   ØØH[U,V][Ø,3,4]3Z

See Appendix L for Procedure Combinations
⊞   ØØHØØMZ
⊞   ØØHØ[3,4]MZ
⊞   ØØH[6,E,U,V][Ø,3,4]MZ

Ø Medical and Surgical
Ø Central Nervous System and Cranial Nerves
J Inspection   Definition: Visually and/or manually exploring a body part

Explanation: Visual exploration may be performed with or without optical instrumentation. Manual exploration may be performed directly or through intervening body layers.

Body Part Character 4	Approach Character 5	Device Character 6	Qualifier Character 7
Ø Brain Cerebrum Corpus callosum Encephalon **E Cranial Nerve** **U Spinal Canal** Epidural space, spinal Extradural space, spinal Subarachnoid space, spinal Subdural space, spinal Vertebral canal **V Spinal Cord** Dorsal root ganglion	**Ø** Open **3** Percutaneous **4** Percutaneous Endoscopic	**Z** No Device	**Z** No Qualifier

Non-OR	ØØJ[Ø,E,U,V]3ZZ

Ø Medical and Surgical
Ø Central Nervous System and Cranial Nerves
K Map   Definition: Locating the route of passage of electrical impulses and/or locating functional areas in a body part

Explanation: Applicable only to the cardiac conduction mechanism and the central nervous system

Body Part Character 4	Approach Character 5	Device Character 6	Qualifier Character 7
Ø Brain Cerebrum Corpus callosum Encephalon **7 Cerebral Hemisphere** Frontal lobe Occipital lobe Parietal lobe Temporal lobe **8 Basal Ganglia** Basal nuclei Claustrum Corpus striatum Globus pallidus Substantia nigra Subthalamic nucleus **9 Thalamus** Epithalamus Geniculate nucleus Metathalamus Pulvinar **A Hypothalamus** Mammillary body **B Pons** Apneustic center Basis pontis Locus ceruleus Pneumotaxic center Pontine tegmentum Superior olivary nucleus **C Cerebellum** Culmen **D Medulla Oblongata** Myelencephalon	**Ø** Open **3** Percutaneous **4** Percutaneous Endoscopic	**Z** No Device	**Z** No Qualifier

NC Noncovered Procedure   LC Limited Coverage   QA Questionable OB Admit   NT New Tech Add-on   ⊞ Combination Member   ♂ Male   ♀ Female

ICD-10-PCS 2024   143

Central Nervous System and Cranial Nerves

Ø   **Medical and Surgical**
Ø   **Central Nervous System and Cranial Nerves**
N   **Release**   Definition: Freeing a body part from an abnormal physical constraint by cutting or by the use of force
                   Explanation: Some of the restraining tissue may be taken out but none of the body part is taken out

Body Part Character 4		Approach Character 5	Device Character 6	Qualifier Character 7

Ø **Brain**
   Cerebrum
   Corpus callosum
   Encephalon
 1 **Cerebral Meninges**
   Arachnoid mater,
     intracranial
   Leptomeninges,
     intracranial
   Pia mater, intracranial
 2 **Dura Mater**
   Diaphragma sellae
   Dura mater, intracranial
   Falx cerebri
   Tentorium cerebelli
 6 **Cerebral Ventricle**
   Aqueduct of Sylvius
   Cerebral aqueduct
     (Sylvius)
   Choroid plexus
   Ependyma
   Foramen of Monro
     (intraventricular)
   Fourth ventricle
   Interventricular foramen
     (Monro)
   Left lateral ventricle
   Right lateral ventricle
   Third ventricle
 7 **Cerebral Hemisphere**
   Frontal lobe
   Occipital lobe
   Parietal lobe
   Temporal lobe
 8 **Basal Ganglia**
   Basal nuclei
   Claustrum
   Corpus striatum
   Globus pallidus
   Substantia nigra
   Subthalamic nucleus
 9 **Thalamus**
   Epithalamus
   Geniculate nucleus
   Metathalamus
   Pulvinar
 A **Hypothalamus**
   Mammillary body
 B **Pons**
   Apneustic center
   Basis pontis
   Locus ceruleus
   Pneumotaxic center
   Pontine tegmentum
   Superior olivary nucleus
 C **Cerebellum**
   Culmen
 D **Medulla Oblongata**
   Myelencephalon
 F **Olfactory Nerve**
   First cranial nerve
   Olfactory bulb
 G **Optic Nerve**
   Optic chiasma
   Second cranial nerve
	H **Oculomotor Nerve**
	   Third cranial nerve
	 J **Trochlear Nerve**
	   Fourth cranial nerve
	 K **Trigeminal Nerve**
	   Fifth cranial nerve
	   Gasserian ganglion
	   Mandibular nerve
	   Maxillary nerve
	   Ophthalmic nerve
	   Trifacial nerve
	 L **Abducens Nerve**
	   Sixth cranial nerve
	 M **Facial Nerve**
	   Chorda tympani
	   Geniculate ganglion
	   Greater superficial petrosal
	     nerve
	   Nerve to the stapedius
	   Parotid plexus
	   Posterior auricular nerve
	   Seventh cranial nerve
	   Submandibular ganglion
	 N **Acoustic Nerve**
	   Cochlear nerve
	   Eighth cranial nerve
	   Scarpa's (vestibular)
	     ganglion
	   Spiral ganglion
	   Vestibular (Scarpa's)
	     ganglion
	   Vestibular nerve
	   Vestibulocochlear nerve
	 P **Glossopharyngeal Nerve**
	   Carotid sinus nerve
	   Ninth cranial nerve
	   Tympanic nerve
	 Q **Vagus Nerve**
	   Anterior vagal trunk
	   Pharyngeal plexus
	   Pneumogastric nerve
	   Posterior vagal trunk
	   Pulmonary plexus
	   Recurrent laryngeal nerve
	   Superior laryngeal nerve
	   Tenth cranial nerve
	 R **Accessory Nerve**
	   Eleventh cranial nerve
	 S **Hypoglossal Nerve**
	   Twelfth cranial nerve
	 T **Spinal Meninges**
	   Arachnoid mater, spinal
	   Denticulate (dentate)
	     ligament
	   Dura mater, spinal
	   Filum terminale
	   Leptomeninges, spinal
	   Pia mater, spinal
	 W **Cervical Spinal Cord**
	   Dorsal root ganglion
	 X **Thoracic Spinal Cord**
	   Dorsal root ganglion
	 Y **Lumbar Spinal Cord**
	   Cauda equina
	   Conus medullaris
	   Dorsal root ganglion
		Ø **Open**
		 3 **Percutaneous**
		 4 **Percutaneous Endoscopic**
			Z **No Device**	Z **No Qualifier**

0   **Medical and Surgical**
0   **Central Nervous System and Cranial Nerves**
P   **Removal**   Definition: Taking out or off a device from a body part

           Explanation: If a device is taken out and a similar device put in without cutting or puncturing the skin or mucous membrane, the procedure is coded to the root operation CHANGE. Otherwise, the procedure for taking out a device is coded to the root operation REMOVAL.

Body Part Character 4	Approach Character 5	Device Character 6	Qualifier Character 7

0   **Brain**
    Cerebrum
    Corpus callosum
    Encephalon
V   **Spinal Cord**
    Dorsal root ganglion
	0 Open
	3 Percutaneous
	4 Percutaneous Endoscopic
		0 Drainage Device
		2 Monitoring Device
		3 Infusion Device
		7 Autologous Tissue Substitute
		J Synthetic Substitute
		K Nonautologous Tissue Substitute
		M Neurostimulator Lead
		Y Other Device
			Z No Qualifier

0   **Brain**
    Cerebrum
    Corpus callosum
    Encephalon
V   **Spinal Cord**
    Dorsal root ganglion
	X External	**0** Drainage Device
		2 Monitoring Device
		3 Infusion Device
		M Neurostimulator Lead
			Z No Qualifier

6   **Cerebral Ventricle**
    Aqueduct of Sylvius
    Cerebral aqueduct (Sylvius)
    Choroid plexus
    Ependyma
    Foramen of Monro (intraventricular)
    Fourth ventricle
    Interventricular foramen (Monro)
    Left lateral ventricle
    Right lateral ventricle
    Third ventricle
U   **Spinal Canal**
    Epidural space, spinal
    Extradural space, spinal
    Subarachnoid space, spinal
    Subdural space, spinal
    Vertebral canal
	0 Open
	3 Percutaneous
	4 Percutaneous Endoscopic
		0 Drainage Device
		2 Monitoring Device
		3 Infusion Device
		J Synthetic Substitute
		M Neurostimulator Lead
		Y Other Device
			Z No Qualifier

6   **Cerebral Ventricle**
    Aqueduct of Sylvius
    Cerebral aqueduct (Sylvius)
    Choroid plexus
    Ependyma
    Foramen of Monro (intraventricular)
    Fourth ventricle
    Interventricular foramen (Monro)
    Left lateral ventricle
    Right lateral ventricle
    Third ventricle
U   **Spinal Canal**
    Epidural space, spinal
    Extradural space, spinal
    Subarachnoid space, spinal
    Subdural space, spinal
    Vertebral canal
	X External	**0** Drainage Device
		2 Monitoring Device
		3 Infusion Device
		M Neurostimulator Lead
			Z No Qualifier

E **Cranial Nerve**	**0** Open **3** Percutaneous **4** Percutaneous Endoscopic	**0** Drainage Device **2** Monitoring Device **3** Infusion Device **7** Autologous Tissue Substitute **M** Neurostimulator Lead **Y** Other Device	**Z** No Qualifier
E **Cranial Nerve**	**X** External	**0** Drainage Device **2** Monitoring Device **3** Infusion Device **M** Neurostimulator Lead	**Z** No Qualifier

Non-OR	00P[0,V]3[0,2,3]Z
Non-OR	00P[0,V][3,4]YZ
Non-OR	00P[0,V]X[0,2,3,M]Z
Non-OR	00P[6,U]3[0,2,3]Z
Non-OR	00P[6,U][3,4]YZ
Non-OR	00P[6,U]X[0,2,3,M]Z
Non-OR	00PE3[0,2,3]Z
Non-OR	00PE[3,4]YZ
Non-OR	00PEX[0,2,3,M]Z

NC Noncovered Procedure   LC Limited Coverage   QA Questionable OB Admit   NT New Tech Add-on   ➕ Combination Member   ♂ Male   ♀ Female

0 Medical and Surgical
0 Central Nervous System and Cranial Nerves
Q Repair   Definition: Restoring, to the extent possible, a body part to its normal anatomic structure and function
                Explanation: Used only when the method to accomplish the repair is not one of the other root operations

Body Part – Character 4	Approach – Character 5	Device – Character 6	Qualifier – Character 7
0 Brain Cerebrum Corpus callosum Encephalon **1 Cerebral Meninges** Arachnoid mater, intracranial Leptomeninges, intracranial Pia mater, intracranial **2 Dura Mater** Diaphragma sellae Dura mater, intracranial Falx cerebri Tentorium cerebelli **6 Cerebral Ventricle** Aqueduct of Sylvius Cerebral aqueduct (Sylvius) Choroid plexus Ependyma Foramen of Monro (intraventricular) Fourth ventricle Interventricular foramen (Monro) Left lateral ventricle Right lateral ventricle Third ventricle **7 Cerebral Hemisphere** Frontal lobe Occipital lobe Parietal lobe Temporal lobe **8 Basal Ganglia** Basal nuclei Claustrum Corpus striatum Globus pallidus Substantia nigra Subthalamic nucleus **9 Thalamus** Epithalamus Geniculate nucleus Metathalamus Pulvinar **A Hypothalamus** Mammillary body **B Pons** Apneustic center Basis pontis Locus ceruleus Pneumotaxic center Pontine tegmentum Superior olivary nucleus **C Cerebellum** Culmen **D Medulla Oblongata** Myelencephalon **F Olfactory Nerve** First cranial nerve Olfactory bulb **G Optic Nerve** Optic chiasma Second cranial nerve	**H Oculomotor Nerve** Third cranial nerve **J Trochlear Nerve** Fourth cranial nerve **K Trigeminal Nerve** Fifth cranial nerve Gasserian ganglion Mandibular nerve Maxillary nerve Ophthalmic nerve Trifacial nerve **L Abducens Nerve** Sixth cranial nerve **M Facial Nerve** Chorda tympani Geniculate ganglion Greater superficial petrosal nerve Nerve to the stapedius Parotid plexus Posterior auricular nerve Seventh cranial nerve Submandibular ganglion **N Acoustic Nerve** Cochlear nerve Eighth cranial nerve Scarpa's (vestibular) ganglion Spiral ganglion Vestibular (Scarpa's) ganglion Vestibular nerve Vestibulocochlear nerve **P Glossopharyngeal Nerve** Carotid sinus nerve Ninth cranial nerve Tympanic nerve **Q Vagus Nerve** Anterior vagal trunk Pharyngeal plexus Pneumogastric nerve Posterior vagal trunk Pulmonary plexus Recurrent laryngeal nerve Superior laryngeal nerve Tenth cranial nerve **R Accessory Nerve** Eleventh cranial nerve **S Hypoglossal Nerve** Twelfth cranial nerve **T Spinal Meninges** Arachnoid mater, spinal Denticulate (dentate) ligament Dura mater, spinal Filum terminale Leptomeninges, spinal Pia mater, spinal **W Cervical Spinal Cord** Dorsal root ganglion **X Thoracic Spinal Cord** Dorsal root ganglion **Y Lumbar Spinal Cord** Cauda equina Conus medullaris Dorsal root ganglion	**0** Open **3** Percutaneous **4** Percutaneous Endoscopic	**Z** No Device	**Z** No Qualifier

Ø   Medical and Surgical
Ø   Central Nervous System and Cranial Nerves
R   Replacement   Definition: Putting in or on biological or synthetic material that physically takes the place and/or function of all or a portion of a body part

Explanation: The body part may have been taken out or replaced, or may be taken out, physically eradicated, or rendered nonfunctional during the REPLACEMENT procedure. A REMOVAL procedure is coded for taking out the device used in a previous replacement procedure.

Body Part Character 4		Approach Character 5	Device Character 6	Qualifier Character 7

1 Cerebral Meninges
  Arachnoid mater,
    intracranial
  Leptomeninges,
    intracranial
  Pia mater, intracranial
2 Dura Mater
  Diaphragma sellae
  Dura mater, intracranial
  Falx cerebri
  Tentorium cerebelli
6 Cerebral Ventricle
  Aqueduct of Sylvius
  Cerebral aqueduct
    (Sylvius)
  Choroid plexus
  Ependyma
  Foramen of Monro
    (intraventricular)
  Fourth ventricle
  Interventricular foramen
    (Monro)
  Left lateral ventricle
  Right lateral ventricle
  Third ventricle
F Olfactory Nerve
  First cranial nerve
  Olfactory bulb
G Optic Nerve
  Optic chiasma
  Second cranial nerve
H Oculomotor Nerve
  Third cranial nerve
J Trochlear Nerve
  Fourth cranial nerve
K Trigeminal Nerve
  Fifth cranial nerve
  Gasserian ganglion
  Mandibular nerve
  Maxillary nerve
  Ophthalmic nerve
  Trifacial nerve
L Abducens Nerve
  Sixth cranial nerve
	M Facial Nerve
	  Chorda tympani
	  Geniculate ganglion
	  Greater superficial petrosal
	    nerve
	  Nerve to the stapedius
	  Parotid plexus
	  Posterior auricular nerve
	  Seventh cranial nerve
	  Submandibular ganglion
	N Acoustic Nerve
	  Cochlear nerve
	  Eighth cranial nerve
	  Scarpa's (vestibular)
	    ganglion
	  Spiral ganglion
	  Vestibular (Scarpa's)
	    ganglion
	  Vestibular nerve
	  Vestibulocochlear nerve
	P Glossopharyngeal Nerve
	  Carotid sinus nerve
	  Ninth cranial nerve
	  Tympanic nerve
	Q Vagus Nerve
	  Anterior vagal trunk
	  Pharyngeal plexus
	  Pneumogastric nerve
	  Posterior vagal trunk
	  Pulmonary plexus
	  Recurrent laryngeal nerve
	  Superior laryngeal nerve
	  Tenth cranial nerve
	R Accessory Nerve
	  Eleventh cranial nerve
	S Hypoglossal Nerve
	  Twelfth cranial nerve
	T Spinal Meninges
	  Arachnoid mater, spinal
	  Denticulate (dentate)
	    ligament
	  Dura mater, spinal
	  Filum terminale
	  Leptomeninges, spinal
	  Pia mater, spinal
		Ø Open
		4 Percutaneous Endoscopic
			7 Autologous Tissue
			    Substitute
			J Synthetic Substitute
			K Nonautologous Tissue
			    Substitute
				Z No Qualifier

0   Medical and Surgical
0   Central Nervous System and Cranial Nerves
S   Reposition   Definition: Moving to its normal location, or other suitable location, all or a portion of a body part

Explanation: The body part is moved to a new location from an abnormal location, or from a normal location where it is not functioning correctly. The body part may or may not be cut out or off to be moved to the new location.

Body Part Character 4		Approach Character 5	Device Character 6	Qualifier Character 7

F Olfactory Nerve
First cranial nerve
Olfactory bulb
G Optic Nerve
Optic chiasma
Second cranial nerve
H Oculomotor Nerve
Third cranial nerve
J Trochlear Nerve
Fourth cranial nerve
K Trigeminal Nerve
Fifth cranial nerve
Gasserian ganglion
Mandibular nerve
Maxillary nerve
Ophthalmic nerve
Trifacial nerve
L Abducens Nerve
Sixth cranial nerve
M Facial Nerve
Chorda tympani
Geniculate ganglion
Greater superficial petrosal
  nerve
Nerve to the stapedius
Parotid plexus
Posterior auricular nerve
Seventh cranial nerve
Submandibular ganglion
	N Acoustic Nerve
	Cochlear nerve
	Eighth cranial nerve
	Scarpa's (vestibular)
	  ganglion
	Spiral ganglion
	Vestibular (Scarpa's)
	  ganglion
	Vestibular nerve
	Vestibulocochlear nerve
	P Glossopharyngeal Nerve
	Carotid sinus nerve
	Ninth cranial nerve
	Tympanic nerve
	Q Vagus Nerve
	Anterior vagal trunk
	Pharyngeal plexus
	Pneumogastric nerve
	Posterior vagal trunk
	Pulmonary plexus
	Recurrent laryngeal nerve
	Superior laryngeal nerve
	Tenth cranial nerve
	R Accessory Nerve
	Eleventh cranial nerve
	S Hypoglossal Nerve
	Twelfth cranial nerve
	W Cervical Spinal Cord
	Dorsal root ganglion
	X Thoracic Spinal Cord
	Dorsal root ganglion
	Y Lumbar Spinal Cord
	Cauda equina
	Conus medullaris
	Dorsal root ganglion
		0 Open
		3 Percutaneous
		4 Percutaneous Endoscopic
			Z No Device	**Z No Qualifier**

0   Medical and Surgical
0   Central Nervous System and Cranial Nerves
T   Resection   Definition: Cutting out or off, without replacement, all of a body part

Explanation: None

Body Part Character 4	Approach Character 5	Device Character 6	Qualifier Character 7
7 Cerebral Hemisphere Frontal lobe Occipital lobe Parietal lobe Temporal lobe	**0 Open** **3 Percutaneous** **4 Percutaneous Endoscopic**	**Z No Device**	**Z No Qualifier**

Non-OR Procedure   DRG Non-OR Procedure   Valid OR Procedure   HAC Associated Procedure   Combination Only   New/Revised April   New/Revised October

148   ICD-10-PCS 2024

Ø   **Medical and Surgical**
Ø   **Central Nervous System and Cranial Nerves**
U   **Supplement**   Definition: Putting in or on biological or synthetic material that physically reinforces and/or augments the function of a portion of a body part
                    Explanation: The biological material is non-living, or is living and from the same individual. The body part may have been previously replaced, and the SUPPLEMENT procedure is performed to physically reinforce and/or augment the function of the replaced body part.

Body Part Character 4		Approach Character 5	Device Character 6	Qualifier Character 7

1 **Cerebral Meninges**
  Arachnoid mater,
    intracranial
  Leptomeninges,
    intracranial
  Pia mater, intracranial
2 **Dura Mater**
  Diaphragma sellae
  Dura mater, intracranial
  Falx cerebri
  Tentorium cerebelli
6 **Cerebral Ventricle**
  Aqueduct of Sylvius
  Cerebral aqueduct
    (Sylvius)
  Choroid plexus
  Ependyma
  Foramen of Monro
    (intraventricular)
  Fourth ventricle
  Interventricular foramen
    (Monro)
  Left lateral ventricle
  Right lateral ventricle
  Third ventricle
F **Olfactory Nerve**
  First cranial nerve
  Olfactory bulb
G **Optic Nerve**
  Optic chiasma
  Second cranial nerve
H **Oculomotor Nerve**
  Third cranial nerve
J **Trochlear Nerve**
  Fourth cranial nerve
K **Trigeminal Nerve**
  Fifth cranial nerve
  Gasserian ganglion
  Mandibular nerve
  Maxillary nerve
  Ophthalmic nerve
  Trifacial nerve
L **Abducens Nerve**
  Sixth cranial nerve
	M **Facial Nerve**
	  Chorda tympani
	  Geniculate ganglion
	  Greater superficial petrosal
	    nerve
	  Nerve to the stapedius
	  Parotid plexus
	  Posterior auricular nerve
	  Seventh cranial nerve
	  Submandibular ganglion
	N **Acoustic Nerve**
	  Cochlear nerve
	  Eighth cranial nerve
	  Scarpa's (vestibular)
	    ganglion
	  Spiral ganglion
	  Vestibular (Scarpa's)
	    ganglion
	  Vestibular nerve
	  Vestibulocochlear nerve
	P **Glossopharyngeal Nerve**
	  Carotid sinus nerve
	  Ninth cranial nerve
	  Tympanic nerve
	Q **Vagus Nerve**
	  Anterior vagal trunk
	  Pharyngeal plexus
	  Pneumogastric nerve
	  Posterior vagal trunk
	  Pulmonary plexus
	  Recurrent laryngeal nerve
	  Superior laryngeal nerve
	  Tenth cranial nerve
	R **Accessory Nerve**
	  Eleventh cranial nerve
	S **Hypoglossal Nerve**
	  Twelfth cranial nerve
	T **Spinal Meninges**
	  Arachnoid mater, spinal
	  Denticulate (dentate)
	    ligament
	  Dura mater, spinal
	  Filum terminale
	  Leptomeninges, spinal
	  Pia mater, spinal
		Ø **Open**
		3 **Percutaneous**
		4 **Percutaneous Endoscopic**
			7 **Autologous Tissue**
			  Substitute
			J **Synthetic Substitute**
			K **Nonautologous Tissue**
			  Substitute
				Z **No Qualifier**

Central Nervous System and Cranial Nerves

Ø   **Medical and Surgical**
Ø   **Central Nervous System and Cranial Nerves**
W   **Revision**   Definition: Correcting, to the extent possible, a portion of a malfunctioning device or the position of a displaced device

Explanation: Revision can include correcting a malfunctioning or displaced device by taking out or putting in components of the device such as a screw or pin

Body Part Character 4	Approach Character 5	Device Character 6	Qualifier Character 7
Ø **Brain** Cerebrum Corpus callosum Encephalon V **Spinal Cord** Dorsal root ganglion	Ø Open 3 Percutaneous 4 Percutaneous Endoscopic	Ø Drainage Device 2 Monitoring Device 3 Infusion Device 7 Autologous Tissue Substitute J Synthetic Substitute K Nonautologous Tissue Substitute M Neurostimulator Lead Y Other Device	Z No Qualifier
Ø **Brain** Cerebrum Corpus callosum Encephalon V **Spinal Cord** Dorsal root ganglion	X External	Ø Drainage Device 2 Monitoring Device 3 Infusion Device 7 Autologous Tissue Substitute J Synthetic Substitute K Nonautologous Tissue Substitute M Neurostimulator Lead	Z No Qualifier
6 **Cerebral Ventricle** Aqueduct of Sylvius Cerebral aqueduct (Sylvius) Choroid plexus Ependyma Foramen of Monro (intraventricular) Fourth ventricle Interventricular foramen (Monro) Left lateral ventricle Right lateral ventricle Third ventricle U **Spinal Canal** Epidural space, spinal Extradural space, spinal Subarachnoid space, spinal Subdural space, spinal Vertebral canal	Ø Open 3 Percutaneous 4 Percutaneous Endoscopic	Ø Drainage Device 2 Monitoring Device 3 Infusion Device J Synthetic Substitute M Neurostimulator Lead Y Other Device	Z No Qualifier
6 **Cerebral Ventricle** Aqueduct of Sylvius Cerebral aqueduct (Sylvius) Choroid plexus Ependyma Foramen of Monro (intraventricular) Fourth ventricle Interventricular foramen (Monro) Left lateral ventricle Right lateral ventricle Third ventricle U **Spinal Canal** Epidural space, spinal Extradural space, spinal Subarachnoid space, spinal Subdural space, spinal Vertebral canal	X External	Ø Drainage Device 2 Monitoring Device 3 Infusion Device J Synthetic Substitute M Neurostimulator Lead	Z No Qualifier
E **Cranial Nerve**	Ø Open 3 Percutaneous 4 Percutaneous Endoscopic	Ø Drainage Device 2 Monitoring Device 3 Infusion Device 7 Autologous Tissue Substitute M Neurostimulator Lead Y Other Device	Z No Qualifier
E **Cranial Nerve**	X External	Ø Drainage Device 2 Monitoring Device 3 Infusion Device 7 Autologous Tissue Substitute M Neurostimulator Lead	Z No Qualifier

Non-OR   00W[Ø,V][3,4]YZ
Non-OR   00W[Ø,V]X[Ø,2,3,7,J,K,M]Z
Non-OR   00W[6,U][3,4]YZ
Non-OR   00W[6,U]X[Ø,2,3,J,M]Z
Non-OR   00WE[3,4]YZ
Non-OR   00WEX[Ø,2,3,7,M]Z

Non-OR Procedure   DRG Non-OR Procedure   Valid OR Procedure   HAC Associated Procedure   Combination Only   New/Revised April   New/Revised October

Ø   Medical and Surgical
Ø   Central Nervous System and Cranial Nerves
X   Transfer   Definition: Moving, without taking out, all or a portion of a body part to another location to take over the function of all or a portion of a body part

Explanation: The body part transferred remains connected to its vascular and nervous supply

Body Part Character 4	Approach Character 5	Device Character 6	Qualifier Character 7

F   Olfactory Nerve
    First cranial nerve
    Olfactory bulb
G   Optic Nerve
    Optic chiasma
    Second cranial nerve
H   Oculomotor Nerve
    Third cranial nerve
J   Trochlear Nerve
    Fourth cranial nerve
K   Trigeminal Nerve
    Fifth cranial nerve
    Gasserian ganglion
    Mandibular nerve
    Maxillary nerve
    Ophthalmic nerve
    Trifacial nerve
L   Abducens Nerve
    Sixth cranial nerve
M   Facial Nerve
    Chorda tympani
    Geniculate ganglion
    Greater superficial petrosal nerve
    Nerve to the stapedius
    Parotid plexus
    Posterior auricular nerve
    Seventh cranial nerve
    Submandibular ganglion
N   Acoustic Nerve
    Cochlear nerve
    Eighth cranial nerve
    Scarpa's (vestibular) ganglion
    Spiral ganglion
    Vestibular (Scarpa's) ganglion
    Vestibular nerve
    Vestibulocochlear nerve
P   Glossopharyngeal Nerve
    Carotid sinus nerve
    Ninth cranial nerve
    Tympanic nerve
Q   Vagus Nerve
    Anterior vagal trunk
    Pharyngeal plexus
    Pneumogastric nerve
    Posterior vagal trunk
    Pulmonary plexus
    Recurrent laryngeal nerve
    Superior laryngeal nerve
    Tenth cranial nerve
R   Accessory Nerve
    Eleventh cranial nerve
S   Hypoglossal Nerve
    Twelfth cranial nerve
	Ø Open
	4 Percutaneous Endoscopic
		Z No Device	**F Olfactory Nerve**
			G Optic Nerve
			H Oculomotor Nerve
			J Trochlear Nerve
			K Trigeminal Nerve
			L Abducens Nerve
			M Facial Nerve
			N Acoustic Nerve
			P Glossopharyngeal Nerve
			Q Vagus Nerve
			R Accessory Nerve
			S Hypoglossal Nerve

NC Noncovered Procedure   **LC** Limited Coverage   **QA** Questionable OB Admit   **NT** New Tech Add-on   ⊞ Combination Member   ♂ Male   ♀ Female

Peripheral Nervous System Ø12–Ø1X

Character Meanings

This Character Meaning table is provided as a guide to assist the user in the identification of character members that may be found in this section of code tables. It **SHOULD NOT** be used to build a PCS code.

Operation–Character 3	Body Part–Character 4	Approach–Character 5	Device–Character 6	Qualifier–Character 7
2 Change	Ø Cervical Plexus	Ø Open	Ø Drainage Device	1 Cervical Nerve
5 Destruction	1 Cervical Nerve	3 Percutaneous	1 Radioactive Element	2 Phrenic Nerve
8 Division	2 Phrenic Nerve	4 Percutaneous Endoscopic	2 Monitoring Device	4 Ulnar Nerve
9 Drainage	3 Brachial Plexus	X External	7 Autologous Tissue Substitute	5 Median Nerve
B Excision	4 Ulnar Nerve		J Synthetic Substitute	6 Radial Nerve
C Extirpation	5 Median Nerve		K Nonautologous Tissue Substitute	8 Thoracic Nerve
D Extraction	6 Radial Nerve		M Neurostimulator Lead	B Lumbar Nerve
H Insertion	8 Thoracic Nerve		Y Other Device	C Perineal Nerve
J Inspection	9 Lumbar Plexus		Z No Device	D Femoral Nerve
N Release	A Lumbosacral Plexus			F Sciatic Nerve
P Removal	B Lumbar Nerve			G Tibial Nerve
Q Repair	C Pudendal Nerve			H Peroneal Nerve
R Replacement	D Femoral Nerve			X Diagnostic
S Reposition	F Sciatic Nerve			Z No Qualifier
U Supplement	G Tibial Nerve			
W Revision	H Peroneal Nerve			
X Transfer	K Head and Neck Sympathetic Nerve			
	L Thoracic Sympathetic Nerve			
	M Abdominal Sympathetic Nerve			
	N Lumbar Sympathetic Nerve			
	P Sacral Sympathetic Nerve			
	Q Sacral Plexus			
	R Sacral Nerve			
	Y Peripheral Nerve			

AHA Coding Clinic for table Ø1B
2018, 2Q, 22   Excision of synovial cyst
2017, 2Q, 19   Thoracic outlet decompression with sympathectomy

AHA Coding Clinic for table Ø1H
2020, 4Q, 43-44   Insertion of radioactive element

AHA Coding Clinic for table Ø1N
2019, 1Q, 28   Decompressive laminectomy of both spinal cord and nerve roots
2018, 2Q, 22   Excision of synovial cyst
2017, 2Q, 19   Thoracic outlet decompression with sympathectomy
2016, 2Q, 16   Decompressive laminectomy/foraminotomy and lumbar discectomy
2016, 2Q, 17   Removal of longitudinal ligament to decompress cervical nerve root
2016, 2Q, 23   Thoracic outlet syndrome and release of brachial plexus
2015, 2Q, 34   Decompressive laminectomy
2014, 3Q, 33   Radial fracture treatment with open reduction internal fixation, and release of carpal ligament

AHA Coding Clinic for table Ø1Q
2019, 3Q, 32   Breast reconstruction with neurotization

AHA Coding Clinic for table Ø1S
2021, 3Q, 19   Elbow amputation and targeted muscle reinnervation

AHA Coding Clinic for table Ø1U
2019, 3Q, 32   Breast reconstruction with neurotization
2017, 4Q, 62   Added and revised device values - Nerve substitutes

Median and Ulnar Nerves

Peripheral Nervous System

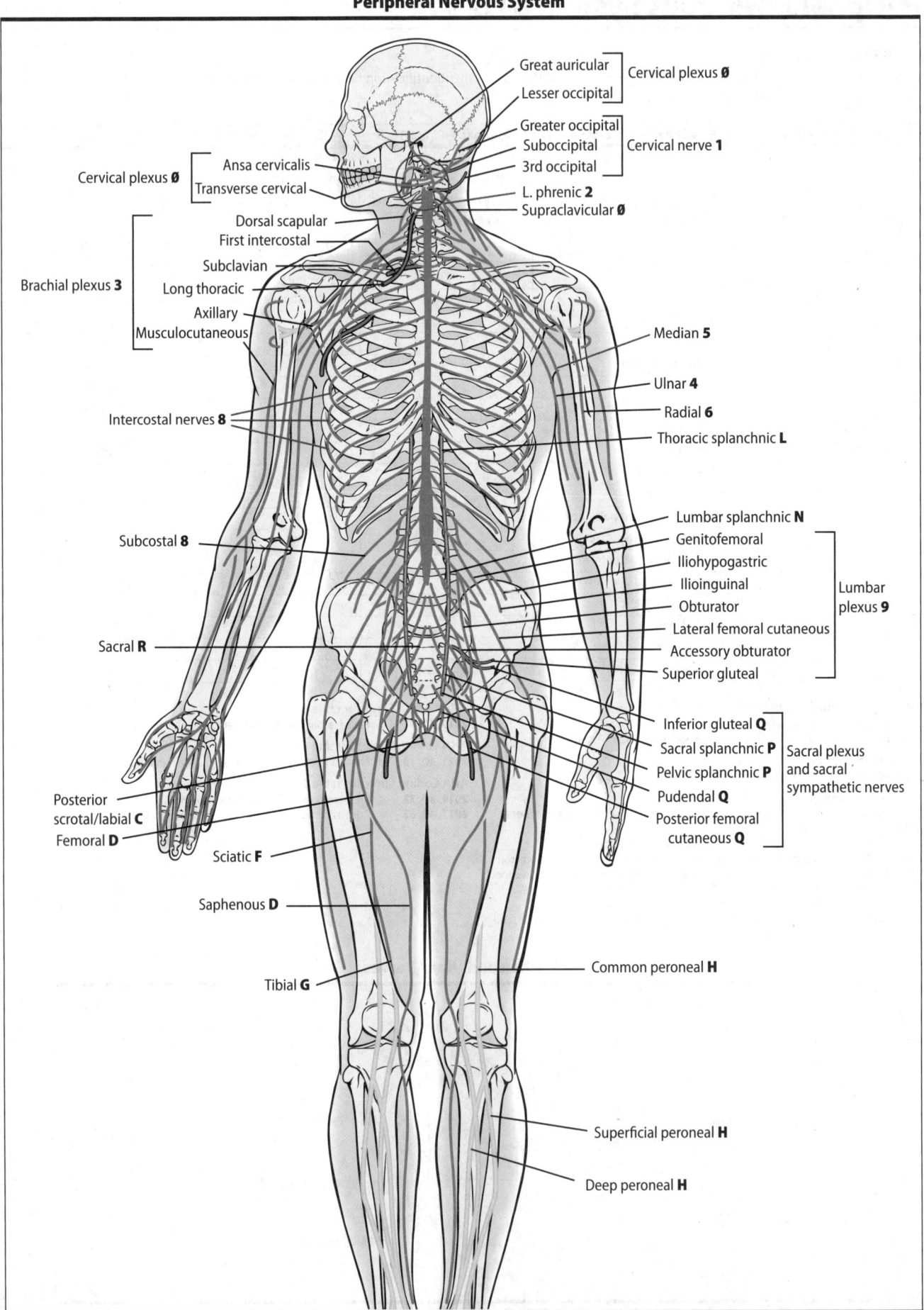

Cervical plexus Ø
- Great auricular
- Lesser occipital

Cervical nerve 1
- Greater occipital
- Suboccipital
- 3rd occipital

L. phrenic 2

Supraclavicular Ø

Cervical plexus Ø
- Ansa cervicalis
- Transverse cervical

Brachial plexus 3
- Dorsal scapular
- First intercostal
- Subclavian
- Long thoracic
- Axillary
- Musculocutaneous

Median 5

Ulnar 4

Radial 6

Thoracic splanchnic L

Intercostal nerves 8

Subcostal 8

Sacral R

Lumbar plexus 9
- Lumbar splanchnic N
- Genitofemoral
- Iliohypogastric
- Ilioinguinal
- Obturator
- Lateral femoral cutaneous
- Accessory obturator
- Superior gluteal

Sacral plexus and sacral sympathetic nerves
- Inferior gluteal Q
- Sacral splanchnic P
- Pelvic splanchnic P
- Pudendal Q
- Posterior femoral cutaneous Q

Posterior scrotal/labial C

Femoral D

Sciatic F

Saphenous D

Tibial G

Common peroneal H

Superficial peroneal H

Deep peroneal H

Ø   **Medical and Surgical**
1   **Peripheral Nervous System**
2   **Change**   Definition: Taking out or off a device from a body part and putting back an identical or similar device in or on the same body part without cutting or puncturing the skin or a mucous membrane
Explanation: All CHANGE procedures are coded using the approach EXTERNAL

Body Part Character 4	Approach Character 5	Device Character 6	Qualifier Character 7
Y Peripheral Nerve	X External	Ø Drainage Device Y Other Device	Z No Qualifier

Non-OR   All body part, approach, device, and qualifier values

Ø   **Medical and Surgical**
1   **Peripheral Nervous System**
5   **Destruction**   Definition: Physical eradication of all or a portion of a body part by the direct use of energy, force, or a destructive agent
Explanation: None of the body part is physically taken out

Body Part Character 4		Approach Character 5	Device Character 6	Qualifier Character 7

Ø Cervical Plexus
  Ansa cervicalis
  Cutaneous (transverse) cervical nerve
  Great auricular nerve
  Lesser occipital nerve
  Supraclavicular nerve
  Transverse (cutaneous) cervical nerve
1 Cervical Nerve
  Greater occipital nerve
  Spinal nerve, cervical
  Suboccipital nerve
  Third occipital nerve
2 Phrenic Nerve
  Accessory phrenic nerve
3 Brachial Plexus
  Axillary nerve
  Dorsal scapular nerve
  First intercostal nerve
  Long thoracic nerve
  Musculocutaneous nerve
  Subclavius nerve
  Suprascapular nerve
4 Ulnar Nerve
  Cubital nerve
5 Median Nerve
  Anterior interosseous nerve
  Palmar cutaneous nerve
6 Radial Nerve
  Dorsal digital nerve
  Musculospiral nerve
  Palmar cutaneous nerve
  Posterior interosseous nerve
8 Thoracic Nerve
  Intercostal nerve
  Intercostobrachial nerve
  Spinal nerve, thoracic
  Subcostal nerve
9 Lumbar Plexus
  Accessory obturator nerve
  Genitofemoral nerve
  Iliohypogastric nerve
  Ilioinguinal nerve
  Lateral femoral cutaneous nerve
  Obturator nerve
  Superior gluteal nerve
A Lumbosacral Plexus
B Lumbar Nerve
  Lumbosacral trunk
  Spinal nerve, lumbar
  Superior clunic (cluneal) nerve
C Pudendal Nerve
  Posterior labial nerve
  Posterior scrotal nerve
D Femoral Nerve
  Anterior crural nerve
  Saphenous nerve
F Sciatic Nerve
  Ischiatic nerve
G Tibial Nerve
  Lateral plantar nerve
  Medial plantar nerve
  Medial popliteal nerve
  Medial sural cutaneous nerve
	H Peroneal Nerve
	  Common fibular nerve
	  Common peroneal nerve
	  External popliteal nerve
	  Lateral sural cutaneous nerve
	K Head and Neck Sympathetic Nerve
	  Cavernous plexus
	  Cervical ganglion
	  Ciliary ganglion
	  Internal carotid plexus
	  Otic ganglion
	  Pterygopalatine (sphenopalatine) ganglion
	  Sphenopalatine (pterygopalatine) ganglion
	  Stellate ganglion
	  Submandibular ganglion
	  Submaxillary ganglion
	L Thoracic Sympathetic Nerve
	  Cardiac plexus
	  Esophageal plexus
	  Greater splanchnic nerve
	  Inferior cardiac nerve
	  Least splanchnic nerve
	  Lesser splanchnic nerve
	  Middle cardiac nerve
	  Pulmonary plexus
	  Superior cardiac nerve
	  Thoracic aortic plexus
	  Thoracic ganglion
	M Abdominal Sympathetic Nerve
	  Abdominal aortic plexus
	  Auerbach's (myenteric) plexus
	  Celiac (solar) plexus
	  Celiac ganglion
	  Gastric plexus
	  Hepatic plexus
	  Inferior hypogastric plexus
	  Inferior mesenteric ganglion
	  Inferior mesenteric plexus
	  Meissner's (submucous) plexus
	  Myenteric (Auerbach's) plexus
	  Pancreatic plexus
	  Pelvic splanchnic nerve
	  Renal nerve
	  Renal plexus
	  Solar (celiac) plexus
	  Splenic plexus
	  Submucous (Meissner's) plexus
	  Superior hypogastric plexus
	  Superior mesenteric ganglion
	  Superior mesenteric plexus
	  Suprarenal plexus
	N Lumbar Sympathetic Nerve
	  Lumbar ganglion
	  Lumbar splanchnic nerve
	P Sacral Sympathetic Nerve
	  Ganglion impar (ganglion of Walther)
	  Pelvic splanchnic nerve
	  Sacral ganglion
	  Sacral splanchnic nerve
	Q Sacral Plexus
	  Inferior gluteal nerve
	  Posterior femoral cutaneous nerve
	  Pudendal nerve
	R Sacral Nerve
	  Spinal nerve, sacral
		Ø Open
		3 Percutaneous
		4 Percutaneous Endoscopic
			Z No Device	Z No Qualifier

Non-OR   Ø15[Ø,2,3,4,5,6,9,A,C,D,F,G,H,Q][Ø,3,4]ZZ   **Non-OR**   Ø15[1,8,B,R]3ZZ

🅝🅒 Noncovered Procedure   🅛🅒 Limited Coverage   🆀🅐 Questionable OB Admit   🅝🅣 New Tech Add-on   ⊞ Combination Member   ♂Male   ♀Female

ICD-10-PCS 2024   155

Peripheral Nervous System

Ø	**Medical and Surgical**
1	**Peripheral Nervous System**
8	**Division**

Definition: Cutting into a body part, without draining fluids and/or gases from the body part, in order to separate or transect a body part

Explanation: All or a portion of the body part is separated into two or more portions

Body Part Character 4		Approach Character 5	Device Character 6	Qualifier Character 7

Ø Cervical Plexus
Ansa cervicalis
Cutaneous (transverse) cervical
nerve
Great auricular nerve
Lesser occipital nerve
Supraclavicular nerve
Transverse (cutaneous) cervical
nervef
1 Cervical Nerve
Greater occipital nerve
Spinal nerve, cervical
Suboccipital nerve
Third occipital nerve
2 Phrenic Nerve
Accessory phrenic nerve
3 Brachial Plexus
Axillary nerve
Dorsal scapular nerve
First intercostal nerve
Long thoracic nerve
Musculocutaneous nerve
Subclavius nerve
Suprascapular nerve
4 Ulnar Nerve
Cubital nerve
5 Median Nerve
Anterior interosseous nerve
Palmar cutaneous nerve
6 Radial Nerve
Dorsal digital nerve
Musculospiral nerve
Palmar cutaneous nerve
Posterior interosseous nerve
8 Thoracic Nerve
Intercostal nerve
Intercostobrachial nerve
Spinal nerve, thoracic
Subcostal nerve
9 Lumbar Plexus
Accessory obturator nerve
Genitofemoral nerve
Iliohypogastric nerve
Ilioinguinal nerve
Lateral femoral cutaneous
nerve
Obturator nerve
Superior gluteal nerve
A Lumbosacral Plexus
B Lumbar Nerve
Lumbosacral trunk
Spinal nerve, lumbar
Superior clunic (cluneal) nerve
C Pudendal Nerve
Posterior labial nerve
Posterior scrotal nerve
D Femoral Nerve
Anterior crural nerve
Saphenous nerve
F Sciatic Nerve
Ischiatic nerve
G Tibial Nerve
Lateral plantar nerve
Medial plantar nerve
Medial popliteal nerve
Medial sural cutaneous nerve
	H Peroneal Nerve
	Common fibular nerve
	Common peroneal nerve
	External popliteal nerve
	Lateral sural cutaneous nerve
	**K Head and Neck Sympathetic
	Nerve**
	Cavernous plexus
	Cervical ganglion
	Ciliary ganglion
	Internal carotid plexus
	Otic ganglion
	Pterygopalatine
	  (sphenopalatine) ganglion
	Sphenopalatine
	  (pterygopalatine) ganglion
	Stellate ganglion
	Submandibular ganglion
	Submaxillary ganglion
	L Thoracic Sympathetic Nerve
	Cardiac plexus
	Esophageal plexus
	Greater splanchnic nerve
	Inferior cardiac nerve
	Least splanchnic nerve
	Lesser splanchnic nerve
	Middle cardiac nerve
	Pulmonary plexus
	Superior cardiac nerve
	Thoracic aortic plexus
	Thoracic ganglion
	**M Abdominal Sympathetic
	Nerve**
	Abdominal aortic plexus
	Auerbach's (myenteric) plexus
	Celiac (solar) plexus
	Celiac ganglion
	Gastric plexus
	Hepatic plexus
	Inferior hypogastric plexus
	Inferior mesenteric ganglion
	Inferior mesenteric plexus
	Meissner's (submucous) plexus
	Myenteric (Auerbach's) plexus
	Pancreatic plexus
	Pelvic splanchnic nerve
	Renal nerve
	Renal plexus
	Solar (celiac) plexus
	Splenic plexus
	Submucous (Meissner's) plexus
	Superior hypogastric plexus
	Superior mesenteric ganglion
	Superior mesenteric plexus
	Suprarenal plexus
	N Lumbar Sympathetic Nerve
	Lumbar ganglion
	Lumbar splanchnic nerve
	P Sacral Sympathetic Nerve
	Ganglion impar (ganglion of
	  Walther)
	Pelvic splanchnic nerve
	Sacral ganglion
	Sacral splanchnic nerve
	Q Sacral Plexus
	Inferior gluteal nerve
	Posterior femoral cutaneous
	  nerve
	Pudendal nerve
	R Sacral Nerve
	Spinal nerve, sacral
		Ø Open
		3 Percutaneous
		4 Percutaneous Endoscopic
			Z No Device	**Z No Qualifier**

Non-OR Procedure   DRG Non-OR Procedure   Valid OR Procedure   HAC Associated Procedure   Combination Only   New/Revised April   New/Revised October

156   ICD-10-PCS 2024

Ø   **Medical and Surgical**
1   **Peripheral Nervous System**
9   **Drainage**   Definition: Taking or letting out fluids and/or gases from a body part
                       Explanation: The qualifier DIAGNOSTIC is used to identify drainage procedures that are biopsies

Body Part Character 4		Approach Character 5	Device Character 6	Qualifier Character 7

Ø   Cervical Plexus
    Ansa cervicalis
    Cutaneous (transverse) cervical
      nerve
    Great auricular nerve
    Lesser occipital nerve
    Supraclavicular nerve
    Transverse (cutaneous) cervical
      nerve
1   Cervical Nerve
    Greater occipital nerve
    Spinal nerve, cervical
    Suboccipital nerve
    Third occipital nerve
2   Phrenic Nerve
    Accessory phrenic nerve
3   Brachial Plexus
    Axillary nerve
    Dorsal scapular nerve
    First intercostal nerve
    Long thoracic nerve
    Musculocutaneous nerve
    Subclavius nerve
    Suprascapular nerve
4   Ulnar Nerve
    Cubital nerve
5   Median Nerve
    Anterior interosseous nerve
    Palmar cutaneous nerve
6   Radial Nerve
    Dorsal digital nerve
    Musculospiral nerve
    Palmar cutaneous nerve
    Posterior interosseous nerve
8   Thoracic Nerve
    Intercostal nerve
    Intercostobrachial nerve
    Spinal nerve, thoracic
    Subcostal nerve
9   Lumbar Plexus
    Accessory obturator nerve
    Genitofemoral nerve
    Iliohypogastric nerve
    Ilioinguinal nerve
    Lateral femoral cutaneous
      nerve
    Obturator nerve
    Superior gluteal nerve
A   Lumbosacral Plexus
B   Lumbar Nerve
    Lumbosacral trunk
    Spinal nerve, lumbar
    Superior clunic (cluneal) nerve
C   Pudendal Nerve
    Posterior labial nerve
    Posterior scrotal nerve
D   Femoral Nerve
    Anterior crural nerve
    Saphenous nerve
F   Sciatic Nerve
    Ischiatic nerve
G   Tibial Nerve
    Lateral plantar nerve
    Medial plantar nerve
    Medial popliteal nerve
    Medial sural cutaneous nerve
	H Peroneal Nerve
	    Common fibular nerve
	    Common peroneal nerve
	    External popliteal nerve
	    Lateral sural cutaneous nerve
	K Head and Neck Sympathetic
	    Nerve
	    Cavernous plexus
	    Cervical ganglion
	    Ciliary ganglion
	    Internal carotid plexus
	    Otic ganglion
	    Pterygopalatine
	      (sphenopalatine) ganglion
	    Sphenopalatine
	      (pterygopalatine) ganglion
	    Stellate ganglion
	    Submandibular ganglion
	    Submaxillary ganglion
	L Thoracic Sympathetic Nerve
	    Cardiac plexus
	    Esophageal plexus
	    Greater splanchnic nerve
	    Inferior cardiac nerve
	    Least splanchnic nerve
	    Lesser splanchnic nerve
	    Middle cardiac nerve
	    Pulmonary plexus
	    Superior cardiac nerve
	    Thoracic aortic plexus
	    Thoracic ganglion
	M Abdominal Sympathetic
	    Nerve
	    Abdominal aortic plexus
	    Auerbach's (myenteric) plexus
	    Celiac (solar) plexus
	    Celiac ganglion
	    Gastric plexus
	    Hepatic plexus
	    Inferior hypogastric plexus
	    Inferior mesenteric ganglion
	    Inferior mesenteric plexus
	    Meissner's (submucous) plexus
	    Myenteric (Auerbach's) plexus
	    Pancreatic plexus
	    Pelvic splanchnic nerve
	    Renal nerve
	    Renal plexus
	    Solar (celiac) plexus
	    Splenic plexus
	    Submucous (Meissner's) plexus
	    Superior hypogastric plexus
	    Superior mesenteric ganglion
	    Superior mesenteric plexus
	    Suprarenal plexus
	N Lumbar Sympathetic Nerve
	    Lumbar ganglion
	    Lumbar splanchnic nerve
	P Sacral Sympathetic Nerve
	    Ganglion impar (ganglion of
	      Walther)
	    Pelvic splanchnic nerve
	    Sacral ganglion
	    Sacral splanchnic nerve
	Q Sacral Plexus
	    Inferior gluteal nerve
	    Posterior femoral cutaneous
	      nerve
	    Pudendal nerve
	R Sacral Nerve
	    Spinal nerve, sacral
		Ø Open
		3 Percutaneous
		4 Percutaneous Endoscopic
			Ø Drainage Device	**Z** No Qualifier

Non-OR   Ø19[Ø,1,2,3,4,5,6,8,9,A,B,C,D,F,G,H,K,L,M,N,P,Q,R]3ØZ

Ø19 Continued on next page

Peripheral Nervous System

Ø   **Medical and Surgical**
1   **Peripheral Nervous System**
9   **Drainage**   Definition: Taking or letting out fluids and/or gases from a body part

Ø19 Continued

Explanation: The qualifier DIAGNOSTIC is used to identify drainage procedures that are biopsies

Body Part Character 4		Approach Character 5	Device Character 6	Qualifier Character 7

Ø **Cervical Plexus**
Ansa cervicalis
Cutaneous (transverse) cervical
   nerve
Great auricular nerve
Lesser occipital nerve
Supraclavicular nerve
Transverse (cutaneous) cervical
   nerve
1 **Cervical Nerve**
Greater occipital nerve
Spinal nerve, cervical
Suboccipital nerve
Third occipital nerve
2 **Phrenic Nerve**
Accessory phrenic nerve
3 **Brachial Plexus**
Axillary nerve
Dorsal scapular nerve
First intercostal nerve
Long thoracic nerve
Musculocutaneous nerve
Subclavius nerve
Suprascapular nerve
4 **Ulnar Nerve**
Cubital nerve
5 **Median Nerve**
Anterior interosseous nerve
Palmar cutaneous nerve
6 **Radial Nerve**
Dorsal digital nerve
Musculospiral nerve
Palmar cutaneous nerve
Posterior interosseous nerve
8 **Thoracic Nerve**
Intercostal nerve
Intercostobrachial nerve
Spinal nerve, thoracic
Subcostal nerve
9 **Lumbar Plexus**
Accessory obturator nerve
Genitofemoral nerve
Iliohypogastric nerve
Ilioinguinal nerve
Lateral femoral cutaneous
   nerve
Obturator nerve
Superior gluteal nerve
A **Lumbosacral Plexus**
B **Lumbar Nerve**
Lumbosacral trunk
Spinal nerve, lumbar
Superior clunic (cluneal) nerve
C **Pudendal Nerve**
Posterior labial nerve
Posterior scrotal nerve
D **Femoral Nerve**
Anterior crural nerve
Saphenous nerve
F **Sciatic Nerve**
Ischiatic nerve
G **Tibial Nerve**
Lateral plantar nerve
Medial plantar nerve
Medial popliteal nerve
Medial sural cutaneous nerve
	H **Peroneal Nerve**
	Common fibular nerve
	Common peroneal nerve
	External popliteal nerve
	Lateral sural cutaneous nerve
	K **Head and Neck Sympathetic**
	Nerve
	Cavernous plexus
	Cervical ganglion
	Ciliary ganglion
	Internal carotid plexus
	Otic ganglion
	Pterygopalatine
	   (sphenopalatine) ganglion
	Sphenopalatine
	   (pterygopalatine) ganglion
	Stellate ganglion
	Submandibular ganglion
	Submaxillary ganglion
	L **Thoracic Sympathetic Nerve**
	Cardiac plexus
	Esophageal plexus
	Greater splanchnic nerve
	Inferior cardiac nerve
	Least splanchnic nerve
	Lesser splanchnic nerve
	Middle cardiac nerve
	Pulmonary plexus
	Superior cardiac nerve
	Thoracic aortic plexus
	Thoracic ganglion
	M **Abdominal Sympathetic**
	Nerve
	Abdominal aortic plexus
	Auerbach's (myenteric) plexus
	Celiac (solar) plexus
	Celiac ganglion
	Gastric plexus
	Hepatic plexus
	Inferior hypogastric plexus
	Inferior mesenteric ganglion
	Inferior mesenteric plexus
	Meissner's (submucous) plexus
	Myenteric (Auerbach's) plexus
	Pancreatic plexus
	Pelvic splanchnic nerve
	Renal nerve
	Renal plexus
	Solar (celiac) plexus
	Splenic plexus
	Submucous (Meissner's) plexus
	Superior hypogastric plexus
	Superior mesenteric ganglion
	Superior mesenteric plexus
	Suprarenal plexus
	N **Lumbar Sympathetic Nerve**
	Lumbar ganglion
	Lumbar splanchnic nerve
	P **Sacral Sympathetic Nerve**
	Ganglion impar (ganglion of
	   Walther)
	Pelvic splanchnic nerve
	Sacral ganglion
	Sacral splanchnic nerve
	Q **Sacral Plexus**
	Inferior gluteal nerve
	Posterior femoral cutaneous
	   nerve
	Pudendal nerve
	R **Sacral Nerve**
	Spinal nerve, sacral
		Ø Open
		3 Percutaneous
		4 Percutaneous Endoscopic
			Z No Device	**X** Diagnostic
				Z No Qualifier

Non-OR   Ø19[Ø,1,2,3,4,5,6,8,9,A,B,C,D,F,G,H,Q,R][3,4]ZX
Non-OR   Ø19[Ø,1,2,3,4,5,6,8,9,A,B,C,D,F,G,H,K,L,M,N,P,Q,R]3ZZ

Ø   Medical and Surgical
1   Peripheral Nervous System
B   Excision   Definition: Cutting out or off, without replacement, a portion of a body part
                         Explanation: The qualifier DIAGNOSTIC is used to identify excision procedures that are biopsies

Body Part Character 4		Approach Character 5	Device Character 6	Qualifier Character 7

Ø Cervical Plexus
Ansa cervicalis
Cutaneous (transverse) cervical
   nerve
Great auricular nerve
Lesser occipital nerve
Supraclavicular nerve
Transverse (cutaneous) cervical
   nerve
1 Cervical Nerve
Greater occipital nerve
Spinal nerve, cervical
Suboccipital nerve
Third occipital nerve
2 Phrenic Nerve
Accessory phrenic nerve
3 Brachial Plexus
Axillary nerve
Dorsal scapular nerve
First intercostal nerve
Long thoracic nerve
Musculocutaneous nerve
Subclavius nerve
Suprascapular nerve
4 Ulnar Nerve
Cubital nerve
5 Median Nerve
Anterior interosseous nerve
Palmar cutaneous nerve
6 Radial Nerve
Dorsal digital nerve
Musculospiral nerve
Palmar cutaneous nerve
Posterior interosseous nerve
8 Thoracic Nerve
Intercostal nerve
Intercostobrachial nerve
Spinal nerve, thoracic
Subcostal nerve
9 Lumbar Plexus
Accessory obturator nerve
Genitofemoral nerve
Iliohypogastric nerve
Ilioinguinal nerve
Lateral femoral cutaneous
   nerve
Obturator nerve
Superior gluteal nerve
A Lumbosacral Plexus
B Lumbar Nerve
Lumbosacral trunk
Spinal nerve, lumbar
Superior clunic (cluneal) nerve
C Pudendal Nerve
Posterior labial nerve
Posterior scrotal nerve
D Femoral Nerve
Anterior crural nerve
Saphenous nerve
F Sciatic Nerve
Ischiatic nerve
G Tibial Nerve
Lateral plantar nerve
Medial plantar nerve
Medial popliteal nerve
Medial sural cutaneous nerve
	H Peroneal Nerve
	Common fibular nerve
	Common peroneal nerve
	External popliteal nerve
	Lateral sural cutaneous nerve
	**K Head and Neck Sympathetic
	    Nerve**
	Cavernous plexus
	Cervical ganglion
	Ciliary ganglion
	Internal carotid plexus
	Otic ganglion
	Pterygopalatine
	   (sphenopalatine) ganglion
	Sphenopalatine
	   (pterygopalatine) ganglion
	Stellate ganglion
	Submandibular ganglion
	Submaxillary ganglion
	**L Thoracic Sympathetic
	    Nerve**
	Cardiac plexus
	Esophageal plexus
	Greater splanchnic nerve
	Inferior cardiac nerve
	Least splanchnic nerve
	Lesser splanchnic nerve
	Middle cardiac nerve
	Pulmonary plexus
	Superior cardiac nerve
	Thoracic aortic plexus
	Thoracic ganglion
	**M Abdominal Sympathetic
	    Nerve**
	Abdominal aortic plexus
	Auerbach's (myenteric) plexus
	Celiac (solar) plexus
	Celiac ganglion
	Gastric plexus
	Hepatic plexus
	Inferior hypogastric plexus
	Inferior mesenteric ganglion
	Inferior mesenteric plexus
	Meissner's (submucous) plexus
	Myenteric (Auerbach's) plexus
	Pancreatic plexus
	Pelvic splanchnic nerve
	Renal nerve
	Renal plexus
	Solar (celiac) plexus
	Splenic plexus
	Submucous (Meissner's) plexus
	Superior hypogastric plexus
	Superior mesenteric ganglion
	Superior mesenteric plexus
	Suprarenal plexus
	N Lumbar Sympathetic Nerve
	Lumbar ganglion
	Lumbar splanchnic nerve
	P Sacral Sympathetic Nerve
	Ganglion impar (ganglion of
	   Walther)
	Pelvic splanchnic nerve
	Sacral ganglion
	Sacral splanchnic nerve
	Q Sacral Plexus
	Inferior gluteal nerve
	Posterior femoral cutaneous
	   nerve
	Pudendal nerve
	R Sacral Nerve
	Spinal nerve, sacral
		Ø Open
		3 Percutaneous
		4 Percutaneous Endoscopic
			Z No Device	**X** Diagnostic
				Z No Qualifier

Non-OR   Ø1B[Ø,1,2,3,4,5,6,8,9,A,B,C,D,F,G,H,Q,R][3,4]ZX

NC Noncovered Procedure   **LC** Limited Coverage   **QA** Questionable OB Admit   **NT** New Tech Add-on   ⊞ Combination Member   ♂ Male   ♀ Female

ICD-10-PCS 2024   **159**

Ø1B–Ø1B

Peripheral Nervous System (side tab)

Ø   **Medical and Surgical**
1   **Peripheral Nervous System**
C   **Extirpation**   Definition: Taking or cutting out solid matter from a body part

Explanation: The solid matter may be an abnormal byproduct of a biological function or a foreign body; it may be imbedded in a body part or in the lumen of a tubular body part. The solid matter may or may not have been previously broken into pieces.

Body Part Character 4		Approach Character 5	Device Character 6	Qualifier Character 7

Ø Cervical Plexus
Ansa cervicalis
Cutaneous (transverse) cervical
  nerve
Great auricular nerve
Lesser occipital nerve
Supraclavicular nerve
Transverse (cutaneous) cervical
  nerve
1 Cervical Nerve
Greater occipital nerve
Spinal nerve, cervical
Suboccipital nerve
Third occipital nerve
2 Phrenic Nerve
Accessory phrenic nerve
3 Brachial Plexus
Axillary nerve
Dorsal scapular nerve
First intercostal nerve
Long thoracic nerve
Musculocutaneous nerve
Subclavius nerve
Suprascapular nerve
4 Ulnar Nerve
Cubital nerve
5 Median Nerve
Anterior interosseous nerve
Palmar cutaneous nerve
6 Radial Nerve
Dorsal digital nerve
Musculospiral nerve
Palmar cutaneous nerve
Posterior interosseous nerve
8 Thoracic Nerve
Intercostal nerve
Intercostobrachial nerve
Spinal nerve, thoracic
Subcostal nerve
9 Lumbar Plexus
Accessory obturator nerve
Genitofemoral nerve
Iliohypogastric nerve
Ilioinguinal nerve
Lateral femoral cutaneous
  nerve
Obturator nerve
Superior gluteal nerve
A Lumbosacral Plexus
B Lumbar Nerve
Lumbosacral trunk
Spinal nerve, lumbar
Superior clunic (cluneal) nerve
C Pudendal Nerve
Posterior labial nerve
Posterior scrotal nerve
D Femoral Nerve
Anterior crural nerve
Saphenous nerve
F Sciatic Nerve
Ischiatic nerve
G Tibial Nerve
Lateral plantar nerve
Medial plantar nerve
Medial popliteal nerve
Medial sural cutaneous nerve
	H Peroneal Nerve
	Common fibular nerve
	Common peroneal nerve
	External popliteal nerve
	Lateral sural cutaneous nerve
	K Head and Neck Sympathetic
	Nerve
	Cavernous plexus
	Cervical ganglion
	Ciliary ganglion
	Internal carotid plexus
	Otic ganglion
	Pterygopalatine
	  (sphenopalatine) ganglion
	Sphenopalatine
	  (pterygopalatine) ganglion
	Stellate ganglion
	Submandibular ganglion
	Submaxillary ganglion
	L Thoracic Sympathetic Nerve
	Cardiac plexus
	Esophageal plexus
	Greater splanchnic nerve
	Inferior cardiac nerve
	Least splanchnic nerve
	Lesser splanchnic nerve
	Middle cardiac nerve
	Pulmonary plexus
	Superior cardiac nerve
	Thoracic aortic plexus
	Thoracic ganglion
	M Abdominal Sympathetic
	Nerve
	Abdominal aortic plexus
	Auerbach's (myenteric) plexus
	Celiac (solar) plexus
	Celiac ganglion
	Gastric plexus
	Hepatic plexus
	Inferior hypogastric plexus
	Inferior mesenteric ganglion
	Inferior mesenteric plexus
	Meissner's (submucous) plexus
	Myenteric (Auerbach's) plexus
	Pancreatic plexus
	Pelvic splanchnic nerve
	Renal nerve
	Renal plexus
	Solar (celiac) plexus
	Splenic plexus
	Submucous (Meissner's) plexus
	Superior hypogastric plexus
	Superior mesenteric ganglion
	Superior mesenteric plexus
	Suprarenal plexus
	N Lumbar Sympathetic Nerve
	Lumbar ganglion
	Lumbar splanchnic nerve
	P Sacral Sympathetic Nerve
	Ganglion impar (ganglion of
	  Walther)
	Pelvic splanchnic nerve
	Sacral ganglion
	Sacral splanchnic nerve
	Q Sacral Plexus
	Inferior gluteal nerve
	Posterior femoral cutaneous
	  nerve
	Pudendal nerve
	R Sacral Nerve
	Spinal nerve, sacral
		Ø Open
		3 Percutaneous
		4 Percutaneous Endoscopic
			Z No Device	**Z No Qualifier**

Non-OR Procedure   DRG Non-OR Procedure   Valid OR Procedure   HAC Associated Procedure   Combination Only   New/Revised April   New/Revised October

0   **Medical and Surgical**
1   **Peripheral Nervous System**
D   **Extraction**   Definition: Pulling or stripping out or off all or a portion of a body part by the use of force
                    Explanation: The qualifier DIAGNOSTIC is used to identify extraction procedures that are biopsies

Body Part Character 4		Approach Character 5	Device Character 6	Qualifier Character 7
0 Cervical Plexus Ansa cervicalis Cutaneous (transverse) cervical nerve Great auricular nerve Lesser occipital nerve Supraclavicular nerve Transverse (cutaneous) cervical nerve **1 Cervical Nerve** Greater occipital nerve Spinal nerve, cervical Suboccipital nerve Third occipital nerve **2 Phrenic Nerve** Accessory phrenic nerve **3 Brachial Plexus** Axillary nerve Dorsal scapular nerve First intercostal nerve Long thoracic nerve Musculocutaneous nerve Subclavius nerve Suprascapular nerve **4 Ulnar Nerve** Cubital nerve **5 Median Nerve** Anterior interosseous nerve Palmar cutaneous nerve **6 Radial Nerve** Dorsal digital nerve Musculospiral nerve Palmar cutaneous nerve Posterior interosseous nerve **8 Thoracic Nerve** Intercostal nerve Intercostobrachial nerve Spinal nerve, thoracic Subcostal nerve **9 Lumbar Plexus** Accessory obturator nerve Genitofemoral nerve Iliohypogastric nerve Ilioinguinal nerve Lateral femoral cutaneous nerve Obturator nerve Superior gluteal nerve **A Lumbosacral Plexus** **B Lumbar Nerve** Lumbosacral trunk Spinal nerve, lumbar Superior clunic (cluneal) nerve **C Pudendal Nerve]** Posterior labial nerve Posterior scrotal nerve **D Femoral Nerve** Anterior crural nerve Saphenous nerve **F Sciatic Nerve** Ischiatic nerve **G Tibial Nerve** Lateral plantar nerve Medial plantar nerve Medial popliteal nerve Medial sural cutaneous nerve	**H Peroneal Nerve** Common fibular nerve Common peroneal nerve External popliteal nerve Lateral sural cutaneous nerve **K Head and Neck Sympathetic Nerve** Cavernous plexus Cervical ganglion Ciliary ganglion Internal carotid plexus Otic ganglion Pterygopalatine (sphenopalatine) ganglion Sphenopalatine (pterygopalatine) ganglion Stellate ganglion Submandibular ganglion Submaxillary ganglion **L Thoracic Sympathetic Nerve** Cardiac plexus Esophageal plexus Greater splanchnic nerve Inferior cardiac nerve Least splanchnic nerve Lesser splanchnic nerve Middle cardiac nerve Pulmonary plexus Superior cardiac nerve Thoracic aortic plexus Thoracic ganglion **M Abdominal Sympathetic Nerve** Abdominal aortic plexus Auerbach's (myenteric) plexus Celiac (solar) plexus Celiac ganglion Gastric plexus Hepatic plexus Inferior hypogastric plexus Inferior mesenteric ganglion Inferior mesenteric plexus Meissner's (submucous) plexus Myenteric (Auerbach's) plexus Pancreatic plexus Pelvic splanchnic nerve Renal nerve Renal plexus Solar (celiac) plexus Splenic plexus Submucous (Meissner's) plexus Superior hypogastric plexus Superior mesenteric ganglion Superior mesenteric plexus Suprarenal plexus **N Lumbar Sympathetic Nerve** Lumbar ganglion Lumbar splanchnic nerve **P Sacral Sympathetic Nerve** Ganglion impar (ganglion of Walther) Pelvic splanchnic nerve Sacral ganglion Sacral splanchnic nerve **Q Sacral Plexus** Inferior gluteal nerve Posterior femoral cutaneous nerve Pudendal nerve **R Sacral Nerve** Spinal nerve, sacral	**0 Open** **3 Percutaneous** **4 Percutaneous Endoscopic**	**Z No Device**	**Z No Qualifier**

NC Noncovered Procedure   **LC** Limited Coverage   **QA** Questionable OB Admit   **NT** New Tech Add-on   ⊞ Combination Member   ♂ Male   ♀ Female

ICD-10-PCS 2024   161

Peripheral Nervous System (side margin)

Ø   Medical and Surgical
1   Peripheral Nervous System
H   Insertion   Definition: Putting in a nonbiological appliance that monitors, assists, performs, or prevents a physiological function but does not physically take the place of a body part

Explanation: None

Body Part Character 4		Approach Character 5	Device Character 6	Qualifier Character 7
Y Peripheral Nerve ⊞		Ø Open 3 Percutaneous 4 Percutaneous Endoscopic	1 Radioactive Element 2 Monitoring Device M Neurostimulator Lead Y Other Device	Z No Qualifier

Non-OR   Ø1HY31Z
Non-OR   Ø1HY[3,4]YZ

See Appendix L for Procedure Combinations
⊞   Ø1HY[Ø,3,4]MZ

Ø   Medical and Surgical
1   Peripheral Nervous System
J   Inspection   Definition: Visually and/or manually exploring a body part

Explanation: Visual exploration may be performed with or without optical instrumentation. Manual exploration may be performed directly or through intervening body layers.

Body Part Character 4		Approach Character 5	Device Character 6	Qualifier Character 7
Y Peripheral Nerve		Ø Open 3 Percutaneous 4 Percutaneous Endoscopic	Z No Device	Z No Qualifier

Non-OR   Ø1JY3ZZ

Non-OR Procedure   DRG Non-OR Procedure   Valid OR Procedure   HAC Associated Procedure   Combination Only   New/Revised April   New/Revised October

Ø   Medical and Surgical
1   Peripheral Nervous System
N   Release   Definition: Freeing a body part from an abnormal physical constraint by cutting or by the use of force
                       Explanation: Some of the restraining tissue may be taken out but none of the body part is taken out

Body Part Character 4	Approach Character 5	Device Character 6	Qualifier Character 7
Ø Cervical Plexus Ansa cervicalis Cutaneous (transverse) cervical nerve Great auricular nerve Lesser occipital nerve Supraclavicular nerve Transverse (cutaneous) cervical nerve **1 Cervical Nerve** Greater occipital nerve Spinal nerve, cervical Suboccipital nerve Third occipital nerve **2 Phrenic Nerve** Accessory phrenic nerve **3 Brachial Plexus** Axillary nerve Dorsal scapular nerve First intercostal nerve Long thoracic nerve Musculocutaneous nerve Subclavius nerve Suprascapular nerve **4 Ulnar Nerve** Cubital nerve **5 Median Nerve** Anterior interosseous nerve Palmar cutaneous nerve **6 Radial Nerve** Dorsal digital nerve Musculospiral nerve Palmar cutaneous nerve Posterior interosseous nerve **8 Thoracic Nerve** Intercostal nerve Intercostobrachial nerve Spinal nerve, thoracic Subcostal nerve **9 Lumbar Plexus** Accessory obturator nerve Genitofemoral nerve Iliohypogastric nerve Ilioinguinal nerve Lateral femoral cutaneous nerve Obturator nerve Superior gluteal nerve **A Lumbosacral Plexus** **B Lumbar Nerve** Lumbosacral trunk Spinal nerve, lumbar Superior clunic (cluneal) nerve **C Pudendal Nerve** Posterior labial nerve Posterior scrotal nerve **D Femoral Nerve** Anterior crural nerve Saphenous nerve **F Sciatic Nerve** Ischiatic nerve **G Tibial Nerve** Lateral plantar nerve Medial plantar nerve Medial popliteal nerve Medial sural cutaneous nerve			
H Peroneal Nerve Common fibular nerve Common peroneal nerve External popliteal nerve Lateral sural cutaneous nerve **K Head and Neck Sympathetic Nerve** Cavernous plexus Cervical ganglion Ciliary ganglion Internal carotid plexus Otic ganglion Pterygopalatine (sphenopalatine) ganglion Sphenopalatine (pterygopalatine) ganglion Stellate ganglion Submandibular ganglion Submaxillary ganglion **L Thoracic Sympathetic Nerve** Cardiac plexus Esophageal plexus Greater splanchnic nerve Inferior cardiac nerve Least splanchnic nerve Lesser splanchnic nerve Middle cardiac nerve Pulmonary plexus Superior cardiac nerve Thoracic aortic plexus Thoracic ganglion **M Abdominal Sympathetic Nerve** Abdominal aortic plexus Auerbach's (myenteric) plexus Celiac (solar) plexus Celiac ganglion Gastric plexus Hepatic plexus Inferior hypogastric plexus Inferior mesenteric ganglion Inferior mesenteric plexus Meissner's (submucous) plexus Myenteric (Auerbach's) plexus Pancreatic plexus Pelvic splanchnic nerve Renal nerve Renal plexus Solar (celiac) plexus Splenic plexus Submucous (Meissner's) plexus Superior hypogastric plexus Superior mesenteric ganglion Superior mesenteric plexus Suprarenal plexus **N Lumbar Sympathetic Nerve** Lumbar ganglion Lumbar splanchnic nerve **P Sacral Sympathetic Nerve** Ganglion impar (ganglion of Walther) Pelvic splanchnic nerve Sacral ganglion Sacral splanchnic nerve **Q Sacral Plexus** Inferior gluteal nerve Posterior femoral cutaneous nerve Pudendal nerve **R Sacral Nerve** Spinal nerve, sacral	**Ø** Open **3** Percutaneous **4** Percutaneous Endoscopic	**Z** No Device	**Z** No Qualifier

NC Noncovered Procedure   **LC** Limited Coverage   **QA** Questionable OB Admit   **NT** New Tech Add-on   ⊞ Combination Member   ♂ Male   ♀ Female

ICD-10-PCS 2024   163

Ø   **Medical and Surgical**
1   **Peripheral Nervous System**
P   **Removal**   Definition: Taking out or off a device from a body part

                     Explanation: If a device is taken out and a similar device put in without cutting or puncturing the skin or mucous membrane, the procedure is coded to the root operation CHANGE. Otherwise, the procedure for taking out a device is coded to the root operation REMOVAL.

Body Part Character 4	Approach Character 5	Device Character 6	Qualifier Character 7
Y Peripheral Nerve	**Ø** Open **3** Percutaneous **4** Percutaneous Endoscopic	**Ø** Drainage Device **2** Monitoring Device **7** Autologous Tissue Substitute **M** Neurostimulator Lead **Y** Other Device	**Z** No Qualifier
Y Peripheral Nerve	**X** External	**Ø** Drainage Device **2** Monitoring Device **M** Neurostimulator Lead	**Z** No Qualifier

Non-OR   Ø1PY3[Ø,2]Z
Non-OR   Ø1PY[3,4]YZ
Non-OR   Ø1PYX[Ø,2,M]Z

Ø   Medical and Surgical
1   Peripheral Nervous System
Q   Repair   Definition: Restoring, to the extent possible, a body part to its normal anatomic structure and function
                 Explanation: Used only when the method to accomplish the repair is not one of the other root operations

Body Part Character 4		Approach Character 5	Device Character 6	Qualifier Character 7
Ø Cervical Plexus Ansa cervicalis Cutaneous (transverse) cervical nerve Great auricular nerve Lesser occipital nerve Supraclavicular nerve Transverse (cutaneous) cervical nerve **1 Cervical Nerve** Greater occipital nerve Spinal nerve, cervical Suboccipital nerve Third occipital nerve **2 Phrenic Nerve** Accessory phrenic nerve **3 Brachial Plexus** Axillary nerve Dorsal scapular nerve First intercostal nerve Long thoracic nerve Musculocutaneous nerve Subclavius nerve Suprascapular nerve **4 Ulnar Nerve** Cubital nerve **5 Median Nerve** Anterior interosseous nerve Palmar cutaneous nerve **6 Radial Nerve** Dorsal digital nerve Musculospiral nerve Palmar cutaneous nerve Posterior interosseous nerve **8 Thoracic Nerve** Intercostal nerve Intercostobrachial nerve Spinal nerve, thoracic Subcostal nerve **9 Lumbar Plexus** Accessory obturator nerve Genitofemoral nerve Iliohypogastric nerve Ilioinguinal nerve Lateral femoral cutaneous nerve Obturator nerve Superior gluteal nerve **A Lumbosacral Plexus** **B Lumbar Nerve** Lumbosacral trunk Spinal nerve, lumbar Superior clunic (cluneal) nerve **C Pudendal Nerve** Posterior labial nerve Posterior scrotal nerve **D Femoral Nerve** Anterior crural nerve Saphenous nerve **F Sciatic Nerve** Ischiatic nerve **G Tibial Nerve** Lateral plantar nerve Medial plantar nerve Medial popliteal nerve Medial sural cutaneous nerve	**H Peroneal Nerve** Common fibular nerve Common peroneal nerve External popliteal nerve Lateral sural cutaneous nerve **K Head and Neck Sympathetic Nerve** Cavernous plexus Cervical ganglion Ciliary ganglion Internal carotid plexus Otic ganglion Pterygopalatine (sphenopalatine) ganglion Sphenopalatine (pterygopalatine) ganglion Stellate ganglion Submandibular ganglion Submaxillary ganglion **L Thoracic Sympathetic Nerve** Cardiac plexus Esophageal plexus Greater splanchnic nerve Inferior cardiac nerve Least splanchnic nerve Lesser splanchnic nerve Middle cardiac nerve Pulmonary plexus Superior cardiac nerve Thoracic aortic plexus Thoracic ganglion **M Abdominal Sympathetic Nerve** Abdominal aortic plexus Auerbach's (myenteric) plexus Celiac (solar) plexus Celiac ganglion Gastric plexus Hepatic plexus Inferior hypogastric plexus Inferior mesenteric ganglion Inferior mesenteric plexus Meissner's (submucous) plexus Myenteric (Auerbach's) plexus Pancreatic plexus Pelvic splanchnic nerve Renal nerve Renal plexus Solar (celiac) plexus Splenic plexus Submucous (Meissner's) plexus Superior hypogastric plexus Superior mesenteric ganglion Superior mesenteric plexus Suprarenal plexus **N Lumbar Sympathetic Nerve** Lumbar ganglion Lumbar splanchnic nerve **P Sacral Sympathetic Nerve** Ganglion impar (ganglion of Walther) Pelvic splanchnic nerve Sacral ganglion Sacral splanchnic nerve **Q Sacral Plexus** Inferior gluteal nerve Posterior femoral cutaneous nerve Pudendal nerve **R Sacral Nerve** Spinal nerve, sacral	**Ø** Open **3** Percutaneous **4** Percutaneous Endoscopic	**Z** No Device	**Z** No Qualifier

NC Noncovered Procedure   **LC** Limited Coverage   **QA** Questionable OB Admit   **NT** New Tech Add-on   ⊞ Combination Member   ♂ Male   ♀ Female

ICD-10-PCS 2024   165

Peripheral Nervous System *(side tab)*

Ø   Medical and Surgical
1   Peripheral Nervous System
R   Replacement   Definition: Putting in or on biological or synthetic material that physically takes the place and/or function of all or a portion of a body part

Explanation: The body part may have been taken out or replaced, or may be taken out, physically eradicated, or rendered nonfunctional during the REPLACEMENT procedure. A REMOVAL procedure is coded for taking out the device used in a previous replacement procedure.

Body Part Character 4	Approach Character 5	Device Character 6	Qualifier Character 7
1 Cervical Nerve Greater occipital nerve Spinal nerve, cervical Suboccipital nerve Third occipital nerve **2 Phrenic Nerve** Accessory phrenic nerve **4 Ulnar Nerve** Cubital nerve **5 Median Nerve** Anterior interosseous nerve Palmar cutaneous nerve **6 Radial Nerve** Dorsal digital nerve Musculospiral nerve Palmar cutaneous nerve Posterior interosseous nerve **8 Thoracic Nerve** Intercostal nerve Intercostobrachial nerve Spinal nerve, thoracic Subcostal nerve **B Lumbar Nerve** Lumbosacral trunk Spinal nerve, lumbar Superior clunic (cluneal) nerve **C Pudendal Nerve** Posterior labial nerve Posterior scrotal nerve **D Femoral Nerve** Anterior crural nerve Saphenous nerve **F Sciatic Nerve** Ischiatic nerve **G Tibial Nerve** Lateral plantar nerve Medial plantar nerve Medial popliteal nerve Medial sural cutaneous nerve **H Peroneal Nerve** Common fibular nerve Common peroneal nerve External popliteal nerve Lateral sural cutaneous nerve **R Sacral Nerve** Spinal nerve, sacral	**Ø Open** **4 Percutaneous Endoscopic**	**7 Autologous Tissue Substitute** **J Synthetic Substitute** **K Nonautologous Tissue Substitute**	**Z No Qualifier**

Ø Medical and Surgical
1 Peripheral Nervous System
S Reposition   Definition: Moving to its normal location, or other suitable location, all or a portion of a body part

Explanation: The body part is moved to a new location from an abnormal location, or from a normal location where it is not functioning correctly. The body part may or may not be cut out or off to be moved to the new location.

Body Part Character 4	Approach Character 5	Device Character 6	Qualifier Character 7
Ø Cervical Plexus Ansa cervicalis Cutaneous (transverse) cervical nerve Great auricular nerve Lesser occipital nerve Supraclavicular nerve Transverse (cutaneous) cervical nerve **1 Cervical Nerve** Greater occipital nerve Spinal nerve, cervical Suboccipital nerve Third occipital nerve **2 Phrenic Nerve** Accessory phrenic nerve **3 Brachial Plexus** Axillary nerve Dorsal scapular nerve First intercostal nerve Long thoracic nerve Musculocutaneous nerve Subclavius nerve Suprascapular nerve **4 Ulnar Nerve** Cubital nerve **5 Median Nerve** Anterior interosseous nerve Palmar cutaneous nerve **6 Radial Nerve** Dorsal digital nerve Musculospiral nerve Palmar cutaneous nerve Posterior interosseous nerve **8 Thoracic Nerve** Intercostal nerve Intercostobrachial nerve Spinal nerve, thoracic Subcostal nerve **9 Lumbar Plexus** Accessory obturator nerve Genitofemoral nerve Iliohypogastric nerve Ilioinguinal nerve Lateral femoral cutaneous nerve Obturator nerve Superior gluteal nerve **A Lumbosacral Plexus** **B Lumbar Nerve** Lumbosacral trunk Spinal nerve, lumbar Superior clunic (cluneal) nerve **C Pudendal Nerve** Posterior labial nerve Posterior scrotal nerve **D Femoral Nerve** Anterior crural nerve Saphenous nerve **F Sciatic Nerve** Ischiatic nerve **G Tibial Nerve** Lateral plantar nerve Medial plantar nerve Medial popliteal nerve Medial sural cutaneous nerve **H Peroneal Nerve** Common fibular nerve Common peroneal nerve External popliteal nerve Lateral sural cutaneous nerve **Q Sacral Plexus** Inferior gluteal nerve Posterior femoral cutaneous nerve Pudendal nerve **R Sacral Nerve** Spinal nerve, sacral	**Ø Open** **3 Percutaneous** **4 Percutaneous Endoscopic**	**Z No Device**	**Z No Qualifier**

NC Noncovered Procedure   **LC** Limited Coverage   **QA** Questionable OB Admit   **NT** New Tech Add-on   ⊞ Combination Member   ♂ Male   ♀ Female

ICD-10-PCS 2024   167

Peripheral Nervous System (side tab)

0   **Medical and Surgical**
1   **Peripheral Nervous System**
U   **Supplement**   Definition: Putting in or on biological or synthetic material that physically reinforces and/or augments the function of a portion of a body part

Explanation: The biological material is non-living, or is living and from the same individual. The body part may have been previously replaced, and the SUPPLEMENT procedure is performed to physically reinforce and/or augment the function of the replaced body part.

Body Part Character 4	Approach Character 5	Device Character 6	Qualifier Character 7
1 Cervical Nerve Greater occipital nerve Spinal nerve, cervical Suboccipital nerve Third occipital nerve **2 Phrenic Nerve** Accessory phrenic nerve **4 Ulnar Nerve** Cubital nerve **5 Median Nerve** Anterior interosseous nerve Palmar cutaneous nerve **6 Radial Nerve** Dorsal digital nerve Musculospiral nerve Palmar cutaneous nerve Posterior interosseous nerve **8 Thoracic Nerve** Intercostal nerve Intercostobrachial nerve Spinal nerve, thoracic Subcostal nerve **B Lumbar Nerve** Lumbosacral trunk Spinal nerve, lumbar Superior clunic (cluneal) nerve **C Pudendal Nerve** Posterior labial nerve Posterior scrotal nerve **D Femoral Nerve** Anterior crural nerve Saphenous nerve **F Sciatic Nerve** Ischiatic nerve **G Tibial Nerve** Lateral plantar nerve Medial plantar nerve Medial popliteal nerve Medial sural cutaneous nerve **H Peroneal Nerve** Common fibular nerve Common peroneal nerve External popliteal nerve Lateral sural cutaneous nerve **R Sacral Nerve** Spinal nerve, sacral	**0** Open **3** Percutaneous **4** Percutaneous Endoscopic	**7** Autologous Tissue Substitute **J** Synthetic Substitute **K** Nonautologous Tissue Substitute	**Z** No Qualifier

0   **Medical and Surgical**
1   **Peripheral Nervous System**
W   **Revision**   Definition: Correcting, to the extent possible, a portion of a malfunctioning device or the position of a displaced device

Explanation: Revision can include correcting a malfunctioning or displaced device by taking out or putting in components of the device such as a screw or pin

Body Part Character 4	Approach Character 5	Device Character 6	Qualifier Character 7
Y Peripheral Nerve	**0** Open **3** Percutaneous **4** Percutaneous Endoscopic	**0** Drainage Device **2** Monitoring Device **7** Autologous Tissue Substitute **M** Neurostimulator Lead **Y** Other Device	**Z** No Qualifier
Y Peripheral Nerve	**X** External	**0** Drainage Device **2** Monitoring Device **7** Autologous Tissue Substitute **M** Neurostimulator Lead	**Z** No Qualifier

Non-OR   01WY[3,4]YZ
Non-OR   01WYX[0,2,7,M]Z

Non-OR Procedure   DRG Non-OR Procedure   Valid OR Procedure   HAC Associated Procedure   Combination Only   New/Revised April   New/Revised October

168   ICD-10-PCS 2024

01U–01W

Ø Medical and Surgical
1 Peripheral Nervous System
X Transfer   Definition: Moving, without taking out, all or a portion of a body part to another location to take over the function of all or a portion of a body part
Explanation: The body part transferred remains connected to its vascular and nervous supply

Body Part Character 4	Approach Character 5	Device Character 6	Qualifier Character 7
1 Cervical Nerve Greater occipital nerve Spinal nerve, cervical Suboccipital nerve Third occipital nerve **2 Phrenic Nerve** Accessory phrenic nerve	**Ø** Open **4** Percutaneous Endoscopic	**Z** No Device	**1** Cervical Nerve **2** Phrenic Nerve
4 Ulnar Nerve Cubital nerve **5 Median Nerve** Anterior interosseous nerve Palmar cutaneous nerve **6 Radial Nerve** Dorsal digital nerve Musculospiral nerve Palmar cutaneous nerve Posterior interosseous nerve	**Ø** Open **4** Percutaneous Endoscopic	**Z** No Device	**4** Ulnar Nerve **5** Median Nerve **6** Radial Nerve
8 Thoracic Nerve Intercostal nerve Intercostobrachial nerve Spinal nerve, thoracic Subcostal nerve	**Ø** Open **4** Percutaneous Endoscopic	**Z** No Device	**8** Thoracic Nerve
B Lumbar Nerve Lumbosacral trunk Spinal nerve, lumbar Superior clunic (cluneal) nerve **C Pudendal Nerve** Posterior labial nerve Posterior scrotal nerve	**Ø** Open **4** Percutaneous Endoscopic	**Z** No Device	**B** Lumbar Nerve **C** Perineal Nerve
D Femoral Nerve Anterior crural nerve Saphenous nerve **F Sciatic Nerve** Ischiatic nerve **G Tibial Nerve** Lateral plantar nerve Medial plantar nerve Medial popliteal nerve Medial sural cutaneous nerve **H Peroneal Nerve** Common fibular nerve Common peroneal nerve External popliteal nerve Lateral sural cutaneous nerve	**Ø** Open **4** Percutaneous Endoscopic	**Z** No Device	**D** Femoral Nerve **F** Sciatic Nerve **G** Tibial Nerve **H** Peroneal Nerve

Heart and Great Vessels Ø21–Ø2Y

Character Meanings

This Character Meaning table is provided as a guide to assist the user in the identification of character members that may be found in this section of code tables. It **SHOULD NOT** be used to build a PCS code.

Operation–Character 3	Body Part–Character 4	Approach–Character 5	Device–Character 6	Qualifier–Character 7
1 Bypass	Ø Coronary Artery, One Artery	Ø Open	Ø Monitoring Device, Pressure Sensor	Ø Allogeneic OR Ultrasonic
4 Creation	1 Coronary Artery, Two Arteries	3 Percutaneous	2 Monitoring Device	1 Syngeneic
5 Destruction	2 Coronary Artery, Three Arteries	4 Percutaneous Endoscopic	3 Infusion Device	2 Zooplastic OR Common Atrioventricular Valve
7 Dilation	3 Coronary Artery, Four or More Arteries	X External	4 Intraluminal Device, Drug-eluting	3 Coronary Artery
8 Division	4 Coronary Vein		5 Intraluminal Device, Drug-eluting, Two	4 Coronary Vein
B Excision	5 Atrial Septum		6 Intraluminal Device, Drug-eluting, Three	5 Coronary Circulation
C Extirpation	6 Atrium, Right		7 Intraluminal Device, Drug-eluting, Four or More OR Autologous Tissue Substitute	6 Bifurcation OR Atrium, Right
F Fragmentation	7 Atrium, Left		8 Zooplastic Tissue	7 Atrium, Left OR Orbital Atherectomy Technique
H Insertion	8 Conduction Mechanism		9 Autologous Venous Tissue	8 Internal Mammary, Right
J Inspection	9 Chordae Tendineae		A Autologous Arterial Tissue	9 Internal Mammary, Left
K Map	A Heart		C Extraluminal Device	A Innominate Artery
L Occlusion	B Heart, Right		D Intraluminal Device	B Subclavian
N Release	C Heart, Left		E Intraluminal Device, Two OR Intraluminal Device, Branched or Fenestrated, One or Two Arteries	C Thoracic Artery
P Removal	D Papillary Muscle		F Intraluminal Device, Three OR Intraluminal Device, Branched or Fenestrated, Three or More Arteries	D Carotid
Q Repair	F Aortic Valve		G Intraluminal Device, Four or More	E Atrioventricular Valve, Left
R Replacement	G Mitral Valve		J Synthetic Substitute OR Cardiac Lead, Pacemaker	F Abdominal Artery
S Reposition	H Pulmonary Valve		K Nonautologous Tissue Substitute OR Cardiac Lead, Defibrillator	G Atrioventricular Valve, Right OR Axillary Artery
T Resection	J Tricuspid Valve		L Biologic with Synthetic Substitute, Autoregulated Electrohydraulic	H Transapical OR Brachial Artery
U Supplement	K Ventricle, Right		M Cardiac Lead OR Synthetic Substitute, Pneumatic	J Truncal Valve OR Temporary OR Intraoperative
V Restriction	L Ventricle, Left		N Intracardiac Pacemaker	K Left Atrial Appendage
W Revision	M Ventricular Septum		Q Implantable Heart Assist System	L In Existing Conduit
Y Transplantation	N Pericardium		R Short-term External Heart Assist System	M Native Site
	P Pulmonary Trunk		T Intraluminal Device, Radioactive	N Rapid Deployment Technique
	Q Pulmonary Artery, Right		Y Other Device	P Pulmonary Trunk
	R Pulmonary Artery, Left		Z No Device	Q Pulmonary Artery, Right
	S Pulmonary Vein, Right			R Pulmonary Artery, Left
	T Pulmonary Vein, Left			S Pulmonary Vein, Right OR Biventricular
	V Superior Vena Cava			T Pulmonary Vein, Left OR Ductus Arteriosus
	W Thoracic Aorta, Descending			U Pulmonary Vein, Confluence
	X Thoracic Aorta, Ascending/Arch			V Lower Extremity Artery
	Y Great Vessel			W Aorta
				X Diagnostic
				Z No Qualifier

Heart and Great Vessels

AHA Coding Clinic for Heart and Great Vessels

2022, 1Q, 10-13	Procedures performed on a continuous vessel, ICD-10-PCS Guideline B4.1c

AHA Coding Clinic for table 021

2023, 2Q, 22	Norwood procedure with excision of thymus
2022, 1Q, 54	Coronary artery bypass graft surgery
2021, 3Q, 22	Left internal mammary artery free graft between obtuse marginal saphenous vein graft and left anterior descending artery
2020, 4Q, 44-45	Atrium bypass qualifier
2020, 1Q, 24	Pulmonary artery unifocalization
2020, 1Q, 37	Bypass of ascending aorta to brachiocephalic artery
2019, 4Q, 23	Bypass thoracic aorta to innominate artery
2019, 3Q, 30	Aortic aneurysm repair with debranching of common carotid and brachiocephalic arteries
2018, 4Q, 45-46	Descending thoracic aorta bypass
2018, 3Q, 8	Coronary artery bypass graft surgery (revision versus total redo)
2018, 3Q, 26	Coronary artery bypass graft surgery with endarterectomy
2017, 4Q, 56	Added approach values - Percutaneous heart valve procedures
2017, 1Q, 19	Norwood Sano procedure
2016, 4Q, 80-81	Thoracic aorta, ascending/arch and descending
2016, 4Q, 82-83	Coronary artery, number of arteries
2016, 4Q, 102-109	Correction of congenital heart defects
2016, 4Q, 144	Repair of atrial septal defect and anomalous pulmonary venous return
2016, 4Q, 145	Modified Warden procedure for repair of septal defect and right partial anomalous pulmonary venous return
2016, 1Q, 27	Aortocoronary bypass graft utilizing Y-graft
2015, 4Q, 22, 24	Congenital heart corrective procedures
2015, 3Q, 16	Revision of previous truncus arteriosus surgery with ventricle to pulmonary artery conduit
2014, 3Q, 3	Blalock-Taussig shunt procedure
2014, 3Q, 8	Coronary artery bypass graft utilizing internal mammary as pedicle graft
2014, 3Q, 20	MAZE procedure performed with coronary artery bypass graft
2014, 3Q, 29	Fontan completion procedure stage II
2014, 3Q, 30	Creation of conduit from right ventricle to pulmonary artery
2014, 1Q, 10	Repair of thoracic aortic aneurysm & coronary artery bypass graft
2013, 2Q, 37	Coronary artery release performed during coronary artery bypass graft

AHA Coding Clinic for table 024

2016, 4Q, 101	Root operation Creation
2016, 4Q, 102-109	Correction of congenital heart defects

AHA Coding Clinic for table 025

2020, 1Q, 32	Ablation convergent procedure (catheter-based and thoracoscopic ablations)
2018, 3Q, 27	Alcohol septal ablation
2016, 4Q, 80-81	Thoracic aorta, ascending/arch and descending
2016, 3Q, 43-44	Peri-pulmonary catheter ablation
2016, 4Q, 44-45	Maze procedure
2016, 2Q, 17	Photodynamic therapy for treatment of malignant mesothelioma
2014, 4Q, 47	Catheter ablation of peripulmonary veins
2014, 3Q, 19	Ablation of ventricular tachycardia with Impella® support
2014, 3Q, 20	MAZE procedure performed with coronary artery bypass graft
2013, 2Q, 38	Catheter ablation to treat atrial fibrillation

AHA Coding Clinic for table 027

2018, 3Q, 7	Coronary brachytherapy with angioplasty
2018, 3Q, 10	Disruption of perma-catheter fibrin sheath via angioplasty of superior vena cava
2018, 2Q, 24	Coronary artery bifurcation
2017, 4Q, 32-33	Corrective surgery of left ventricular outflow tract obstruction
2016, 4Q, 80-81	Thoracic aorta, ascending/arch and descending
2016, 4Q, 82-83	Coronary artery, number of arteries
2016, 4Q, 84-85	Coronary artery, number of stents
2016, 4Q, 86-88	Coronary and peripheral artery bifurcation
2016, 1Q, 16	Pulmonary valvotomy and dilation of annulus
2015, 4Q, 13	New Section X codes—New Technology procedures
2015, 3Q, 9	Failed attempt to treat coronary artery occlusion
2015, 3Q, 10	Coronary angioplasty with unsuccessful stent insertion
2015, 3Q, 16	Revision of previous truncus arteriosus surgery with ventricle to pulmonary artery conduit
2015, 2Q, 3-5	Coronary artery intervention site
2014, 2Q, 4	Coronary angioplasty of bypassed vessel

AHA Coding Clinic for table 02B

2019, 3Q, 32	Endomyocardial biopsy and right heart catheterization
2019, 2Q, 20	Pericardiectomy for constrictive pericarditis
2017, 1Q, 38	Mitral valve repair and chordae tendineae transfer
2016, 4Q, 80-81	Thoracic aorta, ascending/arch and descending
2015, 2Q, 23	Annuloplasty ring

AHA Coding Clinic for table 02C

2021, 4Q, 41	Coronary orbital atherectomy
2019, 4Q, 25	Coronary artery to root operation Supplement
2018, 3Q, 26	Coronary artery bypass graft surgery with endarterectomy
2018, 2Q, 24	Coronary artery bifurcation
2017, 2Q, 23	Thrombectomy via Fogarty catheter
2016, 4Q, 80-81	Thoracic aorta, ascending and descending
2016, 4Q, 82-83	Coronary artery, number of arteries
2016, 4Q, 86-87	Coronary and peripheral artery bifurcation
2016, 2Q, 24	Repair/decalcification of mitral valve
2016, 2Q, 25	Aortic valve surgery with excision of calcium deposits

AHA Coding Clinic for table 02F

2021, 4Q, 41-42	Coronary intravascular lithotripsy
2020, 4Q, 45-49	New fragmentation tables
2020, 4Q, 49-50	Intravascular ultrasound assisted thrombolysis
2020, 4Q, 50	Intravascular lithotripsy

AHA Coding Clinic for table 02H

2022, 3Q, 19	Placement of stent into aorta to secure debris
2022, 2Q, 25	Temporary-permanent pacemaker placement
2021, 2Q, 23	Clarification of lead placement in bundle of HIS
2019, 4Q, 23-24	Coronary artery Body Part to root operation Insertion
2019, 3Q, 19	Insertion of left ventricular catheter
2019, 3Q, 23	Placement of pacemaker lead in Bundle of HIS
2019, 1Q, 24	Replacement of left ventricular assist device with retention of outflow graft
2018, 4Q, 94	Insertion and removal of failed Watchman™ device
2018, 2Q, 3-5	Intra-aortic balloon pump
2018, 2Q, 19	Pacing lead attached to automatic implantable cardioverter defibrillator
2017, 4Q, 42-45	Insertion of external heart assist devices
2017, 4Q, 63-64	Added and revised device values - Vascular access reservoir
2017, 4Q, 104	Placement of Watchman™ left atrial appendage device
2017, 3Q, 11	Placement of peripherally inserted central catheter using 3CG ECG technology
2017, 2Q, 24	Tunneled catheter versus totally implantable catheter
2017, 2Q, 26	Exchange of tunneled catheter
2017, 1Q, 10-11	External heart assist device
2016, 4Q, 80-81	Thoracic aorta, ascending/arch and descending
2016, 4Q, 95	Intracardiac pacemaker
2016, 4Q, 137-138	Heart assist device systems
2016, 2Q, 15	Removal and replacement of tunneled internal jugular catheter
2015, 4Q, 14	New Section X codes—New Technology procedures
2015, 4Q, 26-31	Vascular access devices
2015, 3Q, 35	Swan Ganz catheterization
2015, 2Q, 31	Leadless pacemaker insertion
2015, 2Q, 33	Totally implantable central venous access device (Port-a-Cath)
2013, 3Q, 18	Placement of peripherally inserted central catheter (PICC)

AHA Coding Clinic for table 02J

2015, 3Q, 9	Failed attempt to treat coronary artery occlusion

AHA Coding Clinic for table 02K

2020, 1Q, 32	Ablation convergent procedure (catheter-based and thoracoscopic ablations)

AHA Coding Clinic for table 02L

2023, 1Q, 9	Temporary balloon occlusion of aorta
2018, 4Q, 94	Insertion and removal of failed Watchman™ device
2017, 4Q, 31	Resuscitative endovascular balloon occlusion of the aorta
2017, 4Q, 33-34	Occlusion/ligation of pulmonary trunk & right pulmonary artery
2016, 4Q, 102-109	Correction of congenital heart defects
2016, 2Q, 26	Embolization of pulmonary arteriovenous fistula
2015, 4Q, 23	Congenital heart corrective procedures
2014, 3Q, 20	MAZE procedure performed with coronary artery bypass graft

AHA Coding Clinic for table 02N

2021, 3Q, 26	Cavoatrial junction tear with repair and relief of cardiac tamponade
2019, 2Q, 13	Unroofing of anomalous coronary artery
2019, 2Q, 20	Pericardiectomy for constrictive pericarditis
2017, 4Q, 35	Release of myocardial bridge
2016, 4Q, 80-81	Thoracic aorta, ascending/arch and descending
2014, 3Q, 16	Repair of Tetralogy of Fallot

AHA Coding Clinic for table 02P

2022, 2Q, 25	Temporary-permanent pacemaker placement
2019, 1Q, 24	Replacement of left ventricular assist device with retention of outflow graft
2018, 4Q, 52-54	Percutaneous extracorporeal membrane oxygenation
2018, 4Q, 85	Externalization of lumboatrial shunt
2018, 4Q, 94	Insertion and removal of failed Watchman™ device
2018, 2Q, 3-5	Intra-aortic balloon pump
2017, 4Q, 42-45	Insertion of external heart assist devices
2017, 4Q, 104	Placement of Watchman™ left atrial appendage device
2017, 3Q, 18	Intra-aortic balloon pump removal
2017, 2Q, 24	Tunneled catheter versus totally implantable catheter
2017, 2Q, 26	Exchange of tunneled catheter
2017, 1Q, 11	External heart assist device
2017, 1Q, 13	SynCardia total artificial heart
2016, 4Q, 95-96	Intracardiac pacemaker
2016, 4Q, 137-139	Heart assist device systems
2016, 3Q, 19	Nonoperative removal of peripherally inserted central catheter

AHA Coding Clinic for table 02P (Continued)

2016, 2Q, 15	Removal and replacement of tunneled internal jugular catheter
2015, 4Q, 31	Vascular access devices
2015, 3Q, 33	Approach values for repositioning and removal of cardiac lead

AHA Coding Clinic for table 02Q

2022, 1Q, 40	Repair of common atrioventricular valve using Alfieri stitch
2022, 1Q, 41	Common atrioventricular valve repair with commissuroplasty sutures
2021, 3Q, 26	Cavoatrial junction tear with repair and relief of cardiac tamponade
2018, 1Q, 12	Percutaneous balloon valvuloplasty & cardiac catheterization with ventriculogram
2017, 1Q, 18	Sutureless repair of pulmonary vein stenosis
2016, 4Q, 80-81	Thoracic aorta, ascending/arch and descending
2016, 4Q, 82-83	Coronary artery, number of arteries
2016, 4Q, 101	Root operation Creation
2016, 4Q, 102-109	Correction of congenital heart defects
2015, 4Q, 23	Congenital heart corrective procedures
2015, 3Q, 16	Vascular ring surgery and double aortic arch
2015, 2Q, 23	Annuloplasty ring
2013, 3Q, 26	Transcatheter replacement of heart valve (TAVR) with measurements

AHA Coding Clinic for table 02R

2022, 4Q, 54-55	Rapid deployment technique for replacement of aortic valve using zooplastic tissue
2021, 4Q, 42-43	Total artificial heart systems
2021, 4Q, 43	Transcatheter replacement of pulmonary valve
2020, 1Q, 25	Elephant trunk repair of aortic dissection
2019, 4Q, 24	Coronary artery Body Part to root operation Insertion
2019, 4Q, 46	Cerebral embolic filtration
2019, 3Q, 23	Replacement of atrioventricular valve
2019, 3Q, 24	Valve sparing aortic root replacement with modified Gleason Vascutek® graft to ascending aorta
2019, 1Q, 31	Transcatheter aortic valve in valve replacement
2018, 3Q, 11	Transcatheter aortic valve replacement via transaortic approach
2018, 1Q, 12	Percutaneous balloon valvuloplasty & cardiac catheterization with ventriculogram
2017, 4Q, 55-56	Added approach values - Percutaneous heart valve procedures
2017, 1Q, 13	SynCardia total artificial heart
2016, 4Q, 80-81	Thoracic aorta, ascending/arch and descending
2016, 3Q, 32	Transcatheter tricuspid valve replacement
2014, 1Q, 10	Repair of thoracic aortic aneurysm & coronary artery bypass graft

AHA Coding Clinic for table 02S

2016, 4Q, 80-81	Thoracic aorta, ascending/arch and descending
2016, 4Q, 82-83	Coronary artery, number of arteries
2016, 4Q, 102-109	Correction of congenital heart defects
2015, 4Q, 23	Congenital heart corrective procedures

AHA Coding Clinic for table 02U

2023, 2Q, 21	Placement of Carillon Mitral Contour System®
2023, 2Q, 22	Norwood procedure with excision of thymus
2022, 1Q, 37	Insertion of amplatzer occluder device into atrium
2022, 1Q, 38	Reconstruction of aorto-mitral curtain using bovine pericardium
2021, 3Q, 28	Repair mitral valve with Pascal® system
2020, 4Q, 52	Transapical mitral valve repair with device
2020, 1Q, 24	Pulmonary artery unifocalization
2019, 4Q, 25	Coronary artery to root operation Supplement
2018, 1Q, 12	Percutaneous balloon valvuloplasty & cardiac catheterization with ventriculogram
2017, 4Q, 36	Alfieri stitch procedure
2017, 3Q, 7	Senning procedure (arterial switch)
2017, 1Q, 19	Norwood Sano procedure
2016, 4Q, 80-81	Thoracic aorta, ascending/arch and descending
2016, 4Q, 101	Root operation Creation
2016, 4Q, 102-109	Correction of congenital heart defects
2016, 2Q, 23	Repair of tetralogy of Fallot with autologous pericardial patch graft
2016, 2Q, 26	Aortic valve replacement with aortic root enlargement
2015, 4Q, 22-24	Congenital heart corrective procedures
2015, 3Q, 16	Revision of previous truncus arteriosus surgery with ventricle to pulmonary artery conduit
2015, 2Q, 23	Annuloplasty ring
2014, 3Q, 16	Repair of tetralogy of Fallot

AHA Coding Clinic for table 02V

2022, 1Q, 40	Repair of common atrioventricular valve using Alfieri stitch
2021, 4Q, 44	Restriction of left ventricle
2020, 1Q, 25	Elephant trunk repair of aortic dissection
2017, 4Q, 35-36	Alfieri stitch procedure
2016, 4Q, 80-81	Thoracic aorta, ascending/arch and descending
2016, 4Q, 89-92	Branched and fenestrated endograft repair of aneurysms

AHA Coding Clinic for table 02W

2019, 1Q, 24	Replacement of left ventricular assist device with retention of outflow graft
2018, 3Q, 8	Coronary artery bypass graft surgery (revision versus total redo)
2018, 3Q, 9	Fibrin sheath stripping of malfunctioning port-a-cath
2018, 1Q, 17	Repositioning of Impella short-term external heart assist device
2017, 4Q, 42-45	Insertion of external heart assist devices
2017, 4Q, 55-56	Added approach values - Percutaneous heart valve procedures
2016, 4Q, 85	Coronary artery, number of stents
2016, 4Q, 95-96	Intracardiac pacemaker
2015, 3Q, 32	Approach values for repositioning and removal of cardiac lead
2014, 3Q, 31	Closure of paravalvular leak using Amplatzer® vascular plug

AHA Coding Clinic for table 02Y

2023, 2Q, 32	Preparation of donor organ before transplantation
2013, 3Q, 18	Heart transplant surgery

Heart and Great Vessels

Coronary Arteries

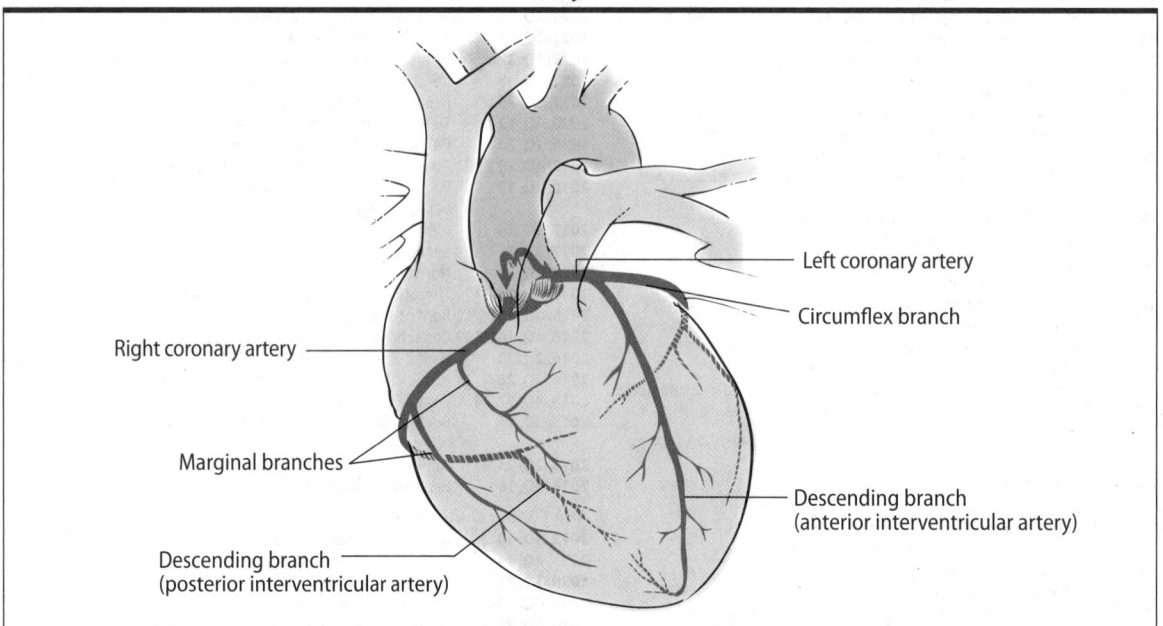

Left coronary artery

Circumflex branch

Right coronary artery

Marginal branches

Descending branch
(anterior interventricular artery)

Descending branch
(posterior interventricular artery)

Heart Anatomy

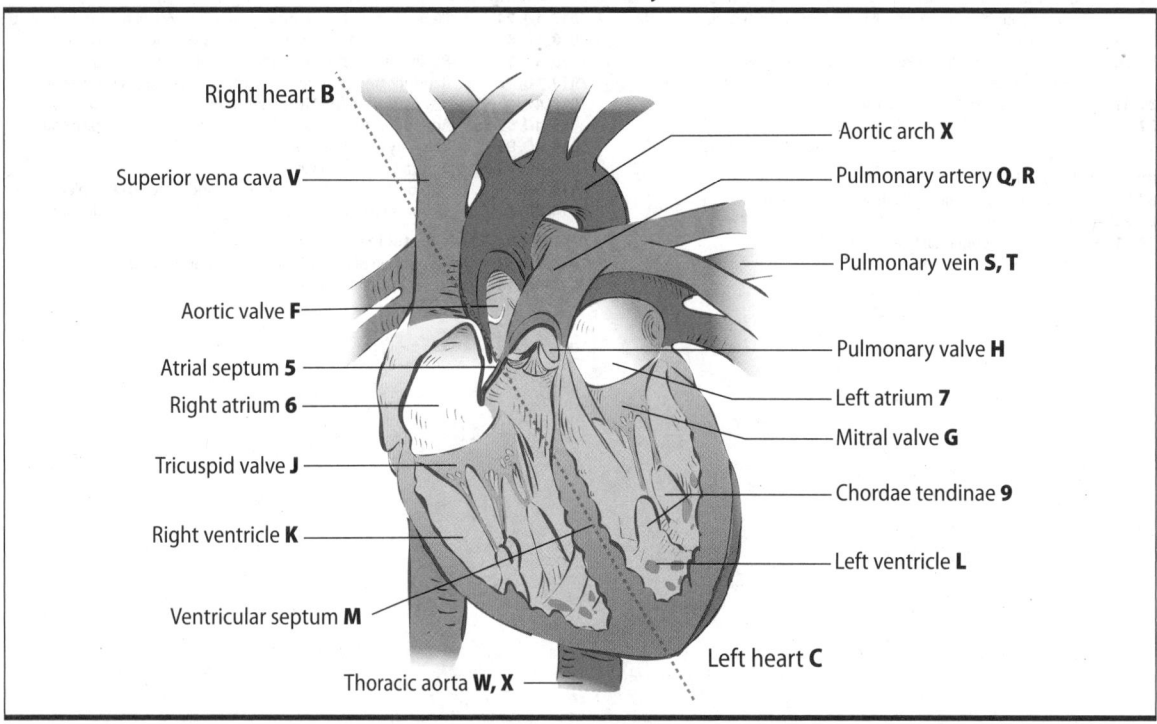

Right heart **B**

Superior vena cava **V**

Aortic valve **F**

Atrial septum **5**

Right atrium **6**

Tricuspid valve **J**

Right ventricle **K**

Ventricular septum **M**

Thoracic aorta **W, X**

Aortic arch **X**

Pulmonary artery **Q, R**

Pulmonary vein **S, T**

Pulmonary valve **H**

Left atrium **7**

Mitral valve **G**

Chordae tendinae **9**

Left ventricle **L**

Left heart **C**

Ø   **Medical and Surgical**
2   **Heart and Great Vessels**
1   **Bypass**   Definition: Altering the route of passage of the contents of a tubular body part

          Explanation: Rerouting contents of a body part to a downstream area of the normal route, to a similar route and body part, or to an abnormal route and dissimilar body part. Includes one or more anastomoses, with or without the use of a device.

Body Part Character 4	Approach Character 5	Device Character 6	Qualifier Character 7
Ø Coronary Artery, One Artery 1 Coronary Artery, Two Arteries 2 Coronary Artery, Three Arteries 3 Coronary Artery, Four or More Arteries	Ø Open	8 Zooplastic Tissue 9 Autologous Venous Tissue A Autologous Arterial Tissue J Synthetic Substitute K Nonautologous Tissue Substitute	3 Coronary Artery 8 Internal Mammary, Right 9 Internal Mammary, Left C Thoracic Artery F Abdominal Artery W Aorta
Ø Coronary Artery, One Artery 1 Coronary Artery, Two Arteries 2 Coronary Artery, Three Arteries 3 Coronary Artery, Four or More Arteries	Ø Open	Z No Device	3 Coronary Artery 8 Internal Mammary, Right 9 Internal Mammary, Left C Thoracic Artery F Abdominal Artery
Ø Coronary Artery, One Artery 1 Coronary Artery, Two Arteries 2 Coronary Artery, Three Arteries 3 Coronary Artery, Four or More Arteries	3 Percutaneous	4 Intraluminal Device, Drug-eluting D Intraluminal Device	4 Coronary Vein
Ø Coronary Artery, One Artery 1 Coronary Artery, Two Arteries 2 Coronary Artery, Three Arteries 3 Coronary Artery, Four or More Arteries	4 Percutaneous Endoscopic	4 Intraluminal Device, Drug-eluting D Intraluminal Device	4 Coronary Vein
Ø Coronary Artery, One Artery 1 Coronary Artery, Two Arteries 2 Coronary Artery, Three Arteries 3 Coronary Artery, Four or More Arteries	4 Percutaneous Endoscopic	8 Zooplastic Tissue 9 Autologous Venous Tissue A Autologous Arterial Tissue J Synthetic Substitute K Nonautologous Tissue Substitute	3 Coronary Artery 8 Internal Mammary, Right 9 Internal Mammary, Left C Thoracic Artery F Abdominal Artery W Aorta
Ø Coronary Artery, One Artery 1 Coronary Artery, Two Arteries 2 Coronary Artery, Three Arteries 3 Coronary Artery, Four or More Arteries	4 Percutaneous Endoscopic	Z No Device	3 Coronary Artery 8 Internal Mammary, Right 9 Internal Mammary, Left C Thoracic Artery F Abdominal Artery

6 Atrium, Right
   Atrium dextrum cordis
   Right auricular appendix
   Sinus venosus
	Ø Open
	4 Percutaneous Endoscopic
		8 Zooplastic Tissue
		9 Autologous Venous Tissue
		A Autologous Arterial Tissue
		J Synthetic Substitute
		K Nonautologous Tissue Substitute
			P Pulmonary Trunk
			Q Pulmonary Artery, Right
			R Pulmonary Artery, Left

6 Atrium, Right
   Atrium dextrum cordis
   Right auricular appendix
   Sinus venosus
	Ø Open
	4 Percutaneous Endoscopic
		Z No Device	7 Atrium, Left
			P Pulmonary Trunk
			Q Pulmonary Artery, Right
			R Pulmonary Artery, Left

6 Atrium, Right
   Atrium dextrum cordis
   Right auricular appendix
   Sinus venosus
	3 Percutaneous	Z No Device	7 Atrium, Left

7 Atrium, Left
   Atrium pulmonale
   Left auricular appendix
	Ø Open
	4 Percutaneous Endoscopic
		8 Zooplastic Tissue
		9 Autologous Venous Tissue
		A Autologous Arterial Tissue
		J Synthetic Substitute
		K Nonautologous Tissue Substitute
		Z No Device
			P Pulmonary Trunk
			Q Pulmonary Artery, Right
			R Pulmonary Artery, Left
			S Pulmonary Vein, Right
			T Pulmonary Vein, Left
			U Pulmonary Vein, Confluence

7 Atrium, Left
   Atrium pulmonale
   Left auricular appendix
	3 Percutaneous	J Synthetic Substitute	6 Atrium, Right

K Ventricle, Right Conus arteriosus L Ventricle, Left	Ø Open 4 Percutaneous Endoscopic	8 Zooplastic Tissue 9 Autologous Venous Tissue A Autologous Arterial Tissue J Synthetic Substitute K Nonautologous Tissue Substitute	P Pulmonary Trunk Q Pulmonary Artery, Right R Pulmonary Artery, Left

HAC   Ø21[Ø,1,2,3]Ø[8,9,A,J,K][3,8,9,C,F,W] when reported with SDx J98.51 or J98.59
HAC   Ø21[Ø,1,2,3]ØZ[3,8,9,C,F] when reported with SDx J98.51 or J98.59
HAC   Ø21[Ø,1,2,3]4[8,9,A,J,K][3,8,9,C,F,W] when reported with SDx J98.51 or J98.59
HAC   Ø21[Ø,1,2,3]4Z[3,8,9,C,F] when reported with SDx J98.51 or J98.59

Ø21 Continued on next page

NC Noncovered Procedure   LC Limited Coverage   OA Questionable OB Admit   NT New Tech Add-on   ⊞ Combination Member   ♂ Male   ♀ Female

Heart and Great Vessels

Ø   Medical and Surgical
2   Heart and Great Vessels
1   Bypass   Definition: Altering the route of passage of the contents of a tubular body part

Ø21 Continued

Explanation: Rerouting contents of a body part to a downstream area of the normal route, to a similar route and body part, or to an abnormal route and dissimilar body part. Includes one or more anastomoses, with or without the use of a device.

Body Part Character 4	Approach Character 5	Device Character 6	Qualifier Character 7
K Ventricle, Right Conus arteriosus L Ventricle, Left	Ø Open 4 Percutaneous Endoscopic	Z No Device	5 Coronary Circulation 8 Internal Mammary, Right 9 Internal Mammary, Left C Thoracic Artery F Abdominal Artery P Pulmonary Trunk Q Pulmonary Artery, Right R Pulmonary Artery, Left W Aorta

P   Pulmonary Trunk
Q   Pulmonary Artery, Right
R   Pulmonary Artery, Left
      Arterial canal (duct)
      Botallo's duct
      Pulmoaortic canal
	Ø Open
	4 Percutaneous Endoscopic
		8 Zooplastic Tissue
		9 Autologous Venous Tissue
		A Autologous Arterial Tissue
		J Synthetic Substitute
		K Nonautologous Tissue Substitute
		Z No Device
			A Innominate Artery
			B Subclavian
			D Carotid

V   Superior Vena Cava
      Cavoatrial junction
      Precava
	Ø Open
	4 Percutaneous Endoscopic
		8 Zooplastic Tissue
		9 Autologous Venous Tissue
		A Autologous Arterial Tissue
		J Synthetic Substitute
		K Nonautologous Tissue Substitute
		Z No Device
			P Pulmonary Trunk
			Q Pulmonary Artery, Right
			R Pulmonary Artery, Left
			S Pulmonary Vein, Right
			T Pulmonary Vein, Left
			U Pulmonary Vein, Confluence

W Thoracic Aorta, Descending	Ø Open	8 Zooplastic Tissue 9 Autologous Venous Tissue A Autologous Arterial Tissue J Synthetic Substitute K Nonautologous Tissue Substitute	A Innominate Artery B Subclavian D Carotid F Abdominal Artery G Axillary Artery H Brachial Artery P Pulmonary Trunk Q Pulmonary Artery, Right R Pulmonary Artery, Left V Lower Extremity Artery
W Thoracic Aorta, Descending	Ø Open	Z No Device	A Innominate Artery B Subclavian D Carotid P Pulmonary Trunk Q Pulmonary Artery, Right R Pulmonary Artery, Left
W Thoracic Aorta, Descending	4 Percutaneous Endoscopic	8 Zooplastic Tissue 9 Autologous Venous Tissue A Autologous Arterial Tissue J Synthetic Substitute K Nonautologous Tissue Substitute Z No Device	A Innominate Artery B Subclavian D Carotid P Pulmonary Trunk Q Pulmonary Artery, Right R Pulmonary Artery, Left

X   Thoracic Aorta, Ascending/Arch
      Aortic arch
      Ascending aorta
	Ø Open
	4 Percutaneous Endoscopic
		8 Zooplastic Tissue
		9 Autologous Venous Tissue
		A Autologous Arterial Tissue
		J Synthetic Substitute
		K Nonautologous Tissue Substitute
		Z No Device
			A Innominate Artery
			B Subclavian
			D Carotid
			P Pulmonary Trunk
			Q Pulmonary Artery, Right
			R Pulmonary Artery, Left

Ø   Medical and Surgical
2   Heart and Great Vessels
4   Creation   Definition: Putting in or on biological or synthetic material to form a new body part that to the extent possible replicates the anatomic structure or function of an absent body part

Explanation: Used for gender reassignment surgery and corrective procedures in individuals with congenital anomalies

Body Part Character 4	Approach Character 5	Device Character 6	Qualifier Character 7
F Aortic Valve Aortic annulus	Ø Open	7 Autologous Tissue 8 Zooplastic Tissue J Synthetic Substitute K Nonautologous Tissue Substitute	J Truncal Valve

G   Mitral Valve
      Bicuspid valve
      Left atrioventricular valve
      Mitral annulus
J   Tricuspid Valve
      Right atrioventricular valve
      Tricuspid annulus
	Ø Open	7 Autologous Tissue
		8 Zooplastic Tissue
		J Synthetic Substitute
		K Nonautologous Tissue Substitute
			2 Common Atrioventricular Valve

Non-OR Procedure   DRG Non-OR Procedure   Valid OR Procedure   HAC Associated Procedure   Combination Only   New/Revised April   New/Revised October

Ø   Medical and Surgical
2   Heart and Great Vessels
5   Destruction   Definition: Physical eradication of all or a portion of a body part by the direct use of energy, force, or a destructive agent
                     Explanation: None of the body part is physically taken out

Body Part Character 4	Approach Character 5	Device Character 6	Qualifier Character 7

4   Coronary Vein
5   Atrial Septum
     Interatrial septum
6   Atrium, Right
     Atrium dextrum cordis
     Right auricular appendix
     Sinus venosus
8   Conduction Mechanism
     Atrioventricular node
     Bundle of His
     Bundle of Kent
     Sinoatrial node
9   Chordae Tendineae
D   Papillary Muscle
F   Aortic Valve
     Aortic annulus
G   Mitral Valve
     Bicuspid valve
     Left atrioventricular valve
     Mitral annulus
H   Pulmonary Valve
     Pulmonary annulus
     Pulmonic valve
J   Tricuspid Valve
     Right atrioventricular valve
     Tricuspid annulus
K   Ventricle, Right
     Conus arteriosus
L   Ventricle, Left
M   Ventricular Septum
     Interventricular septum
N   Pericardium
P   Pulmonary Trunk
Q   Pulmonary Artery, Right
R   Pulmonary Artery, Left
     Arterial canal (duct)
     Botallo's duct
     Pulmoaortic canal
S   Pulmonary Vein, Right
     Right inferior pulmonary vein
     Right superior pulmonary vein
T   Pulmonary Vein, Left
     Left inferior pulmonary vein
     Left superior pulmonary vein
V   Superior Vena Cava
     Cavoatrial junction
     Precava
W   Thoracic Aorta, Descending
X   Thoracic Aorta, Ascending/Arch
     Aortic arch
     Ascending aorta
	Ø Open
	3 Percutaneous
	4 Percutaneous Endoscopic
		Z No Device	Z No Qualifier

7   Atrium, Left
     Atrium pulmonale
     Left auricular appendix
	Ø Open
	3 Percutaneous
	4 Percutaneous Endoscopic
		Z No Device	K Left Atrial Appendage
			Z No Qualifier

DRG Non-OR   Ø257[Ø,3,4]ZK

NC Noncovered Procedure   LC Limited Coverage   QA Questionable OB Admit   NT New Tech Add-on   ⊞ Combination Member   ♂ Male   ♀ Female

ICD-10-PCS 2024   177

Ø   Medical and Surgical
2   Heart and Great Vessels
7   Dilation   Definition: Expanding an orifice or the lumen of a tubular body part

Explanation: The orifice can be a natural orifice or an artificially created orifice. Accomplished by stretching a tubular body part using intraluminal pressure or by cutting part of the orifice or wall of the tubular body part.

Body Part Character 4	Approach Character 5	Device Character 6	Qualifier Character 7
Ø Coronary Artery, One Artery 1 Coronary Artery, Two Arteries 2 Coronary Artery, Three Arteries 3 Coronary Artery, Four or More Arteries	Ø Open 3 Percutaneous 4 Percutaneous Endoscopic	4 Intraluminal Device, Drug-eluting 5 Intraluminal Device, Drug-eluting, Two 6 Intraluminal Device, Drug-eluting, Three 7 Intraluminal Device, Drug-eluting, Four or More D Intraluminal Device E Intraluminal Device, Two F Intraluminal Device, Three G Intraluminal Device, Four or More T Intraluminal Device, Radioactive Z No Device	6 Bifurcation Z No Qualifier

F Aortic Valve
   Aortic annulus
G Mitral Valve
   Bicuspid valve
   Left atrioventricular valve
   Mitral annulus
H Pulmonary Valve
   Pulmonary annulus
   Pulmonic valve
J Tricuspid Valve
   Right atrioventricular valve
   Tricuspid annulus
K Ventricle, Right
   Conus arteriosus
L Ventricle, Left
P Pulmonary Trunk
Q Pulmonary Artery, Right
S Pulmonary Vein, Right
   Right inferior pulmonary vein
   Right superior pulmonary vein
T Pulmonary Vein, Left
   Left inferior pulmonary vein
   Left superior pulmonary vein
V Superior Vena Cava
   Cavoatrial junction
   Precava
W Thoracic Aorta, Descending
X Thoracic Aorta, Ascending/Arch
   Aortic arch
   Ascending aorta
	Ø Open
	3 Percutaneous
	4 Percutaneous Endoscopic
		4 Intraluminal Device, Drug-eluting
		D Intraluminal Device
		Z No Device
			Z No Qualifier

R Pulmonary Artery, Left
   Arterial canal (duct)
   Botallo's duct
   Pulmoaortic canal
	Ø Open
	3 Percutaneous
	4 Percutaneous Endoscopic
		4 Intraluminal Device, Drug-eluting
		D Intraluminal Device
		Z No Device
			T Ductus Arteriosus
			Z No Qualifier

Ø   Medical and Surgical
2   Heart and Great Vessels
8   Division   Definition: Cutting into a body part, without draining fluids and/or gases from the body part, in order to separate or transect a body part

Explanation: All or a portion of the body part is separated into two or more portions

Body Part Character 4	Approach Character 5	Device Character 6	Qualifier Character 7

8 Conduction Mechanism
   Atrioventricular node
   Bundle of His
   Bundle of Kent
   Sinoatrial node
9 Chordae Tendineae
D Papillary Muscle
	Ø Open
	3 Percutaneous
	4 Percutaneous Endoscopic
		Z No Device	Z No Qualifier

Non-OR Procedure   DRG Non-OR Procedure   Valid OR Procedure   HAC Associated Procedure   Combination Only   New/Revised April   New/Revised October

178   ICD-10-PCS 2024

Ø   Medical and Surgical
2   Heart and Great Vessels
B   Excision   Definition: Cutting out or off, without replacement, a portion of a body part
Explanation: The qualifier DIAGNOSTIC is used to identify excision procedures that are biopsies

Body Part Character 4	Approach Character 5	Device Character 6	Qualifier Character 7

4 Coronary Vein
5 Atrial Septum
   Interatrial septum
6 Atrium, Right
   Atrium dextrum cordis
   Right auricular appendix
   Sinus venosus
8 Conduction Mechanism
   Atrioventricular node
   Bundle of His
   Bundle of Kent
   Sinoatrial node
9 Chordae Tendineae
D Papillary Muscle
F Aortic Valve
   Aortic annulus
G Mitral Valve
   Bicuspid valve
   Left atrioventricular valve
   Mitral annulus
H Pulmonary Valve
   Pulmonary annulus
   Pulmonic valve
J Tricuspid Valve
   Right atrioventricular valve
   Tricuspid annulus
K Ventricle, Right NC
   Conus arteriosus
L Ventricle, Left NC
M Ventricular Septum
   Interventricular septum
N Pericardium
P Pulmonary Trunk
Q Pulmonary Artery, Right
R Pulmonary Artery, Left
   Arterial canal (duct)
   Botallo's duct
   Pulmoaortic canal
S Pulmonary Vein, Right
   Right inferior pulmonary vein
   Right superior pulmonary vein
T Pulmonary Vein, Left
   Left inferior pulmonary vein
   Left superior pulmonary vein
V Superior Vena Cava
   Cavoatrial junction
   Precava
W Thoracic Aorta, Descending
X Thoracic Aorta, Ascending/Arch
   Aortic arch
   Ascending aorta
	Ø Open
	3 Percutaneous
	4 Percutaneous Endoscopic
		Z No Device	X Diagnostic
			Z No Qualifier

7 Atrium, Left
   Atrium pulmonale
   Left auricular appendix
	Ø Open
	3 Percutaneous
	4 Percutaneous Endoscopic
		Z No Device	K Left Atrial Appendage
			X Diagnostic
			Z No Qualifier

DRG Non-OR   Ø2B7[Ø,3,4]ZK
Non-OR   Ø2B[4,5,6,8,9,D,F,G,H,J,K,L,M][Ø,3,4]ZX
NC   Ø2B[K,L][Ø,3,4]ZZ

Ø Medical and Surgical
2 Heart and Great Vessels
C Extirpation   Definition: Taking or cutting out solid matter from a body part

Explanation: The solid matter may be an abnormal byproduct of a biological function or a foreign body; it may be imbedded in a body part or in the lumen of a tubular body part. The solid matter may or may not have been previously broken into pieces.

Body Part Character 4	Approach Character 5	Device Character 6	Qualifier Character 7
Ø Coronary Artery, One Artery 1 Coronary Artery, Two Arteries 2 Coronary Artery, Three Arteries 3 Coronary Artery, Four or More Arteries	Ø Open 4 Percutaneous Endoscopic	Z No Device	6 Bifurcation Z No Qualifier
Ø Coronary Artery, One Artery 1 Coronary Artery, Two Arteries 2 Coronary Artery, Three Arteries 3 Coronary Artery, Four or More Arteries	3 Percutaneous	Z No Device	6 Bifurcation 7 Orbital Atherectomy Technique Z No Qualifier

4 Coronary Vein
5 Atrial Septum
   Interatrial septum
6 Atrium, Right
   Atrium dextrum cordis
   Right auricular appendix
   Sinus venosus
7 Atrium, Left
   Atrium pulmonale
   Left auricular appendix
8 Conduction Mechanism
   Atrioventricular node
   Bundle of His
   Bundle of Kent
   Sinoatrial node
9 Chordae Tendineae
D Papillary Muscle
F Aortic Valve
   Aortic annulus
G Mitral Valve
   Bicuspid valve
   Left atrioventricular valve
   Mitral annulus
H Pulmonary Valve
   Pulmonary annulus
   Pulmonic valve
J Tricuspid Valve
   Right atrioventricular valve
   Tricuspid annulus
K Ventricle, Right
   Conus arteriosus
L Ventricle, Left
M Ventricular Septum
   Interventricular septum
N Pericardium
P Pulmonary Trunk
Q Pulmonary Artery, Right
R Pulmonary Artery, Left
   Arterial canal (duct)
   Botallo's duct
   Pulmoaortic canal
S Pulmonary Vein, Right
   Right inferior pulmonary vein
   Right superior pulmonary vein
T Pulmonary Vein, Left
   Left inferior pulmonary vein
   Left superior pulmonary vein
V Superior Vena Cava
   Cavoatrial junction
   Precava
W Thoracic Aorta, Descending
X Thoracic Aorta, Ascending/Arch
   Aortic arch
   Ascending aorta
	Ø Open
	3 Percutaneous
	4 Percutaneous Endoscopic
		Z No Device	Z No Qualifier

Non-OR Procedure   DRG Non-OR Procedure   Valid OR Procedure   HAC Associated Procedure   Combination Only   New/Revised April   New/Revised October

180   ICD-10-PCS 2024

02C–02C

Ø   Medical and Surgical
2   Heart and Great Vessels
F   Fragmentation   Definition: Breaking solid matter in a body part into pieces

Explanation: Physical force (e.g., manual, ultrasonic) applied directly or indirectly is used to break the solid matter into pieces. The solid matter may be an abnormal byproduct of a biological function or a foreign body. The pieces of solid matter are not taken out.

Body Part Character 4	Approach Character 5	Device Character 6	Qualifier Character 7
Ø Coronary Artery, One Artery **1** Coronary Artery, Two Arteries **2** Coronary Artery, Three Arteries **3** Coronary Artery, Four or More Arteries	**3** Percutaneous	**Z** No Device NT	**Z** No Qualifier
N Pericardium NC	**Ø** Open **3** Percutaneous **4** Percutaneous Endoscopic **X** External	**Z** No Device	**Z** No Qualifier

P   Pulmonary Trunk
Q   Pulmonary Artery, Right
R   Pulmonary Artery, Left
      Arterial canal (duct)
      Botallo's duct
      Pulmoaortic canal
S   Pulmonary Vein, Right
      Right inferior pulmonary vein
      Right superior pulmonary vein
T   Pulmonary Vein, Left
      Left inferior pulmonary vein
      Left superior pulmonary vein
	3 Percutaneous	**Z** No Device	**Ø** Ultrasonic
			Z No Qualifier

Non-OR	02FNXZZ
NC	02FNXZZ
NT	02F[Ø,1,2,3]3ZZ for Shockwave Coronary Intravascular Lithotripsy (IVL) System

NC Noncovered Procedure   **LC** Limited Coverage   **QA** Questionable OB Admit   **NT** New Tech Add-on   ⊞ Combination Member   ♂ Male   ♀ Female

ICD-10-PCS 2024   **181**

Heart and Great Vessels *(side tab)*

Ø   **Medical and Surgical**
2   **Heart and Great Vessels**
H   **Insertion**   Definition: Putting in a nonbiological appliance that monitors, assists, performs, or prevents a physiological function but does not physically take the place of a body part
                   Explanation: None

Body Part Character 4	Approach Character 5	Device Character 6	Qualifier Character 7
Ø Coronary Artery, One Artery **1** Coronary Artery, Two Arteries **2** Coronary Artery, Three Arteries **3** Coronary Artery, Four or More Arteries	**Ø** Open **3** Percutaneous **4** Percutaneous Endoscopic	**D** Intraluminal Device **Y** Other Device	**Z** No Qualifier

4 Coronary Vein ⊞
6 Atrium, Right ⊞
    Atrium dextrum cordis
    Right auricular appendix
    Sinus venosus
7 Atrium, Left ⊞
    Atrium pulmonale
    Left auricular appendix
K Ventricle, Right ⊞
    Conus arteriosus
L Ventricle, Left ⊞
	Ø Open
	3 Percutaneous
	4 Percutaneous Endoscopic
		Ø Monitoring Device, Pressure Sensor
		2 Monitoring Device
		3 Infusion Device
		D Intraluminal Device
		J Cardiac Lead, Pacemaker
		K Cardiac Lead, Defibrillator
		M Cardiac Lead
		N Intracardiac Pacemaker
		Y Other Device
			Z No Qualifier

A Heart [NC]	**Ø** Open **3** Percutaneous **4** Percutaneous Endoscopic	**Q** Implantable Heart Assist System **Y** Other Device	**Z** No Qualifier
A Heart ⊞	**Ø** Open **3** Percutaneous **4** Percutaneous Endoscopic	**R** Short-term External Heart Assist System	**J** Intraoperative **S** Biventricular **Z** No Qualifier
N Pericardium ⊞	**Ø** Open **3** Percutaneous **4** Percutaneous Endoscopic	**Ø** Monitoring Device, Pressure Sensor **2** Monitoring Device **J** Cardiac Lead, Pacemaker **K** Cardiac Lead, Defibrillator **M** Cardiac Lead **Y** Other Device	**Z** No Qualifier

P Pulmonary Trunk
Q Pulmonary Artery, Right
R Pulmonary Artery, Left
    Arterial canal (duct)
    Botallo's duct
    Pulmoaortic canal
S Pulmonary Vein, Right
    Right inferior pulmonary vein
    Right superior pulmonary vein
T Pulmonary Vein, Left
    Left inferior pulmonary vein
    Left superior pulmonary vein
V Superior Vena Cava
    Cavoatrial junction
    Precava
	Ø Open
	3 Percutaneous
	4 Percutaneous Endoscopic
		Ø Monitoring Device, Pressure Sensor
		2 Monitoring Device
		3 Infusion Device
		D Intraluminal Device
		Y Other Device
			Z No Qualifier

W Thoracic Aorta, Descending	**Ø** Open **4** Percutaneous Endoscopic	**Ø** Monitoring Device, Pressure Sensor **2** Monitoring Device **3** Infusion Device **D** Intraluminal Device **Y** Other Device	**Z** No Qualifier
W Thoracic Aorta, Descending	**3** Percutaneous	**Ø** Monitoring Device, Pressure Sensor **2** Monitoring Device **3** Infusion Device **D** Intraluminal Device **R** Short-term External Heart Assist System **Y** Other Device	**Z** No Qualifier

DRG Non-OR	02H[4,6,7,K,L][0,3,4][J,M]Z	HAC	02H43[J,K,M]Z when reported with SDx K68.11 or T81.40-T81.49, T82.7 with 7th character A
DRG Non-OR	02HK32Z	HAC	02H[6,K]33Z when reported with SDx J95.811
DRG Non-OR	02HN[0,3,4][J,M]Z	HAC	02H[6,7]3[J,M]Z when reported with SDx K68.11 or T81.40-T81.49, T82.7 with 7th character A
Non-OR	02H[4,6,7,L]3[2,3]Z		
Non-OR	02H[6,7]3MZ	HAC	02H[K,L]3JZ when reported with SDx K68.11 or T81.40-T81.49, T82.7 with 7th character A
Non-OR	02HK3[0,3]Z		
Non-OR	02HN32Z	HAC	02HN[0,3,4][J,M]Z when reported with SDx K68.11 or T81.40-T81.49, T82.7 with 7th character A
Non-OR	02HP[0,3,4][0,2,3]Z		
Non-OR	02H[Q,R][0,3,4][2,3]Z	HAC	02H[S,T,V][3,4]3Z when reported with SDx J95.811
Non-OR	02H[S,T,V][0,3,4]3Z		**See Appendix L for Procedure Combinations**
Non-OR	02H[S,T,V]32Z	⊞	02H[4,6,7,K,L][0,3,4][J,K,M]Z
Non-OR	02HWØ[0,3]Z	⊞	02HA[0,4]R[S,Z]
Non-OR	02HW43Z	⊞	02HA3RS
Non-OR	02HW3[0,2,3]Z	⊞	02HN[0,3,4][J,K,M]Z
[NC]	02HA[3,4]QZ		

Ø2H Continued on next page

Non-OR Procedure   DRG Non-OR Procedure   Valid OR Procedure   HAC Associated Procedure   Combination Only   New/Revised April   New/Revised October

182   ICD-10-PCS 2024

Ø Medical and Surgical
2 Heart and Great Vessels
H Insertion   Definition: Putting in a nonbiological appliance that monitors, assists, performs, or prevents a physiological function but does not physically take the place of a body part

Explanation: None

Ø2H Continued

Body Part Character 4	Approach Character 5	Device Character 6	Qualifier Character 7

X Thoracic Aorta, Ascending/Arch
   Aortic arch
   Ascending aorta
	Ø Open
	3 Percutaneous
	4 Percutaneous Endoscopic
		Ø Monitoring Device, Pressure Sensor
		2 Monitoring Device
		3 Infusion Device
		D Intraluminal Device
			Z No Qualifier

Non-OR   Ø2HX[Ø,3,4][Ø,3]Z

Ø Medical and Surgical
2 Heart and Great Vessels
J Inspection   Definition: Visually and/or manually exploring a body part

Explanation: Visual exploration may be performed with or without optical instrumentation. Manual exploration may be performed directly or through intervening body layers.

Body Part Character 4	Approach Character 5	Device Character 6	Qualifier Character 7
A Heart **Y** Great Vessel	**Ø** Open **3** Percutaneous **4** Percutaneous Endoscopic	**Z** No Device	**Z** No Qualifier

Non-OR   Ø2J[A,Y]3ZZ

Ø Medical and Surgical
2 Heart and Great Vessels
K Map   Definition: Locating the route of passage of electrical impulses and/or locating functional areas in a body part

Explanation: Applicable only to the cardiac conduction mechanism and the central nervous system

Body Part Character 4	Approach Character 5	Device Character 6	Qualifier Character 7

8 Conduction Mechanism
   Atrioventricular node
   Bundle of His
   Bundle of Kent
   Sinoatrial node
	Ø Open
	3 Percutaneous
	4 Percutaneous Endoscopic
		Z No Device	**Z** No Qualifier

DRG Non-OR   Ø2K8[Ø,3,4]ZZ

Ø Medical and Surgical
2 Heart and Great Vessels
L Occlusion   Definition: Completely closing an orifice or the lumen of a tubular body part

Explanation: The orifice can be a natural orifice or an artificially created orifice

Body Part Character 4	Approach Character 5	Device Character 6	Qualifier Character 7

7 Atrium, Left
   Atrium pulmonale
   Left auricular appendix
	Ø Open
	3 Percutaneous
	4 Percutaneous Endoscopic
		C Extraluminal Device
		D Intraluminal Device
		Z No Device
			K Left Atrial Appendage

H Pulmonary Valve
   Pulmonary annulus
   Pulmonic valve
P Pulmonary Trunk
Q Pulmonary Artery, Right
S Pulmonary Vein, Right
   Right inferior pulmonary vein
   Right superior pulmonary vein
T Pulmonary Vein, Left
   Left inferior pulmonary vein
   Left superior pulmonary vein
V Superior Vena Cava
   Cavoatrial junction
   Precava
	Ø Open
	3 Percutaneous
	4 Percutaneous Endoscopic
		C Extraluminal Device
		D Intraluminal Device
		Z No Device
			Z No Qualifier

R Pulmonary Artery, Left
   Arterial canal (duct)
   Botallo's duct
   Pulmoaortic canal
	Ø Open
	3 Percutaneous
	4 Percutaneous Endoscopic
		C Extraluminal Device
		D Intraluminal Device
		Z No Device
			T Ductus Arteriosus
			Z No Qualifier

W Thoracic Aorta, Descending	**Ø** Open **3** Percutaneous	**D** Intraluminal Device	**J** Temporary

DRG Non-OR   Ø2L7[Ø,3,4][C,D,Z]K

NC Noncovered Procedure   **LC** Limited Coverage   **QA** Questionable OB Admit   **NT** New Tech Add-on   ⊞ Combination Member   ♂ Male   ♀ Female

ICD-10-PCS 2024   183

Heart and Great Vessels (left margin, vertical)

Ø   **Medical and Surgical**
2   **Heart and Great Vessels**
N   **Release**   Definition: Freeing a body part from an abnormal physical constraint by cutting or by the use of force
                          Explanation: Some of the restraining tissue may be taken out but none of the body part is taken out

Body Part Character 4	Approach Character 5	Device Character 6	Qualifier Character 7

Ø Coronary Artery, One Artery
1 Coronary Artery, Two Arteries
2 Coronary Artery, Three Arteries
3 Coronary Artery, Four or More Arteries
4 Coronary Vein
5 Atrial Septum
   Interatrial septum
6 Atrium, Right
   Atrium dextrum cordis
   Right auricular appendix
   Sinus venosus
7 Atrium, Left
   Atrium pulmonale
   Left auricular appendix
8 Conduction Mechanism
   Atrioventricular node
   Bundle of His
   Bundle of Kent
   Sinoatrial node
9 Chordae Tendineae
D Papillary Muscle
F Aortic Valve
   Aortic annulus
G Mitral Valve
   Bicuspid valve
   Left atrioventricular valve
   Mitral annulus
H Pulmonary Valve
   Pulmonary annulus
   Pulmonic valve
J Tricuspid Valve
   Right atrioventricular valve
   Tricuspid annulus
K Ventricle, Right
   Conus arteriosus
L Ventricle, Left
M Ventricular Septum
   Interventricular septum
N Pericardium
P Pulmonary Trunk
Q Pulmonary Artery, Right
R Pulmonary Artery, Left
   Arterial canal (duct)
   Botallo's duct
   Pulmoaortic canal
S Pulmonary Vein, Right
   Right inferior pulmonary vein
   Right superior pulmonary vein
T Pulmonary Vein, Left
   Left inferior pulmonary vein
   Left superior pulmonary vein
V Superior Vena Cava
   Cavoatrial junction
   Precava
W Thoracic Aorta, Descending
X Thoracic Aorta, Ascending/Arch
   Aortic arch
   Ascending aorta
	Ø Open
	3 Percutaneous
	4 Percutaneous Endoscopic
		Z No Device	Z No Qualifier

0   Medical and Surgical
2   Heart and Great Vessels
P   Removal   Definition: Taking out or off a device from a body part

Explanation: If a device is taken out and a similar device put in without cutting or puncturing the skin or mucous membrane, the procedure is coded to the root operation CHANGE. Otherwise, the procedure for taking out a device is coded to the root operation REMOVAL.

Body Part Character 4	Approach Character 5	Device Character 6	Qualifier Character 7
A Heart	0 Open 3 Percutaneous 4 Percutaneous Endoscopic	2 Monitoring Device 3 Infusion Device 7 Autologous Tissue Substitute 8 Zooplastic Tissue C Extraluminal Device D Intraluminal Device J Synthetic Substitute K Nonautologous Tissue Substitute M Cardiac Lead N Intracardiac Pacemaker Q Implantable Heart Assist System Y Other Device	Z No Qualifier
A Heart ⊞	0 Open 3 Percutaneous 4 Percutaneous Endoscopic	R Short-term External Heart Assist System	S Biventricular Z No Qualifier
A Heart	X External	2 Monitoring Device 3 Infusion Device D Intraluminal Device M Cardiac Lead	Z No Qualifier
W Thoracic Aorta, Descending	3 Percutaneous	R Short-term External Heart Assist System	Z No Qualifier
Y Great Vessel	0 Open 3 Percutaneous 4 Percutaneous Endoscopic	2 Monitoring Device 3 Infusion Device 7 Autologous Tissue Substitute 8 Zooplastic Tissue C Extraluminal Device D Intraluminal Device J Synthetic Substitute K Nonautologous Tissue Substitute Y Other Device	Z No Qualifier
Y Great Vessel	X External	2 Monitoring Device 3 Infusion Device D Intraluminal Device	Z No Qualifier

Non-OR 02PA3[2,3,D]Z	**See Appendix L for Procedure Combinations**
Non-OR 02PA[3,4]YZ	⊞ 02PA[0,3,4]RZ
Non-OR 02PAX[2,3,D,M]Z	
Non-OR 02PY3[2,3,D]Z	
Non-OR 02PY[3,4]YZ	
Non-OR 02PYX[2,3,D]Z	
HAC 02PA[0,3,4]MZ when reported with SDx K68.11 or T81.40-T81.49, T82.7 with 7th character A	
HAC 02PAXMZ when reported with SDx K68.11 or T81.40-T81.49, T82.7 with 7th character A	

NC Noncovered Procedure   **LC** Limited Coverage   **QA** Questionable OB Admit   **NT** New Tech Add-on   ⊞ Combination Member   ♂ Male   ♀ Female

ICD-10-PCS 2024   185

Heart and Great Vessels

0   **Medical and Surgical**
2   **Heart and Great Vessels**
Q   **Repair**   Definition: Restoring, to the extent possible, a body part to its normal anatomic structure and function
                     Explanation: Used only when the method to accomplish the repair is not one of the other root operations

Body Part Character 4	Approach Character 5	Device Character 6	Qualifier Character 7

0 Coronary Artery, One Artery
1 Coronary Artery, Two Arteries
2 Coronary Artery, Three Arteries
3 Coronary Artery, Four or More
    Arteries
4 Coronary Vein
5 Atrial Septum
    Interatrial septum
6 Atrium, Right
    Atrium dextrum cordis
    Right auricular appendix
    Sinus venosus
7 Atrium, Left
    Atrium pulmonale
    Left auricular appendix
8 Conduction Mechanism
    Atrioventricular node
    Bundle of His
    Bundle of Kent
    Sinoatrial node
9 Chordae Tendineae
A Heart
B Heart, Right
    Right coronary sulcus
C Heart, Left
    Left coronary sulcus
    Obtuse margin
D Papillary Muscle
H Pulmonary Valve
    Pulmonary annulus
    Pulmonic valve
K Ventricle, Right
    Conus arteriosus
L Ventricle, Left
M Ventricular Septum
    Interventricular septum
N Pericardium
P Pulmonary Trunk
Q Pulmonary Artery, Right
R Pulmonary Artery, Left
    Arterial canal (duct)
    Botallo's duct
    Pulmoaortic canal
S Pulmonary Vein, Right
    Right inferior pulmonary vein
    Right superior pulmonary vein
T Pulmonary Vein, Left
    Left inferior pulmonary vein
    Left superior pulmonary vein
V Superior Vena Cava
    Cavoatrial junction
    Precava
W Thoracic Aorta, Descending
X Thoracic Aorta, Ascending/Arch
    Aortic arch
    Ascending aorta
	0 Open
	3 Percutaneous
	4 Percutaneous Endoscopic
		Z No Device	**Z** No Qualifier

F Aortic Valve Aortic annulus	**0** Open **3** Percutaneous **4** Percutaneous Endoscopic	**Z** No Device	**J** Truncal Valve **Z** No Qualifier

G Mitral Valve
    Bicuspid valve
    Left atrioventricular valve
    Mitral annulus
	0 Open
	3 Percutaneous
	4 Percutaneous Endoscopic
		Z No Device	**E** Atrioventricular Valve, Left
			Z No Qualifier

J Tricuspid Valve
    Right atrioventricular valve
    Tricuspid annulus
	0 Open
	3 Percutaneous
	4 Percutaneous Endoscopic
		Z No Device	**G** Atrioventricular Valve, Right
			Z No Qualifier

Non-OR Procedure   DRG Non-OR Procedure   Valid OR Procedure   HAC Associated Procedure   Combination Only   New/Revised April   New/Revised October

186   ICD-10-PCS 2024

0   **Medical and Surgical**
2   **Heart and Great Vessels**
R   **Replacement**   Definition: Putting in or on biological or synthetic material that physically takes the place and/or function of all or a portion of a body part
                Explanation: The body part may have been taken out or replaced, or may be taken out, physically eradicated, or rendered nonfunctional during the REPLACEMENT procedure. A REMOVAL procedure is coded for taking out the device used in a previous replacement procedure.

Body Part Character 4		Approach Character 5	Device Character 6	Qualifier Character 7

5 Atrial Septum
  Interatrial septum
6 Atrium, Right
  Atrium dextrum cordis
  Right auricular appendix
  Sinus venosus
7 Atrium, Left
  Atrium pulmonale
  Left auricular appendix
9 Chordae Tendineae
D Papillary Muscle
K Ventricle, Right ⊞
  Conus arteriosus
L Ventricle, Left ⊞
M Ventricular Septum
  Interventricular septum
N Pericardium
P Pulmonary Trunk
Q Pulmonary Artery, Right
	R Pulmonary Artery, Left
	  Arterial canal (duct)
	  Botallo's duct
	  Pulmoaortic canal
	S Pulmonary Vein, Right
	  Right inferior pulmonary vein
	  Right superior pulmonary vein
	T Pulmonary Vein, Left
	  Left inferior pulmonary vein
	  Left superior pulmonary vein
	V Superior Vena Cava
	  Cavoatrial junction
	  Precava
	W Thoracic Aorta, Descending
	X Thoracic Aorta, Ascending/Arch
	  Aortic arch
	  Ascending aorta
		0 Open
		4 Percutaneous Endoscopic
			7 Autologous Tissue Substitute
			8 Zooplastic Tissue
			J Synthetic Substitute
			K Nonautologous Tissue Substitute
				Z No Qualifier

A Heart		**0** Open	**L** Biologic with Synthetic Substitute, Autoregulated Electrohydraulic **M** Synthetic Substitute, Pneumatic	**Z** No Qualifier
F Aortic Valve Aortic annulus		**0** Open **4** Percutaneous Endoscopic	**7** Autologous Tissue Substitute **J** Synthetic Substitute **K** Nonautologous Tissue Substitute	**Z** No Qualifier
F Aortic Valve Aortic annulus		**0** Open **4** Percutaneous Endoscopic	**8** Zooplastic Tissue	**N** Rapid Deployment Technique **Z** No Qualifier
F Aortic Valve Aortic annulus		**3** Percutaneous	**7** Autologous Tissue Substitute **J** Synthetic Substitute **K** Nonautologous Tissue Substitute	**H** Transapical **Z** No Qualifier
F Aortic Valve Aortic annulus		**3** Percutaneous	**8** Zooplastic Tissue	**H** Transapical **N** Rapid Deployment Technique **Z** No Qualifier

G Mitral Valve
  Bicuspid valve
  Left atrioventricular valve
  Mitral annulus
J Tricuspid Valve
  Right atrioventricular valve
  Tricuspid annulus
		0 Open
		4 Percutaneous Endoscopic
			7 Autologous Tissue Substitute
			8 Zooplastic Tissue
			J Synthetic Substitute
			K Nonautologous Tissue Substitute
				Z No Qualifier

G Mitral Valve
  Bicuspid valve
  Left atrioventricular valve
  Mitral annulus
J Tricuspid Valve
  Right atrioventricular valve
  Tricuspid annulus
		3 Percutaneous	**7** Autologous Tissue Substitute
			8 Zooplastic Tissue
			J Synthetic Substitute
			K Nonautologous Tissue Substitute
				H Transapical
				Z No Qualifier

H Pulmonary Valve
  Pulmonary annulus
  Pulmonic valve
		0 Open
		4 Percutaneous Endoscopic
			7 Autologous Tissue Substitute
			8 Zooplastic Tissue
			J Synthetic Substitute
			K Nonautologous Tissue Substitute
				Z No Qualifier

H Pulmonary Valve
  Pulmonary annulus
  Pulmonic valve
		3 Percutaneous	**7** Autologous Tissue Substitute
			J Synthetic Substitute
			K Nonautologous Tissue Substitute
				H Transapical
				Z No Qualifier

H Pulmonary Valve
  Pulmonary annulus
  Pulmonic valve
		3 Percutaneous	**8** Zooplastic Tissue **NT**	**H** Transapical
				L In Existing Conduit
				M Native Site
				Z No Qualifier

NT   02RH38M for Harmony™ Transcatheter Pulmonary Valve (TPV) System   **See Appendix L for Procedure Combinations**
                                                             ⊞   02R[K,L]0JZ

NC Noncovered Procedure   **LC** Limited Coverage   **QA** Questionable OB Admit   **NT** New Tech Add-on   ⊞ Combination Member   ♂ Male   ♀ Female

ICD-10-PCS 2024   187

02R–02R

Ø   Medical and Surgical
2   Heart and Great Vessels
S   Reposition   Definition: Moving to its normal location, or other suitable location, all or a portion of a body part
                            Explanation: The body part is moved to a new location from an abnormal location, or from a normal location where it is not functioning correctly. The body part may or may not be cut out or off to be moved to the new location.

Body Part Character 4	Approach Character 5	Device Character 6	Qualifier Character 7

Ø   Coronary Artery, One Artery
1   Coronary Artery, Two Arteries
P   Pulmonary Trunk
Q   Pulmonary Artery, Right
R   Pulmonary Artery, Left
    Arterial canal (duct)
    Botallo's duct
    Pulmoaortic canal
S   Pulmonary Vein, Right
    Right inferior pulmonary vein
    Right superior pulmonary vein
T   Pulmonary Vein, Left
    Left inferior pulmonary vein
    Left superior pulmonary vein
V   Superior Vena Cava
    Cavoatrial junction
    Precava
W   Thoracic Aorta, Descending
X   Thoracic Aorta, Ascending/Arch
    Aortic arch
    Ascending aorta
	Ø Open	Z No Device	Z No Qualifier

Ø   Medical and Surgical
2   Heart and Great Vessels
T   Resection   Definition: Cutting out or off, without replacement, all of a body part
                           Explanation: None

Body Part Character 4	Approach Character 5	Device Character 6	Qualifier Character 7

5   Atrial Septum
    Interatrial septum
8   Conduction Mechanism
    Atrioventricular node
    Bundle of His
    Bundle of Kent
    Sinoatrial node
9   Chordae Tendineae
D   Papillary Muscle
H   Pulmonary Valve
    Pulmonary annulus
    Pulmonic valve
M   Ventricular Septum
    Interventricular septum
N   Pericardium
	Ø Open
	3 Percutaneous
	4 Percutaneous Endoscopic
		Z No Device	Z No Qualifier

0   **Medical and Surgical**
2   **Heart and Great Vessels**
U   **Supplement**   Definition: Putting in or on biological or synthetic material that physically reinforces and/or augments the function of a portion of a body part

Explanation: The biological material is non-living, or is living and from the same individual. The body part may have been previously replaced, and the SUPPLEMENT procedure is performed to physically reinforce and/or augment the function of the replaced body part.

Body Part Character 4	Approach Character 5	Device Character 6	Qualifier Character 7

0 Coronary Artery, One Artery
1 Coronary Artery, Two Arteries
2 Coronary Artery, Three Arteries
3 Coronary Artery, Four or More Arteries
5 Atrial Septum
   Interatrial septum
6 Atrium, Right
   Atrium dextrum cordis
   Right auricular appendix
   Sinus venosus
7 Atrium, Left
   Atrium pulmonale
   Left auricular appendix
9 Chordae Tendineae
A Heart
D Papillary Muscle
H Pulmonary Valve
   Pulmonary annulus
   Pulmonic valve
K Ventricle, Right
   Conus arteriosus
L Ventricle, Left
M Ventricular Septum
   Interventricular septum
N Pericardium
P Pulmonary Trunk
Q Pulmonary Artery, Right
R Pulmonary Artery, Left
   Arterial canal (duct)
   Botallo's duct
   Pulmoaortic canal
S Pulmonary Vein, Right
   Right inferior pulmonary vein
   Right superior pulmonary vein
T Pulmonary Vein, Left
   Left inferior pulmonary vein
   Left superior pulmonary vein
V Superior Vena Cava
   Cavoatrial junction
   Precava
W Thoracic Aorta, Descending
X Thoracic Aorta, Ascending/Arch
   Aortic arch
   Ascending aorta
	0 Open
	3 Percutaneous
	4 Percutaneous Endoscopic
		7 Autologous Tissue Substitute
		8 Zooplastic Tissue
		J Synthetic Substitute
		K Nonautologous Tissue Substitute
			Z No Qualifier

F Aortic Valve Aortic annulus	**0** Open **3** Percutaneous **4** Percutaneous Endoscopic	**7** Autologous Tissue Substitute **8** Zooplastic Tissue **J** Synthetic Substitute **K** Nonautologous Tissue Substitute	**J** Truncal Valve **Z** No Qualifier

G Mitral Valve
   Bicuspid valve
   Left atrioventricular valve
   Mitral annulus
	0 Open
	4 Percutaneous Endoscopic
		7 Autologous Tissue Substitute
		8 Zooplastic Tissue
		J Synthetic Substitute
		K Nonautologous Tissue Substitute
			E Atrioventricular Valve, Left
			Z No Qualifier

G Mitral Valve
   Bicuspid valve
   Left atrioventricular valve
   Mitral annulus
	3 Percutaneous	**7** Autologous Tissue Substitute
		8 Zooplastic Tissue
		K Nonautologous Tissue Substitute
			E Atrioventricular Valve, Left
			Z No Qualifier

G Mitral Valve
   Bicuspid valve
   Left atrioventricular valve
   Mitral annulus
	3 Percutaneous	**J** Synthetic Substitute	**E** Atrioventricular Valve, Left
			H Transapical
			Z No Qualifier

J Tricuspid Valve
   Right atrioventricular valve
   Tricuspid annulus
	0 Open
	3 Percutaneous
	4 Percutaneous Endoscopic
		7 Autologous Tissue Substitute
		8 Zooplastic Tissue
		J Synthetic Substitute
		K Nonautologous Tissue Substitute
			G Atrioventricular Valve, Right
			Z No Qualifier

DRG Non-OR   02U7[3,4]JZ

NC Noncovered Procedure   **LC** Limited Coverage   **QA** Questionable OB Admit   **NT** New Tech Add-on   ⊞ Combination Member   ♂ Male   ♀ Female

ICD-10-PCS 2024   189

02U–02U

Heart and Great Vessels

Ø   **Medical and Surgical**
2   **Heart and Great Vessels**
V   **Restriction**   Definition: Partially closing an orifice or the lumen of a tubular body part
                        Explanation: The orifice can be a natural orifice or an artificially created orifice

Body Part Character 4	Approach Character 5	Device Character 6	Qualifier Character 7
A Heart	**Ø** Open **3** Percutaneous **4** Percutaneous Endoscopic	**C** Extraluminal Device **Z** No Device	**Z** No Qualifier

G **Mitral Valve**
    Bicuspid valve
    Left atrioventricular valve
    Mitral annulus
	Ø Open
	3 Percutaneous
	4 Percutaneous Endoscopic
		Z No Device	**Z** No Qualifier

L **Ventricle, Left**
P **Pulmonary Trunk**
Q **Pulmonary Artery, Right**
S **Pulmonary Vein, Right**
    Right inferior pulmonary vein
    Right superior pulmonary vein
T **Pulmonary Vein, Left**
    Left inferior pulmonary vein
    Left superior pulmonary vein
V **Superior Vena Cava**
    Cavoatrial junction
    Precava
	Ø Open
	3 Percutaneous
	4 Percutaneous Endoscopic
		C Extraluminal Device
		D Intraluminal Device
		Z No Device
			Z No Qualifier

R **Pulmonary Artery, Left**
    Arterial canal (duct)
    Botallo's duct
    Pulmoaortic canal
	Ø Open
	3 Percutaneous
	4 Percutaneous Endoscopic
		C Extraluminal Device
		D Intraluminal Device
		Z No Device
			T Ductus Arteriosus
			Z No Qualifier

W **Thoracic Aorta, Descending**
X **Thoracic Aorta, Ascending/Arch**
    Aortic arch
    Ascending aorta
	Ø Open
	3 Percutaneous
	4 Percutaneous Endoscopic
		C Extraluminal Device
		D Intraluminal Device `NT`
		E Intraluminal Device, Branched `NT`
		    or Fenestrated, One or Two Arteries
		F Intraluminal Device, Branched or
		    Fenestrated, Three or More Arteries
		Z No Device
			Z No Qualifier

`NT`   Ø2VW3DZ with Ø2VX3EZ for GORE® TAG® Thoracic Branch Endoprosthesis

Non-OR Procedure   DRG Non-OR Procedure   Valid OR Procedure   HAC Associated Procedure   Combination Only   New/Revised April   New/Revised October

190   ICD-10-PCS 2024

Ø Medical and Surgical
2 Heart and Great Vessels
W Revision   Definition: Correcting, to the extent possible, a portion of a malfunctioning device or the position of a displaced device

Explanation: Revision can include correcting a malfunctioning or displaced device by taking out or putting in components of the device such as a screw or pin

Body Part Character 4	Approach Character 5	Device Character 6	Qualifier Character 7
5 Atrial Septum Interatrial septum **M Ventricular Septum** Interventricular septum	**Ø** Open **4** Percutaneous Endoscopic	**J** Synthetic Substitute	**Z** No Qualifier
A Heart [LC] [+]	**Ø** Open **3** Percutaneous **4** Percutaneous Endoscopic	**2** Monitoring Device **3** Infusion Device **7** Autologous Tissue Substitute **8** Zooplastic Tissue **C** Extraluminal Device **D** Intraluminal Device **J** Synthetic Substitute **K** Nonautologous Tissue Substitute **M** Cardiac Lead **N** Intracardiac Pacemaker **Q** Implantable Heart Assist System **Y** Other Device	**Z** No Qualifier
A Heart [+]	**Ø** Open **3** Percutaneous **4** Percutaneous Endoscopic	**R** Short-term External Heart Assist System	**S** Biventricular **Z** No Qualifier
A Heart	**X** External	**2** Monitoring Device **3** Infusion Device **7** Autologous Tissue Substitute **8** Zooplastic Tissue **C** Extraluminal Device **D** Intraluminal Device **J** Synthetic Substitute **K** Nonautologous Tissue Substitute **M** Cardiac Lead **N** Intracardiac Pacemaker **Q** Implantable Heart Assist System	**Z** No Qualifier
A Heart	**X** External	**R** Short-term External Heart Assist System	**S** Biventricular **Z** No Qualifier
F Aortic Valve Aortic annulus **G Mitral Valve** Bicuspid valve Left atrioventricular valve Mitral annulus **H Pulmonary Valve** Pulmonary annulus Pulmonic valve **J Tricuspid Valve** Right atrioventricular valve Tricuspid annulus	**Ø** Open **3** Percutaneous **4** Percutaneous Endoscopic	**7** Autologous Tissue Substitute **8** Zooplastic Tissue **J** Synthetic Substitute **K** Nonautologous Tissue Substitute	**Z** No Qualifier
W Thoracic Aorta, Descending	**3** Percutaneous	**R** Short-term External Heart Assist System	**Z** No Qualifier
Y Great Vessel	**Ø** Open **3** Percutaneous **4** Percutaneous Endoscopic	**2** Monitoring Device **3** Infusion Device **7** Autologous Tissue Substitute **8** Zooplastic Tissue **C** Extraluminal Device **D** Intraluminal Device **J** Synthetic Substitute **K** Nonautologous Tissue Substitute **Y** Other Device	**Z** No Qualifier
Y Great Vessel	**X** External	**2** Monitoring Device **3** Infusion Device **7** Autologous Tissue Substitute **8** Zooplastic Tissue **C** Extraluminal Device **D** Intraluminal Device **J** Synthetic Substitute **K** Nonautologous Tissue Substitute	**Z** No Qualifier

Non-OR 02WA3[2,3,D]Z	**HAC** 02WA[0,3,4]MZ when reported with T81.4Ø–T81.49, T82.7 with 7th character A
Non-OR 02WA[3,4]YZ	[LC] 02WA[3,4]QZ
Non-OR 02WAX[2,3,7,8,C,D,J,K,M,N,Q]Z	
Non-OR 02WAXRZ	**See Appendix L for Procedure Combinations**
Non-OR 02WY3[2,3]Z	[+] 02WA[0,3,4]QZ
Non-OR 02WY[3,4]YZ	[+] 02WA[0,3,4]RZ
Non-OR 02WYX[2,3,7,8,C,D,J,K]Z	

[NC] Noncovered Procedure   [LC] Limited Coverage   [QA] Questionable OB Admit   [NT] New Tech Add-on   [+] Combination Member   ♂ Male   ♀ Female

ICD-10-PCS 2024   191

02W–02W

Heart and Great Vessels

0   **Medical and Surgical**
2   **Heart and Great Vessels**
Y   **Transplantation**   Definition: Putting in or on all or a portion of a living body part taken from another individual or animal to physically take the place and/or function of all or a portion of a similar body part

                 Explanation: The native body part may or may not be taken out, and the transplanted body part may take over all or a portion of its function

Body Part Character 4	Approach Character 5	Device Character 6	Qualifier Character 7
A Heart ^{LC}	0 Open	Z No Device	0 Allogeneic 1 Syngeneic 2 Zooplastic

     ^{LC}   02YA0Z[0,1,2]

Non-OR Procedure   DRG Non-OR Procedure   Valid OR Procedure   HAC Associated Procedure   Combination Only   New/Revised April   New/Revised October

192   ICD-10-PCS 2024

02Y–02Y

Upper Arteries Ø31–Ø3W

Character Meanings

This Character Meaning table is provided as a guide to assist the user in the identification of character members that may be found in this section of code tables. It **SHOULD NOT** be used to build a PCS code.

Operation–Character 3	Body Part–Character 4	Approach–Character 5	Device–Character 6	Qualifier–Character 7
1 Bypass	Ø Internal Mammary Artery, Right	Ø Open	Ø Drainage Device	Ø Upper Arm Artery, Right OR Ultrasonic
5 Destruction	1 Internal Mammary Artery, Left	3 Percutaneous	2 Monitoring Device	1 Upper Arm Artery, Left OR Drug-Coated Balloon
7 Dilation	2 Innominate Artery	4 Percutaneous Endoscopic	3 Infusion Device	2 Upper Arm Artery, Bilateral
9 Drainage	3 Subclavian Artery, Right	X External	4 Intraluminal Device, Drug-eluting	3 Lower Arm Artery, Right
B Excision	4 Subclavian Artery, Left		5 Intraluminal Device, Drug-eluting, Two	4 Lower Arm Artery, Left
C Extirpation	5 Axillary Artery, Right		6 Intraluminal Device, Drug-eluting, Three	5 Lower Arm Artery, Bilateral
F Fragmentation	6 Axillary Artery, Left		7 Intraluminal Device, Drug-eluting, Four or More OR Autologous Tissue Substitute	6 Upper Leg Artery, Right
H Insertion	7 Brachial Artery, Right		9 Autologous Venous Tissue	7 Upper Leg Artery, Left OR Stent Retriever
J Inspection	8 Brachial Artery, Left		A Autologous Arterial Tissue	8 Upper Leg Artery, Bilateral
L Occlusion	9 Ulnar Artery, Right		B Intraluminal Device, Bioactive	9 Lower Leg Artery, Right
N Release	A Ulnar Artery, Left		C Extraluminal Device	B Lower Leg Artery, Left
P Removal	B Radial Artery, Right		D Intraluminal Device	C Lower Leg Artery, Bilateral
Q Repair	C Radial Artery, Left		E Intraluminal Device, Two	D Upper Arm Vein
R Replacement	D Hand Artery, Right		F Intraluminal Device, Three	F Lower Arm Vein
S Reposition	F Hand Artery, Left		G Intraluminal Device, Four or More	G Intracranial Artery
U Supplement	G Intracranial Artery		H Intraluminal Device, Flow Diverter	J Extracranial Artery, Right
V Restriction	H Common Carotid Artery, Right		J Synthetic Substitute	K Extracranial Artery, Left
W Revision	J Common Carotid Artery, Left		K Nonautologous Tissue Substitute	M Pulmonary Artery, Right
	K Internal Carotid Artery, Right		M Stimulator Lead	N Pulmonary Artery, Left
	L Internal Carotid Artery, Left		Y Other Device	T Abdominal Artery
	M External Carotid Artery, Right		Z No Device	V Superior Vena Cava
	N External Carotid Artery, Left			W Lower Extremity Vein
	P Vertebral Artery, Right			X Diagnostic
	Q Vertebral Artery, Left			Y Upper Artery
	R Face Artery			Z No Qualifier
	S Temporal Artery, Right			
	T Temporal Artery, Left			
	U Thyroid Artery, Right			
	V Thyroid Artery, Left			
	Y Upper Artery			

AHA Coding Clinic for Upper Arteries
2022, 1Q, 10-13	Procedures performed on a continuous vessel, ICD-10-PCS Guideline B4.1c

AHA Coding Clinic for table Ø31
2021, 4Q, 45-46	Percutaneous bypass of brachial artery for arteriovenous fistula creation
2021, 3Q, 14	Arteriovenous fistula revision with graft to cephalic vein stump
2019, 4Q, 26	Upper artery bypass Qualifier
2019, 4Q, 26	Percutaneous approach upper artery bypass
2017, 4Q, 64-65	New qualifier values - Left to right carotid bypass
2017, 2Q, 22	Carotid artery to subclavian artery transposition
2017, 1Q, 31	Left to right common carotid artery bypass
2016, 3Q, 37	Insertion of arteriovenous graft using HeRO device
2016, 3Q, 39	Revision of arteriovenous graft
2013, 4Q, 125	Stage II cephalic vein transposition (superficialization) of arteriovenous fistula
2013, 1Q, 27	Creation of radial artery fistula

AHA Coding Clinic for table Ø37
2020, 4Q, 70-71	Cerebral embolic filtration extracorporeal flow reversal circuit
2019, 4Q, 27	Bifurcation Qualifier
2019, 3Q, 29	Transcarotid arterial catheterization
2018, 2Q, 24	Coronary artery bifurcation
2016, 4Q, 86	Peripheral artery, number of stents
2016, 4Q, 86-87	Coronary and peripheral artery bifurcation
2015, 1Q, 32	Deployment of stent for herniated/migrated coil in basilar artery

AHA Coding Clinic for table Ø3B
2016, 2Q, 12	Resection of malignant neoplasm of infratemporal fossa

AHA Coding Clinic for table Ø3C
2022, 1Q, 43	Cerebral thrombectomy with failed stent retriever deployment and aspiration of thrombus
2021, 2Q, 13	Thromboendarterectomy with deconstruction of internal carotid artery
2020, 3Q, 38	Thrombectomy of arteriovenous fistula with angioplasty and stent placement
2019, 4Q, 27	Bifurcation Qualifier
2018, 4Q, 47-48	Endovascular thrombectomy with stent retriever
2018, 2Q, 24	Coronary artery bifurcation
2017, 4Q, 64-65	New qualifier values - Left to right carotid bypass
2017, 2Q, 23	Thrombectomy via Fogarty catheter
2016, 4Q, 86-87	Coronary and peripheral artery bifurcation
2016, 2Q, 11	Carotid endarterectomy with patch angioplasty
2015, 1Q, 29	Discontinued carotid endarterectomy

AHA Coding Clinic for table Ø3F
2021, 4Q, 46	Fragmentation of intracranial artery
2020, 4Q, 45-49	New fragmentation tables
2020, 4Q, 49-50	Intravascular ultrasound assisted thrombolysis
2020, 4Q, 50	Intravascular lithotripsy

AHA Coding Clinic for table Ø3H
2020, 1Q, 25	Elephant trunk repair of aortic dissection
2016, 2Q, 32	Arterial catheter placement

AHA Coding Clinic for table Ø3J
2021, 1Q, 16	Placement of Sentinel™ embolic protection device with deployment of single filter
2015, 1Q, 29	Discontinued carotid endarterectomy

AHA Coding Clinic for table Ø3L
2021, 2Q, 13	Thromboendarterectomy with deconstruction of internal carotid artery
2016, 2Q, 30	Clipping (occlusion) of cerebral artery, decompressive craniectomy and storage of bone flap in abdominal wall
2014, 4Q, 20	Control of epistaxis
2014, 4Q, 37	Endovascular embolization of arteriovenous malformation using Onyx-18 liquid

AHA Coding Clinic for table Ø3Q
2017, 1Q, 31	Left to right common carotid artery bypass

AHA Coding Clinic for table Ø3S
2017, 2Q, 22	Carotid artery to subclavian artery transposition
2015, 3Q, 27	Moyamoya disease and hemispheric pial synangiosis with craniotomy

AHA Coding Clinic for table Ø3U
2023, 1Q, 35	Carotid artery endarterectomy with imbrication
2019, 1Q, 22	Cerebral artery fusiform aneurysm repair via wrapping
2016, 2Q, 11	Carotid endarterectomy with patch angioplasty

AHA Coding Clinic for table Ø3V
2023, 1Q, 34	Carotid artery pseudoaneurysm embolization using flow diverter stent and coils
2019, 4Q, 27-28	Aneurysm treatment using flow diverter stent
2019, 1Q, 22	Cerebral artery fusiform aneurysm repair via wrapping
2016, 1Q, 19	Embolization of superior hypophyseal aneurysm using stent-assisted coil

AHA Coding Clinic for table Ø3W
2016, 3Q, 39	Revision of arteriovenous graft
2015, 1Q, 32	Deployment of stent for herniated/migrated coil in basilar artery

Upper Arteries

Middle temporal **S, T**
Transverse facial **S, T**
Superficial temporal **S, T**
Face **R**
External carotid **M, N**
Internal carotid **K, L**
Common carotid **H, J**
Superior thyroid **U, V**
Vertebral **P, Q**
Inferior thyroid **U, V**
Subclavian **3, 4**
Innominate **2**
Axillary **5, 6**
Internal thoracic (mammary) **Ø, 1**
Brachial **7, 8**
Radial **B, C**
Ulnar **9, A**
Deep palmar arch **D, F**
Superficial palmar arch **D, F**

Head and Neck Arteries

Middle cerebral **G**
Anterior cerebral **G**
Posterior communicating **G**
Anterior communicating **G**
Posterior cerebral **G**
Ophthalmic **G**
Basilar **G**
Internal carotid **K,L**
External carotid **M,N**
Vertebral **P,Q**
Common carotid **H,J**

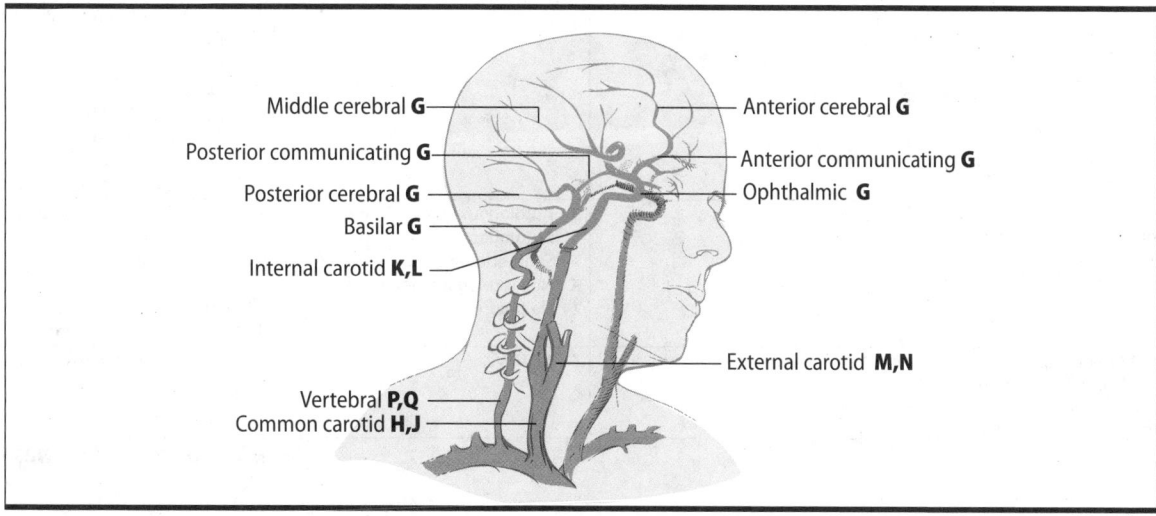

Ø   Medical and Surgical
3   Upper Arteries
1   Bypass   Definition: Altering the route of passage of the contents of a tubular body part

Explanation: Rerouting contents of a body part to a downstream area of the normal route, to a similar route and body part, or to an abnormal route and dissimilar body part. Includes one or more anastomoses, with or without the use of a device.

Body Part Character 4	Approach Character 5	Device Character 6	Qualifier Character 7
2 Innominate Artery Brachiocephalic artery Brachiocephalic trunk	Ø Open	9 Autologous Venous Tissue A Autologous Arterial Tissue J Synthetic Substitute K Nonautologous Tissue Substitute Z No Device	Ø Upper Arm Artery, Right 1 Upper Arm Artery, Left 2 Upper Arm Artery, Bilateral 3 Lower Arm Artery, Right 4 Lower Arm Artery, Left 5 Lower Arm Artery, Bilateral 6 Upper Leg Artery, Right 7 Upper Leg Artery, Left 8 Upper Leg Artery, Bilateral 9 Lower Leg Artery, Right B Lower Leg Artery, Left C Lower Leg Artery, Bilateral D Upper Arm Vein F Lower Arm Vein J Extracranial Artery, Right K Extracranial Artery, Left W Lower Extremity Vein
3 Subclavian Artery, Right Costocervical trunk Dorsal scapular artery Internal thoracic artery **4 Subclavian Artery, Left** *See 3 Subclavian Artery, Right*	Ø Open	9 Autologous Venous Tissue A Autologous Arterial Tissue J Synthetic Substitute K Nonautologous Tissue Substitute Z No Device	Ø Upper Arm Artery, Right 1 Upper Arm Artery, Left 2 Upper Arm Artery, Bilateral 3 Lower Arm Artery, Right 4 Lower Arm Artery, Left 5 Lower Arm Artery, Bilateral 6 Upper Leg Artery, Right 7 Upper Leg Artery, Left 8 Upper Leg Artery, Bilateral 9 Lower Leg Artery, Right B Lower Leg Artery, Left C Lower Leg Artery, Bilateral D Upper Arm Vein F Lower Arm Vein J Extracranial Artery, Right K Extracranial Artery, Left M Pulmonary Artery, Right N Pulmonary Artery, Left W Lower Extremity Vein
5 Axillary Artery, Right Anterior circumflex humeral artery Lateral thoracic artery Posterior circumflex humeral artery Subscapular artery Superior thoracic artery Thoracoacromial artery **6 Axillary Artery, Left** *See 5 Axillary Artery, Right*	Ø Open	9 Autologous Venous Tissue A Autologous Arterial Tissue J Synthetic Substitute K Nonautologous Tissue Substitute Z No Device	Ø Upper Arm Artery, Right 1 Upper Arm Artery, Left 2 Upper Arm Artery, Bilateral 3 Lower Arm Artery, Right 4 Lower Arm Artery, Left 5 Lower Arm Artery, Bilateral 6 Upper Leg Artery, Right 7 Upper Leg Artery, Left 8 Upper Leg Artery, Bilateral 9 Lower Leg Artery, Right B Lower Leg Artery, Left C Lower Leg Artery, Bilateral D Upper Arm Vein F Lower Arm Vein J Extracranial Artery, Right K Extracranial Artery, Left T Abdominal Artery V Superior Vena Cava W Lower Extremity Vein
7 Brachial Artery, Right Inferior ulnar collateral artery Profunda brachii Superior ulnar collateral artery	Ø Open	9 Autologous Venous Tissue A Autologous Arterial Tissue J Synthetic Substitute K Nonautologous Tissue Substitute Z No Device	Ø Upper Arm Artery, Right 3 Lower Arm Artery, Right D Upper Arm Vein F Lower Arm Vein V Superior Vena Cava W Lower Extremity Vein
7 Brachial Artery, Right Inferior ulnar collateral artery Profunda brachii Superior ulnar collateral artery	3 Percutaneous	Z No Device	F Lower Arm Vein

Ø31 Continued on next page

Non-OR Procedure   DRG Non-OR Procedure   Valid OR Procedure   HAC Associated Procedure   Combination Only   New/Revised April   New/Revised October

196   ICD-10-PCS 2024

Ø31–Ø31

Ø   **Medical and Surgical**   *Ø31 Continued*
3   **Upper Arteries**
1   **Bypass**   Definition: Altering the route of passage of the contents of a tubular body part

                      Explanation: Rerouting contents of a body part to a downstream area of the normal route, to a similar route and body part, or to an abnormal route and dissimilar body part. Includes one or more anastomoses, with or without the use of a device.

Body Part Character 4	Approach Character 5	Device Character 6	Qualifier Character 7

8 Brachial Artery, Left
  Inferior ulnar collateral artery
  Profunda brachii
  Superior ulnar collateral artery
	Ø Open	**9** Autologous Venous Tissue
		A Autologous Arterial Tissue
		J Synthetic Substitute
		K Nonautologous Tissue Substitute
		Z No Device
			1 Upper Arm Artery, Left
			4 Lower Arm Artery, Left
			D Upper Arm Vein
			F Lower Arm Vein
			V Superior Vena Cava
			W Lower Extremity Vein

8 Brachial Artery, Left
  Inferior ulnar collateral artery
  Profunda brachii
  Superior ulnar collateral artery
	3 Percutaneous	**Z** No Device	**F** Lower Arm Vein

9 Ulnar Artery, Right
  Anterior ulnar recurrent artery
  Common interosseous artery
  Posterior ulnar recurrent artery
B Radial Artery, Right
  Radial recurrent artery
	Ø Open	**9** Autologous Venous Tissue
		A Autologous Arterial Tissue
		J Synthetic Substitute
		K Nonautologous Tissue Substitute
		Z No Device
			3 Lower Arm Artery, Right
			F Lower Arm Vein

9 Ulnar Artery, Right
  Anterior ulnar recurrent artery
  Common interosseous artery
  Posterior ulnar recurrent artery
B Radial Artery, Right
  Radial recurrent artery
	3 Percutaneous	**Z** No Device	**F** Lower Arm Vein

A Ulnar Artery, Left
  Anterior ulnar recurrent artery
  Common interosseous artery
  Posterior ulnar recurrent artery
C Radial Artery, Left
  Radial recurrent artery
	Ø Open	**9** Autologous Venous Tissue
		A Autologous Arterial Tissue
		J Synthetic Substitute
		K Nonautologous Tissue Substitute
		Z No Device
			4 Lower Arm Artery, Left
			F Lower Arm Vein

A Ulnar Artery, Left
  Anterior ulnar recurrent artery
  Common interosseous artery
  Posterior ulnar recurrent artery
C Radial Artery, Left
  Radial recurrent artery
	3 Percutaneous	**Z** No Device	**F** Lower Arm Vein

G Intracranial Artery
  Anterior cerebral artery
  Anterior choroidal artery
  Anterior communicating artery
  Basilar artery
  Circle of Willis
  Internal carotid artery, intracranial
    portion
  Middle cerebral artery
  Middle meningeal artery, intracranial
    portion
  Ophthalmic artery
  Posterior cerebral artery
  Posterior communicating artery
  Posterior inferior cerebellar artery
    (PICA)
  Vertebral artery, intracranial portion
S Temporal Artery, Right
  Middle temporal artery
  Superficial temporal artery
  Transverse facial artery
T Temporal Artery, Left
  See S Temporal Artery, Right
	Ø Open	**9** Autologous Venous Tissue
		A Autologous Arterial Tissue
		J Synthetic Substitute
		K Nonautologous Tissue Substitute
		Z No Device
			G Intracranial Artery

H Common Carotid Artery, Right **J** Common Carotid Artery, Left	**Ø** Open	**9** Autologous Venous Tissue **A** Autologous Arterial Tissue **J** Synthetic Substitute **K** Nonautologous Tissue Substitute **Z** No Device	**G** Intracranial Artery **J** Extracranial Artery, Right **K** Extracranial Artery, Left **Y** Upper Artery

Ø31 Continued on next page

NC Noncovered Procedure   **LC** Limited Coverage   **QA** Questionable OB Admit   **NT** New Tech Add-on   ⊞ Combination Member   ♂ Male   ♀ Female

ICD-10-PCS 2024   197

Ø31–Ø31

Ø   Medical and Surgical
3   Upper Arteries
1   Bypass   Definition: Altering the route of passage of the contents of a tubular body part

Ø31 Continued

Explanation: Rerouting contents of a body part to a downstream area of the normal route, to a similar route and body part, or to an abnormal route and dissimilar body part. Includes one or more anastomoses, with or without the use of a device.

Body Part Character 4	Approach Character 5	Device Character 6	Qualifier Character 7

K **Internal Carotid Artery, Right**
    Caroticotympanic artery
    Carotid sinus
L **Internal Carotid Artery, Left**
    Caroticotympanic artery
    Carotid sinus
M **External Carotid Artery, Right**
    Ascending pharyngeal artery
    Internal maxillary artery
    Lingual artery
    Maxillary artery
    Occipital artery
    Posterior auricular artery
    Superior thyroid artery
N **External Carotid Artery, Left**
    Ascending pharyngeal artery
    Internal maxillary artery
    Lingual artery
    Maxillary artery
    Occipital artery
    Posterior auricular artery
    Superior thyroid artery
	Ø Open	**9** Autologous Venous Tissue
		A Autologous Arterial Tissue
		J Synthetic Substitute
		K Nonautologous Tissue Substitute
		Z No Device
			J Extracranial Artery, Right
			K Extracranial Artery, Left

Non-OR Procedure   DRG Non-OR Procedure   Valid OR Procedure   HAC Associated Procedure   Combination Only   New/Revised April   New/Revised October

198   ICD-10-PCS 2024

Ø31–Ø31

Ø   Medical and Surgical
3   Upper Arteries
5   Destruction   Definition: Physical eradication of all or a portion of a body part by the direct use of energy, force, or a destructive agent
                        Explanation: None of the body part is physically taken out

Body Part Character 4		Approach Character 5	Device Character 6	Qualifier Character 7
Ø Internal Mammary Artery, Right Anterior intercostal artery Internal thoracic artery Musculophrenic artery Pericardiophrenic artery Superior epigastric artery **1 Internal Mammary Artery, Left** *See Ø Internal Mammary Artery, Right* **2 Innominate Artery** Brachiocephalic artery Brachiocephalic trunk **3 Subclavian Artery, Right** Costocervical trunk Dorsal scapular artery Internal thoracic artery **4 Subclavian Artery, Left** *See 3 Subclavian Artery, Right* **5 Axillary Artery, Right** Anterior circumflex humeral artery Lateral thoracic artery Posterior circumflex humeral artery Subscapular artery Superior thoracic artery Thoracoacromial artery **6 Axillary Artery, Left** *See 5 Axillary Artery, Right* **7 Brachial Artery, Right** Inferior ulnar collateral artery Profunda brachii Superior ulnar collateral artery **8 Brachial Artery, Left** *See 7 Brachial Artery, Right* **9 Ulnar Artery, Right** Anterior ulnar recurrent artery Common interosseous artery Posterior ulnar recurrent artery **A Ulnar Artery, Left** *See 9 Ulnar Artery, Right* **B Radial Artery, Right** Radial recurrent artery **C Radial Artery, Left** *See B Radial Artery, Right* **D Hand Artery, Right** Deep palmar arch Princeps pollicis artery Radialis indicis Superficial palmar arch **F Hand Artery, Left** *See D Hand Artery, Right* **G Intracranial Artery** Anterior cerebral artery Anterior choroidal artery Anterior communicating artery Basilar artery Circle of Willis Internal carotid artery, intracranial portion Middle cerebral artery Middle meningeal artery, intracranial portion Ophthalmic artery Posterior cerebral artery Posterior communicating artery Posterior inferior cerebellar artery (PICA) Vertebral artery, intracranial portion	**H Common Carotid Artery, Right** **J Common Carotid Artery, Left** **K Internal Carotid Artery, Right** Caroticotympanic artery Carotid sinus **L Internal Carotid Artery, Left** *See K Internal Carotid Artery, Right* **M External Carotid Artery, Right** Ascending pharyngeal artery Internal maxillary artery Lingual artery Maxillary artery Occipital artery Posterior auricular artery Superior thyroid artery **N External Carotid Artery, Left** *See M External Carotid Artery, Right* **P Vertebral Artery, Right** Anterior spinal artery Posterior spinal artery **Q Vertebral Artery, Left** *See P Vertebral Artery, Right* **R Face Artery** Angular artery Ascending palatine artery External maxillary artery Facial artery Inferior labial artery Submental artery Superior labial artery **S Temporal Artery, Right** Middle temporal artery Superficial temporal artery Transverse facial artery **T Temporal Artery, Left** *See S Temporal Artery, Right* **U Thyroid Artery, Right** Cricothyroid artery Hyoid artery Sternocleidomastoid artery Superior laryngeal artery Superior thyroid artery Thyrocervical trunk **V Thyroid Artery, Left** *See U Thyroid Artery, Right* **Y Upper Artery** Aortic intercostal artery Bronchial artery Esophageal artery Subcostal artery	**Ø Open** **3 Percutaneous** **4 Percutaneous Endoscopic**	**Z No Device**	**Z No Qualifier**

NC Noncovered Procedure   **LC** Limited Coverage   **QA** Questionable OB Admit   **NT** New Tech Add-on   ⊞ Combination Member   ♂ Male   ♀ Female

ICD-10-PCS 2024   **199**

Ø Medical and Surgical
3 Upper Arteries
7 Dilation   Definition: Expanding an orifice or the lumen of a tubular body part

Explanation: The orifice can be a natural orifice or an artificially created orifice. Accomplished by stretching a tubular body part using intraluminal pressure or by cutting part of the orifice or wall of the tubular body part.

Body Part Character 4		Approach Character 5	Device Character 6	Qualifier Character 7
Ø Internal Mammary Artery, Right Anterior intercostal artery Internal thoracic artery Musculophrenic artery Pericardiophrenic artery Superior epigastric artery **1 Internal Mammary Artery, Left** *See Ø Internal Mammary Artery, Right* **2 Innominate Artery** Brachiocephalic artery Brachiocephalic trunk **3 Subclavian Artery, Right** Costocervical trunk Dorsal scapular artery Internal thoracic artery **4 Subclavian Artery, Left** *See 3 Subclavian Artery, Right* **5 Axillary Artery, Right** Anterior circumflex humeral artery Lateral thoracic artery Posterior circumflex humeral artery Subscapular artery Superior thoracic artery Thoracoacromial artery	**6 Axillary Artery, Left** *See 5 Axillary Artery, Right* **7 Brachial Artery, Right** Inferior ulnar collateral artery Profunda brachii Superior ulnar collateral artery **8 Brachial Artery, Left** *See 7 Brachial Artery, Right* **9 Ulnar Artery, Right** Anterior ulnar recurrent artery Common interosseous artery Posterior ulnar recurrent artery **A Ulnar Artery, Left** *See 9 Ulnar Artery, Right* **B Radial Artery, Right** Radial recurrent artery **C Radial Artery, Left** *See B Radial Artery, Right*	**Ø Open** **3 Percutaneous** **4 Percutaneous Endoscopic**	**4 Intraluminal Device, Drug-eluting** **5 Intraluminal Device, Drug-eluting, Two** **6 Intraluminal Device, Drug-eluting, Three** **7 Intraluminal Device, Drug-eluting, Four or More** **E Intraluminal Device, Two** **F Intraluminal Device, Three** **G Intraluminal Device, Four or More**	**Z No Qualifier**
Ø Internal Mammary Artery, Right Anterior intercostal artery Internal thoracic artery Musculophrenic artery Pericardiophrenic artery Superior epigastric artery **1 Internal Mammary Artery, Left** *See Ø Internal Mammary Artery, Right* **2 Innominate Artery** Brachiocephalic artery Brachiocephalic trunk **3 Subclavian Artery, Right** Costocervical trunk Dorsal scapular artery Internal thoracic artery **4 Subclavian Artery, Left** *See 3 Subclavian Artery, Right* **5 Axillary Artery, Right** Anterior circumflex humeral artery Lateral thoracic artery Posterior circumflex humeral artery Subscapular artery Superior thoracic artery Thoracoacromial artery	**6 Axillary Artery, Left** *See 5 Axillary Artery, Right* **7 Brachial Artery, Right** Inferior ulnar collateral artery Profunda brachii Superior ulnar collateral artery **8 Brachial Artery, Left** *See 7 Brachial Artery, Right* **9 Ulnar Artery, Right** Anterior ulnar recurrent artery Common interosseous artery Posterior ulnar recurrent artery **A Ulnar Artery, Left** *See 9 Ulnar Artery, Right* **B Radial Artery, Right** Radial recurrent artery **C Radial Artery, Left** *See B Radial Artery, Right*	**Ø Open** **3 Percutaneous** **4 Percutaneous Endoscopic**	**D Intraluminal Device** **Z No Device**	**1 Drug-Coated Balloon** **Z No Qualifier**

Ø37 Continued on next page

Non-OR Procedure   DRG Non-OR Procedure   Valid OR Procedure   HAC Associated Procedure   Combination Only   New/Revised April   New/Revised October

Ø   **Medical and Surgical**   *Ø37 Continued*
3   **Upper Arteries**
7   **Dilation**   Definition: Expanding an orifice or the lumen of a tubular body part

Explanation: The orifice can be a natural orifice or an artificially created orifice. Accomplished by stretching a tubular body part using intraluminal pressure or by cutting part of the orifice or wall of the tubular body part.

Body Part Character 4		Approach Character 5	Device Character 6	Qualifier Character 7

D Hand Artery, Right
Deep palmar arch
Princeps pollicis artery
Radialis indicis
Superficial palmar arch
F Hand Artery, Left
See D Hand Artery, Right
G Intracranial Artery NC
Anterior cerebral artery
Anterior choroidal artery
Anterior communicating
   artery
Basilar artery
Circle of Willis
Internal carotid artery,
   intracranial portion
Middle cerebral artery
Middle meningeal artery,
   intracranial portion
Ophthalmic artery
Posterior cerebral artery
Posterior communicating
   artery
Posterior inferior cerebellar
   artery (PICA)
Vertebral artery, intracranial
   portion
**H Common Carotid Artery,
   Right**
J Common Carotid Artery, Left
K Internal Carotid Artery, Right
Caroticotympanic artery
Carotid sinus
L Internal Carotid Artery, Left
*See K Internal Carotid Artery,
   Right*
M External Carotid Artery, Right
Ascending pharyngeal artery
Internal maxillary artery
Lingual artery
Maxillary artery
Occipital artery
Posterior auricular artery
Superior thyroid artery
	N External Carotid Artery, Left
	*See M External Carotid Artery,
	   Right*
	P Vertebral Artery, Right
	Anterior spinal artery
	Posterior spinal artery
	Q Vertebral Artery, Left
	See P Vertebral Artery, Right
	R Face Artery
	Angular artery
	Ascending palatine artery
	External maxillary artery
	Facial artery
	Inferior labial artery
	Submental artery
	Superior labial artery
	S Temporal Artery, Right
	Middle temporal artery
	Superficial temporal artery
	Transverse facial artery
	T Temporal Artery, Left
	See S Temporal Artery, Right
	U Thyroid Artery, Right
	Cricothyroid artery
	Hyoid artery
	Sternocleidomastoid artery
	Superior laryngeal artery
	Superior thyroid artery
	Thyrocervical trunk
	V Thyroid Artery, Left
	See U Thyroid Artery, Right
	Y Upper Artery
	Aortic intercostal artery
	Bronchial artery
	Esophageal artery
	Subcostal artery
		Ø Open
		3 Percutaneous
		4 Percutaneous Endoscopic
			**4 Intraluminal Device,
			   Drug-eluting**
			**5 Intraluminal Device, Drug-
			   eluting, Two**
			**6 Intraluminal Device, Drug-
			   eluting, Three**
			**7 Intraluminal Device, Drug-
			   eluting, Four or More**
			D Intraluminal Device
			E Intraluminal Device, Two
			F Intraluminal Device, Three
			**G Intraluminal Device, Four
			   or More**
			Z No Device
				Z No Qualifier

NC   Ø37G[3,4]ZZ

NC Noncovered Procedure   LC Limited Coverage   QA Questionable OB Admit   NT New Tech Add-on   ⊞ Combination Member   ♂ Male   ♀ Female

ICD-10-PCS 2024   201

Ø37–Ø37

Ø   Medical and Surgical
3   Upper Arteries
9   Drainage   Definition: Taking or letting out fluids and/or gases from a body part

Explanation: The qualifier DIAGNOSTIC is used to identify drainage procedures that are biopsies

Body Part Character 4		Approach Character 5	Device Character 6	Qualifier Character 7
Ø Internal Mammary Artery, Right Anterior intercostal artery Internal thoracic artery Musculophrenic artery Pericardiophrenic artery Superior epigastric artery **1 Internal Mammary Artery, Left** *See Ø Internal Mammary Artery, Right above* **2 Innominate Artery** Brachiocephalic artery Brachiocephalic trunk **3 Subclavian Artery, Right** Costocervical trunk Dorsal scapular artery Internal thoracic artery **4 Subclavian Artery, Left** *See 3 Subclavian Artery, Right* **5 Axillary Artery, Right** Anterior circumflex humeral artery Lateral thoracic artery Posterior circumflex humeral artery Subscapular artery Superior thoracic artery Thoracoacromial artery **6 Axillary Artery, Left** *See 5 Axillary Artery, Right* **7 Brachial Artery, Right** Inferior ulnar collateral artery Profunda brachii Superior ulnar collateral artery **8 Brachial Artery, Left** *See 7 Brachial Artery, Right* **9 Ulnar Artery, Right** Anterior ulnar recurrent artery Common interosseous artery Posterior ulnar recurrent artery **A Ulnar Artery, Left** *See 9 Ulnar Artery, Right* **B Radial Artery, Right** Radial recurrent artery **C Radial Artery, Left** *See B Radial Artery, Right* **D Hand Artery, Right** Deep palmar arch Princeps pollicis artery Radialis indicis Superficial palmar arch **F Hand Artery, Left** *See D Hand Artery, Right* **G Intracranial Artery** Anterior cerebral artery Anterior choroidal artery Anterior communicating artery Basilar artery Circle of Willis Internal carotid artery, intracranial portion Middle cerebral artery Middle meningeal artery, intracranial portion Ophthalmic artery Posterior cerebral artery Posterior communicating artery Posterior inferior cerebellar artery (PICA) Vertebral artery, intracranial portion	**H Common Carotid Artery, Right** **J Common Carotid Artery, Left** **K Internal Carotid Artery, Right** Caroticotympanic artery Carotid sinus **L Internal Carotid Artery, Left** *See K Internal Carotid Artery, Right* **M External Carotid Artery, Right** Ascending pharyngeal artery Internal maxillary artery Lingual artery Maxillary artery Occipital artery Posterior auricular artery Superior thyroid artery **N External Carotid Artery, Left** *See M External Carotid Artery, Right* **P Vertebral Artery, Right** Anterior spinal artery Posterior spinal artery **Q Vertebral Artery, Left** *See P Vertebral Artery, Right* **R Face Artery** Angular artery Ascending palatine artery External maxillary artery Facial artery Inferior labial artery Submental artery Superior labial artery **S Temporal Artery, Right** Middle temporal artery Superficial temporal artery Transverse facial artery **T Temporal Artery, Left** *See S Temporal Artery, Right* **U Thyroid Artery, Right** Cricothyroid artery Hyoid artery Sternocleidomastoid artery Superior laryngeal artery Superior thyroid artery Thyrocervical trunk **V Thyroid Artery, Left** *See U Thyroid Artery, Right* **Y Upper Artery** Aortic intercostal artery Bronchial artery Esophageal artery Subcostal artery	**Ø Open** **3 Percutaneous** **4 Percutaneous Endoscopic**	**Ø Drainage Device**	**Z No Qualifier**

Non-OR   Ø39[Ø,1,2,3,4,5,6,7,8,9,A,B,C,D,F,G,H,J,K,L,M,N,P,Q,R,S,T,U,V,Y][Ø,3,4]ØZ

Ø39 Continued on next page

Non-OR Procedure   DRG Non-OR Procedure   Valid OR Procedure   HAC Associated Procedure   Combination Only   New/Revised April   New/Revised October

0　Medical and Surgical
3　Upper Arteries
9　Drainage　　Definition: Taking or letting out fluids and/or gases from a body part

039 Continued

Explanation: The qualifier DIAGNOSTIC is used to identify drainage procedures that are biopsies

Body Part — Character 4	Approach — Character 5	Device — Character 6	Qualifier — Character 7
0 Internal Mammary Artery, Right Anterior intercostal artery Internal thoracic artery Musculophrenic artery Pericardiophrenic artery Superior epigastric artery **1** Internal Mammary Artery, Left *See 0 Internal Mammary Artery, Right* **2** Innominate Artery Brachiocephalic artery Brachiocephalic trunk **3** Subclavian Artery, Right Costocervical trunk Dorsal scapular artery Internal thoracic artery **4** Subclavian Artery, Left *See 3 Subclavian Artery, Right* **5** Axillary Artery, Right Anterior circumflex humeral artery Lateral thoracic artery Posterior circumflex humeral artery Subscapular artery Superior thoracic artery Thoracoacromial artery **6** Axillary Artery, Left *See 5 Axillary Artery, Right* **7** Brachial Artery, Right Inferior ulnar collateral artery Profunda brachii Superior ulnar collateral artery **8** Brachial Artery, Left *See 7 Brachial Artery, Right* **9** Ulnar Artery, Right Anterior ulnar recurrent artery Common interosseous artery Posterior ulnar recurrent artery **A** Ulnar Artery, Left *See 9 Ulnar Artery, Right* **B** Radial Artery, Right Radial recurrent artery **C** Radial Artery, Left *See B Radial Artery, Right* **D** Hand Artery, Right Deep palmar arch Princeps pollicis artery Radialis indicis Superficial palmar arch **F** Hand Artery, Left *See D Hand Artery, Right* **G** Intracranial Artery Anterior cerebral artery Anterior choroidal artery Anterior communicating artery Basilar artery Circle of Willis Internal carotid artery, intracranial portion Middle cerebral artery Middle meningeal artery, intracranial portion Ophthalmic artery Posterior cerebral artery Posterior communicating artery Posterior inferior cerebellar artery (PICA) Vertebral artery, intracranial portion **H** Common Carotid Artery, Right **J** Common Carotid Artery, Left **K** Internal Carotid Artery, Right Caroticotympanic artery Carotid sinus **L** Internal Carotid Artery, Left *See K Internal Carotid Artery, Right* **M** External Carotid Artery, Right Ascending pharyngeal artery Internal maxillary artery Lingual artery Maxillary artery Occipital artery Posterior auricular artery Superior thyroid artery **N** External Carotid Artery, Left *See M External Carotid Artery, Right* **P** Vertebral Artery, Right Anterior spinal artery Posterior spinal artery **Q** Vertebral Artery, Left *See P Vertebral Artery, Right* **R** Face Artery Angular artery Ascending palatine artery External maxillary artery Facial artery Inferior labial artery Submental artery Superior labial artery **S** Temporal Artery, Right Middle temporal artery Superficial temporal artery Transverse facial artery **T** Temporal Artery, Left *See S Temporal Artery, Right* **U** Thyroid Artery, Right Cricothyroid artery Hyoid artery Sternocleidomastoid artery Superior laryngeal artery Superior thyroid artery Thyrocervical trunk **V** Thyroid Artery, Left *See U Thyroid Artery, Right* **Y** Upper Artery Aortic intercostal artery Bronchial artery Esophageal artery Subcostal artery	**0** Open **3** Percutaneous **4** Percutaneous Endoscopic	**Z** No Device	**X** Diagnostic **Z** No Qualifier

Non-OR 039[0,1,2,3,4,5,6,7,8,9,A,B,C,D,F,G,H,J,K,L,M,N,P,Q,R,S,T,U,V,Y]3ZX
Non-OR 039[0,1,2,3,4,5,6,7,8,9,A,B,C,D,F,G,H,J,K,L,M,N,P,Q,R,S,T,U,V,Y][0,3,4]ZZ

Upper Arteries

Ø **Medical and Surgical**
3 **Upper Arteries**
B **Excision**   Definition: Cutting out or off, without replacement, a portion of a body part
                 Explanation: The qualifier DIAGNOSTIC is used to identify excision procedures that are biopsies

Body Part Character 4		Approach Character 5	Device Character 6	Qualifier Character 7
Ø **Internal Mammary Artery, Right** Anterior intercostal artery Internal thoracic artery Musculophrenic artery Pericardiophrenic artery Superior epigastric artery 1 **Internal Mammary Artery, Left** *See* Ø *Internal Mammary Artery, Right* 2 **Innominate Artery** Brachiocephalic artery Brachiocephalic trunk 3 **Subclavian Artery, Right** Costocervical trunk Dorsal scapular artery Internal thoracic artery 4 **Subclavian Artery, Left** *See* 3 *Subclavian Artery, Right* 5 **Axillary Artery, Right** Anterior circumflex humeral artery Lateral thoracic artery Posterior circumflex humeral artery Subscapular artery Superior thoracic artery Thoracoacromial artery 6 **Axillary Artery, Left** *See* 5 *Axillary Artery, Right* 7 **Brachial Artery, Right** Inferior ulnar collateral artery Profunda brachii Superior ulnar collateral artery 8 **Brachial Artery, Left** *See* 7 *Brachial Artery, Right* 9 **Ulnar Artery, Right** Anterior ulnar recurrent artery Common interosseous artery Posterior ulnar recurrent artery A **Ulnar Artery, Left** *See* 9 *Ulnar Artery, Right* B **Radial Artery, Right** Radial recurrent artery C **Radial Artery, Left** *See* B *Radial Artery, Right* D **Hand Artery, Right** Deep palmar arch Princeps pollicis artery Radialis indicis Superficial palmar arch F **Hand Artery, Left** *See* D *Hand Artery, Right* G **Intracranial Artery** Anterior cerebral artery Anterior choroidal artery Anterior communicating artery Basilar artery Circle of Willis Internal carotid artery, intracranial portion Middle cerebral artery Middle meningeal artery, intracranial portion Ophthalmic artery Posterior cerebral artery Posterior communicating artery Posterior inferior cerebellar artery (PICA) Vertebral artery, intracranial portion	H **Common Carotid Artery, Right** J **Common Carotid Artery, Left** K **Internal Carotid Artery, Right** Caroticotympanic artery Carotid sinus L **Internal Carotid Artery, Left** *See* K *Internal Carotid Artery, Right* M **External Carotid Artery, Right** Ascending pharyngeal artery Internal maxillary artery Lingual artery Maxillary artery Occipital artery Posterior auricular artery Superior thyroid artery N **External Carotid Artery, Left** *See* M *External Carotid Artery, Right* P **Vertebral Artery, Right** Anterior spinal artery Posterior spinal artery Q **Vertebral Artery, Left** *See* P *Vertebral Artery, Right* R **Face Artery** Angular artery Ascending palatine artery External maxillary artery Facial artery Inferior labial artery Submental artery Superior labial artery S **Temporal Artery, Right** Middle temporal artery Superficial temporal artery Transverse facial artery T **Temporal Artery, Left** *See* S *Temporal Artery, Right* U **Thyroid Artery, Right** Cricothyroid artery Hyoid artery Sternocleidomastoid artery Superior laryngeal artery Superior thyroid artery Thyrocervical trunk V **Thyroid Artery, Left** *See* U *Thyroid Artery, Right* Y **Upper Artery** Aortic intercostal artery Bronchial artery Esophageal artery Subcostal artery	Ø Open 3 Percutaneous 4 Percutaneous Endoscopic	Z No Device	X Diagnostic Z No Qualifier

Non-OR Procedure   DRG Non-OR Procedure   Valid OR Procedure   HAC Associated Procedure   Combination Only   New/Revised April   New/Revised October

204   ICD-10-PCS 2024

Ø   **Medical and Surgical**
3   **Upper Arteries**
C   **Extirpation**   Definition: Taking or cutting out solid matter from a body part

Explanation: The solid matter may be an abnormal byproduct of a biological function or a foreign body; it may be imbedded in a body part or in the lumen of a tubular body part. The solid matter may or may not have been previously broken into pieces.

Body Part — Character 4		Approach — Character 5	Device — Character 6	Qualifier — Character 7
Ø **Internal Mammary Artery, Right** Anterior intercostal artery Internal thoracic artery Musculophrenic artery Pericardiophrenic artery Superior epigastric artery **1** **Internal Mammary Artery, Left** *See Ø Internal Mammary Artery, Right* **2** **Innominate Artery** Brachiocephalic artery Brachiocephalic trunk **3** **Subclavian Artery, Right** Costocervical trunk Dorsal scapular artery Internal thoracic artery **4** **Subclavian Artery, Left** *See 3 Subclavian Artery, Right* **5** **Axillary Artery, Right** Anterior circumflex humeral artery Lateral thoracic artery Posterior circumflex humeral artery Subscapular artery Superior thoracic artery Thoracoacromial artery **6** **Axillary Artery, Left** *See 5 Axillary Artery, Right* **7** **Brachial Artery, Right** Inferior ulnar collateral artery Profunda brachii Superior ulnar collateral artery **8** **Brachial Artery, Left** *See 7 Brachial Artery, Right* **9** **Ulnar Artery, Right** Anterior ulnar recurrent artery Common interosseous artery Posterior ulnar recurrent artery	**A** **Ulnar Artery, Left** *See 9 Ulnar Artery, Right* **B** **Radial Artery, Right** Radial recurrent artery **C** **Radial Artery, Left** *See B Radial Artery, Right* **D** **Hand Artery, Right** Deep palmar arch Princeps pollicis artery Radialis indicis Superficial palmar arch **F** **Hand Artery, Left** *See D Hand Artery, Right* **R** **Face Artery** Angular artery Ascending palatine artery External maxillary artery Facial artery Inferior labial artery Submental artery Superior labial artery **S** **Temporal Artery, Right** Middle temporal artery Superficial temporal artery Transverse facial artery **T** **Temporal Artery, Left** *See S Temporal Artery, Right* **U** **Thyroid Artery, Right** Cricothyroid artery Hyoid artery Sternocleidomastoid artery Superior laryngeal artery Superior thyroid artery Thyrocervical trunk **V** **Thyroid Artery, Left** *See U Thyroid Artery, Right* **Y** **Upper Artery** Aortic intercostal artery Bronchial artery Esophageal artery Subcostal artery	**Ø** Open **3** Percutaneous **4** Percutaneous Endoscopic	**Z** No Device	**Z** No Qualifier
G **Intracranial Artery** Anterior cerebral artery Anterior choroidal artery Anterior communicating artery Basilar artery Circle of Willis Internal carotid artery, intracranial portion Middle cerebral artery Middle meningeal artery, intracranial portion Ophthalmic artery Posterior cerebral artery Posterior communicating artery Posterior inferior cerebellar artery (PICA) Vertebral artery, intracranial portion **H** **Common Carotid Artery, Right** **J** **Common Carotid Artery, Left** **K** **Internal Carotid Artery, Right** Caroticotympanic artery Carotid sinus	**L** **Internal Carotid Artery, Left** *See K Internal Carotid Artery, Right* **M** **External Carotid Artery, Right** Ascending pharyngeal artery Internal maxillary artery Lingual artery Maxillary artery Occipital artery Posterior auricular artery Superior thyroid artery **N** **External Carotid Artery, Left** *See M External Carotid Artery, Right* **P** **Vertebral Artery, Right** Anterior spinal artery Posterior spinal artery **Q** **Vertebral Artery, Left** *See P Vertebral Artery, Right*	**Ø** Open **4** Percutaneous Endoscopic	**Z** No Device	**Z** No Qualifier

03C Continued on next page

NC Noncovered Procedure   **LC** Limited Coverage   **QA** Questionable OB Admit   **NT** New Tech Add-on   ⊞ Combination Member   ♂ Male   ♀ Female

ICD-10-PCS 2024   205

03C–03C

0   **Medical and Surgical**   *03C Continued*
3   **Upper Arteries**
C   **Extirpation**   Definition: Taking or cutting out solid matter from a body part

Explanation: The solid matter may be an abnormal byproduct of a biological function or a foreign body; it may be imbedded in a body part or in the lumen of a tubular body part. The solid matter may or may not have been previously broken into pieces.

Body Part Character 4		Approach Character 5	Device Character 6	Qualifier Character 7

G **Intracranial Artery**
  Anterior cerebral artery
  Anterior choroidal artery
  Anterior communicating
    artery
  Basilar artery
  Circle of Willis
  Internal carotid artery,
    intracranial portion
  Middle cerebral artery
  Middle meningeal artery,
    intracranial portion
  Ophthalmic artery
  Posterior cerebral artery
  Posterior communicating
    artery
  Posterior inferior cerebellar
    artery (PICA)
  Vertebral artery, intracranial
    portion
H **Common Carotid Artery,
    Right**
J **Common Carotid Artery, Left**
K **Internal Carotid Artery, Right**
  Caroticotympanic artery
  Carotid sinus
	L **Internal Carotid Artery, Left**
	  *See K Internal Carotid Artery,
	    Right*
	M **External Carotid Artery, Right**
	  Ascending pharyngeal artery
	  Internal maxillary artery
	  Lingual artery
	  Maxillary artery
	  Occipital artery
	  Posterior auricular artery
	  Superior thyroid artery
	N **External Carotid Artery, Left**
	  *See M External Carotid Artery,
	    Right*
	P **Vertebral Artery, Right**
	  Anterior spinal artery
	  Posterior spinal artery
	Q **Vertebral Artery, Left**
	  See P Vertebral Artery, Right
		3 Percutaneous	**Z** No Device	**7** Stent Retriever
				Z No Qualifier

0   **Medical and Surgical**
3   **Upper Arteries**
F   **Fragmentation**   Definition: Breaking solid matter in a body part into pieces

Explanation: Physical force (e.g., manual, ultrasonic) applied directly or indirectly is used to break the solid matter into pieces. The solid matter may be an abnormal byproduct of a biological function or a foreign body. The pieces of solid matter are not taken out.

Body Part Character 4		Approach Character 5	Device Character 6	Qualifier Character 7

2 **Innominate Artery**
  Brachiocephalic artery
  Brachiocephalic trunk
3 **Subclavian Artery, Right**
  Costocervical trunk
  Dorsal scapular artery
  Internal thoracic artery
4 **Subclavian Artery, Left**
  See 3 Subclavian Artery, Right
5 **Axillary Artery, Right**
  Anterior circumflex humeral
    artery
  Lateral thoracic artery
  Posterior circumflex humeral
    artery
  Subscapular artery
  Superior thoracic artery
  Thoracoacromial artery
6 **Axillary Artery, Left**
  See 5 Axillary Artery, Right
7 **Brachial Artery, Right**
  Inferior ulnar collateral artery
  Profunda brachii
  Superior ulnar collateral artery
8 **Brachial Artery, Left**
  See 7 Brachial Artery, Right
9 **Ulnar Artery, Right**
  Anterior ulnar recurrent artery
  Common interosseous artery
  Posterior ulnar recurrent
    artery
	A **Ulnar Artery, Left**
	  See 9 Ulnar Artery, Right
	B **Radial Artery, Right**
	  Radial recurrent artery
	C **Radial Artery, Left**
	  See B Radial Artery, Right
	G **Intracranial Artery**
	  Anterior cerebral artery
	  Anterior choroidal artery
	  Anterior communicating artery
	  Basilar artery
	  Circle of Willis
	  Internal carotid artery,
	    intracranial portion
	  Middle cerebral artery
	  Middle meningeal artery,
	    intracranial portion
	  Ophthalmic artery
	  Posterior cerebral artery
	  Posterior communicating
	    artery
	  Posterior inferior cerebellar
	    artery (PICA)
	  Vertebral artery, intracranial
	    portion
	Y **Upper Artery**
	  Aortic intercostal artery
	  Bronchial artery
	  Esophageal artery
	  Subcostal artery
		3 Percutaneous	**Z** No Device	**0** Ultrasonic
				Z No Qualifier

Non-OR Procedure   DRG Non-OR Procedure   Valid OR Procedure   HAC Associated Procedure   Combination Only   New/Revised April   New/Revised October

206   ICD-10-PCS 2024

Ø   Medical and Surgical
3   Upper Arteries
H   Insertion

Definition: Putting in a nonbiological appliance that monitors, assists, performs, or prevents a physiological function but does not physically take the place of a body part

Explanation: None

Body Part Character 4		Approach Character 5	Device Character 6	Qualifier Character 7
Ø Internal Mammary Artery, Right Anterior intercostal artery Internal thoracic artery Musculophrenic artery Pericardiophrenic artery Superior epigastric artery **1 Internal Mammary Artery, Left** *See Ø Internal Mammary Artery, Right* **2 Innominate Artery** Brachiocephalic artery Brachiocephalic trunk **3 Subclavian Artery, Right** Costocervical trunk Dorsal scapular artery Internal thoracic artery **4 Subclavian Artery, Left** *See 3 Subclavian Artery, Right* **5 Axillary Artery, Right** Anterior circumflex humeral artery Lateral thoracic artery Posterior circumflex humeral artery Subscapular artery Superior thoracic artery Thoracoacromial artery **6 Axillary Artery, Left** *See 5 Axillary Artery, Right* **7 Brachial Artery, Right** Inferior ulnar collateral artery Profunda brachii Superior ulnar collateral artery **8 Brachial Artery, Left** *See 7 Brachial Artery, Right* **9 Ulnar Artery, Right** Anterior ulnar recurrent artery Common interosseous artery Posterior ulnar recurrent artery **A Ulnar Artery, Left** *See 9 Ulnar Artery, Right* **B Radial Artery, Right** Radial recurrent artery **C Radial Artery, Left** *See B Radial Artery, Right* **D Hand Artery, Right** Deep palmar arch Princeps pollicis artery Radialis indicis Superficial palmar arch **F Hand Artery, Left** *See D Hand Artery, Right*	**G Intracranial Artery** Anterior cerebral artery Anterior choroidal artery Anterior communicating artery Basilar artery Circle of Willis Internal carotid artery, intracranial portion Middle cerebral artery Middle meningeal artery, intracranial portion Ophthalmic artery Posterior cerebral artery Posterior communicating artery Posterior inferior cerebellar artery (PICA) Vertebral artery, intracranial portion **H Common Carotid Artery, Right** **J Common Carotid Artery, Left** **M External Carotid Artery, Right** Ascending pharyngeal artery Internal maxillary artery Lingual artery Maxillary artery Occipital artery Posterior auricular artery Superior thyroid artery **N External Carotid Artery, Left** *See M External Carotid Artery, Right* **P Vertebral Artery, Right** Anterior spinal artery Posterior spinal artery **Q Vertebral Artery, Left** *See P Vertebral Artery, Right* **R Face Artery** Angular artery Ascending palatine artery External maxillary artery Facial artery Inferior labial artery Submental artery Superior labial artery **S Temporal Artery, Right** Middle temporal artery Superficial temporal artery Transverse facial artery **T Temporal Artery, Left** *See S Temporal Artery, Right* **U Thyroid Artery, Right** Cricothyroid artery Hyoid artery Sternocleidomastoid artery Superior laryngeal artery Superior thyroid artery Thyrocervical trunk **V Thyroid Artery, Left** *See U Thyroid Artery, Right*	**Ø Open** **3 Percutaneous** **4 Percutaneous Endoscopic**	**3 Infusion Device** **D Intraluminal Device**	**Z No Qualifier**

Non-OR	Ø3H[Ø,1,2,3,4,5,6,7,8,9,A,B,C,D,F,G,H,J,M,N,P,Q,R,S,T,U,V][Ø,3,4]3Z

Ø3H Continued on next page

NC Noncovered Procedure   LC Limited Coverage   QA Questionable OB Admit   NT New Tech Add-on   ⊞ Combination Member   ♂ Male   ♀ Female

ICD-10-PCS 2024   207

Ø3H–Ø3H

Ø Medical and Surgical
3 Upper Arteries
H Insertion

Ø3H Continued

Definition: Putting in a nonbiological appliance that monitors, assists, performs, or prevents a physiological function but does not physically take the place of a body part

Explanation: None

Body Part Character 4	Approach Character 5	Device Character 6	Qualifier Character 7
K Internal Carotid Artery, Right Caroticotympanic artery Carotid sinus L Internal Carotid Artery, Left *See K Internal Carotid Artery, Right*	Ø Open 3 Percutaneous 4 Percutaneous Endoscope	3 Infusion Device D Intraluminal Device M Stimulator Lead	Z No Qualifier
Y Upper Artery Aortic intercostal artery Bronchial artery Esophageal artery Subcostal artery	Ø Open 3 Percutaneous 4 Percutaneous Endoscopic	2 Monitoring Device 3 Infusion Device D Intraluminal Device Y Other Device	Z No Qualifier

Non-OR	Ø3H[K,L][Ø,3,4]3Z
Non-OR	Ø3HY[Ø,3,4]3Z
Non-OR	Ø3HY32Z
Non-OR	Ø3HY[3,4]YZ

Ø Medical and Surgical
3 Upper Arteries
J Inspection

Definition: Visually and/or manually exploring a body part

Explanation: Visual exploration may be performed with or without optical instrumentation. Manual exploration may be performed directly or through intervening body layers.

Body Part Character 4	Approach Character 5	Device Character 6	Qualifier Character 7
Y Upper Artery Aortic intercostal artery Bronchial artery Esophageal artery Subcostal artery	Ø Open 3 Percutaneous 4 Percutaneous Endoscopic X External	Z No Device	Z No Qualifier

Non-OR	Ø3JY[3,4,X]ZZ

Non-OR Procedure   DRG Non-OR Procedure   Valid OR Procedure   HAC Associated Procedure   Combination Only   New/Revised April   New/Revised October

208

ICD-10-PCS 2024

0 Medical and Surgical
3 Upper Arteries
L Occlusion   Definition: Completely closing an orifice or the lumen of a tubular body part
           Explanation: The orifice can be a natural orifice or an artificially created orifice

Body Part Character 4		Approach Character 5	Device Character 6	Qualifier Character 7
0 Internal Mammary Artery, Right Anterior intercostal artery Internal thoracic artery Musculophrenic artery Pericardiophrenic artery Superior epigastric artery **1 Internal Mammary Artery, Left** *See 0 Internal Mammary Artery, Left* **2 Innominate Artery** Brachiocephalic artery Brachiocephalic trunk **3 Subclavian Artery, Right** Costocervical trunk Dorsal scapular artery Internal thoracic artery **4 Subclavian Artery, Left** *See 3 Subclavian Artery, Right* **5 Axillary Artery, Right** Anterior circumflex humeral artery Lateral thoracic artery Posterior circumflex humeral artery Subscapular artery Superior thoracic artery Thoracoacromial artery **6 Axillary Artery, Left** *See 5 Axillary Artery, Right* **7 Brachial Artery, Right** Inferior ulnar collateral artery Profunda brachii Superior ulnar collateral artery **8 Brachial Artery, Left** *See 7 Brachial Artery, Right* **9 Ulnar Artery, Right** Anterior ulnar recurrent artery Common interosseous artery Posterior ulnar recurrent artery	**A Ulnar Artery, Left** *See 9 Ulnar Artery, Right* **B Radial Artery, Right** Radial recurrent artery **C Radial Artery, Left** *See B Radial Artery, Right* **D Hand Artery, Right** Deep palmar arch Princeps pollicis artery Radialis indicis Superficial palmar arch **F Hand Artery, Left** *See D Hand Artery, Right* **R Face Artery** Angular artery Ascending palatine artery External maxillary artery Facial artery Inferior labial artery Submental artery Superior labial artery **S Temporal Artery, Right** Middle temporal artery Superficial temporal artery Transverse facial artery **T Temporal Artery, Left** *See S Temporal Artery, Right* **U Thyroid Artery, Right** Cricothyroid artery Hyoid artery Sternocleidomastoid artery Superior laryngeal artery Superior thyroid artery Thyrocervical trunk **V Thyroid Artery, Left** *See U Thyroid Artery, Right* **Y Upper Artery** Aortic intercostal artery Bronchial artery Esophageal artery Subcostal artery	**0 Open** **3 Percutaneous** **4 Percutaneous Endoscopic**	**C Extraluminal Device** **D Intraluminal Device** **Z No Device**	**Z No Qualifier**
G Intracranial Artery Anterior cerebral artery Anterior choroidal artery Anterior communicating artery Basilar artery Circle of Willis Internal carotid artery, intracranial portion Middle cerebral artery Middle meningeal artery, intracranial portion Ophthalmic artery Posterior cerebral artery Posterior communicating artery Posterior inferior cerebellar artery (PICA) Vertebral artery, intracranial portion **H Common Carotid Artery, Right** **J Common Carotid Artery, Left** **K Internal Carotid Artery, Right** Caroticotympanic artery Carotid sinus	**L Internal Carotid Artery, Left** *See K Internal Carotid Artery, Right* **M External Carotid Artery, Right** Ascending pharyngeal artery Internal maxillary artery Lingual artery Maxillary artery Occipital artery Posterior auricular artery Superior thyroid artery **N External Carotid Artery, Left** *See M External Carotid Artery, Right* **P Vertebral Artery, Right** Anterior spinal artery Posterior spinal artery **Q Vertebral Artery, Left** *See P Vertebral Artery, Right*	**0 Open** **3 Percutaneous** **4 Percutaneous Endoscopic**	**B Intraluminal Device, Bioactive** **C Extraluminal Device** **D Intraluminal Device** **Z No Device**	**Z No Qualifier**

NC Noncovered Procedure   LC Limited Coverage   OA Questionable OB Admit   NT New Tech Add-on   ⊞ Combination Member   ♂ Male   ♀ Female

ICD-10-PCS 2024   209

03L–03L

Ø Medical and Surgical
3 Upper Arteries
N Release   Definition: Freeing a body part from an abnormal physical constraint by cutting or by the use of force

Explanation: Some of the restraining tissue may be taken out but none of the body part is taken out

Body Part Character 4		Approach Character 5	Device Character 6	Qualifier Character 7
Ø Internal Mammary Artery, Right Anterior intercostal artery Internal thoracic artery Musculophrenic artery Pericardiophrenic artery Superior epigastric artery	**H Common Carotid Artery, Right** **J Common Carotid Artery, Left** **K Internal Carotid Artery, Right** Caroticotympanic artery Carotid sinus	**Ø Open** **3 Percutaneous** **4 Percutaneous Endoscopic**	**Z No Device**	**Z No Qualifier**
1 Internal Mammary Artery, Left *See Ø Internal Mammary Artery, Right*	**L Internal Carotid Artery, Left** *See K Internal Carotid Artery, Right*			
2 Innominate Artery Brachiocephalic artery Brachiocephalic trunk	**M External Carotid Artery, Right** Ascending pharyngeal artery Internal maxillary artery Lingual artery Maxillary artery Occipital artery Posterior auricular artery Superior thyroid artery			
3 Subclavian Artery, Right Costocervical trunk Dorsal scapular artery Internal thoracic artery	**N External Carotid Artery, Left** *See M External Carotid Artery, Right*			
4 Subclavian Artery, Left *See 3 Subclavian Artery, Right*	**P Vertebral Artery, Right** Anterior spinal artery Posterior spinal artery			
5 Axillary Artery, Right Anterior circumflex humeral artery Lateral thoracic artery Posterior circumflex humeral artery Subscapular artery Superior thoracic artery Thoracoacromial artery	**Q Vertebral Artery, Left** *See P Vertebral Artery, Right* **R Face Artery** Angular artery Ascending palatine artery External maxillary artery Facial artery Inferior labial artery Submental artery Superior labial artery			
6 Axillary Artery, Left *See 5 Axillary Artery, Right*	**S Temporal Artery, Right** Middle temporal artery Superficial temporal artery Transverse facial artery			
7 Brachial Artery, Right Inferior ulnar collateral artery Profunda brachii Superior ulnar collateral artery	**T Temporal Artery, Left** *See S Temporal Artery, Right*			
8 Brachial Artery, Left *See 7 Brachial Artery, Right*	**U Thyroid Artery, Right** Cricothyroid artery Hyoid artery Sternocleidomastoid artery Superior laryngeal artery Superior thyroid artery Thyrocervical trunk			
9 Ulnar Artery, Right Anterior ulnar recurrent artery Common interosseous artery Posterior ulnar recurrent artery				
A Ulnar Artery, Left *See 9 Ulnar Artery, Right*	**V Thyroid Artery, Left** *See U Thyroid Artery, Right*			
B Radial Artery, Right Radial recurrent artery	**Y Upper Artery** Aortic intercostal artery Bronchial artery Esophageal artery Subcostal artery			
C Radial Artery, Left *See B Radial Artery, Right*				
D Hand Artery, Right Deep palmar arch Princeps pollicis artery Radialis indicis Superficial palmar arch				
F Hand Artery, Left *See D Hand Artery, Right*				
G Intracranial Artery Anterior cerebral artery Anterior choroidal artery Anterior communicating artery Basilar artery Circle of Willis Internal carotid artery, intracranial portion Middle cerebral artery Middle meningeal artery, intracranial portion Ophthalmic artery Posterior cerebral artery Posterior communicating artery Posterior inferior cerebellar artery (PICA) Vertebral artery, intracranial portion				

Non-OR Procedure   DRG Non-OR Procedure   Valid OR Procedure   HAC Associated Procedure   Combination Only   New/Revised April   New/Revised October

210   ICD-10-PCS 2024

Ø3N–Ø3N

Ø   **Medical and Surgical**
3   **Upper Arteries**
P   **Removal**   Definition: Taking out or off a device from a body part

Explanation: If a device is taken out and a similar device put in without cutting or puncturing the skin or mucous membrane, the procedure is coded to the root operation CHANGE. Otherwise, the procedure for taking out a device is coded to the root operation REMOVAL.

Body Part Character 4	Approach Character 5	Device Character 6	Qualifier Character 7
Y **Upper Artery** Aortic intercostal artery Bronchial artery Esophageal artery Subcostal artery	Ø Open 3 Percutaneous 4 Percutaneous Endoscopic	Ø Drainage Device 2 Monitoring Device 3 Infusion Device 7 Autologous Tissue Substitute C Extraluminal Device D Intraluminal Device J Synthetic Substitute K Nonautologous Tissue Substitute M Stimulator Lead Y Other Device	Z No Qualifier
Y **Upper Artery** Aortic intercostal artery Bronchial artery Esophageal artery Subcostal artery	X External	Ø Drainage Device 2 Monitoring Device 3 Infusion Device D Intraluminal Device M Stimulator Lead	Z No Qualifier

Non-OR	03PY3[0,2,3,D]Z
Non-OR	03PY[3,4]YZ
Non-OR	03PYX[0,2,3,D,M]Z

NC Noncovered Procedure   **LC** Limited Coverage   **QA** Questionable OB Admit   **NT** New Tech Add-on   ⊞ Combination Member   ♂ Male   ♀ Female

ICD-10-PCS 2024   211

Ø   Medical and Surgical
3   Upper Arteries
Q   Repair   Definition: Restoring, to the extent possible, a body part to its normal anatomic structure and function

Explanation: Used only when the method to accomplish the repair is not one of the other root operations

Body Part Character 4		Approach Character 5	Device Character 6	Qualifier Character 7
Ø Internal Mammary Artery, Right Anterior intercostal artery Internal thoracic artery Musculophrenic artery Pericardiophrenic artery Superior epigastric artery **1 Internal Mammary Artery, Left** *See Ø Internal Mammary Artery, Right* **2 Innominate Artery** Brachiocephalic artery Brachiocephalic trunk **3 Subclavian Artery, Right** Costocervical trunk Dorsal scapular artery Internal thoracic artery **4 Subclavian Artery, Left** *See 3 Subclavian Artery, Right* **5 Axillary Artery, Right** Anterior circumflex humeral artery Lateral thoracic artery Posterior circumflex humeral artery Subscapular artery Superior thoracic artery Thoracoacromial artery **6 Axillary Artery, Left** *See 5 Axillary Artery, Right* **7 Brachial Artery, Right** Inferior ulnar collateral artery Profunda brachii Superior ulnar collateral artery **8 Brachial Artery, Left** *See 7 Brachial Artery, Right* **9 Ulnar Artery, Right** Anterior ulnar recurrent artery Common interosseous artery Posterior ulnar recurrent artery **A Ulnar Artery, Left** *See 9 Ulnar Artery, Right* **B Radial Artery, Right** Radial recurrent artery **C Radial Artery, Left** *See B Radial Artery, Right* **D Hand Artery, Right** Deep palmar arch Princeps pollicis artery Radialis indicis Superficial palmar arch **F Hand Artery, Left** *See D Hand Artery, Right* **G Intracranial Artery** Anterior cerebral artery Anterior choroidal artery Anterior communicating artery Basilar artery Circle of Willis Internal carotid artery, intracranial portion Middle cerebral artery Middle meningeal artery, intracranial portion Ophthalmic artery Posterior cerebral artery Posterior communicating artery Posterior inferior cerebellar artery (PICA) Vertebral artery, intracranial portion	**H Common Carotid Artery, Right** **J Common Carotid Artery, Left** **K Internal Carotid Artery, Right** Caroticotympanic artery Carotid sinus **L Internal Carotid Artery, Left** *See K Internal Carotid Artery, Right* **M External Carotid Artery, Right** Ascending pharyngeal artery Internal maxillary artery Lingual artery Maxillary artery Occipital artery Posterior auricular artery Superior thyroid artery **N External Carotid Artery, Left** *See M External Carotid Artery, Right* **P Vertebral Artery, Right** Anterior spinal artery Posterior spinal artery **Q Vertebral Artery, Left** *See P Vertebral Artery, Right* **R Face Artery** Angular artery Ascending palatine artery External maxillary artery Facial artery Inferior labial artery Submental artery Superior labial artery **S Temporal Artery, Right** Middle temporal artery Superficial temporal artery Transverse facial artery **T Temporal Artery, Left** *See S Temporal Artery, Right* **U Thyroid Artery, Right** Cricothyroid artery Hyoid artery Sternocleidomastoid artery Superior laryngeal artery Superior thyroid artery Thyrocervical trunk **V Thyroid Artery, Left** *See U Thyroid Artery, Right* **Y Upper Artery** Aortic intercostal artery Bronchial artery Esophageal artery Subcostal artery	**Ø Open** **3 Percutaneous** **4 Percutaneous Endoscopic**	**Z No Device**	**Z No Qualifier**

Non-OR Procedure   DRG Non-OR Procedure   Valid OR Procedure   HAC Associated Procedure   Combination Only   New/Revised April   New/Revised October

212   ICD-10-PCS 2024

Ø   **Medical and Surgical**
3   **Upper Arteries**
R   **Replacement**   Definition: Putting in or on biological or synthetic material that physically takes the place and/or function of all or a portion of a body part
                     Explanation: The body part may have been taken out or replaced, or may be taken out, physically eradicated, or rendered nonfunctional during the REPLACEMENT procedure. A REMOVAL procedure is coded for taking out the device used in a previous replacement procedure.

Body Part Character 4		Approach Character 5	Device Character 6	Qualifier Character 7

Ø Internal Mammary Artery, Right
  Anterior intercostal artery
  Internal thoracic artery
  Musculophrenic artery
  Pericardiophrenic artery
  Superior epigastric artery
1 Internal Mammary Artery, Left
  See Ø Internal Mammary Artery, Right
2 Innominate Artery
  Brachiocephalic artery
  Brachiocephalic trunk
3 Subclavian Artery, Right
  Costocervical trunk
  Dorsal scapular artery
  Internal thoracic artery
4 Subclavian Artery, Left
  See 3 Subclavian Artery, Right
5 Axillary Artery, Right
  Anterior circumflex humeral artery
  Lateral thoracic artery
  Posterior circumflex humeral artery
  Subscapular artery
  Superior thoracic artery
  Thoracoacromial artery
6 Axillary Artery, Left
  See 5 Axillary Artery, Right
7 Brachial Artery, Right
  Inferior ulnar collateral artery
  Profunda brachii
  Superior ulnar collateral artery
8 Brachial Artery, Left
  See 7 Brachial Artery, Right
9 Ulnar Artery, Right
  Anterior ulnar recurrent artery
  Common interosseous artery
  Posterior ulnar recurrent artery
A Ulnar Artery, Left
  See 9 Ulnar Artery, Right
B Radial Artery, Right
  Radial recurrent artery
C Radial Artery, Left
  See B Radial Artery, Right
D Hand Artery, Right
  Deep palmar arch
  Princeps pollicis artery
  Radialis indicis
  Superficial palmar arch
F Hand Artery, Left
  See D Hand Artery, Right
G Intracranial Artery
  Anterior cerebral artery
  Anterior choroidal artery
  Anterior communicating artery
  Basilar artery
  Circle of Willis
  Internal carotid artery, intracranial portion
  Middle cerebral artery
  Middle meningeal artery, intracranial portion
  Ophthalmic artery
  Posterior cerebral artery
  Posterior communicating artery
  Posterior inferior cerebellar artery (PICA)
  Vertebral artery, intracranial portion
	H Common Carotid Artery, Right
	J Common Carotid Artery, Left
	K Internal Carotid Artery, Right
	  Caroticotympanic artery
	  Carotid sinus
	L Internal Carotid Artery, Left
	  See K Internal Carotid Artery, Right
	M External Carotid Artery, Right
	  Ascending pharyngeal artery
	  Internal maxillary artery
	  Lingual artery
	  Maxillary artery
	  Occipital artery
	  Posterior auricular artery
	  Superior thyroid artery
	N External Carotid Artery, Left
	  See M External Carotid Artery, Right
	P Vertebral Artery, Right
	  Anterior spinal artery
	  Posterior spinal artery
	Q Vertebral Artery, Left
	  See P Vertebral Artery, Right
	R Face Artery
	  Angular artery
	  Ascending palatine artery
	  External maxillary artery
	  Facial artery
	  Inferior labial artery
	  Submental artery
	  Superior labial artery
	S Temporal Artery, Right
	  Middle temporal artery
	  Superficial temporal artery
	  Transverse facial artery
	T Temporal Artery, Left
	  See S Temporal Artery, Right
	U Thyroid Artery, Right
	  Cricothyroid artery
	  Hyoid artery
	  Sternocleidomastoid artery
	  Superior laryngeal artery
	  Superior thyroid artery
	  Thyrocervical trunk
	V Thyroid Artery, Left
	  See U Thyroid Artery, Right
	Y Upper Artery
	  Aortic intercostal artery
	  Bronchial artery
	  Esophageal artery
	  Subcostal artery
		Ø Open
		4 Percutaneous Endoscopic
			7 Autologous Tissue Substitute
			J Synthetic Substitute
			K Nonautologous Tissue Substitute
				Z No Qualifier

NC Noncovered Procedure   LC Limited Coverage   QA Questionable OB Admit   NT New Tech Add-on   ⊞ Combination Member   ♂ Male   ♀ Female

Ø   **Medical and Surgical**
3   **Upper Arteries**
S   **Reposition**   Definition: Moving to its normal location, or other suitable location, all or a portion of a body part

Explanation: The body part is moved to a new location from an abnormal location, or from a normal location where it is not functioning correctly. The body part may or may not be cut out or off to be moved to the new location.

Body Part Character 4		Approach Character 5	Device Character 6	Qualifier Character 7

Ø **Internal Mammary Artery, Right**
   Anterior intercostal artery
   Internal thoracic artery
   Musculophrenic artery
   Pericardiophrenic artery
   Superior epigastric artery
1 **Internal Mammary Artery, Left**
   See Ø Internal Mammary Artery, Right
2 **Innominate Artery**
   Brachiocephalic artery
   Brachiocephalic trunk
3 **Subclavian Artery, Right**
   Costocervical trunk
   Dorsal scapular artery
   Internal thoracic artery
4 **Subclavian Artery, Left**
   See 3 Subclavian Artery, Right
5 **Axillary Artery, Right**
   Anterior circumflex humeral artery
   Lateral thoracic artery
   Posterior circumflex humeral artery
   Subscapular artery
   Superior thoracic artery
   Thoracoacromial artery
6 **Axillary Artery, Left**
   See 5 Axillary Artery, Right
7 **Brachial Artery, Right**
   Inferior ulnar collateral artery
   Profunda brachii
   Superior ulnar collateral artery
8 **Brachial Artery, Left**
   See 7 Brachial Artery, Right
9 **Ulnar Artery, Right**
   Anterior ulnar recurrent artery
   Common interosseous artery
   Posterior ulnar recurrent artery
A **Ulnar Artery, Left**
   See 9 Ulnar Artery, Right
B **Radial Artery, Right**
   Radial recurrent artery
C **Radial Artery, Left**
   See B Radial Artery, Right
D **Hand Artery, Right**
   Deep palmar arch
   Princeps pollicis artery
   Radialis indicis
   Superficial palmar arch
F **Hand Artery, Left**
   See D Hand Artery, Right
G **Intracranial Artery**
   Anterior cerebral artery
   Anterior choroidal artery
   Anterior communicating artery
   Basilar artery
   Circle of Willis
   Internal carotid artery, intracranial portion
   Middle cerebral artery
   Middle meningeal artery, intracranial portion
   Ophthalmic artery
   Posterior cerebral artery
   Posterior communicating artery
   Posterior inferior cerebellar artery (PICA)
   Vertebral artery, intracranial portion
	H **Common Carotid Artery, Right**
	J **Common Carotid Artery, Left**
	K **Internal Carotid Artery, Right**
	   Caroticotympanic artery
	   Carotid sinus
	L **Internal Carotid Artery, Left**
	   See K Internal Carotid Artery, Right
	M **External Carotid Artery, Right**
	   Ascending pharyngeal artery
	   Internal maxillary artery
	   Lingual artery
	   Maxillary artery
	   Occipital artery
	   Posterior auricular artery
	   Superior thyroid artery
	N **External Carotid Artery, Left**
	   See M External Carotid Artery, Right
	P **Vertebral Artery, Right**
	   Anterior spinal artery
	   Posterior spinal artery
	Q **Vertebral Artery, Left**
	   See P Vertebral Artery, Right
	R **Face Artery**
	   Angular artery
	   Ascending palatine artery
	   External maxillary artery
	   Facial artery
	   Inferior labial artery
	   Submental artery
	   Superior labial artery
	S **Temporal Artery, Right**
	   Middle temporal artery
	   Superficial temporal artery
	   Transverse facial artery
	T **Temporal Artery, Left**
	   See S Temporal Artery, Right
	U **Thyroid Artery, Right**
	   Cricothyroid artery
	   Hyoid artery
	   Sternocleidomastoid artery
	   Superior laryngeal artery
	   Superior thyroid artery
	   Thyrocervical trunk
	V **Thyroid Artery, Left**
	   See U Thyroid Artery, Right
	Y **Upper Artery**
	   Aortic intercostal artery
	   Bronchial artery
	   Esophageal artery
	   Subcostal artery
		Ø Open
		3 Percutaneous
		4 Percutaneous Endoscopic
			Z No Device	Z No Qualifier

Non-OR Procedure   DRG Non-OR Procedure   Valid OR Procedure   HAC Associated Procedure   Combination Only   New/Revised April   New/Revised October

Ø   Medical and Surgical
3   Upper Arteries
U   Supplement   Definition: Putting in or on biological or synthetic material that physically reinforces and/or augments the function of a portion of a body part
                        Explanation: The biological material is non-living, or is living and from the same individual. The body part may have been previously replaced, and the SUPPLEMENT procedure is performed to physically reinforce and/or augment the function of the replaced body part.

Body Part Character 4		Approach Character 5	Device Character 6	Qualifier Character 7
Ø Internal Mammary Artery, Right Anterior intercostal artery Internal thoracic artery Musculophrenic artery Pericardiophrenic artery Superior epigastric artery **1 Internal Mammary Artery, Left** *See Ø Internal Mammary Artery, Right* **2 Innominate Artery** Brachiocephalic artery Brachiocephalic trunk **3 Subclavian Artery, Right** Costocervical trunk Dorsal scapular artery Internal thoracic artery **4 Subclavian Artery, Left** *See 3 Subclavian Artery, Right* **5 Axillary Artery, Right** Anterior circumflex humeral artery Lateral thoracic artery Posterior circumflex humeral artery Subscapular artery Superior thoracic artery Thoracoacromial artery **6 Axillary Artery, Left** *See 5 Axillary Artery, Right* **7 Brachial Artery, Right** Inferior ulnar collateral artery Profunda brachii Superior ulnar collateral artery **8 Brachial Artery, Left** *See 7 Brachial Artery, Right* **9 Ulnar Artery, Right** Anterior ulnar recurrent artery Common interosseous artery Posterior ulnar recurrent artery **A Ulnar Artery, Left** *See 9 Ulnar Artery, Right* **B Radial Artery, Right** Radial recurrent artery **C Radial Artery, Left** *See B Radial Artery, Right* **D Hand Artery, Right** Deep palmar arch Princeps pollicis artery Radialis indicis Superficial palmar arch **F Hand Artery, Left** *See D Hand Artery, Right* **G Intracranial Artery** Anterior cerebral artery Anterior choroidal artery Anterior communicating artery Basilar artery Circle of Willis Internal carotid artery, intracranial portion Middle cerebral artery Middle meningeal artery, intracranial portion Ophthalmic artery Posterior cerebral artery Posterior communicating artery Posterior inferior cerebellar artery (PICA) Vertebral artery, intracranial portion	**H Common Carotid Artery, Right** **J Common Carotid Artery, Left** **K Internal Carotid Artery, Right** Caroticotympanic artery Carotid sinus **L Internal Carotid Artery, Left** *See K Internal Carotid Artery, Right* **M External Carotid Artery, Right** Ascending pharyngeal artery Internal maxillary artery Lingual artery Maxillary artery Occipital artery Posterior auricular artery Superior thyroid artery **N External Carotid Artery, Left** *See M External Carotid Artery, Right* **P Vertebral Artery, Right** Anterior spinal artery Posterior spinal artery **Q Vertebral Artery, Left** *See P Vertebral Artery, Right* **R Face Artery** Angular artery Ascending palatine artery External maxillary artery Facial artery Inferior labial artery Submental artery Superior labial artery **S Temporal Artery, Right** Middle temporal artery Superficial temporal artery Transverse facial artery **T Temporal Artery, Left** *See S Temporal Artery, Right* **U Thyroid Artery, Right** Cricothyroid artery Hyoid artery Sternocleidomastoid artery Superior laryngeal artery Superior thyroid artery Thyrocervical trunk **V Thyroid Artery, Left** *See U Thyroid Artery, Right* **Y Upper Artery** Aortic intercostal artery Bronchial artery Esophageal artery Subcostal artery	**Ø Open** **3 Percutaneous** **4 Percutaneous Endoscopic**	**7 Autologous Tissue Substitute** **J Synthetic Substitute** **K Nonautologous Tissue Substitute**	**Z No Qualifier**

NC Noncovered Procedure   LC Limited Coverage   QA Questionable OB Admit   NT New Tech Add-on   ⊞ Combination Member   ♂ Male   ♀ Female

Ø   Medical and Surgical
3   Upper Arteries
V   Restriction   Definition: Partially closing an orifice or the lumen of a tubular body part
                    Explanation: The orifice can be a natural orifice or an artificially created orifice

Body Part Character 4		Approach Character 5	Device Character 6	Qualifier Character 7

Ø **Internal Mammary Artery, Right**
Anterior intercostal artery
Internal thoracic artery
Musculophrenic artery
Pericardiophrenic artery
Superior epigastric artery
1 **Internal Mammary Artery, Left**
See Ø Internal Mammary Artery, Right
2 **Innominate Artery**
Brachiocephalic artery
Brachiocephalic trunk
3 **Subclavian Artery, Right**
Costocervical trunk
Dorsal scapular artery
Internal thoracic artery
4 **Subclavian Artery, Left**
See 3 Subclavian Artery, Right
5 **Axillary Artery, Right**
Anterior circumflex humeral
   artery
Lateral thoracic artery
Posterior circumflex humeral
   artery
Subscapular artery
Superior thoracic artery
Thoracoacromial artery
6 **Axillary Artery, Left**
See 5 Axillary Artery, Right
7 **Brachial Artery, Right**
Inferior ulnar collateral artery
Profunda brachii
Superior ulnar collateral artery
8 **Brachial Artery, Left**
See 7 Brachial Artery, Right
9 **Ulnar Artery, Right**
Anterior ulnar recurrent artery
Common interosseous artery
Posterior ulnar recurrent artery
A **Ulnar Artery, Left**
See 9 Ulnar Artery, Right
	B **Radial Artery, Right**
	Radial recurrent artery
	C **Radial Artery, Left**
	See B Radial Artery, Right
	D **Hand Artery, Right**
	Deep palmar arch
	Princeps pollicis artery
	Radialis indicis
	Superficial palmar arch
	F **Hand Artery, Left**
	See D Hand Artery, Right
	R **Face Artery**
	Angular artery
	Ascending palatine artery
	External maxillary artery
	Facial artery
	Inferior labial artery
	Submental artery
	Superior labial artery
	S **Temporal Artery, Right**
	Middle temporal artery
	Superficial temporal artery
	Transverse facial artery
	T **Temporal Artery, Left**
	See S Temporal Artery, Right
	U **Thyroid Artery, Right**
	Cricothyroid artery
	Hyoid artery
	Sternocleidomastoid artery
	Superior laryngeal artery
	Superior thyroid artery
	Thyrocervical trunk
	V **Thyroid Artery, Left**
	See U Thyroid Artery, Right
	Y **Upper Artery**
	Aortic intercostal artery
	Bronchial artery
	Esophageal artery
	Subcostal artery
		Ø Open
		3 Percutaneous
		4 Percutaneous
		   Endoscopic
			C Extraluminal Device
			D Intraluminal Device
			Z No Device
				Z No Qualifier

G **Intracranial Artery**
Anterior cerebral artery
Anterior choroidal artery
Anterior communicating artery
Basilar artery
Circle of Willis
Internal carotid artery,
   intracranial portion
Middle cerebral artery
Middle meningeal artery,
   intracranial portion
Ophthalmic artery
Posterior cerebral artery
Posterior communicating artery
Posterior inferior cerebellar artery
   (PICA)
Vertebral artery, intracranial
   portion
H **Common Carotid Artery, Right**
J **Common Carotid Artery, Left**
K **Internal Carotid Artery, Right**
Caroticotympanic artery
Carotid sinus
	L **Internal Carotid Artery, Left**
	See K Internal Carotid Artery, Right
	M **External Carotid Artery, Right**
	Ascending pharyngeal artery
	Internal maxillary artery
	Lingual artery
	Maxillary artery
	Occipital artery
	Posterior auricular artery
	Superior thyroid artery
	N **External Carotid Artery, Left**
	See M External Carotid Artery, Right
	P **Vertebral Artery, Right**
	Anterior spinal artery
	Posterior spinal artery
	Q **Vertebral Artery, Left**
	See P Vertebral Artery, Right
		Ø Open
		3 Percutaneous
		4 Percutaneous
		   Endoscopic
			B Intraluminal Device,
			   Bioactive
			C Extraluminal Device
			D Intraluminal Device
			H Intraluminal Device,
			   Flow Diverter
			Z No Device
				Z No Qualifier

Non-OR Procedure   DRG Non-OR Procedure   Valid OR Procedure   HAC Associated Procedure   Combination Only   New/Revised April   New/Revised October

216   ICD-10-PCS 2024

Ø3V–Ø3V

0   **Medical and Surgical**
3   **Upper Arteries**
W   **Revision**   Definition: Correcting, to the extent possible, a portion of a malfunctioning device or the position of a displaced device
                        Explanation: Revision can include correcting a malfunctioning or displaced device by taking out or putting in components of the device such as a screw or pin

Body Part Character 4	Approach Character 5	Device Character 6	Qualifier Character 7

Y   Upper Artery
     Aortic intercostal artery
     Bronchial artery
     Esophageal artery
     Subcostal artery
	0 Open
	3 Percutaneous
	4 Percutaneous Endoscopic
		0 Drainage Device
		2 Monitoring Device
		3 Infusion Device
		7 Autologous Tissue Substitute
		C Extraluminal Device
		D Intraluminal Device
		J Synthetic Substitute
		K Nonautologous Tissue Substitute
		M Stimulator Lead
		Y Other Device
			Z No Qualifier

Y   Upper Artery
     Aortic intercostal artery
     Bronchial artery
     Esophageal artery
     Subcostal artery
	X External	**0** Drainage Device
		2 Monitoring Device
		3 Infusion Device
		7 Autologous Tissue Substitute
		C Extraluminal Device
		D Intraluminal Device
		J Synthetic Substitute
		K Nonautologous Tissue Substitute
		M Stimulator Lead
			Z No Qualifier

Non-OR   03WY3[0,2,3]Z
Non-OR   03WY[3,4]YZ
Non-OR   03WYX[0,2,3,7,C,D,J,K,M]Z

Lower Arteries Ø41–Ø4W

Character Meanings

This Character Meaning table is provided as a guide to assist the user in the identification of character members that may be found in this section of code tables. It **SHOULD NOT** be used to build a PCS code.

Operation–Character 3	Body Part–Character 4	Approach–Character 5	Device–Character 6	Qualifier–Character 7
1 Bypass	Ø Abdominal Aorta	Ø Open	Ø Drainage Device	Ø Abdominal Aorta OR Ultrasonic
5 Destruction	1 Celiac Artery	3 Percutaneous	1 Radioactive Element	1 Celiac Artery OR Drug-Coated Balloon
7 Dilation	2 Gastric Artery	4 Percutaneous Endoscopic	2 Monitoring Device	2 Mesenteric Artery
9 Drainage	3 Hepatic Artery	X External	3 Infusion Device	3 Renal Artery, Right
B Excision	4 Splenic Artery		4 Intraluminal Device, Drug-eluting	4 Renal Artery, Left
C Extirpation	5 Superior Mesenteric Artery		5 Intraluminal Device, Drug-eluting, Two	5 Renal Artery, Bilateral
F Fragmentation	6 Colic Artery, Right		6 Intraluminal Device, Drug-eluting, Three	6 Common Iliac Artery, Right
H Insertion	7 Colic Artery, Left		7 Intraluminal Device, Drug-eluting, Four or More OR Autologous Tissue Substitute	7 Common Iliac Artery, Left
J Inspection	8 Colic Artery, Middle		9 Autologous Venous Tissue	8 Common Iliac Arteries, Bilateral
L Occlusion	9 Renal Artery, Right		A Autologous Arterial Tissue	9 Internal Iliac Artery, Right
N Release	A Renal Artery, Left		C Extraluminal Device	B Internal Iliac Artery, Left
P Removal	B Inferior Mesenteric Artery		D Intraluminal Device	C Internal Iliac Arteries, Bilateral
Q Repair	C Common Iliac Artery, Right		E Intraluminal Device, Two OR Intraluminal Device, Branched or Fenestrated, One or Two Arteries	D External Iliac Artery, Right
R Replacement	D Common Iliac Artery, Left		F Intraluminal Device, Three OR Intraluminal Device, Branched or Fenestrated, Three or More Arteries	F External Iliac Artery, Left
S Reposition	E Internal Iliac Artery, Right		G Intraluminal Device, Four or More	G External Iliac Arteries, Bilateral
U Supplement	F Internal Iliac Artery, Left		J Synthetic Substitute	H Femoral Artery, Right
V Restriction	H External Iliac Artery, Right		K Nonautologous Tissue Substitute	J Femoral Artery, Left OR Temporary
W Revision	J External Iliac Artery, Left		Y Other Device	K Femoral Arteries, Bilateral
	K Femoral Artery, Right		Z No Device	L Popliteal Artery
	L Femoral Artery, Left			M Peroneal Artery
	M Popliteal Artery, Right			N Posterior Tibial Artery
	N Popliteal Artery, Left			P Foot Artery
	P Anterior Tibial Artery, Right			Q Lower Extremity Artery
	Q Anterior Tibial Artery, Left			R Lower Artery
	R Posterior Tibial Artery, Right			S Lower Extremity Vein
	S Posterior Tibial Artery, Left			T Uterine Artery, Right
	T Peroneal Artery, Right			U Uterine Artery, Left
	U Peroneal Artery, Left			V Prostatic Artery, Right
	V Foot Artery, Right			W Prostatic Artery, Left
	W Foot Artery, Left			X Diagnostic
	Y Lower Artery			Z No Qualifier

AHA Coding Clinic for Lower Arteries

2022, 1Q, 10-13	Procedures performed on a continuous vessel, ICD-10-PCS Guideline B4.1c

AHA Coding Clinic for table Ø41

2022, 3Q, 5	Aortoiliac aneurysm repair
2019, 1Q, 23	Endovascular repair of shaggy aorta and deployment of chimney stent grafts
2018, 3Q, 25	Femoral artery to tibioperoneal trunk bypass
2017, 4Q, 46-47	New and revised body part values - Bypass hepatic artery to renal artery
2017, 3Q, 5	Femoral artery to posterior tibial artery bypass using autologous and synthetic grafts
2017, 3Q, 16	Abdominal aortic debranching with bypass of external iliac artery to bilateral renal arteries and superior mesenteric artery
2017, 1Q, 32	Peroneal artery to dorsalis pedis artery bypass using saphenous vein graft
2016, 2Q, 18	Femoral-tibial artery bypass and saphenous vein graft
2015, 3Q, 28	Bilateral renal artery bypass

AHA Coding Clinic for table Ø47

2020, 4Q, 50	Intravascular lithotripsy
2019, 4Q, 27	Bifurcation Qualifier
2019, 2Q, 14	Revision of occluded femoral-popliteal bypass graft
2018, 2Q, 24	Coronary artery bifurcation
2016, 4Q, 86	Peripheral artery, number of stents
2016, 4Q, 86-88	Coronary and peripheral artery bifurcation
2016, 3Q, 39	Infrarenal abdominal aortic aneurysm repair with iliac graft extension
2015, 4Q, 4-7, 15	Drug-coated balloon angioplasty in peripheral vessels
2015, 3Q, 9	Aborted endovascular stenting of superficial femoral artery

AHA Coding Clinic for table Ø4C

2021, 1Q, 15	Iliofemoral endarterectomy and furthest point of entry
2019, 4Q, 27	Bifurcation Qualifier
2019, 1Q, 23	Endovascular repair of shaggy aorta and deployment of chimney stent grafts
2018, 2Q, 24	Coronary artery bifurcation
2017, 2Q, 23	Thrombectomy via Fogarty catheter
2016, 4Q, 86-88	Coronary and peripheral artery bifurcation
2016, 1Q, 31	Iliofemoral endarterectomy with patch repair
2015, 1Q, 29	Discontinued carotid endarterectomy
2015, 1Q, 36	Percutaneous mechanical thrombectomy of femoropopliteal bypass graft

AHA Coding Clinic for table Ø4F

2020, 4Q, 45-49	New fragmentation tables
2020, 4Q, 49-50	Intravascular ultrasound assisted thrombolysis
2020, 4Q, 50-51	Intravascular lithotripsy

AHA Coding Clinic for table Ø4H

2022, 3Q, 19	Placement of stent into aorta to secure debris
2019, 3Q, 20	Removal and revision of ECMO component
2019, 1Q, 23	Endovascular repair of shaggy aorta and deployment of chimney stent grafts
2017, 1Q, 30	Insertion of umbilical artery catheter

AHA Coding Clinic for table Ø4J

2022, 4Q, 56	Embolization of prostatic artery

AHA Coding Clinic for table Ø4L

2023, 1Q, 9	Temporary balloon occlusion of aorta
2022, 4Q, 55-56	Embolization of prostatic artery
2020, 3Q, 43	Staged laparoscopic gastric conduit and placement of feeding tube
2018, 2Q, 18	Transverse rectus abdominis myocutaneous (TRAM) delay
2017, 4Q, 31	Resuscitative endovascular balloon occlusion of the aorta
2015, 2Q, 27	Uterine artery embolization using Gelfoam
2014, 3Q, 26	Coil embolization of gastroduodenal artery with chemoembolization of hepatic artery
2014, 1Q, 24	Endovascular embolization for gastrointestinal bleeding

AHA Coding Clinic for table Ø4N

2015, 2Q, 28	Release and replacement of celiac artery

AHA Coding Clinic for table Ø4P

2019, 3Q, 20	Removal and revision of ECMO component

AHA Coding Clinic for table Ø4Q

2014, 1Q, 21	Repair of femoral artery pseudoaneurysm

AHA Coding Clinic for table Ø4R

2022, 3Q, 5	Aortoiliac aneurysm repair
2019, 1Q, 22	Abdominal aortic aneurysm repair using tube graft
2015, 2Q, 28	Release and replacement of celiac artery

AHA Coding Clinic for table Ø4U

2019, 1Q, 22	Abdominal aortic aneurysm repair using tube graft
2016, 2Q, 18	Femoral-tibial artery bypass and saphenous vein graft
2016, 1Q, 31	Iliofemoral endarterectomy with patch repair
2014, 4Q, 37	Bovine patch arterioplasty
2014, 1Q, 22	Repair of pseudoaneurysm of femoral-popliteal bypass graft

AHA Coding Clinic for table Ø4V

2021, 3Q, 23	Transcatheter embolization of splenic artery
2019, 4Q, 27	Bifurcation Qualifier
2019, 1Q, 22	Abdominal aortic aneurysm repair using tube graft
2018, 2Q, 24	Coronary artery bifurcation
2016, 4Q, 86-87	Coronary and peripheral artery bifurcation
2016, 4Q, 89-93	Branched and fenestrated endograft repair of aneurysms
2016, 3Q, 39	Infrarenal abdominal aortic aneurysm repair with iliac graft extension
2014, 1Q, 9	Endovascular repair of abdominal aortic aneurysm

AHA Coding Clinic for table Ø4W

2020, 3Q, 5	Types of endoleaks following endovascular aneurysm repair
2019, 2Q, 14	Revision of occluded femoral-popliteal bypass graft
2015, 1Q, 36	Revision of femoropopliteal bypass graft
2014, 1Q, 9	Endovascular repair of endoleak
2014, 1Q, 22	Repair of pseudoaneurysm of femoral-popliteal bypass graft

Lower Arteries

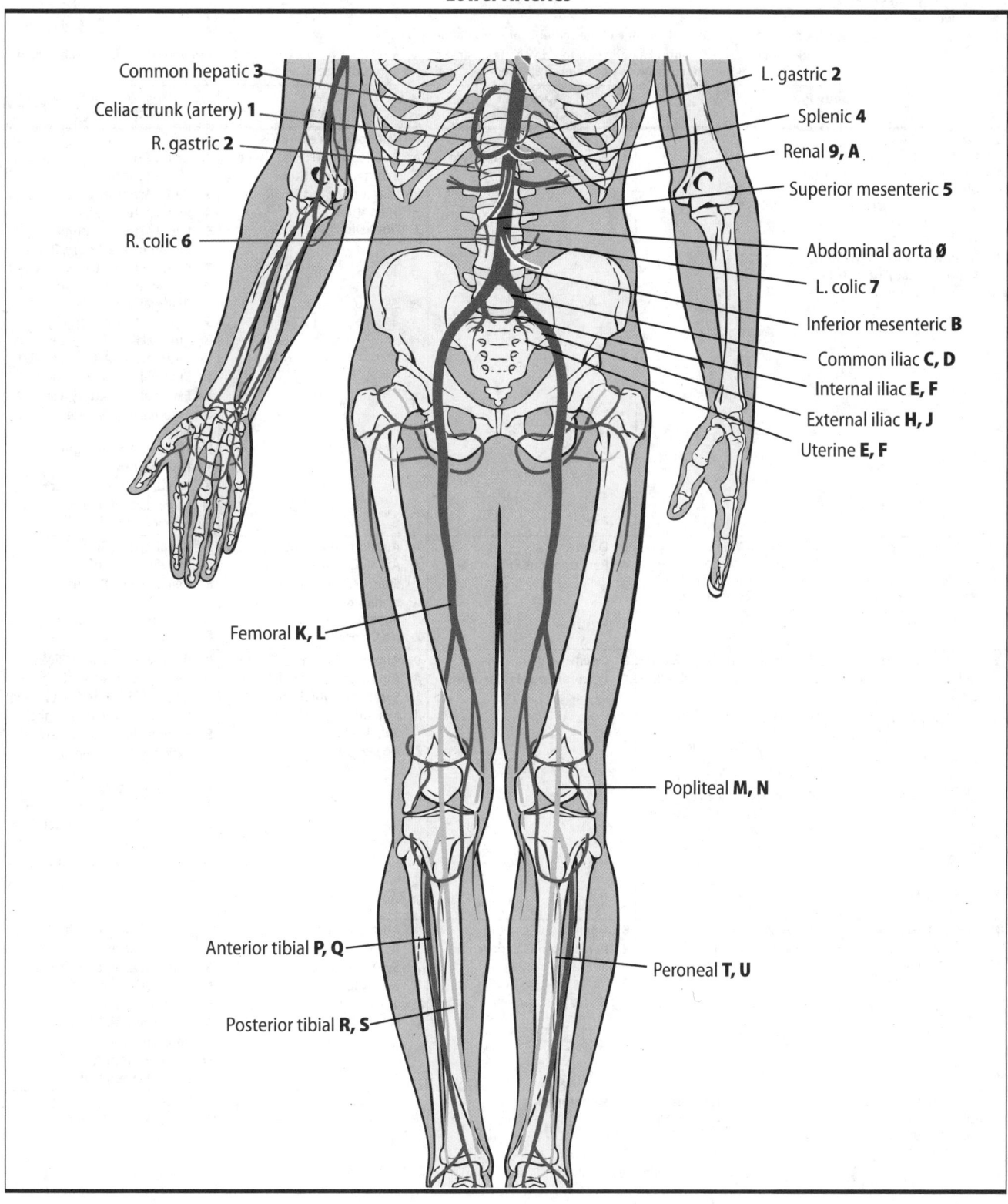

Common hepatic **3**

Celiac trunk (artery) **1**

R. gastric **2**

R. colic **6**

L. gastric **2**

Splenic **4**

Renal **9, A**

Superior mesenteric **5**

Abdominal aorta **Ø**

L. colic **7**

Inferior mesenteric **B**

Common iliac **C, D**

Internal iliac **E, F**

External iliac **H, J**

Uterine **E, F**

Femoral **K, L**

Popliteal **M, N**

Anterior tibial **P, Q**

Peroneal **T, U**

Posterior tibial **R, S**

Lower Arteries (side tab)

0   Medical and Surgical
4   Lower Arteries
1   Bypass   Definition: Altering the route of passage of the contents of a tubular body part

Explanation: Rerouting contents of a body part to a downstream area of the normal route, to a similar route and body part, or to an abnormal route and dissimilar body part. Includes one or more anastomoses, with or without the use of a device.

Body Part Character 4		Approach Character 5	Device Character 6	Qualifier Character 7
0 **Abdominal Aorta** Inferior phrenic artery Lumbar artery Median sacral artery Middle suprarenal artery Ovarian artery Testicular artery C **Common Iliac Artery, Right** D **Common Iliac Artery, Left**		0 Open 4 Percutaneous Endoscopic	9 Autologous Venous Tissue A Autologous Arterial Tissue J Synthetic Substitute K Nonautologous Tissue Substitute Z No Device	0 Abdominal Aorta 1 Celiac Artery 2 Mesenteric Artery 3 Renal Artery, Right 4 Renal Artery, Left 5 Renal Artery, Bilateral 6 Common Iliac Artery, Right 7 Common Iliac Artery, Left 8 Common Iliac Arteries, Bilateral 9 Internal Iliac Artery, Right B Internal Iliac Artery, Left C Internal Iliac Arteries, Bilateral D External Iliac Artery, Right F External Iliac Artery, Left G External Iliac Arteries, Bilateral H Femoral Artery, Right J Femoral Artery, Left K Femoral Arteries, Bilateral Q Lower Extremity Artery R Lower Artery
3 **Hepatic Artery** Common hepatic artery Gastroduodenal artery Hepatic artery proper	4 **Splenic Artery** Left gastroepiploic artery Pancreatic artery Short gastric artery	0 Open 4 Percutaneous Endoscopic	9 Autologous Venous Tissue A Autologous Arterial Tissue J Synthetic Substitute K Nonautologous Tissue Substitute Z No Device	3 Renal Artery, Right 4 Renal Artery, Left 5 Renal Artery, Bilateral
E **Internal Iliac Artery, Right** Deferential artery Hypogastric artery Iliolumbar artery Inferior gluteal artery Inferior vesical artery Internal pudendal artery Lateral sacral artery Middle rectal artery Obturator artery Prostatic artery Superior gluteal artery Superior vesical artery Umbilical artery Uterine artery Vaginal artery	F **Internal Iliac Artery, Left** *See E Internal Iliac Artery, Right* H **External Iliac Artery, Right** Deep circumflex iliac artery Inferior epigastric artery J **External Iliac Artery, Left** *See H External Iliac Artery, Right*	0 Open 4 Percutaneous Endoscopic	9 Autologous Venous Tissue A Autologous Arterial Tissue J Synthetic Substitute K Nonautologous Tissue Substitute Z No Device	9 Internal Iliac Artery, Right B Internal Iliac Artery, Left C Internal Iliac Arteries, Bilateral D External Iliac Artery, Right F External Iliac Artery, Left G External Iliac Arteries, Bilateral H Femoral Artery, Right J Femoral Artery, Left K Femoral Arteries, Bilateral P Foot Artery Q Lower Extremity Artery
K **Femoral Artery, Right** Circumflex iliac artery Deep femoral artery Descending genicular artery External pudendal artery Superficial epigastric artery	L **Femoral Artery, Left** *See K Femoral Artery, Right*	0 Open 4 Percutaneous Endoscopic	9 Autologous Venous Tissue A Autologous Arterial Tissue J Synthetic Substitute K Nonautologous Tissue Substitute Z No Device	H Femoral Artery, Right J Femoral Artery, Left K Femoral Arteries, Bilateral L Popliteal Artery M Peroneal Artery N Posterior Tibial Artery P Foot Artery Q Lower Extremity Artery S Lower Extremity Vein
K **Femoral Artery, Right** Circumflex iliac artery Deep femoral artery Descending genicular artery External pudendal artery Superficial epigastric artery	L **Femoral Artery, Left** *See K Femoral Artery, Right*	3 Percutaneous	J Synthetic Substitute	Q Lower Extremity Artery S Lower Extremity Vein
M **Popliteal Artery, Right** Inferior genicular artery Middle genicular artery Superior genicular artery Sural artery Tibioperoneal trunk	N **Popliteal Artery, Left** *See M Popliteal Artery, Right*	0 Open 4 Percutaneous Endoscopic	9 Autologous Venous Tissue A Autologous Arterial Tissue J Synthetic Substitute K Nonautologous Tissue Substitute Z No Device	L Popliteal Artery M Peroneal Artery P Foot Artery Q Lower Extremity Artery S Lower Extremity Vein

041 Continued on next page

Non-OR Procedure   DRG Non-OR Procedure   Valid OR Procedure   HAC Associated Procedure   Combination Only   New/Revised April   New/Revised October

Ø   Medical and Surgical
4   Lower Arteries
1   Bypass   *Definition: Altering the route of passage of the contents of a tubular body part*

041 Continued

Explanation: Rerouting contents of a body part to a downstream area of the normal route, to a similar route and body part, or to an abnormal route and dissimilar body part. Includes one or more anastomoses, with or without the use of a device.

Body Part Character 4	Approach Character 5	Device Character 6	Qualifier Character 7

M   **Popliteal Artery, Right**
   Inferior genicular artery
   Middle genicular artery
   Superior genicular artery
   Sural artery
   Tibioperoneal trunk
N   **Popliteal Artery, Left**
   See M Popliteal Artery, Right
	3 Percutaneous	**J** Synthetic Substitute	**Q** Lower Extremity Artery
			S Lower Extremity Vein

P   **Anterior Tibial Artery, Right**
   Anterior lateral malleolar artery
   Anterior medial malleolar artery
   Anterior tibial recurrent artery
   Dorsalis pedis artery
   Posterior tibial recurrent artery
Q   **Anterior Tibial Artery, Left**
   See P Anterior Tibial Artery, Right
R   **Posterior Tibial Artery, Right**
S   **Posterior Tibial Artery, Left**
	Ø Open
	3 Percutaneous
	4 Percutaneous Endoscopic
		J Synthetic Substitute	**Q** Lower Extremity Artery
			S Lower Extremity Vein

T   **Peroneal Artery, Right**
   Fibular artery
U   **Peroneal Artery, Left**
   See T Peroneal Artery, Right
V   **Foot Artery, Right**
   Arcuate artery
   Dorsal metatarsal artery
   Lateral plantar artery
   Lateral tarsal artery
   Medial plantar artery
W   **Foot Artery, Left**
   See V Foot Artery, Right
	Ø Open
	4 Percutaneous Endoscopic
		9 Autologous Venous Tissue
		A Autologous Arterial Tissue
		J Synthetic Substitute
		K Nonautologous Tissue Substitute
		Z No Device
			P Foot Artery
			Q Lower Extremity Artery
			S Lower Extremity Vein

T   **Peroneal Artery, Right**
   Fibular artery
U   **Peroneal Artery, Left**
   See T Peroneal Artery, Right
V   **Foot Artery, Right**
   Arcuate artery
   Dorsal metatarsal artery
   Lateral plantar artery
   Lateral tarsal artery
   Medial plantar artery
W   **Foot Artery, Left**
   See V Foot Artery, Right
	3 Percutaneous	**J** Synthetic Substitute	**Q** Lower Extremity Artery
			S Lower Extremity Vein

NC Noncovered Procedure   **LC** Limited Coverage   **QA** Questionable OB Admit   **NT** New Tech Add-on   ⊞ Combination Member   ♂ Male   ♀ Female

ICD-10-PCS 2024   223

Lower Arteries *(left margin)*

Ø Medical and Surgical
4 Lower Arteries
5 Destruction Definition: Physical eradication of all or a portion of a body part by the direct use of energy, force, or a destructive agent
Explanation: None of the body part is physically taken out

Body Part Character 4		Approach Character 5	Device Character 6	Qualifier Character 7

Ø Abdominal Aorta
  Inferior phrenic artery
  Lumbar artery
  Median sacral artery
  Middle suprarenal artery
  Ovarian artery
  Testicular artery
1 Celiac Artery
  Celiac trunk
2 Gastric Artery
  Left gastric artery
  Right gastric artery
3 Hepatic Artery
  Common hepatic artery
  Gastroduodenal artery
  Hepatic artery proper
4 Splenic Artery
  Left gastroepiploic artery
  Pancreatic artery
  Short gastric artery
5 Superior Mesenteric Artery
  Ileal artery
  Ileocolic artery
  Inferior pancreaticoduodenal
    artery
  Jejunal artery
6 Colic Artery, Right
7 Colic Artery, Left
8 Colic Artery, Middle
9 Renal Artery, Right
  Inferior suprarenal artery
  Renal segmental artery
A Renal Artery, Left
  See 9 Renal Artery, Right
B Inferior Mesenteric Artery
  Sigmoid artery
  Superior rectal artery
C Common Iliac Artery, Right
D Common Iliac Artery, Left
E Internal Iliac Artery, Right
  Deferential artery
  Hypogastric artery
  Iliolumbar artery
  Inferior gluteal artery
  Inferior vesical artery
  Internal pudendal artery
  Lateral sacral artery
  Middle rectal artery
  Obturator artery
  Prostatic artery
  Superior gluteal artery
  Superior vesical artery
  Umbilical artery
  Uterine artery
  Vaginal artery
	F Internal Iliac Artery, Left
	  See E Internal Iliac Artery, Right
	H External Iliac Artery, Right
	  Deep circumflex iliac artery
	  Inferior epigastric artery
	J External Iliac Artery, Left
	  See H External Iliac Artery, Right
	K Femoral Artery, Right
	  Circumflex iliac artery
	  Deep femoral artery
	  Descending genicular artery
	  External pudendal artery
	  Superficial epigastric artery
	L Femoral Artery, Left
	  See K Femoral Artery, Right
	M Popliteal Artery, Right
	  Inferior genicular artery
	  Middle genicular artery
	  Superior genicular artery
	  Sural artery
	  Tibioperoneal trunk
	N Popliteal Artery, Left
	  See M Popliteal Artery, Right
	P Anterior Tibial Artery, Right
	  Anterior lateral malleolar
	    artery
	  Anterior medial malleolar
	    artery
	  Anterior tibial recurrent artery
	  Dorsalis pedis artery
	  Posterior tibial recurrent artery
	Q Anterior Tibial Artery, Left
	  *See P Anterior Tibial Artery,
	    Right*
	R Posterior Tibial Artery, Right
	S Posterior Tibial Artery, Left
	T Peroneal Artery, Right
	  Fibular artery
	U Peroneal Artery, Left
	  See T Peroneal Artery, Right
	V Foot Artery, Right
	  Arcuate artery
	  Dorsal metatarsal artery
	  Lateral plantar artery
	  Lateral tarsal artery
	  Medial plantar artery
	W Foot Artery, Left
	  See V Foot Artery, Right
	Y Lower Artery
	  Umbilical artery
		Ø Open
		3 Percutaneous
		4 Percutaneous Endoscopic
			Z No Device	**Z No Qualifier**

045–045 *(left margin bottom)*

Ø   Medical and Surgical
4   Lower Arteries
7   Dilation   Definition: Expanding an orifice or the lumen of a tubular body part

Explanation: The orifice can be a natural orifice or an artificially created orifice. Accomplished by stretching a tubular body part using intraluminal pressure or by cutting part of the orifice or wall of the tubular body part.

Body Part Character 4		Approach Character 5	Device Character 6	Qualifier Character 7

Ø Abdominal Aorta
Inferior phrenic artery
Lumbar artery
Median sacral artery
Middle suprarenal artery
Ovarian artery
Testicular artery
1 Celiac Artery
Celiac trunk
2 Gastric Artery
Left gastric artery
Right gastric artery
3 Hepatic Artery
Common hepatic artery
Gastroduodenal artery
Hepatic artery proper
4 Splenic Artery
Left gastroepiploic artery
Pancreatic artery
Short gastric artery
5 Superior Mesenteric Artery
Ileal artery
Ileocolic artery
Inferior pancreaticoduodenal
   artery
Jejunal artery
6 Colic Artery, Right
7 Colic Artery, Left
8 Colic Artery, Middle
9 Renal Artery, Right
Inferior suprarenal artery
Renal segmental artery
A Renal Artery, Left
See 9 Renal Artery, Right
B Inferior Mesenteric Artery
Sigmoid artery
Superior rectal artery
C Common Iliac Artery, Right
D Common Iliac Artery, Left
E Internal Iliac Artery, Right
Deferential artery
Hypogastric artery
Iliolumbar artery
Inferior gluteal artery
Inferior vesical artery
Internal pudendal artery
Lateral sacral artery
Middle rectal artery
Obturator artery
Prostatic artery
Superior gluteal artery
Superior vesical artery
Umbilical artery
Uterine artery
Vaginal artery
	F Internal Iliac Artery, Left
	See E Internal Iliac Artery, Right
	H External Iliac Artery, Right
	Deep circumflex iliac artery
	Inferior epigastric artery
	J External Iliac Artery, Left
	See H External Iliac Artery, Right
	K Femoral Artery, Right
	Circumflex iliac artery
	Deep femoral artery
	Descending genicular artery
	External pudendal artery
	Superficial epigastric artery
	L Femoral Artery, Left
	See K Femoral Artery, Right
	M Popliteal Artery, Right
	Inferior genicular artery
	Middle genicular artery
	Superior genicular artery
	Sural artery
	Tibioperoneal trunk
	N Popliteal Artery, Left
	See M Popliteal Artery, Right
	P Anterior Tibial Artery, Right
	Anterior lateral malleolar
	   artery
	Anterior medial malleolar
	   artery
	Anterior tibial recurrent artery
	Dorsalis pedis artery
	Posterior tibial recurrent artery
	Q Anterior Tibial Artery, Left
	See P Anterior Tibial Artery,
	Right
	R Posterior Tibial Artery, Right
	S Posterior Tibial Artery, Left
	T Peroneal Artery, Right
	Fibular artery
	U Peroneal Artery, Left
	See T Peroneal Artery, Right
	V Foot Artery, Right
	Arcuate artery
	Dorsal metatarsal artery
	Lateral plantar artery
	Lateral tarsal artery
	Medial plantar artery
	W Foot Artery, Left
	See V Foot Artery, Right
	Y Lower Artery
	Umbilical artery
		Ø Open
		3 Percutaneous
		4 Percutaneous Endoscopic
			**4 Intraluminal Device,
			   Drug-eluting**
			D Intraluminal Device
			Z No Device
				1 Drug-Coated Balloon
				Z No Qualifier

Ø47 Continued on next page

NC Noncovered Procedure   LC Limited Coverage   QA Questionable OB Admit   NT New Tech Add-on   ⊞ Combination Member   ♂ Male   ♀ Female

ICD-10-PCS 2024   225

Ø   Medical and Surgical   *Ø47 Continued*
4   Lower Arteries
7   Dilation   Definition: Expanding an orifice or the lumen of a tubular body part
                        Explanation: The orifice can be a natural orifice or an artificially created orifice. Accomplished by stretching a tubular body part using
                        intraluminal pressure or by cutting part of the orifice or wall of the tubular body part.

Body Part Character 4		Approach Character 5	Device Character 6	Qualifier Character 7

Ø Abdominal Aorta
 Inferior phrenic artery
 Lumbar artery
 Median sacral artery
 Middle suprarenal artery
 Ovarian artery
 Testicular artery
 1 Celiac Artery
 Celiac trunk
 2 Gastric Artery
 Left gastric artery
 Right gastric artery
 3 Hepatic Artery
 Common hepatic artery
 Gastroduodenal artery
 Hepatic artery proper
 4 Splenic Artery
 Left gastroepiploic artery
 Pancreatic artery
 Short gastric artery
 5 Superior Mesenteric Artery
 Ileal artery
 Ileocolic artery
 Inferior pancreaticoduodenal
    artery
 Jejunal artery
 6 Colic Artery, Right
 7 Colic Artery, Left
 8 Colic Artery, Middle
 9 Renal Artery, Right
 Inferior suprarenal artery
 Renal segmental artery
 A Renal Artery, Left
 See 9 Renal Artery, Right
 B Inferior Mesenteric Artery
 Sigmoid artery
 Superior rectal artery
 C Common Iliac Artery, Right
 D Common Iliac Artery, Left
 E Internal Iliac Artery, Right
 Deferential artery
 Hypogastric artery
 Iliolumbar artery
 Inferior gluteal artery
 Inferior vesical artery
 Internal pudendal artery
 Lateral sacral artery
 Middle rectal artery
 Obturator artery
 Prostatic artery
 Superior gluteal artery
 Superior vesical artery
 Umbilical artery
 Uterine artery
 Vaginal artery
	F Internal Iliac Artery, Left
	 See E Internal Iliac Artery, Right
	 H External Iliac Artery, Right
	 Deep circumflex iliac artery
	 Inferior epigastric artery
	 J External Iliac Artery, Left
	 See H External Iliac Artery, Right
	 K Femoral Artery, Right
	 Circumflex iliac artery
	 Deep femoral artery
	 Descending genicular artery
	 External pudendal artery
	 Superficial epigastric artery
	 L Femoral Artery, Left
	 See K Femoral Artery, Right
	 M Popliteal Artery, Right
	 Inferior genicular artery
	 Middle genicular artery
	 Superior genicular artery
	 Sural artery
	 Tibioperoneal trunk
	 N Popliteal Artery, Left
	 See M Popliteal Artery, Right
	 P Anterior Tibial Artery, Right
	 Anterior lateral malleolar
	    artery
	 Anterior medial malleolar
	    artery
	 Anterior tibial recurrent artery
	 Dorsalis pedis artery
	 Posterior tibial recurrent artery
	 Q Anterior Tibial Artery, Left
	 See P Anterior Tibial Artery, Right
	 R Posterior Tibial Artery, Right
	 S Posterior Tibial Artery, Left
	 T Peroneal Artery, Right
	 Fibular artery
	 U Peroneal Artery, Left
	 See T Peroneal Artery, Right
	 V Foot Artery, Right
	 Arcuate artery
	 Dorsal metatarsal artery
	 Lateral plantar artery
	 Lateral tarsal artery
	 Medial plantar artery
	 W Foot Artery, Left
	 See V Foot Artery, Right
	 Y Lower Artery
	 Umbilical artery
		Ø Open
		 3 Percutaneous
		 4 Percutaneous Endoscopic
			5 Intraluminal Device, Drug-eluting, Two
			 6 Intraluminal Device, Drug-eluting, Three
			 7 Intraluminal Device, Drug-eluting, Four or More
			 E Intraluminal Device, Two
			 F Intraluminal Device, Three
			 G Intraluminal Device, Four or More
				Z No Qualifier

Non-OR Procedure   DRG Non-OR Procedure   Valid OR Procedure   HAC Associated Procedure   Combination Only   New/Revised April   New/Revised October

226   ICD-10-PCS 2024

0   **Medical and Surgical**
4   **Lower Arteries**
9   **Drainage**   Definition: Taking or letting out fluids and/or gases from a body part

                     Explanation: The qualifier DIAGNOSTIC is used to identify drainage procedures that are biopsies

Body Part Character 4		Approach Character 5	Device Character 6	Qualifier Character 7

0 Abdominal Aorta
Inferior phrenic artery
Lumbar artery
Median sacral artery
Middle suprarenal artery
Ovarian artery
Testicular artery
1 Celiac Artery
Celiac trunk
2 Gastric Artery
Left gastric artery
Right gastric artery
3 Hepatic Artery
Common hepatic artery
Gastroduodenal artery
Hepatic artery proper
4 Splenic Artery
Left gastroepiploic artery
Pancreatic artery
Short gastric artery
5 Superior Mesenteric Artery
Ileal artery
Ileocolic artery
Inferior pancreaticoduodenal
   artery
Jejunal artery
6 Colic Artery, Right
7 Colic Artery, Left
8 Colic Artery, Middle
9 Renal Artery, Right
Inferior suprarenal artery
Renal segmental artery
A Renal Artery, Left
See 9 Renal Artery, Right
B Inferior Mesenteric Artery
Sigmoid artery
Superior rectal artery
C Common Iliac Artery, Right
D Common Iliac Artery, Left
E Internal Iliac Artery, Right
Deferential artery
Hypogastric artery
Iliolumbar artery
Inferior gluteal artery
Inferior vesical artery
Internal pudendal artery
Lateral sacral artery
Middle rectal artery
Obturator artery
Prostatic artery
Superior gluteal artery
Superior vesical artery
Umbilical artery
Uterine artery
Vaginal artery
	F Internal Iliac Artery, Left
	See E Internal Iliac Artery, Right
	H External Iliac Artery, Right
	Deep circumflex iliac artery
	Inferior epigastric artery
	J External Iliac Artery, Left
	See H External Iliac Artery, Right
	K Femoral Artery, Right
	Circumflex iliac artery
	Deep femoral artery
	Descending genicular artery
	External pudendal artery
	Superficial epigastric artery
	L Femoral Artery, Left
	See K Femoral Artery, Right
	M Popliteal Artery, Right
	Inferior genicular artery
	Middle genicular artery
	Superior genicular artery
	Sural artery
	Tibioperoneal trunk
	N Popliteal Artery, Left
	See M Popliteal Artery, Right
	P Anterior Tibial Artery, Right
	Anterior lateral malleolar
	   artery
	Anterior medial malleolar
	   artery
	Anterior tibial recurrent artery
	Dorsalis pedis artery
	Posterior tibial recurrent artery
	Q Anterior Tibial Artery, Left
	See P Anterior Tibial Artery,
	Right
	R Posterior Tibial Artery, Right
	S Posterior Tibial Artery, Left
	T Peroneal Artery, Right
	Fibular artery
	U Peroneal Artery, Left
	See T Peroneal Artery, Right
	V Foot Artery, Right
	Arcuate artery
	Dorsal metatarsal artery
	Lateral plantar artery
	Lateral tarsal artery
	Medial plantar artery
	W Foot Artery, Left
	See V Foot Artery, Right
	Y Lower Artery
	Umbilical artery
		0 Open
		3 Percutaneous
		4 Percutaneous Endoscopic
			0 Drainage Device	**Z No Qualifier**

Non-OR   049[0,1,2,3,4,5,6,7,8,9,A,B,C,D,E,F,H,J,K,L,M,N,P,Q,R,S,T,U,V,W,Y][0,3,4]0Z

049 Continued on next page

NC Noncovered Procedure   LC Limited Coverage   QA Questionable OB Admit   NT New Tech Add-on   ⊞ Combination Member   ♂ Male   ♀ Female

Ø   **Medical and Surgical**   *Ø49 Continued*
4   **Lower Arteries**
9   **Drainage**   Definition: Taking or letting out fluids and/or gases from a body part
                      Explanation: The qualifier DIAGNOSTIC is used to identify drainage procedures that are biopsies

Body Part Character 4		Approach Character 5	Device Character 6	Qualifier Character 7

Ø Abdominal Aorta
  Inferior phrenic artery
  Lumbar artery
  Median sacral artery
  Middle suprarenal artery
  Ovarian artery
  Testicular artery
1 Celiac Artery
  Celiac trunk
2 Gastric Artery
  Left gastric artery
  Right gastric artery
3 Hepatic Artery
  Common hepatic artery
  Gastroduodenal artery
  Hepatic artery proper
4 Splenic Artery
  Left gastroepiploic artery
  Pancreatic artery
  Short gastric artery
5 Superior Mesenteric Artery
  Ileal artery
  Ileocolic artery
  Inferior pancreaticoduodenal
    artery
  Jejunal artery
6 Colic Artery, Right
7 Colic Artery, Left
8 Colic Artery, Middle
9 Renal Artery, Right
  Inferior suprarenal artery
  Renal segmental artery
A Renal Artery, Left
  See 9 Renal Artery, Right
B Inferior Mesenteric Artery
  Sigmoid artery
  Superior rectal artery
C Common Iliac Artery, Right
D Common Iliac Artery, Left
E Internal Iliac Artery, Right
  Deferential artery
  Hypogastric artery
  Iliolumbar artery
  Inferior gluteal artery
  Inferior vesical artery
  Internal pudendal artery
  Lateral sacral artery
  Middle rectal artery
  Obturator artery
  Prostatic artery
  Superior gluteal artery
  Superior vesical artery
  Umbilical artery
  Uterine artery
  Vaginal artery
	F Internal Iliac Artery, Left
	  See E Internal Iliac Artery, Right
	H External Iliac Artery, Right
	  Deep circumflex iliac artery
	  Inferior epigastric artery
	J External Iliac Artery, Left
	  See H External Iliac Artery, Right
	K Femoral Artery, Right
	  Circumflex iliac artery
	  Deep femoral artery
	  Descending genicular artery
	  External pudendal artery
	  Superficial epigastric artery
	L Femoral Artery, Left
	  See K Femoral Artery, Right
	M Popliteal Artery, Right
	  Inferior genicular artery
	  Middle genicular artery
	  Superior genicular artery
	  Sural artery
	  Tibioperoneal trunk
	N Popliteal Artery, Left
	  See M Popliteal Artery, Right
	P Anterior Tibial Artery, Right
	  Anterior lateral malleolar
	    artery
	  Anterior medial malleolar
	    artery
	  Anterior tibial recurrent artery
	  Dorsalis pedis artery
	  Posterior tibial recurrent artery
	Q Anterior Tibial Artery, Left
	  See P Anterior Tibial Artery,
	    Right
	R Posterior Tibial Artery, Right
	S Posterior Tibial Artery, Left
	T Peroneal Artery, Right
	  Fibular artery
	U Peroneal Artery, Left
	  See T Peroneal Artery, Right
	V Foot Artery, Right
	  Arcuate artery
	  Dorsal metatarsal artery
	  Lateral plantar artery
	  Lateral tarsal artery
	  Medial plantar artery
	W Foot Artery, Left
	  See V Foot Artery, Right
	Y Lower Artery
	  Umbilical artery
		Ø Open
		3 Percutaneous
		4 Percutaneous Endoscopic
			Z No Device	**X Diagnostic**
				Z No Qualifier

Non-OR   049[Ø,1,2,3,4,5,6,7,8,9,A,B,C,D,E,F,H,J,K,L,M,N,P,Q,R,S,T,U,V,W,Y]3ZX
Non-OR   049[Ø,1,2,3,4,5,6,7,8,9,A,B,C,D,E,F,H,J,K,L,M,N,P,Q,R,S,T,U,V,W,Y][Ø,3,4]ZZ

Ø49–Ø49

Non-OR Procedure   DRG Non-OR Procedure   Valid OR Procedure   HAC Associated Procedure   Combination Only   New/Revised April   New/Revised October
228   ICD-10-PCS 2024

0   Medical and Surgical
4   Lower Arteries
B   Excision   Definition: Cutting out or off, without replacement, a portion of a body part

                Explanation: The qualifier DIAGNOSTIC is used to identify excision procedures that are biopsies

Body Part Character 4		Approach Character 5	Device Character 6	Qualifier Character 7

0 Abdominal Aorta
  Inferior phrenic artery
  Lumbar artery
  Median sacral artery
  Middle suprarenal artery
  Ovarian artery
  Testicular artery
1 Celiac Artery
  Celiac trunk
2 Gastric Artery
  Left gastric artery
  Right gastric artery
3 Hepatic Artery
  Common hepatic artery
  Gastroduodenal artery
  Hepatic artery proper
4 Splenic Artery
  Left gastroepiploic artery
  Pancreatic artery
  Short gastric artery
5 Superior Mesenteric Artery
  Ileal artery
  Ileocolic artery
  Inferior pancreaticoduodenal
    artery
  Jejunal artery
6 Colic Artery, Right
7 Colic Artery, Left
8 Colic Artery, Middle
9 Renal Artery, Right
  Inferior suprarenal artery
  Renal segmental artery
A Renal Artery, Left
  See 9 Renal Artery, Right
B Inferior Mesenteric Artery
  Sigmoid artery
  Superior rectal artery
C Common Iliac Artery, Right
D Common Iliac Artery, Left
E Internal Iliac Artery, Right
  Deferential artery
  Hypogastric artery
  Iliolumbar artery
  Inferior gluteal artery
  Inferior vesical artery
  Internal pudendal artery
  Lateral sacral artery
  Middle rectal artery
  Obturator artery
  Prostatic artery
  Superior gluteal artery
  Superior vesical artery
  Umbilical artery
  Uterine artery
  Vaginal artery
	F Internal Iliac Artery, Left
	  See E Internal Iliac Artery, Right
	H External Iliac Artery, Right
	  Deep circumflex iliac artery
	  Inferior epigastric artery
	J External Iliac Artery, Left
	  See H External Iliac Artery, Right
	K Femoral Artery, Right
	  Circumflex iliac artery
	  Deep femoral artery
	  Descending genicular artery
	  External pudendal artery
	  Superficial epigastric artery
	L Femoral Artery, Left
	  See K Femoral Artery, Right
	M Popliteal Artery, Right
	  Inferior genicular artery
	  Middle genicular artery
	  Superior genicular artery
	  Sural artery
	  Tibioperoneal trunk
	N Popliteal Artery, Left
	  See M Popliteal Artery, Right
	P Anterior Tibial Artery, Right
	  Anterior lateral malleolar
	    artery
	  Anterior medial malleolar
	    artery
	  Anterior tibial recurrent artery
	  Dorsalis pedis artery
	  Posterior tibial recurrent artery
	Q Anterior Tibial Artery, Left
	  See P Anterior Tibial Artery,
	    Right
	R Posterior Tibial Artery, Right
	S Posterior Tibial Artery, Left
	T Peroneal Artery, Right
	  Fibular artery
	U Peroneal Artery, Left
	  See T Peroneal Artery, Right
	V Foot Artery, Right
	  Arcuate artery
	  Dorsal metatarsal artery
	  Lateral plantar artery
	  Lateral tarsal artery
	  Medial plantar artery
	W Foot Artery, Left
	  See V Foot Artery, Right
	Y Lower Artery
	  Umbilical artery
		0 Open
		3 Percutaneous
		4 Percutaneous Endoscopic
			Z No Device	**X** Diagnostic
				Z No Qualifier

NC Noncovered Procedure   **LC** Limited Coverage   **QA** Questionable OB Admit   **NT** New Tech Add-on   ⊞ Combination Member   ♂ Male   ♀ Female

ICD-10-PCS 2024   **229**

04B–04B

Ø Medical and Surgical
4 Lower Arteries
C Extirpation   Definition: Taking or cutting out solid matter from a body part

Explanation: The solid matter may be an abnormal byproduct of a biological function or a foreign body; it may be imbedded in a body part or in the lumen of a tubular body part. The solid matter may or may not have been previously broken into pieces.

Body Part Character 4		Approach Character 5	Device Character 6	Qualifier Character 7

Ø Abdominal Aorta
Inferior phrenic artery
Lumbar artery
Median sacral artery
Middle suprarenal artery
Ovarian artery
Testicular artery
1 Celiac Artery
Celiac trunk
2 Gastric Artery
Left gastric artery
Right gastric artery
3 Hepatic Artery
Common hepatic artery
Gastroduodenal artery
Hepatic artery proper
4 Splenic Artery
Left gastroepiploic artery
Pancreatic artery
Short gastric artery
5 Superior Mesenteric Artery
Ileal artery
Ileocolic artery
Inferior pancreaticoduodenal
    artery
Jejunal artery
6 Colic Artery, Right
7 Colic Artery, Left
8 Colic Artery, Middle
9 Renal Artery, Right
Inferior suprarenal artery
Renal segmental artery
A Renal Artery, Left
See 9 Renal Artery, Right
B Inferior Mesenteric Artery
Sigmoid artery
Superior rectal artery
C Common Iliac Artery, Right
D Common Iliac Artery, Left
E Internal Iliac Artery, Right
Deferential artery
Hypogastric artery
Iliolumbar artery
Inferior gluteal artery
Inferior vesical artery
Internal pudendal artery
Lateral sacral artery
Middle rectal artery
Obturator artery
Prostatic artery
Superior gluteal artery
Superior vesical artery
Umbilical artery
Uterine artery
Vaginal artery
	F Internal Iliac Artery, Left
	See E Internal Iliac Artery, Right
	H External Iliac Artery, Right
	Deep circumflex iliac artery
	Inferior epigastric artery
	J External Iliac Artery, Left
	See H External Iliac Artery, Right
	K Femoral Artery, Right
	Circumflex iliac artery
	Deep femoral artery
	Descending genicular artery
	External pudendal artery
	Superficial epigastric artery
	L Femoral Artery, Left
	See K Femoral Artery, Right
	M Popliteal Artery, Right
	Inferior genicular artery
	Middle genicular artery
	Superior genicular artery
	Sural artery
	Tibioperoneal trunk
	N Popliteal Artery, Left
	See M Popliteal Artery, Right
	P Anterior Tibial Artery, Right
	Anterior lateral malleolar
	    artery
	Anterior medial malleolar
	    artery
	Anterior tibial recurrent artery
	Dorsalis pedis artery
	Posterior tibial recurrent artery
	Q Anterior Tibial Artery, Left
	See P Anterior Tibial Artery,
	* Right*
	R Posterior Tibial Artery, Right
	S Posterior Tibial Artery, Left
	T Peroneal Artery, Right
	Fibular artery
	U Peroneal Artery, Left
	See T Peroneal Artery, Right
	V Foot Artery, Right
	Arcuate artery
	Dorsal metatarsal artery
	Lateral plantar artery
	Lateral tarsal artery
	Medial plantar artery
	W Foot Artery, Left
	See V Foot Artery, Right
	Y Lower Artery
	Umbilical artery
		Ø Open
		3 Percutaneous
		4 Percutaneous Endoscopic
			Z No Device	**Z No Qualifier**

Non-OR Procedure   DRG Non-OR Procedure   Valid OR Procedure   HAC Associated Procedure   Combination Only   New/Revised April   New/Revised October

230   ICD-10-PCS 2024

Ø4C–Ø4C

Ø   Medical and Surgical
4   Lower Arteries
F   Fragmentation   Definition: Breaking solid matter in a body part into pieces

Explanation: Physical force (e.g., manual, ultrasonic) applied directly or indirectly is used to break the solid matter into pieces. The solid matter may be an abnormal byproduct of a biological function or a foreign body. The pieces of solid matter are not taken out.

Body Part Character 4	Approach Character 5	Device Character 6	Qualifier Character 7

C Common Iliac Artery, Right
D Common Iliac Artery, Left
E Internal Iliac Artery, Right
   Deferential artery
   Hypogastric artery
   Iliolumbar artery
   Inferior gluteal artery
   Inferior vesical artery
   Internal pudendal artery
   Lateral sacral artery
   Middle rectal artery
   Obturator artery
   Prostatic artery
   Superior gluteal artery
   Superior vesical artery
   Umbilical artery
   Uterine artery
   Vaginal artery
F Internal Iliac Artery, Left
   See E Internal Iliac Artery, Right
H External Iliac Artery, Right
   Deep circumflex iliac artery
   Inferior epigastric artery
J External Iliac Artery, Left
   See H External Iliac Artery, Right
K Femoral Artery, Right
   Circumflex iliac artery
   Deep femoral artery
   Descending genicular artery
   External pudendal artery
   Superficial epigastric artery
L Femoral Artery, Left
   See K Femoral Artery, Right
M Popliteal Artery, Right
   Inferior genicular artery
   Middle genicular artery
   Superior genicular artery
   Sural artery
   Tibioperoneal trunk
N Popliteal Artery, Left
   See M Popliteal Artery, Right
P Anterior Tibial Artery, Right
   Anterior lateral malleolar artery
   Anterior medial malleolar artery
   Anterior tibial recurrent artery
   Dorsalis pedis artery
   Posterior tibial recurrent artery
Q Anterior Tibial Artery, Left
   See P Anterior Tibial Artery, Right
R Posterior Tibial Artery, Right
S Posterior Tibial Artery, Left
T Peroneal Artery, Right
   Fibular artery
U Peroneal Artery, Left
   See T Peroneal Artery, Right
Y Lower Artery
   Umbilical artery
	3 Percutaneous	**Z** No Device	**Ø** Ultrasonic
			Z No Qualifier

NC Noncovered Procedure   **LC** Limited Coverage   **QA** Questionable OB Admit   **NT** New Tech Add-on   ✚ Combination Member   ♂Male   ♀Female

ICD-10-PCS 2024   231

04F–04F

Lower Arteries

0   **Medical and Surgical**
4   **Lower Arteries**
H   **Insertion**   Definition: Putting in a nonbiological appliance that monitors, assists, performs, or prevents a physiological function but does not physically take the place of a body part
                     Explanation: None

Body Part Character 4	Approach Character 5	Device Character 6	Qualifier Character 7

0 Abdominal Aorta
  Inferior phrenic artery
  Lumbar artery
  Median sacral artery
  Middle suprarenal artery
  Ovarian artery
  Testicular artery
	0 Open
	3 Percutaneous
	4 Percutaneous Endoscopic
		2 Monitoring Device
		3 Infusion Device
		D Intraluminal Device
			Z No Qualifier

1 Celiac Artery
  Celiac trunk
2 Gastric Artery
  Left gastric artery
  Right gastric artery
3 Hepatic Artery
  Common hepatic artery
  Gastroduodenal artery
  Hepatic artery proper
4 Splenic Artery
  Left gastroepiploic artery
  Pancreatic artery
  Short gastric artery
5 Superior Mesenteric Artery
  Ileal artery
  Ileocolic artery
  Inferior pancreaticoduodenal
    artery
  Jejunal artery
6 Colic Artery, Right
7 Colic Artery, Left
8 Colic Artery, Middle
9 Renal Artery, Right
  Inferior suprarenal artery
  Renal segmental artery
A Renal Artery, Left
  See 9 Renal Artery, Right
B Inferior Mesenteric Artery
  Sigmoid artery
  Superior rectal artery
C Common Iliac Artery, Right
D Common Iliac Artery, Left
E Internal Iliac Artery, Right
  Deferential artery
  Hypogastric artery
  Iliolumbar artery
  Inferior gluteal artery
  Inferior vesical artery
  Internal pudendal artery
  Lateral sacral artery
  Middle rectal artery
  Obturator artery
  Prostatic artery
  Superior gluteal artery
  Superior vesical artery
  Umbilical artery
  Uterine artery
  Vaginal artery
	F Internal Iliac Artery, Left
	  See E Internal Iliac Artery, Right
	H External Iliac Artery, Right
	  Deep circumflex iliac artery
	  Inferior epigastric artery
	J External Iliac Artery, Left
	  See H External Iliac Artery, Right
	K Femoral Artery, Right
	  Circumflex iliac artery
	  Deep femoral artery
	  Descending genicular artery
	  External pudendal artery
	  Superficial epigastric artery
	L Femoral Artery, Left
	  See K Femoral Artery, Right
	M Popliteal Artery, Right
	  Inferior genicular artery
	  Middle genicular artery
	  Superior genicular artery
	  Sural artery
	  Tibioperoneal trunk
	N Popliteal Artery, Left
	  See M Popliteal Artery, Right
	P Anterior Tibial Artery, Right
	  Anterior lateral malleolar
	    artery
	  Anterior medial malleolar
	    artery
	  Anterior tibial recurrent artery
	  Dorsalis pedis artery
	  Posterior tibial recurrent artery
	Q Anterior Tibial Artery, Left
	  *See P Anterior Tibial Artery,
	    Right*
	R Posterior Tibial Artery, Right
	S Posterior Tibial Artery, Left
	T Peroneal Artery, Right
	  Fibular artery
	U Peroneal Artery, Left
	  See T Peroneal Artery, Right
	V Foot Artery, Right
	  Arcuate artery
	  Dorsal metatarsal artery
	  Lateral plantar artery
	  Lateral tarsal artery
	  Medial plantar artery
	W Foot Artery, Left
	  See V Foot Artery, Right
		0 Open
		3 Percutaneous
		4 Percutaneous Endoscopic
			3 Infusion Device
			D Intraluminal Device
				Z No Qualifier

Y Lower Artery Umbilical artery	**0** Open **3** Percutaneous **4** Percutaneous Endoscopic	**2** Monitoring Device **3** Infusion Device **D** Intraluminal Device **Y** Other Device	**Z** No Qualifier

Non-OR   04H0[0,3,4][2,3]Z
Non-OR   04H[1,2,3,4,5,6,7,8,9,A,B,C,D,E,F,H,J,K,L,M,N,P,Q,R,S,T,U,V,W][0,3,4]3Z
Non-OR   04HY32Z
Non-OR   04HY[0,3,4]3Z
Non-OR   04HY[3,4]YZ

Non-OR Procedure   DRG Non-OR Procedure   Valid OR Procedure   HAC Associated Procedure   Combination Only   New/Revised April   New/Revised October

232   ICD-10-PCS 2024

04H–04H

0   **Medical and Surgical**
4   **Lower Arteries**
J   **Inspection**   Definition: Visually and/or manually exploring a body part

Explanation: Visual exploration may be performed with or without optical instrumentation. Manual exploration may be performed directly or through intervening body layers.

Body Part Character 4	Approach Character 5	Device Character 6	Qualifier Character 7
Y Lower Artery Umbilical artery	**0** Open **3** Percutaneous **4** Percutaneous Endoscopic **X** External	**Z** No Device	**Z** No Qualifier

Non-OR   04JY[3,4,X]ZZ

0   **Medical and Surgical**
4   **Lower Arteries**
L   **Occlusion**   Definition: Completely closing an orifice or the lumen of a tubular body part

Explanation: The orifice can be a natural orifice or an artificially created orifice

Body Part Character 4	Approach Character 5	Device Character 6	Qualifier Character 7

0   Abdominal Aorta
    Inferior phrenic artery
    Lumbar artery
    Median sacral artery
    Middle suprarenal artery
    Ovarian artery
    Testicular artery
	0 Open
	3 Percutaneous
		C Extraluminal Device
		Z No Device
			Z No Qualifier

0   Abdominal Aorta
    Inferior phrenic artery
    Lumbar artery
    Median sacral artery
    Middle suprarenal artery
    Ovarian artery
    Testicular artery
	0 Open
	3 Percutaneous
		D Intraluminal Device	**J** Temporary
			Z No Qualifier

0   Abdominal Aorta
    Inferior phrenic artery
    Lumbar artery
    Median sacral artery
    Middle suprarenal artery
    Ovarian artery
    Testicular artery
	4 Percutaneous Endoscopic	**C** Extraluminal Device
		D Intraluminal Device
		Z No Device
			Z No Qualifier

04L Continued on next page

NC Noncovered Procedure   **LC** Limited Coverage   **QA** Questionable OB Admit   **NT** New Tech Add-on   ✚ Combination Member   ♂ Male   ♀ Female

ICD-10-PCS 2024   233

0   **Medical and Surgical**   *04L Continued*
4   **Lower Arteries**
L   **Occlusion**   Definition: Completely closing an orifice or the lumen of a tubular body part
                   Explanation: The orifice can be a natural orifice or an artificially created orifice

Body Part Character 4		Approach Character 5	Device Character 6	Qualifier Character 7

1 Celiac Artery
   Celiac trunk
2 Gastric Artery
   Left gastric artery
   Right gastric artery
3 Hepatic Artery
   Common hepatic artery
   Gastroduodenal artery
   Hepatic artery proper
4 Splenic Artery
   Left gastroepiploic artery
   Pancreatic artery
   Short gastric artery
5 Superior Mesenteric Artery
   Ileal artery
   Ileocolic artery
   Inferior pancreaticoduodenal
     artery
   Jejunal artery
6 Colic Artery, Right
7 Colic Artery, Left
8 Colic Artery, Middle
9 Renal Artery, Right
   Inferior suprarenal artery
   Renal segmental artery
A Renal Artery, Left
   See 9 Renal Artery, Right
B Inferior Mesenteric Artery
   Sigmoid artery
   Superior rectal artery
C Common Iliac Artery, Right
D Common Iliac Artery, Left
H External Iliac Artery, Right
   Deep circumflex iliac artery
   Inferior epigastric artery
J External Iliac Artery, Left
   See H External Iliac Artery,
    Right
	K Femoral Artery, Right
	   Circumflex iliac artery
	   Deep femoral artery
	   Descending genicular artery
	   External pudendal artery
	   Superficial epigastric artery
	L Femoral Artery, Left
	   See K Femoral Artery, Right
	M Popliteal Artery, Right
	   Inferior genicular artery
	   Middle genicular artery
	   Superior genicular artery
	   Sural artery
	   Tibioperoneal trunk
	N Popliteal Artery, Left
	   See M Popliteal Artery, Right
	P Anterior Tibial Artery, Right
	   Anterior lateral malleolar artery
	   Anterior medial malleolar artery
	   Anterior tibial recurrent artery
	   Dorsalis pedis artery
	   Posterior tibial recurrent artery
	Q Anterior Tibial Artery, Left
	   See P Anterior Tibial Artery, Right
	R Posterior Tibial Artery, Right
	S Posterior Tibial Artery, Left
	T Peroneal Artery, Right
	   Fibular artery
	U Peroneal Artery, Left
	   See T Peroneal Artery, Right
	V Foot Artery, Right
	   Arcuate artery
	   Dorsal metatarsal artery
	   Lateral plantar artery
	   Lateral tarsal artery
	   Medial plantar artery
	W Foot Artery, Left
	   See V Foot Artery, Right
	Y Lower Artery
	   Umbilical artery
		0 Open
		3 Percutaneous
		4 Percutaneous Endoscopic
			C Extraluminal Device
			D Intraluminal Device
			Z No Device
				Z No Qualifier

E Internal Iliac Artery, Right
   Deferential artery
   Hypogastric artery
   Iliolumbar artery
   Inferior gluteal artery
   Inferior vesical artery
   Internal pudendal artery
   Lateral sacral artery
   Middle rectal artery
   Obturator artery
   Prostatic artery
   Superior gluteal artery
   Superior vesical artery
   Umbilical artery
   Uterine artery
   Vaginal artery
		0 Open
		3 Percutaneous
		4 Percutaneous Endoscopic
			C Extraluminal Device
			D Intraluminal Device
			Z No Device
				T Uterine Artery, Right ♀
				V Prostatic Artery, Right ♂
				Z No Qualifier

F Internal Iliac Artery, Left
   Deferential artery
   Hypogastric artery
   Iliolumbar artery
   Inferior gluteal artery
   Inferior vesical artery
   Internal pudendal artery
   Lateral sacral artery
   Middle rectal artery
   Obturator artery
   Prostatic artery
   Superior gluteal artery
   Superior vesical artery
   Umbilical artery
   Uterine artery
   Vaginal artery
		0 Open
		3 Percutaneous
		4 Percutaneous Endoscopic
			C Extraluminal Device
			D Intraluminal Device
			Z No Device
				U Uterine Artery, Left ♀
				W Prostatic Artery, Left ♂
				Z No Qualifier

♀   04LE[0,3,4][C,D,Z]T
♀   04LF[0,3,4][C,D,Z]U
♂   04LE[0,3,4][C,D,Z]V
♂   04LF[0,3,4][C,D,Z]W

Non-OR Procedure   DRG Non-OR Procedure   Valid OR Procedure   HAC Associated Procedure   Combination Only   New/Revised April   New/Revised October

234   ICD-10-PCS 2024

04L–04L

Ø Medical and Surgical
4 Lower Arteries
N Release   Definition: Freeing a body part from an abnormal physical constraint by cutting or by the use of force
                                      Explanation: Some of the restraining tissue may be taken out but none of the body part is taken out

Body Part Character 4		Approach Character 5	Device Character 6	Qualifier Character 7

Ø Abdominal Aorta
  Inferior phrenic artery
  Lumbar artery
  Median sacral artery
  Middle suprarenal artery
  Ovarian artery
  Testicular artery
1 Celiac Artery
  Celiac trunk
2 Gastric Artery
  Left gastric artery
  Right gastric artery
3 Hepatic Artery
  Common hepatic artery
  Gastroduodenal artery
  Hepatic artery proper
4 Splenic Artery
  Left gastroepiploic artery
  Pancreatic artery
  Short gastric artery
5 Superior Mesenteric Artery
  Ileal artery
  Ileocolic artery
  Inferior pancreaticoduodenal
    artery
  Jejunal artery
6 Colic Artery, Right
7 Colic Artery, Left
8 Colic Artery, Middle
9 Renal Artery, Right
  Inferior suprarenal artery
  Renal segmental artery
A Renal Artery, Left
  See 9 Renal Artery, Right
B Inferior Mesenteric Artery
  Sigmoid artery
  Superior rectal artery
C Common Iliac Artery, Right
D Common Iliac Artery, Left
E Internal Iliac Artery, Right
  Deferential artery
  Hypogastric artery
  Iliolumbar artery
  Inferior gluteal artery
  Inferior vesical artery
  Internal pudendal artery
  Lateral sacral artery
  Middle rectal artery
  Obturator artery
  Prostatic artery
  Superior gluteal artery
  Superior vesical artery
  Umbilical artery
  Uterine artery
  Vaginal artery
	F Internal Iliac Artery, Left
	  See E Internal Iliac Artery,
	    Right
	H External Iliac Artery, Right
	  Deep circumflex iliac artery
	  Inferior epigastric artery
	J External Iliac Artery, Left
	  See H External Iliac Artery,
	    Right
	K Femoral Artery, Right
	  Circumflex iliac artery
	  Deep femoral artery
	  Descending genicular artery
	  External pudendal artery
	  Superficial epigastric artery
	L Femoral Artery, Left
	  See K Femoral Artery, Right
	M Popliteal Artery, Right
	  Inferior genicular artery
	  Middle genicular artery
	  Superior genicular artery
	  Sural artery
	  Tibioperoneal trunk
	N Popliteal Artery, Left
	  See M Popliteal Artery, Right
	P Anterior Tibial Artery, Right
	  Anterior lateral malleolar
	    artery
	  Anterior medial malleolar
	    artery
	  Anterior tibial recurrent
	    artery
	  Dorsalis pedis artery
	  Posterior tibial recurrent
	    artery
	Q Anterior Tibial Artery, Left
	  See P Anterior Tibial Artery,
	    Right
	R Posterior Tibial Artery,
	  Right
	S Posterior Tibial Artery, Left
	T Peroneal Artery, Right
	  Fibular artery
	U Peroneal Artery, Left
	  See T Peroneal Artery, Right
	V Foot Artery, Right
	  Arcuate artery
	  Dorsal metatarsal artery
	  Lateral plantar artery
	  Lateral tarsal artery
	  Medial plantar artery
	W Foot Artery, Left
	  See V Foot Artery, Right
	Y Lower Artery
	  Umbilical artery
		Ø Open
		3 Percutaneous
		4 Percutaneous Endoscopic
			Z No Device	**Z No Qualifier**

NC Noncovered Procedure   LC Limited Coverage   QA Questionable OB Admit   NT New Tech Add-on   ⊞ Combination Member   ♂ Male   ♀ Female

Lower Arteries

Ø   **Medical and Surgical**
4   **Lower Arteries**
P   **Removal**   Definition: Taking out or off a device from a body part

Explanation: If a device is taken out and a similar device put in without cutting or puncturing the skin or mucous membrane, the procedure is coded to the root operation CHANGE. Otherwise, the procedure for taking out a device is coded to the root operation REMOVAL.

Body Part Character 4	Approach Character 5	Device Character 6	Qualifier Character 7
Y Lower Artery Umbilical artery	Ø Open 3 Percutaneous 4 Percutaneous Endoscopic	Ø Drainage Device 2 Monitoring Device 3 Infusion Device 7 Autologous Tissue Substitute C Extraluminal Device D Intraluminal Device J Synthetic Substitute K Nonautologous Tissue Substitute Y Other Device	Z No Qualifier
Y Lower Artery Umbilical artery	X External	Ø Drainage Device 1 Radioactive Element 2 Monitoring Device 3 Infusion Device D Intraluminal Device	Z No Qualifier

Non-OR   04PY3[0,2,3,D]Z
Non-OR   04PY[3,4]YZ
Non-OR   04PYX[0,1,2,3,D]Z

Lower Arteries

0   **Medical and Surgical**
4   **Lower Arteries**
Q   **Repair**   Definition: Restoring, to the extent possible, a body part to its normal anatomic structure and function
                    Explanation: Used only when the method to accomplish the repair is not one of the other root operations

Body Part Character 4		Approach Character 5	Device Character 6	Qualifier Character 7

0 Abdominal Aorta
    Inferior phrenic artery
    Lumbar artery
    Median sacral artery
    Middle suprarenal artery
    Ovarian artery
    Testicular artery
1 Celiac Artery
    Celiac trunk
2 Gastric Artery
    Left gastric artery
    Right gastric artery
3 Hepatic Artery
    Common hepatic artery
    Gastroduodenal artery
    Hepatic artery proper
4 Splenic Artery
    Left gastroepiploic artery
    Pancreatic artery
    Short gastric artery
5 Superior Mesenteric Artery
    Ileal artery
    Ileocolic artery
    Inferior pancreaticoduodenal
      artery
    Jejunal artery
6 Colic Artery, Right
7 Colic Artery, Left
8 Colic Artery, Middle
9 Renal Artery, Right
    Inferior suprarenal artery
    Renal segmental artery
A Renal Artery, Left
    See 9 Renal Artery, Right
B Inferior Mesenteric Artery
    Sigmoid artery
    Superior rectal artery
C Common Iliac Artery, Right
D Common Iliac Artery, Left
E Internal Iliac Artery, Right
    Deferential artery
    Hypogastric artery
    Iliolumbar artery
    Inferior gluteal artery
    Inferior vesical artery
    Internal pudendal artery
    Lateral sacral artery
    Middle rectal artery
    Obturator artery
    Prostatic artery
    Superior gluteal artery
    Superior vesical artery
    Umbilical artery
    Uterine artery
    Vaginal artery
	F Internal Iliac Artery, Left
	    See E Internal Iliac Artery,
	     Right
	H External Iliac Artery, Right
	    Deep circumflex iliac artery
	    Inferior epigastric artery
	J External Iliac Artery, Left
	    See H External Iliac Artery,
	     Right
	K Femoral Artery, Right
	    Circumflex iliac artery
	    Deep femoral artery
	    Descending genicular artery
	    External pudendal artery
	    Superficial epigastric artery
	L Femoral Artery, Left
	    See K Femoral Artery, Right
	M Popliteal Artery, Right
	    Inferior genicular artery
	    Middle genicular artery
	    Superior genicular artery
	    Sural artery
	    Tibioperoneal trunk
	N Popliteal Artery, Left
	    See M Popliteal Artery, Right
	P Anterior Tibial Artery, Right
	    Anterior lateral malleolar
	     artery
	    Anterior medial malleolar
	     artery
	    Anterior tibial recurrent
	     artery
	    Dorsalis pedis artery
	    Posterior tibial recurrent
	     artery
	Q Anterior Tibial Artery, Left
	    See P Anterior Tibial Artery,
	     Right
	R Posterior Tibial Artery,
	    Right
	S Posterior Tibial Artery, Left
	T Peroneal Artery, Right
	    Fibular artery
	U Peroneal Artery, Left
	    See T Peroneal Artery, Right
	V Foot Artery, Right
	    Arcuate artery
	    Dorsal metatarsal artery
	    Lateral plantar artery
	    Lateral tarsal artery
	    Medial plantar artery
	W Foot Artery, Left
	    See V Foot Artery, Right
	Y Lower Artery
	    Umbilical artery
		0 Open
		3 Percutaneous
		4 Percutaneous Endoscopic
			Z No Device	**Z** No Qualifier

Lower Arteries (side tab)

0   Medical and Surgical
4   Lower Arteries
R   Replacement

Definition: Putting in or on biological or synthetic material that physically takes the place and/or function of all or a portion of a body part

Explanation: The body part may have been taken out or replaced, or may be taken out, physically eradicated, or rendered nonfunctional during the REPLACEMENT procedure. A REMOVAL procedure is coded for taking out the device used in a previous replacement procedure.

Body Part — Character 4	Approach — Character 5	Device — Character 6	Qualifier — Character 7
0 Abdominal Aorta Inferior phrenic artery Lumbar artery Median sacral artery Middle suprarenal artery Ovarian artery Testicular artery **1** Celiac Artery Celiac trunk **2** Gastric Artery Left gastric artery Right gastric artery **3** Hepatic Artery Common hepatic artery Gastroduodenal artery Hepatic artery proper **4** Splenic Artery Left gastroepiploic artery Pancreatic artery Short gastric artery **5** Superior Mesenteric Artery Ileal artery Ileocolic artery Inferior pancreaticoduodenal artery Jejunal artery **6** Colic Artery, Right **7** Colic Artery, Left **8** Colic Artery, Middle **9** Renal Artery, Right Inferior suprarenal artery Renal segmental artery **A** Renal Artery, Left *See 9 Renal Artery, Right* **B** Inferior Mesenteric Artery Sigmoid artery Superior rectal artery **C** Common Iliac Artery, Right **D** Common Iliac Artery, Left **E** Internal Iliac Artery, Right Deferential artery Hypogastric artery Iliolumbar artery Inferior gluteal artery Inferior vesical artery Internal pudendal artery Lateral sacral artery Middle rectal artery Obturator artery Prostatic artery Superior gluteal artery Superior vesical artery Umbilical artery Uterine artery Vaginal artery	**F** Internal Iliac Artery, Left *See E Internal Iliac Artery, Right* **H** External Iliac Artery, Right Deep circumflex iliac artery Inferior epigastric artery **J** External Iliac Artery, Left *See H External Iliac Artery, Right* **K** Femoral Artery, Right Circumflex iliac artery Deep femoral artery Descending genicular artery External pudendal artery Superficial epigastric artery **L** Femoral Artery, Left *See K Femoral Artery, Right* **M** Popliteal Artery, Right Inferior genicular artery Middle genicular artery Superior genicular artery Sural artery Tibioperoneal trunk **N** Popliteal Artery, Left *See M Popliteal Artery, Right* **P** Anterior Tibial Artery, Right Anterior lateral malleolar artery Anterior medial malleolar artery Anterior tibial recurrent artery Dorsalis pedis artery Posterior tibial recurrent artery **Q** Anterior Tibial Artery, Left *See P Anterior Tibial Artery, Right* **R** Posterior Tibial Artery, Right **S** Posterior Tibial Artery, Left **T** Peroneal Artery, Right Fibular artery **U** Peroneal Artery, Left *See T Peroneal Artery, Right* **V** Foot Artery, Right Arcuate artery Dorsal metatarsal artery Lateral plantar artery Lateral tarsal artery Medial plantar artery **W** Foot Artery, Left *See V Foot Artery, Right* **Y** Lower Artery Umbilical artery	**0** Open **4** Percutaneous Endoscopic	**7** Autologous Tissue Substitute **J** Synthetic Substitute **K** Nonautologous Tissue Substitute	**Z** No Qualifier

Ø   **Medical and Surgical**
4   **Lower Arteries**
S   **Reposition**   Definition: Moving to its normal location, or other suitable location, all or a portion of a body part

Explanation: The body part is moved to a new location from an abnormal location, or from a normal location where it is not functioning correctly. The body part may or may not be cut out or off to be moved to the new location.

Body Part Character 4		Approach Character 5	Device Character 6	Qualifier Character 7

Ø Abdominal Aorta
Inferior phrenic artery
Lumbar artery
Median sacral artery
Middle suprarenal artery
Ovarian artery
Testicular artery
1 Celiac Artery
Celiac trunk
2 Gastric Artery
Left gastric artery
Right gastric artery
3 Hepatic Artery
Common hepatic artery
Gastroduodenal artery
Hepatic artery proper
4 Splenic Artery
Left gastroepiploic artery
Pancreatic artery
Short gastric artery
5 Superior Mesenteric Artery
Ileal artery
Ileocolic artery
Inferior pancreaticoduodenal
   artery
Jejunal artery
6 Colic Artery, Right
7 Colic Artery, Left
8 Colic Artery, Middle
9 Renal Artery, Right
Inferior suprarenal artery
Renal segmental artery
A Renal Artery, Left
See 9 Renal Artery, Right
B Inferior Mesenteric Artery
Sigmoid artery
Superior rectal artery
C Common Iliac Artery, Right
D Common Iliac Artery, Left
E Internal Iliac Artery, Right
Deferential artery
Hypogastric artery
Iliolumbar artery
Inferior gluteal artery
Inferior vesical artery
Internal pudendal artery
Lateral sacral artery
Middle rectal artery
Obturator artery
Prostatic artery
Superior gluteal artery
Superior vesical artery
Umbilical artery
Uterine artery
Vaginal artery
	F Internal Iliac Artery, Left
	See E Internal Iliac Artery, Right
	H External Iliac Artery, Right
	Deep circumflex iliac artery
	Inferior epigastric artery
	J External Iliac Artery, Left
	See H External Iliac Artery, Right
	K Femoral Artery, Right
	Circumflex iliac artery
	Deep femoral artery
	Descending genicular artery
	External pudendal artery
	Superficial epigastric artery
	L Femoral Artery, Left
	See K Femoral Artery, Right
	M Popliteal Artery, Right
	Inferior genicular artery
	Middle genicular artery
	Superior genicular artery
	Sural artery
	Tibioperoneal trunk
	N Popliteal Artery, Left
	See M Popliteal Artery, Right
	P Anterior Tibial Artery, Right
	Anterior lateral malleolar
	   artery
	Anterior medial malleolar
	   artery
	Anterior tibial recurrent artery
	Dorsalis pedis artery
	Posterior tibial recurrent artery
	Q Anterior Tibial Artery, Left
	*See P Anterior Tibial Artery,
	  Right*
	R Posterior Tibial Artery, Right
	S Posterior Tibial Artery, Left
	T Peroneal Artery, Right
	Fibular artery
	U Peroneal Artery, Left
	See T Peroneal Artery, Right
	V Foot Artery, Right
	Arcuate artery
	Dorsal metatarsal artery
	Lateral plantar artery
	Lateral tarsal artery
	Medial plantar artery
	W Foot Artery, Left
	See V Foot Artery, Right
	Y Lower Artery
	Umbilical artery
		Ø Open
		3 Percutaneous
		4 Percutaneous Endoscopic
			Z No Device	**Z** No Qualifier

NC Noncovered Procedure   **LC** Limited Coverage   **QA** Questionable OB Admit   **NT** New Tech Add-on   ⊞ Combination Member   ♂ Male   ♀ Female

ICD-10-PCS 2024   **239**

Ø   Medical and Surgical
4   Lower Arteries
U   Supplement   Definition: Putting in or on biological or synthetic material that physically reinforces and/or augments the function of a portion of a body part

Explanation: The biological material is non-living, or is living and from the same individual. The body part may have been previously replaced, and the SUPPLEMENT procedure is performed to physically reinforce and/or augment the function of the replaced body part.

Body Part Character 4		Approach Character 5	Device Character 6	Qualifier Character 7
Ø Abdominal Aorta Inferior phrenic artery Lumbar artery Median sacral artery Middle suprarenal artery Ovarian artery Testicular artery	**F Internal Iliac Artery, Left** *See E Internal Iliac Artery, Right* **H External Iliac Artery, Right** Deep circumflex iliac artery Inferior epigastric artery	**Ø Open** **3 Percutaneous** **4 Percutaneous Endoscopic**	**7 Autologous Tissue Substitute** **J Synthetic Substitute** **K Nonautologous Tissue Substitute**	**Z No Qualifier**
1 Celiac Artery Celiac trunk	**J External Iliac Artery, Left** *See H External Iliac Artery, Right*			
2 Gastric Artery Left gastric artery Right gastric artery	**K Femoral Artery, Right** Circumflex iliac artery Deep femoral artery Descending genicular artery External pudendal artery Superficial epigastric artery			
3 Hepatic Artery Common hepatic artery Gastroduodenal artery Hepatic artery proper	**L Femoral Artery, Left** *See K Femoral Artery, Right*			
4 Splenic Artery Left gastroepiploic artery Pancreatic artery Short gastric artery	**M Popliteal Artery, Right** Inferior genicular artery Middle genicular artery Superior genicular artery Sural artery Tibioperoneal trunk			
5 Superior Mesenteric Artery Ileal artery Ileocolic artery Inferior pancreaticoduodenal artery Jejunal artery	**N Popliteal Artery, Left** *See M Popliteal Artery, Right* **P Anterior Tibial Artery, Right** Anterior lateral malleolar artery Anterior medial malleolar artery Anterior tibial recurrent artery Dorsalis pedis artery Posterior tibial recurrent artery			
6 Colic Artery, Right				
7 Colic Artery, Left				
8 Colic Artery, Middle				
9 Renal Artery, Right Inferior suprarenal artery Renal segmental artery	**Q Anterior Tibial Artery, Left** *See P Anterior Tibial Artery, Right*			
A Renal Artery, Left *See 9 Renal Artery, Right*	**R Posterior Tibial Artery, Right**			
B Inferior Mesenteric Artery Sigmoid artery Superior rectal artery	**S Posterior Tibial Artery, Left** **T Peroneal Artery, Right** Fibular artery			
C Common Iliac Artery, Right	**U Peroneal Artery, Left** *See T Peroneal Artery, Right*			
D Common Iliac Artery, Left	**V Foot Artery, Right** Arcuate artery Dorsal metatarsal artery Lateral plantar artery Lateral tarsal artery Medial plantar artery			
E Internal Iliac Artery, Right Deferential artery Hypogastric artery Iliolumbar artery Inferior gluteal artery Inferior vesical artery Internal pudendal artery Lateral sacral artery Middle rectal artery Obturator artery Prostatic artery Superior gluteal artery Superior vesical artery Umbilical artery Uterine artery Vaginal artery	**W Foot Artery, Left** *See V Foot Artery, Right* **Y Lower Artery** Umbilical artery			

Non-OR Procedure   DRG Non-OR Procedure   Valid OR Procedure   HAC Associated Procedure   Combination Only   New/Revised April   New/Revised October

240   ICD-10-PCS 2024

Ø4U–Ø4U

Ø　Medical and Surgical
4　Lower Arteries
V　Restriction　　Definition: Partially closing an orifice or the lumen of a tubular body part
　　　　　　　　　　　Explanation: The orifice can be a natural orifice or an artificially created orifice

Body Part Character 4		Approach Character 5	Device Character 6	Qualifier Character 7
Ø Abdominal Aorta Inferior phrenic artery Lumbar artery Median sacral artery Middle suprarenal artery Ovarian artery Testicular artery		**Ø** Open **3** Percutaneous **4** Percutaneous Endoscopic	**C** Extraluminal Device **E** Intraluminal Device, Branched or Fenestrated, One or Two Arteries **F** Intraluminal Device, Branched or Fenestrated, Three or More Arteries **Z** No Device	**Z** No Qualifier
Ø Abdominal Aorta Inferior phrenic artery Lumbar artery Median sacral artery Middle suprarenal artery Ovarian artery Testicular artery		**Ø** Open **3** Percutaneous **4** Percutaneous Endoscopic	**D** Intraluminal Device	**J** Temporary **Z** No Qualifier
1 Celiac Artery Celiac trunk **2 Gastric Artery** Left gastric artery Right gastric artery **3 Hepatic Artery** Common hepatic artery Gastroduodenal artery Hepatic artery proper **4 Splenic Artery** Left gastroepiploic artery Pancreatic artery Short gastric artery **5 Superior Mesenteric Artery** Ileal artery Ileocolic artery Inferior pancreaticoduodenal artery Jejunal artery **6 Colic Artery, Right** **7 Colic Artery, Left** **8 Colic Artery, Middle** **9 Renal Artery, Right** Inferior suprarenal artery Renal segmental artery **A Renal Artery, Left** *See 9 Renal Artery, Right* **B Inferior Mesenteric Artery** Sigmoid artery Superior rectal artery **E Internal Iliac Artery, Right** Deferential artery Hypogastric artery Iliolumbar artery Inferior gluteal artery Inferior vesical artery Internal pudendal artery Lateral sacral artery Middle rectal artery Obturator artery Prostatic artery Superior gluteal artery Superior vesical artery Umbilical artery Uterine artery Vaginal artery **F Internal Iliac Artery, Left** *See E Internal Iliac Artery, Right*	**H External Iliac Artery, Right** Deep circumflex iliac artery Inferior epigastric artery **J External Iliac Artery, Left** *See H External Iliac Artery, Right* **K Femoral Artery, Right** Circumflex iliac artery Deep femoral artery Descending genicular artery External pudendal artery Superficial epigastric artery **L Femoral Artery, Left** *See K Femoral Artery, Right* **M Popliteal Artery, Right** Inferior genicular artery Middle genicular artery Superior genicular artery Sural artery Tibioperoneal trunk **N Popliteal Artery, Left** *See M Popliteal Artery, Right* **P Anterior Tibial Artery, Right** Anterior lateral malleolar artery Anterior medial malleolar artery Anterior tibial recurrent artery Dorsalis pedis artery Posterior tibial recurrent artery **Q Anterior Tibial Artery, Left** *See P Anterior Tibial Artery, Right* **R Posterior Tibial Artery, Right** **S Posterior Tibial Artery, Left** **T Peroneal Artery, Right** Fibular artery **U Peroneal Artery, Left** *See T Peroneal Artery, Right* **V Foot Artery, Right** Arcuate artery Dorsal metatarsal artery Lateral plantar artery Lateral tarsal artery Medial plantar artery **W Foot Artery, Left** *See V Foot Artery, Right* **Y Lower Artery** Umbilical artery	**Ø** Open **3** Percutaneous **4** Percutaneous Endoscopic	**C** Extraluminal Device **D** Intraluminal Device **Z** No Device	**Z** No Qualifier
C Common Iliac Artery, Right **D Common Iliac Artery, Left**		**Ø** Open **3** Percutaneous **4** Percutaneous Endoscopic	**C** Extraluminal Device **D** Intraluminal Device **E** Intraluminal Device, Branched or Fenestrated, One or Two Arteries **Z** No Device	**Z** No Qualifier

NC Noncovered Procedure　　**LC** Limited Coverage　　**QA** Questionable OB Admit　　**NT** New Tech Add-on　　✚ Combination Member　　♂ Male　　♀ Female
ICD-10-PCS 2024　　　241

Ø4V–Ø4V

Ø   Medical and Surgical
4   Lower Arteries
W   Revision

Definition: Correcting, to the extent possible, a portion of a malfunctioning device or the position of a displaced device

Explanation: Revision can include correcting a malfunctioning or displaced device by taking out or putting in components of the device such as a screw or pin

Body Part Character 4	Approach Character 5	Device Character 6	Qualifier Character 7

Y Lower Artery
  Umbilical artery
	Ø Open
	3 Percutaneous
	4 Percutaneous Endoscopic
		Ø Drainage Device
		2 Monitoring Device
		3 Infusion Device
		7 Autologous Tissue
		  Substitute
		C Extraluminal Device
		D Intraluminal Device
		J Synthetic Substitute
		K Nonautologous Tissue
		  Substitute
		Y Other Device
			Z No Qualifier

Y Lower Artery
  Umbilical artery
	X External	Ø Drainage Device
		2 Monitoring Device
		3 Infusion Device
		7 Autologous Tissue
		  Substitute
		C Extraluminal Device
		D Intraluminal Device
		J Synthetic Substitute
		K Nonautologous Tissue
		  Substitute
			Z No Qualifier

Non-OR   Ø4WY3[Ø,2,3]Z
Non-OR   Ø4WY[3,4]YZ
Non-OR   Ø4WYX[Ø,2,3,7,C,D,J,K]Z

Upper Veins Ø51–Ø5W

Character Meanings

This Character Meaning table is provided as a guide to assist the user in the identification of character members that may be found in this section of code tables. It **SHOULD NOT** be used to build a PCS code.

Operation–Character 3		Body Part–Character 4		Approach–Character 5		Device–Character 6		Qualifier–Character 7	
1	Bypass	Ø	Azygos Vein	Ø	Open	Ø	Drainage Device	Ø	Ultrasonic
5	Destruction	1	Hemiazygos Vein	3	Percutaneous	2	Monitoring Device	1	Drug-Coated Balloon
7	Dilation	3	Innominate Vein, Right	4	Percutaneous Endoscopic	3	Infusion Device	X	Diagnostic
9	Drainage	4	Innominate Vein, Left	X	External	7	Autologous Tissue Substitute	Y	Upper Vein
B	Excision	5	Subclavian Vein, Right			9	Autologous Venous Tissue	Z	No Qualifier
C	Extirpation	6	Subclavian Vein, Left			A	Autologous Arterial Tissue		
D	Extraction	7	Axillary Vein, Right			C	Extraluminal Device		
F	Fragmentation	8	Axillary Vein, Left			D	Intraluminal Device		
H	Insertion	9	Brachial Vein, Right			J	Synthetic Substitute		
J	Inspection	A	Brachial Vein, Left			K	Nonautologous Tissue Substitute		
L	Occlusion	B	Basilic Vein, Right			M	Neurostimulator Lead		
N	Release	C	Basilic Vein, Left			Y	Other Device		
P	Removal	D	Cephalic Vein, Right			Z	No Device		
Q	Repair	F	Cephalic Vein, Left						
R	Replacement	G	Hand Vein, Right						
S	Reposition	H	Hand Vein, Left						
U	Supplement	L	Intracranial Vein						
V	Restriction	M	Internal Jugular Vein, Right						
W	Revision	N	Internal Jugular Vein, Left						
		P	External Jugular Vein, Right						
		Q	External Jugular Vein, Left						
		R	Vertebral Vein, Right						
		S	Vertebral Vein, Left						
		T	Face Vein, Right						
		V	Face Vein, Left						
		Y	Upper Vein						

AHA Coding Clinic for Upper Veins
2022, 1Q, 10-13　　Procedures performed on a continuous vessel, ICD-10-PCS Guideline B4.1c

AHA Coding Clinic for table Ø51
2020, 1Q, 28　　Free flap microvascular breast reconstruction
2017, 3Q, 15　　Bypass of innominate vein to atrial appendage

AHA Coding Clinic for table Ø57
2020, 3Q, 38　　Thrombectomy of arteriovenous fistula with angioplasty and stent placement

AHA Coding Clinic for table Ø59
2018, 3Q, 7　　Catheter placement for treatment of congestive heart failure

AHA Coding Clinic for table Ø5B
2021, 2Q, 15　　Excision of pituitary macroadenoma within cavernous sinus
2020, 3Q, 40　　Excision of ulceration of arteriovenous fistula
2020, 1Q, 24　　Resection of vascular malformation, likely cavernoma
2016, 2Q, 12　　Resection of malignant neoplasm of infratemporal fossa

AHA Coding Clinic for table Ø5C
2020, 3Q, 37　　Repair of aneurysm of arteriovenous fistula with endovenectomy
2020, 3Q, 38　　Thrombectomy of arteriovenous fistula with angioplasty and stent placement

AHA Coding Clinic for table Ø5F
2020, 4Q, 45-49　　New fragmentation tables
2020, 4Q, 49-50　　Intravascular ultrasound assisted thrombolysis
2020, 4Q, 50　　Intravascular lithotripsy

AHA Coding Clinic for table Ø5H
2016, 4Q, 97-98　　Phrenic neurostimulator

AHA Coding Clinic for table Ø5P
2016, 4Q, 97-98　　Phrenic neurostimulator

AHA Coding Clinic for table Ø5Q
2017, 3Q, 15　　Bypass of innominate vein to atrial appendage

AHA Coding Clinic for table Ø5S
2013, 4Q, 125　　Stage II cephalic vein transposition (superficialization) of arteriovenous fistula

AHA Coding Clinic for table Ø5V
2020, 3Q, 37　　Repair of aneurysm of arteriovenous fistula with endovenectomy

AHA Coding Clinic for table Ø5W
2016, 4Q, 97-98　　Phrenic neurostimulator

Head and Neck Veins

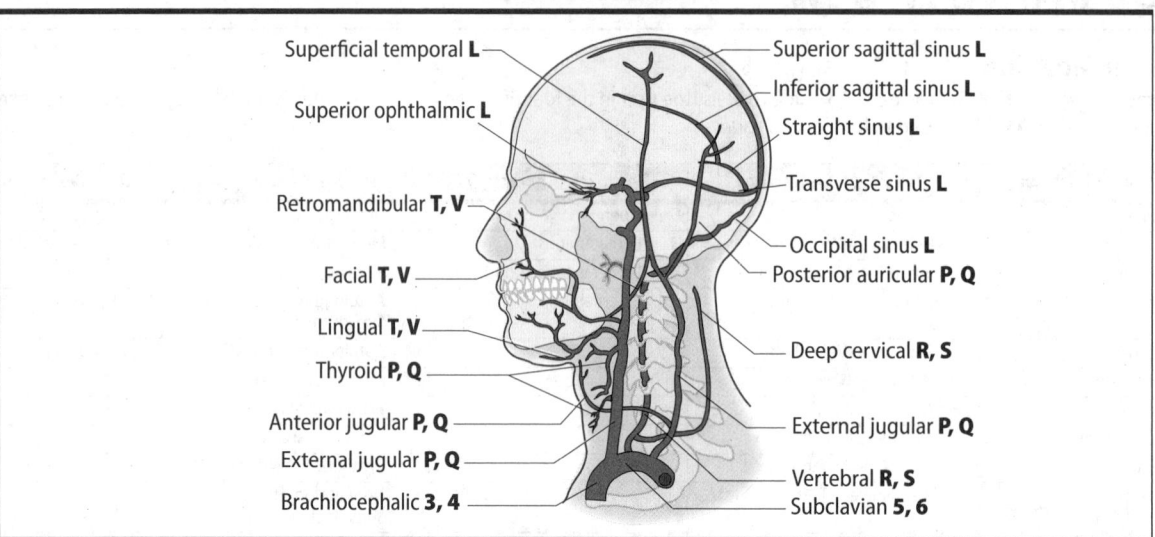

Superficial temporal **L**
Superior ophthalmic **L**
Retromandibular **T, V**
Facial **T, V**
Lingual **T, V**
Thyroid **P, Q**
Anterior jugular **P, Q**
External jugular **P, Q**
Brachiocephalic **3, 4**

Superior sagittal sinus **L**
Inferior sagittal sinus **L**
Straight sinus **L**
Transverse sinus **L**
Occipital sinus **L**
Posterior auricular **P, Q**
Deep cervical **R, S**
External jugular **P, Q**
Vertebral **R, S**
Subclavian **5, 6**

Upper Veins

Superficial temporal **L**
Vertebral **R, S**
Internal jugular **M, N**
External jugular **P, Q**
Subclavian **5, 6**
Innominate **3, 4**
Azygos **Ø**
Axillary **7, 8**
Hemiazygos **1**
Brachial **9, A**
Cephalic **D, F**
Basilic **B, C**
Radial **9, A**
Ulnar **9, A**
Digital **G, H**

Ø   **Medical and Surgical**
5   **Upper Veins**
1   **Bypass**   Definition: Altering the route of passage of the contents of a tubular body part

                          Explanation: Rerouting contents of a body part to a downstream area of the normal route, to a similar route and body part, or to an abnormal route and dissimilar body part. Includes one or more anastomoses, with or without the use of a device.

Body Part Character 4	Approach Character 5	Device Character 6	Qualifier Character 7

Ø **Azygos Vein**
    Right ascending lumbar vein
    Right subcostal vein
1 **Hemiazygos Vein**
    Left ascending lumbar vein
    Left subcostal vein
3 **Innominate Vein, Right**
    Brachiocephalic vein
    Inferior thyroid vein
4 **Innominate Vein, Left**
    See 3 Innominate Vein, Right
5 **Subclavian Vein, Right**
6 **Subclavian Vein, Left**
7 **Axillary Vein, Right**
8 **Axillary Vein, Left**
9 **Brachial Vein, Right**
    Radial vein
    Ulnar vein
A **Brachial Vein, Left**
    See 9 Brachial Vein, Right
B **Basilic Vein, Right**
    Median antebrachial vein
    Median cubital vein
C **Basilic Vein, Left**
    See B Basilic Vein, Right
D **Cephalic Vein, Right**
    Accessory cephalic vein
F **Cephalic Vein, Left**
    See D Cephalic Vein, Right
G **Hand Vein, Right**
    Dorsal metacarpal vein
    Palmar (volar) digital vein
    Palmar (volar) metacarpal vein
    Superficial palmar venous arch
    Volar (palmar) digital vein
    Volar (palmar) metacarpal vein
H **Hand Vein, Left**
    See G Hand Vein, Right
L **Intracranial Vein**
    Anterior cerebral vein
    Basal (internal) cerebral vein
    Dural venous sinus
    Great cerebral vein
    Inferior cerebellar vein
    Inferior cerebral vein
    Internal (basal) cerebral vein
    Middle cerebral vein
    Ophthalmic vein
    Superior cerebellar vein
    Superior cerebral vein
M **Internal Jugular Vein, Right**
N **Internal Jugular Vein, Left**
P **External Jugular Vein, Right**
    Posterior auricular vein
Q **External Jugular Vein, Left**
    See P External Jugular Vein, Right
R **Vertebral Vein, Right**
    Deep cervical vein
    Suboccipital venous plexus
S **Vertebral Vein, Left**
    See R Vertebral Vein, Right
T **Face Vein, Right**
    Angular vein
    Anterior facial vein
    Common facial vein
    Deep facial vein
    Frontal vein
    Posterior facial (retromandibular) vein
    Supraorbital vein
V **Face Vein, Left**
    See T Face Vein, Right
	Ø Open
	4 Percutaneous Endoscopic
		7 Autologous Tissue Substitute
		9 Autologous Venous Tissue
		A Autologous Arterial Tissue
		J Synthetic Substitute
		K Nonautologous Tissue Substitute
		Z No Device
			Y Upper Vein

Ø   Medical and Surgical
5   Upper Veins
5   Destruction   Definition: Physical eradication of all or a portion of a body part by the direct use of energy, force, or a destructive agent
                   Explanation: None of the body part is physically taken out

Body Part Character 4	Approach Character 5	Device Character 6	Qualifier Character 7
Ø Azygos Vein Right ascending lumbar vein Right subcostal vein **1 Hemiazygos Vein** Left ascending lumbar vein Left subcostal vein **3 Innominate Vein, Right** Brachiocephalic vein Inferior thyroid vein **4 Innominate Vein, Left** *See 3 Innominate Vein, Right* **5 Subclavian Vein, Right** **6 Subclavian Vein, Left** **7 Axillary Vein, Right** **8 Axillary Vein, Left** **9 Brachial Vein, Right** Radial vein Ulnar vein **A Brachial Vein, Left** *See 9 Brachial Vein, Right* **B Basilic Vein, Right** Median antebrachial vein Median cubital vein **C Basilic Vein, Left** *See B Basilic Vein, Right* **D Cephalic Vein, Right** Accessory cephalic vein **F Cephalic Vein, Left** *See D Cephalic Vein, Right* **G Hand Vein, Right** Dorsal metacarpal vein Palmar (volar) digital vein Palmar (volar) metacarpal vein Superficial palmar venous arch Volar (palmar) digital vein Volar (palmar) metacarpal vein **H Hand Vein, Left** *See G Hand Vein, Right* **L Intracranial Vein** Anterior cerebral vein Basal (internal) cerebral vein Dural venous sinus Great cerebral vein Inferior cerebellar vein Inferior cerebral vein Internal (basal) cerebral vein Middle cerebral vein Ophthalmic vein Superior cerebellar vein Superior cerebral vein **M Internal Jugular Vein, Right** **N Internal Jugular Vein, Left** **P External Jugular Vein, Right** Posterior auricular vein **Q External Jugular Vein, Left** *See P External Jugular Vein, Right* **R Vertebral Vein, Right** Deep cervical vein Suboccipital venous plexus **S Vertebral Vein, Left** *See R Vertebral Vein, Right* **T Face Vein, Right** Angular vein Anterior facial vein Common facial vein Deep facial vein Frontal vein Posterior facial (retromandibular) vein Supraorbital vein **V Face Vein, Left** *See T Face Vein, Right* **Y Upper Vein**	**Ø Open** **3 Percutaneous** **4 Percutaneous Endoscopic**	**Z No Device**	**Z No Qualifier**

Non-OR Procedure   DRG Non-OR Procedure   Valid OR Procedure   HAC Associated Procedure   Combination Only   New/Revised April   New/Revised October

Ø   **Medical and Surgical**
5   **Upper Veins**
7   **Dilation**

Definition: Expanding an orifice or the lumen of a tubular body part

Explanation: The orifice can be a natural orifice or an artificially created orifice. Accomplished by stretching a tubular body part using intraluminal pressure or by cutting part of the orifice or wall of the tubular body part.

Body Part Character 4	Approach Character 5	Device Character 6	Qualifier Character 7
Ø **Azygos Vein** Right ascending lumbar vein Right subcostal vein **1** **Hemiazygos Vein** Left ascending lumbar vein Left subcostal vein **G** **Hand Vein, Right** Dorsal metacarpal vein Palmar (volar) digital vein Palmar (volar) metacarpal vein Superficial palmar venous arch Volar (palmar) digital vein Volar (palmar) metacarpal vein **H** **Hand Vein, Left** *See G Hand Vein, Right* **L** **Intracranial Vein** NC Anterior cerebral vein Basal (internal) cerebral vein Dural venous sinus Great cerebral vein Inferior cerebellar vein Inferior cerebral vein Internal (basal) cerebral vein Middle cerebral vein Ophthalmic vein Superior cerebellar vein Superior cerebral vein **M** **Internal Jugular Vein, Right** **N** **Internal Jugular Vein, Left** **P** **External Jugular Vein, Right** Posterior auricular vein **Q** **External Jugular Vein, Left** *See P External Jugular Vein, Right* **R** **Vertebral Vein, Right** Deep cervical vein Suboccipital venous plexus **S** **Vertebral Vein, Left** *See R Vertebral Vein, Right* **T** **Face Vein, Right** Angular vein Anterior facial vein Common facial vein Deep facial vein Frontal vein Posterior facial (retromandibular) vein Supraorbital vein **V** **Face Vein, Left** *See T Face Vein, Right* **Y** **Upper Vein**	**Ø** Open **3** Percutaneous **4** Percutaneous Endoscopic	**D** Intraluminal Device **Z** No Device	**Z** No Qualifier
3 **Innominate Vein, Right** Brachiocephalic vein Inferior thyroid vein **4** **Innominate Vein, Left** *See 3 Innominate Vein, Right* **5** **Subclavian Vein, Right** **6** **Subclavian Vein, Left** **7** **Axillary Vein, Right** **8** **Axillary Vein, Left** **9** **Brachial Vein, Right** Radial vein Ulnar vein **A** **Brachial Vein, Left** *See 9 Brachial Vein, Right* **B** **Basilic Vein, Right** Median antebrachial vein Median cubital vein **C** **Basilic Vein, Left** *See B Basilic Vein, Right* **D** **Cephalic Vein, Right** Accessory cephalic vein **F** **Cephalic Vein, Left** *See D Cephalic Vein, Right*	**Ø** Open **3** Percutaneous **4** Percutaneous Endoscopic	**D** Intraluminal Device **Z** No Device	**1** Drug-Coated Balloon **Z** No Qualifier

NC   Ø57L[3,4]ZZ

NC Noncovered Procedure   LC Limited Coverage   QA Questionable OB Admit   NT New Tech Add-on   ⊞ Combination Member   ♂ Male   ♀ Female

ICD-10-PCS 2024   **247**

Upper Veins

Ø   **Medical and Surgical**
5   **Upper Veins**
9   **Drainage**   Definition: Taking or letting out fluids and/or gases from a body part
                       Explanation: The qualifier DIAGNOSTIC is used to identify drainage procedures that are biopsies

Body Part Character 4		Approach Character 5	Device Character 6	Qualifier Character 7
Ø **Azygos Vein** Right ascending lumbar vein Right subcostal vein 1 **Hemiazygos Vein** Left ascending lumbar vein Left subcostal vein 3 **Innominate Vein, Right** Brachiocephalic vein Inferior thyroid vein 4 **Innominate Vein, Left** *See 3 Innominate Vein, Right* 5 **Subclavian Vein, Right** 6 **Subclavian Vein, Left** 7 **Axillary Vein, Right** 8 **Axillary Vein, Left** 9 **Brachial Vein, Right** Radial vein Ulnar vein A **Brachial Vein, Left** *See 9 Brachial Vein, Right* B **Basilic Vein, Right** Median antebrachial vein Median cubital vein C **Basilic Vein, Left** *See B Basilic Vein, Right* D **Cephalic Vein, Right** Accessory cephalic vein F **Cephalic Vein, Left** *See D Cephalic Vein, Right* G **Hand Vein, Right** Dorsal metacarpal vein Palmar (volar) digital vein Palmar (volar) metacarpal vein Superficial palmar venous arch Volar (palmar) digital vein Volar (palmar) metacarpal vein	H **Hand Vein, Left** *See G Hand Vein, Right* L **Intracranial Vein** Anterior cerebral vein Basal (internal) cerebral vein Dural venous sinus Great cerebral vein Inferior cerebellar vein Inferior cerebral vein Internal (basal) cerebral vein Middle cerebral vein Ophthalmic vein Superior cerebellar vein Superior cerebral vein M **Internal Jugular Vein, Right** N **Internal Jugular Vein, Left** P **External Jugular Vein, Right** Posterior auricular vein Q **External Jugular Vein, Left** *See P External Jugular Vein, Right* R **Vertebral Vein, Right** Deep cervical vein Suboccipital venous plexus S **Vertebral Vein, Left** *See R Vertebral Vein, Right* T **Face Vein, Right** Angular vein Anterior facial vein Common facial vein Deep facial vein Frontal vein Posterior facial (retromandibular) vein Supraorbital vein V **Face Vein, Left** *See T Face Vein, Right* Y **Upper Vein**	Ø Open 3 Percutaneous 4 Percutaneous Endoscopic	Ø Drainage Device	Z No Qualifier
Ø **Azygos Vein** Right ascending lumbar vein Right subcostal vein 1 **Hemiazygos Vein** Left ascending lumbar vein Left subcostal vein 3 **Innominate Vein, Right** Brachiocephalic vein Inferior thyroid vein 4 **Innominate Vein, Left** *See 3 Innominate Vein, Right* 5 **Subclavian Vein, Right** 6 **Subclavian Vein, Left** 7 **Axillary Vein, Right** 8 **Axillary Vein, Left** 9 **Brachial Vein, Right** Radial vein Ulnar vein A **Brachial Vein, Left** *See 9 Brachial Vein, Right* B **Basilic Vein, Right** Median antebrachial vein Median cubital vein C **Basilic Vein, Left** *See B Basilic Vein, Right* D **Cephalic Vein, Right** Accessory cephalic vein F **Cephalic Vein, Left** *See D Cephalic Vein, Right* G **Hand Vein, Right** Dorsal metacarpal vein Palmar (volar) digital vein Palmar (volar) metacarpal vein Superficial palmar venous arch Volar (palmar) digital vein Volar (palmar) metacarpal vein	H **Hand Vein, Left** *See G Hand Vein, Right* L **Intracranial Vein** Anterior cerebral vein Basal (internal) cerebral vein Dural venous sinus Great cerebral vein Inferior cerebellar vein Inferior cerebral vein Internal (basal) cerebral vein Middle cerebral vein Ophthalmic vein Superior cerebellar vein Superior cerebral vein M **Internal Jugular Vein, Right** N **Internal Jugular Vein, Left** P **External Jugular Vein, Right** Posterior auricular vein Q **External Jugular Vein, Left** *See P External Jugular Vein, Right* R **Vertebral Vein, Right** Deep cervical vein Suboccipital venous plexus S **Vertebral Vein, Left** *See R Vertebral Vein, Right* T **Face Vein, Right** Angular vein Anterior facial vein Common facial vein Deep facial vein Frontal vein Posterior facial (retromandibular) vein Supraorbital vein V **Face Vein, Left** *See T Face Vein, Right* Y **Upper Vein**	Ø Open 3 Percutaneous 4 Percutaneous Endoscopic	Z No Device	X Diagnostic Z No Qualifier

Non-OR   Ø59[Ø,1,3,4,5,6,7,8,9,A,B,C,D,F,G,H,L,M,N,P,Q,R,S,T,V,Y][Ø,3,4]ØZ
Non-OR   Ø59[Ø,1,3,4,5,6,7,8,9,A,B,C,D,F,G,H,L,M,N,P,Q,R,S,T,V,Y]3ZX
Non-OR   Ø59[Ø,1,3,4,5,6,7,8,9,A,B,C,D,F,G,H,L,M,N,P,Q,R,S,T,V,Y][Ø,3,4]ZZ

Non-OR Procedure   DRG Non-OR Procedure   Valid OR Procedure   HAC Associated Procedure   Combination Only   New/Revised April   New/Revised October

Ø　Medical and Surgical
5　Upper Veins
B　Excision　　Definition: Cutting out or off, without replacement, a portion of a body part
　　　　　　　　　　　Explanation: The qualifier DIAGNOSTIC is used to identify excision procedures that are biopsies

Body Part Character 4	Approach Character 5	Device Character 6	Qualifier Character 7
Ø　Azygos Vein 　　Right ascending lumbar vein 　　Right subcostal vein **1　Hemiazygos Vein** 　　Left ascending lumbar vein 　　Left subcostal vein **3　Innominate Vein, Right** 　　Brachiocephalic vein 　　Inferior thyroid vein **4　Innominate Vein, Left** 　　*See 3 Innominate Vein, Right* **5　Subclavian Vein, Right** **6　Subclavian Vein, Left** **7　Axillary Vein, Right** **8　Axillary Vein, Left** **9　Brachial Vein, Right** 　　Radial vein 　　Ulnar vein **A　Brachial Vein, Left** 　　*See 9 Brachial Vein, Right* **B　Basilic Vein, Right** 　　Median antebrachial vein 　　Median cubital vein **C　Basilic Vein, Left** 　　*See B Basilic Vein, Right* **D　Cephalic Vein, Right** 　　Accessory cephalic vein **F　Cephalic Vein, Left** 　　*See D Cephalic Vein, Right* **G　Hand Vein, Right** 　　Dorsal metacarpal vein 　　Palmar (volar) digital vein 　　Palmar (volar) metacarpal vein 　　Superficial palmar venous arch 　　Volar (palmar) digital vein 　　Volar (palmar) metacarpal vein **H　Hand Vein, Left** 　　*See G Hand Vein, Right* **L　Intracranial Vein** 　　Anterior cerebral vein 　　Basal (internal) cerebral vein 　　Dural venous sinus 　　Great cerebral vein 　　Inferior cerebellar vein 　　Inferior cerebral vein 　　Internal (basal) cerebral vein 　　Middle cerebral vein 　　Ophthalmic vein 　　Superior cerebellar vein 　　Superior cerebral vein **M　Internal Jugular Vein, Right** **N　Internal Jugular Vein, Left** **P　External Jugular Vein, Right** 　　Posterior auricular vein **Q　External Jugular Vein, Left** 　　*See P External Jugular Vein, Right* **R　Vertebral Vein, Right** 　　Deep cervical vein 　　Suboccipital venous plexus **S　Vertebral Vein, Left** 　　*See R Vertebral Vein, Right* **T　Face Vein, Right** 　　Angular vein 　　Anterior facial vein 　　Common facial vein 　　Deep facial vein 　　Frontal vein 　　Posterior facial (retromandibular) vein 　　Supraorbital vein **V　Face Vein, Left** 　　*See T Face Vein, Right* **Y　Upper Vein**	**Ø　Open** **3　Percutaneous** **4　Percutaneous Endoscopic**	**Z　No Device**	**X　Diagnostic** **Z　No Qualifier**

NC Noncovered Procedure　　LC Limited Coverage　　QA Questionable OB Admit　　NT New Tech Add-on　　⊞ Combination Member　　♂Male　　♀Female

Ø   **Medical and Surgical**
5   **Upper Veins**
C   **Extirpation**   Definition: Taking or cutting out solid matter from a body part

Explanation: The solid matter may be an abnormal byproduct of a biological function or a foreign body; it may be imbedded in a body part or in the lumen of a tubular body part. The solid matter may or may not have been previously broken into pieces.

Body Part Character 4	Approach Character 5	Device Character 6	Qualifier Character 7

Ø **Azygos Vein**
   Right ascending lumbar vein
   Right subcostal vein
1 **Hemiazygos Vein**
   Left ascending lumbar vein
   Left subcostal vein
3 **Innominate Vein, Right**
   Brachiocephalic vein
   Inferior thyroid vein
4 **Innominate Vein, Left**
   See 3 Innominate Vein, Right
5 **Subclavian Vein, Right**
6 **Subclavian Vein, Left**
7 **Axillary Vein, Right**
8 **Axillary Vein, Left**
9 **Brachial Vein, Right**
   Radial vein
   Ulnar vein
A **Brachial Vein, Left**
   See 9 Brachial Vein, Right
B **Basilic Vein, Right**
   Median antebrachial vein
   Median cubital vein
C **Basilic Vein, Left**
   See B Basilic Vein, Right
D **Cephalic Vein, Right**
   Accessory cephalic vein
F **Cephalic Vein, Left**
   See D Cephalic Vein, Right
G **Hand Vein, Right**
   Dorsal metacarpal vein
   Palmar (volar) digital vein
   Palmar (volar) metacarpal vein
   Superficial palmar venous arch
   Volar (palmar) digital vein
   Volar (palmar) metacarpal vein
H **Hand Vein, Left**
   See G Hand Vein, Right
L **Intracranial Vein**
   Anterior cerebral vein
   Basal (internal) cerebral vein
   Dural venous sinus
   Great cerebral vein
   Inferior cerebellar vein
   Inferior cerebral vein
   Internal (basal) cerebral vein
   Middle cerebral vein
   Ophthalmic vein
   Superior cerebellar vein
   Superior cerebral vein
M **Internal Jugular Vein, Right**
N **Internal Jugular Vein, Left**
P **External Jugular Vein, Right**
   Posterior auricular vein
Q **External Jugular Vein, Left**
   See P External Jugular Vein, Right
R **Vertebral Vein, Right**
   Deep cervical vein
   Suboccipital venous plexus
S **Vertebral Vein, Left**
   See R Vertebral Vein, Right
T **Face Vein, Right**
   Angular vein
   Anterior facial vein
   Common facial vein
   Deep facial vein
   Frontal vein
   Posterior facial (retromandibular) vein
   Supraorbital vein
V **Face Vein, Left**
   See T Face Vein, Right
Y **Upper Vein**
	Ø Open
	3 Percutaneous
	4 Percutaneous Endoscopic
		Z No Device	**Z** No Qualifier

Non-OR Procedure   DRG Non-OR Procedure   Valid OR Procedure   HAC Associated Procedure   Combination Only   New/Revised April   New/Revised October

250   ICD-10-PCS 2024

Ø   Medical and Surgical
5   Upper Veins
D   Extraction   Definition: Pulling or stripping out or off all or a portion of a body part by the use of force
                 Explanation: The qualifier DIAGNOSTIC is used to identify extraction procedures that are biopsies

Body Part Character 4	Approach Character 5	Device Character 6	Qualifier Character 7

9   Brachial Vein, Right
    Radial vein
    Ulnar vein
A   Brachial Vein, Left
    See 9 Brachial Vein, Right
B   Basilic Vein, Right
    Median antebrachial vein
    Median cubital vein
C   Basilic Vein, Left
    See B Basilic Vein, Right
D   Cephalic Vein, Right
    Accessory cephalic vein
F   Cephalic Vein, Left
    See D Cephalic Vein, Right
G   Hand Vein, Right
    Dorsal metacarpal vein
    Palmar (volar) digital vein
    Palmar (volar) metacarpal vein
    Superficial palmar venous arch
    Volar (palmar) digital vein
    Volar (palmar) metacarpal vein
H   Hand Vein, Left
    See G Hand Vein, Right
Y   Upper Vein
	Ø Open
	3 Percutaneous
		Z No Device	**Z No Qualifier**

Ø   Medical and Surgical
5   Upper Veins
F   Fragmentation   Definition: Breaking solid matter in a body part into pieces
                 Explanation: Physical force (e.g., manual, ultrasonic) applied directly or indirectly is used to break the solid matter into pieces. The solid matter may be an abnormal byproduct of a biological function or a foreign body. The pieces of solid matter are not taken out.

Body Part Character 4	Approach Character 5	Device Character 6	Qualifier Character 7

3   Innominate Vein, Right
    Brachiocephalic vein
    Inferior thyroid vein
4   Innominate Vein, Left
    See 3 Innominate Vein, Right
5   Subclavian Vein, Right
6   Subclavian Vein, Left
7   Axillary Vein, Right
8   Axillary Vein, Left
9   Brachial Vein, Right
    Radial vein
    Ulnar vein
A   Brachial Vein, Left
    See 9 Brachial Vein, Right
B   Basilic Vein, Right
    Median antebrachial vein
    Median cubital vein
C   Basilic Vein, Left
    See B Basilic Vein, Right
D   Cephalic Vein, Right
    Accessory cephalic vein
F   Cephalic Vein, Left
    See D Cephalic Vein, Right
Y   Upper Vein
	3 Percutaneous	**Z No Device**	**Ø Ultrasonic**
			Z No Qualifier

NC Noncovered Procedure   **LC** Limited Coverage   **QA** Questionable OB Admit   **NT** New Tech Add-on   ✛ Combination Member   ♂ Male   ♀ Female

ICD-10-PCS 2024   251

Ø5D–Ø5F

Ø   Medical and Surgical
5   Upper Veins
H   Insertion   Definition: Putting in a nonbiological appliance that monitors, assists, performs, or prevents a physiological function but does not physically take the place of a body part

              Explanation: None

Body Part Character 4		Approach Character 5	Device Character 6	Qualifier Character 7
Ø Azygos Vein ⊞ Right ascending lumbar vein Right subcostal vein		Ø Open 3 Percutaneous 4 Percutaneous Endoscopic	2 Monitoring Device 3 Infusion Device D Intraluminal Device M Neurostimulator Lead	Z No Qualifier
1 Hemiazygos Vein Left ascending lumbar vein Left subcostal vein **5 Subclavian Vein, Right** **6 Subclavian Vein, Left** **7 Axillary Vein, Right** **8 Axillary Vein, Left** **9 Brachial Vein, Right** Radial vein Ulnar vein **A Brachial Vein, Left** *See 9 Brachial Vein, Right* **B Basilic Vein, Right** Median antebrachial vein Median cubital vein **C Basilic Vein, Left** *See B Basilic Vein, Right* **D Cephalic Vein, Right** Accessory cephalic vein **F Cephalic Vein, Left** *See D Cephalic Vein, Right* **G Hand Vein, Right** Dorsal metacarpal vein Palmar (volar) digital vein Palmar (volar) metacarpal vein Superficial palmar venous arch Volar (palmar) digital vein Volar (palmar) metacarpal vein **H Hand Vein, Left** *See G Hand Vein, Right*	**L Intracranial Vein** Anterior cerebral vein Basal (internal) cerebral vein Dural venous sinus Great cerebral vein Inferior cerebellar vein Inferior cerebral vein Internal (basal) cerebral vein Middle cerebral vein Ophthalmic vein Superior cerebellar vein Superior cerebral vein **M Internal Jugular Vein, Right** **N Internal Jugular Vein, Left** **P External Jugular Vein, Right** Posterior auricular vein **Q External Jugular Vein, Left** *See P External Jugular Vein, Right* **R Vertebral Vein, Right** Deep cervical vein Suboccipital venous plexus **S Vertebral Vein, Left** *See R Vertebral Vein, Right* **T Face Vein, Right** Angular vein Anterior facial vein Common facial vein Deep facial vein Frontal vein Posterior facial (retromandibular) vein Supraorbital vein **V Face Vein, Left** *See T Face Vein, Right*	Ø Open 3 Percutaneous 4 Percutaneous Endoscopic	3 Infusion Device D Intraluminal Device	Z No Qualifier
3 Innominate Vein, Right ⊞ Brachiocephalic vein Inferior thyroid vein **4 Innominate Vein, Left** ⊞ *See 3 Innominate Vein, Right*		Ø Open 3 Percutaneous 4 Percutaneous Endoscopic	3 Infusion Device D Intraluminal Device M Neurostimulator Lead	Z No Qualifier
Y Upper Vein		Ø Open 3 Percutaneous 4 Percutaneous Endoscopic	2 Monitoring Device 3 Infusion Device D Intraluminal Device Y Other Device	Z No Qualifier

Non-OR	Ø5HØ[Ø,3,4]3Z
Non-OR	Ø5H[1,5,6,7,8,9,A,B,C,D,F,G,H,L,M,N,P,Q,R,S,T,V][Ø,3,4]3Z
Non-OR	Ø5H[3,4][Ø,3,4]3Z
Non-OR	Ø5HY[Ø,3,4]3Z
Non-OR	Ø5HY32Z
Non-OR	Ø5HY[3,4]YZ
HAC	Ø5HØ[3,4]3Z when reported with SDx J95.811
HAC	Ø5H[1,5,6][3,4]3Z when reported with SDx J95.811
HAC	Ø5H[M,N,P,Q]33Z when reported with SDx J95.811
HAC	Ø5H[3,4][3,4]3Z when reported with SDx J95.811

See Appendix L for Procedure Combinations
⊞   Ø5HØ[Ø,3,4]MZ
⊞   Ø5H[3,4][Ø,3,4]MZ

Ø   Medical and Surgical
5   Upper Veins
J   Inspection   Definition: Visually and/or manually exploring a body part

              Explanation: Visual exploration may be performed with or without optical instrumentation. Manual exploration may be performed directly or through intervening body layers.

Body Part Character 4	Approach Character 5	Device Character 6	Qualifier Character 7
Y Upper Vein	Ø Open 3 Percutaneous 4 Percutaneous Endoscopic X External	Z No Device	Z No Qualifier

Non-OR	Ø5JY[3,X]ZZ

Non-OR Procedure   DRG Non-OR Procedure   Valid OR Procedure   HAC Associated Procedure   Combination Only   New/Revised April   New/Revised October

Ø Medical and Surgical
5 Upper Veins
L Occlusion   Definition: Completely closing an orifice or the lumen of a tubular body part
          Explanation: The orifice can be a natural orifice or an artificially created orifice

Body Part Character 4	Approach Character 5	Device Character 6	Qualifier Character 7
Ø Azygos Vein Right ascending lumbar vein Right subcostal vein **1 Hemiazygos Vein** Left ascending lumbar vein Left subcostal vein **3 Innominate Vein, Right** Brachiocephalic vein Inferior thyroid vein **4 Innominate Vein, Left** *See 3 Innominate Vein, Right* **5 Subclavian Vein, Right** **6 Subclavian Vein, Left** **7 Axillary Vein, Right** **8 Axillary Vein, Left** **9 Brachial Vein, Right** Radial vein Ulnar vein **A Brachial Vein, Left** *See 9 Brachial Vein, Right* **B Basilic Vein, Right** Median antebrachial vein Median cubital vein **C Basilic Vein, Left** *See B Basilic Vein, Right* **D Cephalic Vein, Right** Accessory cephalic vein **F Cephalic Vein, Left** *See D Cephalic Vein, Right* **G Hand Vein, Right** Dorsal metacarpal vein Palmar (volar) digital vein Palmar (volar) metacarpal vein Superficial palmar venous arch Volar (palmar) digital vein Volar (palmar) metacarpal vein **H Hand Vein, Left** *See G Hand Vein, Right* **L Intracranial Vein** Anterior cerebral vein Basal (internal) cerebral vein Dural venous sinus Great cerebral vein Inferior cerebellar vein Inferior cerebral vein Internal (basal) cerebral vein Middle cerebral vein Ophthalmic vein Superior cerebellar vein Superior cerebral vein **M Internal Jugular Vein, Right** **N Internal Jugular Vein, Left** **P External Jugular Vein, Right** Posterior auricular vein **Q External Jugular Vein, Left** *See P External Jugular Vein, Right* **R Vertebral Vein, Right** Deep cervical vein Suboccipital venous plexus **S Vertebral Vein, Left** *See R Vertebral Vein, Right* **T Face Vein, Right** Angular vein Anterior facial vein Common facial vein Deep facial vein Frontal vein Posterior facial (retromandibular) vein Supraorbital vein **V Face Vein, Left** *See T Face Vein, Right* **Y Upper Vein**	**Ø** Open **3** Percutaneous **4** Percutaneous Endoscopic	**C** Extraluminal Device **D** Intraluminal Device **Z** No Device	**Z** No Qualifier

NC Noncovered Procedure   LC Limited Coverage   QA Questionable OB Admit   NT New Tech Add-on   ⊞ Combination Member   ♂ Male   ♀ Female

ICD-10-PCS 2024   253   Ø5L–Ø5L

Ø   Medical and Surgical
5   Upper Veins
N   Release   Definition: Freeing a body part from an abnormal physical constraint by cutting or by the use of force
                      Explanation: Some of the restraining tissue may be taken out but none of the body part is taken out

Body Part Character 4	Approach Character 5	Device Character 6	Qualifier Character 7
Ø Azygos Vein Right ascending lumbar vein Right subcostal vein **1 Hemiazygos Vein** Left ascending lumbar vein Left subcostal vein **3 Innominate Vein, Right** Brachiocephalic vein Inferior thyroid vein **4 Innominate Vein, Left** *See 3 Innominate Vein, Right* **5 Subclavian Vein, Right** **6 Subclavian Vein, Left** **7 Axillary Vein, Right** **8 Axillary Vein, Left** **9 Brachial Vein, Right** Radial vein Ulnar vein **A Brachial Vein, Left** *See 9 Brachial Vein, Right* **B Basilic Vein, Right** Median antebrachial vein Median cubital vein **C Basilic Vein, Left** *See B Basilic Vein, Right* **D Cephalic Vein, Right** Accessory cephalic vein **F Cephalic Vein, Left** *See D Cephalic Vein, Right* **G Hand Vein, Right** Dorsal metacarpal vein Palmar (volar) digital vein Palmar (volar) metacarpal vein Superficial palmar venous arch Volar (palmar) digital vein Volar (palmar) metacarpal vein **H Hand Vein, Left** *See G Hand Vein, Right* **L Intracranial Vein** Anterior cerebral vein Basal (internal) cerebral vein Dural venous sinus Great cerebral vein Inferior cerebellar vein Inferior cerebral vein Internal (basal) cerebral vein Middle cerebral vein Ophthalmic vein Superior cerebellar vein Superior cerebral vein **M Internal Jugular Vein, Right** **N Internal Jugular Vein, Left** **P External Jugular Vein, Right** Posterior auricular vein **Q External Jugular Vein, Left** *See P External Jugular Vein, Right* **R Vertebral Vein, Right** Deep cervical vein Suboccipital venous plexus **S Vertebral Vein, Left** *See R Vertebral Vein, Right* **T Face Vein, Right** Angular vein Anterior facial vein Common facial vein Deep facial vein Frontal vein Posterior facial (retromandibular) vein Supraorbital vein **V Face Vein, Left** *See T Face Vein, Right* **Y Upper Vein**	**Ø Open** **3 Percutaneous** **4 Percutaneous Endoscopic**	**Z No Device**	**Z No Qualifier**

Ø   Medical and Surgical
5   Upper Veins
P   Removal   Definition: Taking out or off a device from a body part

Explanation: If a device is taken out and a similar device put in without cutting or puncturing the skin or mucous membrane, the procedure is coded to the root operation CHANGE. Otherwise, the procedure for taking out a device is coded to the root operation REMOVAL.

Body Part Character 4	Approach Character 5	Device Character 6	Qualifier Character 7
Ø Azygos Vein Right ascending lumbar vein Right subcostal vein	**Ø** Open **3** Percutaneous **4** Percutaneous Endoscopic **X** External	**2** Monitoring Device **M** Neurostimulator Lead	**Z** No Qualifier
3 Innominate Vein, Right Brachiocephalic vein Inferior thyroid vein **4** Innominate Vein, Left *See 3 Innominate Vein, Right*	**Ø** Open **3** Percutaneous **4** Percutaneous Endoscopic **X** External	**M** Neurostimulator Lead	**Z** No Qualifier
Y Upper Vein	**Ø** Open **3** Percutaneous **4** Percutaneous Endoscopic	**Ø** Drainage Device **2** Monitoring Device **3** Infusion Device **7** Autologous Tissue Substitute **C** Extraluminal Device **D** Intraluminal Device **J** Synthetic Substitute **K** Nonautologous Tissue Substitute **Y** Other Device	**Z** No Qualifier
Y Upper Vein	**X** External	**Ø** Drainage Device **2** Monitoring Device **3** Infusion Device **D** Intraluminal Device	**Z** No Qualifier

Non-OR	Ø5PØ[Ø,3,4,X]2Z
Non-OR	Ø5PY3[Ø,2,3]Z
Non-OR	Ø5PY[3,4]YZ
Non-OR	Ø5PYX[Ø,2,3,D]Z

NC Noncovered Procedure   LC Limited Coverage   QA Questionable OB Admit   NT New Tech Add-on   ✛ Combination Member   ♂ Male   ♀ Female

ICD-10-PCS 2024   255

Ø5P–Ø5P

Ø   Medical and Surgical
5   Upper Veins
Q   Repair   Definition: Restoring, to the extent possible, a body part to its normal anatomic structure and function

Explanation: Used only when the method to accomplish the repair is not one of the other root operations

Body Part Character 4	Approach Character 5	Device Character 6	Qualifier Character 7
Ø Azygos Vein Right ascending lumbar vein Right subcostal vein	**Ø Open** **3 Percutaneous** **4 Percutaneous Endoscopic**	**Z No Device**	**Z No Qualifier**

Ø   Azygos Vein
   Right ascending lumbar vein
   Right subcostal vein
1   Hemiazygos Vein
   Left ascending lumbar vein
   Left subcostal vein
3   Innominate Vein, Right
   Brachiocephalic vein
   Inferior thyroid vein
4   Innominate Vein, Left
   See 3 Innominate Vein, Right
5   Subclavian Vein, Right
6   Subclavian Vein, Left
7   Axillary Vein, Right
8   Axillary Vein, Left
9   Brachial Vein, Right
   Radial vein
   Ulnar vein
A   Brachial Vein, Left
   See 9 Brachial Vein, Right
B   Basilic Vein, Right
   Median antebrachial vein
   Median cubital vein
C   Basilic Vein, Left
   See B Basilic Vein, Right
D   Cephalic Vein, Right
   Accessory cephalic vein
F   Cephalic Vein, Left
   See D Cephalic Vein, Right
G   Hand Vein, Right
   Dorsal metacarpal vein
   Palmar (volar) digital vein
   Palmar (volar) metacarpal vein
   Superficial palmar venous arch
   Volar (palmar) digital vein
   Volar (palmar) metacarpal vein
H   Hand Vein, Left
   See G Hand Vein, Right
L   Intracranial Vein
   Anterior cerebral vein
   Basal (internal) cerebral vein
   Dural venous sinus
   Great cerebral vein
   Inferior cerebellar vein
   Inferior cerebral vein
   Internal (basal) cerebral vein
   Middle cerebral vein
   Ophthalmic vein
   Superior cerebellar vein
   Superior cerebral vein
M   Internal Jugular Vein, Right
N   Internal Jugular Vein, Left
P   External Jugular Vein, Right
   Posterior auricular vein
Q   External Jugular Vein, Left
   See P External Jugular Vein, Right
R   Vertebral Vein, Right
   Deep cervical vein
   Suboccipital venous plexus
S   Vertebral Vein, Left
   See R Vertebral Vein, Right
T   Face Vein, Right
   Angular vein
   Anterior facial vein
   Common facial vein
   Deep facial vein
   Frontal vein
   Posterior facial (retromandibular) vein
   Supraorbital vein
V   Face Vein, Left
   See T Face Vein, Right
Y   Upper Vein

Non-OR Procedure   DRG Non-OR Procedure   Valid OR Procedure   HAC Associated Procedure   Combination Only   New/Revised April   New/Revised October

0   **Medical and Surgical**
5   **Upper Veins**
R   **Replacement**   Definition: Putting in or on biological or synthetic material that physically takes the place and/or function of all or a portion of a body part

Explanation: The body part may have been taken out or replaced, or may be taken out, physically eradicated, or rendered nonfunctional during the REPLACEMENT procedure. A REMOVAL procedure is coded for taking out the device used in a previous replacement procedure.

Body Part Character 4	Approach Character 5	Device Character 6	Qualifier Character 7
0 **Azygos Vein** Right ascending lumbar vein Right subcostal vein **1** **Hemiazygos Vein** Left ascending lumbar vein Left subcostal vein **3** **Innominate Vein, Right** Brachiocephalic vein Inferior thyroid vein **4** **Innominate Vein, Left** *See 3 Innominate Vein, Right* **5** **Subclavian Vein, Right** **6** **Subclavian Vein, Left** **7** **Axillary Vein, Right** **8** **Axillary Vein, Left** **9** **Brachial Vein, Right** Radial vein Ulnar vein **A** **Brachial Vein, Left** *See 9 Brachial Vein, Right* **B** **Basilic Vein, Right** Median antebrachial vein Median cubital vein **C** **Basilic Vein, Left** *See B Basilic Vein, Right* **D** **Cephalic Vein, Right** Accessory cephalic vein **F** **Cephalic Vein, Left** *See D Cephalic Vein, Right* **G** **Hand Vein, Right** Dorsal metacarpal vein Palmar (volar) digital vein Palmar (volar) metacarpal vein Superficial palmar venous arch Volar (palmar) digital vein Volar (palmar) metacarpal vein **H** **Hand Vein, Left** *See G Hand Vein, Right* **L** **Intracranial Vein** Anterior cerebral vein Basal (internal) cerebral vein Dural venous sinus Great cerebral vein Inferior cerebellar vein Inferior cerebral vein Internal (basal) cerebral vein Middle cerebral vein Ophthalmic vein Superior cerebellar vein Superior cerebral vein **M** **Internal Jugular Vein, Right** **N** **Internal Jugular Vein, Left** **P** **External Jugular Vein, Right** Posterior auricular vein **Q** **External Jugular Vein, Left** *See P External Jugular Vein, Right* **R** **Vertebral Vein, Right** Deep cervical vein Suboccipital venous plexus **S** **Vertebral Vein, Left** *See R Vertebral Vein, Right* **T** **Face Vein, Right** Angular vein Anterior facial vein Common facial vein Deep facial vein Frontal vein Posterior facial (retromandibular) vein Supraorbital vein **V** **Face Vein, Left** *See T Face Vein, Right* **Y** **Upper Vein**	**0** Open **4** Percutaneous Endoscopic	**7** Autologous Tissue Substitute **J** Synthetic Substitute **K** Nonautologous Tissue Substitute	**Z** No Qualifier

NC Noncovered Procedure   **LC** Limited Coverage   **QA** Questionable OB Admit   **NT** New Tech Add-on   ⊞ Combination Member   ♂ Male   ♀ Female

ICD-10-PCS 2024   257

05R–05R

0   **Medical and Surgical**
5   **Upper Veins**
S   **Reposition**   Definition: Moving to its normal location, or other suitable location, all or a portion of a body part

Explanation: The body part is moved to a new location from an abnormal location, or from a normal location where it is not functioning correctly. The body part may or may not be cut out or off to be moved to the new location.

Body Part Character 4	Approach Character 5	Device Character 6	Qualifier Character 7
0 Azygos Vein Right ascending lumbar vein Right subcostal vein **1** Hemiazygos Vein Left ascending lumbar vein Left subcostal vein **3** Innominate Vein, Right Brachiocephalic vein Inferior thyroid vein **4** Innominate Vein, Left *See 3 Innominate Vein, Right* **5** Subclavian Vein, Right **6** Subclavian Vein, Left **7** Axillary Vein, Right **8** Axillary Vein, Left **9** Brachial Vein, Right Radial vein Ulnar vein **A** Brachial Vein, Left *See 9 Brachial Vein, Right* **B** Basilic Vein, Right Median antebrachial vein Median cubital vein **C** Basilic Vein, Left *See B Basilic Vein, Right* **D** Cephalic Vein, Right Accessory cephalic vein **F** Cephalic Vein, Left *See D Cephalic Vein, Right* **G** Hand Vein, Right Dorsal metacarpal vein Palmar (volar) digital vein Palmar (volar) metacarpal vein Superficial palmar venous arch Volar (palmar) digital vein Volar (palmar) metacarpal vein **H** Hand Vein, Left *See G Hand Vein, Right* **L** Intracranial Vein Anterior cerebral vein Basal (internal) cerebral vein Dural venous sinus Great cerebral vein Inferior cerebellar vein Inferior cerebral vein Internal (basal) cerebral vein Middle cerebral vein Ophthalmic vein Superior cerebellar vein Superior cerebral vein **M** Internal Jugular Vein, Right **N** Internal Jugular Vein, Left **P** External Jugular Vein, Right Posterior auricular vein **Q** External Jugular Vein, Left *See P External Jugular Vein, Right* **R** Vertebral Vein, Right Deep cervical vein Suboccipital venous plexus **S** Vertebral Vein, Left *See R Vertebral Vein, Right* **T** Face Vein, Right Angular vein Anterior facial vein Common facial vein Deep facial vein Frontal vein Posterior facial (retromandibular) vein Supraorbital vein **V** Face Vein, Left *See T Face Vein, Right* **Y** Upper Vein	**0** Open **3** Percutaneous **4** Percutaneous Endoscopic	**Z** No Device	**Z** No Qualifier

Non-OR Procedure   DRG Non-OR Procedure   Valid OR Procedure   HAC Associated Procedure   Combination Only   New/Revised April   New/Revised October

258   ICD-10-PCS 2024

Ø   Medical and Surgical
5   Upper Veins
U   Supplement   Definition: Putting in or on biological or synthetic material that physically reinforces and/or augments the function of a portion of a body part

Explanation: The biological material is non-living, or is living and from the same individual. The body part may have been previously replaced, and the SUPPLEMENT procedure is performed to physically reinforce and/or augment the function of the replaced body part.

Body Part Character 4	Approach Character 5	Device Character 6	Qualifier Character 7

Ø   Azygos Vein
    Right ascending lumbar vein
    Right subcostal vein
1   Hemiazygos Vein
    Left ascending lumbar vein
    Left subcostal vein
3   Innominate Vein, Right
    Brachiocephalic vein
    Inferior thyroid vein
4   Innominate Vein, Left
    See 3 Innominate Vein, Right
5   Subclavian Vein, Right
6   Subclavian Vein, Left
7   Axillary Vein, Right
8   Axillary Vein, Left
9   Brachial Vein, Right
    Radial vein
    Ulnar vein
A   Brachial Vein, Left
    See 9 Brachial Vein, Right
B   Basilic Vein, Right
    Median antebrachial vein
    Median cubital vein
C   Basilic Vein, Left
    See B Basilic Vein, Right
D   Cephalic Vein, Right
    Accessory cephalic vein
F   Cephalic Vein, Left
    See D Cephalic Vein, Right
G   Hand Vein, Right
    Dorsal metacarpal vein
    Palmar (volar) digital vein
    Palmar (volar) metacarpal vein
    Superficial palmar venous arch
    Volar (palmar) digital vein
    Volar (palmar) metacarpal vein
H   Hand Vein, Left
    See G Hand Vein, Right
L   Intracranial Vein
    Anterior cerebral vein
    Basal (internal) cerebral vein
    Dural venous sinus
    Great cerebral vein
    Inferior cerebellar vein
    Inferior cerebral vein
    Internal (basal) cerebral vein
    Middle cerebral vein
    Ophthalmic vein
    Superior cerebellar vein
    Superior cerebral vein
M   Internal Jugular Vein, Right
N   Internal Jugular Vein, Left
P   External Jugular Vein, Right
    Posterior auricular vein
Q   External Jugular Vein, Left
    See P External Jugular Vein, Right
R   Vertebral Vein, Right
    Deep cervical vein
    Suboccipital venous plexus
S   Vertebral Vein, Left
    See R Vertebral Vein, Right
T   Face Vein, Right
    Angular vein
    Anterior facial vein
    Common facial vein
    Deep facial vein
    Frontal vein
    Posterior facial (retromandibular) vein
    Supraorbital vein
V   Face Vein, Left
    See T Face Vein, Right
Y   Upper Vein
	Ø Open
	3 Percutaneous
	4 Percutaneous Endoscopic
		7 Autologous Tissue Substitute
		J Synthetic Substitute
		K Nonautologous Tissue Substitute
			Z No Qualifier

NC Noncovered Procedure   **LC** Limited Coverage   **QA** Questionable OB Admit   **NT** New Tech Add-on   ⊞ Combination Member   ♂ Male   ♀ Female

ICD-10-PCS 2024   **259**

Ø5U–Ø5U

Ø   **Medical and Surgical**
5   **Upper Veins**
V   **Restriction**   Definition: Partially closing an orifice or the lumen of a tubular body part

                         Explanation: The orifice can be a natural orifice or an artificially created orifice

Body Part Character 4	Approach Character 5	Device Character 6	Qualifier Character 7
Ø **Azygos Vein** Right ascending lumbar vein Right subcostal vein 1 **Hemiazygos Vein** Left ascending lumbar vein Left subcostal vein 3 **Innominate Vein, Right** Brachiocephalic vein Inferior thyroid vein 4 **Innominate Vein, Left** *See 3 Innominate Vein, Right* 5 **Subclavian Vein, Right** 6 **Subclavian Vein, Left** 7 **Axillary Vein, Right** 8 **Axillary Vein, Left** 9 **Brachial Vein, Right** Radial vein Ulnar vein A **Brachial Vein, Left** *See 9 Brachial Vein, Right* B **Basilic Vein, Right** Median antebrachial vein Median cubital vein C **Basilic Vein, Left** *See B Basilic Vein, Right* D **Cephalic Vein, Right** Accessory cephalic vein F **Cephalic Vein, Left** *See D Cephalic Vein, Right* G **Hand Vein, Right** Dorsal metacarpal vein Palmar (volar) digital vein Palmar (volar) metacarpal vein Superficial palmar venous arch Volar (palmar) digital vein Volar (palmar) metacarpal vein H **Hand Vein, Left** *See G Hand Vein, Right* L **Intracranial Vein** Anterior cerebral vein Basal (internal) cerebral vein Dural venous sinus Great cerebral vein Inferior cerebellar vein Inferior cerebral vein Internal (basal) cerebral vein Middle cerebral vein Ophthalmic vein Superior cerebellar vein Superior cerebral vein M **Internal Jugular Vein, Right** N **Internal Jugular Vein, Left** P **External Jugular Vein, Right** Posterior auricular vein Q **External Jugular Vein, Left** *See P External Jugular Vein, Right* R **Vertebral Vein, Right** Deep cervical vein Suboccipital venous plexus S **Vertebral Vein, Left** *See R Vertebral Vein, Right* T **Face Vein, Right** Angular vein Anterior facial vein Common facial vein Deep facial vein Frontal vein Posterior facial (retromandibular) vein Supraorbital vein V **Face Vein, Left** *See T Face Vein, Right* Y **Upper Vein**	Ø **Open** 3 **Percutaneous** 4 **Percutaneous Endoscopic**	C **Extraluminal Device** D **Intraluminal Device** Z **No Device**	Z **No Qualifier**

Non-OR Procedure   DRG Non-OR Procedure   Valid OR Procedure   HAC Associated Procedure   Combination Only   New/Revised April   New/Revised October

260   ICD-10-PCS 2024

Ø5V–Ø5V

Ø   Medical and Surgical
5   Upper Veins
W   Revision   Definition: Correcting, to the extent possible, a portion of a malfunctioning device or the position of a displaced device

                            Explanation: Revision can include correcting a malfunctioning or displaced device by taking out or putting in components of the device such as a screw or pin

Body Part Character 4	Approach Character 5	Device Character 6	Qualifier Character 7

Ø   Azygos Vein
     Right ascending lumbar vein
     Right subcostal vein
	Ø Open
	3 Percutaneous
	4 Percutaneous Endoscopic
	X External
		2 Monitoring Device
		M Neurostimulator Lead
			Z No Qualifier

3   Innominate Vein, Right
     Brachiocephalic vein
     Inferior thyroid vein
4   Innominate Vein, Left
     See 3 Innominate Vein, Right
	Ø Open
	3 Percutaneous
	4 Percutaneous Endoscopic
	X External
		M Neurostimulator Lead	**Z** No Qualifier

Y Upper Vein	**Ø** Open **3** Percutaneous **4** Percutaneous Endoscopic	**Ø** Drainage Device **2** Monitoring Device **3** Infusion Device **7** Autologous Tissue Substitute **C** Extraluminal Device **D** Intraluminal Device **J** Synthetic Substitute **K** Nonautologous Tissue Substitute **Y** Other Device	**Z** No Qualifier
Y Upper Vein	**X** External	**Ø** Drainage Device **2** Monitoring Device **3** Infusion Device **7** Autologous Tissue Substitute **C** Extraluminal Device **D** Intraluminal Device **J** Synthetic Substitute **K** Nonautologous Tissue Substitute	**Z** No Qualifier

Non-OR	Ø5WØXMZ
Non-OR	Ø5W[3,4]XMZ
Non-OR	Ø5WY3[Ø,2,3]Z
Non-OR	Ø5WY[3,4]YZ
Non-OR	Ø5WYX[Ø,2,3,7,C,D,J,K]Z

NC Noncovered Procedure   **LC** Limited Coverage   **QA** Questionable OB Admit   **NT** New Tech Add-on   ⊞ Combination Member   ♂ Male   ♀ Female

ICD-10-PCS 2024   **261**

Lower Veins Ø61–Ø6W

Character Meanings

This Character Meaning table is provided as a guide to assist the user in the identification of character members that may be found in this section of code tables. It **SHOULD NOT** be used to build a PCS code.

Operation–Character 3		Body Part–Character 4		Approach–Character 5		Device–Character 6		Qualifier–Character 7	
1	Bypass	Ø	Inferior Vena Cava	Ø	Open	Ø	Drainage Device	Ø	Ultrasonic
5	Destruction	1	Splenic Vein	3	Percutaneous	2	Monitoring Device	4	Hepatic Vein
7	Dilation	2	Gastric Vein	4	Percutaneous Endoscopic	3	Infusion Device	5	Superior Mesenteric Vein
9	Drainage	3	Esophageal Vein	7	Via Natural or Artificial Opening	7	Autologous Tissue Substitute	6	Inferior Mesenteric Vein
B	Excision	4	Hepatic Vein	8	Via Natural or Artificial Opening Endoscopic	9	Autologous Venous Tissue	9	Renal Vein, Right
C	Extirpation	5	Superior Mesenteric Vein	X	External	A	Autologous Arterial Tissue	B	Renal Vein, Left
D	Extraction	6	Inferior Mesenteric Vein			C	Extraluminal Device	C	Hemorrhoidal Plexus
F	Fragmentation	7	Colic Vein			D	Intraluminal Device	P	Pulmonary Trunk
H	Insertion	8	Portal Vein			J	Synthetic Substitute	Q	Pulmonary Artery, Right
J	Inspection	9	Renal Vein, Right			K	Nonautologous Tissue Substitute	R	Pulmonary Artery, Left
L	Occlusion	B	Renal Vein, Left			Y	Other Device	T	Via Umbilical Vein
N	Release	C	Common Iliac Vein, Right			Z	No Device	X	Diagnostic
P	Removal	D	Common Iliac Vein, Left					Y	Lower Vein
Q	Repair	F	External Iliac Vein, Right					Z	No Qualifier
R	Replacement	G	External Iliac Vein, Left						
S	Reposition	H	Hypogastric Vein, Right						
U	Supplement	J	Hypogastric Vein, Left						
V	Restriction	M	Femoral Vein, Right						
W	Revision	N	Femoral Vein, Left						
		P	Saphenous Vein, Right						
		Q	Saphenous Vein, Left						
		T	Foot Vein, Right						
		V	Foot Vein, Left						
		Y	Lower Vein						

AHA Coding Clinic for Lower Veins
2022, 1Q, 10-13   Procedures performed on a continuous vessel, ICD-10-PCS Guideline B4.1c

AHA Coding Clinic for table Ø61
2017, 4Q, 36-38   Fontan completion procedure
2017, 4Q, 66-67   New qualifier values - Portal to hepatic shunt

AHA Coding Clinic for table Ø6B
2020, 1Q, 28   Free flap microvascular breast reconstruction
2017, 3Q, 5   Femoral artery to posterior tibial artery bypass using autologous and synthetic grafts
2017, 1Q, 31   Left to right common carotid artery bypass
2017, 1Q, 32   Peroneal artery to dorsalis pedis artery bypass using saphenous vein graft
2016, 3Q, 31   Femoral to peroneal artery bypass with in-situ saphenous vein graft and lysis of valves
2016, 2Q, 18   Femoral-tibial artery bypass and saphenous vein graft
2016, 1Q, 27   Aortocoronary bypass graft utilizing Y-graft
2014, 3Q, 8   Excision of saphenous vein for coronary artery bypass graft
2014, 3Q, 20   MAZE procedure performed with coronary artery bypass graft
2014, 1Q, 10   Repair of thoracic aortic aneurysm & coronary artery bypass graft

AHA Coding Clinic for table Ø6F
2020, 4Q, 45-49   New fragmentation tables
2020, 4Q, 49-50   Intravascular ultrasound assisted thrombolysis
2020, 4Q, 50   Intravascular lithotripsy

AHA Coding Clinic for table Ø6H
2021, 3Q, 18   Placement and removal of cannulas for extracorporeal membrane oxygenation
2017, 3Q, 11   Placement of peripherally inserted central catheter using 3CG ECG technology
2017, 1Q, 31   Umbilical vein catheterization
2017, 1Q, 31   Central catheter placement in femoral vein
2013, 3Q, 18   Heart transplant surgery

AHA Coding Clinic for table Ø6L
2021, 4Q, 47   Endoscopic banding of hemorrhoidal plexus
2021, 4Q, 49   Division of liver for staged hepatectomy
2020, 3Q, 44   Cardiophrenic vein embolization
2019, 4Q, 28   Transorifice occlusion of gastric varices
2018, 2Q, 18   Transverse rectus abdominis myocutaneous (TRAM) delay
2017, 4Q, 57-58   Added approach values - Transorifice esophageal vein banding
2013, 4Q, 112   Endoscopic banding of esophageal varices

AHA Coding Clinic for table Ø6P
2021, 3Q, 18   Placement and removal of cannulas for extracorporeal membrane oxygenation

AHA Coding Clinic for table Ø6V
2018, 3Q, 11   Transvenous transcatheter placement of valve in inferior vena cava
2018, 1Q, 10   Revision of transjugular intrahepatic portosystemic shunt

AHA Coding Clinic for table Ø6W
2019, 2Q, 39   Transjugular intrahepatic portosystemic shunt revision
2018, 1Q, 10   Revision of transjugular intrahepatic portosystemic shunt
2014, 3Q, 25   Revision of transjugular intrahepatic portosystemic shunt (TIPS)

Lower Veins

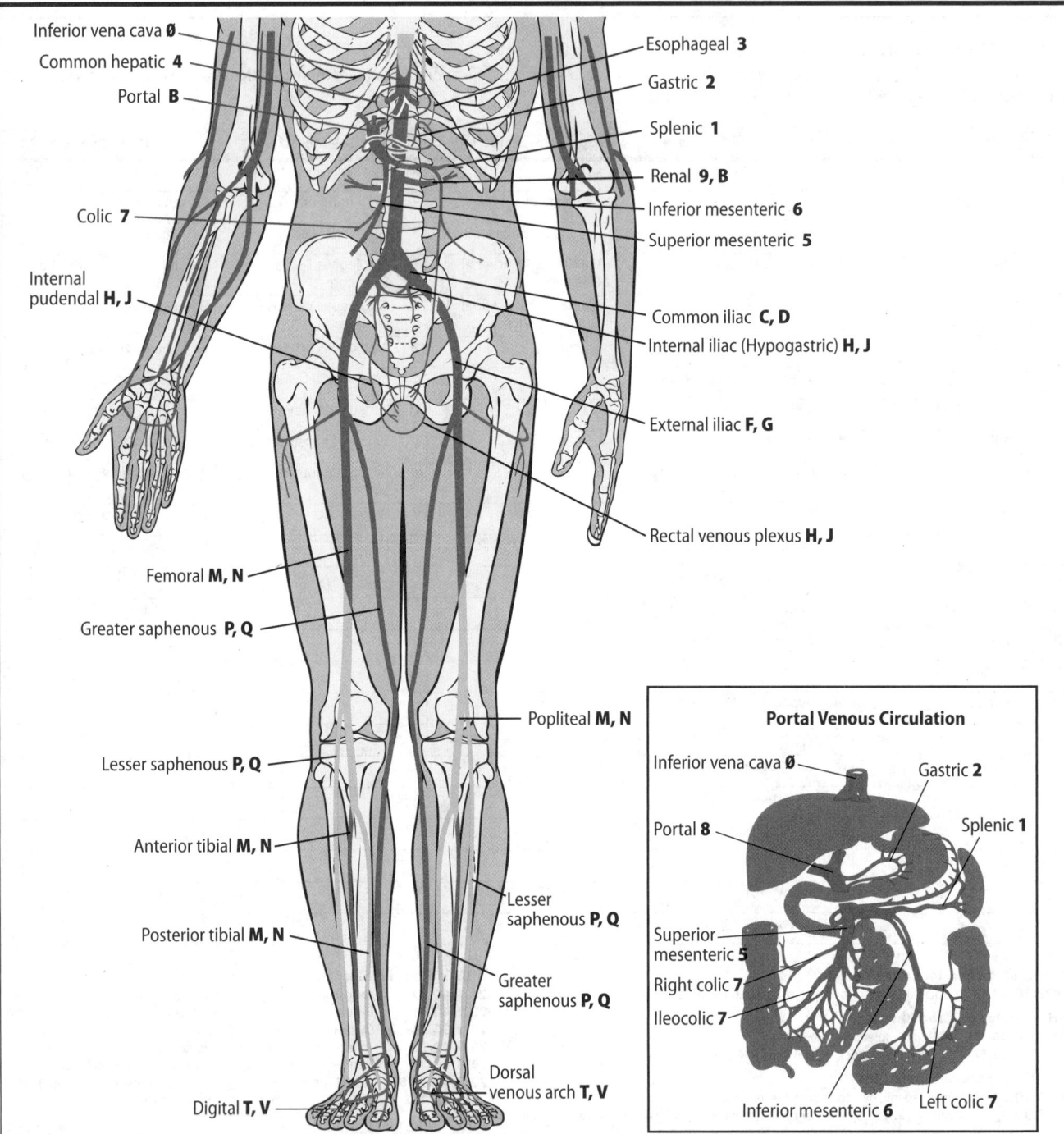

Inferior vena cava **Ø**
Common hepatic **4**
Portal **B**
Colic **7**
Internal pudendal **H, J**
Femoral **M, N**
Greater saphenous **P, Q**
Lesser saphenous **P, Q**
Anterior tibial **M, N**
Posterior tibial **M, N**
Digital **T, V**

Esophageal **3**
Gastric **2**
Splenic **1**
Renal **9, B**
Inferior mesenteric **6**
Superior mesenteric **5**
Common iliac **C, D**
Internal iliac (Hypogastric) **H, J**
External iliac **F, G**
Rectal venous plexus **H, J**
Popliteal **M, N**
Lesser saphenous **P, Q**
Greater saphenous **P, Q**
Dorsal venous arch **T, V**

Portal Venous Circulation

Inferior vena cava **Ø**
Portal **8**
Superior mesenteric **5**
Right colic **7**
Ileocolic **7**
Inferior mesenteric **6**
Gastric **2**
Splenic **1**
Left colic **7**

Ø   Medical and Surgical
6   Lower Veins
1   Bypass   Definition: Altering the route of passage of the contents of a tubular body part

Explanation: Rerouting contents of a body part to a downstream area of the normal route, to a similar route and body part, or to an abnormal route and dissimilar body part. Includes one or more anastomoses, with or without the use of a device.

Body Part Character 4		Approach Character 5	Device Character 6	Qualifier Character 7
Ø Inferior Vena Cava Postcava Right inferior phrenic vein Right ovarian vein Right second lumbar vein Right suprarenal vein Right testicular vein		**Ø** Open **4** Percutaneous Endoscopic	**7** Autologous Tissue Substitute **9** Autologous Venous Tissue **A** Autologous Arterial Tissue **J** Synthetic Substitute **K** Nonautologous Tissue Substitute **Z** No Device	**5** Superior Mesenteric Vein **6** Inferior Mesenteric Vein **P** Pulmonary Trunk **Q** Pulmonary Artery, Right **R** Pulmonary Artery, Left **Y** Lower Vein
1 Splenic Vein Left gastroepiploic vein Pancreatic vein		**Ø** Open **4** Percutaneous Endoscopic	**7** Autologous Tissue Substitute **9** Autologous Venous Tissue **A** Autologous Arterial Tissue **J** Synthetic Substitute **K** Nonautologous Tissue Substitute **Z** No Device	**9** Renal Vein, Right **B** Renal Vein, Left **Y** Lower Vein
2 Gastric Vein **3 Esophageal Vein** **4 Hepatic Vein** **5 Superior Mesenteric Vein** Right gastroepiploic vein **6 Inferior Mesenteric Vein** Sigmoid vein Superior rectal vein **7 Colic Vein** Ileocolic vein Left colic vein Middle colic vein Right colic vein **9 Renal Vein, Right** **B Renal Vein, Left** Left inferior phrenic vein Left ovarian vein Left second lumbar vein Left suprarenal vein Left testicular vein **C Common Iliac Vein, Right** **D Common Iliac Vein, Left** **F External Iliac Vein, Right** **G External Iliac Vein, Left** **H Hypogastric Vein, Right** Gluteal vein Internal iliac vein Internal pudendal vein Lateral sacral vein Middle hemorrhoidal vein Obturator vein Uterine vein Vaginal vein Vesical vein	**J Hypogastric Vein, Left** *See H Hypogastric Vein, Right* **M Femoral Vein, Right** Deep femoral (profunda femoris) vein Popliteal vein Profunda femoris (deep femoral) vein **N Femoral Vein, Left** *See M Femoral Vein, Right* **P Saphenous Vein, Right** External pudendal vein Great(er) saphenous vein Lesser saphenous vein Small saphenous vein Superficial circumflex iliac vein Superficial epigastric vein **Q Saphenous Vein, Left** *See P Saphenous Vein, Right* **T Foot Vein, Right** Common digital vein Dorsal metatarsal vein Dorsal venous arch Plantar digital vein Plantar metatarsal vein Plantar venous arch **V Foot Vein, Left** *See T Foot Vein, Right*	**Ø** Open **4** Percutaneous Endoscopic	**7** Autologous Tissue Substitute **9** Autologous Venous Tissue **A** Autologous Arterial Tissue **J** Synthetic Substitute **K** Nonautologous Tissue Substitute **Z** No Device	**Y** Lower Vein
8 Portal Vein Hepatic portal vein		**Ø** Open	**7** Autologous Tissue Substitute **9** Autologous Venous Tissue **A** Autologous Arterial Tissue **J** Synthetic Substitute **K** Nonautologous Tissue Substitute **Z** No Device	**9** Renal Vein, Right **B** Renal Vein, Left **Y** Lower Vein
8 Portal Vein Hepatic portal vein		**3** Percutaneous	**J** Synthetic Substitute	**4** Hepatic Vein **Y** Lower Vein
8 Portal Vein Hepatic portal vein		**4** Percutaneous Endoscopic	**7** Autologous Tissue Substitute **9** Autologous Venous Tissue **A** Autologous Arterial Tissue **K** Nonautologous Tissue Substitute **Z** No Device	**9** Renal Vein, Right **B** Renal Vein, Left **Y** Lower Vein
8 Portal Vein Hepatic portal vein		**4** Percutaneous Endoscopic	**J** Synthetic Substitute	**4** Hepatic Vein **9** Renal Vein, Right **B** Renal Vein, Left **Y** Lower Vein

Lower Veins *(left margin)*

Ø **Medical and Surgical**
6 **Lower Veins**
5 **Destruction**　　Definition: Physical eradication of all or a portion of a body part by the direct use of energy, force, or a destructive agent
　　　　　　　　　　Explanation: None of the body part is physically taken out

Body Part Character 4	Approach Character 5	Device Character 6	Qualifier Character 7
Ø Inferior Vena Cava Postcava Right inferior phrenic vein Right ovarian vein Right second lumbar vein Right suprarenal vein Right testicular vein 1 Splenic Vein Left gastroepiploic vein Pancreatic vein 2 Gastric Vein 3 Esophageal Vein 4 Hepatic Vein 5 Superior Mesenteric Vein Right gastroepiploic vein 6 Inferior Mesenteric Vein Sigmoid vein Superior rectal vein 7 Colic Vein Ileocolic vein Left colic vein Middle colic vein Right colic vein 8 Portal Vein Hepatic portal vein 9 Renal Vein, Right B Renal Vein, Left Left inferior phrenic vein Left ovarian vein Left second lumbar vein Left suprarenal vein Left testicular vein C Common Iliac Vein, Right D Common Iliac Vein, Left F External Iliac Vein, Right G External Iliac Vein, Left H Hypogastric Vein, Right Gluteal vein Internal iliac vein Internal pudendal vein Lateral sacral vein Middle hemorrhoidal vein Obturator vein Uterine vein Vaginal vein Vesical vein J Hypogastric Vein, Left *See H Hypogastric Vein, Right* M Femoral Vein, Right Deep femoral (profunda femoris) vein Popliteal vein Profunda femoris (deep femoral) vein N Femoral Vein, Left *See M Femoral Vein, Right* P Saphenous Vein, Right External pudendal vein Great(er) saphenous vein Lesser saphenous vein Small saphenous vein Superficial circumflex iliac vein Superficial epigastric vein Q Saphenous Vein, Left *See P Saphenous Vein, Right* T Foot Vein, Right Common digital vein Dorsal metatarsal vein Dorsal venous arch Plantar digital vein Plantar metatarsal vein Plantar venous arch V Foot Vein, Left *See T Foot Vein, Right*	Ø Open 3 Percutaneous 4 Percutaneous Endoscopic	Z No Device	Z No Qualifier
Y Lower Vein	Ø Open 3 Percutaneous 4 Percutaneous Endoscopic	Z No Device	C Hemorrhoidal Plexus Z No Qualifier

Ø **Medical and Surgical**
6 **Lower Veins**
7 **Dilation**　　Definition: Expanding an orifice or the lumen of a tubular body part

Explanation: The orifice can be a natural orifice or an artificially created orifice. Accomplished by stretching a tubular body part using intraluminal pressure or by cutting part of the orifice or wall of the tubular body part.

Body Part Character 4	Approach Character 5	Device Character 6	Qualifier Character 7
Ø **Inferior Vena Cava** 　Postcava 　Right inferior phrenic vein 　Right ovarian vein 　Right second lumbar vein 　Right suprarenal vein 　Right testicular vein **1** **Splenic Vein** 　Left gastroepiploic vein 　Pancreatic vein **2** **Gastric Vein** **3** **Esophageal Vein** **4** **Hepatic Vein** **5** **Superior Mesenteric Vein** 　Right gastroepiploic vein **6** **Inferior Mesenteric Vein** 　Sigmoid vein 　Superior rectal vein **7** **Colic Vein** 　Ileocolic vein 　Left colic vein 　Middle colic vein 　Right colic vein **8** **Portal Vein** 　Hepatic portal vein **9** **Renal Vein, Right** **B** **Renal Vein, Left** 　Left inferior phrenic vein 　Left ovarian vein 　Left second lumbar vein 　Left suprarenal vein 　Left testicular vein **C** **Common Iliac Vein, Right** **D** **Common Iliac Vein, Left** **F** **External Iliac Vein, Right** **G** **External Iliac Vein, Left** **H** **Hypogastric Vein, Right** 　Gluteal vein 　Internal iliac vein 　Internal pudendal vein 　Lateral sacral vein 　Middle hemorrhoidal vein 　Obturator vein 　Uterine vein 　Vaginal vein 　Vesical vein **J** **Hypogastric Vein, Left** 　*See* H Hypogastric Vein, Right **M** **Femoral Vein, Right** 　Deep femoral (profunda femoris) vein 　Popliteal vein 　Profunda femoris (deep femoral) vein **N** **Femoral Vein, Left** 　*See* M Femoral Vein, Right **P** **Saphenous Vein, Right** 　External pudendal vein 　Great(er) saphenous vein 　Lesser saphenous vein 　Small saphenous vein 　Superficial circumflex iliac vein 　Superficial epigastric vein **Q** **Saphenous Vein, Left** 　*See* P Saphenous Vein, Right **T** **Foot Vein, Right** 　Common digital vein 　Dorsal metatarsal vein 　Dorsal venous arch 　Plantar digital vein 　Plantar metatarsal vein 　Plantar venous arch **V** **Foot Vein, Left** 　*See* T Foot Vein, Right **Y** **Lower Vein**	**Ø** Open **3** Percutaneous **4** Percutaneous Endoscopic	**D** Intraluminal Device **Z** No Device	**Z** No Qualifier

NC Noncovered Procedure　　**LC** Limited Coverage　　**QA** Questionable OB Admit　　**NT** New Tech Add-on　　⊞ Combination Member　　♂ Male　　♀ Female

ICD-10-PCS 2024

267

067–067

Ø   **Medical and Surgical**
6   **Lower Veins**
9   **Drainage**   Definition: Taking or letting out fluids and/or gases from a body part
                    Explanation: The qualifier DIAGNOSTIC is used to identify drainage procedures that are biopsies

Body Part Character 4	Approach Character 5	Device Character 6	Qualifier Character 7
Ø Inferior Vena Cava Postcava Right inferior phrenic vein Right ovarian vein Right second lumbar vein Right suprarenal vein Right testicular vein **1 Splenic Vein** Left gastroepiploic vein Pancreatic vein **2 Gastric Vein** **3 Esophageal Vein** **4 Hepatic Vein** **5 Superior Mesenteric Vein** Right gastroepiploic vein **6 Inferior Mesenteric Vein** Sigmoid vein Superior rectal vein **7 Colic Vein** Ileocolic vein Left colic vein Middle colic vein Right colic vein **8 Portal Vein** Hepatic portal vein **9 Renal Vein, Right** **B Renal Vein, Left** Left inferior phrenic vein Left ovarian vein Left second lumbar vein Left suprarenal vein Left testicular vein **C Common Iliac Vein, Right** **D Common Iliac Vein, Left** **F External Iliac Vein, Right** **G External Iliac Vein, Left** **H Hypogastric Vein, Right** Gluteal vein Internal iliac vein Internal pudendal vein Lateral sacral vein Middle hemorrhoidal vein Obturator vein Uterine vein Vaginal vein Vesical vein **J Hypogastric Vein, Left** *See* H Hypogastric Vein, Right **M Femoral Vein, Right** Deep femoral (profunda femoris) vein Popliteal vein Profunda femoris (deep femoral) vein **N Femoral Vein, Left** *See* M Femoral Vein, Right **P Saphenous Vein, Right** External pudendal vein Great(er) saphenous vein Lesser saphenous vein Small saphenous vein Superficial circumflex iliac vein Superficial epigastric vein **Q Saphenous Vein, Left** *See* P Saphenous Vein, Right **T Foot Vein, Right** Common digital vein Dorsal metatarsal vein Dorsal venous arch Plantar digital vein Plantar metatarsal vein Plantar venous arch **V Foot Vein, Left** *See* T Foot Vein, Right **Y Lower Vein**	**Ø Open** **3 Percutaneous** **4 Percutaneous Endoscopic**	**Ø Drainage Device**	**Z No Qualifier**

Non-OR   Ø69[Ø,1,2,4,5,6,7,8,9,B,C,D,F,G,H,J,M,N,P,Q,T,V,Y][Ø,3,4]ØZ
Non-OR   Ø69330Z

Ø69 Continued on next page

Non-OR Procedure   DRG Non-OR Procedure   Valid OR Procedure   HAC Associated Procedure   Combination Only   New/Revised April   New/Revised October

Ø69 Continued

Ø	**Medical and Surgical**	
6	**Lower Veins**	
9	**Drainage**	Definition: Taking or letting out fluids and/or gases from a body part
		Explanation: The qualifier DIAGNOSTIC is used to identify drainage procedures that are biopsies

Body Part Character 4	Approach Character 5	Device Character 6	Qualifier Character 7
Ø Inferior Vena Cava Postcava Right inferior phrenic vein Right ovarian vein Right second lumbar vein Right suprarenal vein Right testicular vein **1 Splenic Vein** Left gastroepiploic vein Pancreatic vein **2 Gastric Vein** **3 Esophageal Vein** **4 Hepatic Vein** **5 Superior Mesenteric Vein** Right gastroepiploic vein **6 Inferior Mesenteric Vein** Sigmoid vein Superior rectal vein **7 Colic Vein** Ileocolic vein Left colic vein Middle colic vein Right colic vein **8 Portal Vein** Hepatic portal vein **9 Renal Vein, Right** **B Renal Vein, Left** Left inferior phrenic vein Left ovarian vein Left second lumbar vein Left suprarenal vein Left testicular vein **C Common Iliac Vein, Right** **D Common Iliac Vein, Left** **F External Iliac Vein, Right** **G External Iliac Vein, Left** **H Hypogastric Vein, Right** Gluteal vein Internal iliac vein Internal pudendal vein Lateral sacral vein Middle hemorrhoidal vein Obturator vein Uterine vein Vaginal vein Vesical vein **J Hypogastric Vein, Left** *See H Hypogastric Vein, Right* **M Femoral Vein, Right** Deep femoral (profunda femoris) vein Popliteal vein Profunda femoris (deep femoral) vein **N Femoral Vein, Left** *See M Femoral Vein, Right* **P Saphenous Vein, Right** External pudendal vein Great(er) saphenous vein Lesser saphenous vein Small saphenous vein Superficial circumflex iliac vein Superficial epigastric vein **Q Saphenous Vein, Left** *See P Saphenous Vein, Right* **T Foot Vein, Right** Common digital vein Dorsal metatarsal vein Dorsal venous arch Plantar digital vein Plantar metatarsal vein Plantar venous arch **V Foot Vein, Left** *See T Foot Vein, Right* **Y Lower Vein**	**Ø Open** **3 Percutaneous** **4 Percutaneous Endoscopic**	**Z No Device**	**X Diagnostic** **Z No Qualifier**

Non-OR	Ø69[Ø,1,2,3,4,5,6,7,8,9,B,C,D,F,G,H,J,M,N,P,Q,T,V,Y]3ZX
Non-OR	Ø69[Ø,1,2,4,5,6,7,8,9,B,C,D,F,G,H,J,M,N,P,Q,T,V,Y][Ø,3,4]ZZ
Non-OR	Ø6933ZZ

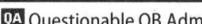

NC Noncovered Procedure   **LC** Limited Coverage   **QA** Questionable OB Admit   **NT** New Tech Add-on   ⊞ Combination Member   ♂ Male   ♀ Female

Ø Medical and Surgical
6 Lower Veins
B Excision Definition: Cutting out or off, without replacement, a portion of a body part

Explanation: The qualifier DIAGNOSTIC is used to identify excision procedures that are biopsies

Body Part Character 4	Approach Character 5	Device Character 6	Qualifier Character 7
Ø Inferior Vena Cava Postcava Right inferior phrenic vein Right ovarian vein Right second lumbar vein Right suprarenal vein Right testicular vein **1 Splenic Vein** Left gastroepiploic vein Pancreatic vein **2 Gastric Vein** **3 Esophageal Vein** **4 Hepatic Vein** **5 Superior Mesenteric Vein** Right gastroepiploic vein **6 Inferior Mesenteric Vein** Sigmoid vein Superior rectal vein **7 Colic Vein** Ileocolic vein Left colic vein Middle colic vein Right colic vein **8 Portal Vein** Hepatic portal vein **9 Renal Vein, Right** **B Renal Vein, Left** Left inferior phrenic vein Left ovarian vein Left second lumbar vein Left suprarenal vein Left testicular vein **C Common Iliac Vein, Right** **D Common Iliac Vein, Left** **F External Iliac Vein, Right** **G External Iliac Vein, Left** **H Hypogastric Vein, Right** Gluteal vein Internal iliac vein Internal pudendal vein Lateral sacral vein Middle hemorrhoidal vein Obturator vein Uterine vein Vaginal vein Vesical vein **J Hypogastric Vein, Left** *See H Hypogastric Vein, Right* **M Femoral Vein, Right** Deep femoral (profunda femoris) vein Popliteal vein Profunda femoris (deep femoral) vein **N Femoral Vein, Left** *See M Femoral Vein, Right* **P Saphenous Vein, Right** External pudendal vein Great(er) saphenous vein Lesser saphenous vein Small saphenous vein Superficial circumflex iliac vein Superficial epigastric vein **Q Saphenous Vein, Left** *See P Saphenous Vein, Right* **T Foot Vein, Right** Common digital vein Dorsal metatarsal vein Dorsal venous arch Plantar digital vein Plantar metatarsal vein Plantar venous arch **V Foot Vein, Left** *See T Foot Vein, Right*	**Ø Open** **3 Percutaneous** **4 Percutaneous Endoscopic**	**Z No Device**	**X Diagnostic** **Z No Qualifier**
Y Lower Vein	**Ø Open** **3 Percutaneous** **4 Percutaneous Endoscopic**	**Z No Device**	**C Hemorrhoidal Plexus** **X Diagnostic** **Z No Qualifier**

Non-OR Procedure DRG Non-OR Procedure Valid OR Procedure HAC Associated Procedure Combination Only New/Revised April New/Revised October

Ø   Medical and Surgical
6   Lower Veins
C   Extirpation   Definition: Taking or cutting out solid matter from a body part

Explanation: The solid matter may be an abnormal byproduct of a biological function or a foreign body; it may be imbedded in a body part or in the lumen of a tubular body part. The solid matter may or may not have been previously broken into pieces.

Body Part Character 4	Approach Character 5	Device Character 6	Qualifier Character 7
Ø Inferior Vena Cava Postcava Right inferior phrenic vein Right ovarian vein Right second lumbar vein Right suprarenal vein Right testicular vein **1 Splenic Vein** Left gastroepiploic vein Pancreatic vein **2 Gastric Vein** **3 Esophageal Vein** **4 Hepatic Vein** **5 Superior Mesenteric Vein** Right gastroepiploic vein **6 Inferior Mesenteric Vein** Sigmoid vein Superior rectal vein **7 Colic Vein** Ileocolic vein Left colic vein Middle colic vein Right colic vein **8 Portal Vein** Hepatic portal vein **9 Renal Vein, Right** **B Renal Vein, Left** Left inferior phrenic vein Left ovarian vein Left second lumbar vein Left suprarenal vein Left testicular vein **C Common Iliac Vein, Right** **D Common Iliac Vein, Left** **F External Iliac Vein, Right** **G External Iliac Vein, Left** **H Hypogastric Vein, Right** Gluteal vein Internal iliac vein Internal pudendal vein Lateral sacral vein Middle hemorrhoidal vein Obturator vein Uterine vein Vaginal vein Vesical vein **J Hypogastric Vein, Left** *See H Hypogastric Vein, Right* **M Femoral Vein, Right** Deep femoral (profunda femoris) vein Popliteal vein Profunda femoris (deep femoral) vein **N Femoral Vein, Left** *See M Femoral Vein, Right* **P Saphenous Vein, Right** External pudendal vein Great(er) saphenous vein Lesser saphenous vein Small saphenous vein Superficial circumflex iliac vein Superficial epigastric vein **Q Saphenous Vein, Left** *See P Saphenous Vein, Right* **T Foot Vein, Right** Common digital vein Dorsal metatarsal vein Dorsal venous arch Plantar digital vein Plantar metatarsal vein Plantar venous arch **V Foot Vein, Left** *See T Foot Vein, Right* **Y Lower Vein**	**Ø Open** **3 Percutaneous** **4 Percutaneous Endoscopic**	**Z No Device**	**Z No Qualifier**

NC Noncovered Procedure   **LC** Limited Coverage   **QA** Questionable OB Admit   **NT** New Tech Add-on   ⊞ Combination Member   ♂ Male   ♀ Female

ICD-10-PCS 2024   271

Ø6C–Ø6C

0   Medical and Surgical
6   Lower Veins
D   Extraction   Definition: Pulling or stripping out or off all or a portion of a body part by the use of force

Explanation: The qualifier DIAGNOSTIC is used to identify extraction procedures that are biopsies

Body Part Character 4	Approach Character 5	Device Character 6	Qualifier Character 7
M Femoral Vein, Right Deep femoral (profunda femoris) vein Popliteal vein Profunda femoris (deep femoral) vein **N** Femoral Vein, Left *See M Femoral Vein, Right* **P** Saphenous Vein, Right External pudendal vein Great(er) saphenous vein Lesser saphenous vein Small saphenous vein Superficial circumflex iliac vein Superficial epigastric vein **Q** Saphenous Vein, Left *See P Saphenous Vein, Right* **T** Foot Vein, Right Common digital vein Dorsal metatarsal vein Dorsal venous arch Plantar digital vein Plantar metatarsal vein Plantar venous arch **V** Foot Vein, Left *See T Foot Vein, Right* **Y** Lower Vein	**0** Open **3** Percutaneous **4** Percutaneous Endoscopic	**Z** No Device	**Z** No Qualifier

0   Medical and Surgical
6   Lower Veins
F   Fragmentation   Definition: Breaking solid matter in a body part into pieces

Explanation: Physical force (e.g., manual, ultrasonic) applied directly or indirectly is used to break the solid matter into pieces. The solid matter may be an abnormal byproduct of a biological function or a foreign body. The pieces of solid matter are not taken out.

Body Part Character 4	Approach Character 5	Device Character 6	Qualifier Character 7
C Common Iliac Vein, Right **D** Common Iliac Vein, Left **F** External Iliac Vein, Right **G** External Iliac Vein, Left **H** Hypogastric Vein, Right Gluteal vein Internal iliac vein Internal pudendal vein Lateral sacral vein Middle hemorrhoidal vein Obturator vein Uterine vein Vaginal vein Vesical vein **J** Hypogastric Vein, Left *See H Hypogastric Vein, Right* **M** Femoral Vein, Right Deep femoral (profunda femoris) vein Popliteal vein Profunda femoris (deep femoral) vein **N** Femoral Vein, Left *See M Femoral Vein, Right* **P** Saphenous Vein, Right External pudendal vein Great(er) saphenous vein Lesser saphenous vein Small saphenous vein Superficial circumflex iliac vein Superficial epigastric vein **Q** Saphenous Vein, Left *See P Saphenous Vein, Right* **Y** Lower Vein	**3** Percutaneous	**Z** No Device	**0** Ultrasonic **Z** No Qualifier

Non-OR Procedure   DRG Non-OR Procedure   Valid OR Procedure   HAC Associated Procedure   Combination Only   New/Revised April   New/Revised October

272   ICD-10-PCS 2024

06D–06F

0   **Medical and Surgical**
6   **Lower Veins**
H   **Insertion**   Definition: Putting in a nonbiological appliance that monitors, assists, performs, or prevents a physiological function but does not physically take the place of a body part

Explanation: None

Body Part Character 4		Approach Character 5	Device Character 6	Qualifier Character 7
0 Inferior Vena Cava Postcava Right inferior phrenic vein Right ovarian vein Right second lumbar vein Right suprarenal vein Right testicular vein		**0** Open **3** Percutaneous	**3** Infusion Device	**T** Via Umbilical Vein **Z** No Qualifier
0 Inferior Vena Cava Postcava Right inferior phrenic vein Right ovarian vein Right second lumbar vein Right suprarenal vein Right testicular vein		**0** Open **3** Percutaneous	**D** Intraluminal Device	**Z** No Qualifier
0 Inferior Vena Cava Postcava Right inferior phrenic vein Right ovarian vein Right second lumbar vein Right suprarenal vein Right testicular vein		**4** Percutaneous Endoscopic	**3** Infusion Device **D** Intraluminal Device	**Z** No Qualifier

1 Splenic Vein
  Left gastroepiploic vein
  Pancreatic vein
2 Gastric Vein
3 Esophageal Vein
4 Hepatic Vein
5 Superior Mesenteric Vein
  Right gastroepiploic vein
6 Inferior Mesenteric Vein
  Sigmoid vein
  Superior rectal vein
7 Colic Vein
  Ileocolic vein
  Left colic vein
  Middle colic vein
  Right colic vein
8 Portal Vein
  Hepatic portal vein
9 Renal Vein, Right
B Renal Vein, Left
  Left inferior phrenic vein
  Left ovarian vein
  Left second lumbar vein
  Left suprarenal vein
  Left testicular vein
C Common Iliac Vein, Right
D Common Iliac Vein, Left
F External Iliac Vein, Right
G External Iliac Vein, Left
	H Hypogastric Vein, Right
	  Gluteal vein
	  Internal iliac vein
	  Internal pudendal vein
	  Lateral sacral vein
	  Middle hemorrhoidal vein
	  Obturator vein
	  Uterine vein
	  Vaginal vein
	  Vesical vein
	J Hypogastric Vein, Left
	  See H Hypogastric Vein, Right
	M Femoral Vein, Right
	  Deep femoral (profunda femoris) vein
	  Popliteal vein
	  Profunda femoris (deep femoral) vein
	N Femoral Vein, Left
	  See M Femoral Vein, Right
	P Saphenous Vein, Right
	  External pudendal vein
	  Great(er) saphenous vein
	  Lesser saphenous vein
	  Small saphenous vein
	  Superficial circumflex iliac vein
	  Superficial epigastric vein
	Q Saphenous Vein, Left
	  See P Saphenous Vein, Right
	T Foot Vein, Right
	  Common digital vein
	  Dorsal metatarsal vein
	  Dorsal venous arch
	  Plantar digital vein
	  Plantar metatarsal vein
	  Plantar venous arch
	V Foot Vein, Left
	  See T Foot Vein, Right
		0 Open
		3 Percutaneous
		4 Percutaneous Endoscopic
			3 Infusion Device
			D Intraluminal Device
				Z No Qualifier

Y Lower Vein		**0** Open **3** Percutaneous **4** Percutaneous Endoscopic	**2** Monitoring Device **3** Infusion Device **D** Intraluminal Device **Y** Other Device	**Z** No Qualifier

Non-OR	06H0[0,3]3[T,Z]
Non-OR	06H03DZ
Non-OR	06H043Z
Non-OR	06H[1,2,3,4,5,6,7,8,9,B,C,D,F,G,H,J,M,N,P,Q,T,V][0,3,4]3Z
Non-OR	06HY[0,3,4]3Z
Non-OR	06HY32Z
Non-OR	06HY[3,4]YZ

NC Noncovered Procedure   **LC** Limited Coverage   **QA** Questionable OB Admit   **NT** New Tech Add-on   ⊞ Combination Member   ♂ Male   ♀ Female

ICD-10-PCS 2024   273

06H–06H

Ø   Medical and Surgical
6   Lower Veins
J   Inspection   Definition: Visually and/or manually exploring a body part

Explanation: Visual exploration may be performed with or without optical instrumentation. Manual exploration may be performed directly or through intervening body layers.

Body Part Character 4	Approach Character 5	Device Character 6	Qualifier Character 7
Y Lower Vein	Ø Open 3 Percutaneous 4 Percutaneous Endoscopic X External	Z No Device	Z No Qualifier

Non-OR   06JY[3,X]ZZ

Ø   Medical and Surgical
6   Lower Veins
L   Occlusion   Definition: Completely closing an orifice or the lumen of a tubular body part

Explanation: The orifice can be a natural orifice or an artificially created orifice

Body Part Character 4	Approach Character 5	Device Character 6	Qualifier Character 7

Ø   Inferior Vena Cava
    Postcava
    Right inferior phrenic vein
    Right ovarian vein
    Right second lumbar vein
    Right suprarenal vein
    Right testicular vein
1   Splenic Vein
    Left gastroepiploic vein
    Pancreatic vein
4   Hepatic Vein
5   Superior Mesenteric Vein
    Right gastroepiploic vein
6   Inferior Mesenteric Vein
    Sigmoid vein
    Superior rectal vein
7   Colic Vein
    Ileocolic vein
    Left colic vein
    Middle colic vein
    Right colic vein
8   Portal Vein
    Hepatic portal vein
9   Renal Vein, Right
B   Renal Vein, Left
    Left inferior phrenic vein
    Left ovarian vein
    Left second lumbar vein
    Left suprarenal vein
    Left testicular vein
C   Common Iliac Vein, Right
D   Common Iliac Vein, Left
F   External Iliac Vein, Right
G   External Iliac Vein, Left
	H Hypogastric Vein, Right
	    Gluteal vein
	    Internal iliac vein
	    Internal pudendal vein
	    Lateral sacral vein
	    Middle hemorrhoidal vein
	    Obturator vein
	    Uterine vein
	    Vaginal vein
	    Vesical vein
	J Hypogastric Vein, Left
	    See H Hypogastric Vein, Right
	M Femoral Vein, Right
	    Deep femoral (profunda
	     femoris) vein
	    Popliteal vein
	    Profunda femoris (deep
	     femoral) vein
	N Femoral Vein, Left
	    See M Femoral Vein, Right
	P Saphenous Vein, Right
	    External pudendal vein
	    Great(er) saphenous vein
	    Lesser saphenous vein
	    Small saphenous vein
	    Superficial circumflex iliac vein
	    Superficial epigastric vein
	Q Saphenous Vein, Left
	    See P Saphenous Vein, Right
	T Foot Vein, Right
	    Common digital vein
	    Dorsal metatarsal vein
	    Dorsal venous arch
	    Plantar digital vein
	    Plantar metatarsal vein
	    Plantar venous arch
	V Foot Vein, Left
	    See T Foot Vein, Right
		Ø Open
		3 Percutaneous
		4 Percutaneous Endoscopic
			C Extraluminal Device
			D Intraluminal Device
			Z No Device
				Z No Qualifier

2   Gastric Vein
3   Esophageal Vein
		Ø Open
		3 Percutaneous
		4 Percutaneous Endoscopic
		7 Via Natural or Artificial
		    Opening
		8 Via Natural or Artificial
		    Opening Endoscopic
			C Extraluminal Device
			D Intraluminal Device
			Z No Device
				Z No Qualifier

Y Lower Vein		Ø Open
		3 Percutaneous
		4 Percutaneous Endoscopic
		7 Via Natural or Artificial
		    Opening
		8 Via Natural or Artificial
		    Opening Endoscopic
			C Extraluminal Device
			D Intraluminal Device
			Z No Device
				C Hemorrhoidal Plexus
				Z No Qualifier

Non-OR   06L2[7,8][C,D,Z]Z
Non-OR   06L3[3,4,7,8][C,D,Z]Z

Non-OR Procedure   DRG Non-OR Procedure   Valid OR Procedure   HAC Associated Procedure   Combination Only   New/Revised April   New/Revised October

274   ICD-10-PCS 2024

06J–06L

0　Medical and Surgical
6　Lower Veins
N　Release　　Definition: Freeing a body part from an abnormal physical constraint by cutting or by the use of force

Explanation: Some of the restraining tissue may be taken out but none of the body part is taken out

Body Part Character 4		Approach Character 5	Device Character 6	Qualifier Character 7
0　Inferior Vena Cava 　　Postcava 　　Right inferior phrenic vein 　　Right ovarian vein 　　Right second lumbar vein 　　Right suprarenal vein 　　Right testicular vein **1　Splenic Vein** 　　Left gastroepiploic vein 　　Pancreatic vein **2　Gastric Vein** **3　Esophageal Vein** **4　Hepatic Vein** **5　Superior Mesenteric Vein** 　　Right gastroepiploic vein **6　Inferior Mesenteric Vein** 　　Sigmoid vein 　　Superior rectal vein **7　Colic Vein** 　　Ileocolic vein 　　Left colic vein 　　Middle colic vein 　　Right colic vein **8　Portal Vein** 　　Hepatic portal vein **9　Renal Vein, Right** **B　Renal Vein, Left** 　　Left inferior phrenic vein 　　Left ovarian vein 　　Left second lumbar vein 　　Left suprarenal vein 　　Left testicular vein **C　Common Iliac Vein, Right** **D　Common Iliac Vein, Left** **F　External Iliac Vein, Right** **G　External Iliac Vein, Left**	**H　Hypogastric Vein, Right** 　　Gluteal vein 　　Internal iliac vein 　　Internal pudendal vein 　　Lateral sacral vein 　　Middle hemorrhoidal vein 　　Obturator vein 　　Uterine vein 　　Vaginal vein 　　Vesical vein **J　Hypogastric Vein, Left** 　　*See H Hypogastric Vein, Right* **M　Femoral Vein, Right** 　　Deep femoral (profunda 　　　femoris) vein 　　Popliteal vein 　　Profunda femoris (deep 　　　femoral) vein **N　Femoral Vein, Left** 　　*See M Femoral Vein, Right* **P　Saphenous Vein, Right** 　　External pudendal vein 　　Great(er) saphenous vein 　　Lesser saphenous vein 　　Small saphenous vein 　　Superficial circumflex iliac vein 　　Superficial epigastric vein **Q　Saphenous Vein, Left** 　　*See P Saphenous Vein, Right* **T　Foot Vein, Right** 　　Common digital vein 　　Dorsal metatarsal vein 　　Dorsal venous arch 　　Plantar digital vein 　　Plantar metatarsal vein 　　Plantar venous arch **V　Foot Vein, Left** 　　*See T Foot Vein, Right* **Y　Lower Vein**	**0　Open** **3　Percutaneous** **4　Percutaneous Endoscopic**	**Z　No Device**	**Z　No Qualifier**

0　Medical and Surgical
6　Lower Veins
P　Removal　　Definition: Taking out or off a device from a body part

Explanation: If a device is taken out and a similar device put in without cutting or puncturing the skin or mucous membrane, the procedure is coded to the root operation CHANGE. Otherwise, the procedure for taking out a device is coded to the root operation REMOVAL.

Body Part Character 4	Approach Character 5	Device Character 6	Qualifier Character 7
Y　Lower Vein	**0　Open** **3　Percutaneous** **4　Percutaneous Endoscopic**	**0　Drainage Device** **2　Monitoring Device** **3　Infusion Device** **7　Autologous Tissue 　　Substitute** **C　Extraluminal Device** **D　Intraluminal Device** **J　Synthetic Substitute** **K　Nonautologous Tissue 　　Substitute** **Y　Other Device**	**Z　No Qualifier**
Y　Lower Vein	**X　External**	**0　Drainage Device** **2　Monitoring Device** **3　Infusion Device** **D　Intraluminal Device**	**Z　No Qualifier**

Non-OR	06PY3[0,2,3]Z
Non-OR	06PY[3,4]YZ
Non-OR	06PYX[0,2,3,D]Z

NC Noncovered Procedure　　**LC** Limited Coverage　　**QA** Questionable OB Admit　　**NT** New Tech Add-on　　✚ Combination Member　　♂ Male　　♀ Female

ICD-10-PCS 2024　　275

06N–06P

Lower Veins

Ø   **Medical and Surgical**
6   **Lower Veins**
Q   **Repair**   Definition: Restoring, to the extent possible, a body part to its normal anatomic structure and function
                     Explanation: Used only when the method to accomplish the repair is not one of the other root operations

Body Part Character 4	Approach Character 5	Device Character 6	Qualifier Character 7

Ø **Inferior Vena Cava**
  Postcava
  Right inferior phrenic vein
  Right ovarian vein
  Right second lumbar vein
  Right suprarenal vein
  Right testicular vein
1 **Splenic Vein**
  Left gastroepiploic vein
  Pancreatic vein
2 **Gastric Vein**
3 **Esophageal Vein**
4 **Hepatic Vein**
5 **Superior Mesenteric Vein**
  Right gastroepiploic vein
6 **Inferior Mesenteric Vein**
  Sigmoid vein
  Superior rectal vein
7 **Colic Vein**
  Ileocolic vein
  Left colic vein
  Middle colic vein
  Right colic vein
8 **Portal Vein**
  Hepatic portal vein
9 **Renal Vein, Right**
B **Renal Vein, Left**
  Left inferior phrenic vein
  Left ovarian vein
  Left second lumbar vein
  Left suprarenal vein
  Left testicular vein
C **Common Iliac Vein, Right**
D **Common Iliac Vein, Left**
F **External Iliac Vein, Right**
G **External Iliac Vein, Left**
H **Hypogastric Vein, Right**
  Gluteal vein
  Internal iliac vein
  Internal pudendal vein
  Lateral sacral vein
  Middle hemorrhoidal vein
  Obturator vein
  Uterine vein
  Vaginal vein
  Vesical vein
J **Hypogastric Vein, Left**
  See H Hypogastric Vein, Right
M **Femoral Vein, Right**
  Deep femoral (profunda femoris) vein
  Popliteal vein
  Profunda femoris (deep femoral) vein
N **Femoral Vein, Left**
  See M Femoral Vein, Right
P **Saphenous Vein, Right**
  External pudendal vein
  Great(er) saphenous vein
  Lesser saphenous vein
  Small saphenous vein
  Superficial circumflex iliac vein
  Superficial epigastric vein
Q **Saphenous Vein, Left**
  See P Saphenous Vein, Right
T **Foot Vein, Right**
  Common digital vein
  Dorsal metatarsal vein
  Dorsal venous arch
  Plantar digital vein
  Plantar metatarsal vein
  Plantar venous arch
V **Foot Vein, Left**
  See T Foot Vein, Right
Y **Lower Vein**
	Ø Open
	3 Percutaneous
	4 Percutaneous Endoscopic
		Z No Device	Z No Qualifier

Non-OR Procedure   DRG Non-OR Procedure   Valid OR Procedure   HAC Associated Procedure   Combination Only   New/Revised April   New/Revised October

276   ICD-10-PCS 2024

06Q–06Q

Ø   Medical and Surgical
6   Lower Veins
R   Replacement   Definition: Putting in or on biological or synthetic material that physically takes the place and/or function of all or a portion of a body part

Explanation: The body part may have been taken out or replaced, or may be taken out, physically eradicated, or rendered nonfunctional during the REPLACEMENT procedure. A REMOVAL procedure is coded for taking out the device used in a previous replacement procedure.

Body Part Character 4	Approach Character 5	Device Character 6	Qualifier Character 7

Ø   Inferior Vena Cava
    Postcava
    Right inferior phrenic vein
    Right ovarian vein
    Right second lumbar vein
    Right suprarenal vein
    Right testicular vein
1   Splenic Vein
    Left gastroepiploic vein
    Pancreatic vein
2   Gastric Vein
3   Esophageal Vein
4   Hepatic Vein
5   Superior Mesenteric Vein
    Right gastroepiploic vein
6   Inferior Mesenteric Vein
    Sigmoid vein
    Superior rectal vein
7   Colic Vein
    Ileocolic vein
    Left colic vein
    Middle colic vein
    Right colic vein
8   Portal Vein
    Hepatic portal vein
9   Renal Vein, Right
B   Renal Vein, Left
    Left inferior phrenic vein
    Left ovarian vein
    Left second lumbar vein
    Left suprarenal vein
    Left testicular vein
C   Common Iliac Vein, Right
D   Common Iliac Vein, Left
F   External Iliac Vein, Right
G   External Iliac Vein, Left
H   Hypogastric Vein, Right
    Gluteal vein
    Internal iliac vein
    Internal pudendal vein
    Lateral sacral vein
    Middle hemorrhoidal vein
    Obturator vein
    Uterine vein
    Vaginal vein
    Vesical vein
J   Hypogastric Vein, Left
    See H Hypogastric Vein, Right
M   Femoral Vein, Right
    Deep femoral (profunda femoris) vein
    Popliteal vein
    Profunda femoris (deep femoral) vein
N   Femoral Vein, Left
    See M Femoral Vein, Right
P   Saphenous Vein, Right
    External pudendal vein
    Great(er) saphenous vein
    Lesser saphenous vein
    Small saphenous vein
    Superficial circumflex iliac vein
    Superficial epigastric vein
Q   Saphenous Vein, Left
    See P Saphenous Vein, Right
T   Foot Vein, Right
    Common digital vein
    Dorsal metatarsal vein
    Dorsal venous arch
    Plantar digital vein
    Plantar metatarsal vein
    Plantar venous arch
V   Foot Vein, Left
    See T Foot Vein, Right
Y   Lower Vein
	Ø Open
	4 Percutaneous Endoscopic
		7 Autologous Tissue Substitute
		J Synthetic Substitute
		K Nonautologous Tissue Substitute
			Z No Qualifier

NC Noncovered Procedure   **LC** Limited Coverage   **QA** Questionable OB Admit   **NT** New Tech Add-on   ⊞ Combination Member   ♂ Male   ♀ Female

ICD-10-PCS 2024   277

Ø   **Medical and Surgical**
6   **Lower Veins**
S   **Reposition**   Definition: Moving to its normal location, or other suitable location, all or a portion of a body part

Explanation: The body part is moved to a new location from an abnormal location, or from a normal location where it is not functioning correctly. The body part may or may not be cut out or off to be moved to the new location.

Body Part Character 4	Approach Character 5	Device Character 6	Qualifier Character 7

Ø **Inferior Vena Cava**
   Postcava
   Right inferior phrenic vein
   Right ovarian vein
   Right second lumbar vein
   Right suprarenal vein
   Right testicular vein
1 **Splenic Vein**
   Left gastroepiploic vein
   Pancreatic vein
2 **Gastric Vein**
3 **Esophageal Vein**
4 **Hepatic Vein**
5 **Superior Mesenteric Vein**
   Right gastroepiploic vein
6 **Inferior Mesenteric Vein**
   Sigmoid vein
   Superior rectal vein
7 **Colic Vein**
   Ileocolic vein
   Left colic vein
   Middle colic vein
   Right colic vein
8 **Portal Vein**
   Hepatic portal vein
9 **Renal Vein, Right**
B **Renal Vein, Left**
   Left inferior phrenic vein
   Left ovarian vein
   Left second lumbar vein
   Left suprarenal vein
   Left testicular vein
C **Common Iliac Vein, Right**
D **Common Iliac Vein, Left**
F **External Iliac Vein, Right**
G **External Iliac Vein, Left**
H **Hypogastric Vein, Right**
   Gluteal vein
   Internal iliac vein
   Internal pudendal vein
   Lateral sacral vein
   Middle hemorrhoidal vein
   Obturator vein
   Uterine vein
   Vaginal vein
   Vesical vein
J **Hypogastric Vein, Left**
   See H Hypogastric Vein, Right
M **Femoral Vein, Right**
   Deep femoral (profunda femoris) vein
   Popliteal vein
   Profunda femoris (deep femoral) vein
N **Femoral Vein, Left**
   See M Femoral Vein, Right
P **Saphenous Vein, Right**
   External pudendal vein
   Great(er) saphenous vein
   Lesser saphenous vein
   Small saphenous vein
   Superficial circumflex iliac vein
   Superficial epigastric vein
Q **Saphenous Vein, Left**
   See P Saphenous Vein, Right
T **Foot Vein, Right**
   Common digital vein
   Dorsal metatarsal vein
   Dorsal venous arch
   Plantar digital vein
   Plantar metatarsal vein
   Plantar venous arch
V **Foot Vein, Left**
   See T Foot Vein, Right
Y **Lower Vein**
	Ø Open
	3 Percutaneous
	4 Percutaneous Endoscopic
		Z No Device	**Z** No Qualifier

Non-OR Procedure   DRG Non-OR Procedure   Valid OR Procedure   HAC Associated Procedure   Combination Only   New/Revised April   New/Revised October

278   ICD-10-PCS 2024

06S–06S

Ø   **Medical and Surgical**
6   **Lower Veins**
U   **Supplement**   Definition: Putting in or on biological or synthetic material that physically reinforces and/or augments the function of a portion of a body part
                    Explanation: The biological material is non-living, or is living and from the same individual. The body part may have been previously replaced, and the SUPPLEMENT procedure is performed to physically reinforce and/or augment the function of the replaced body part.

Body Part Character 4	Approach Character 5	Device Character 6	Qualifier Character 7
Ø Inferior Vena Cava Postcava Right inferior phrenic vein Right ovarian vein Right second lumbar vein Right suprarenal vein Right testicular vein **1** Splenic Vein Left gastroepiploic vein Pancreatic vein **2** Gastric Vein **3** Esophageal Vein **4** Hepatic Vein **5** Superior Mesenteric Vein Right gastroepiploic vein **6** Inferior Mesenteric Vein Sigmoid vein Superior rectal vein **7** Colic Vein Ileocolic vein Left colic vein Middle colic vein Right colic vein **8** Portal Vein Hepatic portal vein **9** Renal Vein, Right **B** Renal Vein, Left Left inferior phrenic vein Left ovarian vein Left second lumbar vein Left suprarenal vein Left testicular vein **C** Common Iliac Vein, Right **D** Common Iliac Vein, Left **F** External Iliac Vein, Right **G** External Iliac Vein, Left **H** Hypogastric Vein, Right Gluteal vein Internal iliac vein Internal pudendal vein Lateral sacral vein Middle hemorrhoidal vein Obturator vein Uterine vein Vaginal vein Vesical vein **J** Hypogastric Vein, Left *See H Hypogastric Vein, Right* **M** Femoral Vein, Right Deep femoral (profunda femoris) vein Popliteal vein Profunda femoris (deep femoral) vein **N** Femoral Vein, Left *See M Femoral Vein, Right* **P** Saphenous Vein, Right External pudendal vein Great(er) saphenous vein Lesser saphenous vein Small saphenous vein Superficial circumflex iliac vein Superficial epigastric vein **Q** Saphenous Vein, Left *See P Saphenous Vein, Right* **T** Foot Vein, Right Common digital vein Dorsal metatarsal vein Dorsal venous arch Plantar digital vein Plantar metatarsal vein Plantar venous arch **V** Foot Vein, Left *See T Foot Vein, Right* **Y** Lower Vein	**Ø** Open **3** Percutaneous **4** Percutaneous Endoscopic	**7** Autologous Tissue Substitute **J** Synthetic Substitute **K** Nonautologous Tissue Substitute	**Z** No Qualifier

NC Noncovered Procedure   **LC** Limited Coverage   **QA** Questionable OB Admit   **NT** New Tech Add-on   ⊞ Combination Member   ♂ Male   ♀ Female

ICD-10-PCS 2024   279

Ø6U–Ø6U

Ø Medical and Surgical
6 Lower Veins
V Restriction   Definition: Partially closing an orifice or the lumen of a tubular body part

                Explanation: The orifice can be a natural orifice or an artificially created orifice

Body Part Character 4	Approach Character 5	Device Character 6	Qualifier Character 7
Ø Inferior Vena Cava Postcava Right inferior phrenic vein Right ovarian vein Right second lumbar vein Right suprarenal vein Right testicular vein **1 Splenic Vein** Left gastroepiploic vein Pancreatic vein **2 Gastric Vein** **3 Esophageal Vein** **4 Hepatic Vein** **5 Superior Mesenteric Vein** Right gastroepiploic vein **6 Inferior Mesenteric Vein** Sigmoid vein Superior rectal vein **7 Colic Vein** Ileocolic vein Left colic vein Middle colic vein Right colic vein **8 Portal Vein** Hepatic portal vein **9 Renal Vein, Right** **B Renal Vein, Left** Left inferior phrenic vein Left ovarian vein Left second lumbar vein Left suprarenal vein Left testicular vein **C Common Iliac Vein, Right** **D Common Iliac Vein, Left** **F External Iliac Vein, Right** **G External Iliac Vein, Left** **H Hypogastric Vein, Right** Gluteal vein Internal iliac vein Internal pudendal vein Lateral sacral vein Middle hemorrhoidal vein Obturator vein Uterine vein Vaginal vein Vesical vein **J Hypogastric Vein, Left** *See H Hypogastric Vein, Right* **M Femoral Vein, Right** Deep femoral (profunda femoris) vein Popliteal vein Profunda femoris (deep femoral) vein **N Femoral Vein, Left** *See M Femoral Vein, Right* **P Saphenous Vein, Right** External pudendal vein Great(er) saphenous vein Lesser saphenous vein Small saphenous vein Superficial circumflex iliac vein Superficial epigastric vein **Q Saphenous Vein, Left** *See P Saphenous Vein, Right* **T Foot Vein, Right** Common digital vein Dorsal metatarsal vein Dorsal venous arch Plantar digital vein Plantar metatarsal vein Plantar venous arch **V Foot Vein, Left** *See T Foot Vein, Right* **Y Lower Vein**	**Ø Open** **3 Percutaneous** **4 Percutaneous Endoscopic**	**C Extraluminal Device** **D Intraluminal Device** **Z No Device**	**Z No Qualifier**

Non-OR Procedure   DRG Non-OR Procedure   Valid OR Procedure   HAC Associated Procedure   Combination Only   New/Revised April   New/Revised October

280   ICD-10-PCS 2024

Ø **Medical and Surgical**
6 **Lower Veins**
W **Revision**   Definition: Correcting, to the extent possible, a portion of a malfunctioning device or the position of a displaced device

Explanation: Revision can include correcting a malfunctioning or displaced device by taking out or putting in components of the device such as a screw or pin

Body Part Character 4	Approach Character 5	Device Character 6	Qualifier Character 7
Y Lower Vein	Ø Open 3 Percutaneous 4 Percutaneous Endoscopic	Ø Drainage Device 2 Monitoring Device 3 Infusion Device 7 Autologous Tissue Substitute C Extraluminal Device D Intraluminal Device J Synthetic Substitute K Nonautologous Tissue Substitute Y Other Device	Z No Qualifier
Y Lower Vein	X External	Ø Drainage Device 2 Monitoring Device 3 Infusion Device 7 Autologous Tissue Substitute C Extraluminal Device D Intraluminal Device J Synthetic Substitute K Nonautologous Tissue Substitute	Z No Qualifier

Non-OR	Ø6WY3[Ø,2,3]Z
Non-OR	Ø6WY[3,4]YZ
Non-OR	Ø6WYX[Ø,2,3,7,C,D,J,K]Z

NC Noncovered Procedure   LC Limited Coverage   QA Questionable OB Admit   NT New Tech Add-on   ⊞ Combination Member   ♂ Male   ♀ Female

ICD-10-PCS 2024   281

06W–06W

Lymphatic and Hemic Systems Ø72–Ø7Y

Character Meanings*

This Character Meaning table is provided as a guide to assist the user in the identification of character members that may be found in this section of code tables. It **SHOULD NOT** be used to build a PCS code.

Operation–Character 3		Body Part–Character 4		Approach–Character 5		Device–Character 6		Qualifier–Character 7	
2	Change	Ø	Lymphatic, Head	Ø	Open	Ø	Drainage Device	Ø	Allogeneic
5	Destruction	1	Lymphatic, Right Neck	3	Percutaneous	1	Radioactive Element	1	Syngeneic
9	Drainage	2	Lymphatic, Left Neck	4	Percutaneous Endoscopic	3	Infusion Device	2	Zooplastic
B	Excision	3	Lymphatic, Right Upper Extremity	8	Via Natural or Artificial Opening Endoscopic	7	Autologous Tissue Substitute	X	Diagnostic
C	Extirpation	4	Lymphatic, Left Upper Extremity	X	External	C	Extraluminal Device	Z	No Qualifier
D	Extraction	5	Lymphatic, Right Axillary			D	Intraluminal Device		
H	Insertion	6	Lymphatic, Left Axillary			J	Synthetic Substitute		
J	Inspection	7	Lymphatic, Thorax			K	Nonautologous Tissue Substitute		
L	Occlusion	8	Lymphatic, Internal Mammary, Right			Y	Other Device		
N	Release	9	Lymphatic, Internal Mammary, Left			Z	No Device		
P	Removal	B	Lymphatic, Mesenteric						
Q	Repair	C	Lymphatic, Pelvis						
S	Reposition	D	Lymphatic, Aortic						
T	Resection	F	Lymphatic, Right Lower Extremity						
U	Supplement	G	Lymphatic, Left Lower Extremity						
V	Restriction	H	Lymphatic, Right Inguinal						
W	Revision	J	Lymphatic, Left Inguinal						
Y	Transplantation	K	Thoracic Duct						
		L	Cisterna Chyli						
		M	Thymus						
		N	Lymphatic						
		P	Spleen						
		Q	Bone Marrow, Sternum						
		R	Bone Marrow, Iliac						
		S	Bone Marrow, Vertebral						
		T	Bone Marrow						

* Includes lymph vessels and lymph nodes.

AHA Coding Clinic for table Ø79

2021, 4Q, 47	Extraction of bone marrow from other sites
2018, 4Q, 84	Fine needle aspiration biopsy of lymphatic tissue
2017, 1Q, 34	Lymphovenous bypass following mastectomy
2014, 1Q, 26	Transbronchial needle aspiration lymph node biopsy
2013, 4Q, 111	Transbronchial needle aspiration lymph node biopsy

AHA Coding Clinic for table Ø7B

2022, 1Q, 14	Reduction mammoplasty for breast symmetry
2019, 1Q, 3-8	Whipple procedure
2018, 4Q, 84	Fine needle aspiration biopsy of lymphatic tissue
2018, 1Q, 22	Resection of lymph node chains
2016, 1Q, 30	Axillary lymph node resection with modified radical mastectomy
2014, 3Q, 10	Selective excision of paratracheal lymph nodes
2014, 1Q, 20	Fiducial marker placement
2014, 1Q, 26	Transbronchial endoscopic lymph node aspiration biopsy

AHA Coding Clinic for table Ø7D

2022, 1Q, 54	Extraction of bone marrow from other sites
2021, 4Q, 47	Extraction of bone marrow from other sites
2018, 4Q, 84	Fine needle aspiration biopsy of lymphatic tissue
2013, 4Q, 111	Root operation for bone marrow biopsy

AHA Coding Clinic for table Ø7H

| 2020, 4Q, 43-44 | Insertion of radioactive element |
| 2020, 4Q, 53 | Bone marrow body part |

AHA Coding Clinic for table Ø7Q

| 2017, 1Q, 34 | Lymphovenous bypass following mastectomy |

AHA Coding Clinic for table Ø7S

| 2019, 3Q, 29 | Thymus transplant for T-Cell production |

AHA Coding Clinic for table Ø7T

2023, 2Q, 22	Norwood procedure with excision of thymus
2018, 1Q, 22	Resection of lymph node chains
2016, 2Q, 12	Resection of malignant neoplasm of infratemporal fossa
2016, 1Q, 30	Axillary lymph node resection with modified radical mastectomy
2015, 4Q, 13	New Section X codes—New Technology procedures
2014, 3Q, 9	Radical resection of level I lymph nodes
2014, 3Q, 16	Repair of Tetralogy of Fallot

AHA Coding Clinic for table Ø7Y

| 2023, 2Q, 32 | Preparation of donor organ before transplantation |
| 2019, 3Q, 29 | Thymus transplant for T-Cell production |

Lymphatic System

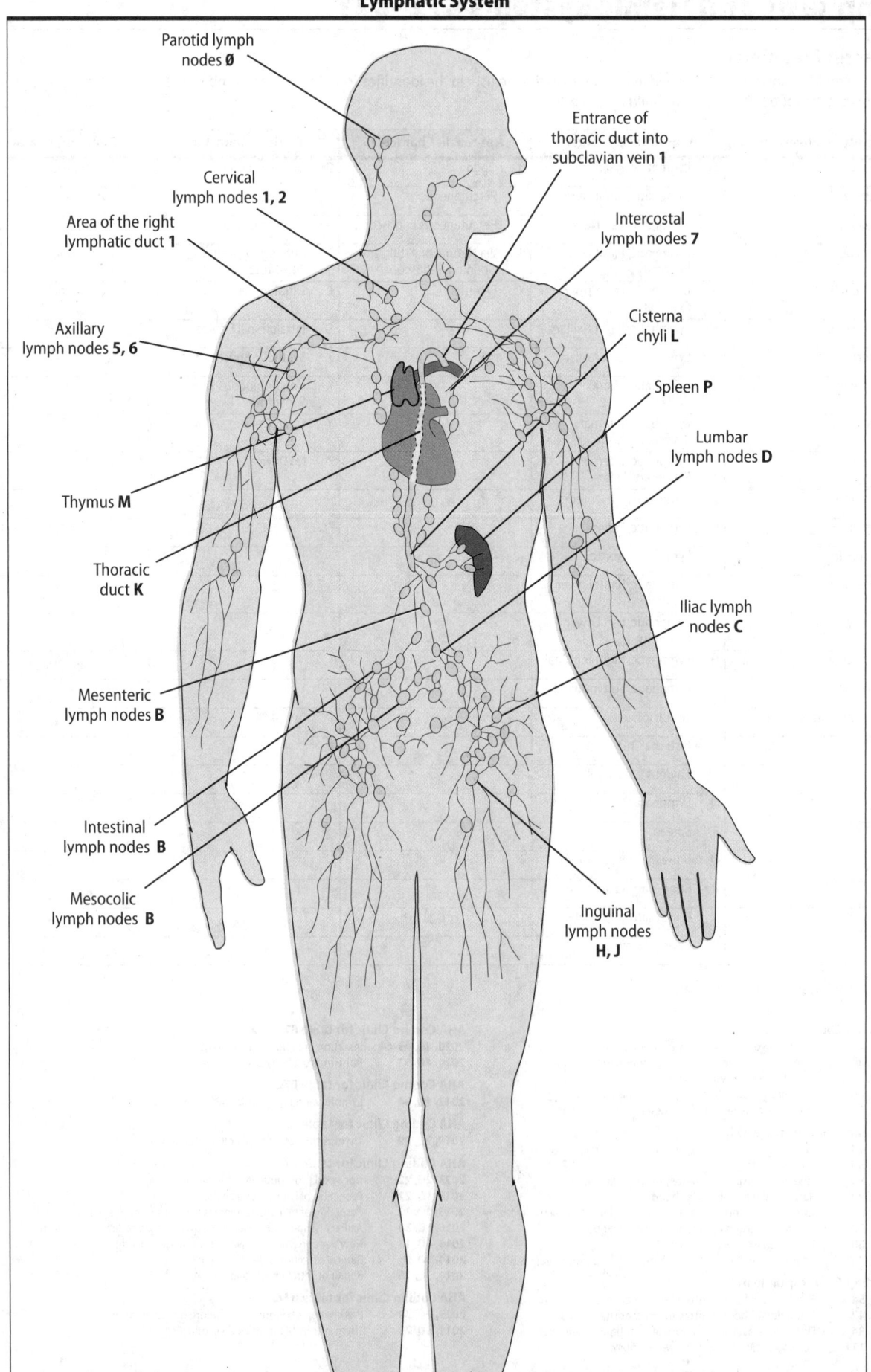

Parotid lymph nodes **Ø**

Cervical lymph nodes **1, 2**

Area of the right lymphatic duct **1**

Axillary lymph nodes **5, 6**

Thymus **M**

Thoracic duct **K**

Mesenteric lymph nodes **B**

Intestinal lymph nodes **B**

Mesocolic lymph nodes **B**

Entrance of thoracic duct into subclavian vein **1**

Intercostal lymph nodes **7**

Cisterna chyli **L**

Spleen **P**

Lumbar lymph nodes **D**

Iliac lymph nodes **C**

Inguinal lymph nodes **H, J**

Ø   **Medical and Surgical**
7   **Lymphatic and Hemic Systems**
2   **Change**   Definition: Taking out or off a device from a body part and putting back an identical or similar device in or on the same body part without cutting or puncturing the skin or a mucous membrane
                Explanation: All CHANGE procedures are coded using the approach EXTERNAL

Body Part Character 4		Approach Character 5	Device Character 6	Qualifier Character 7

K Thoracic Duct
    Left jugular trunk
    Left subclavian trunk
L Cisterna Chyli
    Intestinal lymphatic trunk
    Lumbar lymphatic trunk
	M Thymus
	    Thymus gland
	N Lymphatic
	P Spleen
	    Accessory spleen
	T Bone Marrow
		X External	**Ø** Drainage Device
			Y Other Device
				Z No Qualifier

Non-OR   All body part, approach, device, and qualifier values

Ø   **Medical and Surgical**
7   **Lymphatic and Hemic Systems**
5   **Destruction**   Definition: Physical eradication of all or a portion of a body part by the direct use of energy, force, or a destructive agent
                      Explanation: None of the body part is physically taken out

Body Part Character 4		Approach Character 5	Device Character 6	Qualifier Character 7

Ø Lymphatic, Head
    Buccinator lymph node
    Infraauricular lymph node
    Infraparotid lymph node
    Parotid lymph node
    Preauricular lymph node
    Submandibular lymph node
    Submaxillary lymph node
    Submental lymph node
    Subparotid lymph node
    Suprahyoid lymph node
1 Lymphatic, Right Neck
    Cervical lymph node
    Jugular lymph node
    Mastoid (postauricular) lymph node
    Occipital lymph node
    Postauricular (mastoid) lymph node
    Retropharyngeal lymph node
    Right jugular trunk
    Right lymphatic duct
    Right subclavian trunk
    Supraclavicular (Virchow's) lymph node
    Virchow's (supraclavicular) lymph node
2 Lymphatic, Left Neck
    Cervical lymph node
    Jugular lymph node
    Mastoid (postauricular) lymph node
    Occipital lymph node
    Postauricular (mastoid) lymph node
    Retropharyngeal lymph node
    Supraclavicular (Virchow's) lymph node
    Virchow's (supraclavicular) lymph node
3 Lymphatic, Right Upper Extremity
    Cubital lymph node
    Deltopectoral (infraclavicular) lymph
      node
    Epitrochlear lymph node
    Infraclavicular (deltopectoral) lymph
      node
    Supratrochlear lymph node
4 Lymphatic, Left Upper Extremity
    See 3 Lymphatic, Right Upper Extremity
5 Lymphatic, Right Axillary
    Anterior (pectoral) lymph node
    Apical (subclavicular) lymph node
    Brachial (lateral) lymph node
    Central axillary lymph node
    Lateral (brachial) lymph node
    Pectoral (anterior) lymph node
    Posterior (subscapular) lymph node
    Subclavicular (apical) lymph node
    Subscapular (posterior) lymph node
	6 Lymphatic, Left Axillary
	    See 5 Lymphatic, Right Axillary
	7 Lymphatic, Thorax
	    Intercostal lymph node
	    Mediastinal lymph node
	    Parasternal lymph node
	    Paratracheal lymph node
	    Tracheobronchial lymph node
	8 Lymphatic, Internal Mammary, Right
	9 Lymphatic, Internal Mammary, Left
	B Lymphatic, Mesenteric
	    Inferior mesenteric lymph node
	    Pararectal lymph node
	    Superior mesenteric lymph node
	C Lymphatic, Pelvis
	    Common iliac (subaortic) lymph node
	    Gluteal lymph node
	    Iliac lymph node
	    Inferior epigastric lymph node
	    Obturator lymph node
	    Sacral lymph node
	    Subaortic (common iliac) lymph node
	    Suprainguinal lymph node
	D Lymphatic, Aortic
	    Celiac lymph node
	    Gastric lymph node
	    Hepatic lymph node
	    Lumbar lymph node
	    Pancreaticosplenic lymph node
	    Paraaortic lymph node
	    Retroperitoneal lymph node
	F Lymphatic, Right Lower Extremity
	    Femoral lymph node
	    Popliteal lymph node
	G Lymphatic, Left Lower Extremity
	    See F Lymphatic, Right Lower Extremity
	H Lymphatic, Right Inguinal
	J Lymphatic, Left Inguinal
	K Thoracic Duct
	    Left jugular trunk
	    Left subclavian trunk
	L Cisterna Chyli
	    Intestinal lymphatic trunk
	    Lumbar lymphatic trunk
	M Thymus
	    Thymus gland
	P Spleen
	    Accessory spleen
		Ø Open
		3 Percutaneous
		4 Percutaneous
		    Endoscopic
			Z No Device	**Z** No Qualifier

NC Noncovered Procedure   **LC** Limited Coverage   **QA** Questionable OB Admit   **NT** New Tech Add-on   ⊞ Combination Member   ♂ Male   ♀ Female

ICD-10-PCS 2024   285

Lymphatic and Hemic Systems

Ø	Medical and Surgical
7	Lymphatic and Hemic Systems
9	Drainage

Definition: Taking or letting out fluids and/or gases from a body part

Explanation: The qualifier DIAGNOSTIC is used to identify drainage procedures that are biopsies

Body Part Character 4		Approach Character 5	Device Character 6	Qualifier Character 7

Ø Lymphatic, Head
Buccinator lymph node
Infraauricular lymph node
Infraparotid lymph node
Parotid lymph node
Preauricular lymph node
Submandibular lymph node
Submaxillary lymph node
Submental lymph node
Subparotid lymph node
Suprahyoid lymph node
1 Lymphatic, Right Neck
Cervical lymph node
Jugular lymph node
Mastoid (postauricular) lymph node
Occipital lymph node
Postauricular (mastoid) lymph node
Retropharyngeal lymph node
Right jugular trunk
Right lymphatic duct
Right subclavian trunk
Supraclavicular (Virchow's) lymph
   node
Virchow's (supraclavicular) lymph
   node
2 Lymphatic, Left Neck
Cervical lymph node
Jugular lymph node
Mastoid (postauricular) lymph node
Occipital lymph node
Postauricular (mastoid) lymph node
Retropharyngeal lymph node
Supraclavicular (Virchow's) lymph
   node
Virchow's (supraclavicular) lymph
   node
3 Lymphatic, Right Upper Extremity
Cubital lymph node
Deltopectoral (infraclavicular) lymph
   node
Epitrochlear lymph node
Infraclavicular (deltopectoral) lymph
   node
Supratrochlear lymph node
4 Lymphatic, Left Upper Extremity
See 3 Lymphatic, Right Upper Extremity
5 Lymphatic, Right Axillary
Anterior (pectoral) lymph node
Apical (subclavicular) lymph node
Brachial (lateral) lymph node
Central axillary lymph node
Lateral (brachial) lymph node
Pectoral (anterior) lymph node
Posterior (subscapular) lymph node
Subclavicular (apical) lymph node
Subscapular (posterior) lymph node
	6 Lymphatic, Left Axillary
	See 5 Lymphatic, Right Axillary
	7 Lymphatic, Thorax
	Intercostal lymph node
	Mediastinal lymph node
	Parasternal lymph node
	Paratracheal lymph node
	Tracheobronchial lymph node
	8 Lymphatic, Internal Mammary, Right
	9 Lymphatic, Internal Mammary, Left
	B Lymphatic, Mesenteric
	Inferior mesenteric lymph node
	Pararectal lymph node
	Superior mesenteric lymph node
	C Lymphatic, Pelvis
	Common iliac (subaortic) lymph node
	Gluteal lymph node
	Iliac lymph node
	Inferior epigastric lymph node
	Obturator lymph node
	Sacral lymph node
	Subaortic (common iliac) lymph node
	Suprainguinal lymph node
	D Lymphatic, Aortic
	Celiac lymph node
	Gastric lymph node
	Hepatic lymph node
	Lumbar lymph node
	Pancreaticosplenic lymph node
	Paraaortic lymph node
	Retroperitoneal lymph node
	F Lymphatic, Right Lower Extremity
	Femoral lymph node
	Popliteal lymph node
	G Lymphatic, Left Lower Extremity
	See F Lymphatic, Right Lower Extremity
	H Lymphatic, Right Inguinal
	J Lymphatic, Left Inguinal
	K Thoracic Duct
	Left jugular trunk
	Left subclavian trunk
	L Cisterna Chyli
	Intestinal lymphatic trunk
	Lumbar lymphatic trunk
		Ø Open
		3 Percutaneous
		4 Percutaneous Endoscopic
		8 Via Natural or Artificial Opening Endoscopic
			Ø Drainage Device	**Z No Qualifier**

Non-OR   Ø79[Ø,1,2,3,4,5,6,7,8,9,B,C,D,F,G,H,J,K,L][3,8]ØZ

Ø79 Continued on next page

Ø   **Medical and Surgical**
7   **Lymphatic and Hemic Systems**
9   **Drainage**   Definition: Taking or letting out fluids and/or gases from a body part
          Explanation: The qualifier DIAGNOSTIC is used to identify drainage procedures that are biopsies

Ø79 Continued

Body Part Character 4		Approach Character 5	Device Character 6	Qualifier Character 7

Ø **Lymphatic, Head**
Buccinator lymph node
Infraauricular lymph node
Infraparotid lymph node
Parotid lymph node
Preauricular lymph node
Submandibular lymph node
Submaxillary lymph node
Submental lymph node
Subparotid lymph node
Suprahyoid lymph node
1 **Lymphatic, Right Neck**
Cervical lymph node
Jugular lymph node
Mastoid (postauricular) lymph node
Occipital lymph node
Postauricular (mastoid) lymph node
Retropharyngeal lymph node
Right jugular trunk
Right lymphatic duct
Right subclavian trunk
Supraclavicular (Virchow's) lymph
  node
Virchow's (supraclavicular) lymph
  node
2 **Lymphatic, Left Neck**
Cervical lymph node
Jugular lymph node
Mastoid (postauricular) lymph node
Occipital lymph node
Postauricular (mastoid) lymph node
Retropharyngeal lymph node
Supraclavicular (Virchow's) lymph
  node
Virchow's (supraclavicular) lymph
  node
3 **Lymphatic, Right Upper Extremity**
Cubital lymph node
Deltopectoral (infraclavicular) lymph
  node
Epitrochlear lymph node
Infraclavicular (deltopectoral) lymph
  node
Supratrochlear lymph node
4 **Lymphatic, Left Upper Extremity**
See 3 Lymphatic, Right Upper Extremity
5 **Lymphatic, Right Axillary**
Anterior (pectoral) lymph node
Apical (subclavicular) lymph node
Brachial (lateral) lymph node
Central axillary lymph node
Lateral (brachial) lymph node
Pectoral (anterior) lymph node
Posterior (subscapular) lymph node
Subclavicular (apical) lymph node
Subscapular (posterior) lymph node
	6 **Lymphatic, Left Axillary**
	See 5 Lymphatic, Right Axillary
	7 **Lymphatic, Thorax**
	Intercostal lymph node
	Mediastinal lymph node
	Parasternal lymph node
	Paratracheal lymph node
	Tracheobronchial lymph node
	8 **Lymphatic, Internal Mammary, Right**
	9 **Lymphatic, Internal Mammary, Left**
	B **Lymphatic, Mesenteric**
	Inferior mesenteric lymph node
	Pararectal lymph node
	Superior mesenteric lymph node
	C **Lymphatic, Pelvis**
	Common iliac (subaortic) lymph node
	Gluteal lymph node
	Iliac lymph node
	Inferior epigastric lymph node
	Obturator lymph node
	Sacral lymph node
	Subaortic (common iliac) lymph node
	Suprainguinal lymph node
	D **Lymphatic, Aortic**
	Celiac lymph node
	Gastric lymph node
	Hepatic lymph node
	Lumbar lymph node
	Pancreaticosplenic lymph node
	Paraaortic lymph node
	Retroperitoneal lymph node
	F **Lymphatic, Right Lower Extremity**
	Femoral lymph node
	Popliteal lymph node
	G **Lymphatic, Left Lower Extremity**
	See F Lymphatic, Right Lower Extremity
	H **Lymphatic, Right Inguinal**
	J **Lymphatic, Left Inguinal**
	K **Thoracic Duct**
	Left jugular trunk
	Left subclavian trunk
	L **Cisterna Chyli**
	Intestinal lymphatic trunk
	Lumbar lymphatic trunk
		Ø Open
		3 Percutaneous
		4 Percutaneous
		  Endoscopic
		8 Via Natural or
		  Artificial Opening
		  Endoscopic
			Z No Device	X Diagnostic
				Z No Qualifier

M **Thymus** Thymus gland P **Spleen** Accessory spleen T **Bone Marrow**		Ø Open 3 Percutaneous 4 Percutaneous Endoscopic	Ø Drainage Device	Z No Qualifier
M **Thymus** Thymus gland P **Spleen** Accessory spleen T **Bone Marrow**		Ø Open 3 Percutaneous 4 Percutaneous Endoscopic	Z No Device	X Diagnostic Z No Qualifier

Non-OR	Ø79[Ø,1,2,3,4,5,6,7,8,9,B,C,D,F,G,H,J,K,L]8ZX
Non-OR	Ø79[Ø,1,2,3,4,5,6,7,8,9,B,C,D,F,G,H,J,K,L][3,8]ZZ
Non-OR	Ø79M3ØZ
Non-OR	Ø79P[3,4]ØZ
Non-OR	Ø79T[Ø,3,4]ØZ
Non-OR	Ø79M3ZZ
Non-OR	Ø79P[3,4]Z[X,Z]
Non-OR	Ø79T[Ø,3,4]Z[X,Z]

NC Noncovered Procedure   **LC** Limited Coverage   **QA** Questionable OB Admit   **NT** New Tech Add-on   ⊞ Combination Member   ♂ Male   ♀ Female

ICD-10-PCS 2024   **287**

Lymphatic and Hemic Systems

Ø   **Medical and Surgical**
7   **Lymphatic and Hemic Systems**
B   **Excision**   Definition: Cutting out or off, without replacement, a portion of a body part
                Explanation: The qualifier DIAGNOSTIC is used to identify excision procedures that are biopsies

Body Part Character 4	Approach Character 5	Device Character 6	Qualifier Character 7
Ø Lymphatic, Head Buccinator lymph node Infraauricular lymph node Infraparotid lymph node Parotid lymph node Preauricular lymph node Submandibular lymph node Submaxillary lymph node Submental lymph node Subparotid lymph node Suprahyoid lymph node **1 Lymphatic, Right Neck** Cervical lymph node Jugular lymph node Mastoid (postauricular) lymph node Occipital lymph node Postauricular (mastoid) lymph node Retropharyngeal lymph node Right jugular trunk Right lymphatic duct Right subclavian trunk Supraclavicular (Virchow's) lymph node Virchow's (supraclavicular) lymph node **2 Lymphatic, Left Neck** Cervical lymph node Jugular lymph node Mastoid (postauricular) lymph node Occipital lymph node Postauricular (mastoid) lymph node Retropharyngeal lymph node Supraclavicular (Virchow's) lymph node Virchow's (supraclavicular) lymph node **3 Lymphatic, Right Upper Extremity** Cubital lymph node Deltopectoral (infraclavicular) lymph node Epitrochlear lymph node Infraclavicular (deltopectoral) lymph node Supratrochlear lymph node **4 Lymphatic, Left Upper Extremity** *See 3 Lymphatic, Right Upper Extremity* **5 Lymphatic, Right Axillary** Anterior (pectoral) lymph node Apical (subclavicular) lymph node Brachial (lateral) lymph node Central axillary lymph node Lateral (brachial) lymph node Pectoral (anterior) lymph node Posterior (subscapular) lymph node Subclavicular (apical) lymph node Subscapular (posterior) lymph node **6 Lymphatic, Left Axillary** *See 5 Lymphatic, Right Axillary* **7 Lymphatic, Thorax** Intercostal lymph node Mediastinal lymph node Parasternal lymph node Paratracheal lymph node Tracheobronchial lymph node **8 Lymphatic, Internal Mammary, Right** **9 Lymphatic, Internal Mammary, Left** **B Lymphatic, Mesenteric** Inferior mesenteric lymph node Pararectal lymph node Superior mesenteric lymph node **C Lymphatic, Pelvis** Common iliac (subaortic) lymph node Gluteal lymph node Iliac lymph node Inferior epigastric lymph node Obturator lymph node Sacral lymph node Subaortic (common iliac) lymph node Suprainguinal lymph node **D Lymphatic, Aortic** Celiac lymph node Gastric lymph node Hepatic lymph node Lumbar lymph node Pancreaticosplenic lymph node Paraaortic lymph node Retroperitoneal lymph node **F Lymphatic, Right Lower Extremity** Femoral lymph node Popliteal lymph node **G Lymphatic, Left Lower Extremity** *See F Lymphatic, Right Lower Extremity* **H Lymphatic, Right Inguinal** ⊞ **J Lymphatic, Left Inguinal** ⊞ **K Thoracic Duct** Left jugular trunk Left subclavian trunk **L Cisterna Chyli** Intestinal lymphatic trunk Lumbar lymphatic trunk **M Thymus** Thymus gland **P Spleen** Accessory spleen	**Ø Open** **3 Percutaneous** **4 Percutaneous Endoscopic**	**Z No Device**	**X Diagnostic** **Z No Qualifier**

Non-OR   Ø7BP[3,4]ZX

See Appendix L for Procedure Combinations
⊞   Ø7B[H,J][Ø,4]ZZ

Non-OR Procedure   DRG Non-OR Procedure   Valid OR Procedure   HAC Associated Procedure   Combination Only   New/Revised April   New/Revised October

288   ICD-10-PCS 2024

Ø   Medical and Surgical
7   Lymphatic and Hemic Systems
C   Extirpation   Definition: Taking or cutting out solid matter from a body part

Explanation: The solid matter may be an abnormal byproduct of a biological function or a foreign body; it may be imbedded in a body part or in the lumen of a tubular body part. The solid matter may or may not have been previously broken into pieces.

Body Part Character 4	Approach Character 5	Device Character 6	Qualifier Character 7

Ø Lymphatic, Head
    Buccinator lymph node
    Infraauricular lymph node
    Infraparotid lymph node
    Parotid lymph node
    Preauricular lymph node
    Submandibular lymph node
    Submaxillary lymph node
    Submental lymph node
    Subparotid lymph node
    Suprahyoid lymph node
1 Lymphatic, Right Neck
    Cervical lymph node
    Jugular lymph node
    Mastoid (postauricular) lymph node
    Occipital lymph node
    Postauricular (mastoid) lymph node
    Retropharyngeal lymph node
    Right jugular trunk
    Right lymphatic duct
    Right subclavian trunk
    Supraclavicular (Virchow's) lymph
      node
    Virchow's (supraclavicular) lymph
      node
2 Lymphatic, Left Neck
    Cervical lymph node
    Jugular lymph node
    Mastoid (postauricular) lymph node
    Occipital lymph node
    Postauricular (mastoid) lymph node
    Retropharyngeal lymph node
    Supraclavicular (Virchow's) lymph
      node
    Virchow's (supraclavicular) lymph
      node
3 Lymphatic, Right Upper Extremity
    Cubital lymph node
    Deltopectoral (infraclavicular) lymph
      node
    Epitrochlear lymph node
    Infraclavicular (deltopectoral) lymph
      node
    Supratrochlear lymph node
4 Lymphatic, Left Upper Extremity
    See 3 Lymphatic, Right Upper Extremity
5 Lymphatic, Right Axillary
    Anterior (pectoral) lymph node
    Apical (subclavicular) lymph node
    Brachial (lateral) lymph node
    Central axillary lymph node
    Lateral (brachial) lymph node
    Pectoral (anterior) lymph node
    Posterior (subscapular) lymph node
    Subclavicular (apical) lymph node
    Subscapular (posterior) lymph node
	Ø Open
	3 Percutaneous
	**4 Percutaneous
	    Endoscopic**
		Z No Device	**Z No Qualifier**

6 Lymphatic, Left Axillary
    See 5 Lymphatic, Right Axillary
7 Lymphatic, Thorax
    Intercostal lymph node
    Mediastinal lymph node
    Parasternal lymph node
    Paratracheal lymph node
    Tracheobronchial lymph node
8 Lymphatic, Internal Mammary, Right
9 Lymphatic, Internal Mammary, Left
B Lymphatic, Mesenteric
    Inferior mesenteric lymph node
    Pararectal lymph node
    Superior mesenteric lymph node
C Lymphatic, Pelvis
    Common iliac (subaortic) lymph node
    Gluteal lymph node
    Iliac lymph node
    Inferior epigastric lymph node
    Obturator lymph node
    Sacral lymph node
    Subaortic (common iliac) lymph node
    Suprainguinal lymph node
D Lymphatic, Aortic
    Celiac lymph node
    Gastric lymph node
    Hepatic lymph node
    Lumbar lymph node
    Pancreaticosplenic lymph node
    Paraaortic lymph node
    Retroperitoneal lymph node
F Lymphatic, Right Lower Extremity
    Femoral lymph node
    Popliteal lymph node
G Lymphatic, Left Lower Extremity
    See F Lymphatic, Right Lower Extremity
H Lymphatic, Right Inguinal
J Lymphatic, Left Inguinal
K Thoracic Duct
    Left jugular trunk
    Left subclavian trunk
L Cisterna Chyli
    Intestinal lymphatic trunk
    Lumbar lymphatic trunk
M Thymus
    Thymus gland
P Spleen
    Accessory spleen

Non-OR   Ø7CP[3,4]ZZ

NC Noncovered Procedure   **LC** Limited Coverage   **QA** Questionable OB Admit   **NT** New Tech Add-on   ⊞ Combination Member   ♂ Male   ♀ Female

ICD-10-PCS 2024   **289**

Ø **Medical and Surgical**
7 **Lymphatic and Hemic Systems**
D **Extraction** Definition: Pulling or stripping out or off all or a portion of a body part by the use of force
Explanation: The qualifier DIAGNOSTIC is used to identify extraction procedures that are biopsies

Body Part Character 4		Approach Character 5	Device Character 6	Qualifier Character 7

Ø Lymphatic, Head
Buccinator lymph node
Infraauricular lymph node
Infraparotid lymph node
Parotid lymph node
Preauricular lymph node
Submandibular lymph node
Submaxillary lymph node
Submental lymph node
Subparotid lymph node
Suprahyoid lymph node
1 Lymphatic, Right Neck
Cervical lymph node
Jugular lymph node
Mastoid (postauricular) lymph
  node
Occipital lymph node
Postauricular (mastoid) lymph
  node
Retropharyngeal lymph node
Right jugular trunk
Right lymphatic duct
Right subclavian trunk
Supraclavicular (Virchow's)
  lymph node
Virchow's (supraclavicular)
  lymph node
2 Lymphatic, Left Neck
Cervical lymph node
Jugular lymph node
Mastoid (postauricular) lymph
  node
Occipital lymph node
Postauricular (mastoid) lymph
  node
Retropharyngeal lymph node
Supraclavicular (Virchow's)
  lymph node
Virchow's (supraclavicular)
  lymph node
3 Lymphatic, Right Upper Extremity
Cubital lymph node
Deltopectoral (infraclavicular)
  lymph node
Epitrochlear lymph node
Infraclavicular (deltopectoral)
  lymph node
Supratrochlear lymph node
4 Lymphatic, Left Upper Extremity
*See 3 Lymphatic, Right Upper
  Extremity*
5 Lymphatic, Right Axillary
Anterior (pectoral) lymph node
Apical (subclavicular) lymph
  node
Brachial (lateral) lymph node
Central axillary lymph node
Lateral (brachial) lymph node
Pectoral (anterior) lymph node
Posterior (subscapular) lymph
  node
Subclavicular (apical) lymph
  node
Subscapular (posterior) lymph
  node
	6 Lymphatic, Left Axillary
	See 5 Lymphatic, Right Axillary
	7 Lymphatic, Thorax
	Intercostal lymph node
	Mediastinal lymph node
	Parasternal lymph node
	Paratracheal lymph node
	Tracheobronchial lymph node
	8 Lymphatic, Internal Mammary, Right
	9 Lymphatic, Internal Mammary, Left
	B Lymphatic, Mesenteric
	Inferior mesenteric lymph
	  node
	Pararectal lymph node
	Superior mesenteric lymph
	  node
	C Lymphatic, Pelvis
	Common iliac (subaortic)
	  lymph node
	Gluteal lymph node
	Iliac lymph node
	Inferior epigastric lymph node
	Obturator lymph node
	Sacral lymph node
	Subaortic (common iliac)
	  lymph node
	Suprainguinal lymph node
	D Lymphatic, Aortic
	Celiac lymph node
	Gastric lymph node
	Hepatic lymph node
	Lumbar lymph node
	Pancreaticosplenic lymph
	  node
	Paraaortic lymph node
	Retroperitoneal lymph node
	F Lymphatic, Right Lower Extremity
	Femoral lymph node
	Popliteal lymph node
	G Lymphatic, Left Lower Extremity
	*See F Lymphatic, Right Lower
	  Extremity*
	H Lymphatic, Right Inguinal
	J Lymphatic, Left Inguinal
	K Thoracic Duct
	Left jugular trunk
	Left subclavian trunk
	L Cisterna Chyli
	Intestinal lymphatic trunk
	Lumbar lymphatic trunk
		3 Percutaneous
		4 Percutaneous Endoscopic
		8 Via Natural or Artificial Opening Endoscopic
			Z No Device	**X Diagnostic**

M Thymus Thymus gland **P Spleen** Accessory spleen		**3 Percutaneous** **4 Percutaneous Endoscopic**	**Z No Device**	**X Diagnostic**
Q Bone Marrow, Sternum **R Bone Marrow, Iliac** **S Bone Marrow, Vertebral** **T Bone Marrow**		**Ø Open** **3 Percutaneous**	**Z No Device**	**X Diagnostic** **Z No Qualifier**

Non-OR All body part, approach, device, and qualifier values

Non-OR Procedure   DRG Non-OR Procedure   Valid OR Procedure   HAC Associated Procedure   Combination Only   New/Revised April   New/Revised October

290 ICD-10-PCS 2024

Ø   Medical and Surgical
7   Lymphatic and Hemic Systems
H   Insertion   Definition: Putting in a nonbiological appliance that monitors, assists, performs, or prevents a physiological function but does not physically take the place of a body part
                 Explanation: None

Body Part Character 4	Approach Character 5	Device Character 6	Qualifier Character 7

K   Thoracic Duct
     Left jugular trunk
     Left subclavian trunk
L   Cisterna Chyli
     Intestinal lymphatic trunk
     Lumbar lymphatic trunk
M   Thymus
     Thymus gland
N   Lymphatic
P   Spleen
     Accessory spleen
T   Bone Marrow
	Ø Open
	3 Percutaneous
	4 Percutaneous Endoscopic
		1 Radioactive Element
		3 Infusion Device
		Y Other Device
			Z No Qualifier

Non-OR	07H[K,L,M,N,P][Ø,4]3Z
Non-OR	07H[K,L,M,N,P,T]3[1,3,Y]Z
Non-OR	07H[N,P]4YZ
Non-OR	07HT[Ø,4][1,3,Y]Z

Ø   Medical and Surgical
7   Lymphatic and Hemic Systems
J   Inspection   Definition: Visually and/or manually exploring a body part
                 Explanation: Visual exploration may be performed with or without optical instrumentation. Manual exploration may be performed directly or through intervening body layers.

Body Part Character 4	Approach Character 5	Device Character 6	Qualifier Character 7

K   Thoracic Duct
     Left jugular trunk
     Left subclavian trunk
L   Cisterna Chyli
     Intestinal lymphatic trunk
     Lumbar lymphatic trunk
M   Thymus
     Thymus gland
T   Bone Marrow
	Ø Open
	3 Percutaneous
	4 Percutaneous Endoscopic
		Z No Device	Z No Qualifier

N Lymphatic	Ø Open 3 Percutaneous 4 Percutaneous Endoscopic 8 Via Natural or Artificial Opening Endoscopic X External	Z No Device	Z No Qualifier
P Spleen Accessory spleen	Ø Open 3 Percutaneous 4 Percutaneous Endoscopic X External	Z No Device	Z No Qualifier

Non-OR	07J[K,L,M]3ZZ
Non-OR	07JT[Ø,3,4]ZZ
Non-OR	07JN[3,8,X]ZZ
Non-OR	07JP[3,4,X]ZZ

NC Noncovered Procedure   LC Limited Coverage   QA Questionable OB Admit   NT New Tech Add-on   ⊞ Combination Member   ♂ Male   ♀ Female

ICD-10-PCS 2024   291

Lymphatic and Hemic Systems

0 Medical and Surgical
7 Lymphatic and Hemic Systems
L Occlusion   Definition: Completely closing an orifice or the lumen of a tubular body part
             Explanation: The orifice can be a natural orifice or an artificially created orifice

Body Part Character 4	Approach Character 5	Device Character 6	Qualifier Character 7

0 Lymphatic, Head
Buccinator lymph node
Infraauricular lymph node
Infraparotid lymph node
Parotid lymph node
Preauricular lymph node
Submandibular lymph node
Submaxillary lymph node
Submental lymph node
Subparotid lymph node
Suprahyoid lymph node
1 Lymphatic, Right Neck
Cervical lymph node
Jugular lymph node
Mastoid (postauricular) lymph node
Occipital lymph node
Postauricular (mastoid) lymph node
Retropharyngeal lymph node
Right jugular trunk
Right lymphatic duct
Right subclavian trunk
Supraclavicular (Virchow's) lymph
   node
Virchow's (supraclavicular) lymph
   node
2 Lymphatic, Left Neck
Cervical lymph node
Jugular lymph node
Mastoid (postauricular) lymph node
Occipital lymph node
Postauricular (mastoid) lymph node
Retropharyngeal lymph node
Supraclavicular (Virchow's) lymph
   node
Virchow's (supraclavicular) lymph
   node
3 Lymphatic, Right Upper Extremity
Cubital lymph node
Deltopectoral (infraclavicular) lymph
   node
Epitrochlear lymph node
Infraclavicular (deltopectoral) lymph
   node
Supratrochlear lymph node
4 Lymphatic, Left Upper Extremity
See 3 Lymphatic, Right Upper Extremity
5 Lymphatic, Right Axillary
Anterior (pectoral) lymph node
Apical (subclavicular) lymph node
Brachial (lateral) lymph node
Central axillary lymph node
Lateral (brachial) lymph node
Pectoral (anterior) lymph node
Posterior (subscapular) lymph node
Subclavicular (apical) lymph node
Subscapular (posterior) lymph node
	0 Open
	3 Percutaneous
	4 Percutaneous
	   Endoscopic
		C Extraluminal Device
		D Intraluminal Device
		Z No Device
			Z No Qualifier

6 Lymphatic, Left Axillary
   See 5 Lymphatic, Right Axillary
7 Lymphatic, Thorax
   Intercostal lymph node
   Mediastinal lymph node
   Parasternal lymph node
   Paratracheal lymph node
   Tracheobronchial lymph node
8 Lymphatic, Internal Mammary, Right
9 Lymphatic, Internal Mammary, Left
B Lymphatic, Mesenteric
   Inferior mesenteric lymph node
   Pararectal lymph node
   Superior mesenteric lymph node
C Lymphatic, Pelvis
   Common iliac (subaortic) lymph node
   Gluteal lymph node
   Iliac lymph node
   Inferior epigastric lymph node
   Obturator lymph node
   Sacral lymph node
   Subaortic (common iliac) lymph node
   Suprainguinal lymph node
D Lymphatic, Aortic
   Celiac lymph node
   Gastric lymph node
   Hepatic lymph node
   Lumbar lymph node
   Pancreaticosplenic lymph node
   Paraaortic lymph node
   Retroperitoneal lymph node
F Lymphatic, Right Lower Extremity
   Femoral lymph node
   Popliteal lymph node
G Lymphatic, Left Lower Extremity
   See F Lymphatic, Right Lower Extremity
H Lymphatic, Right Inguinal
J Lymphatic, Left Inguinal
K Thoracic Duct
   Left jugular trunk
   Left subclavian trunk
L Cisterna Chyli
   Intestinal lymphatic trunk
   Lumbar lymphatic trunk

Non-OR Procedure   DRG Non-OR Procedure   Valid OR Procedure   HAC Associated Procedure   Combination Only   New/Revised April   New/Revised October

292   ICD-10-PCS 2024

07L–07L

Ø　**Medical and Surgical**
7　**Lymphatic and Hemic Systems**
N　**Release**　　　　Definition: Freeing a body part from an abnormal physical constraint by cutting or by the use of force
　　　　　　　　　　　Explanation: Some of the restraining tissue may be taken out but none of the body part is taken out

Body Part Character 4		Approach Character 5	Device Character 6	Qualifier Character 7
Ø Lymphatic, Head 　Buccinator lymph node 　Infraauricular lymph node 　Infraparotid lymph node 　Parotid lymph node 　Preauricular lymph node 　Submandibular lymph node 　Submaxillary lymph node 　Submental lymph node 　Subparotid lymph node 　Suprahyoid lymph node **1 Lymphatic, Right Neck** 　Cervical lymph node 　Jugular lymph node 　Mastoid (postauricular) lymph node 　Occipital lymph node 　Postauricular (mastoid) lymph node 　Retropharyngeal lymph node 　Right jugular trunk 　Right lymphatic duct 　Right subclavian trunk 　Supraclavicular (Virchow's) lymph 　　node 　Virchow's (supraclavicular) lymph 　　node **2 Lymphatic, Left Neck** 　Cervical lymph node 　Jugular lymph node 　Mastoid (postauricular) lymph node 　Occipital lymph node 　Postauricular (mastoid) lymph node 　Retropharyngeal lymph node 　Supraclavicular (Virchow's) lymph 　　node 　Virchow's (supraclavicular) lymph 　　node **3 Lymphatic, Right Upper Extremity** 　Cubital lymph node 　Deltopectoral (infraclavicular) lymph 　　node 　Epitrochlear lymph node 　Infraclavicular (deltopectoral) lymph 　　node 　Supratrochlear lymph node **4 Lymphatic, Left Upper Extremity** 　*See 3 Lymphatic, Right Upper Extremity* **5 Lymphatic, Right Axillary** 　Anterior (pectoral) lymph node 　Apical (subclavicular) lymph node 　Brachial (lateral) lymph node 　Central axillary lymph node 　Lateral (brachial) lymph node 　Pectoral (anterior) lymph node 　Posterior (subscapular) lymph node 　Subclavicular (apical) lymph node 　Subscapular (posterior) lymph node	**6 Lymphatic, Left Axillary** 　*See 5 Lymphatic, Right Axillary* **7 Lymphatic, Thorax** 　Intercostal lymph node 　Mediastinal lymph node 　Parasternal lymph node 　Paratracheal lymph node 　Tracheobronchial lymph node **8 Lymphatic, Internal Mammary, Right** **9 Lymphatic, Internal Mammary, Left** **B Lymphatic, Mesenteric** 　Inferior mesenteric lymph node 　Pararectal lymph node 　Superior mesenteric lymph node **C Lymphatic, Pelvis** 　Common iliac (subaortic) lymph node 　Gluteal lymph node 　Iliac lymph node 　Inferior epigastric lymph node 　Obturator lymph node 　Sacral lymph node 　Subaortic (common iliac) lymph node 　Suprainguinal lymph node **D Lymphatic, Aortic** 　Celiac lymph node 　Gastric lymph node 　Hepatic lymph node 　Lumbar lymph node 　Pancreaticosplenic lymph node 　Paraaortic lymph node 　Retroperitoneal lymph node **F Lymphatic, Right Lower Extremity** 　Femoral lymph node 　Popliteal lymph node **G Lymphatic, Left Lower Extremity** 　*See F Lymphatic, Right Lower Extremity* **H Lymphatic, Right Inguinal** **J Lymphatic, Left Inguinal** **K Thoracic Duct** 　Left jugular trunk 　Left subclavian trunk **L Cisterna Chyli** 　Intestinal lymphatic trunk 　Lumbar lymphatic trunk **M Thymus** 　Thymus gland **P Spleen** 　Accessory spleen	**Ø Open** **3 Percutaneous** **4 Percutaneous** 　**Endoscopic**	**Z No Device**	**Z No Qualifier**

Ø   Medical and Surgical
7   Lymphatic and Hemic Systems
P   Removal   Definition: Taking out or off a device from a body part

Explanation: If a device is taken out and a similar device put in without cutting or puncturing the skin or mucous membrane, the procedure is coded to the root operation CHANGE. Otherwise, the procedure for taking out a device is coded to the root operation REMOVAL.

Body Part Character 4	Approach Character 5	Device Character 6	Qualifier Character 7

K Thoracic Duct
    Left jugular trunk
    Left subclavian trunk
 L Cisterna Chyli
    Intestinal lymphatic trunk
    Lumbar lymphatic trunk
 N Lymphatic
	Ø Open
	 3 Percutaneous
	 4 Percutaneous Endoscopic
		Ø Drainage Device
		 3 Infusion Device
		 7 Autologous Tissue Substitute
		 C Extraluminal Device
		 D Intraluminal Device
		 J Synthetic Substitute
		 K Nonautologous Tissue Substitute
		 Y Other Device
			Z No Qualifier

K Thoracic Duct
    Left jugular trunk
    Left subclavian trunk
 L Cisterna Chyli
    Intestinal lymphatic trunk
    Lumbar lymphatic trunk
 N Lymphatic
	X External	Ø Drainage Device
		 3 Infusion Device
		 D Intraluminal Device
			Z No Qualifier

M Thymus
    Thymus gland
 P Spleen
    Accessory spleen
	Ø Open
	 3 Percutaneous
	 4 Percutaneous Endoscopic
		Ø Drainage Device
		 3 Infusion Device
		 Y Other Device
			Z No Qualifier

M Thymus
    Thymus gland
 P Spleen
    Accessory spleen
	X External	Ø Drainage Device
		 3 Infusion Device
			Z No Qualifier

T Bone Marrow	Ø Open 3 Percutaneous 4 Percutaneous Endoscopic X External	Ø Drainage Device	Z No Qualifier

Non-OR	Ø7P[K,L,N][3,4]YZ
Non-OR	Ø7P[K,L,N]X[Ø,3,D]Z
Non-OR	Ø7P[M,P][3,4]YZ
Non-OR	Ø7P[M,P]X[Ø,3]Z
Non-OR	Ø7PT[Ø,3,4,X]ØZ

Lymphatic and Hemic Systems

Ø   **Medical and Surgical**
7   **Lymphatic and Hemic Systems**
Q   **Repair**   Definition: Restoring, to the extent possible, a body part to its normal anatomic structure and function
                        Explanation: Used only when the method to accomplish the repair is not one of the other root operations

Body Part Character 4	Approach Character 5	Device Character 6	Qualifier Character 7
Ø Lymphatic, Head Buccinator lymph node Infraauricular lymph node Infraparotid lymph node Parotid lymph node Preauricular lymph node Submandibular lymph node Submaxillary lymph node Submental lymph node Subparotid lymph node Suprahyoid lymph node **1 Lymphatic, Right Neck** Cervical lymph node Jugular lymph node Mastoid (postauricular) lymph node Occipital lymph node Postauricular (mastoid) lymph node Retropharyngeal lymph node Right jugular trunk Right lymphatic duct Right subclavian trunk Supraclavicular (Virchow's) lymph node Virchow's (supraclavicular) lymph node **2 Lymphatic, Left Neck** Cervical lymph node Jugular lymph node Mastoid (postauricular) lymph node Occipital lymph node Postauricular (mastoid) lymph node Retropharyngeal lymph node Supraclavicular (Virchow's) lymph node Virchow's (supraclavicular) lymph node **3 Lymphatic, Right Upper Extremity** Cubital lymph node Deltopectoral (infraclavicular) lymph node Epitrochlear lymph node Infraclavicular (deltopectoral) lymph node Supratrochlear lymph node **4 Lymphatic, Left Upper Extremity** *See 3 Lymphatic, Right Upper Extremity* **5 Lymphatic, Right Axillary** Anterior (pectoral) lymph node Apical (subclavicular) lymph node Brachial (lateral) lymph node Central axillary lymph node Lateral (brachial) lymph node Pectoral (anterior) lymph node Posterior (subscapular) lymph node Subclavicular (apical) lymph node Subscapular (posterior) lymph node **6 Lymphatic, Left Axillary** *See 5 Lymphatic, Right Axillary* **7 Lymphatic, Thorax** Intercostal lymph node Mediastinal lymph node Parasternal lymph node Paratracheal lymph node Tracheobronchial lymph node **8 Lymphatic, Internal Mammary, Right** **9 Lymphatic, Internal Mammary, Left** **B Lymphatic, Mesenteric** Inferior mesenteric lymph node Pararectal lymph node Superior mesenteric lymph node **C Lymphatic, Pelvis** Common iliac (subaortic) lymph node Gluteal lymph node Iliac lymph node Inferior epigastric lymph node Obturator lymph node Sacral lymph node Subaortic (common iliac) lymph node Suprainguinal lymph node **D Lymphatic, Aortic** Celiac lymph node Gastric lymph node Hepatic lymph node Lumbar lymph node Pancreaticosplenic lymph node Paraaortic lymph node Retroperitoneal lymph node **F Lymphatic, Right Lower Extremity** Femoral lymph node Popliteal lymph node **G Lymphatic, Left Lower Extremity** *See F Lymphatic, Right Lower Extremity* **H Lymphatic, Right Inguinal** **J Lymphatic, Left Inguinal** **K Thoracic Duct** Left jugular trunk Left subclavian trunk **L Cisterna Chyli** Intestinal lymphatic trunk Lumbar lymphatic trunk	**Ø** Open **3** Percutaneous **4** Percutaneous Endoscopic **8** Via Natural or Artificial Opening Endoscopic	**Z** No Device	**Z** No Qualifier
M Thymus Thymus gland **P Spleen** Accessory spleen	**Ø** Open **3** Percutaneous **4** Percutaneous Endoscopic	**Z** No Device	**Z** No Qualifier

Lymphatic and Hemic Systems (side margin)

Ø   **Medical and Surgical**
7   **Lymphatic and Hemic Systems**
S   **Reposition**   Definition: Moving to its normal location, or other suitable location, all or a portion of a body part

Explanation: The body part is moved to a new location from an abnormal location, or from a normal location where it is not functioning correctly. The body part may or may not be cut out or off to be moved to the new location.

Body Part Character 4	Approach Character 5	Device Character 6	Qualifier Character 7

M   Thymus
     Thymus gland
P   Spleen
     Accessory spleen
	Ø Open	Z No Device	Z No Qualifier

Ø   **Medical and Surgical**
7   **Lymphatic and Hemic Systems**
T   **Resection**   Definition: Cutting out or off, without replacement, all of a body part

Explanation: None

Body Part Character 4	Approach Character 5	Device Character 6	Qualifier Character 7

Ø   **Lymphatic, Head**
    Buccinator lymph node
    Infraauricular lymph node
    Infraparotid lymph node
    Parotid lymph node
    Preauricular lymph node
    Submandibular lymph node
    Submaxillary lymph node
    Submental lymph node
    Subparotid lymph node
    Suprahyoid lymph node
1   **Lymphatic, Right Neck**
    Cervical lymph node
    Jugular lymph node
    Mastoid (postauricular) lymph node
    Occipital lymph node
    Postauricular (mastoid) lymph node
    Retropharyngeal lymph node
    Right jugular trunk
    Right lymphatic duct
    Right subclavian trunk
    Supraclavicular (Virchow's) lymph
      node
    Virchow's (supraclavicular) lymph
      node
2   **Lymphatic, Left Neck**
    Cervical lymph node
    Jugular lymph node
    Mastoid (postauricular) lymph node
    Occipital lymph node
    Postauricular (mastoid) lymph node
    Retropharyngeal lymph node
    Supraclavicular (Virchow's) lymph
      node
    Virchow's (supraclavicular) lymph
      node
3   **Lymphatic, Right Upper Extremity**
    Cubital lymph node
    Deltopectoral (infraclavicular) lymph
      node
    Epitrochlear lymph node
    Infraclavicular (deltopectoral) lymph
      node
    Supratrochlear lymph node
4   **Lymphatic, Left Upper Extremity**
    See 3 Lymphatic, Right Upper Extremity
5   **Lymphatic, Right Axillary** ⊞
    Anterior (pectoral) lymph node
    Apical (subclavicular) lymph node
    Brachial (lateral) lymph node
    Central axillary lymph node
    Lateral (brachial) lymph node
    Pectoral (anterior) lymph node
    Posterior (subscapular) lymph node
    Subclavicular (apical) lymph node
    Subscapular (posterior) lymph node
 	
6   **Lymphatic, Left Axillary** ⊞
    See 5 Lymphatic, Right Axillary
7   **Lymphatic, Thorax** ⊞
    Intercostal lymph node
    Mediastinal lymph node
    Parasternal lymph node
    Paratracheal lymph node
    Tracheobronchial lymph node
8   **Lymphatic, Internal** ⊞
    Mammary, Right
9   **Lymphatic, Internal** ⊞
    Mammary, Left
B   **Lymphatic, Mesenteric**
    Inferior mesenteric lymph node
    Pararectal lymph node
    Superior mesenteric lymph node
C   **Lymphatic, Pelvis**
    Common iliac (subaortic) lymph node
    Gluteal lymph node
    Iliac lymph node
    Inferior epigastric lymph node
    Obturator lymph node
    Sacral lymph node
    Subaortic (common iliac) lymph node
    Suprainguinal lymph node
D   **Lymphatic, Aortic**
    Celiac lymph node
    Gastric lymph node
    Hepatic lymph node
    Lumbar lymph node
    Pancreaticosplenic lymph node
    Paraaortic lymph node
    Retroperitoneal lymph node
F   **Lymphatic, Right Lower Extremity**
    Femoral lymph node
    Popliteal lymph node
G   **Lymphatic, Left Lower Extremity**
    See F Lymphatic, Right Lower Extremity
H   **Lymphatic, Right Inguinal**
J   **Lymphatic, Left Inguinal**
K   **Thoracic Duct**
    Left jugular trunk
    Left subclavian trunk
L   **Cisterna Chyli**
    Intestinal lymphatic trunk
    Lumbar lymphatic trunk
M   **Thymus**
    Thymus gland
P   **Spleen**
    Accessory spleen
	Ø Open
	4 Percutaneous
	    Endoscopic
		Z No Device	Z No Qualifier

See Appendix L for Procedure Combinations
⊞   07T[5,6,7,8,9]0ZZ

Ø   **Medical and Surgical**
7   **Lymphatic and Hemic Systems**
U   **Supplement**   Definition: Putting in or on biological or synthetic material that physically reinforces and/or augments the function of a portion of a body part
                      Explanation: The biological material is non-living, or is living and from the same individual. The body part may have been previously replaced, and the SUPPLEMENT procedure is performed to physically reinforce and/or augment the function of the replaced body part.

Body Part Character 4		Approach Character 5	Device Character 6	Qualifier Character 7

Ø Lymphatic, Head
  Buccinator lymph node
  Infraauricular lymph node
  Infraparotid lymph node
  Parotid lymph node
  Preauricular lymph node
  Submandibular lymph node
  Submaxillary lymph node
  Submental lymph node
  Subparotid lymph node
  Suprahyoid lymph node
1 Lymphatic, Right Neck
  Cervical lymph node
  Jugular lymph node
  Mastoid (postauricular) lymph node
  Occipital lymph node
  Postauricular (mastoid) lymph node
  Retropharyngeal lymph node
  Right jugular trunk
  Right lymphatic duct
  Right subclavian trunk
  Supraclavicular (Virchow's) lymph
    node
  Virchow's (supraclavicular) lymph
    node
2 Lymphatic, Left Neck
  Cervical lymph node
  Jugular lymph node
  Mastoid (postauricular) lymph node
  Occipital lymph node
  Postauricular (mastoid) lymph node
  Retropharyngeal lymph node
  Supraclavicular (Virchow's) lymph
    node
  Virchow's (supraclavicular) lymph
    node
3 Lymphatic, Right Upper Extremity
  Cubital lymph node
  Deltopectoral (infraclavicular) lymph
    node
  Epitrochlear lymph node
  Infraclavicular (deltopectoral) lymph
    node
  Supratrochlear lymph node
4 Lymphatic, Left Upper Extremity
  See 3 Lymphatic, Right Upper Extremity
5 Lymphatic, Right Axillary
  Anterior (pectoral) lymph node
  Apical (subclavicular) lymph node
  Brachial (lateral) lymph node
  Central axillary lymph node
  Lateral (brachial) lymph node
  Pectoral (anterior) lymph node
  Posterior (subscapular) lymph node
  Subclavicular (apical) lymph node
  Subscapular (posterior) lymph node
	6 Lymphatic, Left Axillary
	  See 5 Lymphatic, Right Axillary
	7 Lymphatic, Thorax
	  Intercostal lymph node
	  Mediastinal lymph node
	  Parasternal lymph node
	  Paratracheal lymph node
	  Tracheobronchial lymph node
	8 Lymphatic, Internal Mammary, Right
	9 Lymphatic, Internal Mammary, Left
	B Lymphatic, Mesenteric
	  Inferior mesenteric lymph node
	  Pararectal lymph node
	  Superior mesenteric lymph node
	C Lymphatic, Pelvis
	  Common iliac (subaortic) lymph node
	  Gluteal lymph node
	  Iliac lymph node
	  Inferior epigastric lymph node
	  Obturator lymph node
	  Sacral lymph node
	  Subaortic (common iliac) lymph node
	  Suprainguinal lymph node
	D Lymphatic, Aortic
	  Celiac lymph node
	  Gastric lymph node
	  Hepatic lymph node
	  Lumbar lymph node
	  Pancreaticosplenic lymph node
	  Paraaortic lymph node
	  Retroperitoneal lymph node
	F Lymphatic, Right Lower Extremity
	  Femoral lymph node
	  Popliteal lymph node
	G Lymphatic, Left Lower Extremity
	  See F Lymphatic, Right Lower Extremity
	H Lymphatic, Right Inguinal
	J Lymphatic, Left Inguinal
	K Thoracic Duct
	  Left jugular trunk
	  Left subclavian trunk
	L Cisterna Chyli
	  Intestinal lymphatic trunk
	  Lumbar lymphatic trunk
		Ø Open
		4 Percutaneous
		    Endoscopic
			7 Autologous Tissue
			    Substitute
			J Synthetic Substitute
			K Nonautologous
			    Tissue Substitute
				Z No Qualifier

Ø Medical and Surgical
7 Lymphatic and Hemic Systems
V Restriction   Definition: Partially closing an orifice or the lumen of a tubular body part
      Explanation: The orifice can be a natural orifice or an artificially created orifice

Body Part Character 4	Approach Character 5	Device Character 6	Qualifier Character 7
Ø Lymphatic, Head Buccinator lymph node Infraauricular lymph node Infraparotid lymph node Parotid lymph node Preauricular lymph node Submandibular lymph node Submaxillary lymph node Submental lymph node Subparotid lymph node Suprahyoid lymph node **1 Lymphatic, Right Neck** Cervical lymph node Jugular lymph node Mastoid (postauricular) lymph node Occipital lymph node Postauricular (mastoid) lymph node Retropharyngeal lymph node Right jugular trunk Right lymphatic duct Right subclavian trunk Supraclavicular (Virchow's) lymph node Virchow's (supraclavicular) lymph node **2 Lymphatic, Left Neck** Cervical lymph node Jugular lymph node Mastoid (postauricular) lymph node Occipital lymph node Postauricular (mastoid) lymph node Retropharyngeal lymph node Supraclavicular (Virchow's) lymph node Virchow's (supraclavicular) lymph node **3 Lymphatic, Right Upper Extremity** Cubital lymph node Deltopectoral (infraclavicular) lymph node Epitrochlear lymph node Infraclavicular (deltopectoral) lymph node Supratrochlear lymph node **4 Lymphatic, Left Upper Extremity** See 3 Lymphatic, Right Upper Extremity **5 Lymphatic, Right Axillary** Anterior (pectoral) lymph node Apical (subclavicular) lymph node Brachial (lateral) lymph node Central axillary lymph node Lateral (brachial) lymph node Pectoral (anterior) lymph node Posterior (subscapular) lymph node Subclavicular (apical) lymph node Subscapular (posterior) lymph node **6 Lymphatic, Left Axillary** See 5 Lymphatic, Right Axillary **7 Lymphatic, Thorax** Intercostal lymph node Mediastinal lymph node Parasternal lymph node Paratracheal lymph node Tracheobronchial lymph node **8 Lymphatic, Internal Mammary, Right** **9 Lymphatic, Internal Mammary, Left** **B Lymphatic, Mesenteric** Inferior mesenteric lymph node Pararectal lymph node Superior mesenteric lymph node **C Lymphatic, Pelvis** Common iliac (subaortic) lymph node Gluteal lymph node Iliac lymph node Inferior epigastric lymph node Obturator lymph node Sacral lymph node Subaortic (common iliac) lymph node Suprainguinal lymph node **D Lymphatic, Aortic** Celiac lymph node Gastric lymph node Hepatic lymph node Lumbar lymph node Pancreaticosplenic lymph node Paraaortic lymph node Retroperitoneal lymph node **F Lymphatic, Right Lower Extremity** Femoral lymph node Popliteal lymph node **G Lymphatic, Left Lower Extremity** See F Lymphatic, Right Lower Extremity **H Lymphatic, Right Inguinal** **J Lymphatic, Left Inguinal** **K Thoracic Duct** Left jugular trunk Left subclavian trunk **L Cisterna Chyli** Intestinal lymphatic trunk Lumbar lymphatic trunk	**Ø** Open **3** Percutaneous **4** Percutaneous Endoscopic	**C** Extraluminal Device **D** Intraluminal Device **Z** No Device	**Z** No Qualifier

Ø   Medical and Surgical
7   Lymphatic and Hemic Systems
W   Revision   Definition: Correcting, to the extent possible, a portion of a malfunctioning device or the position of a displaced device

Explanation: Revision can include correcting a malfunctioning or displaced device by taking out or putting in components of the device such as a screw or pin

Body Part Character 4	Approach Character 5	Device Character 6	Qualifier Character 7

K Thoracic Duct
  Left jugular trunk
  Left subclavian trunk
L Cisterna Chyli
  Intestinal lymphatic trunk
  Lumbar lymphatic trunk
N Lymphatic
	Ø Open
	3 Percutaneous
	4 Percutaneous Endoscopic
		Ø Drainage Device
		3 Infusion Device
		7 Autologous Tissue
		  Substitute
		C Extraluminal Device
		D Intraluminal Device
		J Synthetic Substitute
		K Nonautologous Tissue
		  Substitute
		Y Other Device
			Z No Qualifier

K Thoracic Duct
  Left jugular trunk
  Left subclavian trunk
L Cisterna Chyli
  Intestinal lymphatic trunk
  Lumbar lymphatic trunk
N Lymphatic
	X External	Ø Drainage Device
		3 Infusion Device
		7 Autologous Tissue
		  Substitute
		C Extraluminal Device
		D Intraluminal Device
		J Synthetic Substitute
		K Nonautologous Tissue
		  Substitute
			Z No Qualifier

M Thymus
  Thymus gland
P Spleen
  Accessory spleen
	Ø Open
	3 Percutaneous
	4 Percutaneous Endoscopic
		Ø Drainage Device
		3 Infusion Device
		Y Other Device
			Z No Qualifier

M Thymus
  Thymus gland
P Spleen
  Accessory spleen
	X External	Ø Drainage Device
		3 Infusion Device
			Z No Qualifier

T Bone Marrow	Ø Open 3 Percutaneous 4 Percutaneous Endoscopic X External	Ø Drainage Device	Z No Qualifier

Non-OR   07W[K,L,N][3,4]YZ
Non-OR   07W[K,L,N]X[Ø,3,7,C,D,J,K]Z
Non-OR   07W[M,P][3,4]YZ
Non-OR   07W[M,P]X[Ø,3]Z
Non-OR   07WT[Ø,3,4,X]ØZ

Ø   Medical and Surgical
7   Lymphatic and Hemic Systems
Y   Transplantation   Definition: Putting in or on all or a portion of a living body part taken from another individual or animal to physically take the place and/or function of all or a portion of a similar body part

Explanation: The native body part may or may not be taken out, and the transplanted body part may take over all or a portion of its function

Body Part Character 4	Approach Character 5	Device Character 6	Qualifier Character 7

M Thymus
  Thymus gland
P Spleen
  Accessory spleen
	Ø Open	Z No Device	Ø Allogeneic
			1 Syngeneic
			2 Zooplastic

Eye Ø8Ø–Ø8X

Character Meanings

This Character Meaning table is provided as a guide to assist the user in the identification of character members that may be found in this section of code tables. It **SHOULD NOT** be used to build a PCS code.

Operation–Character 3	Body Part–Character 4	Approach–Character 5	Device–Character 6	Qualifier–Character 7
Ø Alteration	Ø Eye, Right	Ø Open	Ø Drainage Device OR Synthetic Substitute, Intraocular Telescope	3 Nasal Cavity
1 Bypass	1 Eye, Left	3 Percutaneous	1 Radioactive Element	4 Sclera
2 Change	2 Anterior Chamber, Right	7 Via Natural or Artificial Opening	3 Infusion Device	X Diagnostic
5 Destruction	3 Anterior Chamber, Left	8 Via Natural or Artificial Opening Endoscopic	5 Epiretinal Visual Prosthesis	Z No Qualifier
7 Dilation	4 Vitreous, Right	X External	7 Autologous Tissue Substitute	
9 Drainage	5 Vitreous, Left		C Extraluminal Device	
B Excision	6 Sclera, Right		D Intraluminal Device	
C Extirpation	7 Sclera, Left		J Synthetic Substitute	
D Extraction	8 Cornea, Right		K Nonautologous Tissue Substitute	
F Fragmentation	9 Cornea, Left		Y Other Device	
H Insertion	A Choroid, Right		Z No Device	
J Inspection	B Choroid, Left			
L Occlusion	C Iris, Right			
M Reattachment	D Iris, Left			
N Release	E Retina, Right			
P Removal	F Retina, Left			
Q Repair	G Retinal Vessel, Right			
R Replacement	H Retinal Vessel, Left			
S Reposition	J Lens, Right			
T Resection	K Lens, Left			
U Supplement	L Extraocular Muscle, Right			
V Restriction	M Extraocular Muscle, Left			
W Revision	N Upper Eyelid, Right			
X Transfer	P Upper Eyelid, Left			
	Q Lower Eyelid, Right			
	R Lower Eyelid, Left			
	S Conjunctiva, Right			
	T Conjunctiva, Left			
	V Lacrimal Gland, Right			
	W Lacrimal Gland, Left			
	X Lacrimal Duct, Right			
	Y Lacrimal Duct, Left			

AHA Coding Clinic for table Ø81
2019, 1Q, 27   Glaucoma tube shunt

AHA Coding Clinic for table Ø89
2016, 2Q, 21   Laser trabeculoplasty

AHA Coding Clinic for table Ø8B
2014, 4Q, 35   Vitrectomy with air/fluid exchange
2014, 4Q, 36   Pars plans vitrectomy without mention of instillation of oil, air or fluid

AHA Coding Clinic for table Ø8J
2015, 1Q, 35   Attempted removal of foreign body from cornea

AHA Coding Clinic for table Ø8N
2015, 2Q, 24   Penetrating keratoplasty and anterior segment reconstruction

AHA Coding Clinic for table Ø8Q
2018, 3Q, 13   Repair of ruptured globe

AHA Coding Clinic for table Ø8R
2015, 2Q, 24   Penetrating keratoplasty and anterior segment reconstruction
2015, 2Q, 25   Penetrating keratoplasty and placement of viscoelastic eye with paracentesis

AHA Coding Clinic for table Ø8T
2015, 2Q, 12   Orbital exenteration

AHA Coding Clinic for table Ø8U
2014, 3Q, 31   Corneal amniotic membrane transplantation

Eye

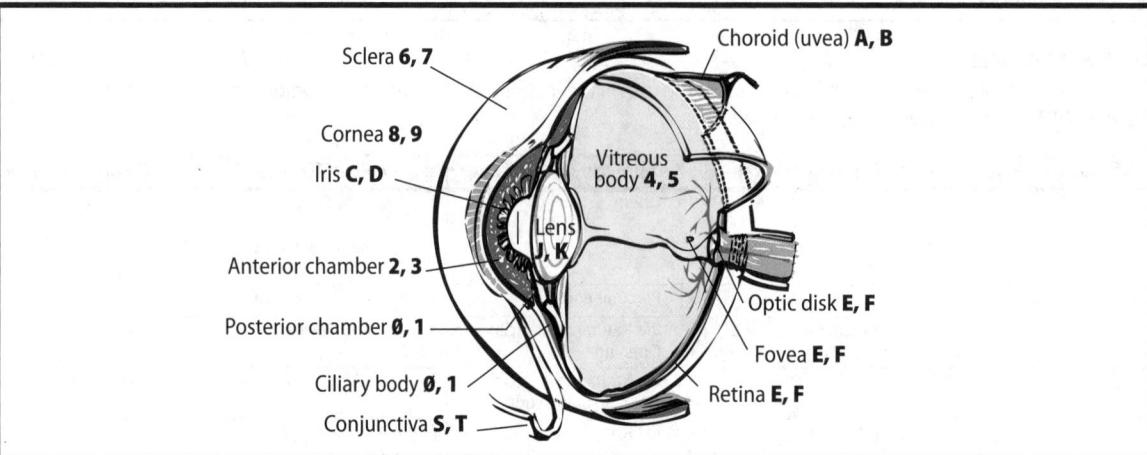

Sclera **6, 7**
Cornea **8, 9**
Iris **C, D**
Lens **J, K**
Anterior chamber **2, 3**
Posterior chamber **Ø, 1**
Ciliary body **Ø, 1**
Conjunctiva **S, T**
Choroid (uvea) **A, B**
Vitreous body **4, 5**
Optic disk **E, F**
Fovea **E, F**
Retina **E, F**

Eye Musculature

Superior rectus
Superior oblique
Lateral rectus
Medial rectus
Inferior oblique
Inferior rectus

Muscles and actions (right eye) **L, M**

Lacrimal System

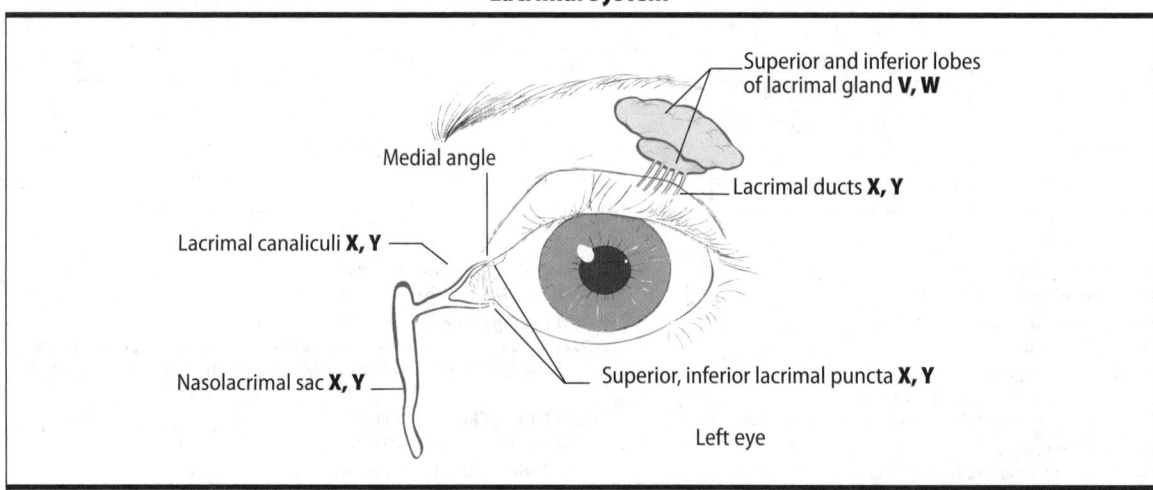

Superior and inferior lobes of lacrimal gland **V, W**
Medial angle
Lacrimal ducts **X, Y**
Lacrimal canaliculi **X, Y**
Nasolacrimal sac **X, Y**
Superior, inferior lacrimal puncta **X, Y**

Left eye

Ø Medical and Surgical
8 Eye
Ø Alteration   Definition: Modifying the anatomic structure of a body part without affecting the function of the body part

Explanation: Principal purpose is to improve appearance

Body Part Character 4	Approach Character 5	Device Character 6	Qualifier Character 7
N Upper Eyelid, Right Lateral canthus Levator palpebrae superioris muscle Orbicularis oculi muscle Superior tarsal plate P Upper Eyelid, Left *See N Upper Eyelid, Right* Q Lower Eyelid, Right Inferior tarsal plate Medial canthus R Lower Eyelid, Left *See Q Lower Eyelid, Right*	Ø Open 3 Percutaneous X External	7 Autologous Tissue Substitute J Synthetic Substitute K Nonautologous Tissue Substitute Z No Device	Z No Qualifier

Non-OR   All body part, approach, device, and qualifier values

Ø Medical and Surgical
8 Eye
1 Bypass   Definition: Altering the route of passage of the contents of a tubular body part

Explanation: Rerouting contents of a body part to a downstream area of the normal route, to a similar route and body part, or to an abnormal route and dissimilar body part. Includes one or more anastomoses, with or without the use of a device.

Body Part Character 4	Approach Character 5	Device Character 6	Qualifier Character 7
2 Anterior Chamber, Right Aqueous humour 3 Anterior Chamber, Left *See 2 Anterior Chamber, Right*	3 Percutaneous	J Synthetic Substitute K Nonautologous Tissue Substitute Z No Device	4 Sclera
X Lacrimal Duct, Right Lacrimal canaliculus Lacrimal punctum Lacrimal sac Nasolacrimal duct Y Lacrimal Duct, Left *See X Lacrimal Duct, Right*	Ø Open 3 Percutaneous	J Synthetic Substitute K Nonautologous Tissue Substitute Z No Device	3 Nasal Cavity

Ø Medical and Surgical
8 Eye
2 Change   Definition: Taking out or off a device from a body part and putting back an identical or similar device in or on the same body part without cutting or puncturing the skin or a mucous membrane

Explanation: All CHANGE procedures are coded using the approach EXTERNAL

Body Part Character 4	Approach Character 5	Device Character 6	Qualifier Character 7
Ø Eye, Right Ciliary body Posterior chamber 1 Eye, Left *See Ø Eye, Right*	X External	Ø Drainage Device Y Other Device	Z No Qualifier

Non-OR   All body part, approach, device, and qualifier values

Ø Medical and Surgical
8 Eye
5 Destruction   Definition: Physical eradication of all or a portion of a body part by the direct use of energy, force, or a destructive agent

Explanation: None of the body part is physically taken out

Body Part Character 4		Approach Character 5	Device Character 6	Qualifier Character 7

Ø Eye, Right
  Ciliary body
  Posterior chamber
1 Eye, Left
  See Ø Eye, Right
6 Sclera, Right
7 Sclera, Left
	8 Cornea, Right
	9 Cornea, Left
	S Conjunctiva, Right
	  Plica semilunaris
	T Conjunctiva, Left
	  See S Conjunctiva, Right
		X External	**Z** No Device	**Z** No Qualifier

2 Anterior Chamber, Right
  Aqueous humour
3 Anterior Chamber, Left
  See 2 Anterior Chamber, Right
4 Vitreous, Right
  Vitreous body
5 Vitreous, Left
  See 4 Vitreous, Right
C Iris, Right
D Iris, Left
	E Retina, Right
	  Fovea
	  Macula
	  Optic disc
	F Retina, Left
	  See E Retina, Right
	G Retinal Vessel, Right
	H Retinal Vessel, Left
	J Lens, Right
	  Zonule of Zinn
	K Lens, Left
	  See J Lens, Right
		3 Percutaneous	**Z** No Device	**Z** No Qualifier

A Choroid, Right
B Choroid, Left
L Extraocular Muscle, Right
  Inferior oblique muscle
  Inferior rectus muscle
  Lateral rectus muscle
  Medial rectus muscle
  Superior oblique muscle
  Superior rectus muscle
	M Extraocular Muscle, Left
	  See L Extraocular Muscle, Right
	V Lacrimal Gland, Right
	W Lacrimal Gland, Left
		Ø Open
		3 Percutaneous
			Z No Device	**Z** No Qualifier

N Upper Eyelid, Right
  Lateral canthus
  Levator palpebrae superioris
   muscle
  Orbicularis oculi muscle
  Superior tarsal plate
P Upper Eyelid, Left
  See N Upper Eyelid, Right
	Q Lower Eyelid, Right
	  Inferior tarsal plate
	  Medial canthus
	R Lower Eyelid, Left
	  See Q Lower Eyelid, Right
		Ø Open
		3 Percutaneous
		X External
			Z No Device	**Z** No Qualifier

X Lacrimal Duct, Right
  Lacrimal canaliculus
  Lacrimal punctum
  Lacrimal sac
  Nasolacrimal duct
	Y Lacrimal Duct, Left
	  See X Lacrimal Duct, Right
		Ø Open
		3 Percutaneous
		7 Via Natural or Artificial
		   Opening
		8 Via Natural or Artificial
		   Opening Endoscopic
			Z No Device	**Z** No Qualifier

Non-OR   Ø85[E,F]3ZZ

Ø Medical and Surgical
8 Eye
7 Dilation   Definition: Expanding an orifice or the lumen of a tubular body part

Explanation: The orifice can be a natural orifice or an artificially created orifice. Accomplished by stretching a tubular body part using intraluminal pressure or by cutting part of the orifice or wall of the tubular body part.

Body Part Character 4	Approach Character 5	Device Character 6	Qualifier Character 7

X Lacrimal Duct, Right
  Lacrimal canaliculus
  Lacrimal punctum
  Lacrimal sac
  Nasolacrimal duct
Y Lacrimal Duct, Left
  See X Lacrimal Duct, Right
	Ø Open
	3 Percutaneous
	7 Via Natural or Artificial
	   Opening
	8 Via Natural or Artificial
	   Opening Endoscopic
		D Intraluminal Device
		Z No Device
			Z No Qualifier

Non-OR Procedure   DRG Non-OR Procedure   Valid OR Procedure   HAC Associated Procedure   Combination Only   New/Revised April   New/Revised October

304   ICD-10-PCS 2024

085–087

Ø   Medical and Surgical
8   Eye
9   Drainage   Definition: Taking or letting out fluids and/or gases from a body part

Explanation: The qualifier DIAGNOSTIC is used to identify drainage procedures that are biopsies

Body Part Character 4		Approach Character 5	Device Character 6	Qualifier Character 7

Ø Eye, Right
  Ciliary body
  Posterior chamber
1 Eye, Left
  See Ø Eye, Right
6 Sclera, Right
7 Sclera, Left
	8 Cornea, Right
	9 Cornea, Left
	S Conjunctiva, Right
	  Plica semilunaris
	T Conjunctiva, Left
	  See S Conjunctiva, Right
		X External	Ø Drainage Device	Z No Qualifier

Ø Eye, Right
  Ciliary body
  Posterior chamber
1 Eye, Left
  See Ø Eye, Right
6 Sclera, Right
7 Sclera, Left
	8 Cornea, Right
	9 Cornea, Left
	S Conjunctiva, Right
	  Plica semilunaris
	T Conjunctiva, Left
	  See S Conjunctiva, Right
		X External	Z No Device	X Diagnostic
				Z No Qualifier

2 Anterior Chamber, Right
  Aqueous humour
3 Anterior Chamber, Left
  See 2 Anterior Chamber, Right
4 Vitreous, Right
  Vitreous body
5 Vitreous, Left
  See 4 Vitreous, Right
C Iris, Right
D Iris, Left
	E Retina, Right
	  Fovea
	  Macula
	  Optic disc
	F Retina, Left
	  See E Retina, Right
	G Retinal Vessel, Right
	H Retinal Vessel, Left
	J Lens, Right
	  Zonule of Zinn
	K Lens, Left
	  See J Lens, Right
		3 Percutaneous	Ø Drainage Device	Z No Qualifier

2 Anterior Chamber, Right
  Aqueous humour
3 Anterior Chamber, Left
  See 2 Anterior Chamber, Right
4 Vitreous, Right
  Vitreous body
5 Vitreous, Left
  See 4 Vitreous, Right
C Iris, Right
D Iris, Left
	E Retina, Right
	  Fovea
	  Macula
	  Optic disc
	F Retina, Left
	  See E Retina, Right
	G Retinal Vessel, Right
	H Retinal Vessel, Left
	J Lens, Right
	  Zonule of Zinn
	K Lens, Left
	  See J Lens, Right
		3 Percutaneous	Z No Device	X Diagnostic
				Z No Qualifier

A Choroid, Right
B Choroid, Left
L Extraocular Muscle, Right
  Inferior oblique muscle
  Inferior rectus muscle
  Lateral rectus muscle
  Medial rectus muscle
  Superior oblique muscle
  Superior rectus muscle
	M Extraocular Muscle, Left
	  See L Extraocular Muscle, Right
	V Lacrimal Gland, Right
	W Lacrimal Gland, Left
		Ø Open
		3 Percutaneous
			Ø Drainage Device	Z No Qualifier

A Choroid, Right
B Choroid, Left
L Extraocular Muscle, Right
  Inferior oblique muscle
  Inferior rectus muscle
  Lateral rectus muscle
  Medial rectus muscle
  Superior oblique muscle
  Superior rectus muscle
	M Extraocular Muscle, Left
	  See L Extraocular Muscle, Right
	V Lacrimal Gland, Right
	W Lacrimal Gland, Left
		Ø Open
		3 Percutaneous
			Z No Device	X Diagnostic
				Z No Qualifier

N Upper Eyelid, Right
  Lateral canthus
  Levator palpebrae superioris
    muscle
  Orbicularis oculi muscle
  Superior tarsal plate
P Upper Eyelid, Left
  See N Upper Eyelid, Right
	Q Lower Eyelid, Right
	  Inferior tarsal plate
	  Medial canthus
	R Lower Eyelid, Left
	  See Q Lower Eyelid, Right
		Ø Open
		3 Percutaneous
		X External
			Ø Drainage Device	Z No Qualifier

Non-OR	Ø89[Ø,1,6,7,8,9,S,T]XZ[X,Z]
Non-OR	Ø89[N,P,Q,R][Ø,3,X]ØZ

Ø89 Continued on next page

NC Noncovered Procedure   LC Limited Coverage   QA Questionable OB Admit   NT New Tech Add-on   ⊞ Combination Member   ♂ Male   ♀ Female

Ø	**Medical and Surgical**
8	**Eye**
9	**Drainage**

Ø89 Continued

Definition: Taking or letting out fluids and/or gases from a body part
Explanation: The qualifier DIAGNOSTIC is used to identify drainage procedures that are biopsies

Body Part Character 4		Approach Character 5	Device Character 6	Qualifier Character 7
N Upper Eyelid, Right Lateral canthus Levator palpebrae superioris muscle Orbicularis oculi muscle Superior tarsal plate **P** Upper Eyelid, Left *See N Upper Eyelid, Right*	**Q** Lower Eyelid, Right Inferior tarsal plate Medial canthus **R** Lower Eyelid, Left *See Q Lower Eyelid, Right*	**Ø** Open **3** Percutaneous **X** External	**Z** No Device	**X** Diagnostic **Z** No Qualifier

X Lacrimal Duct, Right
Lacrimal canaliculus
Lacrimal punctum
Lacrimal sac
Nasolacrimal duct
	Y Lacrimal Duct, Left
	See X Lacrimal Duct, Right
		Ø Open
		3 Percutaneous
		7 Via Natural or Artificial
		   Opening
		8 Via Natural or Artificial
		   Opening Endoscopic
			Ø Drainage Device	**Z** No Qualifier

X Lacrimal Duct, Right
Lacrimal canaliculus
Lacrimal punctum
Lacrimal sac
Nasolacrimal duct
	Y Lacrimal Duct, Left
	See X Lacrimal Duct, Right
		Ø Open
		3 Percutaneous
		7 Via Natural or Artificial
		   Opening
		8 Via Natural or Artificial
		   Opening Endoscopic
			Z No Device	**X** Diagnostic
				Z No Qualifier

Non-OR	Ø89[N,P,Q,R]ØZZ
Non-OR	Ø89[N,P,Q,R][3,X]Z[X,Z]

Ø	**Medical and Surgical**
8	**Eye**
B	**Excision**

Definition: Cutting out or off, without replacement, a portion of a body part
Explanation: The qualifier DIAGNOSTIC is used to identify excision procedures that are biopsies

Body Part Character 4		Approach Character 5	Device Character 6	Qualifier Character 7
Ø Eye, Right Ciliary body Posterior chamber **1** Eye, Left *See Ø Eye, Right* **N** Upper Eyelid, Right Lateral canthus Levator palpebrae superioris muscle Orbicularis oculi muscle Superior tarsal plate	**P** Upper Eyelid, Left *See N Upper Eyelid, Right* **Q** Lower Eyelid, Right Inferior tarsal plate Medial canthus **R** Lower Eyelid, Left *See Q Lower Eyelid, Right*	**Ø** Open **3** Percutaneous **X** External	**Z** No Device	**X** Diagnostic **Z** No Qualifier
4 Vitreous, Right Vitreous body **5** Vitreous, Left *See 4 Vitreous, Right* **C** Iris, Right **D** Iris, Left **E** Retina, Right Fovea Macula Optic disc	**F** Retina, Left *See E Retina, Right* **J** Lens, Right Zonule of Zinn **K** Lens, Left *See J Lens, Right*	**3** Percutaneous	**Z** No Device	**X** Diagnostic **Z** No Qualifier
6 Sclera, Right **7** Sclera, Left **8** Cornea, Right **9** Cornea, Left	**S** Conjunctiva, Right Plica semilunaris **T** Conjunctiva, Left *See S Conjunctiva, Right*	**X** External	**Z** No Device	**X** Diagnostic **Z** No Qualifier
A Choroid, Right **B** Choroid, Left **L** Extraocular Muscle, Right Inferior oblique muscle Inferior rectus muscle Lateral rectus muscle Medial rectus muscle Superior oblique muscle Superior rectus muscle	**M** Extraocular Muscle, Left *See L Extraocular Muscle, Right* **V** Lacrimal Gland, Right **W** Lacrimal Gland, Left	**Ø** Open **3** Percutaneous	**Z** No Device	**X** Diagnostic **Z** No Qualifier

X Lacrimal Duct, Right
Lacrimal canaliculus
Lacrimal punctum
Lacrimal sac
Nasolacrimal duct
	Y Lacrimal Duct, Left
	See X Lacrimal Duct, Right
		Ø Open
		3 Percutaneous
		7 Via Natural or Artificial
		   Opening
		8 Via Natural or Artificial
		   Opening Endoscopic
			Z No Device	**X** Diagnostic
				Z No Qualifier

Non-OR Procedure   DRG Non-OR Procedure   Valid OR Procedure   HAC Associated Procedure   Combination Only   New/Revised April   New/Revised October

Ø   **Medical and Surgical**
8   **Eye**
C   **Extirpation**   Definition: Taking or cutting out solid matter from a body part

Explanation: The solid matter may be an abnormal byproduct of a biological function or a foreign body; it may be imbedded in a body part or in the lumen of a tubular body part. The solid matter may or may not have been previously broken into pieces.

Body Part Character 4	Approach Character 5	Device Character 6	Qualifier Character 7

Ø   **Eye, Right**
   Ciliary body
   Posterior chamber
1   **Eye, Left**
   See Ø Eye, Right
6   **Sclera, Right**
7   **Sclera, Left**
8   **Cornea, Right**
9   **Cornea, Left**
S   **Conjunctiva, Right**
   Plica semilunaris
T   **Conjunctiva, Left**
   See S Conjunctiva, Right
	X External	**Z** No Device	**Z** No Qualifier

2   **Anterior Chamber, Right**
   Aqueous humour
3   **Anterior Chamber, Left**
   See 2 Anterior Chamber, Right
4   **Vitreous, Right**
   Vitreous body
5   **Vitreous, Left**
   See 4 Vitreous, Right
C   **Iris, Right**
D   **Iris, Left**
E   **Retina, Right**
   Fovea
   Macula
   Optic disc
F   **Retina, Left**
   See E Retina, Right
G   **Retinal Vessel, Right**
H   **Retinal Vessel, Left**
J   **Lens, Right**
   Zonule of Zinn
K   **Lens, Left**
   See J Lens, Right
	3 Percutaneous
	X External
		Z No Device	**Z** No Qualifier

A   **Choroid, Right**
B   **Choroid, Left**
L   **Extraocular Muscle, Right**
   Inferior oblique muscle
   Inferior rectus muscle
   Lateral rectus muscle
   Medial rectus muscle
   Superior oblique muscle
   Superior rectus muscle
M   **Extraocular Muscle, Left**
   See L Extraocular Muscle, Right
N   **Upper Eyelid, Right**
   Lateral canthus
   Levator palpebrae superioris muscle
   Orbicularis oculi muscle
   Superior tarsal plate
P   **Upper Eyelid, Left**
   See N Upper Eyelid, Right
Q   **Lower Eyelid, Right**
   Inferior tarsal plate
   Medial canthus
R   **Lower Eyelid, Left**
   See Q Lower Eyelid, Right
V   **Lacrimal Gland, Right**
W   **Lacrimal Gland, Left**
	Ø Open
	3 Percutaneous
	X External
		Z No Device	**Z** No Qualifier

X   **Lacrimal Duct, Right**
   Lacrimal canaliculus
   Lacrimal punctum
   Lacrimal sac
   Nasolacrimal duct
Y   **Lacrimal Duct, Left**
   See X Lacrimal Duct, Right
	Ø Open
	3 Percutaneous
	7 Via Natural or Artificial Opening
	8 Via Natural or Artificial Opening
	     Endoscopic
		Z No Device	**Z** No Qualifier

Non-OR	Ø8C[Ø,1,6,7,S,T]XZZ
Non-OR	Ø8C[2,3]XZZ
Non-OR	Ø8C[N,P,Q,R][Ø,3,X]ZZ

NC Noncovered Procedure   **LC** Limited Coverage   **QA** Questionable OB Admit   **NT** New Tech Add-on   ⊞ Combination Member   ♂ Male   ♀ Female

Ø   Medical and Surgical
8   Eye
D   Extraction   Definition: Pulling or stripping out or off all or a portion of a body part by the use of force
                             Explanation: The qualifier DIAGNOSTIC is used to identify extraction procedures that are biopsies

Body Part Character 4	Approach Character 5	Device Character 6	Qualifier Character 7
8 Cornea, Right 9 Cornea, Left	X External	Z No Device	X Diagnostic Z No Qualifier

J Lens, Right
   Zonule of Zinn
K Lens, Left
   See J Lens, Right
	3 Percutaneous	Z No Device	Z No Qualifier

Ø   Medical and Surgical
8   Eye
F   Fragmentation   Definition: Breaking solid matter in a body part into pieces
                             Explanation: Physical force (e.g., manual, ultrasonic) applied directly or indirectly is used to break the solid matter into pieces. The solid matter may be an abnormal byproduct of a biological function or a foreign body. The pieces of solid matter are not taken out.

Body Part Character 4	Approach Character 5	Device Character 6	Qualifier Character 7

4 Vitreous, Right   **NC**
   Vitreous body
5 Vitreous, Left   **NC**
   See 4 Vitreous, Right
	3 Percutaneous
	X External
		Z No Device	Z No Qualifier

Non-OR   Ø8F[4,5]XZZ
NC   Ø8F[4,5]XZZ

Ø   Medical and Surgical
8   Eye
H   Insertion   Definition: Putting in a nonbiological appliance that monitors, assists, performs, or prevents a physiological function but does not physically take the place of a body part
                            Explanation: None

Body Part Character 4	Approach Character 5	Device Character 6	Qualifier Character 7

Ø Eye, Right
   Ciliary body
   Posterior chamber
1 Eye, Left
   See Ø Eye, Right
	Ø Open	5 Epiretinal Visual Prosthesis
		Y Other Device
			Z No Qualifier

Ø Eye, Right
   Ciliary body
   Posterior chamber
1 Eye, Left
   See Ø Eye, Right
	3 Percutaneous	1 Radioactive Element
		3 Infusion Device
		Y Other Device
			Z No Qualifier

Ø Eye, Right
   Ciliary body
   Posterior chamber
1 Eye, Left
   See Ø Eye, Right
	7 Via Natural or Artificial Opening
	8 Via Natural or Artificial Opening Endoscopic
		Y Other Device	Z No Qualifier

Ø Eye, Right
   Ciliary body
   Posterior chamber
1 Eye, Left
   See Ø Eye, Right
	X External	1 Radioactive Element
		3 Infusion Device
			Z No Qualifier

Non-OR   Ø8H[Ø,1]3YZ
Non-OR   Ø8H[Ø,1][7,8]YZ

Non-OR Procedure   DRG Non-OR Procedure   Valid OR Procedure   HAC Associated Procedure   Combination Only   New/Revised April   New/Revised October

Ø Medical and Surgical
8 Eye
J Inspection   Definition: Visually and/or manually exploring a body part

Explanation: Visual exploration may be performed with or without optical instrumentation. Manual exploration may be performed directly or through intervening body layers.

Body Part Character 4	Approach Character 5	Device Character 6	Qualifier Character 7
Ø Eye, Right Ciliary body Posterior chamber **1 Eye, Left** *See Ø Eye, Right* **J Lens, Right** Zonule of Zinn **K Lens, Left** *See J Lens, Right*	**X External**	**Z No Device**	**Z No Qualifier**
L Extraocular Muscle, Right Inferior oblique muscle Inferior rectus muscle Lateral rectus muscle Medial rectus muscle Superior oblique muscle Superior rectus muscle **M Extraocular Muscle, Left** *See L Extraocular Muscle, Right*	**Ø Open** **X External**	**Z No Device**	**Z No Qualifier**

Non-OR   Ø8J[Ø,1,J,K]XZZ
Non-OR   Ø8J[L,M]XZZ

Ø Medical and Surgical
8 Eye
L Occlusion   Definition: Completely closing an orifice or the lumen of a tubular body part

Explanation: The orifice can be a natural orifice or an artificially created orifice

Body Part Character 4	Approach Character 5	Device Character 6	Qualifier Character 7
X Lacrimal Duct, Right Lacrimal canaliculus Lacrimal punctum Lacrimal sac Nasolacrimal duct **Y Lacrimal Duct, Left** *See X Lacrimal Duct, Right*	**Ø Open** **3 Percutaneous**	**C Extraluminal Device** **D Intraluminal Device** **Z No Device**	**Z No Qualifier**
X Lacrimal Duct, Right Lacrimal canaliculus Lacrimal punctum Lacrimal sac Nasolacrimal duct **Y Lacrimal Duct, Left** *See X Lacrimal Duct, Right*	**7 Via Natural or Artificial Opening** **8 Via Natural or Artificial Opening Endoscopic**	**D Intraluminal Device** **Z No Device**	**Z No Qualifier**

Ø Medical and Surgical
8 Eye
M Reattachment   Definition: Putting back in or on all or a portion of a separated body part to its normal location or other suitable location

Explanation: Vascular circulation and nervous pathways may or may not be reestablished

Body Part Character 4	Approach Character 5	Device Character 6	Qualifier Character 7
N Upper Eyelid, Right Lateral canthus Levator palpebrae superioris muscle Orbicularis oculi muscle Superior tarsal plate **P Upper Eyelid, Left** *See N Upper Eyelid, Right* **Q Lower Eyelid, Right** Inferior tarsal plate Medial canthus **R Lower Eyelid, Left** *See Q Lower Eyelid, Right*	**X External**	**Z No Device**	**Z No Qualifier**

NC Noncovered Procedure   **LC** Limited Coverage   **QA** Questionable OB Admit   **NT** New Tech Add-on   ⊞ Combination Member   ♂ Male   ♀ Female

ICD-10-PCS 2024   309

08J–08M

Ø   Medical and Surgical
8   Eye
N   Release   Definition: Freeing a body part from an abnormal physical constraint by cutting or by the use of force
                    Explanation: Some of the restraining tissue may be taken out but none of the body part is taken out

Body Part Character 4	Approach Character 5	Device Character 6	Qualifier Character 7
Ø Eye, Right Ciliary body Posterior chamber **1 Eye, Left** *See Ø Eye, Right* **6 Sclera, Right** **7 Sclera, Left** **8 Cornea, Right** **9 Cornea, Left** **S Conjunctiva, Right** Plica semilunaris **T Conjunctiva, Left** *See S Conjunctiva, Right*	**X External**	**Z No Device**	**Z No Qualifier**
2 Anterior Chamber, Right Aqueous humour **3 Anterior Chamber, Left** *See 2 Anterior Chamber, Right* **4 Vitreous, Right** Vitreous body **5 Vitreous, Left** *See 4 Vitreous, Right* **C Iris, Right** **D Iris, Left** **E Retina, Right** Fovea Macula Optic disc **F Retina, Left** *See E Retina, Right* **G Retinal Vessel, Right** **H Retinal Vessel, Left** **J Lens, Right** Zonule of Zinn **K Lens, Left** *See J Lens, Right*	**3 Percutaneous**	**Z No Device**	**Z No Qualifier**
A Choroid, Right **B Choroid, Left** **L Extraocular Muscle, Right** Inferior oblique muscle Inferior rectus muscle Lateral rectus muscle Medial rectus muscle Superior oblique muscle Superior rectus muscle **M Extraocular Muscle, Left** *See L Extraocular Muscle, Right* **V Lacrimal Gland, Right** **W Lacrimal Gland, Left**	**Ø Open** **3 Percutaneous**	**Z No Device**	**Z No Qualifier**
N Upper Eyelid, Right Lateral canthus Levator palpebrae superioris muscle Orbicularis oculi muscle Superior tarsal plate **P Upper Eyelid, Left** *See N Upper Eyelid, Right* **Q Lower Eyelid, Right** Inferior tarsal plate Medial canthus **R Lower Eyelid, Left** *See Q Lower Eyelid, Right*	**Ø Open** **3 Percutaneous** **X External**	**Z No Device**	**Z No Qualifier**
X Lacrimal Duct, Right Lacrimal canaliculus Lacrimal punctum Lacrimal sac Nasolacrimal duct **Y Lacrimal Duct, Left** *See X Lacrimal Duct, Right*	**Ø Open** **3 Percutaneous** **7 Via Natural or Artificial Opening** **8 Via Natural or Artificial Opening Endoscopic**	**Z No Device**	**Z No Qualifier**

Ø8N–Ø8N

Non-OR Procedure   DRG Non-OR Procedure   Valid OR Procedure   HAC Associated Procedure   Combination Only   New/Revised April   New/Revised October

310   ICD-10-PCS 2024

Ø   **Medical and Surgical**
8   **Eye**
P   **Removal**   Definition: Taking out or off a device from a body part

Explanation: If a device is taken out and a similar device put in without cutting or puncturing the skin or mucous membrane, the procedure is coded to the root operation CHANGE. Otherwise, the procedure for taking out a device is coded to the root operation REMOVAL.

Body Part Character 4	Approach Character 5	Device Character 6	Qualifier Character 7

Ø   Eye, Right
    Ciliary body
    Posterior chamber
1   Eye, Left
    See Ø Eye, Right
	Ø Open
	3 Percutaneous
	7 Via Natural or Artificial Opening
	8 Via Natural or Artificial Opening Endoscopic
		Ø Drainage Device
		1 Radioactive Element
		3 Infusion Device
		7 Autologous Tissue Substitute
		C Extraluminal Device
		D Intraluminal Device
		J Synthetic Substitute
		K Nonautologous Tissue Substitute
		Y Other Device
			Z No Qualifier

Ø   Eye, Right
    Ciliary body
    Posterior chamber
1   Eye, Left
    See Ø Eye, Right
	X External	Ø Drainage Device
		1 Radioactive Element
		3 Infusion Device
		7 Autologous Tissue Substitute
		C Extraluminal Device
		D Intraluminal Device
		J Synthetic Substitute
		K Nonautologous Tissue Substitute
			Z No Qualifier

J   Lens, Right
    Zonule of Zinn
K   Lens, Left
    See J Lens, Right
	3 Percutaneous	J Synthetic Substitute
		Y Other Device
			Z No Qualifier

L   Extraocular Muscle, Right
    Inferior oblique muscle
    Inferior rectus muscle
    Lateral rectus muscle
    Medial rectus muscle
    Superior oblique muscle
    Superior rectus muscle
M   Extraocular Muscle, Left
    See L Extraocular Muscle, Right
	Ø Open
	3 Percutaneous
		Ø Drainage Device
		7 Autologous Tissue Substitute
		J Synthetic Substitute
		K Nonautologous Tissue Substitute
		Y Other Device
			Z No Qualifier

Non-OR   Ø8P[Ø,1]3YZ
Non-OR   Ø8P[Ø,1][7,8][Ø,3,D,Y]Z
Non-OR   Ø8P[Ø,1]X[Ø,1,3,C,D,J]Z
Non-OR   Ø8P[J,K]3YZ
Non-OR   Ø8P[L,M]3YZ

NC Noncovered Procedure   **LC** Limited Coverage   **QA** Questionable OB Admit   **NT** New Tech Add-on   ⊞ Combination Member   ♂ Male   ♀ Female

ICD-10-PCS 2024   311

Ø8P–Ø8P

0   **Medical and Surgical**
8   **Eye**
Q   **Repair**   Definition: Restoring, to the extent possible, a body part to its normal anatomic structure and function
                      Explanation: Used only when the method to accomplish the repair is not one of the other root operations

Body Part Character 4	Approach Character 5	Device Character 6	Qualifier Character 7

0   **Eye, Right**
    Ciliary body
    Posterior chamber
1   **Eye, Left**
    See 0 Eye, Right
6   **Sclera, Right**
7   **Sclera, Left**
8   **Cornea, Right**   `NC`
9   **Cornea, Left**   `NC`
S   **Conjunctiva, Right**
    Plica semilunaris
T   **Conjunctiva, Left**
    See S Conjunctiva, Right
	X External	**Z** No Device	**Z** No Qualifier

2   **Anterior Chamber, Right**
    Aqueous humour
3   **Anterior Chamber, Left**
    See 2 Anterior Chamber, Right
4   **Vitreous, Right**
    Vitreous body
5   **Vitreous, Left**
    See 4 Vitreous, Right
C   **Iris, Right**
D   **Iris, Left**
E   **Retina, Right**
    Fovea
    Macula
    Optic disc
F   **Retina, Left**
    See E Retina, Right
G   **Retinal Vessel, Right**
H   **Retinal Vessel, Left**
J   **Lens, Right**
    Zonule of Zinn
K   **Lens, Left**
    See J Lens, Right
	3 Percutaneous	**Z** No Device	**Z** No Qualifier

A   **Choroid, Right**
B   **Choroid, Left**
L   **Extraocular Muscle, Right**
    Inferior oblique muscle
    Inferior rectus muscle
    Lateral rectus muscle
    Medial rectus muscle
    Superior oblique muscle
    Superior rectus muscle
M   **Extraocular Muscle, Left**
    See L Extraocular Muscle, Right
V   **Lacrimal Gland, Right**
W   **Lacrimal Gland, Left**
	0 Open
	3 Percutaneous
		Z No Device	**Z** No Qualifier

N   **Upper Eyelid, Right**
    Lateral canthus
    Levator palpebrae superioris muscle
    Orbicularis oculi muscle
    Superior tarsal plate
P   **Upper Eyelid, Left**
    See N Upper Eyelid, Right
Q   **Lower Eyelid, Right**
    Inferior tarsal plate
    Medial canthus
R   **Lower Eyelid, Left**
    See Q Lower Eyelid, Right
	0 Open
	3 Percutaneous
	X External
		Z No Device	**Z** No Qualifier

X   **Lacrimal Duct, Right**
    Lacrimal canaliculus
    Lacrimal punctum
    Lacrimal sac
    Nasolacrimal duct
Y   **Lacrimal Duct, Left**
    See X Lacrimal Duct, Right
	0 Open
	3 Percutaneous
	7 Via Natural or Artificial Opening
	8 Via Natural or Artificial Opening
	    Endoscopic
		Z No Device	**Z** No Qualifier

Non-OR   08Q[N,P,Q,R][0,3,X]ZZ
`NC`   08Q[8,9]XZZ

Non-OR Procedure   DRG Non-OR Procedure   Valid OR Procedure   HAC Associated Procedure   Combination Only   New/Revised April   New/Revised October

312   ICD-10-PCS 2024

Ø   Medical and Surgical
8   Eye
R   Replacement   Definition: Putting in or on biological or synthetic material that physically takes the place and/or function of all or a portion of a body part

                          Explanation: The body part may have been taken out or replaced, or may be taken out, physically eradicated, or rendered nonfunctional during the REPLACEMENT procedure. A REMOVAL procedure is coded for taking out the device used in a previous replacement procedure.

Body Part Character 4	Approach Character 5	Device Character 6	Qualifier Character 7

Ø Eye, Right
    Ciliary body
    Posterior chamber
1 Eye, Left
    See Ø Eye, Right
A Choroid, Right
B Choroid, Left
	Ø Open
	3 Percutaneous
		7 Autologous Tissue Substitute
		J Synthetic Substitute
		K Nonautologous Tissue Substitute
			Z No Qualifier

4 Vitreous, Right
    Vitreous body
5 Vitreous, Left
    See 4 Vitreous, Right
C Iris, Right
D Iris, Left
G Retinal Vessel, Right
H Retinal Vessel, Left
	3 Percutaneous	**7** Autologous Tissue Substitute
		J Synthetic Substitute
		K Nonautologous Tissue Substitute
			Z No Qualifier

6 Sclera, Right
7 Sclera, Left
S Conjunctiva, Right
    Plica semilunaris
T Conjunctiva, Left
    See S Conjunctiva, Right
	X External	**7** Autologous Tissue Substitute
		J Synthetic Substitute
		K Nonautologous Tissue Substitute
			Z No Qualifier

8 Cornea, Right **9** Cornea, Left	**3** Percutaneous **X** External	**7** Autologous Tissue Substitute **J** Synthetic Substitute **K** Nonautologous Tissue Substitute	**Z** No Qualifier

J Lens, Right
    Zonule of Zinn
K Lens, Left
    See J Lens, Right
	3 Percutaneous	**Ø** Synthetic Substitute, Intraocular
		    Telescope
		7 Autologous Tissue Substitute
		J Synthetic Substitute
		K Nonautologous Tissue Substitute
			Z No Qualifier

N Upper Eyelid, Right
    Lateral canthus
    Levator palpebrae superioris muscle
    Orbicularis oculi muscle
    Superior tarsal plate
P Upper Eyelid, Left
    See N Upper Eyelid, Right
Q Lower Eyelid, Right
    Inferior tarsal plate
    Medial canthus
R Lower Eyelid, Left
    See Q Lower Eyelid, Right
	Ø Open
	3 Percutaneous
	X External
		7 Autologous Tissue Substitute
		J Synthetic Substitute
		K Nonautologous Tissue Substitute
			Z No Qualifier

X Lacrimal Duct, Right
    Lacrimal canaliculus
    Lacrimal punctum
    Lacrimal sac
    Nasolacrimal duct
Y Lacrimal Duct, Left
    See X Lacrimal Duct, Right
	Ø Open
	3 Percutaneous
	7 Via Natural or Artificial Opening
	8 Via Natural or Artificial Opening
	    Endoscopic
		7 Autologous Tissue Substitute
		J Synthetic Substitute
		K Nonautologous Tissue Substitute
			Z No Qualifier

NC Noncovered Procedure   **LC** Limited Coverage   **QA** Questionable OB Admit   **NT** New Tech Add-on   ⊞ Combination Member   ♂ Male   ♀ Female

ICD-10-PCS 2024   313

08R–08R

Ø Medical and Surgical
8 Eye
S Reposition   Definition: Moving to its normal location, or other suitable location, all or a portion of a body part

Explanation: The body part is moved to a new location from an abnormal location, or from a normal location where it is not functioning correctly. The body part may or may not be cut out or off to be moved to the new location.

Body Part Character 4	Approach Character 5	Device Character 6	Qualifier Character 7

C Iris, Right
D Iris, Left
G Retinal Vessel, Right
H Retinal Vessel, Left
J Lens, Right
   Zonule of Zinn
K Lens, Left
   See J Lens, Right
	3 Percutaneous	**Z** No Device	**Z** No Qualifier

L Extraocular Muscle, Right
   Inferior oblique muscle
   Inferior rectus muscle
   Lateral rectus muscle
   Medial rectus muscle
   Superior oblique muscle
   Superior rectus muscle
M Extraocular Muscle, Left
   See L Extraocular Muscle, Right
V Lacrimal Gland, Right
W Lacrimal Gland, Left
	Ø Open
	3 Percutaneous
		Z No Device	**Z** No Qualifier

N Upper Eyelid, Right
   Lateral canthus
   Levator palpebrae superioris muscle
   Orbicularis oculi muscle
   Superior tarsal plate
P Upper Eyelid, Left
   See N Upper Eyelid, Right
Q Lower Eyelid, Right
   Inferior tarsal plate
   Medial canthus
R Lower Eyelid, Left
   See Q Lower Eyelid, Right
	Ø Open
	3 Percutaneous
	X External
		Z No Device	**Z** No Qualifier

X Lacrimal Duct, Right
   Lacrimal canaliculus
   Lacrimal punctum
   Lacrimal sac
   Nasolacrimal duct
Y Lacrimal Duct, Left
   See X Lacrimal Duct, Right
	Ø Open
	3 Percutaneous
	7 Via Natural or Artificial Opening
	8 Via Natural or Artificial Opening Endoscopic
		Z No Device	**Z** No Qualifier

Non-OR Procedure   DRG Non-OR Procedure   Valid OR Procedure   HAC Associated Procedure   Combination Only   New/Revised April   New/Revised October

314   ICD-10-PCS 2024

Ø   Medical and Surgical
8   Eye
T   Resection   Definition: Cutting out or off, without replacement, all of a body part
                     Explanation: None

Body Part Character 4	Approach Character 5	Device Character 6	Qualifier Character 7

Ø Eye, Right
    Ciliary body
    Posterior chamber
1 Eye, Left
    See Ø Eye, Right
8 Cornea, Right
9 Cornea, Left
	X External	**Z** No Device	**Z** No Qualifier

4 Vitreous, Right
    Vitreous body
5 Vitreous, Left
    See 4 Vitreous, Right
C Iris, Right
D Iris, Left
J Lens, Right
    Zonule of Zinn
K Lens, Left
    See J Lens, Right
	3 Percutaneous	**Z** No Device	**Z** No Qualifier

L Extraocular Muscle, Right
    Inferior oblique muscle
    Inferior rectus muscle
    Lateral rectus muscle
    Medial rectus muscle
    Superior oblique muscle
    Superior rectus muscle
M Extraocular Muscle, Left
    See L Extraocular Muscle, Right
V Lacrimal Gland, Right
W Lacrimal Gland, Left
	Ø Open
	3 Percutaneous
		Z No Device	**Z** No Qualifier

N Upper Eyelid, Right
    Lateral canthus
    Levator palpebrae superioris muscle
    Orbicularis oculi muscle
    Superior tarsal plate
P Upper Eyelid, Left
    See N Upper Eyelid, Right
Q Lower Eyelid, Right
    Inferior tarsal plate
    Medial canthus
R Lower Eyelid, Left
    See Q Lower Eyelid, Right
	Ø Open
	X External
		Z No Device	**Z** No Qualifier

X Lacrimal Duct, Right
    Lacrimal canaliculus
    Lacrimal punctum
    Lacrimal sac
    Nasolacrimal duct
Y Lacrimal Duct, Left
    See X Lacrimal Duct, Right
	Ø Open
	3 Percutaneous
	7 Via Natural or Artificial Opening
	8 Via Natural or Artificial Opening
	      Endoscopic
		Z No Device	**Z** No Qualifier

NC Noncovered Procedure   **LC** Limited Coverage   **QA** Questionable OB Admit   **NT** New Tech Add-on   ⊞ Combination Member   ♂ Male   ♀ Female

ICD-10-PCS 2024   315

Ø8T–Ø8T

Ø   Medical and Surgical
8   Eye
U   Supplement   Definition: Putting in or on biological or synthetic material that physically reinforces and/or augments the function of a portion of a body part

Explanation: The biological material is non-living, or is living and from the same individual. The body part may have been previously replaced, and the SUPPLEMENT procedure is performed to physically reinforce and/or augment the function of the replaced body part.

Body Part Character 4	Approach Character 5	Device Character 6	Qualifier Character 7

Ø Eye, Right
   Ciliary body
   Posterior chamber
1 Eye, Left
   See Ø Eye, Right
C Iris, Right
D Iris, Left
E Retina, Right
   Fovea
   Macula
   Optic disc
F Retina, Left
   See E Retina, Right
G Retinal Vessel, Right
H Retinal Vessel, Left
L Extraocular Muscle, Right
   Inferior oblique muscle
   Inferior rectus muscle
   Lateral rectus muscle
   Medial rectus muscle
   Superior oblique muscle
   Superior rectus muscle
M Extraocular Muscle, Left
   See L Extraocular Muscle, Right
	Ø Open
	3 Percutaneous
		7 Autologous Tissue Substitute
		J Synthetic Substitute
		K Nonautologous Tissue Substitute
			Z No Qualifier

8 Cornea, Right **NC**
9 Cornea, Left **NC**
N Upper Eyelid, Right
   Lateral canthus
   Levator palpebrae superioris muscle
   Orbicularis oculi muscle
   Superior tarsal plate
P Upper Eyelid, Left
   See N Upper Eyelid, Right
Q Lower Eyelid, Right
   Inferior tarsal plate
   Medial canthus
R Lower Eyelid, Left
   See Q Lower Eyelid, Right
	Ø Open
	3 Percutaneous
	X External
		7 Autologous Tissue Substitute
		J Synthetic Substitute
		K Nonautologous Tissue Substitute
			Z No Qualifier

X Lacrimal Duct, Right
   Lacrimal canaliculus
   Lacrimal punctum
   Lacrimal sac
   Nasolacrimal duct
Y Lacrimal Duct, Left
   See X Lacrimal Duct, Right
	Ø Open
	3 Percutaneous
	7 Via Natural or Artificial Opening
	8 Via Natural or Artificial Opening
	   Endoscopic
		7 Autologous Tissue Substitute
		J Synthetic Substitute
		K Nonautologous Tissue Substitute
			Z No Qualifier

NC Ø8U[8,9][Ø,3,X]KZ

Ø   Medical and Surgical
8   Eye
V   Restriction   Definition: Partially closing an orifice or the lumen of a tubular body part

Explanation: The orifice can be a natural orifice or an artificially created orifice

Body Part Character 4	Approach Character 5	Device Character 6	Qualifier Character 7

X Lacrimal Duct, Right
   Lacrimal canaliculus
   Lacrimal punctum
   Lacrimal sac
   Nasolacrimal duct
Y Lacrimal Duct, Left
   See X Lacrimal Duct, Right
	Ø Open
	3 Percutaneous
		C Extraluminal Device
		D Intraluminal Device
		Z No Device
			Z No Qualifier

X Lacrimal Duct, Right
   Lacrimal canaliculus
   Lacrimal punctum
   Lacrimal sac
   Nasolacrimal duct
Y Lacrimal Duct, Left
   See X Lacrimal Duct, Right
	7 Via Natural or Artificial Opening
	8 Via Natural or Artificial Opening
	   Endoscopic
		D Intraluminal Device
		Z No Device
			Z No Qualifier

Ø8U–Ø8V

Non-OR Procedure   DRG Non-OR Procedure   Valid OR Procedure   HAC Associated Procedure   Combination Only   New/Revised April   New/Revised October

316   ICD-10-PCS 2024

Ø   **Medical and Surgical**
8   **Eye**
W   **Revision**   Definition: Correcting, to the extent possible, a portion of a malfunctioning device or the position of a displaced device

Explanation: Revision can include correcting a malfunctioning or displaced device by taking out or putting in components of the device such as a screw or pin

Body Part Character 4	Approach Character 5	Device Character 6	Qualifier Character 7

Ø   Eye, Right
     Ciliary body
     Posterior chamber
1   Eye, Left
     See Ø Eye, Right
	Ø Open
	3 Percutaneous
	7 Via Natural or Artificial Opening
	8 Via Natural or Artificial Opening
	     Endoscopic
		Ø Drainage Device
		3 Infusion Device
		7 Autologous Tissue Substitute
		C Extraluminal Device
		D Intraluminal Device
		J Synthetic Substitute
		K Nonautologous Tissue Substitute
		Y Other Device
			Z No Qualifier

Ø   Eye, Right
     Ciliary body
     Posterior chamber
1   Eye, Left
     See Ø Eye, Right
	X External	**Ø** Drainage Device
		3 Infusion Device
		7 Autologous Tissue Substitute
		C Extraluminal Device
		D Intraluminal Device
		J Synthetic Substitute
		K Nonautologous Tissue Substitute
			Z No Qualifier

J   Lens, Right
     Zonule of Zinn
K   Lens, Left
     See J Lens, Right
	3 Percutaneous	**J** Synthetic Substitute
		Y Other Device
			Z No Qualifier

J   Lens, Right
     Zonule of Zinn
K   Lens, Left
     See J Lens, Right
	X External	**J** Synthetic Substitute	**Z** No Qualifier

L   Extraocular Muscle, Right
     Inferior oblique muscle
     Inferior rectus muscle
     Lateral rectus muscle
     Medial rectus muscle
     Superior oblique muscle
     Superior rectus muscle
M   Extraocular Muscle, Left
     See L Extraocular Muscle, Right
	Ø Open
	3 Percutaneous
		Ø Drainage Device
		7 Autologous Tissue Substitute
		J Synthetic Substitute
		K Nonautologous Tissue Substitute
		Y Other Device
			Z No Qualifier

Non-OR	Ø8W[Ø,1][3,7,8]YZ
Non-OR	Ø8W[Ø,1]X[Ø,3,7,C,D,J,K]Z
Non-OR	Ø8W[J,K]3YZ
Non-OR	Ø8W[J,K]XJZ
Non-OR	Ø8W[L,M]3YZ

Ø   **Medical and Surgical**
8   **Eye**
X   **Transfer**   Definition: Moving, without taking out, all or a portion of a body part to another location to take over the function of all or a portion of a body part

Explanation: The body part transferred remains connected to its vascular and nervous supply

Body Part Character 4	Approach Character 5	Device Character 6	Qualifier Character 7

L   Extraocular Muscle, Right
     Inferior oblique muscle
     Inferior rectus muscle
     Lateral rectus muscle
     Medial rectus muscle
     Superior oblique muscle
     Superior rectus muscle
M   Extraocular Muscle, Left
     See L Extraocular Muscle, Right
	Ø Open
	3 Percutaneous
		Z No Device	**Z** No Qualifier

NC Noncovered Procedure   **LC** Limited Coverage   **QA** Questionable OB Admit   **NT** New Tech Add-on   ⊞ Combination Member   ♂ Male   ♀ Female

ICD-10-PCS 2024   317

Ear, Nose, Sinus Ø9Ø–Ø9W

Character Meanings*

This Character Meaning table is provided as a guide to assist the user in the identification of character members that may be found in this section of code tables. It **SHOULD NOT** be used to build a PCS code.

Operation–Character 3		Body Part–Character 4		Approach–Character 5		Device–Character 6		Qualifier–Character 7	
Ø	Alteration	Ø	External Ear, Right	Ø	Open	Ø	Drainage Device	Ø	Endolymphatic
1	Bypass	1	External Ear, Left	3	Percutaneous	1	Radioactive Element	X	Diagnostic
2	Change	2	External Ear, Bilateral	4	Percutaneous Endoscopic	4	Hearing Device, Bone Conduction	Z	No Qualifier
3	Control	3	External Auditory Canal, Right	7	Via Natural or Artificial Opening	5	Hearing Device, Single Channel Cochlear Prosthesis		
5	Destruction	4	External Auditory Canal, Left	8	Via Natural or Artificial Opening Endoscopic	6	Hearing Device, Multiple Channel Cochlear Prosthesis		
7	Dilation	5	Middle Ear, Right	X	External	7	Autologous Tissue Substitute		
8	Division	6	Middle Ear, Left			B	Intraluminal Device, Airway		
9	Drainage	7	Tympanic Membrane, Right			D	Intraluminal Device		
B	Excision	8	Tympanic Membrane, Left			J	Synthetic Substitute		
C	Extirpation	9	Auditory Ossicle, Right			K	Nonautologous Tissue Substitute		
D	Extraction	A	Auditory Ossicle, Left			S	Hearing Device		
H	Insertion	B	Mastoid Sinus, Right			Y	Other Device		
J	Inspection	C	Mastoid Sinus, Left			Z	No Device		
M	Reattachment	D	Inner Ear, Right						
N	Release	E	Inner Ear, Left						
P	Removal	F	Eustachian Tube, Right						
Q	Repair	G	Eustachian Tube, Left						
R	Replacement	H	Ear, Right						
S	Reposition	J	Ear, Left						
T	Resection	K	Nasal Mucosa and Soft Tissue						
U	Supplement	L	Nasal Turbinate						
W	Revision	M	Nasal Septum						
		N	Nasopharynx						
		P	Accessory Sinus						
		Q	Maxillary Sinus, Right						
		R	Maxillary Sinus, Left						
		S	Frontal Sinus, Right						
		T	Frontal Sinus, Left						
		U	Ethmoid Sinus, Right						
		V	Ethmoid Sinus, Left						
		W	Sphenoid Sinus, Right						
		X	Sphenoid Sinus, Left						
		Y	Sinus						

* Includes sinus ducts.

AHA Coding Clinic for table Ø93
2018, 4Q, 38   Control of epistaxis

AHA Coding Clinic for table Ø95
2018, 1Q, 19   Control of epistaxis via silver nitrate cauterization

AHA Coding Clinic for table Ø9B
2023, 2Q, 19   Sigmoid sinus dehiscence with mastoidectomy with resurfacing

AHA Coding Clinic for table Ø9H
2022, 2Q, 17   Congenital nasal pyriform aperture stenosis and repair
2020, 4Q, 43-44   Insertion of radioactive element

AHA Coding Clinic for table Ø9Q
2018, 1Q, 19   Control of epistaxis via silver nitrate cauterization
2017, 4Q, 106   Control of bleeding of external naris using suture
2014, 4Q, 20   Control of epistaxis
2014, 3Q, 22   Transsphenoidal removal of pituitary tumor and fat graft placement
2013, 4Q, 114   Balloon sinuplasty

AHA Coding Clinic for table Ø9U
2022, 1Q, 48   Repair of facial fractures of frontal sinus and orbital roof
2019, 4Q, 28-29   Sinus supplement

Ear, Nose, Sinus

Ear Anatomy

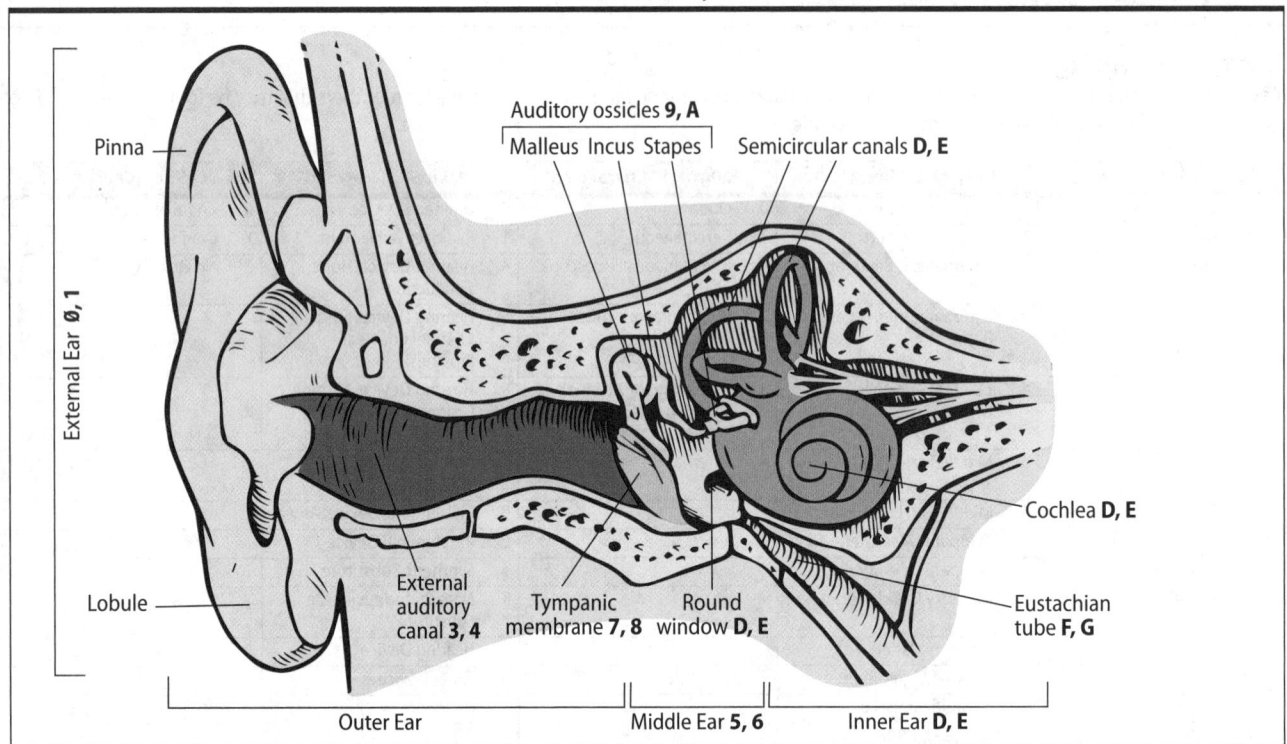

Pinna

External Ear **Ø, 1**

Lobule

Auditory ossicles **9, A**
Malleus Incus Stapes

Semicircular canals **D, E**

Cochlea **D, E**

External auditory canal **3, 4**

Tympanic membrane **7, 8**

Round window **D, E**

Eustachian tube **F, G**

Outer Ear

Middle Ear **5, 6**

Inner Ear **D, E**

Nasal Turbinates

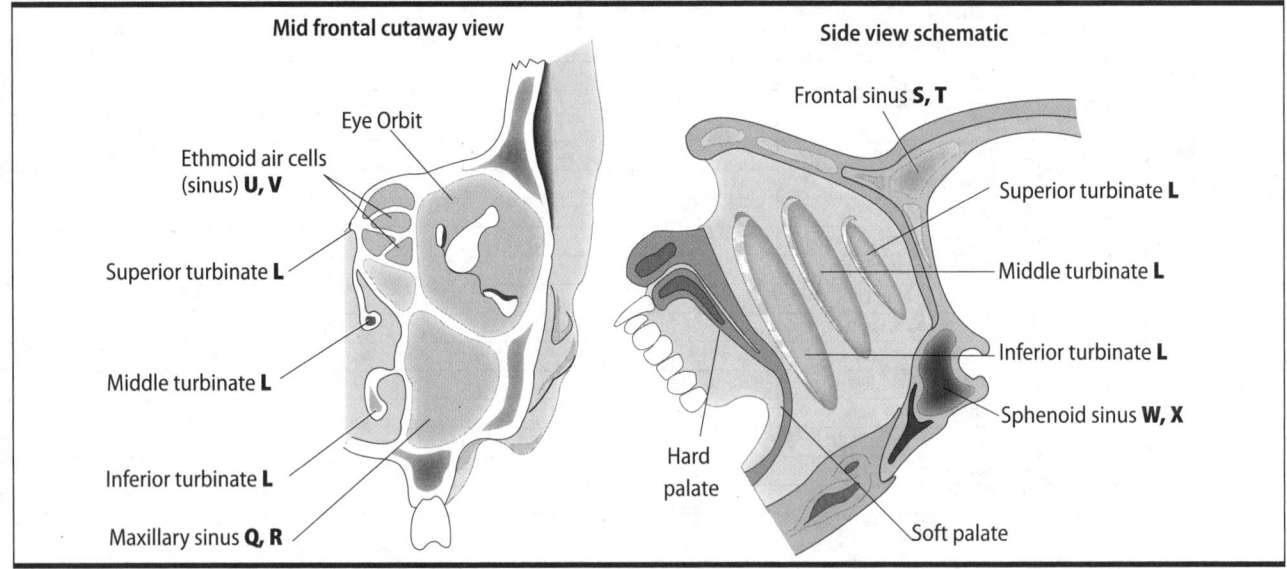

Mid frontal cutaway view

Eye Orbit

Ethmoid air cells (sinus) **U, V**

Superior turbinate **L**

Middle turbinate **L**

Inferior turbinate **L**

Maxillary sinus **Q, R**

Side view schematic

Frontal sinus **S, T**

Superior turbinate **L**

Middle turbinate **L**

Inferior turbinate **L**

Sphenoid sinus **W, X**

Hard palate

Soft palate

Paranasal Sinuses

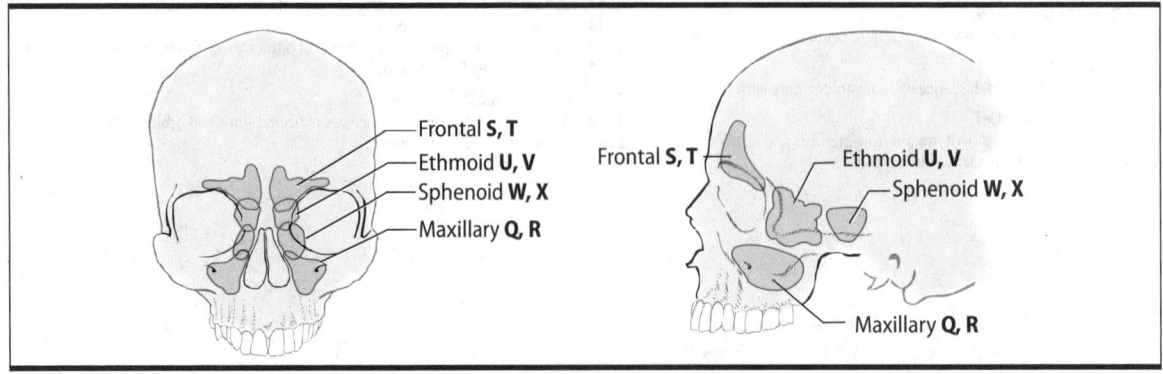

Frontal **S, T**
Ethmoid **U, V**
Sphenoid **W, X**
Maxillary **Q, R**

Frontal **S, T**
Ethmoid **U, V**
Sphenoid **W, X**
Maxillary **Q, R**

Ø Medical and Surgical
9 Ear, Nose, Sinus
Ø Alteration   Definition: Modifying the anatomic structure of a body part without affecting the function of the body part

Explanation: Principal purpose is to improve appearance

Body Part Character 4		Approach Character 5	Device Character 6	Qualifier Character 7
Ø External Ear, Right Antihelix Antitragus Auricle Earlobe Helix Pinna Tragus **1** External Ear, Left *See Ø External Ear, Right*	**2** External Ear, Bilateral *See Ø External Ear, Right* **K** Nasal Mucosa and Soft Tissue Columella External naris Greater alar cartilage Internal naris Lateral nasal cartilage Lesser alar cartilage Nasal cavity Nostril	**Ø** Open **3** Percutaneous **4** Percutaneous Endoscopic **X** External	**7** Autologous Tissue Substitute **J** Synthetic Substitute **K** Nonautologous Tissue Substitute **Z** No Device	**Z** No Qualifier

Ø Medical and Surgical
9 Ear, Nose, Sinus
1 Bypass   Definition: Altering the route of passage of the contents of a tubular body part

Explanation: Rerouting contents of a body part to a downstream area of the normal route, to a similar route and body part, or to an abnormal route and dissimilar body part. Includes one or more anastomoses, with or without the use of a device.

Body Part Character 4	Approach Character 5	Device Character 6	Qualifier Character 7
D Inner Ear, Right Bony labyrinth Bony vestibule Cochlea Round window Semicircular canal **E** Inner Ear, Left *See D Inner Ear, Right*	**Ø** Open	**7** Autologous Tissue Substitute **J** Synthetic Substitute **K** Nonautologous Tissue Substitute **Z** No Device	**Ø** Endolymphatic

Ø Medical and Surgical
9 Ear, Nose, Sinus
2 Change   Definition: Taking out or off a device from a body part and putting back an identical or similar device in or on the same body part without cutting or puncturing the skin or a mucous membrane

Explanation: All CHANGE procedures are coded using the approach EXTERNAL

Body Part Character 4	Approach Character 5	Device Character 6	Qualifier Character 7
H Ear, Right **J** Ear, Left **K** Nasal Mucosa and Soft Tissue Columella External naris Greater alar cartilage Internal naris Lateral nasal cartilage Lesser alar cartilage Nasal cavity Nostril **Y** Sinus	**X** External	**Ø** Drainage Device **Y** Other Device	**Z** No Qualifier

Non-OR   All body part, approach, device, and qualifier values

Ø Medical and Surgical
9 Ear, Nose, Sinus
3 Control   Definition: Stopping, or attempting to stop, postprocedural or other acute bleeding

Explanation: None

Body Part Character 4	Approach Character 5	Device Character 6	Qualifier Character 7
K Nasal Mucosa and Soft Tissue Columella External naris Greater alar cartilage Internal naris Lateral nasal cartilage Lesser alar cartilage Nasal cavity Nostril	**7** Via Natural or Artificial Opening **8** Via Natural or Artificial Opening Endoscopic	**Z** No Device	**Z** No Qualifier

Non-OR   Ø93K[7,8]ZZ

Ear, Nose, Sinus

Ø Medical and Surgical
9 Ear, Nose, Sinus
5 Destruction   Definition: Physical eradication of all or a portion of a body part by the direct use of energy, force, or a destructive agent
                 Explanation: None of the body part is physically taken out

Body Part Character 4		Approach Character 5	Device Character 6	Qualifier Character 7
Ø External Ear, Right Antihelix Antitragus Auricle Earlobe Helix Pinna Tragus	**1 External Ear, Left** *See Ø External Ear, Right*	**Ø** Open **3** Percutaneous **4** Percutaneous Endoscopic **X** External	**Z** No Device	**Z** No Qualifier
3 External Auditory Canal, Right External auditory meatus	**4 External Auditory Canal, Left** *See 3 External Auditory Canal, Right*	**Ø** Open **3** Percutaneous **4** Percutaneous Endoscopic **7** Via Natural or Artificial Opening **8** Via Natural or Artificial Opening Endoscopic **X** External	**Z** No Device	**Z** No Qualifier
5 Middle Ear, Right Oval window Tympanic cavity **6 Middle Ear, Left** *See 5 Middle Ear, Right* **9 Auditory Ossicle, Right** Incus Malleus Stapes **A Auditory Ossicle, Left** *See 9 Auditory Ossicle, Right*	**D Inner Ear, Right** Bony labyrinth Bony vestibule Cochlea Round window Semicircular canal **E Inner Ear, Left** *See D Inner Ear, Right*	**Ø** Open **8** Via Natural or Artificial Opening Endoscopic	**Z** No Device	**Z** No Qualifier
7 Tympanic Membrane, Right Pars flaccida **8 Tympanic Membrane, Left** *See 7 Tympanic Membrane, Right* **F Eustachian Tube, Right** Auditory tube Pharyngotympanic tube **G Eustachian Tube, Left** *See F Eustachian Tube, Right*	**L Nasal Turbinate** Inferior turbinate Middle turbinate Nasal concha Superior turbinate **N Nasopharynx** Choana Fossa of Rosenmuller Pharyngeal recess Rhinopharynx	**Ø** Open **3** Percutaneous **4** Percutaneous Endoscopic **7** Via Natural or Artificial Opening **8** Via Natural or Artificial Opening Endoscopic	**Z** No Device	**Z** No Qualifier
B Mastoid Sinus, Right Mastoid air cells **C Mastoid Sinus, Left** *See B Mastoid Sinus, Right* **M Nasal Septum** Quadrangular cartilage Septal cartilage Vomer bone **P Accessory Sinus** **Q Maxillary Sinus, Right** Antrum of Highmore	**R Maxillary Sinus, Left** *See Q Maxillary Sinus, Right* **S Frontal Sinus, Right** **T Frontal Sinus, Left** **U Ethmoid Sinus, Right** Ethmoidal air cell **V Ethmoid Sinus, Left** *See U Ethmoid Sinus, Right* **W Sphenoid Sinus, Right** **X Sphenoid Sinus, Left**	**Ø** Open **3** Percutaneous **4** Percutaneous Endoscopic **8** Via Natural or Artificial Opening Endoscopic	**Z** No Device	**Z** No Qualifier
K Nasal Mucosa and Soft Tissue Columella External naris Greater alar cartilage Internal naris Lateral nasal cartilage Lesser alar cartilage Nasal cavity Nostril		**Ø** Open **3** Percutaneous **4** Percutaneous Endoscopic **8** Via Natural or Artificial Opening Endoscopic **X** External	**Z** No Device	**Z** No Qualifier

Non-OR	Ø95[Ø,1][Ø,3,4,X]ZZ
Non-OR	Ø95[3,4][Ø,3,4,7,8,X]ZZ
Non-OR	Ø95[F,G][Ø,3,4,7,8]ZZ
Non-OR	Ø95M[Ø,3,4,8]ZZ
Non-OR	Ø95K[Ø,3,4,8,X]ZZ

Non-OR Procedure   DRG Non-OR Procedure   Valid OR Procedure   HAC Associated Procedure   Combination Only   New/Revised April   New/Revised October

Ø   **Medical and Surgical**
9   **Ear, Nose, Sinus**
7   **Dilation**   Definition: Expanding an orifice or the lumen of a tubular body part

Explanation: The orifice can be a natural orifice or an artificially created orifice. Accomplished by stretching a tubular body part using intraluminal pressure or by cutting part of the orifice or wall of the tubular body part.

Body Part Character 4	Approach Character 5	Device Character 6	Qualifier Character 7
F Eustachian Tube, Right Auditory tube Pharyngotympanic tube **G** Eustachian Tube, Left *See F Eustachian Tube, Right*	**Ø** Open **7** Via Natural or Artificial Opening **8** Via Natural or Artificial Opening Endoscopic	**D** Intraluminal Device **Z** No Device	**Z** No Qualifier
F Eustachian Tube, Right Auditory tube Pharyngotympanic tube **G** Eustachian Tube, Left *See F Eustachian Tube, Right*	**3** Percutaneous **4** Percutaneous Endoscopic	**Z** No Device	**Z** No Qualifier

Non-OR   All body part, approach, device, and qualifier values

Ø   **Medical and Surgical**
9   **Ear, Nose, Sinus**
8   **Division**   Definition: Cutting into a body part, without draining fluids and/or gases from the body part, in order to separate or transect a body part

Explanation: All or a portion of the body part is separated into two or more portions

Body Part Character 4	Approach Character 5	Device Character 6	Qualifier Character 7
L Nasal Turbinate Inferior turbinate Middle turbinate Nasal concha Superior turbinate	**Ø** Open **3** Percutaneous **4** Percutaneous Endoscopic **7** Via Natural or Artificial Opening **8** Via Natural or Artificial Opening Endoscopic	**Z** No Device	**Z** No Qualifier

NC Noncovered Procedure   **LC** Limited Coverage   **QA** Questionable OB Admit   **NT** New Tech Add-on   ⊞ Combination Member   ♂ Male   ♀ Female

ICD-10-PCS 2024   323

Ear, Nose, Sinus

Ø Medical and Surgical
9 Ear, Nose, Sinus
9 Drainage   Definition: Taking or letting out fluids and/or gases from a body part
                Explanation: The qualifier DIAGNOSTIC is used to identify drainage procedures that are biopsies

Body Part Character 4		Approach Character 5	Device Character 6	Qualifier Character 7
Ø External Ear, Right Antihelix Antitragus Auricle Earlobe Helix Pinna Tragus	1 External Ear, Left *See Ø External Ear, Right*	Ø Open 3 Percutaneous 4 Percutaneous Endoscopic X External	Ø Drainage Device	Z No Qualifier
Ø External Ear, Right Antihelix Antitragus Auricle Earlobe Helix Pinna Tragus	1 External Ear, Left *See Ø External Ear, Right*	Ø Open 3 Percutaneous 4 Percutaneous Endoscopic X External	Z No Device	X Diagnostic Z No Qualifier
3 External Auditory Canal, Right External auditory meatus 4 External Auditory Canal, Left *See 3 External Auditory Canal, Right*	K Nasal Mucosa and Soft Tissue Columella External naris Greater alar cartilage Internal naris Lateral nasal cartilage Lesser alar cartilage Nasal cavity Nostril	Ø Open 3 Percutaneous 4 Percutaneous Endoscopic 7 Via Natural or Artificial Opening 8 Via Natural or Artificial Opening Endoscopic X External	Ø Drainage Device	Z No Qualifier
3 External Auditory Canal, Right External auditory meatus 4 External Auditory Canal, Left *See 3 External Auditory Canal, Right*	K Nasal Mucosa and Soft Tissue Columella External naris Greater alar cartilage Internal naris Lateral nasal cartilage Lesser alar cartilage Nasal cavity Nostril	Ø Open 3 Percutaneous 4 Percutaneous Endoscopic 7 Via Natural or Artificial Opening 8 Via Natural or Artificial Opening Endoscopic X External	Z No Device	X Diagnostic Z No Qualifier
5 Middle Ear, Right Oval window Tympanic cavity 6 Middle Ear, Left *See 5 Middle Ear, Right* 9 Auditory Ossicle, Right Incus Malleus Stapes	A Auditory Ossicle, Left *See 9 Auditory Ossicle, Right* D Inner Ear, Right Bony labyrinth Bony vestibule Cochlea Round window Semicircular canal E Inner Ear, Left *See D Inner Ear, Right*	Ø Open 7 Via Natural or Artificial Opening 8 Via Natural or Artificial Opening Endoscopic	Ø Drainage Device	Z No Qualifier
5 Middle Ear, Right Oval window Tympanic cavity 6 Middle Ear, Left *See 5 Middle Ear, Right* 9 Auditory Ossicle, Right Incus Malleus Stapes	A Auditory Ossicle, Left *See 9 Auditory Ossicle, Right* D Inner Ear, Right Bony labyrinth Bony vestibule Cochlea Round window Semicircular canal E Inner Ear, Left *See D Inner Ear, Right*	Ø Open 7 Via Natural or Artificial Opening 8 Via Natural or Artificial Opening Endoscopic	Z No Device	X Diagnostic Z No Qualifier

Non-OR   Ø99[Ø,1][Ø,3,4,X]ØZ
Non-OR   Ø99[Ø,1][Ø,3,4,X]Z[X,Z]
Non-OR   Ø99[3,4,K][Ø,3,4,7,8,X]ØZ
Non-OR   Ø99[3,4,K][Ø,3,4,7,8,X]Z[X,Z]
Non-OR   Ø99[5,6]8ØZ
Non-OR   Ø99[9,A,D,E][7,8]ØZ
Non-OR   Ø99[5,6]ØZZ
Non-OR   Ø99[5,6,9,A,D,E][7,8]Z[X,Z]

Ø99 Continued on next page

Non-OR Procedure   DRG Non-OR Procedure   Valid OR Procedure   HAC Associated Procedure   Combination Only   New/Revised April   New/Revised October

Ø Medical and Surgical
9 Ear, Nose, Sinus
9 Drainage   Definition: Taking or letting out fluids and/or gases from a body part

Ø99 Continued

Explanation: The qualifier DIAGNOSTIC is used to identify drainage procedures that are biopsies

Body Part Character 4		Approach Character 5	Device Character 6	Qualifier Character 7
7 Tympanic Membrane, Right Pars flaccida **8 Tympanic Membrane, Left** *See 7 Tympanic Membrane, Right* **B Mastoid Sinus, Right** Mastoid air cells **C Mastoid Sinus, Left** *See B Mastoid Sinus, Right* **F Eustachian Tube, Right** Auditory tube Pharyngotympanic tube **G Eustachian Tube, Left** *See F Eustachian Tube, Right* **L Nasal Turbinate** Inferior turbinate Middle turbinate Nasal concha Superior turbinate **M Nasal Septum** Quadrangular cartilage Septal cartilage Vomer bone	**N Nasopharynx** Choana Fossa of Rosenmuller Pharyngeal recess Rhinopharynx **P Accessory Sinus** **Q Maxillary Sinus, Right** Antrum of Highmore **R Maxillary Sinus, Left** *See Q Maxillary Sinus, Right* **S Frontal Sinus, Right** **T Frontal Sinus, Left** **U Ethmoid Sinus, Right** Ethmoidal air cell **V Ethmoid Sinus, Left** *See U Ethmoid Sinus, Right* **W Sphenoid Sinus, Right** **X Sphenoid Sinus, Left**	**Ø Open** **3 Percutaneous** **4 Percutaneous Endoscopic** **7 Via Natural or Artificial Opening** **8 Via Natural or Artificial Opening Endoscopic**	**Ø Drainage Device**	**Z No Qualifier**
7 Tympanic Membrane, Right Pars flaccida **8 Tympanic Membrane, Left** *See 7 Tympanic Membrane, Right* **B Mastoid Sinus, Right** Mastoid air cells **C Mastoid Sinus, Left** *See B Mastoid Sinus, Right* **F Eustachian Tube, Right** Auditory tube Pharyngotympanic tube **G Eustachian Tube, Left** *See F Eustachian Tube, Right* **L Nasal Turbinate** Inferior turbinate Middle turbinate Nasal concha Superior turbinate **M Nasal Septum** Quadrangular cartilage Septal cartilage Vomer bone	**N Nasopharynx** Choana Fossa of Rosenmuller Pharyngeal recess Rhinopharynx **P Accessory Sinus** **Q Maxillary Sinus, Right** Antrum of Highmore **R Maxillary Sinus, Left** *See Q Maxillary Sinus, Right* **S Frontal Sinus, Right** **T Frontal Sinus, Left** **U Ethmoid Sinus, Right** Ethmoidal air cell **V Ethmoid Sinus, Left** *See U Ethmoid Sinus, Right* **W Sphenoid Sinus, Right** **X Sphenoid Sinus, Left**	**Ø Open** **3 Percutaneous** **4 Percutaneous Endoscopic** **7 Via Natural or Artificial Opening** **8 Via Natural or Artificial Opening Endoscopic**	**Z No Device**	**X Diagnostic** **Z No Qualifier**

Non-OR	Ø99[B,C][3,7,8]ØZ
Non-OR	Ø99[F,G,L,M][Ø,3,4,7,8]ØZ
Non-OR	Ø99N3ØZ
Non-OR	Ø99[P,Q,R,S,T,U,V,W,X][3,4,7,8]ØZ
Non-OR	Ø99[7,8][Ø,3,4,7,8]ZZ
Non-OR	Ø99[7,8][7,8]ZX
Non-OR	Ø99[B,C]3ZZ
Non-OR	Ø99[B,C][7,8]Z[X,Z]
Non-OR	Ø99[F,G][Ø,3,4,7,8]ZZ
Non-OR	Ø99[F,G][7,8]ZX
Non-OR	Ø99[L,M][Ø,3,4,7,8]Z[X,Z]
Non-OR	Ø99N[Ø,3,4,7,8]ZX
Non-OR	Ø99N3ZZ
Non-OR	Ø99[P,Q,R,S,T,U,V,W,X][3,4,7,8]Z[X,Z]

NC Noncovered Procedure   LC Limited Coverage   QA Questionable OB Admit   NT New Tech Add-on   ⊞ Combination Member   ♂ Male   ♀ Female

ICD-10-PCS 2024   325

Ø   **Medical and Surgical**
9   **Ear, Nose, Sinus**
B   **Excision**   Definition: Cutting out or off, without replacement, a portion of a body part
                    Explanation: The qualifier DIAGNOSTIC is used to identify excision procedures that are biopsies

Body Part Character 4		Approach Character 5	Device Character 6	Qualifier Character 7
Ø External Ear, Right Antihelix Antitragus Auricle Earlobe Helix Pinna Tragus	**1 External Ear, Left** *See Ø External Ear, Right*	**Ø** Open **3** Percutaneous **4** Percutaneous Endoscopic **X** External	**Z** No Device	**X** Diagnostic **Z** No Qualifier
3 External Auditory Canal, Right External auditory meatus	**4 External Auditory Canal, Left** *See 3 External Auditory Canal, Right*	**Ø** Open **3** Percutaneous **4** Percutaneous Endoscopic **7** Via Natural or Artificial Opening **8** Via Natural or Artificial Opening Endoscopic **X** External	**Z** No Device	**X** Diagnostic **Z** No Qualifier
5 Middle Ear, Right Oval window Tympanic cavity **6 Middle Ear, Left** *See 5 Middle Ear, Right* **9 Auditory Ossicle, Right** Incus Malleus Stapes	**A Auditory Ossicle, Left** *See 9 Auditory Ossicle, Right* **D Inner Ear, Right** Bony labyrinth Bony vestibule Cochlea Round window Semicircular canal **E Inner Ear, Left** *See D Inner Ear, Right*	**Ø** Open **8** Via Natural or Artificial Opening Endoscopic	**Z** No Device	**X** Diagnostic **Z** No Qualifier
7 Tympanic Membrane, Right Pars flaccida **8 Tympanic Membrane, Left** *See 7 Tympanic Membrane, Right* **F Eustachian Tube, Right** Auditory tube Pharyngotympanic tube **G Eustachian Tube, Left** *See F Eustachian Tube, Right*	**L Nasal Turbinate** Inferior turbinate Middle turbinate Nasal concha Superior turbinate **N Nasopharynx** Choana Fossa of Rosenmuller Pharyngeal recess Rhinopharynx	**Ø** Open **3** Percutaneous **4** Percutaneous Endoscopic **7** Via Natural or Artificial Opening **8** Via Natural or Artificial Opening Endoscopic	**Z** No Device	**X** Diagnostic **Z** No Qualifier
B Mastoid Sinus, Right Mastoid air cells **C Mastoid Sinus, Left** *See B Mastoid Sinus, Right* **M Nasal Septum** Quadrangular cartilage Septal cartilage Vomer bone **P Accessory Sinus** **Q Maxillary Sinus, Right** Antrum of Highmore	**R Maxillary Sinus, Left** *See Q Maxillary Sinus, Right* **S Frontal Sinus, Right** **T Frontal Sinus, Left** **U Ethmoid Sinus, Right** Ethmoidal air cell **V Ethmoid Sinus, Left** *See U Ethmoid Sinus, Right* **W Sphenoid Sinus, Right** **X Sphenoid Sinus, Left**	**Ø** Open **3** Percutaneous **4** Percutaneous Endoscopic **8** Via Natural or Artificial Opening Endoscopic	**Z** No Device	**X** Diagnostic **Z** No Qualifier
K Nasal Mucosa and Soft Tissue Columella External naris Greater alar cartilage Internal naris Lateral nasal cartilage Lesser alar cartilage Nasal cavity Nostril		**Ø** Open **3** Percutaneous **4** Percutaneous Endoscopic **8** Via Natural or Artificial Opening Endoscopic **X** External	**Z** No Device	**X** Diagnostic **Z** No Qualifier

Non-OR   09B[Ø,1][Ø,3,4,X]Z[X,Z]
Non-OR   09B[3,4][Ø,3,4,7,8,X]Z[X,Z]
Non-OR   09B[F,G,L,N][Ø,3,4,7,8]Z[X,Z]
Non-OR   09BM[Ø,3,4,8]ZX
Non-OR   09B[P,Q,R,S,T,U,V,W,X][3,4,8]ZX
Non-OR   09BK8Z[X,Z]

Non-OR Procedure   DRG Non-OR Procedure   Valid OR Procedure   HAC Associated Procedure   Combination Only   New/Revised April   New/Revised October

Ø   Medical and Surgical
9   Ear, Nose, Sinus
C   Extirpation   Definition: Taking or cutting out solid matter from a body part

Explanation: The solid matter may be an abnormal byproduct of a biological function or a foreign body; it may be imbedded in a body part or in the lumen of a tubular body part. The solid matter may or may not have been previously broken into pieces.

Body Part Character 4		Approach Character 5	Device Character 6	Qualifier Character 7
Ø External Ear, Right Antihelix Antitragus Auricle Earlobe Helix Pinna Tragus	**1 External Ear, Left** *See Ø External Ear, Right*	**Ø** Open **3** Percutaneous **4** Percutaneous Endoscopic **X** External	**Z** No Device	**Z** No Qualifier
3 External Auditory Canal, Right External auditory meatus	**4 External Auditory Canal, Left** *See 3 External Auditory Canal, Right*	**Ø** Open **3** Percutaneous **4** Percutaneous Endoscopic **7** Via Natural or Artificial Opening **8** Via Natural or Artificial Opening Endoscopic **X** External	**Z** No Device	**Z** No Qualifier
5 Middle Ear, Right Oval window Tympanic cavity **6 Middle Ear, Left** *See 5 Middle Ear, Right* **9 Auditory Ossicle, Right** Incus Malleus Stapes	**A Auditory Ossicle, Left** *See 9 Auditory Ossicle, Right* **D Inner Ear, Right** Bony labyrinth Bony vestibule Cochlea Round window Semicircular canal **E Inner Ear, Left** *See D Inner Ear, Right*	**Ø** Open **8** Via Natural or Artificial Opening Endoscopic	**Z** No Device	**Z** No Qualifier
7 Tympanic Membrane, Right Pars flaccida **8 Tympanic Membrane, Left** *See 7 Tympanic Membrane, Right* **F Eustachian Tube, Right** Auditory tube Pharyngotympanic tube **G Eustachian Tube, Left** *See F Eustachian Tube, Right*	**L Nasal Turbinate** Inferior turbinate Middle turbinate Nasal concha Superior turbinate **N Nasopharynx** Choana Fossa of Rosenmuller Pharyngeal recess Rhinopharynx	**Ø** Open **3** Percutaneous **4** Percutaneous Endoscopic **7** Via Natural or Artificial Opening **8** Via Natural or Artificial Opening Endoscopic	**Z** No Device	**Z** No Qualifier
B Mastoid Sinus, Right Mastoid air cells **C Mastoid Sinus, Left** *See B Mastoid Sinus, Right* **M Nasal Septum** Quadrangular cartilage Septal cartilage Vomer bone **P Accessory Sinus** **Q Maxillary Sinus, Right** Antrum of Highmore	**R Maxillary Sinus, Left** *See Q Maxillary Sinus, Right* **S Frontal Sinus, Right** **T Frontal Sinus, Left** **U Ethmoid Sinus, Right** Ethmoidal air cell **V Ethmoid Sinus, Left** *See U Ethmoid Sinus, Right* **W Sphenoid Sinus, Right** **X Sphenoid Sinus, Left**	**Ø** Open **3** Percutaneous **4** Percutaneous Endoscopic **8** Via Natural or Artificial Opening Endoscopic	**Z** No Device	**Z** No Qualifier
K Nasal Mucosa and Soft Tissue Columella External naris Greater alar cartilage Internal naris Lateral nasal cartilage Lesser alar cartilage Nasal cavity Nostril		**Ø** Open **3** Percutaneous **4** Percutaneous Endoscopic **8** Via Natural or Artificial Opening Endoscopic **X** External	**Z** No Device	**Z** No Qualifier

Non-OR   Ø9C[Ø,1][Ø,3,4,X]ZZ
Non-OR   Ø9C[3,4][Ø,3,4,7,8,X]ZZ
Non-OR   Ø9C[7,8,F,G,L][Ø,3,4,7,8]ZZ
Non-OR   Ø9CM[Ø,3,4,8]ZZ
Non-OR   Ø9CK8ZZ

NC Noncovered Procedure   **LC** Limited Coverage   **QA** Questionable OB Admit   **NT** New Tech Add-on   ⊞ Combination Member   ♂ Male   ♀ Female

ICD-10-PCS 2024   327

Ø   **Medical and Surgical**
9   **Ear, Nose, Sinus**
D   **Extraction**   Definition: Pulling or stripping out or off all or a portion of a body part by the use of force

Explanation: The qualifier DIAGNOSTIC is used to identify extraction procedures that are biopsies

Body Part Character 4	Approach Character 5	Device Character 6	Qualifier Character 7

7   **Tympanic Membrane, Right**
   Pars flaccida
8   **Tympanic Membrane, Left**
   See 7 Tympanic Membrane, Right
L   **Nasal Turbinate**
   Inferior turbinate
   Middle turbinate
   Nasal concha
   Superior turbinate
	Ø Open
	3 Percutaneous
	4 Percutaneous Endoscopic
	7 Via Natural or Artificial Opening
	8 Via Natural or Artificial Opening
	    Endoscopic
		Z No Device	**Z** No Qualifier

9   **Auditory Ossicle, Right**
   Incus
   Malleus
   Stapes
A   **Auditory Ossicle, Left**
   See 9 Auditory Ossicle, Right
	Ø Open	**Z** No Device	**Z** No Qualifier

B   **Mastoid Sinus, Right**
   Mastoid air cells
C   **Mastoid Sinus, Left**
   See B Mastoid Sinus, Right
M   **Nasal Septum**
   Quadrangular cartilage
   Septal cartilage
   Vomer bone
P   **Accessory Sinus**
Q   **Maxillary Sinus, Right**
   Antrum of Highmore
R   **Maxillary Sinus, Left**
   See Q Maxillary Sinus, Right
S   **Frontal Sinus, Right**
T   **Frontal Sinus, Left**
U   **Ethmoid Sinus, Right**
   Ethmoidal air cell
V   **Ethmoid Sinus, Left**
   See U Ethmoid Sinus, Right
W   **Sphenoid Sinus, Right**
X   **Sphenoid Sinus, Left**
	Ø Open
	3 Percutaneous
	4 Percutaneous Endoscopic
		Z No Device	**Z** No Qualifier

Ø   **Medical and Surgical**
9   **Ear, Nose, Sinus**
H   **Insertion**   Definition: Putting in a nonbiological appliance that monitors, assists, performs, or prevents a physiological function but does not physically take the place of a body part

Explanation: None

Body Part Character 4	Approach Character 5	Device Character 6	Qualifier Character 7

D   **Inner Ear, Right**
   Bony labyrinth
   Bony vestibule
   Cochlea
   Round window
   Semicircular canal
E   **Inner Ear, Left**
   See D Inner Ear, Right
	Ø Open
	3 Percutaneous
	4 Percutaneous Endoscopic
		1 Radioactive Element
		4 Hearing Device, Bone Conduction
		5 Hearing Device, Single Channel
		    Cochlear Prosthesis
		6 Hearing Device, Multiple Channel
		    Cochlear Prosthesis
		S Hearing Device
			Z No Qualifier

H   **Ear, Right**
J   **Ear, Left**
K   **Nasal Mucosa and Soft Tissue**
   Columella
   External naris
   Greater alar cartilage
   Internal naris
   Lateral nasal cartilage
   Lesser alar cartilage
   Nasal cavity
   Nostril
Y   **Sinus**
	Ø Open
	3 Percutaneous
	4 Percutaneous Endoscopic
	7 Via Natural or Artificial Opening
	8 Via Natural or Artificial Opening
	    Endoscopic
		1 Radioactive Element
		Y Other Device
			Z No Qualifier

N   **Nasopharynx**
   Choana
   Fossa of Rosenmuller
   Pharyngeal recess
   Rhinopharynx
	7 Via Natural or Artificial Opening
	8 Via Natural or Artificial Opening
	    Endoscopic
		1 Radioactive Element
		B Intraluminal Device, Airway
			Z No Qualifier

Non-OR   Ø9H[H,J,K]Ø1Z
Non-OR   Ø9HKØYZ

Non-OR   Ø9H[H,J,K,Y][3,4,7,8][1,Y]Z
Non-OR   Ø9HN[7,8][1,B]Z

Non-OR Procedure   DRG Non-OR Procedure   Valid OR Procedure   HAC Associated Procedure   Combination Only   New/Revised April   New/Revised October

Ø   Medical and Surgical
9   Ear, Nose, Sinus
J   Inspection   Definition: Visually and/or manually exploring a body part

Explanation: Visual exploration may be performed with or without optical instrumentation. Manual exploration may be performed directly or through intervening body layers.

Body Part Character 4	Approach Character 5	Device Character 6	Qualifier Character 7

7 Tympanic Membrane, Right
   Pars flaccida
8 Tympanic Membrane, Left
   See 7 Tympanic Membrane, Right
H Ear, Right
J Ear, Left
	Ø Open
	3 Percutaneous
	4 Percutaneous Endoscopic
	7 Via Natural or Artificial Opening
	8 Via Natural or Artificial Opening
	   Endoscopic
	X External
		Z No Device	**Z** No Qualifier

D Inner Ear, Right
   Bony labyrinth
   Bony vestibule
   Cochlea
   Round window
   Semicircular canal
E Inner Ear, Left
   See D Inner Ear, Right
K Nasal Mucosa and Soft Tissue
   Columella
   External naris
   Greater alar cartilage
   Internal naris
   Lateral nasal cartilage
   Lesser alar cartilage
   Nasal cavity
   Nostril
Y Sinus
	Ø Open
	3 Percutaneous
	4 Percutaneous Endoscopic
	8 Via Natural or Artificial Opening
	   Endoscopic
	X External
		Z No Device	**Z** No Qualifier

Non-OR	Ø9J[7,8][3,7,8,X]ZZ
Non-OR	Ø9J[H,J][Ø,3,4,7,8,X]ZZ
Non-OR	Ø9J[D,E][3,8,X]ZZ
Non-OR	Ø9J[K,Y][Ø,3,4,8,X]ZZ

Ø   Medical and Surgical
9   Ear, Nose, Sinus
M   Reattachment   Definition: Putting back in or on all or a portion of a separated body part to its normal location or other suitable location

Explanation: Vascular circulation and nervous pathways may or may not be reestablished

Body Part Character 4	Approach Character 5	Device Character 6	Qualifier Character 7

Ø External Ear, Right
   Antihelix
   Antitragus
   Auricle
   Earlobe
   Helix
   Pinna
   Tragus
1 External Ear, Left
   See Ø External Ear, Right
K Nasal Mucosa and Soft Tissue
   Columella
   External naris
   Greater alar cartilage
   Internal naris
   Lateral nasal cartilage
   Lesser alar cartilage
   Nasal cavity
   Nostril
	X External	**Z** No Device	**Z** No Qualifier

NC Noncovered Procedure   **LC** Limited Coverage   **QA** Questionable OB Admit   **NT** New Tech Add-on   ⊞ Combination Member   ♂ Male   ♀ Female

ICD-10-PCS 2024   329

Ear, Nose, Sinus

Ø   **Medical and Surgical**
9   **Ear, Nose, Sinus**
N   **Release**   Definition: Freeing a body part from an abnormal physical constraint by cutting or by the use of force

Explanation: Some of the restraining tissue may be taken out but none of the body part is taken out

Body Part Character 4		Approach Character 5	Device Character 6	Qualifier Character 7
Ø External Ear, Right Antihelix Antitragus Auricle Earlobe Helix Pinna Tragus	**1 External Ear, Left** *See Ø External Ear, Right*	**Ø** Open **3** Percutaneous **4** Percutaneous Endoscopic **X** External	**Z** No Device	**Z** No Qualifier
3 External Auditory Canal, Right External auditory meatus	**4 External Auditory Canal, Left** *See 3 External Auditory Canal, Right*	**Ø** Open **3** Percutaneous **4** Percutaneous Endoscopic **7** Via Natural or Artificial Opening **8** Via Natural or Artificial Opening Endoscopic **X** External	**Z** No Device	**Z** No Qualifier
5 Middle Ear, Right Oval window Tympanic cavity **6 Middle Ear, Left** *See 5 Middle Ear, Right* **9 Auditory Ossicle, Right** Incus Malleus Stapes	**A Auditory Ossicle, Left** *See 9 Auditory Ossicle, Right* **D Inner Ear, Right** Bony labyrinth Bony vestibule Cochlea Round window Semicircular canal **E Inner Ear, Left** *See D Inner Ear, Right*	**Ø** Open **8** Via Natural or Artificial Opening Endoscopic	**Z** No Device	**Z** No Qualifier
7 Tympanic Membrane, Right Pars flaccida **8 Tympanic Membrane, Left** *See 7 Tympanic Membrane, Right* **F Eustachian Tube, Right** Auditory tube Pharyngotympanic tube **G Eustachian Tube, Left** *See F Eustachian Tube, Right*	**L Nasal Turbinate** Inferior turbinate Middle turbinate Nasal concha Superior turbinate **N Nasopharynx** Choana Fossa of Rosenmuller Pharyngeal recess Rhinopharynx	**Ø** Open **3** Percutaneous **4** Percutaneous Endoscopic **7** Via Natural or Artificial Opening **8** Via Natural or Artificial Opening Endoscopic	**Z** No Device	**Z** No Qualifier
B Mastoid Sinus, Right Mastoid air cells **C Mastoid Sinus, Left** *See B Mastoid Sinus, Right* **M Nasal Septum** Quadrangular cartilage Septal cartilage Vomer bone **P Accessory Sinus** **Q Maxillary Sinus, Right** Antrum of Highmore	**R Maxillary Sinus, Left** *See Q Maxillary Sinus, Right* **S Frontal Sinus, Right** **T Frontal Sinus, Left** **U Ethmoid Sinus, Right** Ethmoidal air cell **V Ethmoid Sinus, Left** *See U Ethmoid Sinus, Right* **W Sphenoid Sinus, Right** **X Sphenoid Sinus, Left**	**Ø** Open **3** Percutaneous **4** Percutaneous Endoscopic **8** Via Natural or Artificial Opening Endoscopic	**Z** No Device	**Z** No Qualifier
K Nasal Mucosa and Soft Tissue Columella External naris Greater alar cartilage Internal naris Lateral nasal cartilage Lesser alar cartilage Nasal cavity Nostril		**Ø** Open **3** Percutaneous **4** Percutaneous Endoscopic **8** Via Natural or Artificial Opening Endoscopic **X** External	**Z** No Device	**Z** No Qualifier

Non-OR   Ø9N[Ø,1]XZZ
Non-OR   Ø9N[3,4]XZZ
Non-OR   Ø9N[F,G,L][Ø,3,4,7,8]ZZ
Non-OR   Ø9NM[Ø,3,4,8]ZZ
Non-OR   Ø9NK[Ø,3,4,8,X]ZZ

0   **Medical and Surgical**
9   **Ear, Nose, Sinus**
P   **Removal**   Definition: Taking out or off a device from a body part

Explanation: If a device is taken out and a similar device put in without cutting or puncturing the skin or mucous membrane, the procedure is coded to the root operation CHANGE. Otherwise, the procedure for taking out a device is coded to the root operation REMOVAL.

Body Part Character 4	Approach Character 5	Device Character 6	Qualifier Character 7
7 **Tympanic Membrane, Right** Pars flaccida **8** **Tympanic Membrane, Left** *See 7 Tympanic Membrane, Right*	**0** Open **7** Via Natural or Artificial Opening **8** Via Natural or Artificial Opening Endoscopic **X** External	**0** Drainage Device	**Z** No Qualifier
D **Inner Ear, Right** Bony labyrinth Bony vestibule Cochlea Round window Semicircular canal **E** **Inner Ear, Left** *See D Inner Ear, Right*	**0** Open **7** Via Natural or Artificial Opening **8** Via Natural or Artificial Opening Endoscopic	**S** Hearing Device	**Z** No Qualifier
H **Ear, Right** **J** **Ear, Left** **K** **Nasal Mucosa and Soft Tissue** Columella External naris Greater alar cartilage Internal naris Lateral nasal cartilage Lesser alar cartilage Nasal cavity Nostril	**0** Open **3** Percutaneous **4** Percutaneous Endoscopic **7** Via Natural or Artificial Opening **8** Via Natural or Artificial Opening Endoscopic	**0** Drainage Device **7** Autologous Tissue Substitute **D** Intraluminal Device **J** Synthetic Substitute **K** Nonautologous Tissue Substitute **Y** Other Device	**Z** No Qualifier
H **Ear, Right** **J** **Ear, Left** **K** **Nasal Mucosa and Soft Tissue** Columella External naris Greater alar cartilage Internal naris Lateral nasal cartilage Lesser alar cartilage Nasal cavity Nostril	**X** External	**0** Drainage Device **7** Autologous Tissue Substitute **D** Intraluminal Device **J** Synthetic Substitute **K** Nonautologous Tissue Substitute	**Z** No Qualifier
Y **Sinus**	**0** Open **3** Percutaneous **4** Percutaneous Endoscopic	**0** Drainage Device **Y** Other Device	**Z** No Qualifier
Y **Sinus**	**7** Via Natural or Artificial Opening **8** Via Natural or Artificial Opening Endoscopic	**Y** Other Device	**Z** No Qualifier
Y **Sinus**	**X** External	**0** Drainage Device	**Z** No Qualifier

Non-OR   09P[7,8][0,7,8,X]0Z
Non-OR   09P[H,J][3,4][0,J,K,Y]Z
Non-OR   09P[H,J][7,8][0,D,Y]Z
Non-OR   09PK[0,3,4,7,8][0,7,D,J,K,Y]Z
Non-OR   09P[H,J]X[0,7,D,J,K]Z
Non-OR   09PKX[0,7,D,J,K]Z
Non-OR   09PY[3,4]YZ
Non-OR   09PY[7,8]YZ
Non-OR   09PYX0Z

NC Noncovered Procedure   **LC** Limited Coverage   **QA** Questionable OB Admit   **NT** New Tech Add-on   ⊞ Combination Member   ♂ Male   ♀ Female

ICD-10-PCS 2024   331

09P–09P

Ear, Nose, Sinus

Ø   **Medical and Surgical**
9   **Ear, Nose, Sinus**
Q   **Repair**   Definition: Restoring, to the extent possible, a body part to its normal anatomic structure and function
                     Explanation: Used only when the method to accomplish the repair is not one of the other root operations

Body Part Character 4		Approach Character 5	Device Character 6	Qualifier Character 7

Ø **External Ear, Right**
  Antihelix
  Antitragus
  Auricle
  Earlobe
  Helix
  Pinna
  Tragus
	1 **External Ear, Left**
	  See Ø External Ear, Right
	2 **External Ear, Bilateral**
	  See Ø External Ear, Right
		Ø Open
		3 Percutaneous
		4 Percutaneous Endoscopic
		X External
			Z No Device	Z No Qualifier

3 **External Auditory Canal,**
  Right
  External auditory meatus
4 **External Auditory Canal, Left**
  See 3 External Auditory Canal,
  Right
	F **Eustachian Tube, Right**
	  Auditory tube
	  Pharyngotympanic tube
	G **Eustachian Tube, Left**
	  See F Eustachian Tube, Right
		Ø Open
		3 Percutaneous
		4 Percutaneous Endoscopic
		7 Via Natural or Artificial
		     Opening
		8 Via Natural or Artificial
		     Opening Endoscopic
		X External
			Z No Device	Z No Qualifier

5 **Middle Ear, Right**
  Oval window
  Tympanic cavity
6 **Middle Ear, Left**
  See 5 Middle Ear, Right
9 **Auditory Ossicle, Right**
  Incus
  Malleus
  Stapes
	A **Auditory Ossicle, Left**
	  See 9 Auditory Ossicle, Right
	D **Inner Ear, Right**
	  Bony labyrinth
	  Bony vestibule
	  Cochlea
	  Round window
	  Semicircular canal
	E **Inner Ear, Left**
	  See D Inner Ear, Right
		Ø Open
		8 Via Natural or Artificial
		     Opening Endoscopic
			Z No Device	Z No Qualifier

7 **Tympanic Membrane, Right**
  Pars flaccida
8 **Tympanic Membrane, Left**
  See 7 Tympanic Membrane,
  Right
L **Nasal Turbinate**
  Inferior turbinate
  Middle turbinate
  Nasal concha
  Superior turbinate
	N **Nasopharynx**
	  Choana
	  Fossa of Rosenmuller
	  Pharyngeal recess
	  Rhinopharynx
		Ø Open
		3 Percutaneous
		4 Percutaneous Endoscopic
		7 Via Natural or Artificial
		     Opening
		8 Via Natural or Artificial
		     Opening Endoscopic
			Z No Device	Z No Qualifier

B **Mastoid Sinus, Right**
  Mastoid air cells
C **Mastoid Sinus, Left**
  See B Mastoid Sinus, Right
M **Nasal Septum**
  Quadrangular cartilage
  Septal cartilage
  Vomer bone
P **Accessory Sinus**
Q **Maxillary Sinus, Right**
  Antrum of Highmore
	R **Maxillary Sinus, Left**
	  See Q Maxillary Sinus, Right
	S **Frontal Sinus, Right**
	T **Frontal Sinus, Left**
	U **Ethmoid Sinus, Right**
	  Ethmoidal air cell
	V **Ethmoid Sinus, Left**
	  See U Ethmoid Sinus, Right
	W **Sphenoid Sinus, Right**
	X **Sphenoid Sinus, Left**
		Ø Open
		3 Percutaneous
		4 Percutaneous Endoscopic
		8 Via Natural or Artificial
		     Opening Endoscopic
			Z No Device	Z No Qualifier

K **Nasal Mucosa and Soft Tissue**
  Columella
  External naris
  Greater alar cartilage
  Internal naris
  Lateral nasal cartilage
  Lesser alar cartilage
  Nasal cavity
  Nostril
		Ø Open
		3 Percutaneous
		4 Percutaneous Endoscopic
		8 Via Natural or Artificial
		     Opening Endoscopic
		X External
			Z No Device	Z No Qualifier

Non-OR   Ø9Q[Ø,1,2]XZZ
Non-OR   Ø9Q[3,4]XZZ
Non-OR   Ø9Q[F,G][Ø,3,4,7,8,X]ZZ
Non-OR   Ø9QKXZZ

Ø   **Medical and Surgical**
9   **Ear, Nose, Sinus**
R   **Replacement**   Definition: Putting in or on biological or synthetic material that physically takes the place and/or function of all or a portion of a body part
                        Explanation: The body part may have been taken out or replaced, or may be taken out, physically eradicated, or rendered nonfunctional during
                        the REPLACEMENT procedure. A REMOVAL procedure is coded for taking out the device used in a previous replacement procedure.

Body Part Character 4	Approach Character 5	Device Character 6	Qualifier Character 7
Ø **External Ear, Right** Antihelix Antitragus Auricle Earlobe Helix Pinna Tragus **1** **External Ear, Left** *See Ø External Ear, Right* **2** **External Ear, Bilateral** *See Ø External Ear, Right* **K** **Nasal Mucosa and Soft Tissue** Columella External naris Greater alar cartilage Internal naris Lateral nasal cartilage Lesser alar cartilage Nasal cavity Nostril	**Ø** Open **X** External	**7** Autologous Tissue Substitute **J** Synthetic Substitute **K** Nonautologous Tissue Substitute	**Z** No Qualifier
5 **Middle Ear, Right** Oval window Tympanic cavity **6** **Middle Ear, Left** *See 5 Middle Ear, Right* **9** **Auditory Ossicle, Right** Incus Malleus Stapes **A** **Auditory Ossicle, Left** *See 9 Auditory Ossicle, Right* **D** **Inner Ear, Right** Bony labyrinth Bony vestibule Cochlea Round window Semicircular canal **E** **Inner Ear, Left** *See D Inner Ear, Right*	**Ø** Open	**7** Autologous Tissue Substitute **J** Synthetic Substitute **K** Nonautologous Tissue Substitute	**Z** No Qualifier
7 **Tympanic Membrane, Right** Pars flaccida **8** **Tympanic Membrane, Left** *See 7 Tympanic Membrane, Right* **N** **Nasopharynx** Choana Fossa of Rosenmuller Pharyngeal recess Rhinopharynx	**Ø** Open **7** Via Natural or Artificial Opening **8** Via Natural or Artificial Opening Endoscopic	**7** Autologous Tissue Substitute **J** Synthetic Substitute **K** Nonautologous Tissue Substitute	**Z** No Qualifier
L **Nasal Turbinate** Inferior turbinate Middle turbinate Nasal concha Superior turbinate	**Ø** Open **3** Percutaneous **4** Percutaneous Endoscopic **7** Via Natural or Artificial Opening **8** Via Natural or Artificial Opening Endoscopic	**7** Autologous Tissue Substitute **J** Synthetic Substitute **K** Nonautologous Tissue Substitute	**Z** No Qualifier
M **Nasal Septum** Quadrangular cartilage Septal cartilage Vomer bone	**Ø** Open **3** Percutaneous **4** Percutaneous Endoscopic	**7** Autologous Tissue Substitute **J** Synthetic Substitute **K** Nonautologous Tissue Substitute	**Z** No Qualifier

NC Noncovered Procedure   **LC** Limited Coverage   **QA** Questionable OB Admit   **NT** New Tech Add-on   ⊞ Combination Member   ♂ Male   ♀ Female

ICD-10-PCS 2024   **333**

Ø9R–Ø9R

Ø   Medical and Surgical
9   Ear, Nose, Sinus
S   Reposition   Definition: Moving to its normal location, or other suitable location, all or a portion of a body part

Explanation: The body part is moved to a new location from an abnormal location, or from a normal location where it is not functioning correctly. The body part may or may not be cut out or off to be moved to the new location.

Body Part Character 4	Approach Character 5	Device Character 6	Qualifier Character 7
Ø External Ear, Right Antihelix Antitragus Auricle Earlobe Helix Pinna Tragus **1 External Ear, Left** *See Ø External Ear, Right* **2 External Ear, Bilateral** *See Ø External Ear, Right* **K Nasal Mucosa and Soft Tissue** Columella External naris Greater alar cartilage Internal naris Lateral nasal cartilage Lesser alar cartilage Nasal cavity Nostril	**Ø** Open **4** Percutaneous Endoscopic **X** External	**Z** No Device	**Z** No Qualifier
7 Tympanic Membrane, Right Pars flaccida **8 Tympanic Membrane, Left** *See 7 Tympanic Membrane, Right* **F Eustachian Tube, Right** Auditory tube Pharyngotympanic tube **G Eustachian Tube, Left** *See F Eustachian Tube, Right* **L Nasal Turbinate** Inferior turbinate Middle turbinate Nasal concha Superior turbinate	**Ø** Open **4** Percutaneous Endoscopic **7** Via Natural or Artificial Opening **8** Via Natural or Artificial Opening Endoscopic	**Z** No Device	**Z** No Qualifier
9 Auditory Ossicle, Right Incus Malleus Stapes **A Auditory Ossicle, Left** *See 9 Auditory Ossicle, Right* **M Nasal Septum** Quadrangular cartilage Septal cartilage Vomer bone	**Ø** Open **4** Percutaneous Endoscopic	**Z** No Device	**Z** No Qualifier

Non-OR   09S[F,G][Ø,4,7,8]ZZ

Non-OR Procedure   DRG Non-OR Procedure   Valid OR Procedure   HAC Associated Procedure   Combination Only   New/Revised April   New/Revised October

334   ICD-10-PCS 2024

Ø   Medical and Surgical
9   Ear, Nose, Sinus
T   Resection   Definition: Cutting out or off, without replacement, all of a body part
                       Explanation: None

Body Part Character 4		Approach Character 5	Device Character 6	Qualifier Character 7
Ø External Ear, Right Antihelix Antitragus Auricle Earlobe Helix Pinna Tragus	**1 External Ear, Left** *See Ø External Ear, Right*	**Ø** Open **4** Percutaneous Endoscopic **X** External	**Z** No Device	**Z** No Qualifier
5 Middle Ear, Right Oval window Tympanic cavity **6 Middle Ear, Left** *See 5 Middle Ear, Right* **9 Auditory Ossicle, Right** Incus Malleus Stapes	**A Auditory Ossicle, Left** *See 9 Auditory Ossicle, Right* **D Inner Ear, Right** Bony labyrinth Bony vestibule Cochlea Round window Semicircular canal **E Inner Ear, Left** *See D Inner Ear, Right*	**Ø** Open **8** Via Natural or Artificial Opening Endoscopic	**Z** No Device	**Z** No Qualifier
7 Tympanic Membrane, Right Pars flaccida **8 Tympanic Membrane, Left** *See 7 Tympanic Membrane, Right* **F Eustachian Tube, Right** Auditory tube Pharyngotympanic tube **G Eustachian Tube, Left** *See F Eustachian Tube, Right*	**L Nasal Turbinate** Inferior turbinate Middle turbinate Nasal concha Superior turbinate **N Nasopharynx** Choana Fossa of Rosenmuller Pharyngeal recess Rhinopharynx	**Ø** Open **4** Percutaneous Endoscopic **7** Via Natural or Artificial Opening **8** Via Natural or Artificial Opening Endoscopic	**Z** No Device	**Z** No Qualifier
B Mastoid Sinus, Right Mastoid air cells **C Mastoid Sinus, Left** *See B Mastoid Sinus, Right* **M Nasal Septum** Quadrangular cartilage Septal cartilage Vomer bone **P Accessory Sinus** **Q Maxillary Sinus, Right** Antrum of Highmore	**R Maxillary Sinus, Left** *See Q Maxillary Sinus, Right* **S Frontal Sinus, Right** **T Frontal Sinus, Left** **U Ethmoid Sinus, Right** Ethmoidal air cell **V Ethmoid Sinus, Left** *See U Ethmoid Sinus, Right* **W Sphenoid Sinus, Right** **X Sphenoid Sinus, Left**	**Ø** Open **4** Percutaneous Endoscopic **8** Via Natural or Artificial Opening Endoscopic	**Z** No Device	**Z** No Qualifier
K Nasal Mucosa and Soft Tissue Columella External naris Greater alar cartilage Internal naris Lateral nasal cartilage Lesser alar cartilage Nasal cavity Nostril		**Ø** Open **4** Percutaneous Endoscopic **8** Via Natural or Artificial Opening Endoscopic **X** External	**Z** No Device	**Z** No Qualifier

Non-OR   Ø9T[F,G][Ø,4,7,8]ZZ

NC Noncovered Procedure   **LC** Limited Coverage   **QA** Questionable OB Admit   **NT** New Tech Add-on   ⊞ Combination Member   ♂ Male   ♀ Female
ICD-10-PCS 2024   **335**

09T–09T

Ø   **Medical and Surgical**
9   **Ear, Nose, Sinus**
U   **Supplement**   Definition: Putting in or on biological or synthetic material that physically reinforces and/or augments the function of a portion of a body part
           Explanation: The biological material is non-living, or is living and from the same individual. The body part may have been previously replaced, and the SUPPLEMENT procedure is performed to physically reinforce and/or augment the function of the replaced body part.

Body Part Character 4		Approach Character 5	Device Character 6	Qualifier Character 7
Ø **External Ear, Right** Antihelix Antitragus Auricle Earlobe Helix Pinna Tragus	**1** **External Ear, Left** *See Ø External Ear, Right* **2** **External Ear, Bilateral** *See Ø External Ear, Right*	**Ø** Open **X** External	**7** Autologous Tissue Substitute **J** Synthetic Substitute **K** Nonautologous Tissue Substitute	**Z** No Qualifier
5 **Middle Ear, Right** Oval window Tympanic cavity **6** **Middle Ear, Left** *See 5 Middle Ear, Right* **9** **Auditory Ossicle, Right** Incus Malleus Stapes **A** **Auditory Ossicle, Left** *See 9 Auditory Ossicle, Right*	**D** **Inner Ear, Right** Bony labyrinth Bony vestibule Cochlea Round window Semicircular canal **E** **Inner Ear, Left** *See D Inner Ear, Right*	**Ø** Open **8** Via Natural or Artificial Opening Endoscopic	**7** Autologous Tissue Substitute **J** Synthetic Substitute **K** Nonautologous Tissue Substitute	**Z** No Qualifier
7 **Tympanic Membrane, Right** Pars flaccida **8** **Tympanic Membrane, Left** *See 7 Tympanic Membrane, Right*	**N** **Nasopharynx** Choana Fossa of Rosenmuller Pharyngeal recess Rhinopharynx	**Ø** Open **7** Via Natural or Artificial Opening **8** Via Natural or Artificial Opening Endoscopic	**7** Autologous Tissue Substitute **J** Synthetic Substitute **K** Nonautologous Tissue Substitute	**Z** No Qualifier
B **Mastoid Sinus, Right** Mastoid air cells **C** **Mastoid Sinus, Left** *See B Mastoid Sinus, Right* **L** **Nasal Turbinate** Inferior turbinate Middle turbinate Nasal concha Superior turbinate **P** **Accessory Sinus** **Q** **Maxillary Sinus, Right** Antrum of Highmore	**R** **Maxillary Sinus, Left** *See Q Maxillary Sinus, Right* **S** **Frontal Sinus, Right** **T** **Frontal Sinus, Left** **U** **Ethmoid Sinus, Right** Ethmoidal air cell **V** **Ethmoid Sinus, Left** *See U Ethmoid Sinus, Right* **W** **Sphenoid Sinus, Right** **X** **Sphenoid Sinus, Left**	**Ø** Open **3** Percutaneous **4** Percutaneous Endoscopic **7** Via Natural or Artificial Opening **8** Via Natural or Artificial Opening Endoscopic	**7** Autologous Tissue Substitute **J** Synthetic Substitute **K** Nonautologous Tissue Substitute	**Z** No Qualifier
K **Nasal Mucosa and Soft Tissue** Columella External naris Greater alar cartilage Internal naris Lateral nasal cartilage Lesser alar cartilage Nasal cavity Nostril		**Ø** Open **8** Via Natural or Artificial Opening Endoscopic **X** External	**7** Autologous Tissue Substitute **J** Synthetic Substitute **K** Nonautologous Tissue Substitute	**Z** No Qualifier
M **Nasal Septum** Quadrangular cartilage Septal cartilage Vomer bone		**Ø** Open **3** Percutaneous **4** Percutaneous Endoscopic **8** Via Natural or Artificial Opening Endoscopic	**7** Autologous Tissue Substitute **J** Synthetic Substitute **K** Nonautologous Tissue Substitute	**Z** No Qualifier

Ø Medical and Surgical
9 Ear, Nose, Sinus
W Revision

Definition: Correcting, to the extent possible, a portion of a malfunctioning device or the position of a displaced device

Explanation: Revision can include correcting a malfunctioning or displaced device by taking out or putting in components of the device such as a screw or pin

Body Part Character 4	Approach Character 5	Device Character 6	Qualifier Character 7
7 Tympanic Membrane, Right Pars flaccida **8 Tympanic Membrane, Left** *See 7 Tympanic Membrane, Right* **9 Auditory Ossicle, Right** Incus Malleus Stapes **A Auditory Ossicle, Left** *See 9 Auditory Ossicle, Right*	**Ø** Open **7** Via Natural or Artificial Opening **8** Via Natural or Artificial Opening Endoscopic	**7** Autologous Tissue Substitute **J** Synthetic Substitute **K** Nonautologous Tissue Substitute	**Z** No Qualifier
D Inner Ear, Right Bony labyrinth Bony vestibule Cochlea Round window Semicircular canal **E Inner Ear, Left** *See D Inner Ear, Right*	**Ø** Open **7** Via Natural or Artificial Opening **8** Via Natural or Artificial Opening Endoscopic	**S** Hearing Device	**Z** No Qualifier
H Ear, Right **J Ear, Left** **K Nasal Mucosa and Soft Tissue** Columella External naris Greater alar cartilage Internal naris Lateral nasal cartilage Lesser alar cartilage Nasal cavity Nostril	**Ø** Open **3** Percutaneous **4** Percutaneous Endoscopic **7** Via Natural or Artificial Opening **8** Via Natural or Artificial Opening Endoscopic	**Ø** Drainage Device **7** Autologous Tissue Substitute **D** Intraluminal Device **J** Synthetic Substitute **K** Nonautologous Tissue Substitute **Y** Other Device	**Z** No Qualifier
H Ear, Right **J Ear, Left** **K Nasal Mucosa and Soft Tissue** Columella External naris Greater alar cartilage Internal naris Lateral nasal cartilage Lesser alar cartilage Nasal cavity Nostril	**X** External	**Ø** Drainage Device **7** Autologous Tissue Substitute **D** Intraluminal Device **J** Synthetic Substitute **K** Nonautologous Tissue Substitute	**Z** No Qualifier
Y Sinus	**Ø** Open **3** Percutaneous **4** Percutaneous Endoscopic	**Ø** Drainage Device **Y** Other Device	**Z** No Qualifier
Y Sinus	**7** Via Natural or Artificial Opening **8** Via Natural or Artificial Opening Endoscopic	**Y** Other Device	**Z** No Qualifier
Y Sinus	**X** External	**Ø** Drainage Device	**Z** No Qualifier

Non-OR   Ø9W[H,J][3,4][J,K,Y]Z
Non-OR   Ø9W[H,J][7,8][D,Y]Z
Non-OR   Ø9WK[Ø,3,4,7,8][Ø,7,D,J,K,Y]Z
Non-OR   Ø9W[H,J,K]X[Ø,7,D,J,K]Z
Non-OR   Ø9WY[3,4]YZ
Non-OR   Ø9WY[7,8]YZ
Non-OR   Ø9WYXØZ

Respiratory System ØB1–ØBY

Character Meanings

This Character Meaning table is provided as a guide to assist the user in the identification of character members that may be found in this section of code tables. It **SHOULD NOT** be used to build a PCS code.

Operation–Character 3		Body Part–Character 4		Approach–Character 5		Device–Character 6		Qualifier–Character 7	
1	Bypass	Ø	Tracheobronchial Tree	Ø	Open	Ø	Drainage Device	Ø	Allogeneic
2	Change	1	Trachea	3	Percutaneous	1	Radioactive Element	1	Syngeneic
5	Destruction	2	Carina	4	Percutaneous Endoscopic	2	Monitoring Device	2	Zooplastic
7	Dilation	3	Main Bronchus, Right	7	Via Natural or Artificial Opening	3	Infusion Device	3	Laser Interstitial Thermal Therapy
9	Drainage	4	Upper Lobe Bronchus, Right	8	Via Natural or Artificial Opening Endoscopic	7	Autologous Tissue Substitute	4	Cutaneous
B	Excision	5	Middle Lobe Bronchus, Right	X	External	C	Extraluminal Device	6	Esophagus
C	Extirpation	6	Lower Lobe Bronchus, Right			D	Intraluminal Device	X	Diagnostic
D	Extraction	7	Main Bronchus, Left			E	Intraluminal Device, Endotracheal Airway	Z	No Qualifier
F	Fragmentation	8	Upper Lobe Bronchus, Left			F	Tracheostomy Device		
H	Insertion	9	Lingula Bronchus			G	Intraluminal Device, Endobronchial Valve		
J	Inspection	B	Lower Lobe Bronchus, Left			J	Synthetic Substitute		
L	Occlusion	C	Upper Lung Lobe, Right			K	Nonautologous Tissue Substitute		
M	Reattachment	D	Middle Lung Lobe, Right			M	Diaphragmatic Pacemaker Lead		
N	Release	F	Lower Lung Lobe, Right			Y	Other Device		
P	Removal	G	Upper Lung Lobe, Left			Z	No Device		
Q	Repair	H	Lung Lingula						
R	Replacement	J	Lower Lung Lobe, Left						
S	Reposition	K	Lung, Right						
T	Resection	L	Lung, Left						
U	Supplement	M	Lungs, Bilateral						
V	Restriction	N	Pleura, Right						
W	Revision	P	Pleura, Left						
Y	Transplantation	Q	Pleura						
		T	Diaphragm						

AHA Coding Clinic for table ØB5
2022, 4Q, 53-54   Laser interstitial thermal therapy
2016, 2Q, 17   Photodynamic therapy for treatment of malignant mesothelioma
2015, 2Q, 31   Thoracoscopic talc pleurodesis

AHA Coding Clinic for table ØB7
2020, 3Q, 43   Tracheobronchomalacia with placement of tracheobronchial stent

AHA Coding Clinic for table ØB9
2017, 3Q, 15   Bronchoscopy with suctioning for removal of retained secretions
2017, 1Q, 51   Bronchoalveolar lavage
2016, 1Q, 26   Bronchoalveolar lavage, endobronchial biopsy and transbronchial biopsy
2016, 1Q, 27   Fiberoptic bronchoscopy with brushings and bronchoalveolar lavage

AHA Coding Clinic for table ØBB
2022, 2Q, 19   Transbronchial lung biopsy using alligator forceps
2016, 1Q, 26   Bronchoalveolar lavage, endobronchial biopsy and transbronchial biopsy
2016, 1Q, 27   Fiberoptic bronchoscopy with brushings and bronchoalveolar lavage
2014, 1Q, 20   Fiducial marker placement

AHA Coding Clinic for table ØBC
2017, 3Q, 14   Bronchoscopy with suctioning and washings for removal of mucus plug

AHA Coding Clinic for table ØBD
2020, 3Q, 40   Transbronchial cryobiopsy of upper, middle and lower lobes of lung
2018, 3Q, 28   Lung decortication for empyema

AHA Coding Clinic for table ØBH
2022, 3Q, 22   Approach value for placement of endotracheal tube
2019, 3Q, 33   Insertion of endobronchial valve
2014, 4Q, 3-10   Mechanical ventilation

AHA Coding Clinic for table ØBJ
2015, 2Q, 31   Thoracoscopic talc pleurodesis
2014, 1Q, 20   Fiducial marker placement

AHA Coding Clinic for table ØBL
2019, 3Q, 33   Insertion of endobronchial valve

AHA Coding Clinic for table ØBN
2019, 2Q, 20   Pericardiectomy for constrictive pericarditis
2018, 3Q, 28   Lung decortication
2018, 3Q, 28   Lung decortication for empyema
2015, 3Q, 15   Vascular ring surgery with release of esophagus and trachea

AHA Coding Clinic for table ØBQ
2020, 3Q, 41   Plication of diaphragm
2016, 2Q, 22   Esophageal lengthening Collis gastroplasty with Nissen fundoplication and hiatal hernia
2014, 3Q, 28   Laparoscopic Nissen fundoplication and diaphragmatic hernia repair

AHA Coding Clinic for table ØBU
2020, 3Q, 43   Tracheobronchomalacia with placement of tracheobronchial stent
2015, 1Q, 28   Repair of bronchopleural fistula using omental pedicle graft

AHA Coding Clinic for table ØBV
2020, 3Q, 41   Plication of diaphragm

AHA Coding Clinic for table ØBY
2023, 2Q, 32   Preparation of donor organ before transplantation

Respiratory System

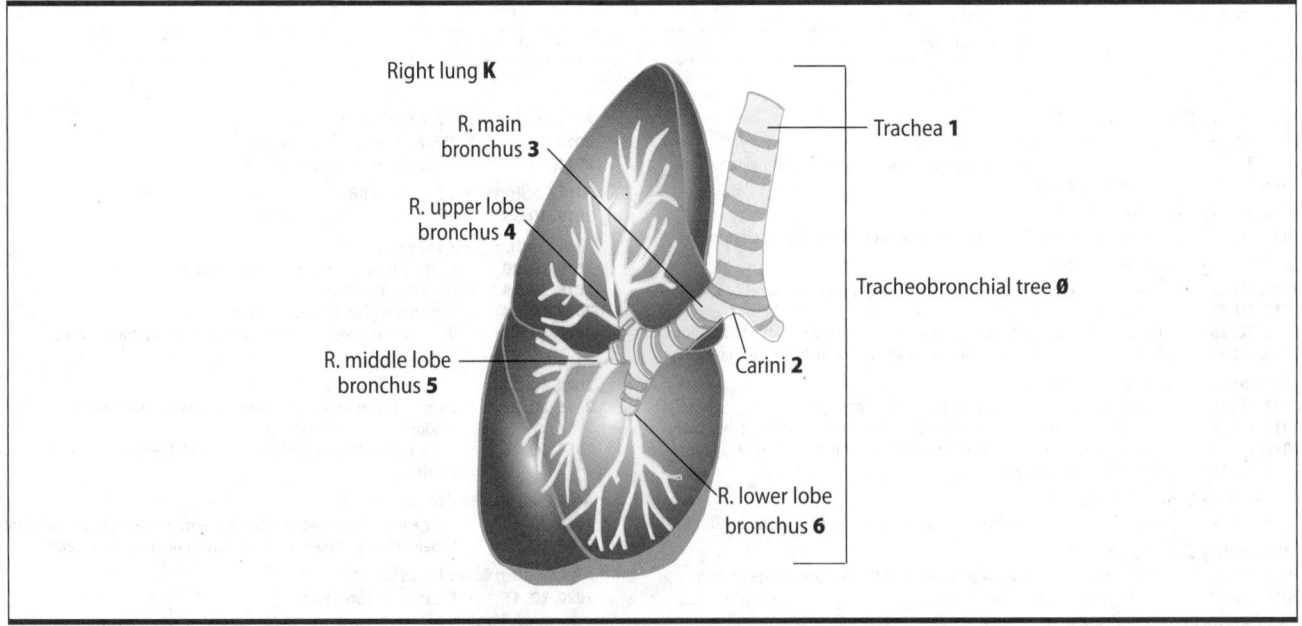

Trachea **1**

Right lung **K**

Right main/ primary bronchus **3**

Diaphragm **T**

Pleura **N, P, Q**

Left lung **L**

Carina of trachea **2**

Left main/ primary bronchus **7**

Right Lung Bronchi

Right lung **K**

R. main bronchus **3**

R. upper lobe bronchus **4**

R. middle lobe bronchus **5**

R. lower lobe bronchus **6**

Trachea **1**

Tracheobronchial tree **Ø**

Carini **2**

Ø   Medical and Surgical
B   Respiratory System
1   Bypass   Definition: Altering the route of passage of the contents of a tubular body part

Explanation: Rerouting contents of a body part to a downstream area of the normal route, to a similar route and body part, or to an abnormal route and dissimilar body part. Includes one or more anastomoses, with or without the use of a device.

Body Part Character 4	Approach Character 5	Device Character 6	Qualifier Character 7
1 Trachea Cricoid cartilage	Ø Open	D Intraluminal Device	6 Esophagus
1 Trachea Cricoid cartilage	Ø Open	F Tracheostomy Device Z No Device	4 Cutaneous
1 Trachea Cricoid cartilage	3 Percutaneous 4 Percutaneous Endoscopic	F Tracheostomy Device Z No Device	4 Cutaneous

DRG Non-OR	ØB113[F,Z]4
Non-OR	ØB110D6

Ø   Medical and Surgical
B   Respiratory System
2   Change   Definition: Taking out or off a device from a body part and putting back an identical or similar device in or on the same body part without cutting or puncturing the skin or a mucous membrane

Explanation: All CHANGE procedures are coded using the approach EXTERNAL

Body Part Character 4	Approach Character 5	Device Character 6	Qualifier Character 7
Ø Tracheobronchial Tree K Lung, Right L Lung, Left Q Pleura T Diaphragm	X External	Ø Drainage Device Y Other Device	Z No Qualifier
1 Trachea Cricoid cartilage	X External	Ø Drainage Device E Intraluminal Device, Endotracheal Airway F Tracheostomy Device Y Other Device	Z No Qualifier

Non-OR	All body part, approach, device, and qualifier values

Respiratory System

Ø Medical and Surgical
B Respiratory System
5 Destruction   Definition: Physical eradication of all or a portion of a body part by the direct use of energy, force, or a destructive agent

                    Explanation: None of the body part is physically taken out

Body Part Character 4	Approach Character 5	Device Character 6	Qualifier Character 7

1 Trachea
  Cricoid cartilage
2 Carina
3 Main Bronchus, Right
  Bronchus intermedius
  Intermediate bronchus
4 Upper Lobe Bronchus, Right
5 Middle Lobe Bronchus, Right
6 Lower Lobe Bronchus, Right
7 Main Bronchus, Left
8 Upper Lobe Bronchus, Left
9 Lingula Bronchus
B Lower Lobe Bronchus, Left
	Ø Open
	3 Percutaneous
	4 Percutaneous Endoscopic
	7 Via Natural or Artificial Opening
	8 Via Natural or Artificial Opening Endoscopic
		Z No Device	Z No Qualifier

C Upper Lung Lobe, Right D Middle Lung Lobe, Right F Lower Lung Lobe, Right G Upper Lung Lobe, Left H Lung Lingula J Lower Lung Lobe, Left K Lung, Right L Lung, Left M Lungs, Bilateral	Ø Open 3 Percutaneous 4 Percutaneous Endoscopic	Z No Device	3 Laser Interstitial Thermal Therapy Z No Qualifier
C Upper Lung Lobe, Right D Middle Lung Lobe, Right F Lower Lung Lobe, Right G Upper Lung Lobe, Left H Lung Lingula J Lower Lung Lobe, Left K Lung, Right L Lung, Left M Lungs, Bilateral	7 Via Natural or Artificial Opening 8 Via Natural or Artificial Opening Endoscopic	Z No Device	Z No Qualifier
N Pleura, Right P Pleura, Left T Diaphragm	Ø Open 3 Percutaneous 4 Percutaneous Endoscopic	Z No Device	Z No Qualifier

Non-OR   ØB5[3,4,5,6,7,8,9,B]4ZZ
Non-OR   ØB5[C,D,F,G,H,J,K,L,M]8ZZ

Ø Medical and Surgical
B Respiratory System
7 Dilation   Definition: Expanding an orifice or the lumen of a tubular body part

                Explanation: The orifice can be a natural orifice or an artificially created orifice. Accomplished by stretching a tubular body part using intraluminal pressure or by cutting part of the orifice or wall of the tubular body part.

Body Part Character 4	Approach Character 5	Device Character 6	Qualifier Character 7

1 Trachea
  Cricoid cartilage
2 Carina
3 Main Bronchus, Right
  Bronchus intermedius
  Intermediate bronchus
4 Upper Lobe Bronchus, Right
5 Middle Lobe Bronchus, Right
6 Lower Lobe Bronchus, Right
7 Main Bronchus, Left
8 Upper Lobe Bronchus, Left
9 Lingula Bronchus
B Lower Lobe Bronchus, Left
	Ø Open
	3 Percutaneous
	4 Percutaneous Endoscopic
	7 Via Natural or Artificial Opening
	8 Via Natural or Artificial Opening Endoscopic
		D Intraluminal Device
		Z No Device
			Z No Qualifier

Non-OR   ØB7[3,4,5,6,7,8,9,B][Ø,3,4,7,8][D,Z]Z

Non-OR Procedure   ~~DRG Non-OR Procedure~~   Valid OR Procedure   HAC Associated Procedure   Combination Only   New/Revised April   New/Revised October

0   **Medical and Surgical**
B   **Respiratory System**
9   **Drainage**   Definition: Taking or letting out fluids and/or gases from a body part
                 Explanation: The qualifier DIAGNOSTIC is used to identify drainage procedures that are biopsies

Body Part Character 4		Approach Character 5	Device Character 6	Qualifier Character 7

1 Trachea
    Cricoid cartilage
2 Carina
3 Main Bronchus, Right
    Bronchus intermedius
    Intermediate bronchus
4 Upper Lobe Bronchus,
    Right
5 Middle Lobe Bronchus,
    Right
6 Lower Lobe Bronchus,
    Right
7 Main Bronchus, Left
	8 Upper Lobe Bronchus, Left
	9 Lingula Bronchus
	B Lower Lobe Bronchus, Left
	C Upper Lung Lobe, Right
	D Middle Lung Lobe, Right
	F Lower Lung Lobe, Right
	G Upper Lung Lobe, Left
	H Lung Lingula
	J Lower Lung Lobe, Left
	K Lung, Right
	L Lung, Left
	M Lungs, Bilateral
		0 Open
		3 Percutaneous
		4 Percutaneous Endoscopic
		7 Via Natural or Artificial
		    Opening
		8 Via Natural or Artificial
		    Opening Endoscopic
			0 Drainage Device	**Z** No Qualifier

1 Trachea
    Cricoid cartilage
2 Carina
3 Main Bronchus, Right
    Bronchus intermedius
    Intermediate bronchus
4 Upper Lobe Bronchus,
    Right
5 Middle Lobe Bronchus,
    Right
6 Lower Lobe Bronchus,
    Right
7 Main Bronchus, Left
	8 Upper Lobe Bronchus, Left
	9 Lingula Bronchus
	B Lower Lobe Bronchus, Left
	C Upper Lung Lobe, Right
	D Middle Lung Lobe, Right
	F Lower Lung Lobe, Right
	G Upper Lung Lobe, Left
	H Lung Lingula
	J Lower Lung Lobe, Left
	K Lung, Right
	L Lung, Left
	M Lungs, Bilateral
		0 Open
		3 Percutaneous
		4 Percutaneous Endoscopic
		7 Via Natural or Artificial
		    Opening
		8 Via Natural or Artificial
		    Opening Endoscopic
			Z No Device	**X** Diagnostic
				Z No Qualifier

N Pleura, Right **P** Pleura, Left		**0** Open **3** Percutaneous **4** Percutaneous Endoscopic **8** Via Natural or Artificial Opening Endoscopic	**0** Drainage Device	**Z** No Qualifier
N Pleura, Right **P** Pleura, Left		**0** Open **3** Percutaneous **4** Percutaneous Endoscopic **8** Via Natural or Artificial Opening Endoscopic	**Z** No Device	**X** Diagnostic **Z** No Qualifier
T Diaphragm		**0** Open **3** Percutaneous **4** Percutaneous Endoscopic	**0** Drainage Device	**Z** No Qualifier
T Diaphragm		**0** Open **3** Percutaneous **4** Percutaneous Endoscopic	**Z** No Device	**X** Diagnostic **Z** No Qualifier

Non-OR	0B9[1,2,3,4,5,6,7,8,9,B][7,8]0Z	**Non-OR**	0B9[N,P][0,3,8]0Z
Non-OR	0B9[1,2,3,4,5,6,7,8,9,B][3,4]ZX	**Non-OR**	0B9[N,P][0,3,8]Z[X,Z]
Non-OR	0B9[1,2,3,4,5,6,7,8,9,B][7,8]Z[X,Z]	**Non-OR**	0B9[N,P]4ZX
Non-OR	0B9[C,D,F,G,H,J,K,L,M][3,4,7]ZX	**Non-OR**	0B9T[3,4]0Z
Non-OR	0B9[C,D,F,G,H,J,K,L,M]8Z[X,Z]	**Non-OR**	0B9T[3,4]Z[X,Z]

NC Noncovered Procedure   **LC** Limited Coverage   **QA** Questionable OB Admit   **NT** New Tech Add-on   ⊞ Combination Member   ♂ Male   ♀ Female

ICD-10-PCS 2024   343

0B9–0B9

Respiratory System

Ø **Medical and Surgical**
B **Respiratory System**
B **Excision**   Definition: Cutting out or off, without replacement, a portion of a body part
               Explanation: The qualifier DIAGNOSTIC is used to identify excision procedures that are biopsies

Body Part Character 4	Approach Character 5	Device Character 6	Qualifier Character 7

1 Trachea
   Cricoid cartilage
2 Carina
3 Main Bronchus, Right
   Bronchus intermedius
   Intermediate bronchus
4 Upper Lobe Bronchus, Right
5 Middle Lobe Bronchus, Right
6 Lower Lobe Bronchus, Right
7 Main Bronchus, Left
8 Upper Lobe Bronchus, Left
9 Lingula Bronchus
B Lower Lobe Bronchus, Left
C Upper Lung Lobe, Right
D Middle Lung Lobe, Right
F Lower Lung Lobe, Right
G Upper Lung Lobe, Left
H Lung Lingula
J Lower Lung Lobe, Left
K Lung, Right
L Lung, Left
M Lungs, Bilateral
	Ø Open
	3 Percutaneous
	4 Percutaneous Endoscopic
	7 Via Natural or Artificial Opening
	8 Via Natural or Artificial Opening
	   Endoscopic
		Z No Device	X Diagnostic
			Z No Qualifier

N Pleura, Right P Pleura, Left	Ø Open 3 Percutaneous 4 Percutaneous Endoscopic 8 Via Natural or Artificial Opening Endoscopic	Z No Device	X Diagnostic Z No Qualifier
T Diaphragm	Ø Open 3 Percutaneous 4 Percutaneous Endoscopic	Z No Device	X Diagnostic Z No Qualifier

Non-OR   ØBB[1,2,3,4,5,6,7,8,9,B][3,4,7,8]ZX
Non-OR   ØBB[3,4,5,6,7,8,9,B,M][4,8]ZZ
Non-OR   ØBB[C,D,F,G,H,J,K,L,M]3ZX
Non-OR   ØBB[C,D,F,G,H,J,K,L]8ZZ
Non-OR   ØBB[N,P]3ZX

Ø **Medical and Surgical**
B **Respiratory System**
C **Extirpation**   Definition: Taking or cutting out solid matter from a body part
               Explanation: The solid matter may be an abnormal byproduct of a biological function or a foreign body; it may be imbedded in a body part or in
               the lumen of a tubular body part. The solid matter may or may not have been previously broken into pieces.

Body Part Character 4	Approach Character 5	Device Character 6	Qualifier Character 7

1 Trachea
   Cricoid cartilage
2 Carina
3 Main Bronchus, Right
   Bronchus intermedius
   Intermediate bronchus
4 Upper Lobe Bronchus, Right
5 Middle Lobe Bronchus, Right
6 Lower Lobe Bronchus, Right
7 Main Bronchus, Left
8 Upper Lobe Bronchus, Left
9 Lingula Bronchus
B Lower Lobe Bronchus, Left
C Upper Lung Lobe, Right
D Middle Lung Lobe, Right
F Lower Lung Lobe, Right
G Upper Lung Lobe, Left
H Lung Lingula
J Lower Lung Lobe, Left
K Lung, Right
L Lung, Left
M Lungs, Bilateral
	Ø Open
	3 Percutaneous
	4 Percutaneous Endoscopic
	7 Via Natural or Artificial Opening
	8 Via Natural or Artificial Opening
	   Endoscopic
		Z No Device	Z No Qualifier

N Pleura, Right P Pleura, Left T Diaphragm	Ø Open 3 Percutaneous 4 Percutaneous Endoscopic	Z No Device	Z No Qualifier

Non-OR   ØBC[1,2,3,4,5,6,7,8,9,B][7,8]ZZ
Non-OR   ØBC[N,P]3ZZ

Non-OR Procedure   DRG Non-OR Procedure   Valid OR Procedure   HAC Associated Procedure   Combination Only   New/Revised April   New/Revised October

Ø	Medical and Surgical
B	Respiratory System
D	Extraction Definition: Pulling or stripping out or off all or a portion of a body part by the use of force

Explanation: The qualifier DIAGNOSTIC is used to identify extraction procedures that are biopsies

Body Part Character 4	Approach Character 5	Device Character 6	Qualifier Character 7

1   Trachea
    Cricoid cartilage
2   Carina
3   Main Bronchus, Right
    Bronchus intermedius
    Intermediate bronchus
4   Upper Lobe Bronchus, Right
5   Middle Lobe Bronchus, Right
6   Lower Lobe Bronchus, Right
7   Main Bronchus, Left
8   Upper Lobe Bronchus, Left
9   Lingula Bronchus
B   Lower Lobe Bronchus, Left
C   Upper Lung Lobe, Right
D   Middle Lung Lobe, Right
F   Lower Lung Lobe, Right
G   Upper Lung Lobe, Left
H   Lung Lingula
J   Lower Lung Lobe, Left
K   Lung, Right
L   Lung, Left
M   Lungs, Bilateral
	4 Percutaneous Endoscopic
	8 Via Natural or Artificial Opening
	    Endoscopic
		Z No Device	X Diagnostic

N Pleura, Right P Pleura, Left	Ø Open 3 Percutaneous 4 Percutaneous Endoscopic	Z No Device	X Diagnostic Z No Qualifier

Non-OR   ØBD[1,2,3,4,5,6,7,8,9,B,C,D,F,G,H,J,K,L,M][4,8]ZX

Ø	Medical and Surgical
B	Respiratory System
F	Fragmentation Definition: Breaking solid matter in a body part into pieces

Explanation: Physical force (e.g., manual, ultrasonic) applied directly or indirectly is used to break the solid matter into pieces. The solid matter may be an abnormal byproduct of a biological function or a foreign body. The pieces of solid matter are not taken out.

Body Part Character 4	Approach Character 5	Device Character 6	Qualifier Character 7

1   Trachea   `NC`
    Cricoid cartilage
2   Carina   `NC`
3   Main Bronchus, Right   `NC`
    Bronchus intermedius
    Intermediate bronchus
4   Upper Lobe Bronchus, Right   `NC`
5   Middle Lobe Bronchus, Right   `NC`
6   Lower Lobe Bronchus, Right   `NC`
7   Main Bronchus, Left   `NC`
8   Upper Lobe Bronchus, Left   `NC`
9   Lingula Bronchus   `NC`
B   Lower Lobe Bronchus, Left   `NC`
	Ø Open
	3 Percutaneous
	4 Percutaneous Endoscopic
	7 Via Natural or Artificial Opening
	8 Via Natural or Artificial Opening
	    Endoscopic
	X External
		Z No Device	Z No Qualifier

Non-OR   ØBF[1,2,3,4,5,6,7,8,9,B]XZZ
Non-OR   ØBF[3,4,5,6,7,8,9,B][7,8]ZZ
`NC`   ØBF[1,2,3,4,5,6,7,8,9,B]XZZ

`NC` Noncovered Procedure   `LC` Limited Coverage   `QA` Questionable OB Admit   `NT` New Tech Add-on   ⊞ Combination Member   ♂ Male   ♀ Female

ICD-10-PCS 2024   345

Ø　Medical and Surgical
B　Respiratory System
H　Insertion　　Definition: Putting in a nonbiological appliance that monitors, assists, performs, or prevents a physiological function but does not physically take the place of a body part
　　　　　　　　　　Explanation: None

Body Part Character 4	Approach Character 5	Device Character 6	Qualifier Character 7
Ø Tracheobronchial Tree	Ø Open 3 Percutaneous 4 Percutaneous Endoscopic 7 Via Natural or Artificial Opening 8 Via Natural or Artificial Opening Endoscopic	1 Radioactive Element 2 Monitoring Device 3 Infusion Device D Intraluminal Device Y Other Device	Z No Qualifier
1 Trachea Cricoid cartilage	Ø Open	2 Monitoring Device D Intraluminal Device Y Other Device	Z No Qualifier
1 Trachea Cricoid cartilage	3 Percutaneous	D Intraluminal Device E Intraluminal Device, Endotracheal Airway Y Other Device	Z No Qualifier
1 Trachea Cricoid cartilage	4 Percutaneous Endoscopic	D Intraluminal Device Y Other Device	Z No Qualifier
1 Trachea Cricoid cartilage	7 Via Natural or Artificial Opening 8 Via Natural or Artificial Opening Endoscopic	2 Monitoring Device D Intraluminal Device E Intraluminal Device, Endotracheal Airway Y Other Device	Z No Qualifier
3 Main Bronchus, Right Bronchus intermedius Intermediate bronchus 4 Upper Lobe Bronchus, Right 5 Middle Lobe Bronchus, Right 6 Lower Lobe Bronchus, Right 7 Main Bronchus, Left 8 Upper Lobe Bronchus, Left 9 Lingula Bronchus B Lower Lobe Bronchus, Left	Ø Open 3 Percutaneous 4 Percutaneous Endoscopic 7 Via Natural or Artificial Opening 8 Via Natural or Artificial Opening Endoscopic	G Intraluminal Device, Endobronchial Valve	Z No Qualifier
K Lung, Right L Lung, Left	Ø Open 3 Percutaneous 4 Percutaneous Endoscopic 7 Via Natural or Artificial Opening 8 Via Natural or Artificial Opening Endoscopic	1 Radioactive Element 2 Monitoring Device 3 Infusion Device Y Other Device	Z No Qualifier
Q Pleura	Ø Open 3 Percutaneous 4 Percutaneous Endoscopic 7 Via Natural or Artificial Opening 8 Via Natural or Artificial Opening Endoscopic	Y Other Device	Z No Qualifier
T Diaphragm	Ø Open 3 Percutaneous 4 Percutaneous Endoscopic	2 Monitoring Device M Diaphragmatic Pacemaker Lead Y Other Device	Z No Qualifier
T Diaphragm	7 Via Natural or Artificial Opening 8 Via Natural or Artificial Opening Endoscopic	Y Other Device	Z No Qualifier

DRG Non-OR	ØBH[3,4,5,6,7,8,9,B]8GZ
Non-OR	ØBH03YZ
Non-OR	ØBHØ[7,8][2,3,D,Y]Z
Non-OR	ØBH13[E,Y]Z
Non-OR	ØBH1[7,8][2,D,E,Y]Z
Non-OR	ØBH[K,L]3YZ
Non-OR	ØBH[K,L]7[2,3,Y]Z
Non-OR	ØBH[K,L]8[2,3]Z
Non-OR	ØBHQ[3,7]YZ
Non-OR	ØBHT3YZ
Non-OR	ØBHT[7,8]YZ

Non-OR Procedure　　DRG Non-OR Procedure　　Valid OR Procedure　　HAC Associated Procedure　　Combination Only　　New/Revised April　　New/Revised October

Ø   Medical and Surgical
B   Respiratory System
J   Inspection   Definition: Visually and/or manually exploring a body part

Explanation: Visual exploration may be performed with or without optical instrumentation. Manual exploration may be performed directly or through intervening body layers.

Body Part Character 4	Approach Character 5	Device Character 6	Qualifier Character 7

Ø   Tracheobronchial Tree
1   Trachea
    Cricoid cartilage
K   Lung, Right
L   Lung, Left
Q   Pleura
T   Diaphragm
	Ø Open
	3 Percutaneous
	4 Percutaneous Endoscopic
	7 Via Natural or Artificial Opening
	8 Via Natural or Artificial Opening
	    Endoscopic
	X External
		Z No Device	Z No Qualifier

Non-OR   ØBJ[Ø,K,L,Q,T][3,7,8,X]ZZ
Non-OR   ØBJ1[3,4,7,8,X]ZZ

Ø   Medical and Surgical
B   Respiratory System
L   Occlusion   Definition: Completely closing an orifice or the lumen of a tubular body part

Explanation: The orifice can be a natural orifice or an artificially created orifice

Body Part Character 4	Approach Character 5	Device Character 6	Qualifier Character 7

1   Trachea
    Cricoid cartilage
2   Carina
3   Main Bronchus, Right
    Bronchus intermedius
    Intermediate bronchus
4   Upper Lobe Bronchus, Right
5   Middle Lobe Bronchus, Right
6   Lower Lobe Bronchus, Right
7   Main Bronchus, Left
8   Upper Lobe Bronchus, Left
9   Lingula Bronchus
B   Lower Lobe Bronchus, Left
	Ø Open
	3 Percutaneous
	4 Percutaneous Endoscopic
		C Extraluminal Device
		D Intraluminal Device
		Z No Device
			Z No Qualifier

1   Trachea
    Cricoid cartilage
2   Carina
3   Main Bronchus, Right
    Bronchus intermedius
    Intermediate bronchus
4   Upper Lobe Bronchus, Right
5   Middle Lobe Bronchus, Right
6   Lower Lobe Bronchus, Right
7   Main Bronchus, Left
8   Upper Lobe Bronchus, Left
9   Lingula Bronchus
B   Lower Lobe Bronchus, Left
	7 Via Natural or Artificial Opening
	8 Via Natural or Artificial Opening
	    Endoscopic
		D Intraluminal Device
		Z No Device
			Z No Qualifier

NC Noncovered Procedure   LC Limited Coverage   QA Questionable OB Admit   NT New Tech Add-on   ⊞ Combination Member   ♂ Male   ♀ Female

ICD-10-PCS 2024   347

Respiratory System

Ø Medical and Surgical
B Respiratory System
M Reattachment   Definition: Putting back in or on all or a portion of a separated body part to its normal location or other suitable location

Explanation: Vascular circulation and nervous pathways may or may not be reestablished

Body Part Character 4	Approach Character 5	Device Character 6	Qualifier Character 7

1   Trachea
     Cricoid cartilage
2   Carina
3   Main Bronchus, Right
     Bronchus intermedius
     Intermediate bronchus
4   Upper Lobe Bronchus, Right
5   Middle Lobe Bronchus, Right
6   Lower Lobe Bronchus, Right
7   Main Bronchus, Left
8   Upper Lobe Bronchus, Left
9   Lingula Bronchus
B   Lower Lobe Bronchus, Left
C   Upper Lung Lobe, Right
D   Middle Lung Lobe, Right
F   Lower Lung Lobe, Right
G   Upper Lung Lobe, Left
H   Lung Lingula
J   Lower Lung Lobe, Left
K   Lung, Right
L   Lung, Left
T   Diaphragm
	Ø Open	Z No Device	Z No Qualifier

Ø Medical and Surgical
B Respiratory System
N Release   Definition: Freeing a body part from an abnormal physical constraint by cutting or by the use of force

Explanation: Some of the restraining tissue may be taken out but none of the body part is taken out

Body Part Character 4	Approach Character 5	Device Character 6	Qualifier Character 7

1   Trachea
     Cricoid cartilage
2   Carina
3   Main Bronchus, Right
     Bronchus intermedius
     Intermediate bronchus
4   Upper Lobe Bronchus, Right
5   Middle Lobe Bronchus, Right
6   Lower Lobe Bronchus, Right
7   Main Bronchus, Left
8   Upper Lobe Bronchus, Left
9   Lingula Bronchus
B   Lower Lobe Bronchus, Left
C   Upper Lung Lobe, Right
D   Middle Lung Lobe, Right
F   Lower Lung Lobe, Right
G   Upper Lung Lobe, Left
H   Lung Lingula
J   Lower Lung Lobe, Left
K   Lung, Right
L   Lung, Left
M   Lungs, Bilateral
	Ø Open
	3 Percutaneous
	4 Percutaneous Endoscopic
	7 Via Natural or Artificial Opening
	8 Via Natural or Artificial Opening
	     Endoscopic
		Z No Device	Z No Qualifier

N Pleura, Right P Pleura, Left T Diaphragm	Ø Open 3 Percutaneous 4 Percutaneous Endoscopic	Z No Device	Z No Qualifier

Non-OR Procedure   DRG Non-OR Procedure   Valid OR Procedure   HAC Associated Procedure   Combination Only   New/Revised April   New/Revised October

348   ICD-10-PCS 2024

Ø   Medical and Surgical
B   Respiratory System
P   Removal   Definition: Taking out or off a device from a body part

Explanation: If a device is taken out and a similar device put in without cutting or puncturing the skin or mucous membrane, the procedure is coded to the root operation CHANGE. Otherwise, the procedure for taking out a device is coded to the root operation REMOVAL.

Body Part Character 4	Approach Character 5	Device Character 6	Qualifier Character 7
Ø Tracheobronchial Tree	Ø Open 3 Percutaneous 4 Percutaneous Endoscopic 7 Via Natural or Artificial Opening 8 Via Natural or Artificial Opening Endoscopic	Ø Drainage Device 1 Radioactive Element 2 Monitoring Device 3 Infusion Device 7 Autologous Tissue Substitute C Extraluminal Device D Intraluminal Device J Synthetic Substitute K Nonautologous Tissue Substitute Y Other Device	Z No Qualifier
Ø Tracheobronchial Tree	X External	Ø Drainage Device 1 Radioactive Element 2 Monitoring Device 3 Infusion Device D Intraluminal Device	Z No Qualifier
1 Trachea Cricoid cartilage	Ø Open 3 Percutaneous 4 Percutaneous Endoscopic 7 Via Natural or Artificial Opening 8 Via Natural or Artificial Opening Endoscopic	Ø Drainage Device 2 Monitoring Device 7 Autologous Tissue Substitute C Extraluminal Device D Intraluminal Device F Tracheostomy Device J Synthetic Substitute K Nonautologous Tissue Substitute	Z No Qualifier
1 Trachea Cricoid cartilage	X External	Ø Drainage Device 2 Monitoring Device D Intraluminal Device F Tracheostomy Device	Z No Qualifier
K Lung, Right L Lung, Left	Ø Open 3 Percutaneous 4 Percutaneous Endoscopic 7 Via Natural or Artificial Opening 8 Via Natural or Artificial Opening Endoscopic	Ø Drainage Device 1 Radioactive Element 2 Monitoring Device 3 Infusion Device Y Other Device	Z No Qualifier
K Lung, Right L Lung, Left	X External	Ø Drainage Device 1 Radioactive Element 2 Monitoring Device 3 Infusion Device	Z No Qualifier
Q Pleura	Ø Open 3 Percutaneous 4 Percutaneous Endoscopic 7 Via Natural or Artificial Opening 8 Via Natural or Artificial Opening Endoscopic	Ø Drainage Device 1 Radioactive Element 2 Monitoring Device Y Other Device	Z No Qualifier
Q Pleura	X External	Ø Drainage Device 1 Radioactive Element 2 Monitoring Device	Z No Qualifier
T Diaphragm	Ø Open 3 Percutaneous 4 Percutaneous Endoscopic 7 Via Natural or Artificial Opening 8 Via Natural or Artificial Opening Endoscopic	Ø Drainage Device 2 Monitoring Device 7 Autologous Tissue Substitute J Synthetic Substitute K Nonautologous Tissue Substitute M Diaphragmatic Pacemaker Lead Y Other Device	Z No Qualifier
T Diaphragm	X External	Ø Drainage Device 2 Monitoring Device M Diaphragmatic Pacemaker Lead	Z No Qualifier

Non-OR	ØBPØ[3,4]YZ	**Non-OR**	ØBPL7[Ø,2,3,Y]Z
Non-OR	ØBPØ[7,8][Ø,2,3,D,Y]Z	**Non-OR**	ØBPL8[Ø,2,3]Z
Non-OR	ØBPØX[Ø,1,2,3,D]Z	**Non-OR**	ØBP[K,L]X[Ø,1,2,3]Z
Non-OR	ØBP1[Ø,3,4]FZ	**Non-OR**	ØBPQ[Ø,3,4,7,8][Ø,1,2,]Z
Non-OR	ØBP1[7,8][Ø,2,D,F]Z	**Non-OR**	ØBPQ[3,7]YZ
Non-OR	ØBP1X[Ø,2,D,F]Z	**Non-OR**	ØBPQX[Ø,1,2]Z
Non-OR	ØBP[K,L]3YZ	**Non-OR**	ØBPT3YZ
Non-OR	ØBPK7[Ø,1,2,3,Y]Z	**Non-OR**	ØBPT[7,8][Ø,2,Y]Z
Non-OR	ØBPK8[Ø,1,2,3]Z	**Non-OR**	ØBPTX[Ø,2,M]Z

NC Noncovered Procedure   LC Limited Coverage   QA Questionable OB Admit   NT New Tech Add-on   ⊞ Combination Member   ♂ Male   ♀ Female

ICD-10-PCS 2024   349

Respiratory System

Ø   **Medical and Surgical**
B   **Respiratory System**
Q   **Repair**   Definition: Restoring, to the extent possible, a body part to its normal anatomic structure and function
                          Explanation: Used only when the method to accomplish the repair is not one of the other root operations

Body Part Character 4	Approach Character 5	Device Character 6	Qualifier Character 7

1 Trachea
    Cricoid cartilage
 2 Carina
 3 Main Bronchus, Right
    Bronchus intermedius
    Intermediate bronchus
 4 Upper Lobe Bronchus, Right
 5 Middle Lobe Bronchus, Right
 6 Lower Lobe Bronchus, Right
 7 Main Bronchus, Left
 8 Upper Lobe Bronchus, Left
 9 Lingula Bronchus
 B Lower Lobe Bronchus, Left
 C Upper Lung Lobe, Right
 D Middle Lung Lobe, Right
 F Lower Lung Lobe, Right
 G Upper Lung Lobe, Left
 H Lung Lingula
 J Lower Lung Lobe, Left
 K Lung, Right
 L Lung, Left
 M Lungs, Bilateral
	Ø Open
	 3 Percutaneous
	 4 Percutaneous Endoscopic
	 7 Via Natural or Artificial Opening
	 8 Via Natural or Artificial Opening Endoscopic
		Z No Device	Z No Qualifier

N Pleura, Right P Pleura, Left T Diaphragm	Ø Open 3 Percutaneous 4 Percutaneous Endoscopic	Z No Device	Z No Qualifier

Ø   **Medical and Surgical**
B   **Respiratory System**
R   **Replacement**   Definition: Putting in or on biological or synthetic material that physically takes the place and/or function of all or a portion of a body part
                          Explanation: The body part may have been taken out or replaced, or may be taken out, physically eradicated, or rendered nonfunctional during the REPLACEMENT procedure. A REMOVAL procedure is coded for taking out the device used in a previous replacement procedure.

Body Part Character 4	Approach Character 5	Device Character 6	Qualifier Character 7

1 Trachea
    Cricoid cartilage
 2 Carina
 3 Main Bronchus, Right
    Bronchus intermedius
    Intermediate bronchus
 4 Upper Lobe Bronchus, Right
 5 Middle Lobe Bronchus, Right
 6 Lower Lobe Bronchus, Right
 7 Main Bronchus, Left
 8 Upper Lobe Bronchus, Left
 9 Lingula Bronchus
 B Lower Lobe Bronchus, Left
 T Diaphragm
	Ø Open
	 4 Percutaneous Endoscopic
		7 Autologous Tissue Substitute
		 J Synthetic Substitute
		 K Nonautologous Tissue Substitute
			Z No Qualifier

Ø   **Medical and Surgical**
B   **Respiratory System**
S   **Reposition**   Definition: Moving to its normal location, or other suitable location, all or a portion of a body part
                        Explanation: The body part is moved to a new location from an abnormal location, or from a normal location where it is not functioning correctly. The body part may or may not be cut out or off to be moved to the new location.

Body Part Character 4	Approach Character 5	Device Character 6	Qualifier Character 7
1 Trachea 　　Cricoid cartilage 2 Carina 3 Main Bronchus, Right 　　Bronchus intermedius 　　Intermediate bronchus 4 Upper Lobe Bronchus, Right 5 Middle Lobe Bronchus, Right 6 Lower Lobe Bronchus, Right 7 Main Bronchus, Left 8 Upper Lobe Bronchus, Left 9 Lingula Bronchus B Lower Lobe Bronchus, Left C Upper Lung Lobe, Right D Middle Lung Lobe, Right F Lower Lung Lobe, Right G Upper Lung Lobe, Left H Lung Lingula J Lower Lung Lobe, Left K Lung, Right L Lung, Left T Diaphragm	Ø Open	Z No Device	Z No Qualifier

Ø   **Medical and Surgical**
B   **Respiratory System**
T   **Resection**   Definition: Cutting out or off, without replacement, all of a body part
                        Explanation: None

Body Part Character 4	Approach Character 5	Device Character 6	Qualifier Character 7
1 Trachea 　　Cricoid cartilage 2 Carina 3 Main Bronchus, Right 　　Bronchus intermedius 　　Intermediate bronchus 4 Upper Lobe Bronchus, Right 5 Middle Lobe Bronchus, Right 6 Lower Lobe Bronchus, Right 7 Main Bronchus, Left 8 Upper Lobe Bronchus, Left 9 Lingula Bronchus B Lower Lobe Bronchus, Left C Upper Lung Lobe, Right D Middle Lung Lobe, Right F Lower Lung Lobe, Right G Upper Lung Lobe, Left H Lung Lingula J Lower Lung Lobe, Left K Lung, Right L Lung, Left M Lungs, Bilateral T Diaphragm	Ø Open 4 Percutaneous Endoscopic	Z No Device	Z No Qualifier

NC Noncovered Procedure   **LC** Limited Coverage   **QA** Questionable OB Admit   **NT** New Tech Add-on   ⊞ Combination Member   ♂ Male   ♀ Female

ICD-10-PCS 2024   351

Respiratory System

Ø   **Medical and Surgical**
B   **Respiratory System**
U   **Supplement**   Definition: Putting in or on biological or synthetic material that physically reinforces and/or augments the function of a portion of a body part
                     Explanation: The biological material is non-living, or is living and from the same individual. The body part may have been previously replaced, and the SUPPLEMENT procedure is performed to physically reinforce and/or augment the function of the replaced body part.

Body Part Character 4	Approach Character 5	Device Character 6	Qualifier Character 7

1 Trachea
   Cricoid cartilage
2 Carina
3 Main Bronchus, Right
   Bronchus intermedius
   Intermediate bronchus
4 Upper Lobe Bronchus, Right
5 Middle Lobe Bronchus, Right
6 Lower Lobe Bronchus, Right
7 Main Bronchus, Left
8 Upper Lobe Bronchus, Left
9 Lingula Bronchus
B Lower Lobe Bronchus, Left
	Ø Open
	4 Percutaneous Endoscopic
	8 Via Natural or Artificial Opening Endoscopic
		7 Autologous Tissue Substitute
		J Synthetic Substitute
		K Nonautologous Tissue Substitute
			Z No Qualifier

T Diaphragm	Ø Open 4 Percutaneous Endoscopic	7 Autologous Tissue Substitute J Synthetic Substitute K Nonautologous Tissue Substitute	Z No Qualifier

Ø   **Medical and Surgical**
B   **Respiratory System**
V   **Restriction**   Definition: Partially closing an orifice or the lumen of a tubular body part
                     Explanation: The orifice can be a natural orifice or an artificially created orifice

Body Part Character 4	Approach Character 5	Device Character 6	Qualifier Character 7

1 Trachea
   Cricoid cartilage
2 Carina
3 Main Bronchus, Right
   Bronchus intermedius
   Intermediate bronchus
4 Upper Lobe Bronchus, Right
5 Middle Lobe Bronchus, Right
6 Lower Lobe Bronchus, Right
7 Main Bronchus, Left
8 Upper Lobe Bronchus, Left
9 Lingula Bronchus
B Lower Lobe Bronchus, Left
	Ø Open
	3 Percutaneous
	4 Percutaneous Endoscopic
		C Extraluminal Device
		D Intraluminal Device
		Z No Device
			Z No Qualifier

1 Trachea
   Cricoid cartilage
2 Carina
3 Main Bronchus, Right
   Bronchus intermedius
   Intermediate bronchus
4 Upper Lobe Bronchus, Right
5 Middle Lobe Bronchus, Right
6 Lower Lobe Bronchus, Right
7 Main Bronchus, Left
8 Upper Lobe Bronchus, Left
9 Lingula Bronchus
B Lower Lobe Bronchus, Left
	7 Via Natural or Artificial Opening
	8 Via Natural or Artificial Opening Endoscopic
		D Intraluminal Device
		Z No Device
			Z No Qualifier

Ø Medical and Surgical
B Respiratory System
W Revision   Definition: Correcting, to the extent possible, a portion of a malfunctioning device or the position of a displaced device
               Explanation: Revision can include correcting a malfunctioning or displaced device by taking out or putting in components of the device such as a screw or pin

Body Part Character 4	Approach Character 5	Device Character 6	Qualifier Character 7
Ø Tracheobronchial Tree	Ø Open 3 Percutaneous 4 Percutaneous Endoscopic 7 Via Natural or Artificial Opening 8 Via Natural or Artificial Opening Endoscopic	Ø Drainage Device 2 Monitoring Device 3 Infusion Device 7 Autologous Tissue Substitute C Extraluminal Device D Intraluminal Device J Synthetic Substitute K Nonautologous Tissue Substitute Y Other Device	Z No Qualifier
Ø Tracheobronchial Tree	X External	Ø Drainage Device 2 Monitoring Device 3 Infusion Device 7 Autologous Tissue Substitute C Extraluminal Device D Intraluminal Device J Synthetic Substitute K Nonautologous Tissue Substitute	Z No Qualifier
1 Trachea Cricoid cartilage	Ø Open 3 Percutaneous 4 Percutaneous Endoscopic 7 Via Natural or Artificial Opening 8 Via Natural or Artificial Opening Endoscopic X External	Ø Drainage Device 2 Monitoring Device 7 Autologous Tissue Substitute C Extraluminal Device D Intraluminal Device F Tracheostomy Device J Synthetic Substitute K Nonautologous Tissue Substitute	Z No Qualifier
K Lung, Right L Lung, Left	Ø Open 3 Percutaneous 4 Percutaneous Endoscopic 7 Via Natural or Artificial Opening 8 Via Natural or Artificial Opening Endoscopic	Ø Drainage Device 2 Monitoring Device 3 Infusion Device Y Other Device	Z No Qualifier
K Lung, Right L Lung, Left	X External	Ø Drainage Device 2 Monitoring Device 3 Infusion Device	Z No Qualifier
Q Pleura	Ø Open 3 Percutaneous 4 Percutaneous Endoscopic 7 Via Natural or Artificial Opening 8 Via Natural or Artificial Opening Endoscopic	Ø Drainage Device 2 Monitoring Device Y Other Device	Z No Qualifier
Q Pleura	X External	Ø Drainage Device 2 Monitoring Device	Z No Qualifier
T Diaphragm	Ø Open 3 Percutaneous 4 Percutaneous Endoscopic 7 Via Natural or Artificial Opening 8 Via Natural or Artificial Opening Endoscopic	Ø Drainage Device 2 Monitoring Device 7 Autologous Tissue Substitute J Synthetic Substitute K Nonautologous Tissue Substitute M Diaphragmatic Pacemaker Lead Y Other Device	Z No Qualifier
T Diaphragm	X External	Ø Drainage Device 2 Monitoring Device 7 Autologous Tissue Substitute J Synthetic Substitute K Nonautologous Tissue Substitute M Diaphragmatic Pacemaker Lead	Z No Qualifier

Non-OR   ØBWØ[3,4]YZ
Non-OR   ØBWØ[7,8][2,3,D,Y]Z
Non-OR   ØBWØX[Ø,2,3,7,C,D,J,K]Z
Non-OR   ØBW1X[Ø,2,7,C,D,F,J,K]Z
Non-OR   ØBW[K,L]3YZ
Non-OR   ØBW[K,L]7[Ø,2,3,Y]Z
Non-OR   ØBW[K,L]8[Ø,2,3]Z
Non-OR   ØBW[K,L]X[Ø,2,3]Z
Non-OR   ØBWQ[Ø,3,4,7,8][Ø,2]Z
Non-OR   ØBWQ[Ø,3,7]YZ
Non-OR   ØBWQX[Ø,2]Z
Non-OR   ØBWT[3,7,8]YZ
Non-OR   ØBWTX[Ø,2,7,J,K,M]Z

NC Noncovered Procedure   LC Limited Coverage   QA Questionable OB Admit   NT New Tech Add-on   ⊞ Combination Member   ♂ Male   ♀ Female

Ø Medical and Surgical
B Respiratory System
Y Transplantation   Definition: Putting in or on all or a portion of a living body part taken from another individual or animal to physically take the place and/or function of all or a portion of a similar body part

                 Explanation: The native body part may or may not be taken out, and the transplanted body part may take over all or a portion of its function

Body Part Character 4	Approach Character 5	Device Character 6	Qualifier Character 7
C Upper Lung Lobe, Right `LC` D Middle Lung Lobe, Right `LC` F Lower Lung Lobe, Right `LC` G Upper Lung Lobe, Left `LC` H Lung Lingula `LC` J Lower Lung Lobe, Left `LC` K Lung, Right `LC` L Lung, Left `LC` M Lungs, Bilateral `LC`	Ø Open	Z No Device	Ø Allogeneic 1 Syngeneic 2 Zooplastic

`LC`   ØBY[C,D,F,G,H,J,K,L,M]ØZ[Ø,1,2]

Non-OR Procedure   DRG Non-OR Procedure   Valid OR Procedure   HAC Associated Procedure   Combination Only   New/Revised April   New/Revised October

354   ICD-10-PCS 2024

Mouth and Throat 0C0–0CX

Character Meanings

This Character Meaning table is provided as a guide to assist the user in the identification of character members that may be found in this section of code tables. It **SHOULD NOT** be used to build a PCS code.

Operation–Character 3		Body Part–Character 4		Approach–Character 5		Device–Character 6		Qualifier–Character 7	
0	Alteration	0	Upper Lip	0	Open	0	Drainage Device	0	Single
2	Change	1	Lower Lip	3	Percutaneous	1	Radioactive Element	1	Multiple
5	Destruction	2	Hard Palate	4	Percutaneous Endoscopic	5	External Fixation Device	2	All
7	Dilation	3	Soft Palate	7	Via Natural or Artificial Opening	7	Autologous Tissue Substitute	X	Diagnostic
9	Drainage	4	Buccal Mucosa	8	Via Natural or Artificial Opening Endoscopic	B	Intraluminal Device, Airway	Z	No Qualifier
B	Excision	5	Upper Gingiva	X	External	C	Extraluminal Device		
C	Extirpation	6	Lower Gingiva			D	Intraluminal Device		
D	Extraction	7	Tongue			J	Synthetic Substitute		
F	Fragmentation	8	Parotid Gland, Right			K	Nonautologous Tissue Substitute		
H	Insertion	9	Parotid Gland, Left			Y	Other Device		
J	Inspection	A	Salivary Gland			Z	No Device		
L	Occlusion	B	Parotid Duct, Right						
M	Reattachment	C	Parotid Duct, Left						
N	Release	D	Sublingual Gland, Right						
P	Removal	F	Sublingual Gland, Left						
Q	Repair	G	Submaxillary Gland, Right						
R	Replacement	H	Submaxillary Gland, Left						
S	Reposition	J	Minor Salivary Gland						
T	Resection	M	Pharynx						
U	Supplement	N	Uvula						
V	Restriction	P	Tonsils						
W	Revision	Q	Adenoids						
X	Transfer	R	Epiglottis						
		S	Larynx						
		T	Vocal Cord, Right						
		V	Vocal Cord, Left						
		W	Upper Tooth						
		X	Lower Tooth						
		Y	Mouth and Throat						

AHA Coding Clinic for table 0C9
2017, 2Q, 16   Incision and drainage of floor of mouth

AHA Coding Clinic for table 0CB
2017, 2Q, 16   Excision of floor of mouth
2016, 3Q, 28   Lingual tonsillectomy, tongue base excision and epiglottopexy
2016, 2Q, 19   Biopsy of the base of tongue
2014, 3Q, 21   Superficial parotidectomy

AHA Coding Clinic for table 0CC
2016, 2Q, 20   Sialendoscopy with stone removal

AHA Coding Clinic for table 0CH
2020, 4Q, 43-44   Insertion of radioactive element

AHA Coding Clinic for table 0CQ
2017, 1Q, 20   Preparatory nasal adhesion repair before definitive cleft palate repair

AHA Coding Clinic for table 0CR
2014, 2Q, 5   Excision of soft palate with placement of surgical obturator
2014, 2Q, 5   Oasis acellular matrix graft
2014, 2Q, 6   Composite grafting (synthetic versus nonautologous tissue substitute)

AHA Coding Clinic for table 0CS
2022, 2Q, 24   Palatoplasty with intravelar veloplasty
2016, 3Q, 28   Lingual tonsillectomy, tongue base excision and epiglottopexy

AHA Coding Clinic for table 0CT
2016, 2Q, 12   Resection of malignant neoplasm of infratemporal fossa
2014, 3Q, 21   Superficial parotidectomy
2014, 3Q, 23   Le Fort I osteotomy

Salivary Glands

Oral Anatomy

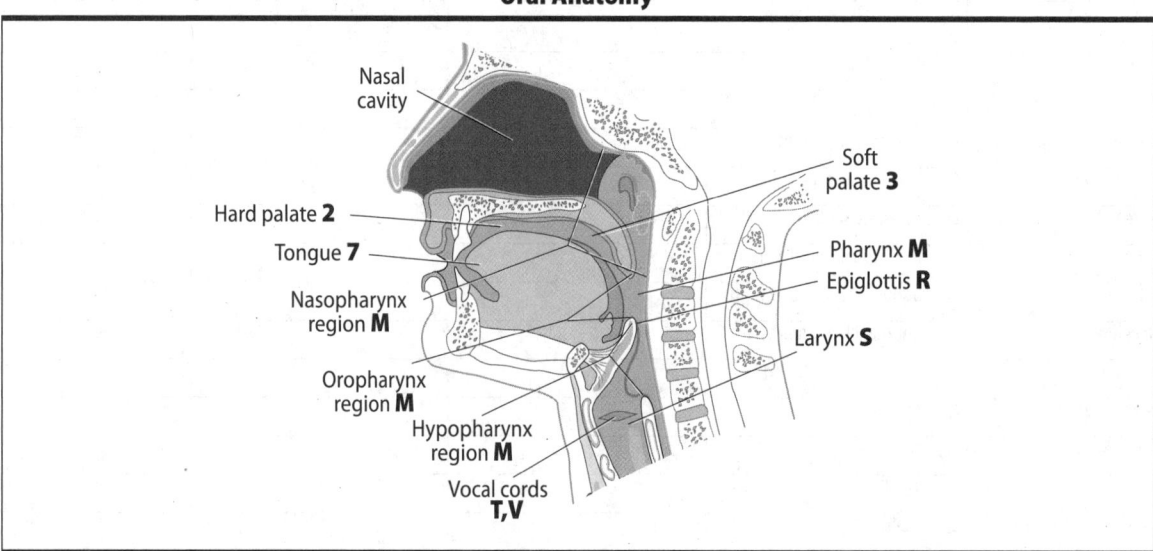

Mouth Frontal View (Upper)

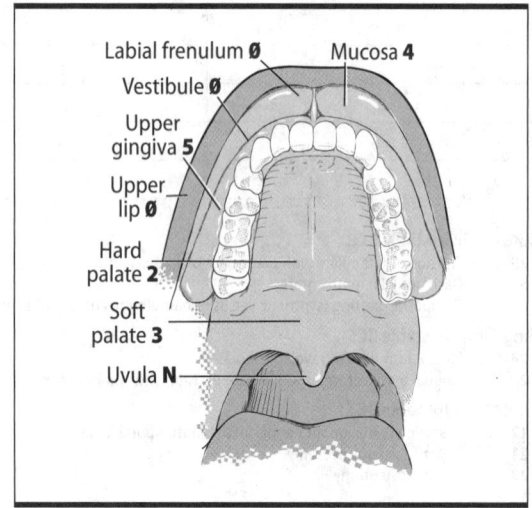

Mouth Frontal View (Lower)

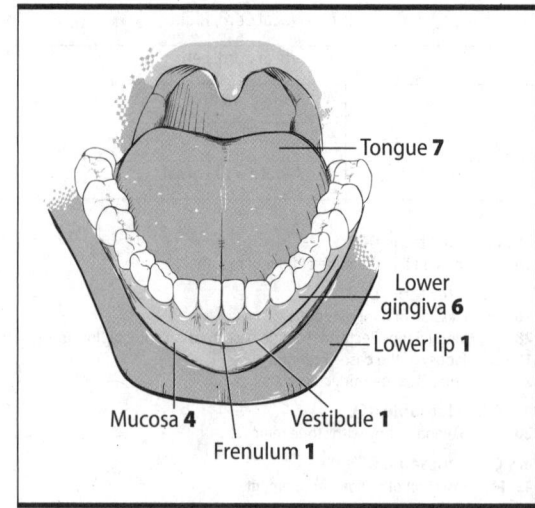

Ø   **Medical and Surgical**
C   **Mouth and Throat**
Ø   **Alteration**   Definition: Modifying the anatomic structure of a body part without affecting the function of the body part
      Explanation: Principal purpose is to improve appearance

Body Part Character 4	Approach Character 5	Device Character 6	Qualifier Character 7

Ø Upper Lip
   Frenulum labii superioris
   Labial gland
   Vermilion border
1 Lower Lip
   Frenulum labii inferioris
   Labial gland
   Vermilion border
	X External	**7** Autologous Tissue Substitute
		J Synthetic Substitute
		K Nonautologous Tissue Substitute
		Z No Device
			Z No Qualifier

Ø   **Medical and Surgical**
C   **Mouth and Throat**
2   **Change**   Definition: Taking out or off a device from a body part and putting back an identical or similar device in or on the same body part without cutting or puncturing the skin or a mucous membrane
      Explanation: All CHANGE procedures are coded using the approach EXTERNAL

Body Part Character 4	Approach Character 5	Device Character 6	Qualifier Character 7

A Salivary Gland
S Larynx
   Aryepiglottic fold
   Arytenoid cartilage
   Corniculate cartilage
   Cuneiform cartilage
   False vocal cord
   Glottis
   Rima glottidis
   Thyroid cartilage
   Ventricular fold
Y Mouth and Throat
	X External	**Ø** Drainage Device
		Y Other Device
			Z No Qualifier

Non-OR   All body part, approach, device, and qualifier values

Mouth and Throat *(side tab)*

0   **Medical and Surgical**
C   **Mouth and Throat**
5   **Destruction**   Definition: Physical eradication of all or a portion of a body part by the direct use of energy, force, or a destructive agent
                       Explanation: None of the body part is physically taken out

Body Part — Character 4	Approach — Character 5	Device — Character 6	Qualifier — Character 7
0 Upper Lip Frenulum labii superioris Labial gland Vermilion border 1 Lower Lip Frenulum labii inferioris Labial gland Vermilion border 2 Hard Palate 3 Soft Palate 4 Buccal Mucosa Buccal gland Molar gland Palatine gland 5 Upper Gingiva 6 Lower Gingiva 7 Tongue Frenulum linguae N Uvula Palatine uvula P Tonsils Palatine tonsil Q Adenoids Pharyngeal tonsil	0 Open 3 Percutaneous X External	Z No Device	Z No Qualifier
8 Parotid Gland, Right 9 Parotid Gland, Left B Parotid Duct, Right Stensen's duct C Parotid Duct, Left See B Parotid Duct, Right D Sublingual Gland, Right F Sublingual Gland, Left G Submaxillary Gland, Right Submandibular gland H Submaxillary Gland, Left See G Submaxillary Gland, Right J Minor Salivary Gland Anterior lingual gland	0 Open 3 Percutaneous	Z No Device	Z No Qualifier
M Pharynx Base of tongue Hypopharynx Laryngopharynx Lingual tonsil Oropharynx Piriform recess (sinus) Tongue, base of R Epiglottis Glossoepiglottic fold S Larynx Aryepiglottic fold Arytenoid cartilage Corniculate cartilage Cuneiform cartilage False vocal cord Glottis Rima glottidis Thyroid cartilage Ventricular fold T Vocal Cord, Right Vocal fold V Vocal Cord, Left See T Vocal Cord, Right	0 Open 3 Percutaneous 4 Percutaneous Endoscopic 7 Via Natural or Artificial Opening 8 Via Natural or Artificial Opening Endoscopic	Z No Device	Z No Qualifier
W Upper Tooth X Lower Tooth	0 Open X External	Z No Device	0 Single 1 Multiple 2 All

Non-OR   0C5[5,6][0,3,X]ZZ
Non-OR   0C5[W,X][0,X]Z[0,1,2]

0   **Medical and Surgical**
C   **Mouth and Throat**
7   **Dilation**   Definition: Expanding an orifice or the lumen of a tubular body part
                   Explanation: The orifice can be a natural orifice or an artificially created orifice. Accomplished by stretching a tubular body part using intraluminal pressure or by cutting part of the orifice or wall of the tubular body part.

Body Part — Character 4	Approach — Character 5	Device — Character 6	Qualifier — Character 7
B Parotid Duct, Right Stensen's duct C Parotid Duct, Left See B Parotid Duct, Right	0 Open 3 Percutaneous 7 Via Natural or Artificial Opening	D Intraluminal Device Z No Device	Z No Qualifier
M Pharynx Base of tongue Hypopharynx Laryngopharynx Lingual tonsil Oropharynx Piriform recess (sinus) Tongue, base of	7 Via Natural or Artificial Opening 8 Via Natural or Artificial Opening Endoscopic	D Intraluminal Device Z No Device	Z No Qualifier
S Larynx Aryepiglottic fold Arytenoid cartilage Corniculate cartilage Cuneiform cartilage False vocal cord Glottis Rima glottidis Thyroid cartilage Ventricular fold	0 Open 3 Percutaneous 4 Percutaneous Endoscopic 7 Via Natural or Artificial Opening 8 Via Natural or Artificial Opening Endoscopic	D Intraluminal Device Z No Device	Z No Qualifier

Non-OR   0C7[B,C][0,3,7][D,Z]Z
Non-OR   0C7M[7,8][D,Z]Z

Non-OR Procedure   DRG Non-OR Procedure   Valid OR Procedure   HAC Associated Procedure   Combination Only   New/Revised April   New/Revised October

0	**Medical and Surgical**
C	**Mouth and Throat**
9	**Drainage** Definition: Taking or letting out fluids and/or gases from a body part
	Explanation: The qualifier DIAGNOSTIC is used to identify drainage procedures that are biopsies

Body Part Character 4		Approach Character 5	Device Character 6	Qualifier Character 7
0 Upper Lip Frenulum labii superioris Labial gland Vermilion border **1 Lower Lip** Frenulum labii inferioris Labial gland Vermilion border **2 Hard Palate** **3 Soft Palate** **4 Buccal Mucosa** Buccal gland Molar gland Palatine gland	**5 Upper Gingiva** **6 Lower Gingiva** **7 Tongue** Frenulum linguae **N Uvula** Palatine uvula **P Tonsils** Palatine tonsil **Q Adenoids** Pharyngeal tonsil	**0 Open** **3 Percutaneous** **X External**	**0 Drainage Device**	**Z No Qualifier**
0 Upper Lip Frenulum labii superioris Labial gland Vermilion border **1 Lower Lip** Frenulum labii inferioris Labial gland Vermilion border **2 Hard Palate** **3 Soft Palate** **4 Buccal Mucosa** Buccal gland Molar gland Palatine gland	**5 Upper Gingiva** **6 Lower Gingiva** **7 Tongue** Frenulum linguae **N Uvula** Palatine uvula **P Tonsils** Palatine tonsil **Q Adenoids** Pharyngeal tonsil	**0 Open** **3 Percutaneous** **X External**	**Z No Device**	**X Diagnostic** **Z No Qualifier**
8 Parotid Gland, Right **9 Parotid Gland, Left** **B Parotid Duct, Right** Stensen's duct **C Parotid Duct, Left** *See B Parotid Duct, Right* **D Sublingual Gland, Right**	**F Sublingual Gland, Left** **G Submaxillary Gland, Right** Submandibular gland **H Submaxillary Gland, Left** *See G Submaxillary Gland, Right* **J Minor Salivary Gland** Anterior lingual gland	**0 Open** **3 Percutaneous**	**0 Drainage Device**	**Z No Qualifier**
8 Parotid Gland, Right **9 Parotid Gland, Left** **B Parotid Duct, Right** Stensen's duct **C Parotid Duct, Left** *See B Parotid Duct, Right*	**D Sublingual Gland, Right** **F Sublingual Gland, Left** **G Submaxillary Gland, Right** Submandibular gland **H Submaxillary Gland, Left** *See G Submaxillary Gland, Right* **J Minor Salivary Gland** Anterior lingual gland	**0 Open** **3 Percutaneous**	**Z No Device**	**X Diagnostic** **Z No Qualifier**
M Pharynx Base of tongue Hypopharynx Laryngopharynx Lingual tonsil Oropharynx Piriform recess (sinus) Tongue, base of **R Epiglottis** Glossoepiglottic fold	**S Larynx** Aryepiglottic fold Arytenoid cartilage Corniculate cartilage Cuneiform cartilage False vocal cord Glottis Rima glottidis Thyroid cartilage Ventricular fold **T Vocal Cord, Right** Vocal fold **V Vocal Cord, Left** *See T Vocal Cord, Right*	**0 Open** **3 Percutaneous** **4 Percutaneous Endoscopic** **7 Via Natural or Artificial Opening** **8 Via Natural or Artificial Opening Endoscopic**	**0 Drainage Device**	**Z No Qualifier**

Non-OR	0C9[0,1,2,3,4,7,N,P,Q]30Z
Non-OR	0C9[5,6][0,3,X]0Z
Non-OR	0C9[0,1,4][0,3,X]ZX
Non-OR	0C9[0,1,2,3,4,7,N,P,Q]3ZZ
Non-OR	0C9[5,6][0,3,X]Z[X,Z]
Non-OR	0C97[3,X]ZX
Non-OR	0C9[8,9,B,C,D,F,G,H,J][0,3]0Z
Non-OR	0C9[8,9,B,C,D,F,G,H,J]3ZX
Non-OR	0C9[8,9,G,H]3ZZ
Non-OR	0C9[B,C,D, F,J][0,3]ZZ
Non-OR	0C9[M,R,S,T,V]30Z

0C9 Continued on next page

NC Noncovered Procedure   LC Limited Coverage   OA Questionable OB Admit   NT New Tech Add-on   ⊞ Combination Member   ♂ Male   ♀ Female

Mouth and Throat

ØC9 Continued

Ø   **Medical and Surgical**
C   **Mouth and Throat**
9   **Drainage**   Definition: Taking or letting out fluids and/or gases from a body part
Explanation: The qualifier DIAGNOSTIC is used to identify drainage procedures that are biopsies

Body Part Character 4		Approach Character 5	Device Character 6	Qualifier Character 7

M Pharynx
  Base of tongue
  Hypopharynx
  Laryngopharynx
  Lingual tonsil
  Oropharynx
  Piriform recess (sinus)
  Tongue, base of
R Epiglottis
  Glossoepiglottic fold
	S Larynx
	  Aryepiglottic fold
	  Arytenoid cartilage
	  Corniculate cartilage
	  Cuneiform cartilage
	  False vocal cord
	  Glottis
	  Rima glottidis
	  Thyroid cartilage
	  Ventricular fold
	T Vocal Cord, Right
	  Vocal fold
	V Vocal Cord, Left
	  See T Vocal Cord, Right
		Ø Open
		3 Percutaneous
		4 Percutaneous Endoscopic
		7 Via Natural or Artificial Opening
		8 Via Natural or Artificial Opening Endoscopic
			Z No Device	X Diagnostic
				Z No Qualifier

W Upper Tooth X Lower Tooth		Ø Open X External	Ø Drainage Device Z No Device	Ø Single 1 Multiple 2 All

Non-OR   ØC9M[Ø,3,4,7,8]ZX
Non-OR   ØC9[M,R,S,T,V]3ZZ
Non-OR   ØC9[R,S,T,V][3,4,7,8]ZZ
Non-OR   ØC9[W,X][Ø,X][Ø,Z][Ø,1,2]

Ø   **Medical and Surgical**
C   **Mouth and Throat**
B   **Excision**   Definition: Cutting out or off, without replacement, a portion of a body part
Explanation: The qualifier DIAGNOSTIC is used to identify excision procedures that are biopsies

Body Part Character 4		Approach Character 5	Device Character 6	Qualifier Character 7

Ø Upper Lip
  Frenulum labii superioris
  Labial gland
  Vermilion border
1 Lower Lip
  Frenulum labii inferioris
  Labial gland
  Vermilion border
2 Hard Palate
3 Soft Palate
4 Buccal Mucosa
  Buccal gland
  Molar gland
  Palatine gland
	5 Upper Gingiva
	6 Lower Gingiva
	7 Tongue
	  Frenulum linguae
	N Uvula
	  Palatine uvula
	P Tonsils
	  Palatine tonsil
	Q Adenoids
	  Pharyngeal tonsil
		Ø Open
		3 Percutaneous
		X External
			Z No Device	X Diagnostic
				Z No Qualifier

8 Parotid Gland, Right
9 Parotid Gland, Left
B Parotid Duct, Right
  Stensen's duct
C Parotid Duct, Left
  See B Parotid Duct, Right
D Sublingual Gland, Right
	F Sublingual Gland, Left
	G Submaxillary Gland, Right
	  Submandibular gland
	H Submaxillary Gland, Left
	  See G Submaxillary Gland, Right
	J Minor Salivary Gland
	  Anterior lingual gland
		Ø Open
		3 Percutaneous
			Z No Device	X Diagnostic
				Z No Qualifier

M Pharynx
  Base of tongue
  Hypopharynx
  Laryngopharynx
  Lingual tonsil
  Oropharynx
  Piriform recess (sinus)
  Tongue, base of
R Epiglottis
  Glossoepiglottic fold
	S Larynx
	  Aryepiglottic fold
	  Arytenoid cartilage
	  Corniculate cartilage
	  Cuneiform cartilage
	  False vocal cord
	  Glottis
	  Rima glottidis
	  Thyroid cartilage
	  Ventricular fold
	T Vocal Cord, Right
	  Vocal fold
	V Vocal Cord, Left
	  See T Vocal Cord, Right
		Ø Open
		3 Percutaneous
		4 Percutaneous Endoscopic
		7 Via Natural or Artificial Opening
		8 Via Natural or Artificial Opening Endoscopic
			Z No Device	X Diagnostic
				Z No Qualifier

W Upper Tooth X Lower Tooth		Ø Open X External	Z No Device	Ø Single 1 Multiple 2 All

Non-OR   ØCB[Ø,1,4][Ø,3,X]ZX
Non-OR   ØCB[5,6][Ø,3,X]Z[X,Z]
Non-OR   ØCB7[3,X]ZX
Non-OR   ØCB[8,9,B,C,D,F,G,H,J]3ZX

Non-OR   ØCBM[Ø,3,4,7,8]ZX
Non-OR   ØCB[R,S,T,V][3,4,7,8]ZX
Non-OR   ØCB[W,X][Ø,X]Z[Ø,1,2]

Ø **Medical and Surgical**
C **Mouth and Throat**
C **Extirpation**　　Definition: Taking or cutting out solid matter from a body part

Explanation: The solid matter may be an abnormal byproduct of a biological function or a foreign body; it may be imbedded in a body part or in the lumen of a tubular body part. The solid matter may or may not have been previously broken into pieces.

Body Part Character 4		Approach Character 5	Device Character 6	Qualifier Character 7
Ø Upper Lip Frenulum labii superioris Labial gland Vermilion border **1 Lower Lip** Frenulum labii inferioris Labial gland Vermilion border **2 Hard Palate** **3 Soft Palate** **4 Buccal Mucosa** Buccal gland Molar gland Palatine gland	**5 Upper Gingiva** **6 Lower Gingiva** **7 Tongue** Frenulum linguae **N Uvula** Palatine uvula **P Tonsils** Palatine tonsil **Q Adenoids** Pharyngeal tonsil	**Ø** Open **3** Percutaneous **X** External	**Z** No Device	**Z** No Qualifier
8 Parotid Gland, Right **9 Parotid Gland, Left** **B Parotid Duct, Right** Stensen's duct **C Parotid Duct, Left** *See B Parotid Duct, Right* **D Sublingual Gland, Right**	**F Sublingual Gland, Left** **G Submaxillary Gland, Right** Submandibular gland **H Submaxillary Gland, Left** *See G Submaxillary Gland, Right* **J Minor Salivary Gland** Anterior lingual gland	**Ø** Open **3** Percutaneous	**Z** No Device	**Z** No Qualifier
M Pharynx Base of tongue Hypopharynx Laryngopharynx Lingual tonsil Oropharynx Piriform recess (sinus) Tongue, base of **R Epiglottis** Glossoepiglottic fold	**S Larynx** Aryepiglottic fold Arytenoid cartilage Corniculate cartilage Cuneiform cartilage False vocal cord Glottis Rima glottidis Thyroid cartilage Ventricular fold **T Vocal Cord, Right** Vocal fold **V Vocal Cord, Left** *See T Vocal Cord, Right*	**Ø** Open **3** Percutaneous **4** Percutaneous Endoscopic **7** Via Natural or Artificial Opening **8** Via Natural or Artificial Opening Endoscopic	**Z** No Device	**Z** No Qualifier
W Upper Tooth **X Lower Tooth**		**Ø** Open **X** External	**Z** No Device	**Ø** Single **1** Multiple **2** All

Non-OR	ØCC[Ø,1,2,3,4,7,N,P,Q]XZZ
Non-OR	ØCC[5,6][Ø,3,X]ZZ
Non-OR	ØCC[8,9,G,H]3ZZ
Non-OR	ØCC[B,C,D,F,J][Ø,3]ZZ
Non-OR	ØCC[M,S][7,8]ZZ
Non-OR	ØCC[W,X][Ø,X]Z[Ø,1,2]

Ø **Medical and Surgical**
C **Mouth and Throat**
D **Extraction**　　Definition: Pulling or stripping out or off all or a portion of a body part by the use of force

Explanation: The qualifier DIAGNOSTIC is used to identify extraction procedures that are biopsies

Body Part Character 4	Approach Character 5	Device Character 6	Qualifier Character 7
T Vocal Cord, Right Vocal fold **V Vocal Cord, Left** *See T Vocal Cord, Right*	**Ø** Open **3** Percutaneous **4** Percutaneous Endoscopic **7** Via Natural or Artificial Opening **8** Via Natural or Artificial Opening Endoscopic	**Z** No Device	**Z** No Qualifier
W Upper Tooth **X Lower Tooth**	**X** External	**Z** No Device	**Ø** Single **1** Multiple **2** All

Non-OR	ØCD[W,X]XZ[Ø,1,2]

Mouth and Throat

Ø   **Medical and Surgical**
C   **Mouth and Throat**
F   **Fragmentation**   Definition: Breaking solid matter in a body part into pieces

           Explanation: Physical force (e.g., manual, ultrasonic) applied directly or indirectly is used to break the solid matter into pieces. The solid matter may be an abnormal byproduct of a biological function or a foreign body. The pieces of solid matter are not taken out.

Body Part Character 4	Approach Character 5	Device Character 6	Qualifier Character 7

B   Parotid Duct, Right   **NC**
     Stensen's duct
C   Parotid Duct, Left   **NC**
     See B Parotid Duct, Right
	Ø Open
	3 Percutaneous
	7 Via Natural or Artificial Opening
	X External
		Z No Device	Z No Qualifier

Non-OR   All body part, approach, device, and qualifier values
NC   ØCF[B,C]XZZ

Ø   **Medical and Surgical**
C   **Mouth and Throat**
H   **Insertion**   Definition: Putting in a nonbiological appliance that monitors, assists, performs, or prevents a physiological function but does not physically take the place of a body part

           Explanation: None

Body Part Character 4	Approach Character 5	Device Character 6	Qualifier Character 7
7 Tongue Frenulum linguae	Ø Open 3 Percutaneous X External	1 Radioactive Element	Z No Qualifier

A   Salivary Gland
S   Larynx
     Aryepiglottic fold
     Arytenoid cartilage
     Corniculate cartilage
     Cuneiform cartilage
     False vocal cord
     Glottis
     Rima glottidis
     Thyroid cartilage
     Ventricular fold
	Ø Open
	3 Percutaneous
	7 Via Natural or Artificial Opening
	8 Via Natural or Artificial Opening Endoscopic
		1 Radioactive Element
		Y Other Device
			Z No Qualifier

Y Mouth and Throat	Ø Open 3 Percutaneous	1 Radioactive Element Y Other Device	Z No Qualifier
Y Mouth and Throat	7 Via Natural or Artificial Opening 8 Via Natural or Artificial Opening Endoscopic	1 Radioactive Element B Intraluminal Device, Airway Y Other Device	Z No Qualifier

Non-OR   ØCH[A,S]Ø1Z
Non-OR   ØCHSØYZ
Non-OR   ØCH[A,S][3,7,8][1,Y]Z
Non-OR   ØCHY[Ø,3][1,Y]Z
Non-OR   ØCHY[7,8][1,B,Y]Z

Ø   **Medical and Surgical**
C   **Mouth and Throat**
J   **Inspection**   Definition: Visually and/or manually exploring a body part

           Explanation: Visual exploration may be performed with or without optical instrumentation. Manual exploration may be performed directly or through intervening body layers.

Body Part Character 4	Approach Character 5	Device Character 6	Qualifier Character 7
A Salivary Gland	Ø Open 3 Percutaneous X External	Z No Device	Z No Qualifier

S   Larynx
     Aryepiglottic fold
     Arytenoid cartilage
     Corniculate cartilage
     Cuneiform cartilage
     False vocal cord
     Glottis
     Rima glottidis
     Thyroid cartilage
     Ventricular fold
Y   Mouth and Throat
	Ø Open
	3 Percutaneous
	4 Percutaneous Endoscopic
	7 Via Natural or Artificial Opening
	8 Via Natural or Artificial Opening Endoscopic
	X External
		Z No Device	Z No Qualifier

Non-OR   All body part, approach, device, and qualifier values

Ø　Medical and Surgical
C　Mouth and Throat
L　Occlusion　　　Definition: Completely closing an orifice or the lumen of a tubular body part
　　　　　　　　　　Explanation: The orifice can be a natural orifice or an artificially created orifice

Body Part Character 4	Approach Character 5	Device Character 6	Qualifier Character 7
B　Parotid Duct, Right 　　Stensen's duct C　Parotid Duct, Left 　　*See B Parotid Duct, Right*	Ø　Open 3　Percutaneous 4　Percutaneous Endoscopic	C　Extraluminal Device D　Intraluminal Device Z　No Device	Z　No Qualifier
B　Parotid Duct, Right 　　Stensen's duct C　Parotid Duct, Left 　　*See B Parotid Duct, Right*	7　Via Natural or Artificial Opening 8　Via Natural or Artificial Opening 　　Endoscopic	D　Intraluminal Device Z　No Device	Z　No Qualifier

Ø　Medical and Surgical
C　Mouth and Throat
M　Reattachment　　Definition: Putting back in or on all or a portion of a separated body part to its normal location or other suitable location
　　　　　　　　　　Explanation: Vascular circulation and nervous pathways may or may not be reestablished

Body Part Character 4	Approach Character 5	Device Character 6	Qualifier Character 7
Ø　Upper Lip 　　Frenulum labii superioris 　　Labial gland 　　Vermilion border 1　Lower Lip 　　Frenulum labii inferioris 　　Labial gland 　　Vermilion border 3　Soft Palate 7　Tongue 　　Frenulum linguae N　Uvula 　　Palatine uvula	Ø　Open	Z　No Device	Z　No Qualifier
W　Upper Tooth X　Lower Tooth	Ø　Open X　External	Z　No Device	Ø　Single 1　Multiple 2　All

Non-OR　ØCM[W,X][Ø,X]Z[Ø,1,2]

NC Noncovered Procedure　　LC Limited Coverage　　QA Questionable OB Admit　　NT New Tech Add-on　　⊞ Combination Member　　♂ Male　　♀ Female

ICD-10-PCS 2024　　　　　　　　　　　　　　　　　　　　　　　　　　　　　　　　　363

Mouth and Throat

Ø **Medical and Surgical**
C **Mouth and Throat**
N **Release**   Definition: Freeing a body part from an abnormal physical constraint by cutting or by the use of force
                   Explanation: Some of the restraining tissue may be taken out but none of the body part is taken out

Body Part Character 4	Approach Character 5	Device Character 6	Qualifier Character 7

Ø Upper Lip
   Frenulum labii superioris
   Labial gland
   Vermilion border
1 Lower Lip
   Frenulum labii inferioris
   Labial gland
   Vermilion border
2 Hard Palate
3 Soft Palate
4 Buccal Mucosa
   Buccal gland
   Molar gland
   Palatine gland
5 Upper Gingiva
6 Lower Gingiva
7 Tongue
   Frenulum linguae
N Uvula
   Palatine uvula
P Tonsils
   Palatine tonsil
Q Adenoids
   Pharyngeal tonsil
	Ø Open
	3 Percutaneous
	X External
		Z No Device	Z No Qualifier

8 Parotid Gland, Right
9 Parotid Gland, Left
B Parotid Duct, Right
   Stensen's duct
C Parotid Duct, Left
   See B Parotid Duct, Right
D Sublingual Gland, Right
F Sublingual Gland, Left
G Submaxillary Gland, Right
   Submandibular gland
H Submaxillary Gland, Left
   See G Submaxillary Gland, Right
J Minor Salivary Gland
   Anterior lingual gland
	Ø Open
	3 Percutaneous
		Z No Device	Z No Qualifier

M Pharynx
   Base of tongue
   Hypopharynx
   Laryngopharynx
   Lingual tonsil
   Oropharynx
   Piriform recess (sinus)
   Tongue, base of
R Epiglottis
   Glossoepiglottic fold
S Larynx
   Aryepiglottic fold
   Arytenoid cartilage
   Corniculate cartilage
   Cuneiform cartilage
   False vocal cord
   Glottis
   Rima glottidis
   Thyroid cartilage
   Ventricular fold
T Vocal Cord, Right
   Vocal fold
V Vocal Cord, Left
   See T Vocal Cord, Right
	Ø Open
	3 Percutaneous
	4 Percutaneous Endoscopic
	7 Via Natural or Artificial Opening
	8 Via Natural or Artificial Opening Endoscopic
		Z No Device	Z No Qualifier

W Upper Tooth X Lower Tooth	Ø Open X External	Z No Device	Ø Single 1 Multiple 2 All

Non-OR   ØCN[Ø,1,5,6,7][Ø,3,X]ZZ
Non-OR   ØCN[W,X][Ø,X]Z[Ø,1,2]

0   Medical and Surgical
C   Mouth and Throat
P   Removal   Definition: Taking out or off a device from a body part

Explanation: If a device is taken out and a similar device put in without cutting or puncturing the skin or mucous membrane, the procedure is coded to the root operation CHANGE. Otherwise, the procedure for taking out a device is coded to the root operation REMOVAL.

Body Part Character 4	Approach Character 5	Device Character 6	Qualifier Character 7
A Salivary Gland	**0** Open **3** Percutaneous	**0** Drainage Device **C** Extraluminal Device **Y** Other Device	**Z** No Qualifier
A Salivary Gland	**7** Via Natural or Artificial Opening **8** Via Natural or Artificial Opening Endoscopic	**Y** Other Device	**Z** No Qualifier

S Larynx
  Aryepiglottic fold
  Arytenoid cartilage
  Corniculate cartilage
  Cuneiform cartilage
  False vocal cord
  Glottis
  Rima glottidis
  Thyroid cartilage
  Ventricular fold
	0 Open
	3 Percutaneous
	7 Via Natural or Artificial Opening
	8 Via Natural or Artificial Opening Endoscopic
		0 Drainage Device
		7 Autologous Tissue Substitute
		D Intraluminal Device
		J Synthetic Substitute
		K Nonautologous Tissue Substitute
		Y Other Device
			Z No Qualifier

S Larynx
  Aryepiglottic fold
  Arytenoid cartilage
  Corniculate cartilage
  Cuneiform cartilage
  False vocal cord
  Glottis
  Rima glottidis
  Thyroid cartilage
  Ventricular fold
	X External	**0** Drainage Device
		7 Autologous Tissue Substitute
		D Intraluminal Device
		J Synthetic Substitute
		K Nonautologous Tissue Substitute
			Z No Qualifier

Y Mouth and Throat	**0** Open **3** Percutaneous **7** Via Natural or Artificial Opening **8** Via Natural or Artificial Opening Endoscopic	**0** Drainage Device **1** Radioactive Element **7** Autologous Tissue Substitute **D** Intraluminal Device **J** Synthetic Substitute **K** Nonautologous Tissue Substitute **Y** Other Device	**Z** No Qualifier
Y Mouth and Throat	**X** External	**0** Drainage Device **1** Radioactive Element **7** Autologous Tissue Substitute **D** Intraluminal Device **J** Synthetic Substitute **K** Nonautologous Tissue Substitute	**Z** No Qualifier

Non-OR   0CPA[0,3][0,C,Y]Z
Non-OR   0CPA[7,8]YZ
Non-OR   0CPS3YZ
Non-OR   0CPS[7,8][0,D,Y]Z
Non-OR   0CPSX[0,7,D,J,K]Z
Non-OR   0CPY3YZ
Non-OR   0CPY[7,8][0,D,Y]Z
Non-OR   0CPYX[0,1,7,D,J,K]Z

Mouth and Throat *(left margin)*

Ø   **Medical and Surgical**
C   **Mouth and Throat**
Q   **Repair**   Definition: Restoring, to the extent possible, a body part to its normal anatomic structure and function

                      Explanation: Used only when the method to accomplish the repair is not one of the other root operations

Body Part Character 4	Approach Character 5	Device Character 6	Qualifier Character 7
Ø Upper Lip Frenulum labii superioris Labial gland Vermilion border 1 Lower Lip Frenulum labii inferioris Labial gland Vermilion border 2 Hard Palate 3 Soft Palate 4 Buccal Mucosa Buccal gland Molar gland Palatine gland 5 Upper Gingiva 6 Lower Gingiva 7 Tongue Frenulum linguae N Uvula Palatine uvula P Tonsils Palatine tonsil Q Adenoids Pharyngeal tonsil	Ø Open 3 Percutaneous X External	Z No Device	Z No Qualifier
8 Parotid Gland, Right 9 Parotid Gland, Left B Parotid Duct, Right Stensen's duct C Parotid Duct, Left See B Parotid Duct, Right D Sublingual Gland, Right F Sublingual Gland, Left G Submaxillary Gland, Right Submandibular gland H Submaxillary Gland, Left See G Submaxillary Gland, Right J Minor Salivary Gland Anterior lingual gland	Ø Open 3 Percutaneous	Z No Device	Z No Qualifier
M Pharynx Base of tongue Hypopharynx Laryngopharynx Lingual tonsil Oropharynx Piriform recess (sinus) Tongue, base of R Epiglottis Glossoepiglottic fold S Larynx Aryepiglottic fold Arytenoid cartilage Corniculate cartilage Cuneiform cartilage False vocal cord Glottis Rima glottidis Thyroid cartilage Ventricular fold T Vocal Cord, Right Vocal fold V Vocal Cord, Left See T Vocal Cord, Right	Ø Open 3 Percutaneous 4 Percutaneous Endoscopic 7 Via Natural or Artificial Opening 8 Via Natural or Artificial Opening Endoscopic	Z No Device	Z No Qualifier
W Upper Tooth X Lower Tooth	Ø Open X External	Z No Device	Ø Single 1 Multiple 2 All

Non-OR   ØCQ[Ø,1,4,7]XZZ
Non-OR   ØCQ[5,6][Ø,3,X]ZZ
Non-OR   ØCQ[W,X][Ø,X]Z[Ø,1,2]

Non-OR Procedure   DRG Non-OR Procedure   Valid OR Procedure   HAC Associated Procedure   Combination Only   New/Revised April   New/Revised October

Ø Medical and Surgical
C Mouth and Throat
R Replacement   Definition: Putting in or on biological or synthetic material that physically takes the place and/or function of all or a portion of a body part

Explanation: The body part may have been taken out or replaced, or may be taken out, physically eradicated, or rendered nonfunctional during the REPLACEMENT procedure. A REMOVAL procedure is coded for taking out the device used in a previous replacement procedure.

Body Part Character 4	Approach Character 5	Device Character 6	Qualifier Character 7
Ø Upper Lip Frenulum labii superioris Labial gland Vermilion border **1 Lower Lip** Frenulum labii inferioris Labial gland Vermilion border **2 Hard Palate** **3 Soft Palate** **4 Buccal Mucosa** Buccal gland Molar gland Palatine gland **5 Upper Gingiva** **6 Lower Gingiva** **7 Tongue** Frenulum linguae **N Uvula** Palatine uvula	**Ø** Open **3** Percutaneous **X** External	**7** Autologous Tissue Substitute **J** Synthetic Substitute **K** Nonautologous Tissue Substitute	**Z** No Qualifier
B Parotid Duct, Right Stensen's duct **C Parotid Duct, Left** *See B Parotid Duct, Right*	**Ø** Open **3** Percutaneous	**7** Autologous Tissue Substitute **J** Synthetic Substitute **K** Nonautologous Tissue Substitute	**Z** No Qualifier
M Pharynx Base of tongue Hypopharynx Laryngopharynx Lingual tonsil Oropharynx Piriform recess (sinus) Tongue, base of **R Epiglottis** Glossoepiglottic fold **S Larynx** Aryepiglottic fold Arytenoid cartilage Corniculate cartilage Cuneiform cartilage False vocal cord Glottis Rima glottidis Thyroid cartilage Ventricular fold **T Vocal Cord, Right** Vocal fold **V Vocal Cord, Left** *See T Vocal Cord, Right*	**Ø** Open **7** Via Natural or Artificial Opening **8** Via Natural or Artificial Opening Endoscopic	**7** Autologous Tissue Substitute **J** Synthetic Substitute **K** Nonautologous Tissue Substitute	**Z** No Qualifier
W Upper Tooth **X Lower Tooth**	**Ø** Open **X** External	**7** Autologous Tissue Substitute **J** Synthetic Substitute **K** Nonautologous Tissue Substitute	**Ø** Single **1** Multiple **2** All

Non-OR   ØCR[W,X][Ø,X][7,J,K][Ø,1,2]

NC Noncovered Procedure   **LC** Limited Coverage   **QA** Questionable OB Admit   **NT** New Tech Add-on   ⊞ Combination Member   ♂ Male   ♀ Female

ICD-10-PCS 2024   367

ØCR–ØCR

Mouth and Throat

Ø   **Medical and Surgical**
C   **Mouth and Throat**
S   **Reposition**   Definition: Moving to its normal location, or other suitable location, all or a portion of a body part

                             Explanation: The body part is moved to a new location from an abnormal location, or from a normal location where it is not functioning correctly. The body part may or may not be cut out or off to be moved to the new location.

Body Part Character 4	Approach Character 5	Device Character 6	Qualifier Character 7

Ø   **Upper Lip**
    Frenulum labii superioris
    Labial gland
    Vermilion border
1   **Lower Lip**
    Frenulum labii inferioris
    Labial gland
    Vermilion border
2   **Hard Palate**
3   **Soft Palate**
7   **Tongue**
    Frenulum linguae
N   **Uvula**
    Palatine uvula
	Ø Open
	X External
		Z No Device	Z No Qualifier

B   **Parotid Duct, Right**
    Stensen's duct
C   **Parotid Duct, Left**
    See B Parotid Duct, Right
	Ø Open
	3 Percutaneous
		Z No Device	Z No Qualifier

R   **Epiglottis**
    Glossoepiglottic fold
S   Larynx
T   **Vocal Cord, Right**
    Vocal fold
V   **Vocal Cord, Left**
    See T Vocal Cord, Right
	Ø Open
	7 Via Natural or Artificial Opening
	8 Via Natural or Artificial Opening
	    Endoscopic
		Z No Device	Z No Qualifier

W Upper Tooth X Lower Tooth	Ø Open X External	5 External Fixation Device Z No Device	Ø Single 1 Multiple 2 All

Non-OR   ØCS[W,X][Ø,X][5,Z][Ø,1,2]

Non-OR Procedure   **DRG Non-OR Procedure**   Valid OR Procedure   HAC Associated Procedure   **Combination Only**   New/Revised April   New/Revised October

368   ICD-10-PCS 2024

Mouth and Throat

Ø   **Medical and Surgical**
C   **Mouth and Throat**
T   **Resection**   Definition: Cutting out or off, without replacement, all of a body part
           Explanation: None

Body Part Character 4	Approach Character 5	Device Character 6	Qualifier Character 7
Ø Upper Lip Frenulum labii superioris Labial gland Vermilion border 1 Lower Lip Frenulum labii inferioris Labial gland Vermilion border 2 Hard Palate 3 Soft Palate 7 Tongue Frenulum linguae N Uvula Palatine uvula P Tonsils Palatine tonsil Q Adenoids Pharyngeal tonsil	Ø Open X External	Z No Device	Z No Qualifier
8 Parotid Gland, Right 9 Parotid Gland, Left B Parotid Duct, Right Stensen's duct C Parotid Duct, Left See B Parotid Duct, Right D Sublingual Gland, Right F Sublingual Gland, Left G Submaxillary Gland, Right Submandibular gland H Submaxillary Gland, Left See G Submaxillary Gland, Right J Minor Salivary Gland Anterior lingual gland	Ø Open	Z No Device	Z No Qualifier
M Pharynx Base of tongue Hypopharynx Laryngopharynx Lingual tonsil Oropharynx Piriform recess (sinus) Tongue, base of R Epiglottis Glossoepiglottic fold S Larynx Aryepiglottic fold Arytenoid cartilage Corniculate cartilage Cuneiform cartilage False vocal cord Glottis Rima glottidis Thyroid cartilage Ventricular fold T Vocal Cord, Right Vocal fold V Vocal Cord, Left See T Vocal Cord, Right	Ø Open 4 Percutaneous Endoscopic 7 Via Natural or Artificial Opening 8 Via Natural or Artificial Opening Endoscopic	Z No Device	Z No Qualifier
W Upper Tooth X Lower Tooth	Ø Open	Z No Device	Ø Single 1 Multiple 2 All

Non-OR   ØCT[W,X]ØZ[Ø,1,2]

Mouth and Throat

Ø   **Medical and Surgical**
C   **Mouth and Throat**
U   **Supplement**   Definition: Putting in or on biological or synthetic material that physically reinforces and/or augments the function of a portion of a body part

                       Explanation: The biological material is non-living, or is living and from the same individual. The body part may have been previously replaced, and the SUPPLEMENT procedure is performed to physically reinforce and/or augment the function of the replaced body part.

Body Part Character 4	Approach Character 5	Device Character 6	Qualifier Character 7

Ø   Upper Lip
    Frenulum labii superioris
    Labial gland
    Vermilion border
1   Lower Lip
    Frenulum labii inferioris
    Labial gland
    Vermilion border
2   Hard Palate
3   Soft Palate
4   Buccal Mucosa
    Buccal gland
    Molar gland
    Palatine gland
5   Upper Gingiva
6   Lower Gingiva
7   Tongue
    Frenulum linguae
N   Uvula
    Palatine uvula
	Ø Open
	3 Percutaneous
	X External
		7 Autologous Tissue Substitute
		J Synthetic Substitute
		K Nonautologous Tissue Substitute
			Z No Qualifier

M   Pharynx
    Base of tongue
    Hypopharynx
    Laryngopharynx
    Lingual tonsil
    Oropharynx
    Piriform recess (sinus)
    Tongue, base of
R   Epiglottis
    Glossoepiglottic fold
S   Larynx
    Aryepiglottic fold
    Arytenoid cartilage
    Corniculate cartilage
    Cuneiform cartilage
    False vocal cord
    Glottis
    Rima glottidis
    Thyroid cartilage
    Ventricular fold
T   Vocal Cord, Right
    Vocal fold
V   Vocal Cord, Left
    See T Vocal Cord, Right
	Ø Open
	7 Via Natural or Artificial Opening
	8 Via Natural or Artificial Opening
	    Endoscopic
		7 Autologous Tissue Substitute
		J Synthetic Substitute
		K Nonautologous Tissue Substitute
			Z No Qualifier

Non-OR   ØCU2[Ø,3]JZ

Ø   **Medical and Surgical**
C   **Mouth and Throat**
V   **Restriction**   Definition: Partially closing an orifice or the lumen of a tubular body part

                       Explanation: The orifice can be a natural orifice or an artificially created orifice

Body Part Character 4	Approach Character 5	Device Character 6	Qualifier Character 7

B   Parotid Duct, Right
    Stensen's duct
C   Parotid Duct, Left
    See B Parotid Duct, Right
	Ø Open
	3 Percutaneous
		C Extraluminal Device
		D Intraluminal Device
		Z No Device
			Z No Qualifier

B   Parotid Duct, Right
    Stensen's duct
C   Parotid Duct, Left
    See B Parotid Duct, Right
	7 Via Natural or Artificial Opening
	8 Via Natural or Artificial Opening
	    Endoscopic
		D Intraluminal Device
		Z No Device
			Z No Qualifier

Ø   Medical and Surgical
C   Mouth and Throat
W   Revision   Definition: Correcting, to the extent possible, a portion of a malfunctioning device or the position of a displaced device

                        Explanation: Revision can include correcting a malfunctioning or displaced device by taking out or putting in components of the device such as a screw or pin

Body Part Character 4	Approach Character 5	Device Character 6	Qualifier Character 7
A Salivary Gland	Ø Open 3 Percutaneous	Ø Drainage Device C Extraluminal Device Y Other Device	Z No Qualifier
A Salivary Gland	7 Via Natural or Artificial Opening 8 Via Natural or Artificial Opening Endoscopic	Y Other Device	Z No Qualifier
A Salivary Gland	X External	Ø Drainage Device C Extraluminal Device	Z No Qualifier

S   Larynx
    Aryepiglottic fold
    Arytenoid cartilage
    Corniculate cartilage
    Cuneiform cartilage
    False vocal cord
    Glottis
    Rima glottidis
    Thyroid cartilage
    Ventricular fold
	Ø Open
	3 Percutaneous
	7 Via Natural or Artificial Opening
	8 Via Natural or Artificial Opening Endoscopic
		Ø Drainage Device
		7 Autologous Tissue Substitute
		D Intraluminal Device
		J Synthetic Substitute
		K Nonautologous Tissue Substitute
		Y Other Device
			Z No Qualifier

S   Larynx
    Aryepiglottic fold
    Arytenoid cartilage
    Corniculate cartilage
    Cuneiform cartilage
    False vocal cord
    Glottis
    Rima glottidis
    Thyroid cartilage
    Ventricular fold
	X External	Ø Drainage Device
		7 Autologous Tissue Substitute
		D Intraluminal Device
		J Synthetic Substitute
		K Nonautologous Tissue Substitute
			Z No Qualifier

Y Mouth and Throat	Ø Open 3 Percutaneous 7 Via Natural or Artificial Opening 8 Via Natural or Artificial Opening Endoscopic	Ø Drainage Device 1 Radioactive Element 7 Autologous Tissue Substitute D Intraluminal Device J Synthetic Substitute K Nonautologous Tissue Substitute Y Other Device	Z No Qualifier
Y Mouth and Throat	X External	Ø Drainage Device 1 Radioactive Element 7 Autologous Tissue Substitute D Intraluminal Device J Synthetic Substitute K Nonautologous Tissue Substitute	Z No Qualifier

Non-OR   ØCWA[Ø,3][Ø,C,Y]Z
Non-OR   ØCWA[7,8]YZ
Non-OR   ØCWAX[Ø,C]Z
Non-OR   ØCWS[3,7,8]YZ
Non-OR   ØCWSX[Ø,7,D,J,K]Z
Non-OR   ØCWYØ7Z
Non-OR   ØCWY[3,7,8]YZ
Non-OR   ØCWYX[Ø,1,7,D,J,K]Z

NC Noncovered Procedure   LC Limited Coverage   QA Questionable OB Admit   NT New Tech Add-on   ⊞ Combination Member   ♂ Male   ♀ Female

ICD-10-PCS 2024   371

Mouth and Throat

Ø   **Medical and Surgical**
C   **Mouth and Throat**
X   **Transfer**   Definition: Moving, without taking out, all or a portion of a body part to another location to take over the function of all or a portion of a body part

                         Explanation: The body part transferred remains connected to its vascular and nervous supply

Body Part Character 4	Approach Character 5	Device Character 6	Qualifier Character 7

Ø **Upper Lip**
    Frenulum labii superioris
    Labial gland
    Vermilion border
1 **Lower Lip**
    Frenulum labii inferioris
    Labial gland
    Vermilion border
3 **Soft Palate**
4 **Buccal Mucosa**
    Buccal gland
    Molar gland
    Palatine gland
5 **Upper Gingiva**
6 **Lower Gingiva**
7 **Tongue**
    Frenulum linguae
	Ø Open
	X External
		Z No Device	Z No Qualifier

Non-OR Procedure   DRG Non-OR Procedure   Valid OR Procedure   HAC Associated Procedure   Combination Only   New/Revised April   New/Revised October

372   ICD-10-PCS 2024

Gastrointestinal System ØD1–ØDY

Character Meanings

This Character Meaning table is provided as a guide to assist the user in the identification of character members that may be found in this section of code tables. It **SHOULD NOT** be used to build a PCS code.

Operation–Character 3		Body Part–Character 4		Approach–Character 5		Device–Character 6		Qualifier–Character 7	
1	Bypass	Ø	Upper Intestinal Tract	Ø	Open	Ø	Drainage Device	Ø	Allogeneic
2	Change	1	Esophagus, Upper	3	Percutaneous	1	Radioactive Element	1	Syngeneic
5	Destruction	2	Esophagus, Middle	4	Percutaneous Endoscopic	2	Monitoring Device	2	Zooplastic
7	Dilation	3	Esophagus, Lower	7	Via Natural or Artificial Opening	3	Infusion Device	3	Vertical OR Laser Interstitial Thermal Therapy
8	Division	4	Esophagogastric Junction	8	Via Natural or Artificial Opening Endoscopic	7	Autologous Tissue Substitute	4	Cutaneous
9	Drainage	5	Esophagus	F	Via Natural or Artificial Opening with Percutaneous Endoscopic Assistance	B	Intraluminal Device, Airway	5	Esophagus
B	Excision	6	Stomach	X	External	C	Extraluminal Device	6	Stomach
C	Extirpation	7	Stomach, Pylorus			D	Intraluminal Device	7	Vagina
D	Extraction	8	Small Intestine			J	Synthetic Substitute OR Magnetic Lengthening Device	8	Small Intestine
F	Fragmentation	9	Duodenum			K	Nonautologous Tissue Substitute	9	Duodenum
H	Insertion	A	Jejunum			L	Artificial Sphincter	A	Jejunum
J	Inspection	B	Ileum			M	Stimulator Lead	B	Ileum OR Bladder
L	Occlusion	C	Ileocecal Valve			U	Feeding Device	C	Ureter, Right
M	Reattachment	D	Lower Intestinal Tract			Y	Other Device	D	Ureter, Left
N	Release	E	Large Intestine			Z	No Device	E	Large Intestine
P	Removal	F	Large Intestine, Right					F	Ureters, Bilateral
Q	Repair	G	Large Intestine, Left					H	Cecum
R	Replacement	H	Cecum					K	Ascending Colon
S	Reposition	J	Appendix					L	Transverse Colon
T	Resection	K	Ascending Colon					M	Descending Colon
U	Supplement	L	Transverse Colon					N	Sigmoid Colon
V	Restriction	M	Descending Colon					P	Rectum
W	Revision	N	Sigmoid Colon					Q	Anus
X	Transfer	P	Rectum					X	Diagnostic
Y	Transplantation	Q	Anus					Z	No Qualifier
		R	Anal Sphincter						
		U	Omentum						
		V	Mesentery						
		W	Peritoneum						

AHA Coding Clinic for Gastrointestinal System

2022, 1Q, 11	Procedures performed on a continuous vessel, ICD-10-PCS Guideline B4.1c

AHA Coding Clinic for table ØD1

2021, 1Q, 19	Kock pouch revision surgery
2019, 4Q, 29	Intestinal bypass
2017, 2Q, 17	Billroth II (distal gastrectomy and gastrojejunostomy)
2016, 2Q, 31	Laparoscopic biliopancreatic diversion with duodenal switch
2014, 4Q, 41	Abdominoperineal resection (APR) with flap closure of perineum and colostomy

AHA Coding Clinic for table ØD2

2022, 1Q, 45	Insertion, removal and replacement of endoluminal vacuum application
2019, 1Q, 26	Exchange of clogged gastrojejunostomy tube

AHA Coding Clinic for table ØD5

2022, 4Q, 53-54	Laser interstitial thermal therapy
2017, 1Q, 34	Debulking of tumor and peritoneum ablation

AHA Coding Clinic for table ØD7

2020, 3Q, 45	Dilation versus drainage of perirectal cyst
2017, 3Q, 23	Laparoscopic pyloromyotomy
2014, 4Q, 40	Dilation of gastrojejunostomy anastomosis stricture

AHA Coding Clinic for table ØD8

2019, 2Q, 15	Reversal of Roux-en-Y bypass
2017, 3Q, 22	Laparoscopic esophagomyotomy (Heller type) and Toupet fundoplication
2017, 3Q, 23	Laparoscopic pyloromyotomy

AHA Coding Clinic for table ØD9

2020, 3Q, 45	Dilation versus drainage of perirectal cyst
2015, 2Q, 29	Insertion of nasogastric tube for drainage and feeding

AHA Coding Clinic for table ØDB

2023, 2Q, 23	V-Y anoplasty and excision of mucosal ectropion
2023, 1Q, 32	Zenker's diverticulectomy
2021, 3Q, 28	Retrieval of capsule via small bowel excision
2021, 2Q, 11	Serosal injury with excision of small intestine
2021, 1Q, 20	Rectal suction biopsy
2021, 1Q, 22	Total proctocolectomy with creation of J-pouch
2019, 2Q, 15	Reversal of Roux-en-Y bypass
2019, 1Q, 3-8	Whipple procedure
2019, 1Q, 27	Excision of pelvic sidewall mass
2017, 2Q, 17	Billroth II (distal gastrectomy and gastrojejunostomy)
2017, 1Q, 16	Hepatic flexure versus transverse colon
2016, 3Q, 3-7	Stoma creation & takedown procedures
2016, 2Q, 31	Laparoscopic biliopancreatic diversion with duodenal switch
2016, 1Q, 22	Perineal proctectomy
2016, 1Q, 24	Endoscopic brush biopsy of esophagus
2014, 4Q, 40	Abdominoperineal resection (APR) with flap closure of perineum and colostomy
2014, 3Q, 28	Ileostomy takedown and parastomal hernia repair
2014, 3Q, 32	Pyloric-sparing Whipple procedure

AHA Coding Clinic for table ØDD

2021, 1Q, 20	Rectal suction biopsy
2017, 4Q, 41-42	Extraction procedures

AHA Coding Clinic for table ØDH

2022, 1Q, 44	Insertion, removal and replacement of endoluminal vacuum application
2020, 4Q, 43-44	Insertion of radioactive element
2020, 3Q, 43	Staged laparoscopic gastric conduit and placement of feeding tube
2019, 2Q, 18	Endoscopic wound VAC placement
2016, 3Q, 26	Insertion of gastrostomy tube
2013, 4Q,117	Percutaneous endoscopic placement of gastrostomy tube

AHA Coding Clinic for table ØDJ

2019, 1Q, 25	Laparoscopic appendectomy converted to open procedure
2019, 1Q, 25	Milking of inspissated material from ileum to colon
2017, 2Q, 15	Low anterior resection with sigmoidoscopy
2016, 2Q, 20	Capsule endoscopy of small intestine
2015, 3Q, 24	Esophagogastroduodenoscopy with epinephrine injection for control of bleeding

AHA Coding Clinic for table ØDL

2013, 4Q, 112	Endoscopic banding of esophageal varices

AHA Coding Clinic for table ØDN

2017, 4Q, 49-50	New and revised body part values - Repositioning of the intestine
2017, 1Q, 35	Lysis of omental and peritoneal adhesions
2015, 3Q, 15	Vascular ring surgery with release of esophagus and trachea
2015, 3Q, 16	Vascular ring surgery and double aortic arch

AHA Coding Clinic for table ØDP

2019, 2Q, 18	Removal of wound VAC

AHA Coding Clinic for table ØDQ

2023, 2Q, 23	V-Y anoplasty and excision of mucosal ectropion
2019, 2Q, 15	Reversal of Roux-en-Y bypass
2018, 2Q, 25	Third and fourth degree obstetric lacerations
2018, 1Q, 11	Repair of internal hernia at Petersen space
2017, 3Q, 17	Posterior sagittal anorectoplasty
2016, 3Q, 3-7	Stoma creation & takedown procedures
2016, 3Q, 26	Insertion of gastrostomy tube
2016, 1Q, 7	Obstetrical perineal laceration repair
2016, 1Q, 8	Obstetrical perineal laceration repair
2014, 4Q, 20	Control of bleeding duodenal ulcer

AHA Coding Clinic for table ØDS

2019, 1Q, 30	Laparoscopic-assisted rectopexy with manual reduction of prolapse
2017, 4Q, 49-50	New and revised body part values - Repositioning of the intestine
2017, 3Q, 9	Ileocolic intussusception reduction via air enema
2017, 3Q, 17	Posterior sagittal anorectoplasty
2016, 3Q, 3-5	Stoma creation & takedown procedures

AHA Coding Clinic for table ØDT

2022, 1Q, 49	Robotic-assisted low anterior resection of colon
2021, 1Q, 22	Total proctocolectomy with creation of J-pouch
2020, 4Q, 100	Robotic-assisted sigmoid colectomy with extension of incision for specimen removal
2019, 1Q, 3-8	Whipple procedure
2019, 1Q, 14	Esophagectomy with colon interposition
2017, 4Q, 49-50	New and revised body part values - Repositioning of the intestine
2014, 4Q, 40	Abdominoperineal resection (APR) with flap closure of perineum and colostomy
2014, 4Q, 42	Right colectomy with side-to-side functional end-to-end anastomosis
2014, 3Q, 6	Ileocecectomy including cecum, terminal ileum and appendix
2014, 3Q, 6	Right colectomy

AHA Coding Clinic for table ØDU

2023, 2Q, 23	V-Y anoplasty and excision of mucosal ectropion
2021, 2Q, 20	Malone antegrade continence enema procedure
2021, 1Q, 22	Total proctocolectomy with creation of J-pouch
2019, 1Q, 30	Laparoscopic-assisted rectopexy with manual reduction of prolapse

AHA Coding Clinic for table ØDV

2017, 3Q, 22	Laparoscopic esophagomyotomy (Heller type) and Toupet fundoplication
2016, 2Q, 22	Esophageal lengthening Collis gastroplasty with Nissen fundoplication and hiatal hernia
2014, 3Q, 28	Laparoscopic Nissen fundoplication and diaphragmatic hernia repair

AHA Coding Clinic for table ØDW

2021, 1Q, 19	Kock pouch revision surgery
2018, 1Q, 20	Adjustment of gastric band

AHA Coding Clinic for table ØDX

2022, 4Q, 56-57	Bladder augmentation
2022, 4Q, 58	Ileal ureter
2019, 4Q, 29-30	Transfer large intestine to vagina
2019, 1Q, 14	Esophagectomy with colon interposition
2017, 2Q, 18	Esophagectomy and esophagogastrectomy with cervical esophagogastrostomy
2016, 2Q, 22	Esophageal lengthening Collis gastroplasty with Nissen fundoplication and hiatal hernia
2015, 1Q, 28	Repair of bronchopleural fistula using omental pedicle graft

AHA Coding Clinic for table ØDY

2023, 2Q, 32	Preparation of donor organ before transplantation

Upper Intestinal Tract (Ø) and Lower Intestinal Tract (D)

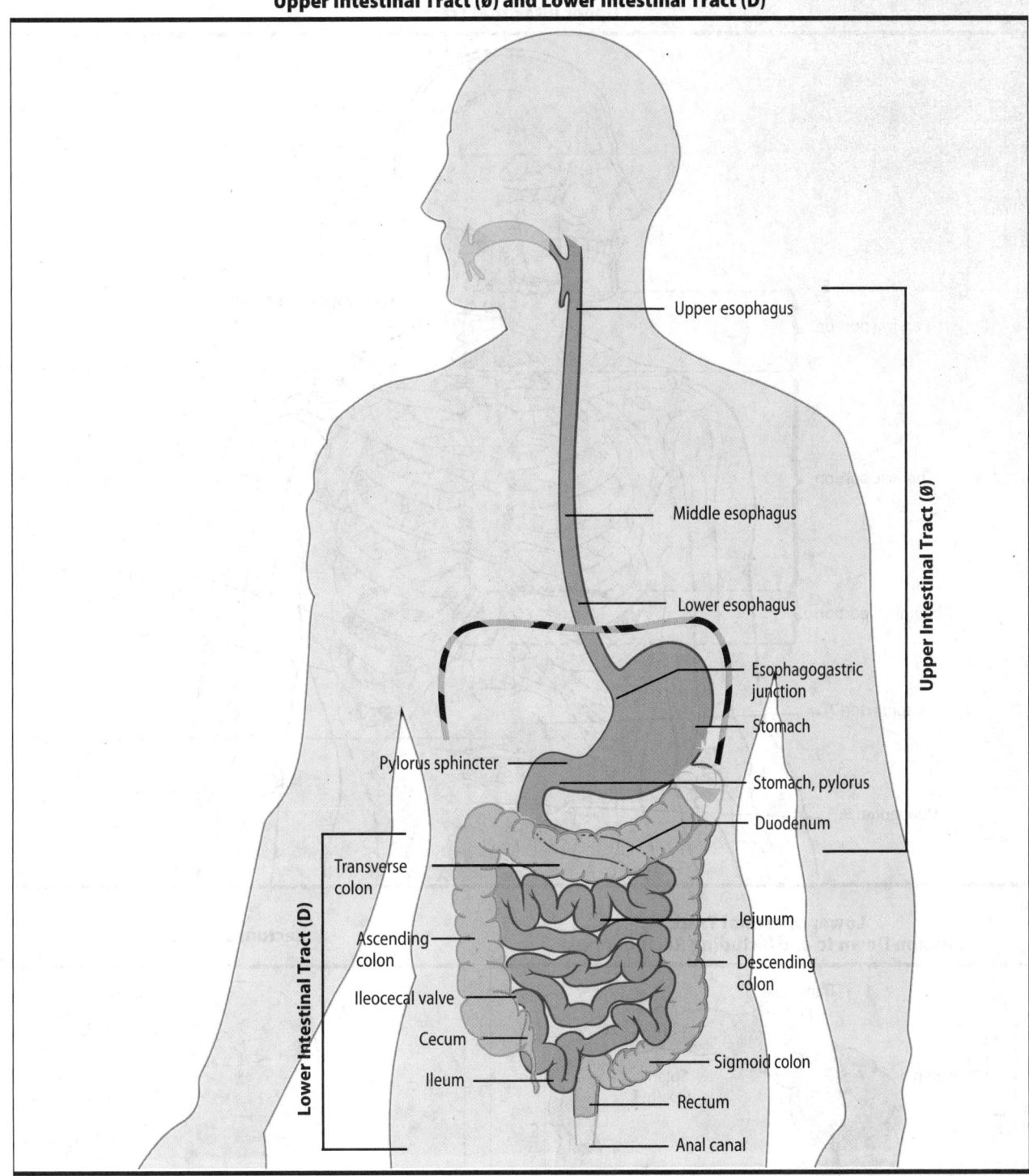

Gastrointestinal System

Upper Intestinal Tract

Esophageal region **5**:

Cervical portion

Thoracic portion

Abdominal portion

Pylorus sphincter **7**

Duodenum **9**

Upper esophagus **1**

Middle esophagus **2**

Lower esophagus **3**

Esophagogastric junction **4**

Stomach **6**

Stomach, pylorus

Lower Intestinal Tract
(Jejunum Down to and Including Rectum/Anus)

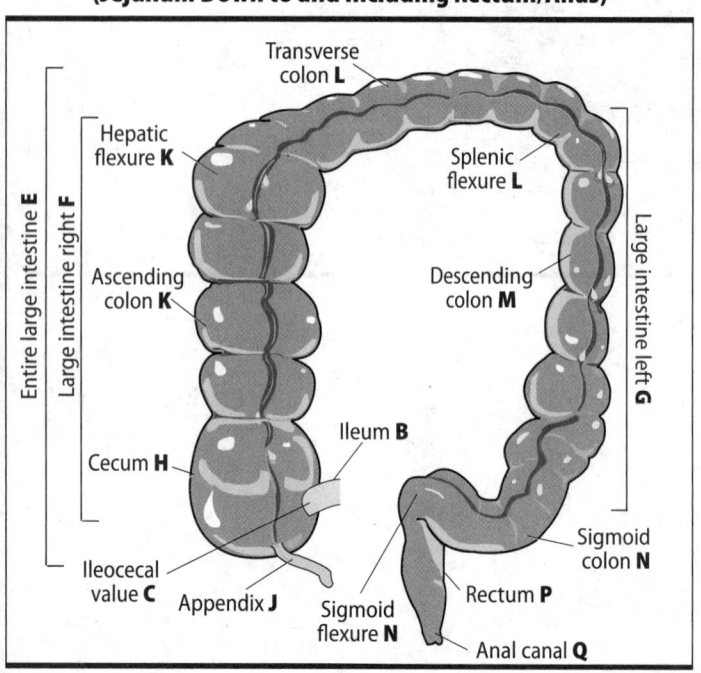

Transverse colon **L**

Hepatic flexure **K**

Splenic flexure **L**

Ascending colon **K**

Descending colon **M**

Entire large intestine **E**

Large intestine right **F**

Large intestine left **G**

Cecum **H**

Ileum **B**

Ileocecal value **C**

Appendix **J**

Sigmoid flexure **N**

Rectum **P**

Sigmoid colon **N**

Anal canal **Q**

Rectum and Anus

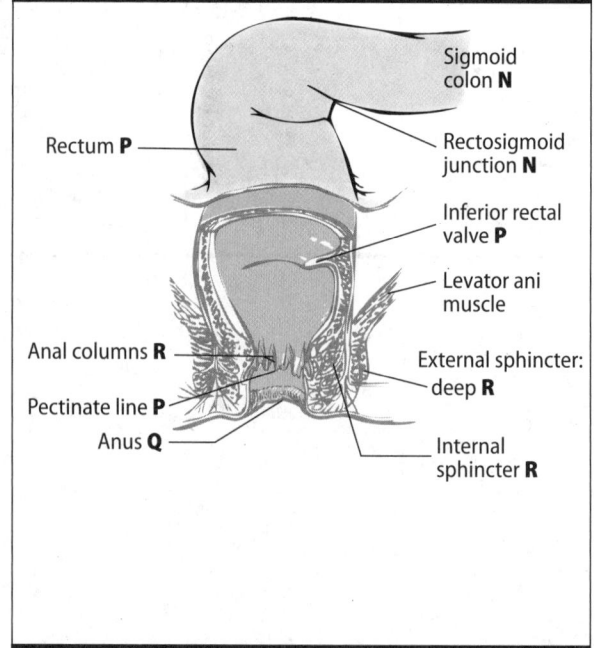

Rectum **P**

Sigmoid colon **N**

Rectosigmoid junction **N**

Inferior rectal valve **P**

Levator ani muscle

Anal columns **R**

External sphincter: deep **R**

Pectinate line **P**

Anus **Q**

Internal sphincter **R**

Ø   **Medical and Surgical**
D   **Gastrointestinal System**
1   **Bypass**   Definition: Altering the route of passage of the contents of a tubular body part

                      Explanation: Rerouting contents of a body part to a downstream area of the normal route, to a similar route and body part, or to an abnormal route and dissimilar body part. Includes one or more anastomoses, with or without the use of a device.

Body Part Character 4	Approach Character 5	Device Character 6	Qualifier Character 7

1 Esophagus, Upper
    Cervical esophagus
2 Esophagus, Middle
    Thoracic esophagus
3 Esophagus, Lower
    Abdominal esophagus
5 Esophagus
	Ø Open
	4 Percutaneous Endoscopic
	8 Via Natural or Artificial Opening Endoscopic
		7 Autologous Tissue Substitute
		J Synthetic Substitute
		K Nonautologous Tissue Substitute
		Z No Device
			4 Cutaneous
			6 Stomach
			9 Duodenum
			A Jejunum
			B Ileum

1 Esophagus, Upper
    Cervical esophagus
2 Esophagus, Middle
    Thoracic esophagus
3 Esophagus, Lower
    Abdominal esophagus
5 Esophagus
	3 Percutaneous	**J** Synthetic Substitute	**4** Cutaneous

6 Stomach **9** Duodenum	**Ø** Open **4** Percutaneous Endoscopic **8** Via Natural or Artificial Opening Endoscopic	**7** Autologous Tissue Substitute **J** Synthetic Substitute **K** Nonautologous Tissue Substitute **Z** No Device	**4** Cutaneous **9** Duodenum **A** Jejunum **B** Ileum **L** Transverse Colon
6 Stomach **9** Duodenum	**3** Percutaneous	**J** Synthetic Substitute	**4** Cutaneous
8 Small Intestine	**Ø** Open **4** Percutaneous Endoscopic **8** Via Natural or Artificial Opening Endoscopic	**7** Autologous Tissue Substitute **J** Synthetic Substitute **K** Nonautologous Tissue Substitute **Z** No Device	**4** Cutaneous **8** Small Intestine **H** Cecum **K** Ascending Colon **L** Transverse Colon **M** Descending Colon **N** Sigmoid Colon **P** Rectum **Q** Anus
A Jejunum Duodenojejunal flexure	**Ø** Open **4** Percutaneous Endoscopic **8** Via Natural or Artificial Opening Endoscopic	**7** Autologous Tissue Substitute **J** Synthetic Substitute **K** Nonautologous Tissue Substitute **Z** No Device	**4** Cutaneous **A** Jejunum **B** Ileum **H** Cecum **K** Ascending Colon **L** Transverse Colon **M** Descending Colon **N** Sigmoid Colon **P** Rectum **Q** Anus
A Jejunum Duodenojejunal flexure	**3** Percutaneous	**J** Synthetic Substitute	**4** Cutaneous
B Ileum	**Ø** Open **4** Percutaneous Endoscopic **8** Via Natural or Artificial Opening Endoscopic	**7** Autologous Tissue Substitute **J** Synthetic Substitute **K** Nonautologous Tissue Substitute **Z** No Device	**4** Cutaneous **B** Ileum **H** Cecum **K** Ascending Colon **L** Transverse Colon **M** Descending Colon **N** Sigmoid Colon **P** Rectum **Q** Anus
B Ileum	**3** Percutaneous	**J** Synthetic Substitute	**4** Cutaneous
E Large Intestine	**Ø** Open **4** Percutaneous Endoscopic **8** Via Natural or Artificial Opening Endoscopic	**7** Autologous Tissue Substitute **J** Synthetic Substitute **K** Nonautologous Tissue Substitute **Z** No Device	**4** Cutaneous **E** Large Intestine **P** Rectum
H Cecum	**Ø** Open **4** Percutaneous Endoscopic **8** Via Natural or Artificial Opening Endoscopic	**7** Autologous Tissue Substitute **J** Synthetic Substitute **K** Nonautologous Tissue Substitute **Z** No Device	**4** Cutaneous **H** Cecum **K** Ascending Colon **L** Transverse Colon **M** Descending Colon **N** Sigmoid Colon **P** Rectum
H Cecum	**3** Percutaneous	**J** Synthetic Substitute	**4** Cutaneous

Non-OR   ØD16[Ø,4,8][7,J,K,Z]4
Non-OR   ØD163J4
HAC   ØD16[Ø,4,8][7,J,K,Z][9,A,B,L] when reported with PDx E66.Ø1 and SDx K68.11, K95.Ø1, K95.81 or T81.4Ø–T81.49 with 7th character A

ØD1 Continued on next page

NC Noncovered Procedure   **LC** Limited Coverage   **QA** Questionable OB Admit   **NT** New Tech Add-on   ⊞ Combination Member   ♂ Male   ♀ Female

Gastrointestinal System

Ø   **Medical and Surgical**
D   **Gastrointestinal System**
1   **Bypass**   Definition: Altering the route of passage of the contents of a tubular body part

Explanation: Rerouting contents of a body part to a downstream area of the normal route, to a similar route and body part, or to an abnormal route and dissimilar body part. Includes one or more anastomoses, with or without the use of a device.

Body Part Character 4	Approach Character 5	Device Character 6	Qualifier Character 7
K Ascending Colon	Ø Open 4 Percutaneous Endoscopic 8 Via Natural or Artificial Opening Endoscopic	7 Autologous Tissue Substitute J Synthetic Substitute K Nonautologous Tissue Substitute Z No Device	4 Cutaneous K Ascending Colon L Transverse Colon M Descending Colon N Sigmoid Colon P Rectum
K Ascending Colon	3 Percutaneous	J Synthetic Substitute	4 Cutaneous

L   Transverse Colon
     Hepatic flexure
     Splenic flexure
	Ø Open
	4 Percutaneous Endoscopic
	8 Via Natural or Artificial Opening Endoscopic
		7 Autologous Tissue Substitute
		J Synthetic Substitute
		K Nonautologous Tissue Substitute
		Z No Device
			4 Cutaneous
			L Transverse Colon
			M Descending Colon
			N Sigmoid Colon
			P Rectum

L   Transverse Colon
     Hepatic flexure
     Splenic flexure
	3 Percutaneous	J Synthetic Substitute	4 Cutaneous

M Descending Colon	Ø Open 4 Percutaneous Endoscopic 8 Via Natural or Artificial Opening Endoscopic	7 Autologous Tissue Substitute J Synthetic Substitute K Nonautologous Tissue Substitute Z No Device	4 Cutaneous M Descending Colon N Sigmoid Colon P Rectum
M Descending Colon	3 Percutaneous	J Synthetic Substitute	4 Cutaneous

N   Sigmoid Colon
     Rectosigmoid junction
     Sigmoid flexure
	Ø Open
	4 Percutaneous Endoscopic
	8 Via Natural or Artificial Opening Endoscopic
		7 Autologous Tissue Substitute
		J Synthetic Substitute
		K Nonautologous Tissue Substitute
		Z No Device
			4 Cutaneous
			N Sigmoid Colon
			P Rectum

N   Sigmoid Colon
     Rectosigmoid junction
     Sigmoid flexure
	3 Percutaneous	J Synthetic Substitute	4 Cutaneous

Ø   **Medical and Surgical**
D   **Gastrointestinal System**
2   **Change**   Definition: Taking out or off a device from a body part and putting back an identical or similar device in or on the same body part without cutting or puncturing the skin or a mucous membrane

Explanation: All CHANGE procedures are coded using the approach EXTERNAL

Body Part Character 4	Approach Character 5	Device Character 6	Qualifier Character 7
Ø Upper Intestinal Tract D Lower Intestinal Tract	X External	Ø Drainage Device U Feeding Device Y Other Device	Z No Qualifier

U   Omentum
     Gastrocolic ligament
     Gastrocolic omentum
     Gastrohepatic omentum
     Gastrophrenic ligament
     Gastrosplenic ligament
     Greater Omentum
     Hepatogastric ligament
     Lesser Omentum
V   Mesentery
     Mesoappendix
     Mesocolon
W   Peritoneum
     Epiploic foramen
	X External	Ø Drainage Device
		Y Other Device
			Z No Qualifier

Non-OR   All body part, approach, device, and qualifier values

Non-OR Procedure   DRG Non-OR Procedure   Valid OR Procedure   HAC Associated Procedure   Combination Only   New/Revised April   New/Revised October

378   ICD-10-PCS 2024

Ø　Medical and Surgical
D　Gastrointestinal System
5　Destruction　　Definition: Physical eradication of all or a portion of a body part by the direct use of energy, force, or a destructive agent
　　　　　　　　　　Explanation: None of the body part is physically taken out

Body Part Character 4		Approach Character 5	Device Character 6	Qualifier Character 7
1 Esophagus, Upper Cervical esophagus **2 Esophagus, Middle** Thoracic esophagus **3 Esophagus, Lower** Abdominal esophagus **4 Esophagogastric Junction** Cardia Cardioesophageal junction Gastroesophageal (GE) junction **5 Esophagus** **6 Stomach** **7 Stomach, Pylorus** Pyloric antrum Pyloric canal Pyloric sphincter **8 Small Intestine** **9 Duodenum** **A Jejunum** Duodenojejunal flexure	**B Ileum** **C Ileocecal Valve** **E Large Intestine** **F Large Intestine, Right** **G Large Intestine, Left** **H Cecum** **J Appendix** Appendiceal orifice Vermiform appendix **K Ascending Colon** **L Transverse Colon** Hepatic flexure Splenic flexure **M Descending Colon** **N Sigmoid Colon** Rectosigmoid junction Sigmoid flexure **P Rectum** Anorectal junction	**Ø Open** **3 Percutaneous** **4 Percutaneous Endoscopic**	**Z No Device**	**3 Laser Interstitial Thermal Therapy** **Z No Qualifier**
1 Esophagus, Upper Cervical esophagus **2 Esophagus, Middle** Thoracic esophagus **3 Esophagus, Lower** Abdominal esophagus **4 Esophagogastric Junction** Cardia Cardioesophageal junction Gastroesophageal (GE) junction **5 Esophagus** **6 Stomach** **7 Stomach, Pylorus** Pyloric antrum Pyloric canal Pyloric sphincter **8 Small Intestine** **9 Duodenum**	**A Jejunum** Duodenojejunal flexure **B Ileum** **C Ileocecal Valve** **E Large Intestine** **F Large Intestine, Right** **G Large Intestine, Left** **H Cecum** **J Appendix** Appendiceal orifice Vermiform appendix **K Ascending Colon** **L Transverse Colon** Hepatic flexure Splenic flexure **M Descending Colon** **N Sigmoid Colon** Rectosigmoid junction Sigmoid flexure **P Rectum** Anorectal junction	**7 Via Natural or Artificial Opening** **8 Via Natural or Artificial Opening Endoscopic**	**Z No Device**	**Z No Qualifier**
Q Anus Anal orifice		**Ø Open** **3 Percutaneous** **4 Percutaneous Endoscopic**	**Z No Device**	**3 Laser Interstitial Thermal Therapy** **Z No Qualifier**
Q Anus Anal orifice		**7 Via Natural or Artificial Opening** **8 Via Natural or Artificial Opening Endoscopic** **X External**	**Z No Device**	**Z No Qualifier**
R Anal Sphincter External anal sphincter Internal anal sphincter **U Omentum** Gastrocolic ligament Gastrocolic omentum Gastrohepatic omentum Gastrophrenic ligament Gastrosplenic ligament Greater Omentum Hepatogastric ligament Lesser Omentum	**V Mesentery** Mesoappendix Mesocolon **W Peritoneum** Epiploic foramen	**Ø Open** **3 Percutaneous** **4 Percutaneous Endoscopic**	**Z No Device**	**Z No Qualifier**

DRG Non-OR	ØD5[1,2,3,4,5,6,7,9,E,F,G,H,K,L,M,N]4Z3	**Non-OR**	ØD5[1,2,3,4,5,6,7,9,E,F,G,H,K,L,M,N]4ZZ
DRG Non-OR	ØD5P[Ø,3,4]Z3	**Non-OR**	ØD5P[Ø,3,4]ZZ
DRG Non-OR	ØD5Q4Z3	**Non-OR**	ØD5[1,2,3,4,5,6,7,8,9,A,B,C,E,F,G,H,K,L,M,N]8ZZ
		Non-OR	ØD5P[7,8]ZZ
		Non-OR	ØD5Q4ZZ
		Non-OR	ØD5Q8ZZ
		Non-OR	ØD5R4ZZ

NC Noncovered Procedure　　**LC** Limited Coverage　　**QA** Questionable OB Admit　　**NT** New Tech Add-on　　⊞ Combination Member　　♂ Male　　♀ Female

ICD-10-PCS 2024　　　　　　　　　　　　　　　　　　　　　　　　　　　　　　　　　　　　　　379

Gastrointestinal System

Ø　**Medical and Surgical**
D　**Gastrointestinal System**
7　**Dilation**　　　Definition: Expanding an orifice or the lumen of a tubular body part

Explanation: The orifice can be a natural orifice or an artificially created orifice. Accomplished by stretching a tubular body part using intraluminal pressure or by cutting part of the orifice or wall of the tubular body part.

Body Part Character 4	Approach Character 5	Device Character 6	Qualifier Character 7
1　Esophagus, Upper 　　Cervical esophagus 2　Esophagus, Middle 　　Thoracic esophagus 3　Esophagus, Lower 　　Abdominal esophagus 4　Esophagogastric Junction 　　Cardia 　　Cardioesophageal junction 　　Gastroesophageal (GE) junction 5　Esophagus 6　Stomach 7　Stomach, Pylorus 　　Pyloric antrum 　　Pyloric canal 　　Pyloric sphincter 8　Small Intestine 9　Duodenum A　Jejunum 　　Duodenojejunal flexure B　Ileum C　Ileocecal Valve E　Large Intestine F　Large Intestine, Right G　Large Intestine, Left H　Cecum K　Ascending Colon L　Transverse Colon 　　Hepatic flexure 　　Splenic flexure M　Descending Colon N　Sigmoid Colon 　　Rectosigmoid junction 　　Sigmoid flexure P　Rectum 　　Anorectal junction Q　Anus 　　Anal orifice	Ø　Open 3　Percutaneous 4　Percutaneous Endoscopic 7　Via Natural or Artificial Opening 8　Via Natural or Artificial Opening 　　Endoscopic	D　Intraluminal Device Z　No Device	Z　No Qualifier

Non-OR　ØD7[1,2,3,4,5,6,8,9,A,B,C,E,F,G,H,K,L,M,N,P,Q][7,8][D,Z]Z
Non-OR　ØD77[4,8]DZ
Non-OR　ØD777[D,Z]Z
Non-OR　ØD7[8,9,A,B,C,E,F,G,H,K,L,M,N][Ø,3,4]DZ

Ø　**Medical and Surgical**
D　**Gastrointestinal System**
8　**Division**　　　Definition: Cutting into a body part, without draining fluids and/or gases from the body part, in order to separate or transect a body part

Explanation: All or a portion of the body part is separated into two or more portions

Body Part Character 4	Approach Character 5	Device Character 6	Qualifier Character 7
4　Esophagogastric Junction 　　Cardia 　　Cardioesophageal junction 　　Gastroesophageal (GE) junction 7　Stomach, Pylorus 　　Pyloric antrum 　　Pyloric canal 　　Pyloric sphincter	Ø　Open 3　Percutaneous 4　Percutaneous Endoscopic 7　Via Natural or Artificial Opening 8　Via Natural or Artificial Opening 　　Endoscopic	Z　No Device	Z　No Qualifier
R　Anal Sphincter 　　External anal sphincter 　　Internal anal sphincter	Ø　Open 3　Percutaneous	Z　No Device	Z　No Qualifier

Ø Medical and Surgical
D Gastrointestinal System
9 Drainage   Definition: Taking or letting out fluids and/or gases from a body part
                    Explanation: The qualifier DIAGNOSTIC is used to identify drainage procedures that are biopsies

Body Part Character 4	Approach Character 5	Device Character 6	Qualifier Character 7

1 Esophagus, Upper
  Cervical esophagus
2 Esophagus, Middle
  Thoracic esophagus
3 Esophagus, Lower
  Abdominal esophagus
4 Esophagogastric Junction
  Cardia
  Cardioesophageal junction
  Gastroesophageal (GE) junction
5 Esophagus
6 Stomach
7 Stomach, Pylorus
  Pyloric antrum
  Pyloric canal
  Pyloric sphincter
8 Small Intestine
9 Duodenum
A Jejunum
  Duodenojejunal flexure
B Ileum
C Ileocecal Valve
E Large Intestine
F Large Intestine, Right
G Large Intestine, Left
H Cecum
J Appendix
  Appendiceal orifice
  Vermiform appendix
K Ascending Colon
L Transverse Colon
  Hepatic flexure
  Splenic flexure
M Descending Colon
N Sigmoid Colon
  Rectosigmoid junction
  Sigmoid flexure
P Rectum
  Anorectal junction
	Ø Open
	3 Percutaneous
	4 Percutaneous Endoscopic
	7 Via Natural or Artificial Opening
	8 Via Natural or Artificial Opening Endoscopic
		Ø Drainage Device	Z No Qualifier

1 Esophagus, Upper
  Cervical esophagus
2 Esophagus, Middle
  Thoracic esophagus
3 Esophagus, Lower
  Abdominal esophagus
4 Esophagogastric Junction
  Cardia
  Cardioesophageal junction
  Gastroesophageal (GE) junction
5 Esophagus
6 Stomach
7 Stomach, Pylorus
  Pyloric antrum
  Pyloric canal
  Pyloric sphincter
8 Small Intestine
9 Duodenum
A Jejunum
  Duodenojejunal flexure
B Ileum
C Ileocecal Valve
E Large Intestine
F Large Intestine, Right
G Large Intestine, Left
H Cecum
J Appendix
  Appendiceal orifice
  Vermiform appendix
K Ascending Colon
L Transverse Colon
  Hepatic flexure
  Splenic flexure
M Descending Colon
N Sigmoid Colon
  Rectosigmoid junction
  Sigmoid flexure
P Rectum
  Anorectal junction
	Ø Open
	3 Percutaneous
	4 Percutaneous Endoscopic
	7 Via Natural or Artificial Opening
	8 Via Natural or Artificial Opening Endoscopic
		Z No Device	X Diagnostic
			Z No Qualifier

Q Anus Anal orifice	Ø Open 3 Percutaneous 4 Percutaneous Endoscopic 7 Via Natural or Artificial Opening 8 Via Natural or Artificial Opening Endoscopic X External	Ø Drainage Device	Z No Qualifier
Q Anus Anal orifice	Ø Open 3 Percutaneous 4 Percutaneous Endoscopic 7 Via Natural or Artificial Opening 8 Via Natural or Artificial Opening Endoscopic X External	Z No Device	X Diagnostic Z No Qualifier

Non-OR	ØD9[1,2,3,4,5,C,J]3ØZ
Non-OR	ØD9[6,7,8,9,A,B,E,F,G,H,K,L,M,N,P][3,7,8]ØZ
Non-OR	ØD9[1,2,3,4,5,6,7,8,9,A,B,C,E,F,G,H,K,L,M,N,P][3,4,7,8]ZX
Non-OR	ØD9[1,2,3,4,5,6,7,8,9,A,B,C,E,F,G,H,J,K,L,M,N,P]3ZZ
Non-OR	ØD9Q3ØZ
Non-OR	ØD9Q[Ø,3,4,7,8,X]ZX
Non-OR	ØD9Q3ZZ

ØD9 Continued on next page

NC Noncovered Procedure   **LC** Limited Coverage   **QA** Questionable OB Admit   **NT** New Tech Add-on   ⊞ Combination Member   ♂ Male   ♀ Female

ICD-10-PCS 2024   381

ØD9–ØD9

Gastrointestinal System

Ø   **Medical and Surgical**
D   **Gastrointestinal System**
9   **Drainage**   Definition: Taking or letting out fluids and/or gases from a body part
                     Explanation: The qualifier DIAGNOSTIC is used to identify drainage procedures that are biopsies

Body Part Character 4	Approach Character 5	Device Character 6	Qualifier Character 7

R   Anal Sphincter
    External anal sphincter
    Internal anal sphincter
U   Omentum
    Gastrocolic ligament
    Gastrocolic omentum
    Gastrohepatic omentum
    Gastrophrenic ligament
    Gastrosplenic ligament
    Greater Omentum
    Hepatogastric ligament
    Lesser Omentum
V   Mesentery
    Mesoappendix
    Mesocolon
W   Peritoneum
    Epiploic foramen
	Ø Open
	3 Percutaneous
	4 Percutaneous Endoscopic
		Ø Drainage Device	**Z** No Qualifier

R   Anal Sphincter
    External anal sphincter
    Internal anal sphincter
U   Omentum
    Gastrocolic ligament
    Gastrocolic omentum
    Gastrohepatic omentum
    Gastrophrenic ligament
    Gastrosplenic ligament
    Greater Omentum
    Hepatogastric ligament
    Lesser Omentum
V   Mesentery
    Mesoappendix
    Mesocolon
W   Peritoneum
    Epiploic foramen
	Ø Open
	3 Percutaneous
	4 Percutaneous Endoscopic
		Z No Device	**X** Diagnostic
			Z No Qualifier

Non-OR	ØD9[R,W]3ØZ
Non-OR	ØD9[U,V][3,4]ØZ
Non-OR	ØD9[R,U,V,W]3Z[X,Z]
Non-OR	ØD9R[Ø,4]ZX
Non-OR	ØD9[U,V]4ZZ

Ø   Medical and Surgical
D   Gastrointestinal System
B   Excision   Definition: Cutting out or off, without replacement, a portion of a body part
                    Explanation: The qualifier DIAGNOSTIC is used to identify excision procedures that are biopsies

Body Part Character 4	Approach Character 5	Device Character 6	Qualifier Character 7

1 Esophagus, Upper
  Cervical esophagus
2 Esophagus, Middle
  Thoracic esophagus
3 Esophagus, Lower
  Abdominal esophagus
4 Esophagogastric
  Junction
  Cardia
  Cardioesophageal
    junction
  Gastroesophageal (GE)
    junction
5 Esophagus
7 Stomach, Pylorus
  Pyloric antrum
  Pyloric canal
  Pyloric sphincter
	8 Small Intestine
	9 Duodenum
	A Jejunum
	  Duodenojejunal flexure
	B Ileum
	C Ileocecal Valve
	E Large Intestine
	F Large Intestine, Right
	H Cecum
	J Appendix
	  Appendiceal orifice
	  Vermiform appendix
	K Ascending Colon
	P Rectum
	  Anorectal junction
		Ø Open
		3 Percutaneous
		4 Percutaneous Endoscopic
		7 Via Natural or Artificial
		   Opening
		8 Via Natural or Artificial
		   Opening Endoscopic
			Z No Device	**X** Diagnostic
				Z No Qualifier

6 Stomach	**Ø** Open
	3 Percutaneous
	4 Percutaneous Endoscopic
	7 Via Natural or Artificial
	   Opening
	8 Via Natural or Artificial
	   Opening Endoscopic
		Z No Device	**3** Vertical
			X Diagnostic
			Z No Qualifier

G Large Intestine, Left
L Transverse Colon
  Hepatic flexure
  Splenic flexure
M Descending Colon
N Sigmoid Colon
  Rectosigmoid junction
  Sigmoid flexure
	Ø Open
	3 Percutaneous
	4 Percutaneous Endoscopic
	7 Via Natural or Artificial
	   Opening
	8 Via Natural or Artificial
	   Opening Endoscopic
		Z No Device	**X** Diagnostic
			Z No Qualifier

G Large Intestine, Left
L Transverse Colon
  Hepatic flexure
  Splenic flexure
M Descending Colon
N Sigmoid Colon
  Rectosigmoid junction
  Sigmoid flexure
	F Via Natural or Artificial
	   Opening with Percutaneous
	   Endoscopic Assistance
		Z No Device	**Z** No Qualifier

Q Anus
  Anal orifice
	Ø Open
	3 Percutaneous
	4 Percutaneous Endoscopic
	7 Via Natural or Artificial
	   Opening
	8 Via Natural or Artificial
	   Opening Endoscopic
	X External
		Z No Device	**X** Diagnostic
			Z No Qualifier

R Anal Sphincter
  External anal sphincter
  Internal anal sphincter
U Omentum
  Gastrocolic ligament
  Gastrocolic omentum
  Gastrohepatic omentum
  Gastrophrenic ligament
  Gastrosplenic ligament
  Greater Omentum
  Hepatogastric ligament
  Lesser Omentum
V Mesentery
  Mesoappendix
  Mesocolon
W Peritoneum
  Epiploic foramen
	Ø Open
	3 Percutaneous
	4 Percutaneous Endoscopic
		Z No Device	**X** Diagnostic
			Z No Qualifier

Non-OR ØDB[1,2,3,4,5,7,8,9,A,B,C,E,F,H,K,P][3,4,7,8]ZX		**Non-OR** ØDB[G,L,M,N]8ZZ	
Non-OR ØDB[1,2,3,5,7,9][4,8]ZZ		**Non-OR** ØDBQ[Ø,3,4,7,8,X]ZX	
Non-OR ØDB[4,E,F,H,K,P]8ZZ		**Non-OR** ØDBQ8ZZ	
Non-OR ØDB6[3,7]ZX		**Non-OR** ØDBR[Ø,3,4]ZX	
Non-OR ØDB68Z[X,Z]		**Non-OR** ØDB[U,V,W][3,4]ZX	
Non-OR ØDB[G,L,M,N][3,4,7,8]ZX			

NC Noncovered Procedure   **LC** Limited Coverage   **QA** Questionable OB Admit   **NT** New Tech Add-on   ⊞ Combination Member   ♂ Male   ♀ Female

ICD-10-PCS 2024   **383**

Gastrointestinal System

Ø   **Medical and Surgical**
D   **Gastrointestinal System**
C   **Extirpation**   Definition: Taking or cutting out solid matter from a body part

           Explanation: The solid matter may be an abnormal byproduct of a biological function or a foreign body; it may be imbedded in a body part or in the lumen of a tubular body part. The solid matter may or may not have been previously broken into pieces.

Body Part Character 4	Approach Character 5	Device Character 6	Qualifier Character 7

1 Esophagus, Upper
   Cervical esophagus
2 Esophagus, Middle
   Thoracic esophagus
3 Esophagus, Lower
   Abdominal esophagus
4 Esophagogastric Junction
   Cardia
   Cardioesophageal junction
   Gastroesophageal (GE) junction
5 Esophagus
6 Stomach
7 Stomach, Pylorus
   Pyloric antrum
   Pyloric canal
   Pyloric sphincter
8 Small Intestine
9 Duodenum
A Jejunum
   Duodenojejunal flexure
B Ileum
C Ileocecal Valve
E Large Intestine
F Large Intestine, Right
G Large Intestine, Left
H Cecum
J Appendix
   Appendiceal orifice
   Vermiform appendix
K Ascending Colon
L Transverse Colon
   Hepatic flexure
   Splenic flexure
M Descending Colon
N Sigmoid Colon
   Rectosigmoid junction
   Sigmoid flexure
P Rectum
   Anorectal junction
	Ø Open
	3 Percutaneous
	4 Percutaneous Endoscopic
	7 Via Natural or Artificial Opening
	8 Via Natural or Artificial Opening Endoscopic
		Z No Device	Z No Qualifier

Q Anus Anal orifice	Ø Open 3 Percutaneous 4 Percutaneous Endoscopic 7 Via Natural or Artificial Opening 8 Via Natural or Artificial Opening Endoscopic X External	Z No Device	Z No Qualifier

R Anal Sphincter
   External anal sphincter
   Internal anal sphincter
U Omentum
   Gastrocolic ligament
   Gastrocolic omentum
   Gastrohepatic omentum
   Gastrophrenic ligament
   Gastrosplenic ligament
   Greater Omentum
   Hepatogastric ligament
   Lesser Omentum
V Mesentery
   Mesoappendix
   Mesocolon
W Peritoneum
   Epiploic foramen
	Ø Open
	3 Percutaneous
	4 Percutaneous Endoscopic
		Z No Device	Z No Qualifier

Non-OR	ØDC[1,2,3,4,5,6,7,8,9,A,B,C,E,F,G,H,K,L,M,N,P][7,8]ZZ
Non-OR	ØDCQ[7,8,X]ZZ

Non-OR Procedure   DRG Non-OR Procedure   Valid OR Procedure   HAC Associated Procedure   Combination Only   New/Revised April   New/Revised October

384   ICD-10-PCS 2024

Ø   **Medical and Surgical**
D   **Gastrointestinal System**
D   **Extraction**   Definition: Pulling or stripping out or off all or a portion of a body part by the use of force
                        Explanation: The qualifier DIAGNOSTIC is used to identify extraction procedures that are biopsies

Body Part Character 4	Approach Character 5	Device Character 6	Qualifier Character 7

1 Esophagus, Upper
   Cervical esophagus
2 Esophagus, Middle
   Thoracic esophagus
3 Esophagus, Lower
   Abdominal esophagus
4 Esophagogastric Junction
   Cardia
   Cardioesophageal junction
   Gastroesophageal (GE) junction
5 Esophagus
6 Stomach
7 Stomach, Pylorus
   Pyloric antrum
   Pyloric canal
   Pyloric sphincter
8 Small Intestine
9 Duodenum
A Jejunum
   Duodenojejunal flexure
B Ileum
C Ileocecal Valve
E Large Intestine
F Large Intestine, Right
G Large Intestine, Left
H Cecum
J Appendix
   Appendiceal orifice
   Vermiform appendix
K Ascending Colon
L Transverse Colon
   Hepatic flexure
   Splenic flexure
M Descending Colon
N Sigmoid Colon
   Rectosigmoid junction
   Sigmoid flexure
P Rectum
   Anorectal junction
	3 Percutaneous
	4 Percutaneous Endoscopic
	8 Via Natural or Artificial Opening
	   Endoscopic
		Z No Device	**X** Diagnostic

Q Anus
   Anal orifice
	3 Percutaneous
	4 Percutaneous Endoscopic
	8 Via Natural or Artificial Opening
	   Endoscopic
	X External
		Z No Device	**X** Diagnostic

Non-OR   ØDD[1,2,3,4,5,6,7,8,9,A,B,C,E,F,G,H,K,L,M,N,P][3,4,8]ZX
Non-OR   ØDDQ[3,4,8,X]ZX

Ø   Medical and Surgical
D   Gastrointestinal System
F   Fragmentation   Definition: Breaking solid matter in a body part into pieces

Explanation: Physical force (e.g., manual, ultrasonic) applied directly or indirectly is used to break the solid matter into pieces. The solid matter may be an abnormal byproduct of a biological function or a foreign body. The pieces of solid matter are not taken out.

Body Part Character 4		Approach Character 5	Device Character 6	Qualifier Character 7
5 Esophagus	NC	Ø Open	Z No Device	Z No Qualifier
6 Stomach	NC	3 Percutaneous		
8 Small Intestine	NC	4 Percutaneous Endoscopic		
9 Duodenum	NC	7 Via Natural or Artificial Opening		
A Jejunum	NC	8 Via Natural or Artificial Opening		
Duodenojejunal flexure		Endoscopic		
B Ileum	NC	X External		
E Large Intestine	NC			
F Large Intestine, Right	NC			
G Large Intestine, Left	NC			
H Cecum	NC			
J Appendix	NC			
Appendiceal orifice				
Vermiform appendix				
K Ascending Colon	NC			
L Transverse Colon	NC			
Hepatic flexure				
Splenic flexure				
M Descending Colon	NC			
N Sigmoid Colon	NC			
Rectosigmoid junction				
Sigmoid flexure				
P Rectum	NC			
Anorectal junction				
Q Anus	NC			
Anal orifice				

Non-OR   ØDF[5,6,8,9,A,B,E,F,G,H,J,K,L,M,N,P,Q]XZZ
NC   ØDF[5,6,8,9,A,B,E,F,G,H,J,K,L,M,N,P,Q]XZZ

Ø   **Medical and Surgical**
D   **Gastrointestinal System**
H   **Insertion**   Definition: Putting in a nonbiological appliance that monitors, assists, performs, or prevents a physiological function but does not physically take the place of a body part
                        Explanation: None

Body Part Character 4	Approach Character 5	Device Character 6	Qualifier Character 7
Ø Upper Intestinal Tract D Lower Intestinal Tract	Ø Open 3 Percutaneous 4 Percutaneous Endoscopic 7 Via Natural or Artificial Opening 8 Via Natural or Artificial Opening Endoscopic	Y Other Device	Z No Qualifier
1 Esophagus, Upper 2 Esophagus, Middle 3 Esophagus, Lower	7 Via Natural or Artificial Opening	J Magnetic Lengthening Device	Z No Qualifier
5 Esophagus	Ø Open 3 Percutaneous 4 Percutaneous Endoscopic	1 Radioactive Element 2 Monitoring Device 3 Infusion Device D Intraluminal Device U Feeding Device Y Other Device	Z No Qualifier
5 Esophagus	7 Via Natural or Artificial Opening 8 Via Natural or Artificial Opening Endoscopic	1 Radioactive Element 2 Monitoring Device 3 Infusion Device B Intraluminal Device, Airway D Intraluminal Device U Feeding Device Y Other Device	Z No Qualifier
6 Stomach ⊞	Ø Open 3 Percutaneous 4 Percutaneous Endoscopic	1 Radioactive Element 2 Monitoring Device 3 Infusion Device D Intraluminal Device M Stimulator Lead U Feeding Device Y Other Device	Z No Qualifier
6 Stomach	7 Via Natural or Artificial Opening 8 Via Natural or Artificial Opening Endoscopic	1 Radioactive Element 2 Monitoring Device 3 Infusion Device D Intraluminal Device U Feeding Device Y Other Device	Z No Qualifier
8 Small Intestine 9 Duodenum A Jejunum Duodenojejunal flexure B Ileum	Ø Open 3 Percutaneous 4 Percutaneous Endoscopic 7 Via Natural or Artificial Opening 8 Via Natural or Artificial Opening Endoscopic	1 Radioactive Element 2 Monitoring Device 3 Infusion Device D Intraluminal Device U Feeding Device	Z No Qualifier
E Large Intestine P Rectum Anorectal junction	Ø Open 3 Percutaneous 4 Percutaneous Endoscopic 7 Via Natural or Artificial Opening 8 Via Natural or Artificial Opening Endoscopic	1 Radioactive Element D Intraluminal Device	Z No Qualifier
Q Anus Anal orifice	Ø Open 3 Percutaneous 4 Percutaneous Endoscopic	D Intraluminal Device L Artificial Sphincter	Z No Qualifier
Q Anus Anal orifice	7 Via Natural or Artificial Opening 8 Via Natural or Artificial Opening Endoscopic	D Intraluminal Device	Z No Qualifier

R Anal Sphincter
   External anal sphincter
   Internal anal sphincter
	Ø Open
	3 Percutaneous
	4 Percutaneous Endoscopic
		M Stimulator Lead	Z No Qualifier

Non-OR   ØDH[Ø,D][Ø,3,4,7,8]YZ
Non-OR   ØDH5[Ø,3,4][D,U]Z
Non-OR   ØDH5[3,4]YZ
Non-OR   ØDH5[7,8][2,3,B,D,U,Y]Z
Non-OR   ØDH631Z
Non-OR   ØDH6[Ø,3,4]UZ
Non-OR   ØDH6[3,4]YZ
Non-OR   ØDH6[7,8][1,2,3,D,U,Y]Z

Non-OR   ØDH[8,9,A,B][Ø,3,4,7,8][1,D,U]Z
Non-OR   ØDH[8,9,A,B][7,8][2,3]Z
Non-OR   ØDHE[Ø,3,4,7,8][1,D]Z
Non-OR   ØDHP[Ø,3,4,7,8]DZ

See Appendix L for Procedure Combinations
    ⊞   ØDH6[Ø,3,4]MZ

Gastrointestinal System

Ø   Medical and Surgical
D   Gastrointestinal System
J   Inspection   Definition: Visually and/or manually exploring a body part

Explanation: Visual exploration may be performed with or without optical instrumentation. Manual exploration may be performed directly or through intervening body layers.

Body Part Character 4	Approach Character 5	Device Character 6	Qualifier Character 7
Ø Upper Intestinal Tract **6** Stomach **D** Lower Intestinal Tract	**Ø** Open **3** Percutaneous **4** Percutaneous Endoscopic **7** Via Natural or Artificial Opening **8** Via Natural or Artificial Opening Endoscopic **X** External	**Z** No Device	**Z** No Qualifier

U Omentum
  Gastrocolic ligament
  Gastrocolic omentum
  Gastrohepatic omentum
  Gastrophrenic ligament
  Gastrosplenic ligament
  Greater Omentum
  Hepatogastric ligament
  Lesser Omentum
V Mesentery
  Mesoappendix
  Mesocolon
W Peritoneum
  Epiploic foramen
	Ø Open
	3 Percutaneous
	4 Percutaneous Endoscopic
	X External
		Z No Device	**Z** No Qualifier

Non-OR	ØDJ[Ø,6,D][3,7,8,X]ZZ
Non-OR	ØDJ[U,V,W][3,X]ZZ

Ø   **Medical and Surgical**
D   **Gastrointestinal System**
L   **Occlusion**   Definition: Completely closing an orifice or the lumen of a tubular body part
                      Explanation: The orifice can be a natural orifice or an artificially created orifice

Body Part Character 4		Approach Character 5	Device Character 6	Qualifier Character 7
1 Esophagus, Upper Cervical esophagus **2** Esophagus, Middle Thoracic esophagus **3** Esophagus, Lower Abdominal esophagus **4** Esophagogastric Junction Cardia Cardioesophageal junction Gastroesophageal (GE) junction **5** Esophagus **6** Stomach **7** Stomach, Pylorus Pyloric antrum Pyloric canal Pyloric sphincter **8** Small Intestine	**9** Duodenum **A** Jejunum Duodenojejunal flexure **B** Ileum **C** Ileocecal Valve **E** Large Intestine **F** Large Intestine, Right **G** Large Intestine, Left **H** Cecum **K** Ascending Colon **L** Transverse Colon Hepatic flexure Splenic flexure **M** Descending Colon **N** Sigmoid Colon Rectosigmoid junction Sigmoid flexure **P** Rectum Anorectal junction	**Ø** Open **3** Percutaneous **4** Percutaneous Endoscopic	**C** Extraluminal Device **D** Intraluminal Device **Z** No Device	**Z** No Qualifier
1 Esophagus, Upper Cervical esophagus **2** Esophagus, Middle Thoracic esophagus **3** Esophagus, Lower Abdominal esophagus **4** Esophagogastric Junction Cardia Cardioesophageal junction Gastroesophageal (GE) junction **5** Esophagus **6** Stomach **7** Stomach, Pylorus Pyloric antrum Pyloric canal Pyloric sphincter **8** Small Intestine	**9** Duodenum **A** Jejunum Duodenojejunal flexure **B** Ileum **C** Ileocecal Valve **E** Large Intestine **F** Large Intestine, Right **G** Large Intestine, Left **H** Cecum **K** Ascending Colon **L** Transverse Colon Hepatic flexure Splenic flexure **M** Descending Colon **N** Sigmoid Colon Rectosigmoid junction Sigmoid flexure **P** Rectum Anorectal junction	**7** Via Natural or Artificial Opening **8** Via Natural or Artificial Opening Endoscopic	**D** Intraluminal Device **Z** No Device	**Z** No Qualifier
Q Anus Anal orifice		**Ø** Open **3** Percutaneous **4** Percutaneous Endoscopic **X** External	**C** Extraluminal Device **D** Intraluminal Device **Z** No Device	**Z** No Qualifier
Q Anus Anal orifice		**7** Via Natural or Artificial Opening **8** Via Natural or Artificial Opening Endoscopic	**D** Intraluminal Device **Z** No Device	**Z** No Qualifier

Non-OR   ØDL[1,2,3,4,5][Ø,3,4][C,D,Z]Z
Non-OR   ØDL[1,2,3,4,5][7,8][D,Z]Z

Gastrointestinal System

Ø   Medical and Surgical
D   Gastrointestinal System
M   Reattachment   Definition: Putting back in or on all or a portion of a separated body part to its normal location or other suitable location

                Explanation: Vascular circulation and nervous pathways may or may not be reestablished

Body Part Character 4	Approach Character 5	Device Character 6	Qualifier Character 7

5 Esophagus
6 Stomach
8 Small Intestine
9 Duodenum
A Jejunum
   Duodenojejunal flexure
B Ileum
E Large Intestine
F Large Intestine, Right
G Large Intestine, Left
H Cecum
K Ascending Colon
L Transverse Colon
   Hepatic flexure
   Splenic flexure
M Descending Colon
N Sigmoid Colon
   Rectosigmoid junction
   Sigmoid flexure
P Rectum
   Anorectal junction
	Ø Open
	4 Percutaneous Endoscopic
		Z No Device	Z No Qualifier

Ø   Medical and Surgical
D   Gastrointestinal System
N   Release   Definition: Freeing a body part from an abnormal physical constraint by cutting or by the use of force

                Explanation: Some of the restraining tissue may be taken out but none of the body part is taken out

Body Part Character 4	Approach Character 5	Device Character 6	Qualifier Character 7

1 Esophagus, Upper
   Cervical esophagus
2 Esophagus, Middle
   Thoracic esophagus
3 Esophagus, Lower
   Abdominal esophagus
4 Esophagogastric
   Junction
   Cardia
   Cardioesophageal
     junction
   Gastroesophageal (GE)
     junction
5 Esophagus
6 Stomach
7 Stomach, Pylorus
   Pyloric antrum
   Pyloric canal
   Pyloric sphincter
8 Small Intestine
9 Duodenum
 	
A Jejunum
   Duodenojejunal flexure
B Ileum
C Ileocecal Valve
E Large Intestine
F Large Intestine, Right
G Large Intestine, Left
H Cecum
J Appendix
   Appendiceal orifice
   Vermiform appendix
K Ascending Colon
L Transverse Colon
   Hepatic flexure
   Splenic flexure
M Descending Colon
N Sigmoid Colon
   Rectosigmoid junction
   Sigmoid flexure
P Rectum
   Anorectal junction
	Ø Open
	3 Percutaneous
	4 Percutaneous Endoscopic
	7 Via Natural or Artificial
	   Opening
	8 Via Natural or Artificial
	   Opening Endoscopic
		Z No Device	Z No Qualifier

Q Anus
   Anal orifice
	Ø Open
	3 Percutaneous
	4 Percutaneous Endoscopic
	7 Via Natural or Artificial
	   Opening
	8 Via Natural or Artificial
	   Opening Endoscopic
	X External
		Z No Device	Z No Qualifier

R Anal Sphincter
   External anal sphincter
   Internal anal sphincter
U Omentum
   Gastrocolic ligament
   Gastrocolic omentum
   Gastrohepatic
     omentum
   Gastrophrenic ligament
   Gastrosplenic ligament
   Greater Omentum
   Hepatogastric ligament
   Lesser Omentum
 	
V Mesentery
   Mesoappendix
   Mesocolon
W Peritoneum
   Epiploic foramen
	Ø Open
	3 Percutaneous
	4 Percutaneous Endoscopic
		Z No Device	Z No Qualifier

Non-OR   ØDN[8,9,A,B,E,F,G,H,K,L,M,N][7,8]ZZ

Non-OR Procedure   DRG Non-OR Procedure   Valid OR Procedure   HAC Associated Procedure   Combination Only   New/Revised April   New/Revised October

390   ICD-10-PCS 2024

Ø　**Medical and Surgical**
D　**Gastrointestinal System**
P　**Removal**　　　Definition: Taking out or off a device from a body part

　　　Explanation: If a device is taken out and a similar device put in without cutting or puncturing the skin or mucous membrane, the procedure is coded to the root operation CHANGE. Otherwise, the procedure for taking out a device is coded to the root operation REMOVAL.

Body Part Character 4	Approach Character 5	Device Character 6	Qualifier Character 7
Ø Upper Intestinal Tract D Lower Intestinal Tract	Ø Open 3 Percutaneous 4 Percutaneous Endoscopic 7 Via Natural or Artificial Opening 8 Via Natural or Artificial Opening Endoscopic	Ø Drainage Device 2 Monitoring Device 3 Infusion Device 7 Autologous Tissue Substitute C Extraluminal Device D Intraluminal Device J Synthetic Substitute K Nonautologous Tissue Substitute U Feeding Device Y Other Device	Z No Qualifier
Ø Upper Intestinal Tract D Lower Intestinal Tract	X External	Ø Drainage Device 2 Monitoring Device 3 Infusion Device D Intraluminal Device U Feeding Device	Z No Qualifier
5 Esophagus	Ø Open 3 Percutaneous 4 Percutaneous Endoscopic	1 Radioactive Element 2 Monitoring Device 3 Infusion Device U Feeding Device Y Other Device	Z No Qualifier
5 Esophagus	7 Via Natural or Artificial Opening 8 Via Natural or Artificial Opening Endoscopic	1 Radioactive Element D Intraluminal Device Y Other Device	Z No Qualifier
5 Esophagus	X External	1 Radioactive Element 2 Monitoring Device 3 Infusion Device D Intraluminal Device U Feeding Device	Z No Qualifier
6 Stomach	Ø Open 3 Percutaneous 4 Percutaneous Endoscopic	Ø Drainage Device 2 Monitoring Device 3 Infusion Device 7 Autologous Tissue Substitute C Extraluminal Device D Intraluminal Device J Synthetic Substitute K Nonautologous Tissue Substitute M Stimulator Lead U Feeding Device Y Other Device	Z No Qualifier
6 Stomach	7 Via Natural or Artificial Opening 8 Via Natural or Artificial Opening Endoscopic	Ø Drainage Device 2 Monitoring Device 3 Infusion Device 7 Autologous Tissue Substitute C Extraluminal Device D Intraluminal Device J Synthetic Substitute K Nonautologous Tissue Substitute U Feeding Device Y Other Device	Z No Qualifier
6 Stomach	X External	Ø Drainage Device 2 Monitoring Device 3 Infusion Device D Intraluminal Device U Feeding Device	Z No Qualifier

Non-OR　ØDP[Ø,D][3,4]YZ
Non-OR　ØDP[Ø,D][7,8][Ø,2,3,D,U,Y]Z
Non-OR　ØDP[Ø,D]X[Ø,2,3,D,U]Z
Non-OR　ØDP5[3,4]YZ
Non-OR　ØDP5[7,8][1,D,Y]Z
Non-OR　ØDP5X[1,2,3,D,U]Z
Non-OR　ØDP6[3,4]YZ
Non-OR　ØDP6[7,8][Ø,2,3,D,U,Y]Z
Non-OR　ØDP6X[Ø,2,3,D,U]Z

ØDP Continued on next page

Gastrointestinal System

ØDP Continued

Ø   **Medical and Surgical**
D   **Gastrointestinal System**
P   **Removal**   Definition: Taking out or off a device from a body part

Explanation: If a device is taken out and a similar device put in without cutting or puncturing the skin or mucous membrane, the procedure is coded to the root operation CHANGE. Otherwise, the procedure for taking out a device is coded to the root operation REMOVAL.

Body Part Character 4	Approach Character 5	Device Character 6	Qualifier Character 7
P Rectum Anorectal junction	**Ø** Open **3** Percutaneous **4** Percutaneous Endoscopic **7** Via Natural or Artificial Opening **8** Via Natural or Artificial Opening Endoscopic **X** External	**1** Radioactive Element	**Z** No Qualifier
Q Anus Anal orifice	**Ø** Open **3** Percutaneous **4** Percutaneous Endoscopic **7** Via Natural or Artificial Opening **8** Via Natural or Artificial Opening Endoscopic	**L** Artificial Sphincter	**Z** No Qualifier

R Anal Sphincter
   External anal sphincter
   Internal anal sphincter
	Ø Open
	3 Percutaneous
	4 Percutaneous Endoscopic
		M Stimulator Lead	**Z** No Qualifier

U Omentum
   Gastrocolic ligament
   Gastrocolic omentum
   Gastrohepatic omentum
   Gastrophrenic ligament
   Gastrosplenic ligament
   Greater Omentum
   Hepatogastric ligament
   Lesser Omentum
V Mesentery
   Mesoappendix
   Mesocolon
W Peritoneum
   Epiploic foramen
	Ø Open
	3 Percutaneous
	4 Percutaneous Endoscopic
		Ø Drainage Device
		1 Radioactive Element
		7 Autologous Tissue Substitute
		J Synthetic Substitute
		K Nonautologous Tissue Substitute
			Z No Qualifier

Non-OR   ØDPP[7,8,X]1Z

Non-OR Procedure   DRG Non-OR Procedure   Valid OR Procedure   HAC Associated Procedure   Combination Only   New/Revised April   New/Revised October

392   ICD-10-PCS 2024

Ø   Medical and Surgical
D   Gastrointestinal System
Q   Repair   Definition: Restoring, to the extent possible, a body part to its normal anatomic structure and function

                     Explanation: Used only when the method to accomplish the repair is not one of the other root operations

Body Part Character 4	Approach Character 5	Device Character 6	Qualifier Character 7

1 Esophagus, Upper
   Cervical esophagus
2 Esophagus, Middle
   Thoracic esophagus
3 Esophagus, Lower
   Abdominal esophagus
4 Esophagogastric Junction
   Cardia
   Cardioesophageal junction
   Gastroesophageal (GE) junction
5 Esophagus
6 Stomach
7 Stomach, Pylorus
   Pyloric antrum
   Pyloric canal
   Pyloric sphincter
8 Small Intestine ⊞
9 Duodenum ⊞
A Jejunum ⊞
   Duodenojejunal flexure
B Ileum ⊞
C Ileocecal Valve
E Large Intestine ⊞
F Large Intestine, Right ⊞
G Large Intestine, Left ⊞
H Cecum ⊞
J Appendix
   Appendiceal orifice
   Vermiform appendix
K Ascending Colon ⊞
L Transverse Colon ⊞
   Hepatic flexure
   Splenic flexure
M Descending Colon ⊞
N Sigmoid Colon ⊞
   Rectosigmoid junction
   Sigmoid flexure
P Rectum
   Anorectal junction
	Ø Open
	3 Percutaneous
	4 Percutaneous Endoscopic
	7 Via Natural or Artificial Opening
	8 Via Natural or Artificial Opening
	   Endoscopic
		Z No Device	Z No Qualifier

Q Anus
   Anal orifice
	Ø Open
	3 Percutaneous
	4 Percutaneous Endoscopic
	7 Via Natural or Artificial Opening
	8 Via Natural or Artificial Opening
	   Endoscopic
	X External
		Z No Device	Z No Qualifier

R Anal Sphincter
   External anal sphincter
   Internal anal sphincter
U Omentum
   Gastrocolic ligament
   Gastrocolic omentum
   Gastrohepatic omentum
   Gastrophrenic ligament
   Gastrosplenic ligament
   Greater Omentum
   Hepatogastric ligament
   Lesser Omentum
V Mesentery
   Mesoappendix
   Mesocolon
W Peritoneum
   Epiploic foramen
	Ø Open
	3 Percutaneous
	4 Percutaneous Endoscopic
		Z No Device	Z No Qualifier

See Appendix L for Procedure Combinations
  ⊞   ØDQ[8,9,A,B,E,F,G,H,K,L,M,N]ØZZ

NC Noncovered Procedure   **LC** Limited Coverage   **QA** Questionable OB Admit   **NT** New Tech Add-on   ⊞ Combination Member   ♂ Male   ♀ Female

ICD-10-PCS 2024   **393**

Gastrointestinal System (side tab)

Ø   **Medical and Surgical**
D   **Gastrointestinal System**
R   **Replacement**   Definition: Putting in or on biological or synthetic material that physically takes the place and/or function of all or a portion of a body part

                          Explanation: The body part may have been taken out or replaced, or may be taken out, physically eradicated, or rendered nonfunctional during the REPLACEMENT procedure. A REMOVAL procedure is coded for taking out the device used in a previous replacement procedure.

Body Part Character 4	Approach Character 5	Device Character 6	Qualifier Character 7
5 Esophagus	Ø Open 4 Percutaneous Endoscopic 7 Via Natural or Artificial Opening 8 Via Natural or Artificial Opening Endoscopic	7 Autologous Tissue Substitute J Synthetic Substitute K Nonautologous Tissue Substitute	Z No Qualifier

R Anal Sphincter
    External anal sphincter
    Internal anal sphincter
U Omentum
    Gastrocolic ligament
    Gastrocolic omentum
    Gastrohepatic omentum
    Gastrophrenic ligament
    Gastrosplenic ligament
    Greater Omentum
    Hepatogastric ligament
    Lesser Omentum
V Mesentery
    Mesoappendix
    Mesocolon
W Peritoneum
    Epiploic foramen
	Ø Open
	4 Percutaneous Endoscopic
		7 Autologous Tissue Substitute
		J Synthetic Substitute
		K Nonautologous Tissue Substitute
			Z No Qualifier

Ø   **Medical and Surgical**
D   **Gastrointestinal System**
S   **Reposition**   Definition: Moving to its normal location, or other suitable location, all or a portion of a body part

                          Explanation: The body part is moved to a new location from an abnormal location, or from a normal location where it is not functioning correctly. The body part may or may not be cut out or off to be moved to the new location.

Body Part Character 4	Approach Character 5	Device Character 6	Qualifier Character 7

5 Esophagus
6 Stomach
9 Duodenum
A Jejunum
    Duodenojejunal flexure
B Ileum
H Cecum
K Ascending Colon
L Transverse Colon
    Hepatic flexure
    Splenic flexure
M Descending Colon
N Sigmoid Colon
    Rectosigmoid junction
    Sigmoid flexure
P Rectum
    Anorectal junction
Q Anus
    Anal orifice
	Ø Open
	4 Percutaneous Endoscopic
	7 Via Natural or Artificial Opening
	8 Via Natural or Artificial Opening Endoscopic
	X External
		Z No Device	Z No Qualifier

8 Small Intestine E Large Intestine	Ø Open 4 Percutaneous Endoscopic 7 Via Natural or Artificial Opening 8 Via Natural or Artificial Opening Endoscopic	Z No Device	Z No Qualifier

Non-OR   ØDS[5,6,9,A,B,H,K,L,M,N,P,Q]XZZ

Non-OR Procedure   DRG Non-OR Procedure   Valid OR Procedure   HAC Associated Procedure   Combination Only   New/Revised April   New/Revised October

Ø   **Medical and Surgical**
D   **Gastrointestinal System**
T   **Resection**   Definition: Cutting out or off, without replacement, all of a body part
                     Explanation: None

Body Part Character 4	Approach Character 5	Device Character 6	Qualifier Character 7

1   **Esophagus, Upper**
    Cervical esophagus
2   **Esophagus, Middle**
    Thoracic esophagus
3   **Esophagus, Lower**
    Abdominal esophagus
4   **Esophagogastric Junction**
    Cardia
    Cardioesophageal junction
    Gastroesophageal (GE) junction
5   **Esophagus**
6   **Stomach**
7   **Stomach, Pylorus**
    Pyloric antrum
    Pyloric canal
    Pyloric sphincter
8   **Small Intestine**
9   **Duodenum**   ⊞
A   **Jejunum**
    Duodenojejunal flexure
B   **Ileum**
C   **Ileocecal Valve**
E   **Large Intestine**
F   **Large Intestine, Right**
H   **Cecum**
J   **Appendix**
    Appendiceal orifice
    Vermiform appendix
K   **Ascending Colon**
P   **Rectum**
    Anorectal junction
Q   **Anus**
    Anal orifice
	Ø Open
	4 Percutaneous Endoscopic
	7 Via Natural or Artificial Opening
	8 Via Natural or Artificial Opening
	    Endoscopic
		Z No Device	**Z** No Qualifier

G   **Large Intestine, Left**
L   **Transverse Colon**
    Hepatic flexure
    Splenic flexure
M   **Descending Colon**
N   **Sigmoid Colon**
    Rectosigmoid junction
    Sigmoid flexure
	Ø Open
	4 Percutaneous Endoscopic
	7 Via Natural or Artificial Opening
	8 Via Natural or Artificial Opening
	    Endoscopic
	F Via Natural or Artificial Opening
	    with Percutaneous Endoscopic
	    Assistance
		Z No Device	**Z** No Qualifier

R   **Anal Sphincter**
    External anal sphincter
    Internal anal sphincter
U   **Omentum**
    Gastrocolic ligament
    Gastrocolic omentum
    Gastrohepatic omentum
    Gastrophrenic ligament
    Gastrosplenic ligament
    Greater Omentum
    Hepatogastric ligament
    Lesser Omentum
	Ø Open
	4 Percutaneous Endoscopic
		Z No Device	**Z** No Qualifier

See Appendix L for Procedure Combinations
   ⊞   ØDT9ØZZ

NC Noncovered Procedure   **LC** Limited Coverage   **QA** Questionable OB Admit   **NT** New Tech Add-on   ⊞ Combination Member   ♂ Male   ♀ Female

ICD-10-PCS 2024   **395**

ØDT–ØDT

Gastrointestinal System *(left margin)*

Ø   Medical and Surgical
D   Gastrointestinal System
U   Supplement   Definition: Putting in or on biological or synthetic material that physically reinforces and/or augments the function of a portion of a body part

Explanation: The biological material is non-living, or is living and from the same individual. The body part may have been previously replaced, and the SUPPLEMENT procedure is performed to physically reinforce and/or augment the function of the replaced body part.

Body Part Character 4	Approach Character 5	Device Character 6	Qualifier Character 7

1 **Esophagus, Upper**
   Cervical esophagus
2 **Esophagus, Middle**
   Thoracic esophagus
3 **Esophagus, Lower**
   Abdominal esophagus
4 **Esophagogastric Junction**
   Cardia
   Cardioesophageal junction
   Gastroesophageal (GE) junction
5 **Esophagus**
6 **Stomach**
7 **Stomach, Pylorus**
   Pyloric antrum
   Pyloric canal
   Pyloric sphincter
8 **Small Intestine**
9 **Duodenum**
A **Jejunum**
   Duodenojejunal flexure
B **Ileum**
C **Ileocecal Valve**
E **Large Intestine**
F **Large Intestine, Right**
G **Large Intestine, Left**
H **Cecum**
K **Ascending Colon**
L **Transverse Colon**
   Hepatic flexure
   Splenic flexure
M **Descending Colon**
N **Sigmoid Colon**
   Rectosigmoid junction
   Sigmoid flexure
P **Rectum**
   Anorectal junction
	Ø **Open**
	4 **Percutaneous Endoscopic**
	7 **Via Natural or Artificial Opening**
	8 **Via Natural or Artificial Opening Endoscopic**
		7 **Autologous Tissue Substitute**
		J **Synthetic Substitute**
		K **Nonautologous Tissue Substitute**
			Z **No Qualifier**

Q **Anus** Anal orifice	Ø **Open** 4 **Percutaneous Endoscopic** 7 **Via Natural or Artificial Opening** 8 **Via Natural or Artificial Opening Endoscopic** X **External**	7 **Autologous Tissue Substitute** J **Synthetic Substitute** K **Nonautologous Tissue Substitute**	Z **No Qualifier**

R **Anal Sphincter**
   External anal sphincter
   Internal anal sphincter
U **Omentum**
   Gastrocolic ligament
   Gastrocolic omentum
   Gastrohepatic omentum
   Gastrophrenic ligament
   Gastrosplenic ligament
   Greater Omentum
   Hepatogastric ligament
   Lesser Omentum
V **Mesentery**
   Mesoappendix
   Mesocolon
W **Peritoneum**
   Epiploic foramen
	Ø **Open**
	4 **Percutaneous Endoscopic**
		7 **Autologous Tissue Substitute**
		J **Synthetic Substitute**
		K **Nonautologous Tissue Substitute**
			Z **No Qualifier**

Non-OR Procedure   DRG Non-OR Procedure   Valid OR Procedure   HAC Associated Procedure   Combination Only   New/Revised April   New/Revised October

Ø   Medical and Surgical
D   Gastrointestinal System
V   Restriction   Definition: Partially closing an orifice or the lumen of a tubular body part
                        Explanation: The orifice can be a natural orifice or an artificially created orifice

Body Part Character 4		Approach Character 5	Device Character 6	Qualifier Character 7

1 Esophagus, Upper
   Cervical esophagus
2 Esophagus, Middle
   Thoracic esophagus
3 Esophagus, Lower
   Abdominal esophagus
4 Esophagogastric
   Junction
   Cardia
   Cardioesophageal
     junction
   Gastroesophageal (GE)
     junction
5 Esophagus
6 Stomach
7 Stomach, Pylorus
   Pyloric antrum
   Pyloric canal
   Pyloric sphincter
8 Small Intestine
	9 Duodenum
	A Jejunum
	   Duodenojejunal flexure
	B Ileum
	C Ileocecal Valve
	E Large Intestine
	F Large Intestine, Right
	G Large Intestine, Left
	H Cecum
	K Ascending Colon
	L Transverse Colon
	   Hepatic flexure
	   Splenic flexure
	M Descending Colon
	N Sigmoid Colon
	   Rectosigmoid junction
	   Sigmoid flexure
	P Rectum
	   Anorectal junction
		Ø Open
		3 Percutaneous
		4 Percutaneous Endoscopic
			C Extraluminal Device
			D Intraluminal Device
			Z No Device
				Z No Qualifier

1 Esophagus, Upper
   Cervical esophagus
2 Esophagus, Middle
   Thoracic esophagus
3 Esophagus, Lower
   Abdominal esophagus
4 Esophagogastric
   Junction
   Cardia
   Cardioesophageal
     junction
   Gastroesophageal (GE)
     junction
5 Esophagus
6 Stomach NC
7 Stomach, Pylorus
   Pyloric antrum
   Pyloric canal
   Pyloric sphincter
8 Small Intestine
	9 Duodenum
	A Jejunum
	   Duodenojejunal flexure
	B Ileum
	C Ileocecal Valve
	E Large Intestine
	F Large Intestine, Right
	G Large Intestine, Left
	H Cecum
	K Ascending Colon
	L Transverse Colon
	   Hepatic flexure
	   Splenic flexure
	M Descending Colon
	N Sigmoid Colon
	   Rectosigmoid junction
	   Sigmoid flexure
	P Rectum
	   Anorectal junction
		7 Via Natural or Artificial
		   Opening
		8 Via Natural or Artificial
		   Opening Endoscopic
			D Intraluminal Device
			Z No Device
				Z No Qualifier

Q Anus Anal orifice		Ø Open 3 Percutaneous 4 Percutaneous Endoscopic X External	C Extraluminal Device D Intraluminal Device Z No Device	Z No Qualifier

Q Anus
   Anal orifice
		7 Via Natural or Artificial
		   Opening
		8 Via Natural or Artificial
		   Opening Endoscopic
			D Intraluminal Device
			Z No Device
				Z No Qualifier

Non-OR   ØDV6[7,8]DZ
HAC   ØDV64CZ when reported with PDx E66.Ø1 and SDx K68.11, K95.Ø1, K95.81, or T81.4Ø–T81.49 with 7th character A
NC   ØDV6[7,8]DZ

NC Noncovered Procedure   LC Limited Coverage   QA Questionable OB Admit   NT New Tech Add-on   ⊞ Combination Member   ♂Male   ♀Female

ICD-10-PCS 2024   397

ØDV–ØDV

Gastrointestinal System

Ø   **Medical and Surgical**
D   **Gastrointestinal System**
W   **Revision**   Definition: Correcting, to the extent possible, a portion of a malfunctioning device or the position of a displaced device
               Explanation: Revision can include correcting a malfunctioning or displaced device by taking out or putting in components of the device such as a screw or pin

Body Part Character 4	Approach Character 5	Device Character 6	Qualifier Character 7
Ø Upper Intestinal Tract D Lower Intestinal Tract	Ø Open 3 Percutaneous 4 Percutaneous Endoscopic 7 Via Natural or Artificial Opening 8 Via Natural or Artificial Opening Endoscopic	Ø Drainage Device 2 Monitoring Device 3 Infusion Device 7 Autologous Tissue Substitute C Extraluminal Device D Intraluminal Device J Synthetic Substitute K Nonautologous Tissue Substitute U Feeding Device Y Other Device	Z No Qualifier
Ø Upper Intestinal Tract D Lower Intestinal Tract	X External	Ø Drainage Device 2 Monitoring Device 3 Infusion Device 7 Autologous Tissue Substitute C Extraluminal Device D Intraluminal Device J Synthetic Substitute K Nonautologous Tissue Substitute U Feeding Device	Z No Qualifier
5 Esophagus	Ø Open 3 Percutaneous 4 Percutaneous Endoscopic	Y Other Device	Z No Qualifier
5 Esophagus	7 Via Natural or Artificial Opening 8 Via Natural or Artificial Opening Endoscopic	D Intraluminal Device Y Other Device	Z No Qualifier
5 Esophagus	X External	D Intraluminal Device	Z No Qualifier
6 Stomach	Ø Open 3 Percutaneous 4 Percutaneous Endoscopic	Ø Drainage Device 2 Monitoring Device 3 Infusion Device 7 Autologous Tissue Substitute C Extraluminal Device D Intraluminal Device J Synthetic Substitute K Nonautologous Tissue Substitute M Stimulator Lead U Feeding Device Y Other Device	Z No Qualifier
6 Stomach	7 Via Natural or Artificial Opening 8 Via Natural or Artificial Opening Endoscopic	Ø Drainage Device 2 Monitoring Device 3 Infusion Device 7 Autologous Tissue Substitute C Extraluminal Device D Intraluminal Device J Synthetic Substitute K Nonautologous Tissue Substitute U Feeding Device Y Other Device	Z No Qualifier
6 Stomach	X External	Ø Drainage Device 2 Monitoring Device 3 Infusion Device 7 Autologous Tissue Substitute C Extraluminal Device D Intraluminal Device J Synthetic Substitute K Nonautologous Tissue Substitute U Feeding Device	Z No Qualifier

Non-OR   ØDW[Ø,D][3,4,7,8]YZ
Non-OR   ØDW[Ø,D]8UZ
Non-OR   ØDW[Ø,D]X[Ø,2,3,7,C,D,J,K,U]Z
Non-OR   ØDW5[Ø,3,4]YZ
Non-OR   ØDW5[7,8]YZ
Non-OR   ØDW5XDZ
Non-OR   ØDW6[3,4]YZ
Non-OR   ØDW68UZ
Non-OR   ØDW6[7,8]YZ
Non-OR   ØDW6X[Ø,2,3,7,C,D,J,K,U]Z

ØDW Continued on next page

Non-OR Procedure   DRG Non-OR Procedure   Valid OR Procedure   HAC Associated Procedure   Combination Only   New/Revised April   New/Revised October

Gastrointestinal System

Ø Medical and Surgical
D Gastrointestinal System
W Revision

ØDW Continued

Definition: Correcting, to the extent possible, a portion of a malfunctioning device or the position of a displaced device

Explanation: Revision can include correcting a malfunctioning or displaced device by taking out or putting in components of the device such as a screw or pin

Body Part Character 4	Approach Character 5	Device Character 6	Qualifier Character 7
8 Small Intestine E Large Intestine	Ø Open 4 Percutaneous Endoscopic 7 Via Natural or Artificial Opening 8 Via Natural or Artificial Opening Endoscopic	7 Autologous Tissue Substitute J Synthetic Substitute K Nonautologous Tissue Substitute	Z No Qualifier
Q Anus Anal orifice	Ø Open 3 Percutaneous 4 Percutaneous Endoscopic 7 Via Natural or Artificial Opening 8 Via Natural or Artificial Opening Endoscopic	L Artificial Sphincter	Z No Qualifier

R Anal Sphincter
  External anal sphincter
  Internal anal sphincter
	Ø Open
	3 Percutaneous
	4 Percutaneous Endoscopic
		M Stimulator Lead	Z No Qualifier

U Omentum
  Gastrocolic ligament
  Gastrocolic omentum
  Gastrohepatic omentum
  Gastrophrenic ligament
  Gastrosplenic ligament
  Greater Omentum
  Hepatogastric ligament
  Lesser Omentum
V Mesentery
  Mesoappendix
  Mesocolon
W Peritoneum
  Epiploic foramen
	Ø Open
	3 Percutaneous
	4 Percutaneous Endoscopic
		Ø Drainage Device
		7 Autologous Tissue Substitute
		J Synthetic Substitute
		K Nonautologous Tissue Substitute
			Z No Qualifier

Non-OR ØDW[U,V,W][Ø,3,4]ØZ

Ø Medical and Surgical
D Gastrointestinal System
X Transfer

Definition: Moving, without taking out, all or a portion of a body part to another location to take over the function of all or a portion of a body part

Explanation: The body part transferred remains connected to its vascular and nervous supply

Body Part Character 4	Approach Character 5	Device Character 6	Qualifier Character 7
6 Stomach	Ø Open 4 Percutaneous Endoscopic	Z No Device	5 Esophagus
8 Small Intestine	Ø Open 4 Percutaneous Endoscopic	Z No Device	5 Esophagus B Bladder C Ureter, Right D Ureter, Left F Ureters, Bilateral
E Large Intestine	Ø Open 4 Percutaneous Endoscopic	Z No Device	5 Esophagus 7 Vagina ♀ B Bladder

♀   ØDXE[Ø,4]Z7

Ø Medical and Surgical
D Gastrointestinal System
Y Transplantation

Definition: Putting in or on all or a portion of a living body part taken from another individual or animal to physically take the place and/or function of all or a portion of a similar body part

Explanation: The native body part may or may not be taken out, and the transplanted body part may take over all or a portion of its function

Body Part Character 4	Approach Character 5	Device Character 6	Qualifier Character 7
5 Esophagus 6 Stomach 8 Small Intestine LC E Large Intestine LC	Ø Open	Z No Device	Ø Allogeneic 1 Syngeneic 2 Zooplastic

Non-OR ØDY5ØZ[Ø,1,2]
LC ØDY[8,E]ØZ[Ø,1,2]

NC Noncovered Procedure   LC Limited Coverage   QA Questionable OB Admit   NT New Tech Add-on   ⊞ Combination Member   ♂ Male   ♀ Female

ICD-10-PCS 2024   399

Hepatobiliary System and Pancreas ØF1–ØFY

Character Meanings

This Character Meaning table is provided as a guide to assist the user in the identification of character members that may be found in this section of code tables. It **SHOULD NOT** be used to build a PCS code.

Operation–Character 3		Body Part–Character 4		Approach–Character 5		Device–Character 6		Qualifier–Character 7	
1	Bypass	Ø	Liver	Ø	Open	Ø	Drainage Device	Ø	Allogeneic
2	Change	1	Liver, Right Lobe	3	Percutaneous	1	Radioactive Element	1	Syngeneic
5	Destruction	2	Liver, Left Lobe	4	Percutaneous Endoscopic	2	Monitoring Device	2	Zooplastic
7	Dilation	4	Gallbladder	7	Via Natural or Artificial Opening	3	Infusion Device	3	Duodenum OR Laser Interstitial Thermal Therapy
8	Division	5	Hepatic Duct, Right	8	Via Natural or Artificial Opening Endoscopic	7	Autologous Tissue Substitute	4	Stomach
9	Drainage	6	Hepatic Duct, Left	X	External	C	Extraluminal Device	5	Hepatic Duct, Right
B	Excision	7	Hepatic Duct, Common			D	Intraluminal Device	6	Hepatic Duct, Left
C	Extirpation	8	Cystic Duct			J	Synthetic Substitute	7	Hepatic Duct, Caudate
D	Extraction	9	Common Bile Duct			K	Nonautologous Tissue Substitute	8	Cystic Duct
F	Fragmentation	B	Hepatobiliary Duct			Y	Other Device	9	Common Bile Duct
H	Insertion	C	Ampulla of Vater			Z	No Device	B	Small Intestine
J	Inspection	D	Pancreatic Duct					C	Large Intestine
L	Occlusion	F	Pancreatic Duct, Accessory					F	Irreversible Electroporation
M	Reattachment	G	Pancreas					X	Diagnostic
N	Release							Z	No Qualifier
P	Removal								
Q	Repair								
R	Replacement								
S	Reposition								
T	Resection								
U	Supplement								
V	Restriction								
W	Revision								
Y	Transplantation								

AHA Coding Clinic for table ØF1
2020, 4Q, 53　　　Bypass pancreatic duct to stomach

AHA Coding Clinic for table ØF5
2022, 4Q, 53-54　　Laser interstitial thermal therapy
2018, 4Q, 39　　　Irreversible electroporation

AHA Coding Clinic for table ØF7
2016, 3Q, 27　　　Endoscopic retrograde cholangiopancreatography with sphincterotomy and insertion of pancreatic stent
2016, 1Q, 25　　　Endoscopic retrograde cholangiopancreatography with brush biopsy of pancreatic and common bile ducts
2015, 1Q, 32　　　Percutaneous transhepatic biliary drainage catheter placement
2014, 3Q, 15　　　Drainage of pancreatic pseudocyst

AHA Coding Clinic for table ØF8
2021, 4Q, 48-49　　Division of liver for staged hepatectomy

AHA Coding Clinic for table ØF9
2023, 2Q, 22　　　Direct endoscopic necrosectomy
2020, 3Q, 34　　　Cystogastrostomy with stent insertion
2015, 1Q, 32　　　Percutaneous transhepatic biliary drainage catheter placement
2014, 3Q, 15　　　Drainage of pancreatic pseudocyst

AHA Coding Clinic for table ØFB
2023, 2Q, 22　　　Direct endoscopic necrosectomy
2023, 1Q, 38　　　Ex-vivo liver tumor resection and autotransplantation
2019, 1Q, 3-8　　　Whipple procedure
2016, 3Q, 41　　　Open cholecystectomy with needle biopsy of liver
2016, 1Q, 23　　　Endoscopic ultrasound with aspiration biopsy of common hepatic duct
2016, 1Q, 25　　　Endoscopic retrograde cholangiopancreatography with brush biopsy of pancreatic and common bile ducts
2014, 3Q, 32　　　Pyloric-sparing Whipple procedure

AHA Coding Clinic for table ØFC
2023, 2Q, 22　　　Direct endoscopic necrosectomy
2016, 3Q, 27　　　Endoscopic retrograde cholangiopancreatography with sphincterotomy and insertion of pancreatic stent

AHA Coding Clinic for table ØFD
2023, 2Q, 22　　　Direct endoscopic necrosectomy

AHA Coding Clinic for table ØFH
2022, 2Q, 26　　　Radioembolization of right hepatic lobe
2020, 4Q, 43-44　　Insertion of radioactive element

AHA Coding Clinic for table ØFQ
2016, 3Q, 27　　　Revision of common bile duct anastomosis
2013, 4Q, 109　　　Separating conjoined twins

AHA Coding Clinic for table ØFT
2021, 4Q, 49　　　Division of liver for staged hepatectomy
2019, 1Q, 3-8　　　Whipple procedure
2012, 4Q, 99　　　Domino liver transplant

AHA Coding Clinic for table ØFY
2023, 2Q, 32　　　Preparation of donor organ before transplantation
2023, 1Q, 38　　　Ex-vivo liver tumor resection and autotransplantation
2014, 3Q, 13　　　Orthotopic liver transplant with end to side cavoplasty
2012, 4Q, 99　　　Domino liver transplant

Liver

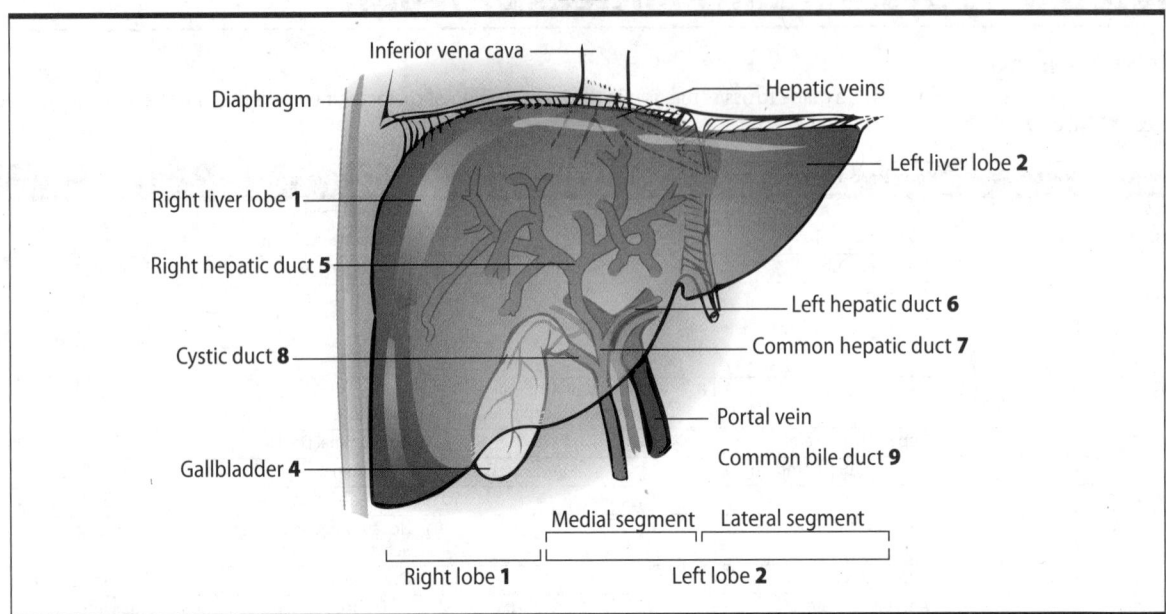

Inferior vena cava

Diaphragm

Hepatic veins

Left liver lobe **2**

Right liver lobe **1**

Right hepatic duct **5**

Left hepatic duct **6**

Common hepatic duct **7**

Cystic duct **8**

Portal vein

Common bile duct **9**

Gallbladder **4**

Medial segment | Lateral segment

Right lobe **1** | Left lobe **2**

Pancreas

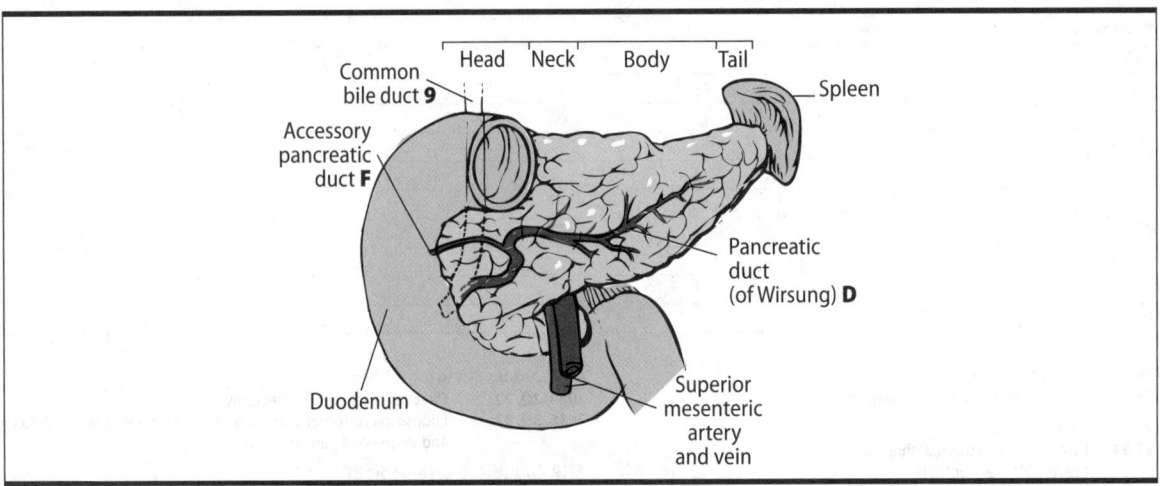

Head Neck Body Tail

Common bile duct **9**

Spleen

Accessory pancreatic duct **F**

Pancreatic duct (of Wirsung) **D**

Duodenum

Superior mesenteric artery and vein

Gallbladder and Ducts

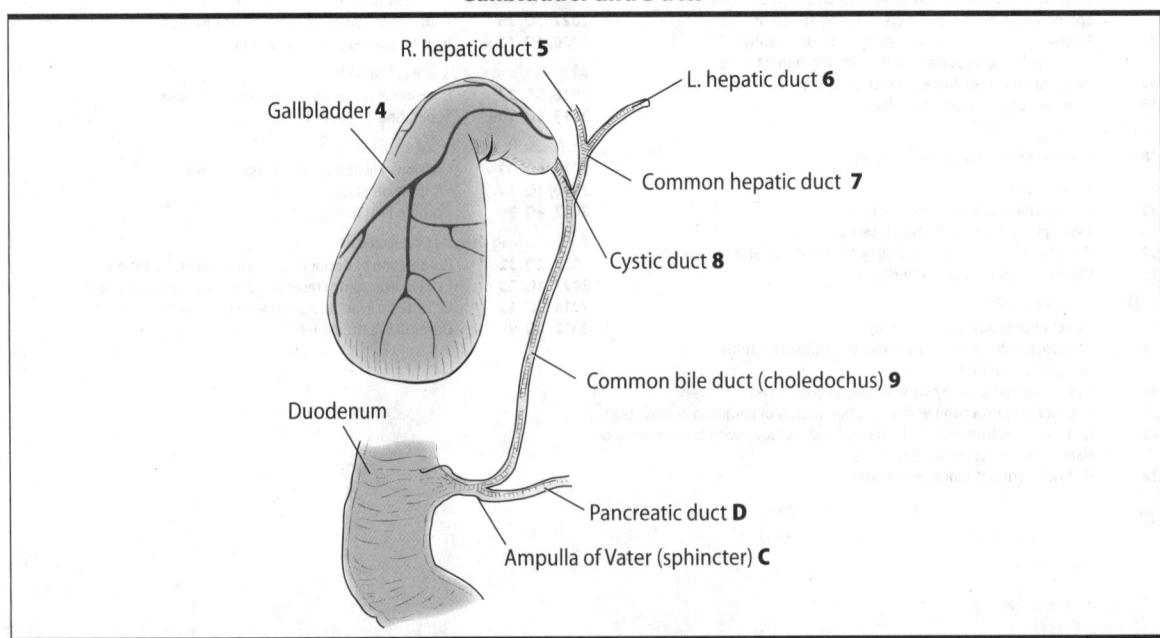

R. hepatic duct **5**

Gallbladder **4**

L. hepatic duct **6**

Common hepatic duct **7**

Cystic duct **8**

Common bile duct (choledochus) **9**

Duodenum

Pancreatic duct **D**

Ampulla of Vater (sphincter) **C**

0   Medical and Surgical
F   Hepatobiliary System and Pancreas
1   Bypass   Definition: Altering the route of passage of the contents of a tubular body part

                     Explanation: Rerouting contents of a body part to a downstream area of the normal route, to a similar route and body part, or to an abnormal route and dissimilar body part. Includes one or more anastomoses, with or without the use of a device.

Body Part Character 4	Approach Character 5	Device Character 6	Qualifier Character 7
4 Gallbladder 5 Hepatic Duct, Right 6 Hepatic Duct, Left 7 Hepatic Duct, Common 8 Cystic Duct 9 Common Bile Duct	0 Open 4 Percutaneous Endoscopic	D Intraluminal Device Z No Device	3 Duodenum 4 Stomach 5 Hepatic Duct, Right 6 Hepatic Duct, Left 7 Hepatic Duct, Caudate 8 Cystic Duct 9 Common Bile Duct B Small Intestine
D Pancreatic Duct Duct of Wirsung	0 Open 4 Percutaneous Endoscopic	D Intraluminal Device Z No Device	3 Duodenum 4 Stomach B Small Intestine C Large Intestine
F Pancreatic Duct, Accessory Duct of Santorini G Pancreas	0 Open 4 Percutaneous Endoscopic	D Intraluminal Device Z No Device	3 Duodenum B Small Intestine C Large Intestine

0   Medical and Surgical
F   Hepatobiliary System and Pancreas
2   Change   Definition: Taking out or off a device from a body part and putting back an identical or similar device in or on the same body part without cutting or puncturing the skin or a mucous membrane

                     Explanation: All CHANGE procedures are coded using the approach EXTERNAL

Body Part Character 4	Approach Character 5	Device Character 6	Qualifier Character 7

0 Liver
   Quadrate lobe
4 Gallbladder
B Hepatobiliary Duct
D Pancreatic Duct
   Duct of Wirsung
G Pancreas
	X External	0 Drainage Device
		Y Other Device
			Z No Qualifier

Non-OR	All body part, approach, device, and qualifier values

Ø Medical and Surgical
F Hepatobiliary System and Pancreas
5 Destruction   Definition: Physical eradication of all or a portion of a body part by the direct use of energy, force, or a destructive agent
                  Explanation: None of the body part is physically taken out

Body Part Character 4	Approach Character 5	Device Character 6	Qualifier Character 7
Ø Liver Quadrate lobe 1 Liver, Right Lobe 2 Liver, Left Lobe	Ø Open 3 Percutaneous 4 Percutaneous Endoscopic	Z No Device	3 Laser Interstitial Thermal Therapy F Irreversible Electroporation Z No Qualifier
4 Gallbladder	Ø Open 3 Percutaneous 4 Percutaneous Endoscopic	Z No Device	3 Laser Interstitial Thermal Therapy Z No Qualifier
4 Gallbladder	8 Via Natural or Artificial Opening Endoscopic	Z No Device	Z No Qualifier

5 Hepatic Duct, Right
6 Hepatic Duct, Left
7 Hepatic Duct, Common
8 Cystic Duct
9 Common Bile Duct
C Ampulla of Vater
   Duodenal ampulla
   Hepatopancreatic ampulla
D Pancreatic Duct
   Duct of Wirsung
F Pancreatic Duct, Accessory
   Duct of Santorini
	Ø Open
	3 Percutaneous
	4 Percutaneous Endoscopic
		Z No Device	3 Laser Interstitial Thermal Therapy
			Z No Qualifier

5 Hepatic Duct, Right
6 Hepatic Duct, Left
7 Hepatic Duct, Common
8 Cystic Duct
9 Common Bile Duct
C Ampulla of Vater
   Duodenal ampulla
   Hepatopancreatic ampulla
D Pancreatic Duct
   Duct of Wirsung
F Pancreatic Duct, Accessory
   Duct of Santorini
	7 Via Natural or Artificial Opening
	8 Via Natural or Artificial Opening Endoscopic
		Z No Device	Z No Qualifier

G Pancreas	Ø Open 3 Percutaneous 4 Percutaneous Endoscopic	Z No Device	3 Laser Interstitial Thermal Therapy F Irreversible Electroporation Z No Qualifier
G Pancreas	8 Via Natural or Artificial Opening Endoscopic	Z No Device	Z No Qualifier

DRG Non-OR	ØF5[5,6,7,8,9,C,D,F]4Z3
DRG Non-OR	ØF5G4Z3
Non-OR	ØF5[5,6,7,8,9,C,D,F]4ZZ
Non-OR	ØF5[5,6,7,8,9,C,D,F]8ZZ
Non-OR	ØF5G4Z[F,Z]
Non-OR	ØF5G8ZZ

Ø Medical and Surgical
F Hepatobiliary System and Pancreas
7 Dilation   Definition: Expanding an orifice or the lumen of a tubular body part
                  Explanation: The orifice can be a natural orifice or an artificially created orifice. Accomplished by stretching a tubular body part using intraluminal pressure or by cutting part of the orifice or wall of the tubular body part.

Body Part Character 4	Approach Character 5	Device Character 6	Qualifier Character 7

5 Hepatic Duct, Right
6 Hepatic Duct, Left
7 Hepatic Duct, Common
8 Cystic Duct
9 Common Bile Duct
C Ampulla of Vater
   Duodenal ampulla
   Hepatopancreatic ampulla
D Pancreatic Duct
   Duct of Wirsung
F Pancreatic Duct, Accessory
   Duct of Santorini
	Ø Open
	3 Percutaneous
	4 Percutaneous Endoscopic
	7 Via Natural or Artificial Opening
	8 Via Natural or Artificial Opening Endoscopic
		D Intraluminal Device
		Z No Device
			Z No Qualifier

Non-OR	ØF7[5,6,7,8,9][3,4,8][D,Z]Z
Non-OR	ØF7[5,6,7,8,9,D]]7DZ
Non-OR	ØF7C8[D,Z]Z
Non-OR	ØF7[D,F][4,8][D,Z]Z

Ø   **Medical and Surgical**
F   **Hepatobiliary System and Pancreas**
8   **Division**   Definition: Cutting into a body part, without draining fluids and/or gases from the body part, in order to separate or transect a body part
                         Explanation: All or a portion of the body part is separated into two or more portions

Body Part Character 4	Approach Character 5	Device Character 6	Qualifier Character 7
Ø Liver 1 Liver, Right Lobe 2 Liver, Left Lobe G Pancreas	Ø Open 3 Percutaneous 4 Percutaneous Endoscopic	Z No Device	Z No Qualifier

Non-OR   ØF8[Ø,1,2]3ZZ

Ø   **Medical and Surgical**
F   **Hepatobiliary System and Pancreas**
9   **Drainage**   Definition: Taking or letting out fluids and/or gases from a body part
                         Explanation: The qualifier DIAGNOSTIC is used to identify drainage procedures that are biopsies

Body Part Character 4	Approach Character 5	Device Character 6	Qualifier Character 7
Ø Liver Quadrate lobe 1 Liver, Right Lobe 2 Liver, Left Lobe	Ø Open 3 Percutaneous 4 Percutaneous Endoscopic	Ø Drainage Device	Z No Qualifier
Ø Liver Quadrate lobe 1 Liver, Right Lobe 2 Liver, Left Lobe	Ø Open 3 Percutaneous 4 Percutaneous Endoscopic	Z No Device	X Diagnostic Z No Qualifier
4 Gallbladder G Pancreas	Ø Open 3 Percutaneous 4 Percutaneous Endoscopic 8 Via Natural or Artificial Opening Endoscopic	Ø Drainage Device	Z No Qualifier
4 Gallbladder G Pancreas	Ø Open 3 Percutaneous 4 Percutaneous Endoscopic 8 Via Natural or Artificial Opening Endoscopic	Z No Device	X Diagnostic Z No Qualifier

5   Hepatic Duct, Right
6   Hepatic Duct, Left
7   Hepatic Duct, Common
8   Cystic Duct
9   Common Bile Duct
C   Ampulla of Vater
     Duodenal ampulla
     Hepatopancreatic ampulla
D   Pancreatic Duct
     Duct of Wirsung
F   Pancreatic Duct, Accessory
     Duct of Santorini
	Ø Open
	3 Percutaneous
	4 Percutaneous Endoscopic
	7 Via Natural or Artificial Opening
	8 Via Natural or Artificial Opening
	     Endoscopic
		Ø Drainage Device	Z No Qualifier

5   Hepatic Duct, Right
6   Hepatic Duct, Left
7   Hepatic Duct, Common
8   Cystic Duct
9   Common Bile Duct
C   Ampulla of Vater
     Duodenal ampulla
     Hepatopancreatic ampulla
D   Pancreatic Duct
     Duct of Wirsung
F   Pancreatic Duct, Accessory
     Duct of Santorini
	Ø Open
	3 Percutaneous
	4 Percutaneous Endoscopic
	7 Via Natural or Artificial Opening
	8 Via Natural or Artificial Opening
	     Endoscopic
		Z No Device	X Diagnostic
			Z No Qualifier

Non-OR ØF9[Ø,1,2][3,4]ØZ	**Non-OR** ØF99[3,8]ØZ
Non-OR ØF9[Ø,1,2][3,4]Z[X,Z]	**Non-OR** ØF9C[3,4,8]ØZ
Non-OR ØF9[4,G]8ØZ	**Non-OR** ØF9[D,F][3,8]ØZ
Non-OR ØF9G3ØZ	**Non-OR** ØF9[5,6,8,9,C,D,F]3Z[X,Z]
Non-OR ØF9[4,G]8Z[X,Z]	**Non-OR** ØF9[5,6,8,9,C,D,F][4,7,8]ZX
Non-OR ØF9G3Z[XZ]	**Non-OR** ØF9[5,6,8,D,F]8ZZ
Non-OR ØF9G4ZX	**Non-OR** ØF97[3,4,7,8]Z[X,Z]
Non-OR ØF9[5,6,8][3,8]ØZ	**Non-OR** ØF99[4,7,8]ZZ
Non-OR ØF97[3,4,7,8]ØZ	**Non-OR** ØF9C[4,8]ZZ

NC Noncovered Procedure   **LC** Limited Coverage   **QA** Questionable OB Admit   **NT** New Tech Add-on   ⊞ Combination Member   ♂Male   ♀Female

ICD-10-PCS 2024   405

Ø **Medical and Surgical**
F **Hepatobiliary System and Pancreas**
B **Excision**   Definition: Cutting out or off, without replacement, a portion of a body part
            Explanation: The qualifier DIAGNOSTIC is used to identify excision procedures that are biopsies

Body Part Character 4	Approach Character 5	Device Character 6	Qualifier Character 7
Ø Liver Quadrate lobe 1 Liver, Right Lobe 2 Liver, Left Lobe	Ø Open 3 Percutaneous 4 Percutaneous Endoscopic	Z No Device	X Diagnostic Z No Qualifier
4 Gallbladder G Pancreas	Ø Open 3 Percutaneous 4 Percutaneous Endoscopic 8 Via Natural or Artificial Opening Endoscopic	Z No Device	X Diagnostic Z No Qualifier

5 Hepatic Duct, Right
6 Hepatic Duct, Left
7 Hepatic Duct, Common
8 Cystic Duct
9 Common Bile Duct
C Ampulla of Vater
   Duodenal ampulla
   Hepatopancreatic ampulla
D Pancreatic Duct
   Duct of Wirsung
F Pancreatic Duct, Accessory
   Duct of Santorini
	Ø Open
	3 Percutaneous
	4 Percutaneous Endoscopic
	7 Via Natural or Artificial Opening
	8 Via Natural or Artificial Opening Endoscopic
		Z No Device	X Diagnostic
			Z No Qualifier

Non-OR ØFB[Ø,1,2]3ZX
Non-OR ØFB[4,G][3,4,8]ZX
Non-OR ØFB[5,6,7,8,9,C,D,F][3,4,7,8]ZX
Non-OR ØFB[5,6,7,8,9,C,D,F][4,8]ZZ

Ø **Medical and Surgical**
F **Hepatobiliary System and Pancreas**
C **Extirpation**   Definition: Taking or cutting out solid matter from a body part
            Explanation: The solid matter may be an abnormal byproduct of a biological function or a foreign body; it may be imbedded in a body part or in the lumen of a tubular body part. The solid matter may or may not have been previously broken into pieces.

Body Part Character 4	Approach Character 5	Device Character 6	Qualifier Character 7
Ø Liver Quadrate lobe 1 Liver, Right Lobe 2 Liver, Left Lobe	Ø Open 3 Percutaneous 4 Percutaneous Endoscopic	Z No Device	Z No Qualifier
4 Gallbladder G Pancreas	Ø Open 3 Percutaneous 4 Percutaneous Endoscopic 8 Via Natural or Artificial Opening Endoscopic	Z No Device	Z No Qualifier

5 Hepatic Duct, Right
6 Hepatic Duct, Left
7 Hepatic Duct, Common
8 Cystic Duct
9 Common Bile Duct
C Ampulla of Vater
   Duodenal ampulla
   Hepatopancreatic ampulla
D Pancreatic Duct
   Duct of Wirsung
F Pancreatic Duct, Accessory
   Duct of Santorini
	Ø Open
	3 Percutaneous
	4 Percutaneous Endoscopic
	7 Via Natural or Artificial Opening
	8 Via Natural or Artificial Opening Endoscopic
		Z No Device	Z No Qualifier

Non-OR ØFC[5,6,7,8][3,4,7,8]ZZ
Non-OR ØFC9[3,7,8]ZZ
Non-OR ØFCC[4,8]ZZ
Non-OR ØFC[D,F][3,4,8]ZZ

Ø **Medical and Surgical**
F **Hepatobiliary System and Pancreas**
D **Extraction**　　Definition: Pulling or stripping out or off all or a portion of a body part by the use of force
　　　　　　　　　　Explanation: The qualifier DIAGNOSTIC is used to identify extraction procedures that are biopsies

Body Part Character 4	Approach Character 5	Device Character 6	Qualifier Character 7
Ø Liver 　　Quadrate lobe **1** Liver, Right Lobe **2** Liver, Left Lobe	**3** Percutaneous **4** Percutaneous Endoscopic	**Z** No Device	**X** Diagnostic
4 Gallbladder **5** Hepatic Duct, Right **6** Hepatic Duct, Left **7** Hepatic Duct, Common **8** Cystic Duct **9** Common Bile Duct **C** Ampulla of Vater 　　Duodenal ampulla 　　Hepatopancreatic ampulla **D** Pancreatic Duct 　　Duct of Wirsung **F** Pancreatic Duct, Accessory 　　Duct of Santorini **G** Pancreas	**3** Percutaneous **4** Percutaneous Endoscopic **8** Via Natural or Artificial Opening 　　Endoscopic	**Z** No Device	**X** Diagnostic

Non-OR ØFD[Ø,1,2]3ZX
Non-OR ØFD[4,5,6,7,8,9,C,D,F,G][3,4,8]ZX

Ø **Medical and Surgical**
F **Hepatobiliary System and Pancreas**
F **Fragmentation**　　Definition: Breaking solid matter in a body part into pieces
　　　　　　　　　　Explanation: Physical force (e.g., manual, ultrasonic) applied directly or indirectly is used to break the solid matter into pieces. The solid matter may be an abnormal byproduct of a biological function or a foreign body. The pieces of solid matter are not taken out.

Body Part Character 4	Approach Character 5	Device Character 6	Qualifier Character 7
4 Gallbladder `NC` **5** Hepatic Duct, Right `NC` **6** Hepatic Duct, Left `NC` **7** Hepatic Duct, Common **8** Cystic Duct `NC` **9** Common Bile Duct `NC` **C** Ampulla of Vater `NC` 　　Duodenal ampulla 　　Hepatopancreatic ampulla **D** Pancreatic Duct `NC` 　　Duct of Wirsung **F** Pancreatic Duct, Accessory `NC` 　　Duct of Santorini	**Ø** Open **3** Percutaneous **4** Percutaneous Endoscopic **7** Via Natural or Artificial Opening **8** Via Natural or Artificial Opening 　　Endoscopic **X** External	**Z** No Device	**Z** No Qualifier

Non-OR ØFF[4,5,6,7,8,9,C,D,F][8,X]ZZ
`NC` ØFF[4,5,6,8,9,C,D,F]XZZ

Ø **Medical and Surgical**
F **Hepatobiliary System and Pancreas**
H **Insertion**　　Definition: Putting in a nonbiological appliance that monitors, assists, performs, or prevents a physiological function but does not physically take the place of a body part
　　　　　　　　　　Explanation: None

Body Part Character 4	Approach Character 5	Device Character 6	Qualifier Character 7
Ø Liver 　　Quadrate lobe **4** Gallbladder **G** Pancreas	**Ø** Open **3** Percutaneous **4** Percutaneous Endoscopic	**1** Radioactive Element **2** Monitoring Device **3** Infusion Device **Y** Other Device	**Z** No Qualifier
1 Liver, Right Lobe **2** Liver, Left Lobe	**Ø** Open **3** Percutaneous **4** Percutaneous Endoscopic	**2** Monitoring Device **3** Infusion Device	**Z** No Qualifier
B Hepatobiliary Duct ⊞ **D** Pancreatic Duct 　　Duct of Wirsung	**Ø** Open **3** Percutaneous **4** Percutaneous Endoscopic **7** Via Natural or Artificial Opening **8** Via Natural or Artificial Opening 　　Endoscopic	**1** Radioactive Element **2** Monitoring Device **3** Infusion Device **D** Intraluminal Device **Y** Other Device	**Z** No Qualifier

Non-OR ØFH[Ø,4,G]31Z	**Non-OR** ØFH[B,D][Ø,3,4]3Z	**See Appendix L for Procedure Combinations**
Non-OR ØFH[Ø,4,G][Ø,3,4]3Z	**Non-OR** ØFH[B,D][4,8]DZ	⊞　　ØFHB7DZ
Non-OR ØFH[Ø,4,G][3,4]YZ	**Non-OR** ØFH[B,D][7,8][2,3]Z	
Non-OR ØFH[1,2][Ø,3,4]3Z	**Non-OR** ØFH[B,D][3,4,7,8]YZ	

`NC` Noncovered Procedure　　`LC` Limited Coverage　　`QA` Questionable OB Admit　　`NT` New Tech Add-on　　⊞ Combination Member　　♂Male　　♀Female

Ø   Medical and Surgical
F   Hepatobiliary System and Pancreas
J   Inspection   Definition: Visually and/or manually exploring a body part

Explanation: Visual exploration may be performed with or without optical instrumentation. Manual exploration may be performed directly or through intervening body layers.

Body Part Character 4	Approach Character 5	Device Character 6	Qualifier Character 7
Ø Liver Quadrate lobe	Ø Open 3 Percutaneous 4 Percutaneous Endoscopic X External	Z No Device	Z No Qualifier
4 Gallbladder G Pancreas	Ø Open 3 Percutaneous 4 Percutaneous Endoscopic 8 Via Natural or Artificial Opening Endoscopic X External	Z No Device	Z No Qualifier

B Hepatobiliary Duct
D Pancreatic Duct
  Duct of Wirsung
	Ø Open
	3 Percutaneous
	4 Percutaneous Endoscopic
	7 Via Natural or Artificial Opening
	8 Via Natural or Artificial Opening
	  Endoscopic
		Z No Device	Z No Qualifier

Non-OR   ØFJØ[3,X]ZZ
Non-OR   ØFJ[4,G][3,8,X]ZZ
Non-OR   ØFJ[B,D][3,7,8]ZZ

Ø   Medical and Surgical
F   Hepatobiliary System and Pancreas
L   Occlusion   Definition: Completely closing an orifice or the lumen of a tubular body part

Explanation: The orifice can be a natural orifice or an artificially created orifice

Body Part Character 4	Approach Character 5	Device Character 6	Qualifier Character 7

5 Hepatic Duct, Right
6 Hepatic Duct, Left
7 Hepatic Duct, Common
8 Cystic Duct
9 Common Bile Duct
C Ampulla of Vater
  Duodenal ampulla
  Hepatopancreatic ampulla
D Pancreatic Duct
  Duct of Wirsung
F Pancreatic Duct, Accessory
  Duct of Santorini
	Ø Open
	3 Percutaneous
	4 Percutaneous Endoscopic
		C Extraluminal Device
		D Intraluminal Device
		Z No Device
			Z No Qualifier

5 Hepatic Duct, Right
6 Hepatic Duct, Left
7 Hepatic Duct, Common
8 Cystic Duct
9 Common Bile Duct
C Ampulla of Vater
  Duodenal ampulla
  Hepatopancreatic ampulla
D Pancreatic Duct
  Duct of Wirsung
F Pancreatic Duct, Accessory
  Duct of Santorini
	7 Via Natural or Artificial Opening
	8 Via Natural or Artificial Opening
	  Endoscopic
		D Intraluminal Device
		Z No Device
			Z No Qualifier

Non-OR   ØFL[5,6,7,8,9][3,4][C,D,Z]Z
Non-OR   ØFL[5,6,7,8,9][7,8][D,Z]Z

Ø Medical and Surgical
F Hepatobiliary System and Pancreas
M Reattachment   Definition: Putting back in or on all or a portion of a separated body part to its normal location or other suitable location

Explanation: Vascular circulation and nervous pathways may or may not be reestablished

Body Part Character 4	Approach Character 5	Device Character 6	Qualifier Character 7

Ø Liver
  Quadrate lobe
1 Liver, Right Lobe
2 Liver, Left Lobe
4 Gallbladder
5 Hepatic Duct, Right
6 Hepatic Duct, Left
7 Hepatic Duct, Common
8 Cystic Duct
9 Common Bile Duct
C Ampulla of Vater
  Duodenal ampulla
  Hepatopancreatic ampulla
D Pancreatic Duct
  Duct of Wirsung
F Pancreatic Duct, Accessory
  Duct of Santorini
G Pancreas
	Ø Open
	4 Percutaneous Endoscopic
		Z No Device	Z No Qualifier

Non-OR   ØFM[4,5,6,7,8,9]4ZZ

Ø Medical and Surgical
F Hepatobiliary System and Pancreas
N Release   Definition: Freeing a body part from an abnormal physical constraint by cutting or by the use of force

Explanation: Some of the restraining tissue may be taken out but none of the body part is taken out

Body Part Character 4	Approach Character 5	Device Character 6	Qualifier Character 7
Ø Liver Quadrate lobe 1 Liver, Right Lobe 2 Liver, Left Lobe	Ø Open 3 Percutaneous 4 Percutaneous Endoscopic	Z No Device	Z No Qualifier
4 Gallbladder G Pancreas	Ø Open 3 Percutaneous 4 Percutaneous Endoscopic 8 Via Natural or Artificial Opening Endoscopic	Z No Device	Z No Qualifier

5 Hepatic Duct, Right
6 Hepatic Duct, Left
7 Hepatic Duct, Common
8 Cystic Duct
9 Common Bile Duct
C Ampulla of Vater
  Duodenal ampulla
  Hepatopancreatic ampulla
D Pancreatic Duct
  Duct of Wirsung
F Pancreatic Duct, Accessory
  Duct of Santorini
	Ø Open
	3 Percutaneous
	4 Percutaneous Endoscopic
	7 Via Natural or Artificial Opening
	8 Via Natural or Artificial Opening Endoscopic
		Z No Device	Z No Qualifier

Ø   **Medical and Surgical**
F   **Hepatobiliary System and Pancreas**
P   **Removal**   Definition: Taking out or off a device from a body part

                Explanation: If a device is taken out and a similar device put in without cutting or puncturing the skin or mucous membrane, the procedure is coded to the root operation CHANGE. Otherwise, the procedure for taking out a device is coded to the root operation REMOVAL.

Body Part Character 4	Approach Character 5	Device Character 6	Qualifier Character 7
Ø Liver Quadrate lobe	**Ø** Open **3** Percutaneous **4** Percutaneous Endoscopic	**Ø** Drainage Device **2** Monitoring Device **3** Infusion Device **Y** Other Device	**Z** No Qualifier
Ø Liver Quadrate lobe	**X** External	**Ø** Drainage Device **2** Monitoring Device **3** Infusion Device	**Z** No Qualifier
4 Gallbladder **G** Pancreas	**Ø** Open **3** Percutaneous **4** Percutaneous Endoscopic	**Ø** Drainage Device **2** Monitoring Device **3** Infusion Device **D** Intraluminal Device **Y** Other Device	**Z** No Qualifier
4 Gallbladder **G** Pancreas	**X** External	**Ø** Drainage Device **2** Monitoring Device **3** Infusion Device **D** Intraluminal Device	**Z** No Qualifier

B   Hepatobiliary Duct
D   Pancreatic Duct
     Duct of Wirsung
	Ø Open
	3 Percutaneous
	4 Percutaneous Endoscopic
	7 Via Natural or Artificial Opening
	8 Via Natural or Artificial Opening
	     Endoscopic
		Ø Drainage Device
		1 Radioactive Element
		2 Monitoring Device
		3 Infusion Device
		7 Autologous Tissue Substitute
		C Extraluminal Device
		D Intraluminal Device
		J Synthetic Substitute
		K Nonautologous Tissue Substitute
		Y Other Device
			Z No Qualifier

B Hepatobiliary Duct **D** Pancreatic Duct Duct of Wirsung	**X** External	**Ø** Drainage Device **1** Radioactive Element **2** Monitoring Device **3** Infusion Device **D** Intraluminal Device	**Z** No Qualifier

Non-OR ØFPØ[3,4]YZ		**See Appendix L for Procedure Combinations**
Non-OR ØFPØX[Ø,2,3]Z		Combo-only ØFP[B,D][7,8]DZ
Non-OR ØFPG3ØZ		Combo-only ØFP[B,D]XDZ
Non-OR ØFP[4,G][3,4]YZ		
Non-OR ØFP4X[Ø,2,3,D]Z		
Non-OR ØFPGX[Ø,2,3]Z		
Non-OR ØFP[B,D][3,4]YZ		
Non-OR ØFP[B,D][7,8][Ø,2,3,D,Y]Z		
Non-OR ØFP[B,D]X[Ø,1,2,3,D]Z		

Non-OR Procedure   DRG Non-OR Procedure   Valid OR Procedure   HAC Associated Procedure   Combination Only   New/Revised April   New/Revised October

410   ICD-10-PCS 2024

Ø   **Medical and Surgical**
F   **Hepatobiliary System and Pancreas**
Q   **Repair**   Definition: Restoring, to the extent possible, a body part to its normal anatomic structure and function

                          Explanation: Used only when the method to accomplish the repair is not one of the other root operations

Body Part Character 4	Approach Character 5	Device Character 6	Qualifier Character 7
Ø Liver Quadrate lobe 1 Liver, Right Lobe 2 Liver, Left Lobe	Ø Open 3 Percutaneous 4 Percutaneous Endoscopic	Z No Device	Z No Qualifier
4 Gallbladder G Pancreas	Ø Open 3 Percutaneous 4 Percutaneous Endoscopic 8 Via Natural or Artificial Opening Endoscopic	Z No Device	Z No Qualifier

5   Hepatic Duct, Right
6   Hepatic Duct, Left
7   Hepatic Duct, Common
8   Cystic Duct
9   Common Bile Duct
C   Ampulla of Vater
     Duodenal ampulla
     Hepatopancreatic ampulla
D   Pancreatic Duct
     Duct of Wirsung
F   Pancreatic Duct, Accessory
     Duct of Santorini
	Ø Open
	3 Percutaneous
	4 Percutaneous Endoscopic
	7 Via Natural or Artificial Opening
	8 Via Natural or Artificial Opening
	     Endoscopic
		Z No Device	Z No Qualifier

Ø   **Medical and Surgical**
F   **Hepatobiliary System and Pancreas**
R   **Replacement**   Definition: Putting in or on biological or synthetic material that physically takes the place and/or function of all or a portion of a body part

                          Explanation: The body part may have been taken out or replaced, or may be taken out, physically eradicated, or rendered nonfunctional during the REPLACEMENT procedure. A REMOVAL procedure is coded for taking out the device used in a previous replacement procedure.

Body Part Character 4	Approach Character 5	Device Character 6	Qualifier Character 7

5   Hepatic Duct, Right
6   Hepatic Duct, Left
7   Hepatic Duct, Common
8   Cystic Duct
9   Common Bile Duct
C   Ampulla of Vater
     Duodenal ampulla
     Hepatopancreatic ampulla
D   Pancreatic Duct
     Duct of Wirsung
F   Pancreatic Duct, Accessory
     Duct of Santorini
	Ø Open
	4 Percutaneous Endoscopic
	8 Via Natural or Artificial Opening
	     Endoscopic
		7 Autologous Tissue Substitute
		J Synthetic Substitute
		K Nonautologous Tissue Substitute
			Z No Qualifier

Ø   **Medical and Surgical**
F   **Hepatobiliary System and Pancreas**
S   **Reposition**   Definition: Moving to its normal location, or other suitable location, all or a portion of a body part

                          Explanation: The body part is moved to a new location from an abnormal location, or from a normal location where it is not functioning correctly. The body part may or may not be cut out or off to be moved to the new location.

Body Part Character 4	Approach Character 5	Device Character 6	Qualifier Character 7

Ø   Liver
     Quadrate lobe
4   Gallbladder
5   Hepatic Duct, Right
6   Hepatic Duct, Left
7   Hepatic Duct, Common
8   Cystic Duct
9   Common Bile Duct
C   Ampulla of Vater
     Duodenal ampulla
     Hepatopancreatic ampulla
D   Pancreatic Duct
     Duct of Wirsung
F   Pancreatic Duct, Accessory
     Duct of Santorini
G   Pancreas
	Ø Open
	4 Percutaneous Endoscopic
		Z No Device	Z No Qualifier

Ø   **Medical and Surgical**
F   **Hepatobiliary System and Pancreas**
T   **Resection**   Definition: Cutting out or off, without replacement, all of a body part
                     Explanation: None

Body Part Character 4	Approach Character 5	Device Character 6	Qualifier Character 7
Ø Liver Quadrate lobe 1 Liver, Right Lobe 2 Liver, Left Lobe 4 Gallbladder G Pancreas ⊞	Ø Open 4 Percutaneous Endoscopic	Z No Device	Z No Qualifier

5 Hepatic Duct, Right
6 Hepatic Duct, Left
7 Hepatic Duct, Common
8 Cystic Duct
9 Common Bile Duct
C Ampulla of Vater
    Duodenal ampulla
    Hepatopancreatic ampulla
D Pancreatic Duct
    Duct of Wirsung
F Pancreatic Duct, Accessory
    Duct of Santorini
	Ø Open
	4 Percutaneous Endoscopic
	7 Via Natural or Artificial Opening
	8 Via Natural or Artificial Opening
	    Endoscopic
		Z No Device	Z No Qualifier

Non-OR   ØFT[D,F][4,8]ZZ

See Appendix L for Procedure Combinations
⊞   ØFTGØZZ

Ø   **Medical and Surgical**
F   **Hepatobiliary System and Pancreas**
U   **Supplement**   Definition: Putting in or on biological or synthetic material that physically reinforces and/or augments the function of a portion of a body part
                     Explanation: The biological material is non-living, or is living and from the same individual. The body part may have been previously replaced, and the SUPPLEMENT procedure is performed to physically reinforce and/or augment the function of the replaced body part.

Body Part Character 4	Approach Character 5	Device Character 6	Qualifier Character 7

5 Hepatic Duct, Right
6 Hepatic Duct, Left
7 Hepatic Duct, Common
8 Cystic Duct
9 Common Bile Duct
C Ampulla of Vater
    Duodenal ampulla
    Hepatopancreatic ampulla
D Pancreatic Duct
    Duct of Wirsung
F Pancreatic Duct, Accessory
    Duct of Santorini
	Ø Open
	3 Percutaneous
	4 Percutaneous Endoscopic
	8 Via Natural or Artificial Opening
	    Endoscopic
		7 Autologous Tissue Substitute
		J Synthetic Substitute
		K Nonautologous Tissue Substitute
			Z No Qualifier

Non-OR Procedure   DRG Non-OR Procedure   Valid OR Procedure   HAC Associated Procedure   Combination Only   New/Revised April   New/Revised October

Ø Medical and Surgical
F Hepatobiliary System and Pancreas
V Restriction　　Definition: Partially closing an orifice or the lumen of a tubular body part
　　　　　　　　　　Explanation: The orifice can be a natural orifice or an artificially created orifice

Body Part Character 4	Approach Character 5	Device Character 6	Qualifier Character 7
5 Hepatic Duct, Right 6 Hepatic Duct, Left 7 Hepatic Duct, Common 8 Cystic Duct 9 Common Bile Duct C Ampulla of Vater 　Duodenal ampulla 　Hepatopancreatic ampulla D Pancreatic Duct 　Duct of Wirsung F Pancreatic Duct, Accessory 　Duct of Santorini	Ø Open 3 Percutaneous 4 Percutaneous Endoscopic	C Extraluminal Device D Intraluminal Device Z No Device	Z No Qualifier
5 Hepatic Duct, Right 6 Hepatic Duct, Left 7 Hepatic Duct, Common 8 Cystic Duct 9 Common Bile Duct C Ampulla of Vater 　Duodenal ampulla 　Hepatopancreatic ampulla D Pancreatic Duct 　Duct of Wirsung F Pancreatic Duct, Accessory 　Duct of Santorini	7 Via Natural or Artificial Opening 8 Via Natural or Artificial Opening Endoscopic	D Intraluminal Device Z No Device	Z No Qualifier

Non-OR ØFV[5,6,7,8,9][3,4][C,D,Z]Z
Non-OR ØFV[5,6,7,8,9][7,8][D,Z]Z

Ø Medical and Surgical
F Hepatobiliary System and Pancreas
W Revision   Definition: Correcting, to the extent possible, a portion of a malfunctioning device or the position of a displaced device

Explanation: Revision can include correcting a malfunctioning or displaced device by taking out or putting in components of the device such as a screw or pin

Body Part Character 4	Approach Character 5	Device Character 6	Qualifier Character 7
Ø Liver Quadrate lobe	Ø Open 3 Percutaneous 4 Percutaneous Endoscopic	Ø Drainage Device 2 Monitoring Device 3 Infusion Device Y Other Device	Z No Qualifier
Ø Liver Quadrate lobe	X External	Ø Drainage Device 2 Monitoring Device 3 Infusion Device	Z No Qualifier
4 Gallbladder G Pancreas	Ø Open 3 Percutaneous 4 Percutaneous Endoscopic	Ø Drainage Device 2 Monitoring Device 3 Infusion Device D Intraluminal Device Y Other Device	Z No Qualifier
4 Gallbladder G Pancreas	X External	Ø Drainage Device 2 Monitoring Device 3 Infusion Device D Intraluminal Device	Z No Qualifier

B Hepatobiliary Duct
D Pancreatic Duct
   Duct of Wirsung
	Ø Open
	3 Percutaneous
	4 Percutaneous Endoscopic
	7 Via Natural or Artificial Opening
	8 Via Natural or Artificial Opening
	   Endoscopic
		Ø Drainage Device
		2 Monitoring Device
		3 Infusion Device
		7 Autologous Tissue Substitute
		C Extraluminal Device
		D Intraluminal Device
		J Synthetic Substitute
		K Nonautologous Tissue Substitute
		Y Other Device
			Z No Qualifier

B Hepatobiliary Duct D Pancreatic Duct Duct of Wirsung	X External	Ø Drainage Device 2 Monitoring Device 3 Infusion Device 7 Autologous Tissue Substitute C Extraluminal Device D Intraluminal Device J Synthetic Substitute K Nonautologous Tissue Substitute	Z No Qualifier

Non-OR	ØFWØ[3,4]YZ
Non-OR	ØFWØX[Ø,2,3]Z
Non-OR	ØFW[4,G][3,4]YZ
Non-OR	ØFW[4,G]X[Ø,2,3,D]Z
Non-OR	ØFW[B,D][3,4,7,8]YZ
Non-OR	ØFW[B,D]X[Ø,2,3,7,C,D,J,K]Z

Ø Medical and Surgical
F Hepatobiliary System and Pancreas
Y Transplantation   Definition: Putting in or on all or a portion of a living body part taken from another individual or animal to physically take the place and/or function of all or a portion of a similar body part

Explanation: The native body part may or may not be taken out, and the transplanted body part may take over all or a portion of its function

Body Part Character 4	Approach Character 5	Device Character 6	Qualifier Character 7
Ø Liver **LC** Quadrate lobe G Pancreas **LC** **NC** ⊞	Ø Open	Z No Device	Ø Allogeneic 1 Syngeneic 2 Zooplastic

LC	ØFYØØZ[Ø,1,2]	**See Appendix L for Procedure Combinations**
LC	ØFYGØZ[Ø,1]	⊞ ØFYGØZ[Ø,1,2]
NC	ØFYGØZ2	
NC	ØFYGØZ[Ø,1] If reported alone without one of the following procedures ØTYØØZ[Ø,1,2], ØTY1ØZ[Ø,1,2] and without one of the following diagnoses E10.10-E10.9, E89.1	

Non-OR Procedure   DRG Non-OR Procedure   Valid OR Procedure   HAC Associated Procedure   Combination Only   New/Revised April   New/Revised October

414   ICD-10-PCS 2024

Endocrine System 0G2–0GW

Character Meanings

This Character Meaning table is provided as a guide to assist the user in the identification of character members that may be found in this section of code tables. It **SHOULD NOT** be used to build a PCS code.

Operation–Character 3		Body Part–Character 4		Approach–Character 5		Device–Character 6		Qualifier–Character 7	
2	Change	0	Pituitary Gland	0	Open	0	Drainage Device	3	Laser Interstitial Thermal Therapy
5	Destruction	1	Pineal Body	3	Percutaneous	1	Radioactive Element	X	Diagnostic
8	Division	2	Adrenal Gland, Left	4	Percutaneous Endoscopic	2	Monitoring Device	Z	No Qualifier
9	Drainage	3	Adrenal Gland, Right	X	External	3	Infusion Device		
B	Excision	4	Adrenal Glands, Bilateral			Y	Other Device		
C	Extirpation	5	Adrenal Gland			Z	No Device		
H	Insertion	6	Carotid Body, Left						
J	Inspection	7	Carotid Body, Right						
M	Reattachment	8	Carotid Bodies, Bilateral						
N	Release	9	Para-aortic Body						
P	Removal	B	Coccygeal Glomus						
Q	Repair	C	Glomus Jugulare						
S	Reposition	D	Aortic Body						
T	Resection	F	Paraganglion Extremity						
W	Revision	G	Thyroid Gland Lobe, Left						
		H	Thyroid Gland Lobe, Right						
		J	Thyroid Gland Isthmus						
		K	Thyroid Gland						
		L	Superior Parathyroid Gland, Right						
		M	Superior Parathyroid Gland, Left						
		N	Inferior Parathyroid Gland, Right						
		P	Inferior Parathyroid Gland, Left						
		Q	Parathyroid Glands, Multiple						
		R	Parathyroid Gland						
		S	Endocrine Gland						

AHA Coding Clinic for table 0G5

2022, 4Q, 53-54   Laser interstitial thermal therapy

AHA Coding Clinic for table 0GB

2021, 2Q, 7   Infrarenal para-aortic paraganglioma with excision
2017, 2Q, 20   Near total thyroidectomy
2014, 3Q, 22   Transsphenoidal removal of pituitary tumor and fat graft placement

AHA Coding Clinic for table 0GH

2020, 4Q, 43-44   Insertion of radioactive element

AHA Coding Clinic for table 0GT

2017, 2Q, 20   Near total thyroidectomy

Endocrine System

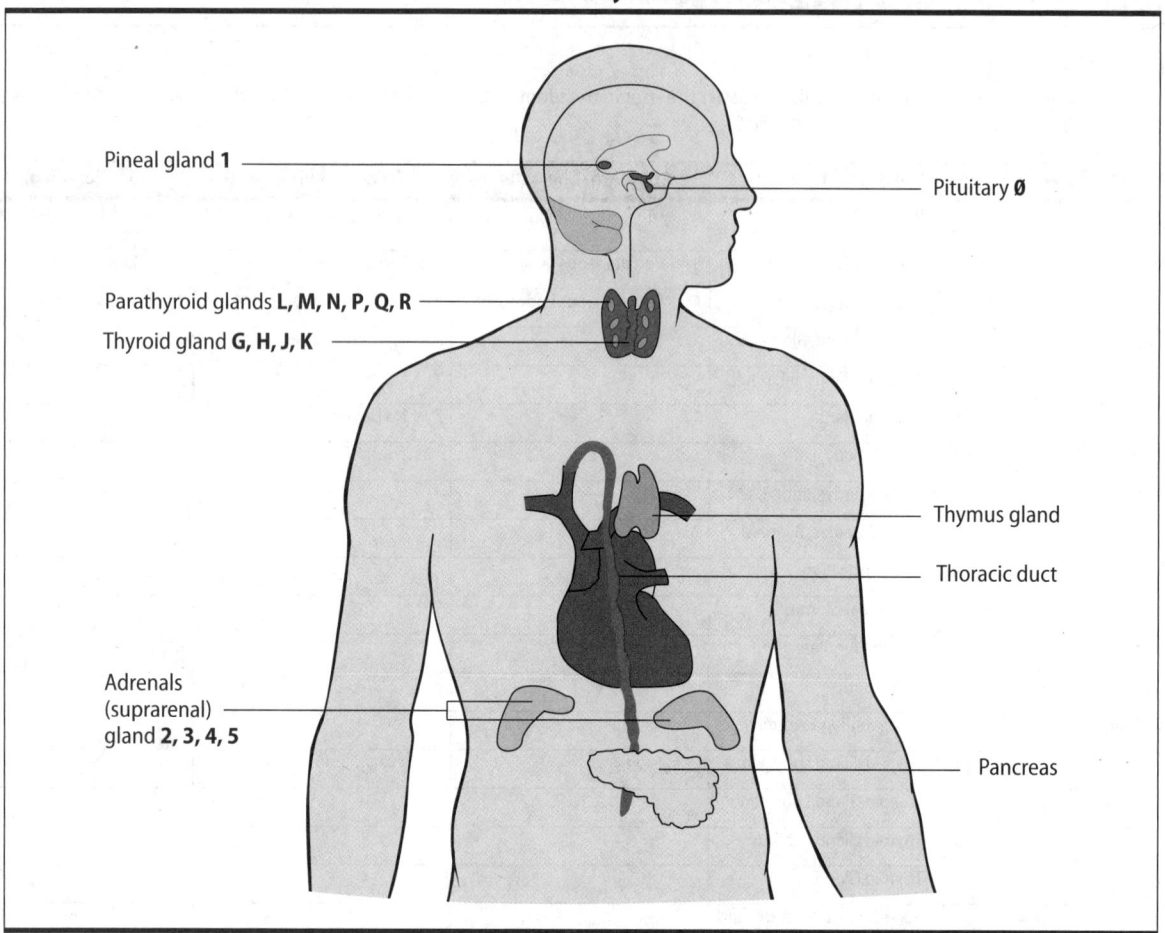

Pineal gland **1**

Pituitary **Ø**

Parathyroid glands **L, M, N, P, Q, R**

Thyroid gland **G, H, J, K**

Thymus gland

Thoracic duct

Adrenals (suprarenal) gland **2, 3, 4, 5**

Pancreas

Left Adrenal Gland

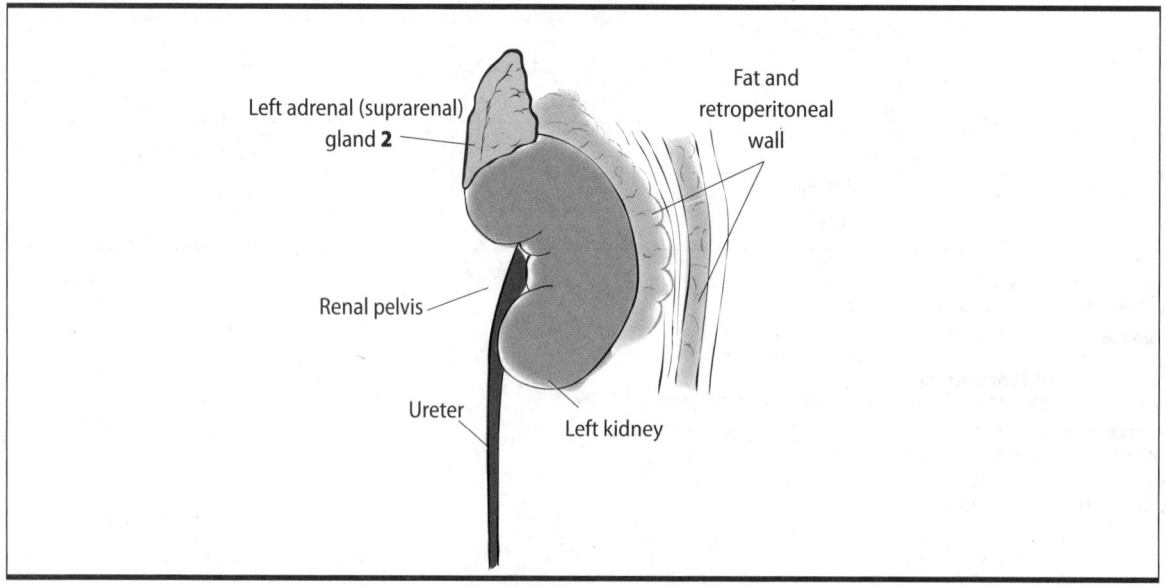

Left adrenal (suprarenal) gland **2**

Fat and retroperitoneal wall

Renal pelvis

Ureter

Left kidney

Thyroid

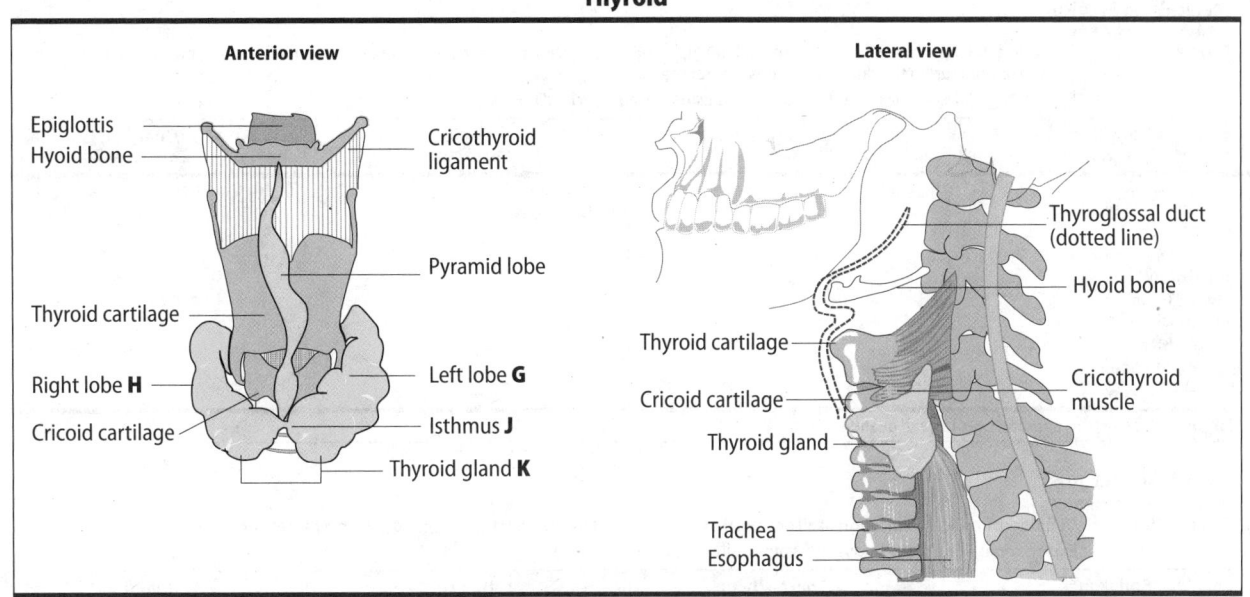

Anterior view

Epiglottis
Hyoid bone
Cricothyroid ligament
Pyramid lobe
Thyroid cartilage
Right lobe **H**
Left lobe **G**
Cricoid cartilage
Isthmus **J**
Thyroid gland **K**

Lateral view

Thyroglossal duct (dotted line)
Hyoid bone
Thyroid cartilage
Cricothyroid muscle
Cricoid cartilage
Thyroid gland
Trachea
Esophagus

Thyroid and Parathyroid Glands

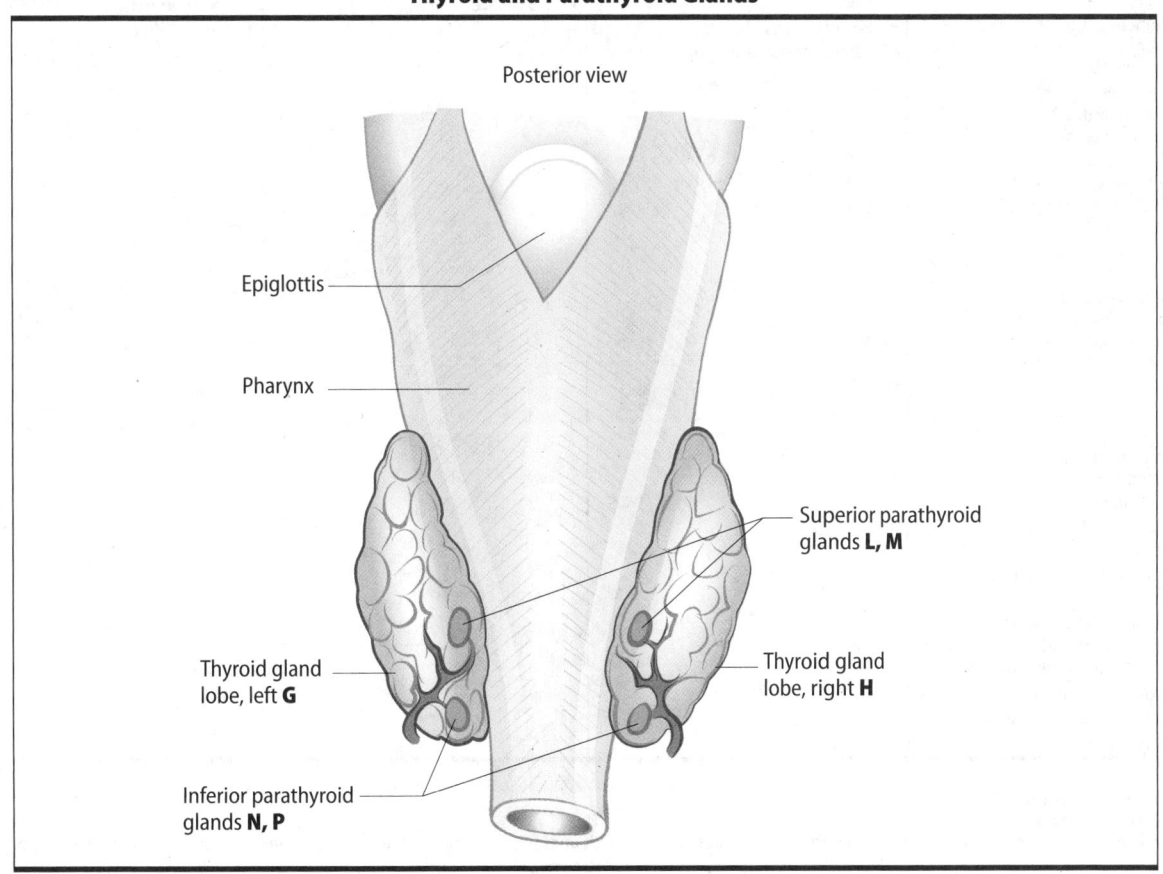

Posterior view

Epiglottis
Pharynx
Superior parathyroid glands **L, M**
Thyroid gland lobe, left **G**
Thyroid gland lobe, right **H**
Inferior parathyroid glands **N, P**

Ø **Medical and Surgical**
G **Endocrine System**
2 **Change**   Definition: Taking out or off a device from a body part and putting back an identical or similar device in or on the same body part without cutting or puncturing the skin or a mucous membrane

                  Explanation: All CHANGE procedures are coded using the approach EXTERNAL

Body Part Character 4	Approach Character 5	Device Character 6	Qualifier Character 7

Ø Pituitary Gland
    Adenohypophysis
    Hypophysis
    Neurohypophysis
1 Pineal Body
5 Adrenal Gland
    Suprarenal gland
K Thyroid Gland
R Parathyroid Gland
S Endocrine Gland
	X External	Ø Drainage Device
		Y Other Device
			Z No Qualifier

Non-OR All body part, approach, device, and qualifier values

Ø **Medical and Surgical**
G **Endocrine System**
5 **Destruction**   Definition: Physical eradication of all or a portion of a body part by the direct use of energy, force, or a destructive agent

                  Explanation: None of the body part is physically taken out

Body Part Character 4	Approach Character 5	Device Character 6	Qualifier Character 7

Ø Pituitary Gland
    Adenohypophysis
    Hypophysis
    Neurohypophysis
1 Pineal Body
2 Adrenal Gland, Left
    Suprarenal gland
3 Adrenal Gland, Right
    See 2 Adrenal Gland, Left
4 Adrenal Glands, Bilateral
    See 2 Adrenal Gland, Left
6 Carotid Body, Left
    Carotid glomus
7 Carotid Body, Right
    See 6 Carotid Body, Left
8 Carotid Bodies, Bilateral
    See 6 Carotid Body, Left
9 Para-aortic Body
B Coccygeal Glomus
    Coccygeal body
C Glomus Jugulare
    Jugular body
D Aortic Body
F Paraganglion Extremity
G Thyroid Gland Lobe, Left
H Thyroid Gland Lobe, Right
K Thyroid Gland
L Superior Parathyroid Gland, Right
M Superior Parathyroid Gland, Left
N Inferior Parathyroid Gland, Right
P Inferior Parathyroid Gland, Left
Q Parathyroid Glands, Multiple
R Parathyroid Gland
	Ø Open
	3 Percutaneous
	4 Percutaneous Endoscopic
		Z No Device	3 Laser Interstitial Thermal Therapy
			Z No Qualifier

Ø **Medical and Surgical**
G **Endocrine System**
8 **Division**   Definition: Cutting into a body part, without draining fluids and/or gases from the body part, in order to separate or transect a body part

                  Explanation: All or a portion of the body part is separated into two or more portions

Body Part Character 4	Approach Character 5	Device Character 6	Qualifier Character 7

Ø Pituitary Gland
    Adenohypophysis
    Hypophysis
    Neurohypophysis
J Thyroid Gland Isthmus
	Ø Open
	3 Percutaneous
	4 Percutaneous Endoscopic
		Z No Device	Z No Qualifier

Non-OR Procedure   DRG Non-OR Procedure   Valid OR Procedure   HAC Associated Procedure   Combination Only   New/Revised April   New/Revised October

418   ICD-10-PCS 2024

ØG2–ØG8

Ø   Medical and Surgical
G   Endocrine System
9   Drainage   Definition: Taking or letting out fluids and/or gases from a body part
                          Explanation: The qualifier DIAGNOSTIC is used to identify drainage procedures that are biopsies

Body Part Character 4	Approach Character 5	Device Character 6	Qualifier Character 7

Ø Pituitary Gland
  Adenohypophysis
  Hypophysis
  Neurohypophysis
1 Pineal Body
2 Adrenal Gland, Left
  Suprarenal gland
3 Adrenal Gland, Right
  See 2 Adrenal Gland, Left
4 Adrenal Glands, Bilateral
  See 2 Adrenal Gland, Left
6 Carotid Body, Left
  Carotid glomus
7 Carotid Body, Right
  See 6 Carotid Body, Left
8 Carotid Bodies, Bilateral
  See 6 Carotid Body, Left
9 Para-aortic Body
B Coccygeal Glomus
  Coccygeal body
C Glomus Jugulare
  Jugular body
D Aortic Body
F Paraganglion Extremity
G Thyroid Gland Lobe, Left
H Thyroid Gland Lobe, Right
K Thyroid Gland
L Superior Parathyroid Gland, Right
M Superior Parathyroid Gland, Left
N Inferior Parathyroid Gland, Right
P Inferior Parathyroid Gland, Left
Q Parathyroid Glands, Multiple
R Parathyroid Gland
	Ø Open
	3 Percutaneous
	4 Percutaneous Endoscopic
		Ø Drainage Device	Z No Qualifier

Ø Pituitary Gland
  Adenohypophysis
  Hypophysis
  Neurohypophysis
1 Pineal Body
2 Adrenal Gland, Left
  Suprarenal gland
3 Adrenal Gland, Right
  See 2 Adrenal Gland, Left
4 Adrenal Glands, Bilateral
  See 2 Adrenal Gland, Left
6 Carotid Body, Left
  Carotid glomus
7 Carotid Body, Right
  See 6 Carotid Body, Left
8 Carotid Bodies, Bilateral
  See 6 Carotid Body, Left
9 Para-aortic Body
B Coccygeal Glomus
  Coccygeal body
C Glomus Jugulare
  Jugular body
D Aortic Body
F Paraganglion Extremity
G Thyroid Gland Lobe, Left
H Thyroid Gland Lobe, Right
K Thyroid Gland
L Superior Parathyroid Gland, Right
M Superior Parathyroid Gland, Left
N Inferior Parathyroid Gland, Right
P Inferior Parathyroid Gland, Left
Q Parathyroid Glands, Multiple
R Parathyroid Gland
	Ø Open
	3 Percutaneous
	4 Percutaneous Endoscopic
		Z No Device	X Diagnostic
			Z No Qualifier

Non-OR	0G9[Ø,1,2,3,4,6,7,8,9,B,C,D,F,G,H,K,L,M,N,P,Q,R]3ØZ
Non-OR	0G9[G,H,K,L,M,N,P,Q,R]4ØZ
Non-OR	0G9[2,3,4,G,H,K][3,4]ZX
Non-OR	0G9[Ø,1,2,3,4,6,7,8,9,B,C,D,F,G,H,K,L,M,N,P,Q,R]3ZZ
Non-OR	0G9[G,H,K,L,M,N,P,Q,R]4ZZ

NC Noncovered Procedure   LC Limited Coverage   OA Questionable OB Admit   NT New Tech Add-on   ⊞ Combination Member   ♂ Male   ♀ Female
ICD-10-PCS 2024   419

0G9–0G9

Endocrine System

Ø   **Medical and Surgical**
G   **Endocrine System**
B   **Excision**   Definition: Cutting out or off, without replacement, a portion of a body part
                            Explanation: The qualifier DIAGNOSTIC is used to identify excision procedures that are biopsies

Body Part Character 4	Approach Character 5	Device Character 6	Qualifier Character 7

Ø Pituitary Gland
    Adenohypophysis
    Hypophysis
    Neurohypophysis
1 Pineal Body
2 Adrenal Gland, Left
    Suprarenal gland
3 Adrenal Gland, Right
    See 2 Adrenal Gland, Left
4 Adrenal Glands, Bilateral
    See 2 Adrenal Gland, Left
6 Carotid Body, Left
    Carotid glomus
7 Carotid Body, Right
    See 6 Carotid Body, Left
8 Carotid Bodies, Bilateral
    See 6 Carotid Body, Left
9 Para-aortic Body
B Coccygeal Glomus
    Coccygeal body
C Glomus Jugulare
    Jugular body
D Aortic Body
F Paraganglion Extremity
G Thyroid Gland Lobe, Left
H Thyroid Gland Lobe, Right
J Thyroid Gland Isthmus
L Superior Parathyroid Gland, Right
M Superior Parathyroid Gland, Left
N Inferior Parathyroid Gland, Right
P Inferior Parathyroid Gland, Left
Q Parathyroid Glands, Multiple
R Parathyroid Gland
	Ø Open
	3 Percutaneous
	4 Percutaneous Endoscopic
		Z No Device	X Diagnostic
			Z No Qualifier

Non-OR   ØGB[2,3,4,G,H,J][3,4]ZX

Ø Medical and Surgical
G Endocrine System
C Extirpation

Definition: Taking or cutting out solid matter from a body part

Explanation: The solid matter may be an abnormal byproduct of a biological function or a foreign body; it may be imbedded in a body part or in the lumen of a tubular body part. The solid matter may or may not have been previously broken into pieces.

Body Part Character 4	Approach Character 5	Device Character 6	Qualifier Character 7

Ø Pituitary Gland
  Adenohypophysis
  Hypophysis
  Neurohypophysis
1 Pineal Body
2 Adrenal Gland, Left
  Suprarenal gland
3 Adrenal Gland, Right
  See 2 Adrenal Gland, Left
4 Adrenal Glands, Bilateral
  See 2 Adrenal Gland, Left
6 Carotid Body, Left
  Carotid glomus
7 Carotid Body, Right
  See 6 Carotid Body, Left
8 Carotid Bodies, Bilateral
  See 6 Carotid Body, Left
9 Para-aortic Body
B Coccygeal Glomus
  Coccygeal body
C Glomus Jugulare
  Jugular body
D Aortic Body
F Paraganglion Extremity
G Thyroid Gland Lobe, Left
H Thyroid Gland Lobe, Right
K Thyroid Gland
L Superior Parathyroid Gland, Right
M Superior Parathyroid Gland, Left
N Inferior Parathyroid Gland, Right
P Inferior Parathyroid Gland, Left
Q Parathyroid Glands, Multiple
R Parathyroid Gland
	Ø Open
	3 Percutaneous
	4 Percutaneous Endoscopic
		Z No Device	Z No Qualifier

Ø Medical and Surgical
G Endocrine System
H Insertion

Definition: Putting in a nonbiological appliance that monitors, assists, performs, or prevents a physiological function but does not physically take the place of a body part

Explanation: None

Body Part Character 4	Approach Character 5	Device Character 6	Qualifier Character 7
S Endocrine Gland	Ø Open 3 Percutaneous 4 Percutaneous Endoscopic	1 Radioactive Element 2 Monitoring Device 3 Infusion Device Y Other Device	Z No Qualifier

Non-OR   ØGHS31Z
Non-OR   ØGHS[3,4]YZ

Ø Medical and Surgical
G Endocrine System
J Inspection

Definition: Visually and/or manually exploring a body part

Explanation: Visual exploration may be performed with or without optical instrumentation. Manual exploration may be performed directly or through intervening body layers.

Body Part Character 4	Approach Character 5	Device Character 6	Qualifier Character 7

Ø Pituitary Gland
  Adenohypophysis
  Hypophysis
  Neurohypophysis
1 Pineal Body
5 Adrenal Gland
  Suprarenal gland
K Thyroid Gland
R Parathyroid Gland
S Endocrine Gland
	Ø Open
	3 Percutaneous
	4 Percutaneous Endoscopic
		Z No Device	Z No Qualifier

Non-OR   ØGJ[Ø,1,5,K,R,S]3ZZ

Ø Medical and Surgical
G Endocrine System
M Reattachment   Definition: Putting back in or on all or a portion of a separated body part to its normal location or other suitable location

Explanation: Vascular circulation and nervous pathways may or may not be reestablished

Body Part Character 4	Approach Character 5	Device Character 6	Qualifier Character 7

2   Adrenal Gland, Left
     Suprarenal gland
3   Adrenal Gland, Right
     See 2 Adrenal Gland, Left
G   Thyroid Gland Lobe, Left
H   Thyroid Gland Lobe, Right
L   Superior Parathyroid Gland, Right
M   Superior Parathyroid Gland, Left
N   Inferior Parathyroid Gland, Right
P   Inferior Parathyroid Gland, Left
Q   Parathyroid Glands, Multiple
R   Parathyroid Gland
	Ø Open
	4 Percutaneous Endoscopic
		Z No Device	Z No Qualifier

Ø Medical and Surgical
G Endocrine System
N Release   Definition: Freeing a body part from an abnormal physical constraint by cutting or by the use of force

Explanation: Some of the restraining tissue may be taken out but none of the body part is taken out

Body Part Character 4	Approach Character 5	Device Character 6	Qualifier Character 7

Ø   Pituitary Gland
     Adenohypophysis
     Hypophysis
     Neurohypophysis
1   Pineal Body
2   Adrenal Gland, Left
     Suprarenal gland
3   Adrenal Gland, Right
     See 2 Adrenal Gland, Left
4   Adrenal Glands, Bilateral
     See 2 Adrenal Gland, Left
6   Carotid Body, Left
     Carotid glomus
7   Carotid Body, Right
     See 6 Carotid Body, Left
8   Carotid Bodies, Bilateral
     See 6 Carotid Body, Left
9   Para-aortic Body
B   Coccygeal Glomus
     Coccygeal body
C   Glomus Jugulare
     Jugular body
D   Aortic Body
F   Paraganglion Extremity
G   Thyroid Gland Lobe, Left
H   Thyroid Gland Lobe, Right
K   Thyroid Gland
L   Superior Parathyroid Gland, Right
M   Superior Parathyroid Gland, Left
N   Inferior Parathyroid Gland, Right
P   Inferior Parathyroid Gland, Left
Q   Parathyroid Glands, Multiple
R   Parathyroid Gland
	Ø Open
	3 Percutaneous
	4 Percutaneous Endoscopic
		Z No Device	Z No Qualifier

Non-OR   ØGN[6,7,8,9,B,C,D,F][Ø,3,4]ZZ

Non-OR Procedure   DRG Non-OR Procedure   Valid OR Procedure   HAC Associated Procedure   Combination Only   New/Revised April   New/Revised October

422   ICD-10-PCS 2024

Ø   **Medical and Surgical**
G   **Endocrine System**
P   **Removal**   Definition: Taking out or off a device from a body part

Explanation: If a device is taken out and a similar device put in without cutting or puncturing the skin or mucous membrane, the procedure is coded to the root operation CHANGE. Otherwise, the procedure for taking out a device is coded to the root operation REMOVAL.

Body Part Character 4	Approach Character 5	Device Character 6	Qualifier Character 7

Ø   Pituitary Gland
     Adenohypophysis
     Hypophysis
     Neurohypophysis
1   Pineal Body
5   Adrenal Gland
     Suprarenal gland
K   Thyroid Gland
R   Parathyroid Gland
	Ø Open
	3 Percutaneous
	4 Percutaneous Endoscopic
	X External
		Ø Drainage Device	Z No Qualifier

S Endocrine Gland	Ø Open 3 Percutaneous 4 Percutaneous Endoscopic	Ø Drainage Device 2 Monitoring Device 3 Infusion Device Y Other Device	Z No Qualifier
S Endocrine Gland	X External	Ø Drainage Device 2 Monitoring Device 3 Infusion Device	Z No Qualifier

Non-OR	ØGP[Ø,1,5,K,R]XØZ
Non-OR	ØGPS[3,4]YZ
Non-OR	ØGPSX[Ø,2,3]Z

Ø   **Medical and Surgical**
G   **Endocrine System**
Q   **Repair**   Definition: Restoring, to the extent possible, a body part to its normal anatomic structure and function

Explanation: Used only when the method to accomplish the repair is not one of the other root operations

Body Part Character 4	Approach Character 5	Device Character 6	Qualifier Character 7

Ø   Pituitary Gland
     Adenohypophysis
     Hypophysis
     Neurohypophysis
1   Pineal Body
2   Adrenal Gland, Left
     Suprarenal gland
3   Adrenal Gland, Right
     See 2 Adrenal Gland, Left
4   Adrenal Glands, Bilateral
     See 2 Adrenal Gland, Left
6   Carotid Body, Left
     Carotid glomus
7   Carotid Body, Right
     See 6 Carotid Body, Left
8   Carotid Bodies, Bilateral
     See 6 Carotid Body, Left
9   Para-aortic Body
B   Coccygeal Glomus
     Coccygeal body
C   Glomus Jugulare
     Jugular body
D   Aortic Body
F   Paraganglion Extremity
G   Thyroid Gland Lobe, Left
H   Thyroid Gland Lobe, Right
J   Thyroid Gland Isthmus
K   Thyroid Gland
L   Superior Parathyroid Gland, Right
M   Superior Parathyroid Gland, Left
N   Inferior Parathyroid Gland, Right
P   Inferior Parathyroid Gland, Left
Q   Parathyroid Glands, Multiple
R   Parathyroid Gland
	Ø Open
	3 Percutaneous
	4 Percutaneous Endoscopic
		Z No Device	Z No Qualifier

NC Noncovered Procedure   **LC** Limited Coverage   **OA** Questionable OB Admit   **NT** New Tech Add-on   ⊞ Combination Member   ♂ Male   ♀ Female

ICD-10-PCS 2024   423

Ø   **Medical and Surgical**
G   **Endocrine System**
S   **Reposition**   Definition: Moving to its normal location, or other suitable location, all or a portion of a body part

Explanation: The body part is moved to a new location from an abnormal location, or from a normal location where it is not functioning correctly. The body part may or may not be cut out or off to be moved to the new location.

Body Part Character 4	Approach Character 5	Device Character 6	Qualifier Character 7

2 Adrenal Gland, Left
   Suprarenal gland
3 Adrenal Gland, Right
   See 2 Adrenal Gland, Left
G Thyroid Gland Lobe, Left
H Thyroid Gland Lobe, Right
L Superior Parathyroid Gland, Right
M Superior Parathyroid Gland, Left
N Inferior Parathyroid Gland, Right
P Inferior Parathyroid Gland, Left
Q Parathyroid Glands, Multiple
R Parathyroid Gland
	Ø Open
	4 Percutaneous Endoscopic
		Z No Device	Z No Qualifier

Ø   **Medical and Surgical**
G   **Endocrine System**
T   **Resection**   Definition: Cutting out or off, without replacement, all of a body part

Explanation: None

Body Part Character 4	Approach Character 5	Device Character 6	Qualifier Character 7

Ø Pituitary Gland
   Adenohypophysis
   Hypophysis
   Neurohypophysis
1 Pineal Body
2 Adrenal Gland, Left
   Suprarenal gland
3 Adrenal Gland, Right
   See 2 Adrenal Gland, Left
4 Adrenal Glands, Bilateral
   See 2 Adrenal Gland, Left
6 Carotid Body, Left
   Carotid glomus
7 Carotid Body, Right
   See 6 Carotid Body, Left
8 Carotid Bodies, Bilateral
   See 6 Carotid Body, Left
9 Para-aortic Body
B Coccygeal Glomus
   Coccygeal body
C Glomus Jugulare
   Jugular body
D Aortic Body
F Paraganglion Extremity
G Thyroid Gland Lobe, Left
H Thyroid Gland Lobe, Right
J Thyroid Gland Isthmus
K Thyroid Gland
L Superior Parathyroid Gland, Right
M Superior Parathyroid Gland, Left
N Inferior Parathyroid Gland, Right
P Inferior Parathyroid Gland, Left
Q Parathyroid Glands, Multiple
R Parathyroid Gland
	Ø Open
	4 Percutaneous Endoscopic
		Z No Device	Z No Qualifier

Non-OR   ØGT[6,7,8,9,B,C,D,F][Ø,4]ZZ

Non-OR Procedure   DRG Non-OR Procedure   Valid OR Procedure   HAC Associated Procedure   Combination Only   New/Revised April   New/Revised October

424   ICD-10-PCS 2024

ØGS–ØGT

0   Medical and Surgical
G   Endocrine System
W   Revision   Definition: Correcting, to the extent possible, a portion of a malfunctioning device or the position of a displaced device

                     Explanation: Revision can include correcting a malfunctioning or displaced device by taking out or putting in components of the device such as a screw or pin

Body Part Character 4	Approach Character 5	Device Character 6	Qualifier Character 7

0 Pituitary Gland
   Adenohypophysis
   Hypophysis
   Neurohypophysis
1 Pineal Body
5 Adrenal Gland
   Suprarenal gland
K Thyroid Gland
R Parathyroid Gland
	0 Open
	3 Percutaneous
	4 Percutaneous Endoscopic
	X External
		0 Drainage Device	**Z** No Qualifier

S Endocrine Gland	**0** Open **3** Percutaneous **4** Percutaneous Endoscopic	**0** Drainage Device **2** Monitoring Device **3** Infusion Device **Y** Other Device	**Z** No Qualifier
S Endocrine Gland	**X** External	**0** Drainage Device **2** Monitoring Device **3** Infusion Device	**Z** No Qualifier

Non-OR   0GW[0,1,5,K,R]X0Z
Non-OR   0GWS[3,4]YZ
Non-OR   0GWSX[0,2,3]Z

NC Noncovered Procedure   LC Limited Coverage   QA Questionable OB Admit   NT New Tech Add-on   ⊞ Combination Member   ♂ Male   ♀ Female

ICD-10-PCS 2024   **425**

Skin and Breast ØHØ–ØHX

Character Meanings*

This Character Meaning table is provided as a guide to assist the user in the identification of character members that may be found in this section of code tables. It **SHOULD NOT** be used to build a PCS code.

Operation–Character 3		Body Part–Character 4		Approach–Character 5		Device–Character 6		Qualifier–Character 7	
Ø	Alteration	Ø	Skin, Scalp	Ø	Open	Ø	Drainage Device	2	Cell Suspension Technique
2	Change	1	Skin, Face	3	Percutaneous	1	Radioactive Element	3	Full Thickness OR Laser Interstitial Thermal Therapy
5	Destruction	2	Skin, Right Ear	7	Via Natural or Artificial Opening	7	Autologous Tissue Substitute	4	Partial Thickness
8	Division	3	Skin, Left Ear	8	Via Natural or Artificial Opening Endoscopic	J	Synthetic Substitute	5	Latissimus Dorsi Myocutaneous Flap
9	Drainage	4	Skin, Neck	X	External	K	Nonautologous Tissue Substitute	6	Transverse Rectus Abdominis Myocutaneous Flap
B	Excision	5	Skin, Chest			N	Tissue Expander	7	Deep Inferior Epigastric Artery Perforator Flap
C	Extirpation	6	Skin, Back			Y	Other Device	8	Superficial Inferior Epigastric Artery Flap
D	Extraction	7	Skin, Abdomen			Z	No Device	9	Gluteal Artery Perforator Flap
H	Insertion	8	Skin, Buttock					D	Multiple
J	Inspection	9	Skin, Perineum					X	Diagnostic
M	Reattachment	A	Skin, Inguinal					Z	No Qualifier
N	Release	B	Skin, Right Upper Arm						
P	Removal	C	Skin, Left Upper Arm						
Q	Repair	D	Skin, Right Lower Arm						
R	Replacement	E	Skin, Left Lower Arm						
S	Reposition	F	Skin, Right Hand						
T	Resection	G	Skin, Left Hand						
U	Supplement	H	Skin, Right Upper Leg						
W	Revision	J	Skin, Left Upper Leg						
X	Transfer	K	Skin, Right Lower Leg						
		L	Skin, Left Lower Leg						
		M	Skin, Right Foot						
		N	Skin, Left Foot						
		P	Skin						
		Q	Finger Nail						
		R	Toe Nail						
		S	Hair						
		T	Breast, Right						
		U	Breast, Left						
		V	Breast, Bilateral						
		W	Nipple, Right						
		X	Nipple, Left						
		Y	Supernumerary Breast						

*   Includes skin and breast glands and ducts.

AHA Coding Clinic for table ØHØ

2022, 1Q, 14	Reduction mammoplasty for breast symmetry
2022, 1Q, 15	Nipple reconstruction and breast reduction
2019, 4Q, 30-31	Breast procedures

AHA Coding Clinic for table ØH5

| 2022, 4Q, 53-54 | Laser interstitial thermal therapy |
| 2019, 4Q, 30-31 | Breast procedures |

AHA Coding Clinic for table ØH9

| 2019, 4Q, 30-31 | Breast procedures |

AHA Coding Clinic for table ØHB

2022, 1Q, 14	Reduction mammoplasty for breast symmetry
2020, 1Q, 31	Repair of buried penis
2019, 4Q, 30-31	Breast procedures
2018, 1Q, 14	Excisional debridement of breast tissue and skin
2016, 3Q, 29	Closure of bilateral alveolar clefts
2015, 3Q, 3-8	Excisional and nonexcisional debridement

AHA Coding Clinic for table ØHC

| 2019, 4Q, 30-31 | Breast procedures |

AHA Coding Clinic for table ØHD

2019, 4Q, 30-31	Breast procedures
2016, 1Q, 40	Nonexcisional debridement of skin and subcutaneous tissue
2015, 3Q, 3-8	Excisional and nonexcisional debridement

AHA Coding Clinic for table ØHH

2019, 4Q, 30-31	Breast procedures
2017, 4Q, 67	New qualifier values - Pedicle flap procedures
2014, 2Q, 12	Pedicle latissimus myocutaneous flap with placement of breast tissue expanders
2013, 4Q, 107	Breast tissue expander placement using acellular dermal matrix

AHA Coding Clinic for table ØHJ

| 2019, 4Q, 30-31 | Breast procedures |

AHA Coding Clinic for table ØHN

| 2019, 4Q, 30-31 | Breast procedures |

AHA Coding Clinic for table ØHP

2022, 3Q, 20	Bilateral breast capsulectomy and tissue expander removal
2019, 4Q, 30-31	Breast procedures
2018, 3Q, 13	Deep inferior epigastric artery perforator flap breast reconstruction
2016, 2Q, 27	Removal of nonviable transverse rectus abdominis myocutaneous (TRAM) flaps

AHA Coding Clinic for table ØHQ

2019, 4Q, 30-31	Breast procedures
2018, 2Q, 25	Third and fourth degree obstetric lacerations
2016, 1Q, 7	Obstetrical perineal laceration repair
2014, 4Q, 31	Delayed wound closure following fracture treatment

AHA Coding Clinic for table ØHR

2023, 2Q, 30	Inframammary fold adjacent tissue transfer and deep inferior epigastric perforator flap breast reconstruction
2022, 1Q, 15	Nipple reconstruction and breast reduction
2020, 1Q, 27	Delayed reconstruction following mastectomy using gracilis musculocutaneous free flap
2020, 1Q, 28	Free flap microvascular breast reconstruction
2020, 1Q, 30	Polarity Skin TE™ application
2019, 4Q, 30-31	Breast procedures
2019, 4Q, 32	Cell suspension epithelial autograft
2019, 3Q, 32	Breast reconstruction with neurotization
2018, 3Q, 13	Deep inferior epigastric artery perforator flap breast reconstruction
2017, 1Q, 35	Epifix® allograft
2014, 3Q, 14	Application of TheraSkin® and excisional debridement

AHA Coding Clinic for table ØHT

2021, 2Q, 16	Goldilocks breast reconstruction
2018, 3Q, 13	Deep inferior epigastric artery perforator flap breast reconstruction
2014, 4Q, 34	Skin-sparing mastectomy

AHA Coding Clinic for table ØHU

| 2019, 4Q, 30-31 | Breast procedures |

AHA Coding Clinic for table ØHW

| 2019, 4Q, 30-31 | Breast procedures |

AHA Coding Clinic for table ØHX

2023, 2Q, 23	V-Y anoplasty and excision of mucosal ectropion
2023, 2Q, 30	Inframammary fold adjacent tissue transfer and deep inferior epigastric perforator flap breast reconstruction
2022, 3Q, 13	Repair of prolapsed neovaginal graft

Integumentary Anatomy

Hair follicle **S**
Hair **S**
Sebaceous gland **Ø-9, A-P**
Arrector pili muscle
Epidermis
Thick-skin epidermis
Dermis
Hair shaft **S**
Pacinian corpuscle
Hair matrix **S**
Hypodermis (subcutaneous layer)
Sweat (eccrine gland) **Ø-9, A-P**
Sensory nerve
Bulb
Blood vessels

Nail Anatomy

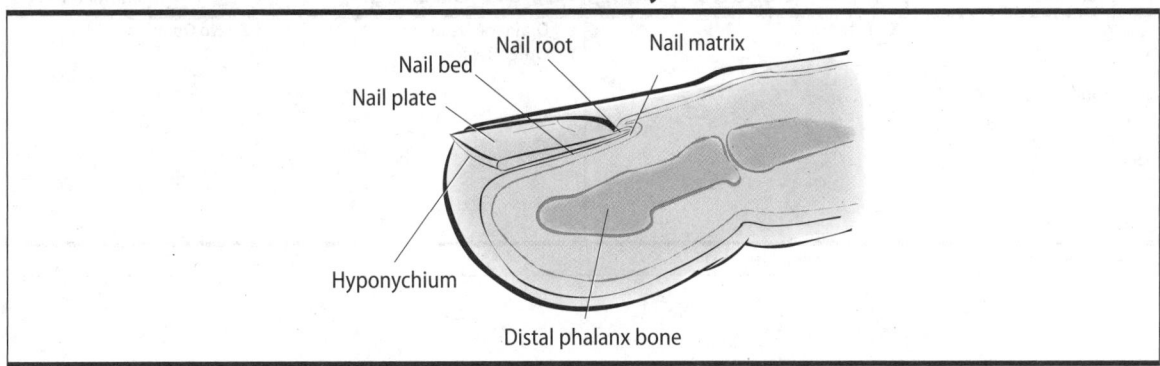

Nail bed
Nail root
Nail matrix
Nail plate
Hyponychium
Distal phalanx bone

Breast

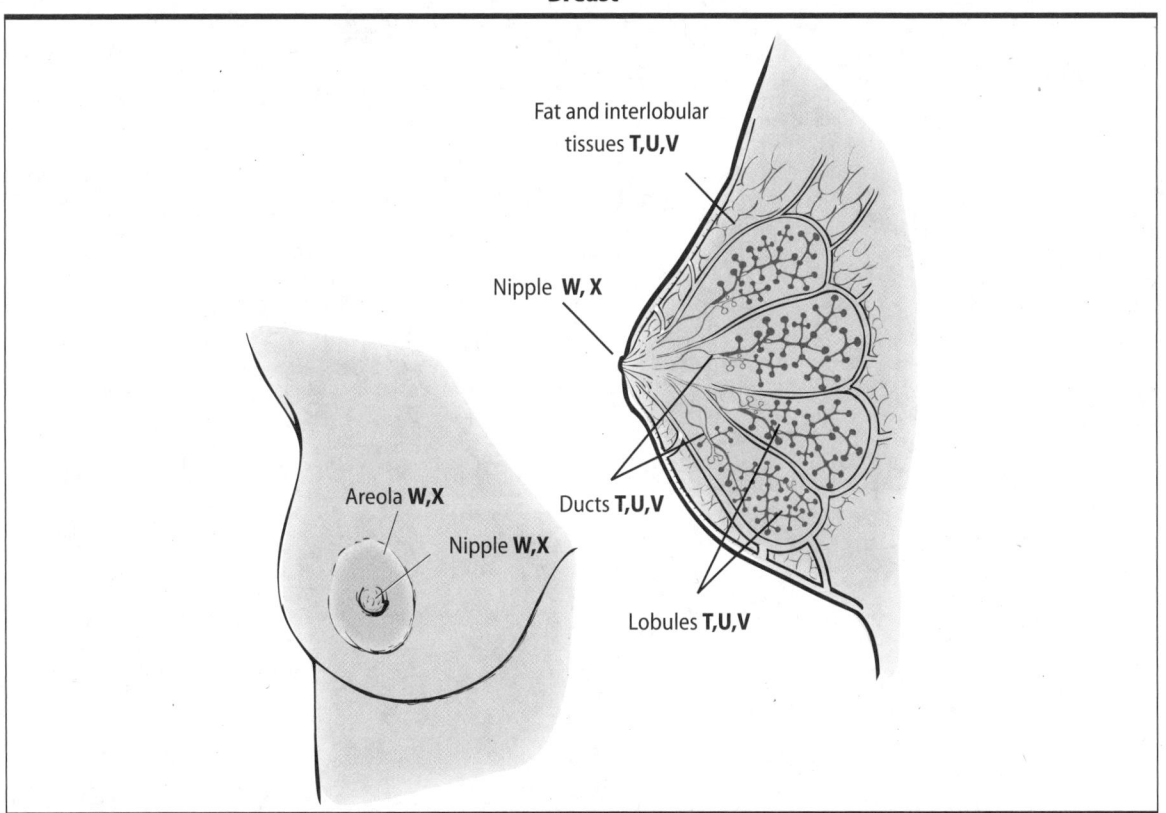

Fat and interlobular tissues **T,U,V**
Nipple **W, X**
Areola **W,X**
Nipple **W,X**
Ducts **T,U,V**
Lobules **T,U,V**

Skin and Breast

Ø   **Medical and Surgical**
H   **Skin and Breast**
Ø   **Alteration**   Definition: Modifying the anatomic structure of a body part without affecting the function of the body part
                        Explanation: Principal purpose is to improve appearance

Body Part Character 4	Approach Character 5	Device Character 6	Qualifier Character 7

T   Breast, Right
    Mammary duct
    Mammary gland
U   Breast, Left
    See T Breast, Right
V   Breast, Bilateral
    See T Breast, Right
	Ø Open
	3 Percutaneous
		7 Autologous Tissue Substitute
		J Synthetic Substitute
		K Nonautologous Tissue Substitute
		Z No Device
			Z No Qualifier

Non-OR   ØHØ[T,U,V]3JZ

Ø   **Medical and Surgical**
H   **Skin and Breast**
2   **Change**   Definition: Taking out or off a device from a body part and putting back an identical or similar device in or on the same body part without cutting or puncturing the skin or a mucous membrane
                        Explanation: All CHANGE procedures are coded using the approach EXTERNAL

Body Part Character 4	Approach Character 5	Device Character 6	Qualifier Character 7

P   Skin
    Dermis
    Epidermis
    Sebaceous gland
    Sweat gland
T   Breast, Right
    Mammary duct
    Mammary gland
U   Breast, Left
    See T Breast, Right
	X External	**Ø** Drainage Device
		Y Other Device
			Z No Qualifier

Non-OR   All body part, approach, device, and qualifier values

---

Non-OR Procedure   DRG Non-OR Procedure   Valid OR Procedure   HAC Associated Procedure   Combination Only   New/Revised April   New/Revised October

Ø　Medical and Surgical
H　Skin and Breast
5　Destruction　　Definition: Physical eradication of all or a portion of a body part by the direct use of energy, force, or a destructive agent
　　　　　　　　　　　Explanation: None of the body part is physically taken out

Body Part Character 4	Approach Character 5	Device Character 6	Qualifier Character 7
Ø　Skin, Scalp 1　Skin, Face 2　Skin, Right Ear 3　Skin, Left Ear 4　Skin, Neck 5　Skin, Chest 　　Breast procedures, skin only 6　Skin, Back 7　Skin, Abdomen 8　Skin, Buttock 9　Skin, Perineum 　　Perianal skin A　Skin, Inguinal B　Skin, Right Upper Arm C　Skin, Left Upper Arm D　Skin, Right Lower Arm E　Skin, Left Lower Arm F　Skin, Right Hand G　Skin, Left Hand H　Skin, Right Upper Leg J　Skin, Left Upper Leg K　Skin, Right Lower Leg L　Skin, Left Lower Leg M　Skin, Right Foot N　Skin, Left Foot	X　External	Z　No Device	D　Multiple Z　No Qualifier
Q　Finger Nail 　　Nail bed 　　Nail plate R　Toe Nail 　　*See Q Finger Nail*	X　External	Z　No Device	Z　No Qualifier
T　Breast, Right 　　Mammary duct 　　Mammary gland U　Breast, Left 　　*See T Breast, Right* V　Breast, Bilateral 　　*See T Breast, Right*	Ø　Open 3　Percutaneous	Z　No Device	3　Laser Interstitial Thermal Therapy Z　No Qualifier
T　Breast, Right 　　Mammary duct 　　Mammary gland U　Breast, Left 　　*See T Breast, Right* V　Breast, Bilateral 　　*See T Breast, Right*	7　Via Natural or Artificial Opening 8　Via Natural or Artificial Opening 　　Endoscopic	Z　No Device	Z　No Qualifier
W　Nipple, Right 　　Areola X　Nipple, Left 　　*See W Nipple, Right*	Ø　Open 3　Percutaneous 7　Via Natural or Artificial Opening 8　Via Natural or Artificial Opening 　　Endoscopic X　External	Z　No Device	Z　No Qualifier

DRG Non-OR　ØH5[Ø,1,4,5,6,7,8,9,A,B,C,D,E,F,G,H,J,K,L,M,N]XZ[D,Z]
DRG Non-OR　ØH5[Q,R]XZZ
Non-OR　　　ØH5[2,3]XZ[D,Z]

NC Noncovered Procedure　　**LC** Limited Coverage　　**QA** Questionable OB Admit　　**NT** New Tech Add-on　　✛ Combination Member　　♂ Male　　♀ Female
ICD-10-PCS 2024　　431

ØH5–ØH5

Skin and Breast

Ø	Medical and Surgical
H	Skin and Breast
8	Division

Definition: Cutting into a body part, without draining fluids and/or gases from the body part, in order to separate or transect a body part

Explanation: All or a portion of the body part is separated into two or more portions

Body Part Character 4	Approach Character 5	Device Character 6	Qualifier Character 7
Ø Skin, Scalp	X External	Z No Device	Z No Qualifier
1 Skin, Face			
2 Skin, Right Ear			
3 Skin, Left Ear			
4 Skin, Neck			
5 Skin, Chest Breast procedures, skin only			
6 Skin, Back			
7 Skin, Abdomen			
8 Skin, Buttock			
9 Skin, Perineum Perianal skin			
A Skin, Inguinal			
B Skin, Right Upper Arm			
C Skin, Left Upper Arm			
D Skin, Right Lower Arm			
E Skin, Left Lower Arm			
F Skin, Right Hand			
G Skin, Left Hand			
H Skin, Right Upper Leg			
J Skin, Left Upper Leg			
K Skin, Right Lower Leg			
L Skin, Left Lower Leg			
M Skin, Right Foot			
N Skin, Left Foot			

Non-OR   All body part, approach, device, and qualifier values

Non-OR Procedure   DRG Non-OR Procedure   Valid OR Procedure   HAC Associated Procedure   Combination Only   New/Revised April   New/Revised October

432   ICD-10-PCS 2024

Ø   **Medical and Surgical**
H   **Skin and Breast**
9   **Drainage**   Definition: Taking or letting out fluids and/or gases from a body part
                           Explanation: The qualifier DIAGNOSTIC is used to identify drainage procedures that are biopsies

Body Part Character 4		Approach Character 5	Device Character 6	Qualifier Character 7

Ø Skin, Scalp
1 Skin, Face
2 Skin, Right Ear
3 Skin, Left Ear
4 Skin, Neck
5 Skin, Chest
    Breast procedures, skin
       only
6 Skin, Back
7 Skin, Abdomen
8 Skin, Buttock
9 Skin, Perineum
    Perianal skin
A Skin, Inguinal
B Skin, Right Upper Arm
C Skin, Left Upper Arm
D Skin, Right Lower Arm
	E Skin, Left Lower Arm
	F Skin, Right Hand
	G Skin, Left Hand
	H Skin, Right Upper Leg
	J Skin, Left Upper Leg
	K Skin, Right Lower Leg
	L Skin, Left Lower Leg
	M Skin, Right Foot
	N Skin, Left Foot
	Q Finger Nail
	    Nail bed
	    Nail plate
	R Toe Nail
	    See Q Finger Nail
		X External	Ø Drainage Device	Z No Qualifier

Ø Skin, Scalp
1 Skin, Face
2 Skin, Right Ear
3 Skin, Left Ear
4 Skin, Neck
5 Skin, Chest
    Breast procedures, skin
       only
6 Skin, Back
7 Skin, Abdomen
8 Skin, Buttock
9 Skin, Perineum
    Perianal skin
A Skin, Inguinal
B Skin, Right Upper Arm
C Skin, Left Upper Arm
D Skin, Right Lower Arm
	E Skin, Left Lower Arm
	F Skin, Right Hand
	G Skin, Left Hand
	H Skin, Right Upper Leg
	J Skin, Left Upper Leg
	K Skin, Right Lower Leg
	L Skin, Left Lower Leg
	M Skin, Right Foot
	N Skin, Left Foot
	Q Finger Nail
	    Nail bed
	    Nail plate
	R Toe Nail
	    See Q Finger Nail
		X External	Z No Device	X Diagnostic
				Z No Qualifier

T Breast, Right
    Mammary duct
    Mammary gland
U Breast, Left
    See T Breast, Right
V Breast, Bilateral
    See T Breast, Right
		Ø Open
		3 Percutaneous
		7 Via Natural or Artificial
		    Opening
		8 Via Natural or Artificial
		    Opening Endoscopic
			Ø Drainage Device	Z No Qualifier

T Breast, Right
    Mammary duct
    Mammary gland
U Breast, Left
    See T Breast, Right
V Breast, Bilateral
    See T Breast, Right
		Ø Open
		3 Percutaneous
		7 Via Natural or Artificial
		    Opening
		8 Via Natural or Artificial
		    Opening Endoscopic
			Z No Device	X Diagnostic
				Z No Qualifier

W Nipple, Right
    Areola
X Nipple, Left
    See W Nipple, Right
		Ø Open
		3 Percutaneous
		7 Via Natural or Artificial
		    Opening
		8 Via Natural or Artificial
		    Opening Endoscopic
		X External
			Ø Drainage Device	Z No Qualifier

W Nipple, Right
    Areola
X Nipple, Left
    See W Nipple, Right
		Ø Open
		3 Percutaneous
		7 Via Natural or Artificial
		    Opening
		8 Via Natural or Artificial
		    Opening Endoscopic
		X External
			Z No Device	X Diagnostic
				Z No Qualifier

Non-OR   ØH9[Ø,1,2,3,4,5,6,7,8,A,B,C,D,E,F,G,H,J,K,L,M,N,Q,R]XØZ
Non-OR   ØH9[Ø,1,2,3,4,5,6,7,8,A,B,C,D,E,F,G,H,J,K,L,M,N,Q,R]XZ[X,Z]
Non-OR   ØH99XZX
Non-OR   ØH9[T,U,V][Ø,3,7,8]ØZ
Non-OR   ØH9[T,U,V][3,7,8]Z[X,Z]
Non-OR   ØH9[W,X][Ø,3,7,8,X]ØZ
Non-OR   ØH9[W,X][3,7,8,X]Z[X,Z]

Ø Medical and Surgical
H Skin and Breast
B Excision   Definition: Cutting out or off, without replacement, a portion of a body part

Explanation: The qualifier DIAGNOSTIC is used to identify excision procedures that are biopsies

Body Part Character 4	Approach Character 5	Device Character 6	Qualifier Character 7

Ø Skin, Scalp
1 Skin, Face
2 Skin, Right Ear
3 Skin, Left Ear
4 Skin, Neck
5 Skin, Chest
   Breast procedures, skin only
6 Skin, Back
7 Skin, Abdomen
8 Skin, Buttock
9 Skin, Perineum
   Perianal skin
A Skin, Inguinal
B Skin, Right Upper Arm
C Skin, Left Upper Arm
D Skin, Right Lower Arm
E Skin, Left Lower Arm
F Skin, Right Hand
G Skin, Left Hand
H Skin, Right Upper Leg
J Skin, Left Upper Leg
K Skin, Right Lower Leg
L Skin, Left Lower Leg
M Skin, Right Foot
N Skin, Left Foot
Q Finger Nail
   Nail bed
   Nail plate
R Toe Nail
   See Q Finger Nail
	X External	**Z** No Device	**X** Diagnostic
			Z No Qualifier

T Breast, Right
   Mammary duct
   Mammary gland
U Breast, Left
   See T Breast, Right
V Breast, Bilateral
   See T Breast, Right
Y Supernumerary Breast
	Ø Open
	3 Percutaneous
	7 Via Natural or Artificial Opening
	8 Via Natural or Artificial Opening Endoscopic
		Z No Device	**X** Diagnostic
			Z No Qualifier

W Nipple, Right
   Areola
X Nipple, Left
   See W Nipple, Right
	Ø Open
	3 Percutaneous
	7 Via Natural or Artificial Opening
	8 Via Natural or Artificial Opening Endoscopic
	X External
		Z No Device	**X** Diagnostic
			Z No Qualifier

DRG Non-OR	ØHB9XZZ
Non-OR	ØHB[Ø,1,2,3,4,5,6,7,8,A,B,C,D,E,F,G,H,J,K,L,M,N,Q,R]XZ[X,Z]
Non-OR	ØHB9XZX
Non-OR	ØHB[T,U,V,Y][3,7,8]ZX
Non-OR	ØHB[W,X][3,7,8,X]ZX

Non-OR Procedure   DRG Non-OR Procedure   Valid OR Procedure   HAC Associated Procedure   Combination Only   New/Revised April   New/Revised October

434   ICD-10-PCS 2024

Ø   **Medical and Surgical**
H   **Skin and Breast**
C   **Extirpation**   Definition: Taking or cutting out solid matter from a body part

                     Explanation: The solid matter may be an abnormal byproduct of a biological function or a foreign body; it may be imbedded in a body part or in the lumen of a tubular body part. The solid matter may or may not have been previously broken into pieces.

Body Part Character 4	Approach Character 5	Device Character 6	Qualifier Character 7

Ø Skin, Scalp
1 Skin, Face
2 Skin, Right Ear
3 Skin, Left Ear
4 Skin, Neck
5 Skin, Chest
    Breast procedures, skin only
6 Skin, Back
7 Skin, Abdomen
8 Skin, Buttock
9 Skin, Perineum
    Perianal skin
A Skin, Inguinal
B Skin, Right Upper Arm
C Skin, Left Upper Arm
D Skin, Right Lower Arm
E Skin, Left Lower Arm
F Skin, Right Hand
G Skin, Left Hand
H Skin, Right Upper Leg
J Skin, Left Upper Leg
K Skin, Right Lower Leg
L Skin, Left Lower Leg
M Skin, Right Foot
N Skin, Left Foot
Q Finger Nail
    Nail bed
    Nail plate
R Toe Nail
    See Q Finger Nail
	X External	**Z** No Device	**Z** No Qualifier

T Breast, Right
    Mammary duct
    Mammary gland
U Breast, Left
    See T Breast, Right
V Breast, Bilateral
    See T Breast, Right
	Ø Open
	3 Percutaneous
	7 Via Natural or Artificial Opening
	8 Via Natural or Artificial Opening
	    Endoscopic
		Z No Device	**Z** No Qualifier

W Nipple, Right
    Areola
X Nipple, Left
    See W Nipple, Right
	Ø Open
	3 Percutaneous
	7 Via Natural or Artificial Opening
	8 Via Natural or Artificial Opening
	    Endoscopic
	X External
		Z No Device	**Z** No Qualifier

     Non-OR   ØHC[Ø,1,2,3,4,5,6,7,8,9,A,B,C,D,E,F,G,H,J,K,L,M,N,Q,R]XZZ
     Non-OR   ØHC[T,U,V][3,7,8]ZZ
     Non-OR   ØHC[W,X][3,7,8,X]ZZ

NC Noncovered Procedure   **LC** Limited Coverage   **QA** Questionable OB Admit   **NT** New Tech Add-on   ⊞ Combination Member   ♂ Male   ♀ Female

ICD-10-PCS 2024   435

Ø   Medical and Surgical
H   Skin and Breast
D   Extraction   Definition: Pulling or stripping out or off all or a portion of a body part by the use of force
                              Explanation: The qualifier DIAGNOSTIC is used to identify extraction procedures that are biopsies

Body Part Character 4	Approach Character 5	Device Character 6	Qualifier Character 7
Ø Skin, Scalp	X External	Z No Device	Z No Qualifier
1 Skin, Face			
2 Skin, Right Ear			
3 Skin, Left Ear			
4 Skin, Neck			
5 Skin, Chest Breast procedures, skin only			
6 Skin, Back			
7 Skin, Abdomen			
8 Skin, Buttock			
9 Skin, Perineum Perianal skin			
A Skin, Inguinal			
B Skin, Right Upper Arm			
C Skin, Left Upper Arm			
D Skin, Right Lower Arm			
E Skin, Left Lower Arm			
F Skin, Right Hand			
G Skin, Left Hand			
H Skin, Right Upper Leg			
J Skin, Left Upper Leg			
K Skin, Right Lower Leg			
L Skin, Left Lower Leg			
M Skin, Right Foot			
N Skin, Left Foot			

Q   Finger Nail
    Nail bed
    Nail plate			

R Toe Nail *See Q Finger Nail*			
S Hair			

T   Breast, Right
    Mammary duct
    Mammary gland
	Ø Open	Z No Device	Z No Qualifier

U Breast, Left *See T Breast, Right*			
V Breast, Bilateral *See T Breast, Right*			
Y Supernumerary Breast			

Non-OR   All body part, approach, device, and qualifier values

Non-OR Procedure   DRG Non-OR Procedure   Valid OR Procedure   HAC Associated Procedure   Combination Only   New/Revised April   New/Revised October

436   ICD-10-PCS 2024

Ø **Medical and Surgical**
H **Skin and Breast**
H **Insertion**　　Definition: Putting in a nonbiological appliance that monitors, assists, performs, or prevents a physiological function but does not physically take the place of a body part
　　　　　　　　　Explanation: None

Body Part Character 4	Approach Character 5	Device Character 6	Qualifier Character 7
P Skin	**X** External	**Y** Other Device	**Z** No Qualifier
T Breast, Right 　Mammary duct 　Mammary gland **U** Breast, Left 　*See T Breast, Right*	**Ø** Open **3** Percutaneous **7** Via Natural or Artificial Opening **8** Via Natural or Artificial Opening Endoscopic	**1** Radioactive Element **N** Tissue Expander **Y** Other Device	**Z** No Qualifier
V Breast, Bilateral 　Mammary duct 　Mammary gland	**Ø** Open **3** Percutaneous **7** Via Natural or Artificial Opening **8** Via Natural or Artificial Opening Endoscopic	**1** Radioactive Element **N** Tissue Expander	**Z** No Qualifier
W Nipple, Right 　Areola **X** Nipple, Left 　*See W Nipple, Right*	**Ø** Open **3** Percutaneous **7** Via Natural or Artificial Opening **8** Via Natural or Artificial Opening Endoscopic	**1** Radioactive Element **N** Tissue Expander	**Z** No Qualifier
W Nipple, Right 　Areola **X** Nipple, Left 　*See W Nipple, Right*	**X** External	**1** Radioactive Element	**Z** No Qualifier

Non-OR　ØHHPXYZ
Non-OR　ØHH[T,U][3,7,8]YZ

Ø **Medical and Surgical**
H **Skin and Breast**
J **Inspection**　　Definition: Visually and/or manually exploring a body part
　　　　　　　　　Explanation: Visual exploration may be performed with or without optical instrumentation. Manual exploration may be performed directly or through intervening body layers.

Body Part Character 4	Approach Character 5	Device Character 6	Qualifier Character 7
P Skin 　Dermis 　Epidermis 　Sebaceous gland 　Sweat gland **Q** Finger Nail 　Nail bed 　Nail plate **R** Toe Nail 　*See Q Finger Nail*	**X** External	**Z** No Device	**Z** No Qualifier
T Breast, Right 　Mammary duct 　Mammary gland **U** Breast, Left 　*See T Breast, Right*	**Ø** Open **3** Percutaneous **7** Via Natural or Artificial Opening **8** Via Natural or Artificial Opening Endoscopic	**Z** No Device	**Z** No Qualifier

Non-OR　All body part, approach, device and qualifier values

NC Noncovered Procedure　　**LC** Limited Coverage　　**QA** Questionable OB Admit　　**NT** New Tech Add-on　　⊞ Combination Member　　♂ Male　　♀ Female

ICD-10-PCS 2024　　　**437**

ØHH–ØHJ

Ø   Medical and Surgical
H   Skin and Breast
M   Reattachment   Definition: Putting back in or on all or a portion of a separated body part to its normal location or other suitable location
Explanation: Vascular circulation and nervous pathways may or may not be reestablished

Body Part Character 4	Approach Character 5	Device Character 6	Qualifier Character 7
Ø Skin, Scalp	X External	Z No Device	Z No Qualifier
1 Skin, Face			
2 Skin, Right Ear			
3 Skin, Left Ear			
4 Skin, Neck			
5 Skin, Chest Breast procedures, skin only			
6 Skin, Back			
7 Skin, Abdomen			
8 Skin, Buttock			
9 Skin, Perineum Perianal skin			
A Skin, Inguinal			
B Skin, Right Upper Arm			
C Skin, Left Upper Arm			
D Skin, Right Lower Arm			
E Skin, Left Lower Arm			
F Skin, Right Hand			
G Skin, Left Hand			
H Skin, Right Upper Leg			
J Skin, Left Upper Leg			
K Skin, Right Lower Leg			
L Skin, Left Lower Leg			
M Skin, Right Foot			
N Skin, Left Foot			

T Breast, Right
   Mammary duct
   Mammary gland			

U Breast, Left *See* T Breast, Right			
V Breast, Bilateral *See* T Breast, Right			
W Nipple, Right Areola			
X Nipple, Left *See* W Nipple, Right			

Non-OR   ØHMØXZZ

Ø   Medical and Surgical
H   Skin and Breast
N   Release   Definition: Freeing a body part from an abnormal physical constraint by cutting or by the use of force
                   Explanation: Some of the restraining tissue may be taken out but none of the body part is taken out

Body Part Character 4	Approach Character 5	Device Character 6	Qualifier Character 7

Ø   Skin, Scalp
1   Skin, Face
2   Skin, Right Ear
3   Skin, Left Ear
4   Skin, Neck
5   Skin, Chest
     Breast procedures, skin only
6   Skin, Back
7   Skin, Abdomen
8   Skin, Buttock
9   Skin, Perineum
     Perianal skin
A   Skin, Inguinal
B   Skin, Right Upper Arm
C   Skin, Left Upper Arm
D   Skin, Right Lower Arm
E   Skin, Left Lower Arm
F   Skin, Right Hand
G   Skin, Left Hand
H   Skin, Right Upper Leg
J   Skin, Left Upper Leg
K   Skin, Right Lower Leg
L   Skin, Left Lower Leg
M   Skin, Right Foot
N   Skin, Left Foot
Q   Finger Nail
     Nail bed
     Nail plate
R   Toe Nail
     See Q Finger Nail
	X External	Z No Device	Z No Qualifier

T   Breast, Right
     Mammary duct
     Mammary gland
U   Breast, Left
     See T Breast, Right
V   Breast, Bilateral
     See T Breast, Right
	Ø Open
	3 Percutaneous
	7 Via Natural or Artificial Opening
	8 Via Natural or Artificial Opening
	     Endoscopic
		Z No Device	Z No Qualifier

W   Nipple, Right
     Areola
X   Nipple, Left
     See W Nipple, Right
	Ø Open
	3 Percutaneous
	7 Via Natural or Artificial Opening
	8 Via Natural or Artificial Opening
	     Endoscopic
	X External
		Z No Device	Z No Qualifier

Ø **Medical and Surgical**
H **Skin and Breast**
P **Removal**   Definition: Taking out or off a device from a body part

Explanation: If a device is taken out and a similar device put in without cutting or puncturing the skin or mucous membrane, the procedure is coded to the root operation CHANGE. Otherwise, the procedure for taking out a device is coded to the root operation REMOVAL.

Body Part Character 4	Approach Character 5	Device Character 6	Qualifier Character 7
P Skin Dermis Epidermis Sebaceous gland Sweat gland	**X** External	**Ø** Drainage Device **7** Autologous Tissue Substitute **J** Synthetic Substitute **K** Nonautologous Tissue Substitute **Y** Other Device	**Z** No Qualifier
Q Finger Nail Nail bed Nail plate **R Toe Nail** *See Q Finger Nail*	**X** External	**Ø** Drainage Device **7** Autologous Tissue Substitute **J** Synthetic Substitute **K** Nonautologous Tissue Substitute	**Z** No Qualifier
S Hair	**X** External	**7** Autologous Tissue Substitute **J** Synthetic Substitute **K** Nonautologous Tissue Substitute	**Z** No Qualifier
T Breast, Right Mammary duct Mammary gland **U Breast, Left** *See T Breast, Right*	**Ø** Open **3** Percutaneous **7** Via Natural or Artificial Opening **8** Via Natural or Artificial Opening Endoscopic	**Ø** Drainage Device **1** Radioactive Element **7** Autologous Tissue Substitute **J** Synthetic Substitute **K** Nonautologous Tissue Substitute **N** Tissue Expander **Y** Other Device	**Z** No Qualifier

Non-OR	ØHPPX[Ø,7,J,K,Y]Z
Non-OR	ØHP[Q,R]X[Ø,7,J,K]Z
Non-OR	ØHPSX[7,J,K]Z
Non-OR	ØHP[T,U]Ø[Ø,1,7,K]Z
Non-OR	ØHP[T,U]3[Ø,1,7,K,Y]Z
Non-OR	ØHP[T,U][7,8][Ø,1,7,J,K,N,Y]Z

Non-OR Procedure   DRG Non-OR Procedure   Valid OR Procedure   HAC Associated Procedure   Combination Only   New/Revised April   New/Revised October

440   ICD-10-PCS 2024

Ø **Medical and Surgical**
H **Skin and Breast**
Q **Repair**　　　Definition: Restoring, to the extent possible, a body part to its normal anatomic structure and function
　　　　　　　　　　Explanation: Used only when the method to accomplish the repair is not one of the other root operations

Body Part Character 4	Approach Character 5	Device Character 6	Qualifier Character 7
Ø Skin, Scalp	**X** External	**Z** No Device	**Z** No Qualifier
1 Skin, Face			
2 Skin, Right Ear			
3 Skin, Left Ear			
4 Skin, Neck			
5 Skin, Chest 　Breast procedures, skin only			
6 Skin, Back			
7 Skin, Abdomen			
8 Skin, Buttock			
9 Skin, Perineum 　Perianal skin			
A Skin, Inguinal			
B Skin, Right Upper Arm			
C Skin, Left Upper Arm			
D Skin, Right Lower Arm			
E Skin, Left Lower Arm			
F Skin, Right Hand			
G Skin, Left Hand			
H Skin, Right Upper Leg			
J Skin, Left Upper Leg			
K Skin, Right Lower Leg			
L Skin, Left Lower Leg			
M Skin, Right Foot			
N Skin, Left Foot			
Q Finger Nail 　Nail bed 　Nail plate			
R Toe Nail 　*See Q Finger Nail*			
T Breast, Right 　Mammary duct 　Mammary gland	**Ø** Open **3** Percutaneous **7** Via Natural or Artificial Opening **8** Via Natural or Artificial Opening 　Endoscopic	**Z** No Device	**Z** No Qualifier
U Breast, Left 　*See T Breast, Right*			
V Breast, Bilateral 　*See T Breast, Right*			
Y Supernumerary Breast			
W Nipple, Right 　Areola	**Ø** Open **3** Percutaneous **7** Via Natural or Artificial Opening **8** Via Natural or Artificial Opening 　Endoscopic **X** External	**Z** No Device	**Z** No Qualifier
X Nipple, Left 　*See W Nipple, Right*			

DRG Non-OR　ØHQ9XZZ
Non-OR　　　ØHQ[Ø,1,2,3,4,5,6,7,8,A,B,C,D,E,F,G,H,J,K,L,M,N]XZZ

Skin and Breast (side tab)

Ø   **Medical and Surgical**
H   **Skin and Breast**
R   **Replacement**   Definition: Putting in or on biological or synthetic material that physically takes the place and/or function of all or a portion of a body part
                     Explanation: The body part may have been taken out or replaced, or may be taken out, physically eradicated, or rendered nonfunctional during the REPLACEMENT procedure. A REMOVAL procedure is coded for taking out the device used in a previous replacement procedure.

Body Part Character 4		Approach Character 5	Device Character 6	Qualifier Character 7

Ø Skin, Scalp
1 Skin, Face
2 Skin, Right Ear
3 Skin, Left Ear
4 Skin, Neck
5 Skin, Chest
   Breast procedures, skin only
6 Skin, Back
7 Skin, Abdomen
8 Skin, Buttock
9 Skin, Perineum
   Perianal skin
A Skin, Inguinal
	B Skin, Right Upper Arm
	C Skin, Left Upper Arm
	D Skin, Right Lower Arm
	E Skin, Left Lower Arm
	F Skin, Right Hand
	G Skin, Left Hand
	H Skin, Right Upper Leg
	J Skin, Left Upper Leg
	K Skin, Right Lower Leg
	L Skin, Left Lower Leg
	M Skin, Right Foot
	N Skin, Left Foot
		X External	7 Autologous Tissue Substitute	2 Cell Suspension Technique
				3 Full Thickness
				4 Partial Thickness

Ø Skin, Scalp
1 Skin, Face
2 Skin, Right Ear
3 Skin, Left Ear
4 Skin, Neck
5 Skin, Chest
   Breast procedures, skin only
6 Skin, Back
7 Skin, Abdomen
8 Skin, Buttock
9 Skin, Perineum
   Perianal skin
A Skin, Inguinal
	B Skin, Right Upper Arm
	C Skin, Left Upper Arm
	D Skin, Right Lower Arm
	E Skin, Left Lower Arm
	F Skin, Right Hand
	G Skin, Left Hand
	H Skin, Right Upper Leg
	J Skin, Left Upper Leg
	K Skin, Right Lower Leg
	L Skin, Left Lower Leg
	M Skin, Right Foot
	N Skin, Left Foot
		X External	J Synthetic Substitute	3 Full Thickness
				4 Partial Thickness
				Z No Qualifier

Ø Skin, Scalp
1 Skin, Face
2 Skin, Right Ear
3 Skin, Left Ear
4 Skin, Neck
5 Skin, Chest
   Breast procedures, skin only
6 Skin, Back
7 Skin, Abdomen
8 Skin Buttock
9 Skin, Perineum
   Perianal skin
A Skin, Inguinal
	B Skin, Right Upper Arm
	C Skin, Left Upper Arm
	D Skin, Right Lower Arm
	E Skin, Left Lower Arm
	F Skin, Right Hand
	G Skin, Left Hand
	H Skin, Right Upper Leg
	J Skin, Left Upper Leg
	K Skin, Right Lower Leg
	L Skin, Left Lower Leg
	M Skin, Right Foot
	N Skin, Left Foot
		X External	K Nonautologous Tissue Substitute	3 Full Thickness
				4 Partial Thickness

Q Finger Nail
   Nail bed
   Nail plate
	R Toe Nail
	   See Q Finger Nail
	S Hair
		X External	7 Autologous Tissue Substitute
			J Synthetic Substitute
			K Nonautologous Tissue Substitute
				Z No Qualifier

T Breast, Right
   Mammary duct
   Mammary gland
	U Breast, Left
	   See T Breast, Right
	V Breast, Bilateral
	   See T Breast, Right
		Ø Open	7 Autologous Tissue Substitute	5 Latissimus Dorsi Myocutaneous Flap
				6 Transverse Rectus Abdominis Myocutaneous Flap
				7 Deep Inferior Epigastric Artery Perforator Flap
				8 Superficial Inferior Epigastric Artery Flap
				9 Gluteal Artery Perforator Flap
				Z No Qualifier

T Breast, Right
   Mammary duct
   Mammary gland
	U Breast, Left
	   See T Breast, Right
	V Breast, Bilateral
	   See T Breast, Right
		Ø Open	J Synthetic Substitute
			K Nonautologous Tissue Substitute
				Z No Qualifier

T Breast, Right ⊞
   Mammary duct
   Mammary gland
U Breast, Left ⊞
   See T Breast, Right
	V Breast, Bilateral ⊞
	   See T Breast, Right
		3 Percutaneous	7 Autologous Tissue Substitute
			J Synthetic Substitute
			K Nonautologous Tissue Substitute
				Z No Qualifier

W Nipple, Right
   Areola
	X Nipple, Left
	   See W Nipple, Right
		Ø Open
		3 Percutaneous
		X External
			7 Autologous Tissue Substitute
			J Synthetic Substitute
			K Nonautologous Tissue Substitute
				Z No Qualifier

Non-OR   ØHRSX7Z

See Appendix L for Procedure Combinations
   ⊞   ØHR[T,U,V]37Z

Non-OR Procedure   DRG Non-OR Procedure   Valid OR Procedure   HAC Associated Procedure   Combination Only   New/Revised April   New/Revised October

Ø   Medical and Surgical
H   Skin and Breast
S   Reposition   Definition: Moving to its normal location, or other suitable location, all or a portion of a body part

Explanation: The body part is moved to a new location from an abnormal location, or from a normal location where it is not functioning correctly. The body part may or may not be cut out or off to be moved to the new location.

Body Part Character 4	Approach Character 5	Device Character 6	Qualifier Character 7

S   Hair
W   Nipple, Right
     Areola
X   Nipple, Left
     See W Nipple, Right
	X External	Z No Device	Z No Qualifier

T   Breast, Right
     Mammary duct
     Mammary gland
U   Breast, Left
     See T Breast, Right
V   Breast, Bilateral
     See T Breast, Right
	Ø Open	Z No Device	Z No Qualifier

Non-OR   ØHSSXZZ

Ø   Medical and Surgical
H   Skin and Breast
T   Resection   Definition: Cutting out or off, without replacement, all of a body part

Explanation: None

Body Part Character 4	Approach Character 5	Device Character 6	Qualifier Character 7

Q   Finger Nail
     Nail bed
     Nail plate
R   Toe Nail
     See Q Finger Nail
W   Nipple, Right
     Areola
X   Nipple, Left
     See W Nipple, Right
	X External	Z No Device	Z No Qualifier

T   Breast, Right ⊞
     Mammary duct
     Mammary gland
U   Breast, Left ⊞
     See T Breast, Right
V   Breast, Bilateral ⊞
     See T Breast, Right
Y   Supernumerary Breast
	Ø Open	Z No Device	Z No Qualifier

Non-OR   ØHT[Q,R]XZZ   **See Appendix L for Procedure Combinations**
                          ⊞   ØHT[T,U,V]ØZZ

Ø   Medical and Surgical
H   Skin and Breast
U   Supplement   Definition: Putting in or on biological or synthetic material that physically reinforces and/or augments the function of a portion of a body part

Explanation: The biological material is non-living, or is living and from the same individual. The body part may have been previously replaced, and the SUPPLEMENT procedure is performed to physically reinforce and/or augment the function of the replaced body part.

Body Part Character 4	Approach Character 5	Device Character 6	Qualifier Character 7

T   Breast, Right
     Mammary duct
     Mammary gland
U   Breast, Left
     See T Breast, Right
V   Breast, Bilateral
     See T Breast, Right
	Ø Open
	3 Percutaneous
	7 Via Natural or Artificial Opening
	8 Via Natural or Artificial Opening Endoscopic
		7 Autologous Tissue Substitute
		J Synthetic Substitute
		K Nonautologous Tissue Substitute
			Z No Qualifier

W   Nipple, Right
     Areola
X   Nipple, Left
     See W Nipple, Right
	Ø Open
	3 Percutaneous
	7 Via Natural or Artificial Opening
	8 Via Natural or Artificial Opening Endoscopic
	X External
		7 Autologous Tissue Substitute
		J Synthetic Substitute
		K Nonautologous Tissue Substitute
			Z No Qualifier

Non-OR   ØHU[T,U,V]3JZ

NC Noncovered Procedure   LC Limited Coverage   QA Questionable OB Admit   NT New Tech Add-on   ⊞ Combination Member   ♂ Male   ♀ Female

ICD-10-PCS 2024   443

ØHS–ØHU

Ø Medical and Surgical
H Skin and Breast
W Revision   Definition: Correcting, to the extent possible, a portion of a malfunctioning device or the position of a displaced device
                         Explanation: Revision can include correcting a malfunctioning or displaced device by taking out or putting in components of the device such as a screw or pin

Body Part Character 4	Approach Character 5	Device Character 6	Qualifier Character 7

P Skin
  Dermis
  Epidermis
  Sebaceous gland
  Sweat gland
	X External	**Ø** Drainage Device
		7 Autologous Tissue Substitute
		J Synthetic Substitute
		K Nonautologous Tissue Substitute
		Y Other Device
			Z No Qualifier

Q Finger Nail
  Nail bed
  Nail plate
R Toe Nail
  See Q Finger Nail
	X External	**Ø** Drainage Device
		7 Autologous Tissue Substitute
		J Synthetic Substitute
		K Nonautologous Tissue Substitute
			Z No Qualifier

S Hair	**X** External	**7** Autologous Tissue Substitute **J** Synthetic Substitute **K** Nonautologous Tissue Substitute	**Z** No Qualifier

T Breast, Right
  Mammary duct
  Mammary gland
U Breast, Left
  See T Breast, Right
	Ø Open
	3 Percutaneous
	7 Via Natural or Artificial Opening
	8 Via Natural or Artificial Opening Endoscopic
		Ø Drainage Device
		7 Autologous Tissue Substitute
		J Synthetic Substitute
		K Nonautologous Tissue Substitute
		N Tissue Expander
		Y Other Device
			Z No Qualifier

Non-OR	ØHWPX[Ø,7,J,K,Y]Z
Non-OR	ØHW[Q,R]X[Ø,7,J,K]Z
Non-OR	ØHWSX[7,J,K]Z
Non-OR	ØHW[T,U]Ø[Ø,7,K,N]Z
Non-OR	ØHW[T,U]3[Ø,7,K,N,Y]Z
Non-OR	ØHW[T,U][7,8][Ø,7,J,K,N,Y]Z

Ø Medical and Surgical
H Skin and Breast
X Transfer   Definition: Moving, without taking out, all or a portion of a body part to another location to take over the function of all or a portion of a body part
                         Explanation: The body part transferred remains connected to its vascular and nervous supply

Body Part Character 4	Approach Character 5	Device Character 6	Qualifier Character 7

Ø Skin, Scalp
1 Skin, Face
2 Skin, Right Ear
3 Skin, Left Ear
4 Skin, Neck
5 Skin, Chest
  Breast procedures, skin only
6 Skin, Back
7 Skin, Abdomen
8 Skin, Buttock
9 Skin, Perineum
  Perianal skin
A Skin, Inguinal
B Skin, Right Upper Arm
C Skin, Left Upper Arm
D Skin, Right Lower Arm
E Skin, Left Lower Arm
F Skin, Right Hand
G Skin, Left Hand
H Skin, Right Upper Leg
J Skin, Left Upper Leg
K Skin, Right Lower Leg
L Skin, Left Lower Leg
M Skin, Right Foot
N Skin, Left Foot
	X External	**Z** No Device	**Z** No Qualifier

Non-OR Procedure   DRG Non-OR Procedure   Valid OR Procedure   HAC Associated Procedure   Combination Only   New/Revised April   New/Revised October

444   ICD-10-PCS 2024

Subcutaneous Tissue and Fascia 0J0–0JX

Character Meanings

This Character Meaning table is provided as a guide to assist the user in the identification of character members that may be found in this section of code tables. It **SHOULD NOT** be used to build a PCS code.

Operation–Character 3		Body Part–Character 4		Approach–Character 5		Device–Character 6		Qualifier–Character 7	
0	Alteration	0	Subcutaneous Tissue and Fascia, Scalp	0	Open	0	Drainage Device OR Monitoring Device, Hemodynamic	B	Skin and Subcutaneous Tissue
2	Change	1	Subcutaneous Tissue and Fascia, Face	3	Percutaneous	1	Radioactive Element	C	Skin, Subcutaneous Tissue and Fascia
5	Destruction	4	Subcutaneous Tissue and Fascia, Right Neck	X	External	2	Monitoring Device	X	Diagnostic
8	Division	5	Subcutaneous Tissue and Fascia, Left Neck			3	Infusion Device	Z	No Qualifier
9	Drainage	6	Subcutaneous Tissue and Fascia, Chest			4	Pacemaker, Single Chamber		
B	Excision	7	Subcutaneous Tissue and Fascia, Back			5	Pacemaker, Single Chamber Rate Responsive		
C	Extirpation	8	Subcutaneous Tissue and Fascia, Abdomen			6	Pacemaker, Dual Chamber		
D	Extraction	9	Subcutaneous Tissue and Fascia, Buttock			7	Autologous Tissue Substitute OR Cardiac Resynchronization Pacemaker Pulse Generator		
H	Insertion	B	Subcutaneous Tissue and Fascia, Perineum			8	Defibrillator Generator		
J	Inspection	C	Subcutaneous Tissue and Fascia, Pelvic Region			9	Cardiac Resynchronization Defibrillator Pulse Generator		
N	Release	D	Subcutaneous Tissue and Fascia, Right Upper Arm			A	Contractility Modulation Device		
P	Removal	F	Subcutaneous Tissue and Fascia, Left Upper Arm			B	Stimulator Generator, Single Array		
Q	Repair	G	Subcutaneous Tissue and Fascia, Right Lower Arm			C	Stimulator Generator, Single Array Rechargeable		
R	Replacement	H	Subcutaneous Tissue and Fascia, Left Lower Arm			D	Stimulator Generator, Multiple Array		
U	Supplement	J	Subcutaneous Tissue and Fascia, Right Hand			E	Stimulator Generator, Multiple Array Rechargeable		
W	Revision	K	Subcutaneous Tissue and Fascia, Left Hand			F	Subcutaneous Defibrillator Lead		
X	Transfer	L	Subcutaneous Tissue and Fascia, Right Upper Leg			H	Contraceptive Device		
		M	Subcutaneous Tissue and Fascia, Left Upper Leg			J	Synthetic Substitute		
		N	Subcutaneous Tissue and Fascia, Right Lower Leg			K	Nonautologous Tissue Substitute		
		P	Subcutaneous Tissue and Fascia, Left Lower Leg			M	Stimulator Generator		
		Q	Subcutaneous Tissue and Fascia, Right Foot			N	Tissue Expander		
		R	Subcutaneous Tissue and Fascia, Left Foot			P	Cardiac Rhythm Related Device		
		S	Subcutaneous Tissue and Fascia, Head and Neck			V	Infusion Device, Pump		
		T	Subcutaneous Tissue and Fascia, Trunk			W	Vascular Access Device, Totally Implantable		
		V	Subcutaneous Tissue and Fascia, Upper Extremity			X	Vascular Access Device, Tunneled		
		W	Subcutaneous Tissue and Fascia, Lower Extremity			Y	Other Device		
						Z	No Device		

AHA Coding Clinic for table ØJ2

| 2018, 3Q, 10 | Disruption of perma-catheter fibrin sheath via angioplasty of superior vena cava |
| 2017, 2Q, 26 | Exchange of tunneled catheter |

AHA Coding Clinic for table ØJ5

| 2019, 3Q, 25 | Endoscopic removal of pilonidal sinus and cyst |

AHA Coding Clinic for table ØJ8

| 2017, 3Q, 11 | Bilateral escharotomy of leg, thigh and foot |

AHA Coding Clinic for table ØJ9

2018, 3Q, 16	Incision and drainage of submandibular space
2018, 3Q, 16	Incision and drainage of neck abscess
2015, 3Q, 23	Incision and drainage of multiple abscess cavities using vessel loop

AHA Coding Clinic for table ØJB

2023, 2Q, 30	Excisional debridement and non-excisional debridement at deeper layer same site
2022, 3Q, 11	Ulceration and soft tissue redundancy at amputation site due to osteo-integrated implant
2020, 1Q, 31	Repair of buried penis
2019, 3Q, 25	Endoscopic removal of pilonidal sinus and cyst
2018, 3Q, 17	Excisional debridement of periosteum
2018, 1Q, 7	Placement of fat graft following lumbar decompression surgery
2015, 3Q, 3-8	Excisional and nonexcisional debridement
2015, 2Q, 13	Transfer of free flap to reconstruct orbital defect
2015, 1Q, 29	Fistulectomy with placement of seton
2014, 4Q, 38	Abdominoplasty and abdominal wall plication for hernia repair
2014, 3Q, 22	Transsphenoidal removal of pituitary tumor and fat graft placement

AHA Coding Clinic for table ØJC

| 2017, 3Q, 22 | Replacement of native skull bone flap |

AHA Coding Clinic for table ØJD

2023, 2Q, 30	Excisional debridement and non-excisional debridement at deeper layer same site
2023, 1Q, 36	Maggot therapy
2016, 3Q, 20	VersaJet™ nonexcisional debridement of leg muscle
2016, 3Q, 21	Nonexcisional debridement of infected lumbar wound
2016, 3Q, 21	Nonexcisional pulsed lavage debridement
2016, 3Q, 22	Debridement of bone and tendon using Tenex ultrasound device
2016, 1Q, 40	Nonexcisional debridement of skin and subcutaneous tissue
2015, 3Q, 3-8	Excisional and nonexcisional debridement
2015, 1Q, 23	Non-Excisional debridement with lavage of wound

AHA Coding Clinic for table ØJH

2020, 4Q, 54	Insertion of other device into subcutaneous tissue and fascia
2020, 4Q, 55	Insertion of subcutaneous pump system for ascites drainage
2020, 2Q, 15	Ommaya reservoir with ventricular catheter placement
2020, 2Q, 16	Ommaya reservoir placement for cerebrospinal fluid infusion therapy
2019, 4Q, 33	Subcutaneous implantable cardioverter defibrillator lead
2017, 4Q, 63-64	Added and revised device values - Vascular access reservoir
2017, 2Q, 24	Tunneled catheter versus totally implantable catheter
2017, 2Q, 26	Exchange of tunneled catheter
2016, 4Q, 97-98	Phrenic neurostimulator
2016, 2Q, 14	Insertion of peritoneal totally implantable venous access device
2016, 2Q, 15	Removal and replacement of tunneled internal jugular catheter
2015, 4Q, 14	New Section X codes—New Technology procedures
2015, 4Q, 30-31	Vascular access devices
2015, 2Q, 33	Totally implantable central venous access device (Port-a-Cath)
2014, 3Q, 19	End of life replacement of Baclofen pump
2013, 4Q, 116	Device character for Port-A-Cath placement
2012, 4Q, 104	Placement of subcutaneous implantable cardioverter defibrillator

AHA Coding Clinic for table ØJN

| 2017, 3Q, 11 | Bilateral escharotomy of leg, thigh and foot |

AHA Coding Clinic for table ØJP

2019, 4Q, 33	Subcutaneous implantable cardioverter defibrillator lead
2018, 4Q, 86	Placement of lumboatrial shunt
2018, 3Q, 29	Decommissioning of left ventricular assist device with exploration of mediastinum
2016, 2Q, 15	Removal and replacement of tunneled internal jugular catheter
2015, 4Q, 31	Vascular access devices
2014, 3Q, 19	End of life replacement of Baclofen pump
2013, 4Q, 109	Separating conjoined twins
2012, 4Q, 104	Placement of subcutaneous implantable cardioverter defibrillator

AHA Coding Clinic for table ØJQ

2022, 3Q, 24	Leakage of cerebrospinal fluid with revision of intrathecal baclofen system
2017, 3Q, 19	Anterior repair of cystocele
2014, 4Q, 44	Posterior colporrhaphy/rectocele repair

AHA Coding Clinic for table ØJR

| 2015, 2Q, 13 | Transfer of free flap to reconstruct orbital defect |

AHA Coding Clinic for table ØJU

| 2018, 2Q, 20 | Prelaminated free flap graft using Alloderm™ |
| 2018, 1Q, 7 | Placement of fat graft following lumbar decompression surgery |

AHA Coding Clinic for table ØJW

2022, 3Q, 24	Leakage of cerebrospinal fluid with revision of intrathecal baclofen system
2019, 4Q, 33	Subcutaneous implantable cardioverter defibrillator lead
2018, 1Q, 8	Ventricular peritoneal shunt ligation
2015, 4Q, 33	Externalization of peritoneal dialysis catheter
2015, 2Q, 9	Revision of ventriculoperitoneal (VP) shunt
2012, 4Q, 104	Placement of subcutaneous implantable cardioverter defibrillator

AHA Coding Clinic for table ØJX

2022, 3Q, 11	Ulceration and soft tissue redundancy at amputation site due to osteo-integrated implant
2022, 1Q, 48	Repair of facial fractures of frontal sinus and orbital roof
2021, 3Q, 19	Elbow amputation and targeted muscle reinnervation
2021, 2Q, 16	Goldilocks breast reconstruction
2018, 1Q, 10	Complex wound closure using pericranial flap
2014, 3Q, 18	Placement of reverse sural fasciocutaneous pedicle flap
2013, 4Q, 109	Separating conjoined twins

Subcutaneous Tissue and Fascia

0　Medical and Surgical
J　Subcutaneous Tissue and Fascia
0　Alteration　　Definition: Modifying the anatomic structure of a body part without affecting the function of the body part
　　　　　　　　　Explanation: Principal purpose is to improve appearance

Body Part Character 4		Approach Character 5	Device Character 6	Qualifier Character 7
1 Subcutaneous Tissue and Fascia, Face Chin Masseteric fascia Orbital fascia Submandibular space **4 Subcutaneous Tissue and Fascia, Right Neck** Deep cervical fascia Pretracheal fascia Prevertebral fascia **5 Subcutaneous Tissue and Fascia, Left Neck** *See 4 Subcutaneous Tissue and Fascia, Right Neck* **6 Subcutaneous Tissue and Fascia, Chest** Pectoral fascia **7 Subcutaneous Tissue and Fascia, Back** **8 Subcutaneous Tissue and Fascia, Abdomen** **9 Subcutaneous Tissue and Fascia, Buttock** **D Subcutaneous Tissue and Fascia, Right Upper Arm** Axillary fascia Deltoid fascia Infraspinatus fascia Subscapular aponeurosis Supraspinatus fascia	**F Subcutaneous Tissue and Fascia, Left Upper Arm** *See D Subcutaneous Tissue and Fascia, Right Upper Arm* **G Subcutaneous Tissue and Fascia, Right Lower Arm** Antebrachial fascia Bicipital aponeurosis **H Subcutaneous Tissue and Fascia, Left Lower Arm** *See G Subcutaneous Tissue and Fascia, Right Lower Arm* **L Subcutaneous Tissue and Fascia, Right Upper Leg** Crural fascia Fascia lata Iliac fascia Iliotibial tract (band) **M Subcutaneous Tissue and Fascia, Left Upper Leg** *See L Subcutaneous Tissue and Fascia, Right Upper Leg* **N Subcutaneous Tissue and Fascia, Right Lower Leg** **P Subcutaneous Tissue and Fascia, Left Lower Leg**	**0 Open** **3 Percutaneous**	**Z No Device**	**Z No Qualifier**

0　Medical and Surgical
J　Subcutaneous Tissue and Fascia
2　Change　　Definition: Taking out or off a device from a body part and putting back an identical or similar device in or on the same body part without cutting or puncturing the skin or a mucous membrane
　　　　　　　　　Explanation: All CHANGE procedures are coded using the approach EXTERNAL

Body Part Character 4	Approach Character 5	Device Character 6	Qualifier Character 7
S Subcutaneous Tissue and Fascia, Head and Neck **T Subcutaneous Tissue and Fascia, Trunk** External oblique aponeurosis Transversalis fascia **V Subcutaneous Tissue and Fascia, Upper Extremity** **W Subcutaneous Tissue and Fascia, Lower Extremity**	**X External**	**0 Drainage Device** **Y Other Device**	**Z No Qualifier**

Non-OR　All body part, approach, device, and qualifier values

NC Noncovered Procedure　　**LC** Limited Coverage　　**QA** Questionable OB Admit　　**NT** New Tech Add-on　　⊞ Combination Member　　♂ Male　　♀ Female

ICD-10-PCS 2024　　　　　　　　　　　　　　　　　　　　　　　　　　　　　　　　　　　　　447

Subcutaneous Tissue and Fascia

Ø   Medical and Surgical
J   Subcutaneous Tissue and Fascia
5   Destruction   Definition: Physical eradication of all or a portion of a body part by the direct use of energy, force, or a destructive agent
                     Explanation: None of the body part is physically taken out

Body Part Character 4		Approach Character 5	Device Character 6	Qualifier Character 7
Ø Subcutaneous Tissue and Fascia, Scalp Galea aponeurotica **1 Subcutaneous Tissue and Fascia, Face** Chin Masseteric fascia Orbital fascia Submandibular space **4 Subcutaneous Tissue and Fascia, Right Neck** Deep cervical fascia Pretracheal fascia Preverterbral fascia **5 Subcutaneous Tissue and Fascia, Left Neck** *See 4 Subcutaneous Tissue and Fascia, Right Neck* **6 Subcutaneous Tissue and Fascia, Chest** Pectoral fascia **7 Subcutaneous Tissue and Fascia, Back** **8 Subcutaneous Tissue and Fascia, Abdomen** **9 Subcutaneous Tissue and Fascia, Buttock** **B Subcutaneous Tissue and Fascia, Perineum** **C Subcutaneous Tissue and Fascia, Pelvic Region** **D Subcutaneous Tissue and Fascia, Right Upper Arm** Axillary fascia Deltoid fascia Infraspinatus fascia Subscapular aponeurosis Supraspinatus fascia **F Subcutaneous Tissue and Fascia, Left Upper Arm** *See D Subcutaneous Tissue and Fascia, Right Upper Arm*	**G Subcutaneous Tissue and Fascia, Right Lower Arm** Antebrachial fascia Bicipital aponeurosis **H Subcutaneous Tissue and Fascia, Left Lower Arm** *See G Subcutaneous Tissue and Fascia, Right Lower Arm* **J Subcutaneous Tissue and Fascia, Right Hand** Palmar fascia (aponeurosis) **K Subcutaneous Tissue and Fascia, Left Hand** *See J Subcutaneous Tissue and Fascia, Right Hand* **L Subcutaneous Tissue and Fascia, Right Upper Leg** Crural fascia Fascia lata Iliac fascia Iliotibial tract (band) **M Subcutaneous Tissue and Fascia, Left Upper Leg** *See L Subcutaneous Tissue and Fascia, Right Upper Leg* **N Subcutaneous Tissue and Fascia, Right Lower Leg** **P Subcutaneous Tissue and Fascia, Left Lower Leg** **Q Subcutaneous Tissue and Fascia, Right Foot** Plantar fascia (aponeurosis) **R Subcutaneous Tissue and Fascia, Left Foot** *See Q Subcutaneous Tissue and Fascia, Right Foot*	**Ø Open** **3 Percutaneous**	**Z No Device**	**Z No Qualifier**

DRG Non-OR   All body part, approach, device, and qualifier values

0   **Medical and Surgical**
J   **Subcutaneous Tissue and Fascia**
8   **Division**   Definition: Cutting into a body part, without draining fluids and/or gases from the body part, in order to separate or transect a body part
                    Explanation: All or a portion of the body part is separated into two or more portions

Body Part Character 4	Approach Character 5	Device Character 6	Qualifier Character 7

0 Subcutaneous Tissue and Fascia, Scalp
  Galea aponeurotica
1 Subcutaneous Tissue and Fascia, Face
  Chin
  Masseteric fascia
  Orbital fascia
  Submandibular space
4 Subcutaneous Tissue and Fascia, Right Neck
  Deep cervical fascia
  Pretracheal fascia
  Prevertebral fascia
5 Subcutaneous Tissue and Fascia, Left Neck
  See 4 *Subcutaneous Tissue and Fascia, Right Neck*
6 Subcutaneous Tissue and Fascia, Chest
  Pectoral fascia
7 Subcutaneous Tissue and Fascia, Back
8 Subcutaneous Tissue and Fascia, Abdomen
9 Subcutaneous Tissue and Fascia, Buttock
B Subcutaneous Tissue and Fascia, Perineum
C Subcutaneous Tissue and Fascia, Pelvic Region
D Subcutaneous Tissue and Fascia, Right Upper Arm
  Axillary fascia
  Deltoid fascia
  Infraspinatus fascia
  Subscapular aponeurosis
  Supraspinatus fascia
F Subcutaneous Tissue and Fascia, Left Upper Arm
  See D *Subcutaneous Tissue and Fascia, Right Upper Arm*
G Subcutaneous Tissue and Fascia, Right Lower Arm
  Antebrachial fascia
  Bicipital aponeurosis
	H Subcutaneous Tissue and Fascia, Left Lower Arm
	  See G *Subcutaneous Tissue and Fascia, Right Lower Arm*
	J Subcutaneous Tissue and Fascia, Right Hand
	  Palmar fascia (aponeurosis)
	K Subcutaneous Tissue and Fascia, Left Hand
	  See J *Subcutaneous Tissue and Fascia, Right Hand*
	L Subcutaneous Tissue and Fascia, Right Upper Leg
	  Crural fascia
	  Fascia lata
	  Iliac fascia
	  Iliotibial tract (band)
	M Subcutaneous Tissue and Fascia, Left Upper Leg
	  See L *Subcutaneous Tissue and Fascia, Right Upper Leg*
	N Subcutaneous Tissue and Fascia, Right Lower Leg
	P Subcutaneous Tissue and Fascia, Left Lower Leg
	Q Subcutaneous Tissue and Fascia, Right Foot
	  Plantar fascia (aponeurosis)
	R Subcutaneous Tissue and Fascia, Left Foot
	  See Q *Subcutaneous Tissue and Fascia, Right Foot*
	S Subcutaneous Tissue and Fascia, Head and Neck
	T Subcutaneous Tissue and Fascia, Trunk
	  External oblique aponeurosis
	  Transversalis fascia
	V Subcutaneous Tissue and Fascia, Upper Extremity
	W Subcutaneous Tissue and Fascia, Lower Extremity
		0 Open
		3 Percutaneous
			Z No Device	**Z** No Qualifier

NC Noncovered Procedure   **LC** Limited Coverage   **QA** Questionable OB Admit   **NT** New Tech Add-on   ⊞ Combination Member   ♂ Male   ♀ Female

ICD-10-PCS 2024   **449**

Ø   Medical and Surgical
J   Subcutaneous Tissue and Fascia
9   Drainage   Definition: Taking or letting out fluids and/or gases from a body part

          Explanation: The qualifier DIAGNOSTIC is used to identify drainage procedures that are biopsies

Body Part Character 4		Approach Character 5	Device Character 6	Qualifier Character 7
Ø Subcutaneous Tissue and Fascia, Scalp Galea aponeurotica **1 Subcutaneous Tissue and Fascia, Face** Chin Masseteric fascia Orbital fascia Submandibular space **4 Subcutaneous Tissue and Fascia, Right Neck** Deep cervical fascia Pretracheal fascia Prevertebral fascia **5 Subcutaneous Tissue and Fascia, Left Neck** *See 4 Subcutaneous Tissue and Fascia, Right Neck* **6 Subcutaneous Tissue and Fascia, Chest** Pectoral fascia **7 Subcutaneous Tissue and Fascia, Back** **8 Subcutaneous Tissue and Fascia, Abdomen** **9 Subcutaneous Tissue and Fascia, Buttock** **B Subcutaneous Tissue and Fascia, Perineum** **C Subcutaneous Tissue and Fascia, Pelvic Region** **D Subcutaneous Tissue and Fascia, Right Upper Arm** Axillary fascia Deltoid fascia Infraspinatus fascia Subscapular aponeurosis Supraspinatus fascia **F Subcutaneous Tissue and Fascia, Left Upper Arm** *See D Subcutaneous Tissue and Fascia, Right Upper Arm*	**G Subcutaneous Tissue and Fascia, Right Lower Arm** Antebrachial fascia Bicipital aponeurosis **H Subcutaneous Tissue and Fascia, Left Lower Arm** *See G Subcutaneous Tissue and Fascia, Right Lower Arm* **J Subcutaneous Tissue and Fascia, Right Hand** Palmar fascia (aponeurosis) **K Subcutaneous Tissue and Fascia, Left Hand** *See J Subcutaneous Tissue and Fascia, Right Hand* **L Subcutaneous Tissue and Fascia, Right Upper Leg** Crural fascia Fascia lata Iliac fascia Iliotibial tract (band) **M Subcutaneous Tissue and Fascia, Left Upper Leg** *See L Subcutaneous Tissue and Fascia, Right Upper Leg* **N Subcutaneous Tissue and Fascia, Right Lower Leg** **P Subcutaneous Tissue and Fascia, Left Lower Leg** **Q Subcutaneous Tissue and Fascia, Right Foot** Plantar fascia (aponeurosis) **R Subcutaneous Tissue and Fascia, Left Foot** *See Q Subcutaneous Tissue and Fascia, Right Foot*	**Ø Open** **3 Percutaneous**	**Ø Drainage Device**	**Z No Qualifier**

Non-OR   All body part, approach, device, and qualifier values

ØJ9 Continued on next page

Ø **Medical and Surgical**
J **Subcutaneous Tissue and Fascia**
9 **Drainage**　　　Definition: Taking or letting out fluids and/or gases from a body part

ØJ9 Continued

Explanation: The qualifier DIAGNOSTIC is used to identify drainage procedures that are biopsies

Body Part Character 4		Approach Character 5	Device Character 6	Qualifier Character 7
Ø Subcutaneous Tissue and Fascia, Scalp Galea aponeurotica	**G** Subcutaneous Tissue and Fascia, Right Lower Arm Antebrachial fascia Bicipital aponeurosis	**Ø** Open **3** Percutaneous	**Z** No Device	**X** Diagnostic **Z** No Qualifier
1 Subcutaneous Tissue and Fascia, Face Chin Masseteric fascia Orbital fascia Submandibular space	**H** Subcutaneous Tissue and Fascia, Left Lower Arm *See G Subcutaneous Tissue and Fascia, Right Lower Arm*			
4 Subcutaneous Tissue and Fascia, Right Neck Deep cervical fascia Pretracheal fascia Prevertebral fascia	**J** Subcutaneous Tissue and Fascia, Right Hand Palmar fascia (aponeurosis)			
5 Subcutaneous Tissue and Fascia, Left Neck *See 4 Subcutaneous Tissue and Fascia, Right Neck*	**K** Subcutaneous Tissue and Fascia, Left Hand *See J Subcutaneous Tissue and Fascia, Right Hand*			
6 Subcutaneous Tissue and Fascia, Chest Pectoral fascia	**L** Subcutaneous Tissue and Fascia, Right Upper Leg Crural fascia Fascia lata Iliac fascia Iliotibial tract (band)			
7 Subcutaneous Tissue and Fascia, Back	**M** Subcutaneous Tissue and Fascia, Left Upper Leg *See L Subcutaneous Tissue and Fascia, Right Upper Leg*			
8 Subcutaneous Tissue and Fascia, Abdomen	**N** Subcutaneous Tissue and Fascia, Right Lower Leg			
9 Subcutaneous Tissue and Fascia, Buttock	**P** Subcutaneous Tissue and Fascia, Left Lower Leg			
B Subcutaneous Tissue and Fascia, Perineum	**Q** Subcutaneous Tissue and Fascia, Right Foot Plantar fascia (aponeurosis)			
C Subcutaneous Tissue and Fascia, Pelvic Region	**R** Subcutaneous Tissue and Fascia, Left Foot *See Q Subcutaneous Tissue and Fascia, Right Foot*			
D Subcutaneous Tissue and Fascia, Right Upper Arm Axillary fascia Deltoid fascia Infraspinatus fascia Subscapular aponeurosis Supraspinatus fascia				
F Subcutaneous Tissue and Fascia, Left Upper Arm *See D Subcutaneous Tissue and Fascia, Right Upper Arm*				

Non-OR All body part, approach, device, and qualifier values

Subcutaneous Tissue and Fascia

Ø   Medical and Surgical
J   Subcutaneous Tissue and Fascia
B   Excision   Definition: Cutting out or off, without replacement, a portion of a body part

               Explanation: The qualifier DIAGNOSTIC is used to identify excision procedures that are biopsies

Body Part Character 4		Approach Character 5	Device Character 6	Qualifier Character 7
Ø Subcutaneous Tissue and Fascia, Scalp Galea aponeurotica **1 Subcutaneous Tissue and Fascia, Face** Chin Masseteric fascia Orbital fascia Submandibular space **4 Subcutaneous Tissue and Fascia, Right Neck** Deep cervical fascia Pretracheal fascia Prevertebral fascia **5 Subcutaneous Tissue and Fascia, Left Neck** *See 4 Subcutaneous Tissue and Fascia, Right Neck* **6 Subcutaneous Tissue and Fascia, Chest** Pectoral fascia **7 Subcutaneous Tissue and Fascia, Back** **8 Subcutaneous Tissue and Fascia, Abdomen** **9 Subcutaneous Tissue and Fascia, Buttock** **B Subcutaneous Tissue and Fascia, Perineum** **C Subcutaneous Tissue and Fascia, Pelvic Region** **D Subcutaneous Tissue and Fascia, Right Upper Arm** Axillary fascia Deltoid fascia Infraspinatus fascia Subscapular aponeurosis Supraspinatus fascia **F Subcutaneous Tissue and Fascia, Left Upper Arm** *See D Subcutaneous Tissue and Fascia, Right Upper Arm*	**G Subcutaneous Tissue and Fascia, Right Lower Arm** Antebrachial fascia Bicipital aponeurosis **H Subcutaneous Tissue and Fascia, Left Lower Arm** *See G Subcutaneous Tissue and Fascia, Right Lower Arm* **J Subcutaneous Tissue and Fascia, Right Hand** Palmar fascia (aponeurosis) **K Subcutaneous Tissue and Fascia, Left Hand** *See J Subcutaneous Tissue and Fascia, Right Hand* **L Subcutaneous Tissue and Fascia, Right Upper Leg** Crural fascia Fascia lata Iliac fascia Iliotibial tract (band) **M Subcutaneous Tissue and Fascia, Left Upper Leg** *See L Subcutaneous Tissue and Fascia, Right Upper Leg* **N Subcutaneous Tissue and Fascia, Right Lower Leg** **P Subcutaneous Tissue and Fascia, Left Lower Leg** **Q Subcutaneous Tissue and Fascia, Right Foot** Plantar fascia (aponeurosis) **R Subcutaneous Tissue and Fascia, Left Foot** *See Q Subcutaneous Tissue and Fascia, Right Foot*	**Ø Open** **3 Percutaneous**	**Z No Device**	**X Diagnostic** **Z No Qualifier**

DRG Non-OR   ØJB[Ø,4,5,6,7,8,9,B,C,D,F,G,H,L,M,N,P,Q,R]3ZZ
Non-OR   ØJB[Ø,1,4,5,6,7,8,9,B,C,D,F,G,H,J,K,L,M,N,P,Q,R][Ø,3]ZX

Ø   **Medical and Surgical**
J   **Subcutaneous Tissue and Fascia**
C   **Extirpation**   Definition: Taking or cutting out solid matter from a body part

Explanation: The solid matter may be an abnormal byproduct of a biological function or a foreign body; it may be imbedded in a body part or in the lumen of a tubular body part. The solid matter may or may not have been previously broken into pieces.

Body Part Character 4		Approach Character 5	Device Character 6	Qualifier Character 7
Ø **Subcutaneous Tissue and Fascia, Scalp** Galea aponeurotica **1** **Subcutaneous Tissue and Fascia, Face** Chin Masseteric fascia Orbital fascia Submandibular space **4** **Subcutaneous Tissue and Fascia, Right Neck** Deep cervical fascia Pretracheal fascia Prevertebral fascia **5** **Subcutaneous Tissue and Fascia, Left Neck** *See* 4 *Subcutaneous Tissue and Fascia, Right Neck* **6** **Subcutaneous Tissue and Fascia, Chest** Pectoral fascia **7** **Subcutaneous Tissue and Fascia, Back** **8** **Subcutaneous Tissue and Fascia, Abdomen** **9** **Subcutaneous Tissue and Fascia, Buttock** **B** **Subcutaneous Tissue and Fascia, Perineum** **C** **Subcutaneous Tissue and Fascia, Pelvic Region** **D** **Subcutaneous Tissue and Fascia, Right Upper Arm** Axillary fascia Deltoid fascia Infraspinatus fascia Subscapular aponeurosis Supraspinatus fascia **F** **Subcutaneous Tissue and Fascia, Left Upper Arm** *See* D *Subcutaneous Tissue and Fascia, Right Upper Arm*	**G** **Subcutaneous Tissue and Fascia, Right Lower Arm** Antebrachial fascia Bicipital aponeurosis **H** **Subcutaneous Tissue and Fascia, Left Lower Arm** *See* G *Subcutaneous Tissue and Fascia, Right Lower Arm* **J** **Subcutaneous Tissue and Fascia, Right Hand** Palmar fascia (aponeurosis) **K** **Subcutaneous Tissue and Fascia, Left Hand** *See* J *Subcutaneous Tissue and Fascia, Right Hand* **L** **Subcutaneous Tissue and Fascia, Right Upper Leg** Crural fascia Fascia lata Iliac fascia Iliotibial tract (band) **M** **Subcutaneous Tissue and Fascia, Left Upper Leg** *See* L *Subcutaneous Tissue and Fascia, Right Upper Leg* **N** **Subcutaneous Tissue and Fascia, Right Lower Leg** **P** **Subcutaneous Tissue and Fascia, Left Lower Leg** **Q** **Subcutaneous Tissue and Fascia, Right Foot** Plantar fascia (aponeurosis) **R** **Subcutaneous Tissue and Fascia, Left Foot** *See* Q *Subcutaneous Tissue and Fascia, Right Foot*	**Ø** Open **3** Percutaneous	**Z** No Device	**Z** No Qualifier

Non-OR   ØJC[Ø,1,4,5,6,7,8,9,B,C,D,F,G,H,J,K,L,M,N,P,Q,R]3ZZ

Ø   **Medical and Surgical**
J   **Subcutaneous Tissue and Fascia**
D   **Extraction**   Definition: Pulling or stripping out or off all or a portion of a body part by the use of force
                      Explanation: The qualifier DIAGNOSTIC is used to identify extraction procedures that are biopsies

Body Part Character 4		Approach Character 5	Device Character 6	Qualifier Character 7
Ø **Subcutaneous Tissue and Fascia, Scalp** Galea aponeurotica **1** **Subcutaneous Tissue and Fascia, Face** Chin Masseteric fascia Orbital fascia Submandibular space **4** **Subcutaneous Tissue and Fascia, Right Neck** Deep cervical fascia Pretracheal fascia Prevertebral fascia **5** **Subcutaneous Tissue and Fascia, Left Neck** *See 4 Subcutaneous Tissue and Fascia, Right Neck* **6** **Subcutaneous Tissue and Fascia, Chest** Pectoral fascia **7** **Subcutaneous Tissue and Fascia, Back** **8** **Subcutaneous Tissue and Fascia, Abdomen** **9** **Subcutaneous Tissue and Fascia, Buttock** **B** **Subcutaneous Tissue and Fascia, Perineum** **C** **Subcutaneous Tissue and Fascia, Pelvic Region** **D** **Subcutaneous Tissue and Fascia, Right Upper Arm** Axillary fascia Deltoid fascia Infraspinatus fascia Subscapular aponeurosis Supraspinatus fascia **F** **Subcutaneous Tissue and Fascia, Left Upper Arm** *See D Subcutaneous Tissue and Fascia, Right Upper Arm*	**G** **Subcutaneous Tissue and Fascia, Right Lower Arm** Antebrachial fascia Bicipital aponeurosis **H** **Subcutaneous Tissue and Fascia, Left Lower Arm** *See G Subcutaneous Tissue and Fascia, Right Lower Arm* **J** **Subcutaneous Tissue and Fascia, Right Hand** Palmar fascia (aponeurosis) **K** **Subcutaneous Tissue and Fascia, Left Hand** *See J Subcutaneous Tissue and Fascia, Right Hand* **L** **Subcutaneous Tissue and Fascia, Right Upper Leg** Crural fascia Fascia lata Iliac fascia Iliotibial tract (band) **M** **Subcutaneous Tissue and Fascia, Left Upper Leg** *See L Subcutaneous Tissue and Fascia, Right Upper Leg* **N** **Subcutaneous Tissue and Fascia, Right Lower Leg** **P** **Subcutaneous Tissue and Fascia, Left Lower Leg** **Q** **Subcutaneous Tissue and Fascia, Right Foot** Plantar fascia (aponeurosis) **R** **Subcutaneous Tissue and Fascia, Left Foot** *See Q Subcutaneous Tissue and Fascia, Right Foot*	**Ø** Open **3** Percutaneous	**Z** No Device	**Z** No Qualifier

Non-OR   ØJD[Ø,1,4,5,B,C,D,F,G,H,J,K,N,P,Q,R]3ZZ

See Appendix L for Procedure Combinations
    Combo-only   ØJD[6,7,8,9,L,M]3ZZ

Ø   Medical and Surgical
J   Subcutaneous Tissue and Fascia
H   Insertion   Definition: Putting in a nonbiological appliance that monitors, assists, performs, or prevents a physiological function but does not physically take the place of a body part
           Explanation: None

Body Part Character 4		Approach Character 5	Device Character 6	Qualifier Character 7

Ø Subcutaneous Tissue and Fascia, Scalp
   Galea aponeurotica
1 Subcutaneous Tissue and Fascia, Face
   Chin
   Masseteric fascia
   Orbital fascia
   Submandibular space
4 Subcutaneous Tissue and Fascia, Right Neck
   Deep cervical fascia
   Pretracheal fascia
   Prevertebral fascia
5 Subcutaneous Tissue and Fascia, Left Neck
   See 4 Subcutaneous Tissue and Fascia, Right Neck
9 Subcutaneous Tissue and Fascia, Buttock
B Subcutaneous Tissue and Fascia, Perineum
	C Subcutaneous Tissue and Fascia, Pelvic Region
	J Subcutaneous Tissue and Fascia, Right Hand
	   Palmar fascia (aponeurosis)
	K Subcutaneous Tissue and Fascia, Left Hand
	   See J Subcutaneous Tissue and Fascia, Right Hand
	Q Subcutaneous Tissue and Fascia, Right Foot
	   Plantar fascia (aponeurosis)
	R Subcutaneous Tissue and Fascia, Left Foot
	   See Q Subcutaneous Tissue and Fascia, Right Foot
		Ø Open
		3 Percutaneous
			N Tissue Expander	**Z** No Qualifier

6 Subcutaneous Tissue and Fascia, Chest ⊞ Pectoral fascia		**Ø** Open **3** Percutaneous	**Ø** Monitoring Device, Hemodynamic **2** Monitoring Device **4** Pacemaker, Single Chamber **5** Pacemaker, Single Chamber Rate Responsive **6** Pacemaker, Dual Chamber **7** Cardiac Resynchronization Pacemaker Pulse Generator **8** Defibrillator Generator **9** Cardiac Resynchronization Defibrillator Pulse Generator **A** Contractility Modulation Device **B** Stimulator Generator, Single Array **C** Stimulator Generator, Single Array Rechargeable **D** Stimulator Generator, Multiple Array **E** Stimulator Generator, Multiple Array Rechargeable **F** Subcutaneous Defibrillator Lead **H** Contraceptive Device **M** Stimulator Generator **N** Tissue Expander **P** Cardiac Rhythm Related Device **V** Infusion Device, Pump **W** Vascular Access Device, Totally Implantable **X** Vascular Access Device, Tunneled **Y** Other Device	**Z** No Qualifier
7 Subcutaneous Tissue and Fascia, Back 🆖 ⊞		**Ø** Open **3** Percutaneous	**B** Stimulator Generator, Single Array **C** Stimulator Generator, Single Array Rechargeable **D** Stimulator Generator, Multiple Array **E** Stimulator Generator, Multiple Array Rechargeable **M** Stimulator Generator **N** Tissue Expander **V** Infusion Device, Pump **Y** Other Device	**Z** No Qualifier

DRG Non-OR	ØJH6[Ø,3][4,5,6,7,H,P,X]Z	
DRG Non-OR	ØJH63WX	
Non-OR	ØJH63YZ	
Non-OR	ØJH73YZ	
HAC	ØJH6[Ø,3][4,5,6,7,8,9,P]Z when reported with SDx K68.11 or T81.4Ø-T81.49, T82.7 with 7th character A	
HAC	ØJH63XZ when reported with SDx J95.811	

🆖   ØJH7[Ø,3]MZ

See Appendix L for Procedure Combinations
⊞   ØJH6[Ø,3][4,5,6,7,8,9,A,B,C,D,E,F,M,P]Z
⊞   ØJH7[Ø,3][B,C,D,E,M]Z

ØJH Continued on next page

🆖 Noncovered Procedure   🄻🄲 Limited Coverage   🅀🄰 Questionable OB Admit   🅽🅃 New Tech Add-on   ⊞ Combination Member   ♂ Male   ♀ Female

Subcutaneous Tissue and Fascia

Ø Medical and Surgical
J Subcutaneous Tissue and Fascia
H Insertion   Definition: Putting in a nonbiological appliance that monitors, assists, performs, or prevents a physiological function but does not physically take the place of a body part
                       Explanation: None

Body Part Character 4	Approach Character 5	Device Character 6	Qualifier Character 7
8 Subcutaneous Tissue and Fascia, Abdomen ᴺᶜ ⊞	Ø Open 3 Percutaneous	Ø Monitoring Device, Hemodynamic 2 Monitoring Device 4 Pacemaker, Single Chamber 5 Pacemaker, Single Chamber Rate Responsive 6 Pacemaker, Dual Chamber 7 Cardiac Resynchronization Pacemaker Pulse Generator 8 Defibrillator Generator 9 Cardiac Resynchronization Defibrillator Pulse Generator A Contractility Modulation Device B Stimulator Generator, Single Array C Stimulator Generator, Single Array Rechargeable D Stimulator Generator, Multiple Array E Stimulator Generator, Multiple Array Rechargeable H Contraceptive Device M Stimulator Generator N Tissue Expander P Cardiac Rhythm Related Device V Infusion Device, Pump W Vascular Access Device, Totally Implantable X Vascular Access Device, Tunneled Y Other Device	Z No Qualifier

D Subcutaneous Tissue and Fascia, Right Upper Arm
   Axillary fascia
   Deltoid fascia
   Infraspinatus fascia
   Subscapular aponeurosis
   Supraspinatus fascia
F Subcutaneous Tissue and Fascia, Left Upper Arm
   See D Subcutaneous Tissue and Fascia, Right Upper Arm
G Subcutaneous Tissue and Fascia, Right Lower Arm
   Antebrachial fascia
   Bicipital aponeurosis
H Subcutaneous Tissue and Fascia, Left Lower Arm
   See G Subcutaneous Tissue and Fascia, Right Lower Arm
L Subcutaneous Tissue and Fascia, Right Upper Leg
   Crural fascia
   Fascia lata
   Iliac fascia
   Iliotibial tract (band)
M Subcutaneous Tissue and Fascia, Left Upper Leg
   See L Subcutaneous Tissue and Fascia, Right Upper Leg
N Subcutaneous Tissue and Fascia, Right Lower Leg
P Subcutaneous Tissue and Fascia, Left Lower Leg
	Ø Open
	3 Percutaneous
		H Contraceptive Device
		N Tissue Expander
		V Infusion Device, Pump
		W Vascular Access Device, Totally Implantable
		X Vascular Access Device, Tunneled
			Z No Qualifier

S Subcutaneous Tissue and Fascia, Head and Neck V Subcutaneous Tissue and Fascia, Upper Extremity W Subcutaneous Tissue and Fascia, Lower Extremity	Ø Open 3 Percutaneous	1 Radioactive Element 3 Infusion Device Y Other Device	Z No Qualifier

T Subcutaneous Tissue and Fascia, Trunk
   External oblique aponeurosis
   Transversalis fascia
	Ø Open
	3 Percutaneous
		1 Radioactive Element
		3 Infusion Device
		V Infusion Device, Pump
		Y Other Device
			Z No Qualifier

DRG Non-OR	ØJH8[Ø,3][2,4,5,6,7,H,P,X]Z	**Non-OR** ØJH83YZ	**HAC** ØJH8[Ø,3][4,5,6,7,8,9,P]Z when reported with SDx K68.11 or
DRG Non-OR	ØJH83WX	**Non-OR** ØJH[D,F,G,H,L,M][Ø,3]HZ	T81.4Ø–T81.49, T82.7 with 7th character A
DRG Non-OR	ØJH[D,F,G,H,L,M,N,P]ØXZ	**Non-OR** ØJHNØHZ	ᴺᶜ ØJH8[Ø,3]MZ
DRG Non-OR	ØJH[D,F,G,H,L,M,N,P]3[W,X]Z	**Non-OR** ØJH[S,V,W]Ø3Z	
DRG Non-OR	ØJHN3HZ	**Non-OR** ØJH[S,V,W]3[3,Y]Z	**See Appendix L for Procedure Combinations**
DRG Non-OR	ØJHP[Ø,3]HZ	**Non-OR** ØJHTØ3Z	⊞ ØJH8[Ø,3][4,5,6,7,8,9,A,B,C,D,E,M,P]Z
		Non-OR ØJHT3[3,Y]Z	

Ø   Medical and Surgical
J   Subcutaneous Tissue and Fascia
J   Inspection   Definition: Visually and/or manually exploring a body part

Explanation: Visual exploration may be performed with or without optical instrumentation. Manual exploration may be performed directly or through intervening body layers.

Body Part Character 4	Approach Character 5	Device Character 6	Qualifier Character 7

S   Subcutaneous Tissue and Fascia, Head and Neck
T   Subcutaneous Tissue and Fascia, Trunk
     External oblique aponeurosis
     Transversalis fascia
V   Subcutaneous Tissue and Fascia, Upper Extremity
W   Subcutaneous Tissue and Fascia, Lower Extremity
	Ø Open
	3 Percutaneous
	X External
		Z No Device	**Z** No Qualifier

Non-OR   All body part, approach, device, and qualifier values

Ø   Medical and Surgical
J   Subcutaneous Tissue and Fascia
N   Release   Definition: Freeing a body part from an abnormal physical constraint by cutting or by the use of force

Explanation: Some of the restraining tissue may be taken out but none of the body part is taken out

Body Part Character 4		Approach Character 5	Device Character 6	Qualifier Character 7

Ø   Subcutaneous Tissue and Fascia, Scalp
     Galea aponeurotica
1   Subcutaneous Tissue and Fascia, Face
     Chin
     Masseteric fascia
     Orbital fascia
     Submandibular space
4   Subcutaneous Tissue and Fascia, Right Neck
     Deep cervical fascia
     Pretracheal fascia
     Prevertebral fascia
5   Subcutaneous Tissue and Fascia, Left Neck
     See 4 Subcutaneous Tissue and Fascia, Right Neck
6   Subcutaneous Tissue and Fascia, Chest
     Pectoral fascia
7   Subcutaneous Tissue and Fascia, Back
8   Subcutaneous Tissue and Fascia, Abdomen
9   Subcutaneous Tissue and Fascia, Buttock
B   Subcutaneous Tissue and Fascia, Perineum
C   Subcutaneous Tissue and Fascia, Pelvic Region
D   Subcutaneous Tissue and Fascia, Right Upper Arm
     Axillary fascia
     Deltoid fascia
     Infraspinatus fascia
     Subscapular aponeurosis
     Supraspinatus fascia
F   Subcutaneous Tissue and Fascia, Left Upper Arm
     See D Subcutaneous Tissue and Fascia, Right Upper Arm
	G Subcutaneous Tissue and Fascia, Right Lower Arm
	     Antebrachial fascia
	     Bicipital aponeurosis
	H Subcutaneous Tissue and Fascia, Left Lower Arm
	     See G Subcutaneous Tissue and Fascia, Right Lower Arm
	J Subcutaneous Tissue and Fascia, Right Hand
	     Palmar fascia (aponeurosis)
	K Subcutaneous Tissue and Fascia, Left Hand
	     See J Subcutaneous Tissue and Fascia, Right Hand
	L Subcutaneous Tissue and Fascia, Right Upper Leg
	     Crural fascia
	     Fascia lata
	     Iliac fascia
	     Iliotibial tract (band)
	M Subcutaneous Tissue and Fascia, Left Upper Leg
	     See L Subcutaneous Tissue and Fascia, Right Upper Leg
	N Subcutaneous Tissue and Fascia, Right Lower Leg
	P Subcutaneous Tissue and Fascia, Left Lower Leg
	Q Subcutaneous Tissue and Fascia, Right Foot
	     Plantar fascia (aponeurosis)
	R Subcutaneous Tissue and Fascia, Left Foot
	     See Q Subcutaneous Tissue and Fascia, Right Foot
		Ø Open
		3 Percutaneous
		X External
			Z No Device	**Z** No Qualifier

Non-OR   ØJN[Ø,1,4,5,6,7,8,9,B,C,D,F,G,H,J,K,L,M,N,P,Q,R]XZZ

Subcutaneous Tissue and Fascia

ØJP–ØJP

Ø   **Medical and Surgical**
J   **Subcutaneous Tissue and Fascia**
P   **Removal**   Definition: Taking out or off a device from a body part

Explanation: If a device is taken out and a similar device put in without cutting or puncturing the skin or mucous membrane, the procedure is coded to the root operation CHANGE. Otherwise, the procedure for taking out a device is coded to the root operation REMOVAL.

Body Part Character 4	Approach Character 5	Device Character 6	Qualifier Character 7
S Subcutaneous Tissue and Fascia, Head and Neck	**Ø** Open **3** Percutaneous	**Ø** Drainage Device **1** Radioactive Element **3** Infusion Device **7** Autologous Tissue Substitute **J** Synthetic Substitute **K** Nonautologous Tissue Substitute **N** Tissue Expander **Y** Other Device	**Z** No Qualifier
S Subcutaneous Tissue and Fascia, Head and Neck	**X** External	**Ø** Drainage Device **1** Radioactive Element **3** Infusion Device	**Z** No Qualifier
T Subcutaneous Tissue and Fascia, Trunk External oblique aponeurosis Transversalis fascia	**Ø** Open **3** Percutaneous	**Ø** Drainage Device **1** Radioactive Element **2** Monitoring Device **3** Infusion Device **7** Autologous Tissue Substitute **F** Subcutaneous Defibrillator Lead **H** Contraceptive Device **J** Synthetic Substitute **K** Nonautologous Tissue Substitute **M** Stimulator Generator **N** Tissue Expander **P** Cardiac Rhythm Related Device **V** Infusion Device, Pump **W** Vascular Access Device, Totally Implantable **X** Vascular Access Device, Tunneled **Y** Other Device	**Z** No Qualifier
T Subcutaneous Tissue and Fascia, Trunk External oblique aponeurosis Transversalis fascia	**X** External	**Ø** Drainage Device **1** Radioactive Element **2** Monitoring Device **3** Infusion Device **H** Contraceptive Device **V** Infusion Device, Pump **X** Vascular Access Device, Tunneled	**Z** No Qualifier
V Subcutaneous Tissue and Fascia, Upper Extremity **W** Subcutaneous Tissue and Fascia, Lower Extremity	**Ø** Open **3** Percutaneous	**Ø** Drainage Device **1** Radioactive Element **3** Infusion Device **7** Autologous Tissue Substitute **H** Contraceptive Device **J** Synthetic Substitute **K** Nonautologous Tissue Substitute **N** Tissue Expander **V** Infusion Device, Pump **W** Vascular Access Device, Totally Implantable **X** Vascular Access Device, Tunneled **Y** Other Device	**Z** No Qualifier
V Subcutaneous Tissue and Fascia, Upper Extremity **W** Subcutaneous Tissue and Fascia, Lower Extremity	**X** External	**Ø** Drainage Device **1** Radioactive Element **3** Infusion Device **H** Contraceptive Device **V** Infusion Device, Pump **X** Vascular Access Device, Tunneled	**Z** No Qualifier

Non-OR	ØJPS[Ø,3][Ø,1,3,7,J,K,N,Y]Z
Non-OR	ØJPSX[Ø,1,3]Z
Non-OR	ØJPT[Ø,3][Ø,1,2,3,7,H,J,K,M,N,V,W,X,Y]Z
Non-OR	ØJPTX[Ø,1,2,3,H,V,X]Z
Non-OR	ØJP[V,W][Ø,3][Ø,1,3,7,H,J,K,N,V,W,X,Y]Z
Non-OR	ØJP[V,W]X[Ø,1,3,H,V,X]Z
HAC	ØJPT[Ø,3][F,P]Z when reported with SDx K68.11 or T81.4Ø-T81.49, T82.7 with 7th character A

Non-OR Procedure   DRG Non-OR Procedure   Valid OR Procedure   HAC Associated Procedure   Combination Only   New/Revised April   New/Revised October

458   ICD-10-PCS 2024

Ø   **Medical and Surgical**
J   **Subcutaneous Tissue and Fascia**
Q   **Repair**   Definition: Restoring, to the extent possible, a body part to its normal anatomic structure and function
                     Explanation: Used only when the method to accomplish the repair is not one of the other root operations

Body Part Character 4		Approach Character 5	Device Character 6	Qualifier Character 7
Ø Subcutaneous Tissue and Fascia, Scalp Galea aponeurotica **1** Subcutaneous Tissue and Fascia, Face Chin Masseteric fascia Orbital fascia Submandibular space **4** Subcutaneous Tissue and Fascia, Right Neck Deep cervical fascia Pretracheal fascia Prevertebral fascia **5** Subcutaneous Tissue and Fascia, Left Neck *See 4 Subcutaneous Tissue and Fascia, Right Neck* **6** Subcutaneous Tissue and Fascia, Chest Pectoral fascia **7** Subcutaneous Tissue and Fascia, Back **8** Subcutaneous Tissue and Fascia, Abdomen **9** Subcutaneous Tissue and Fascia, Buttock **B** Subcutaneous Tissue and Fascia, Perineum **C** Subcutaneous Tissue and Fascia, Pelvic Region **D** Subcutaneous Tissue and Fascia, Right Upper Arm Axillary fascia Deltoid fascia Infraspinatus fascia Subscapular aponeurosis Supraspinatus fascia **F** Subcutaneous Tissue and Fascia, Left Upper Arm *See D Subcutaneous Tissue and Fascia, Right Upper Arm*	**G** Subcutaneous Tissue and Fascia, Right Lower Arm Antebrachial fascia Bicipital aponeurosis **H** Subcutaneous Tissue and Fascia, Left Lower Arm *See G Subcutaneous Tissue and Fascia, Right Lower Arm* **J** Subcutaneous Tissue and Fascia, Right Hand Palmar fascia (aponeurosis) **K** Subcutaneous Tissue and Fascia, Left Hand *See J Subcutaneous Tissue and Fascia, Right Hand* **L** Subcutaneous Tissue and Fascia, Right Upper Leg Crural fascia Fascia lata Iliac fascia Iliotibial tract (band) **M** Subcutaneous Tissue and Fascia, Left Upper Leg *See L Subcutaneous Tissue and Fascia, Right Upper Leg* **N** Subcutaneous Tissue and Fascia, Right Lower Leg **P** Subcutaneous Tissue and Fascia, Left Lower Leg **Q** Subcutaneous Tissue and Fascia, Right Foot Plantar fascia (aponeurosis) **R** Subcutaneous Tissue and Fascia, Left Foot *See Q Subcutaneous Tissue and Fascia, Right Foot*	**Ø** Open **3** Percutaneous	**Z** No Device	**Z** No Qualifier

Non-OR   ØJQ[Ø,1,4,5,6,7,8,9,B,C,D,F,G,H,J,K,L,M,N,P,Q,R]3ZZ

NC Noncovered Procedure   **LC** Limited Coverage   **QA** Questionable OB Admit   **NT** New Tech Add-on   ⊞ Combination Member   ♂ Male   ♀ Female

ICD-10-PCS 2024   **459**

Ø Medical and Surgical
J Subcutaneous Tissue and Fascia
R Replacement   Definition: Putting in or on biological or synthetic material that physically takes the place and/or function of all or a portion of a body part

Explanation: The body part may have been taken out or replaced, or may be taken out, physically eradicated, or rendered nonfunctional during the REPLACEMENT procedure. A REMOVAL procedure is coded for taking out the device used in a previous replacement procedure.

Body Part Character 4		Approach Character 5	Device Character 6	Qualifier Character 7
Ø Subcutaneous Tissue and Fascia, Scalp Galea aponeurotica **1 Subcutaneous Tissue and Fascia, Face** Chin Masseteric fascia Orbital fascia Submandibular space **4 Subcutaneous Tissue and Fascia, Right Neck** Deep cervical fascia Pretracheal fascia Prevertebral fascia **5 Subcutaneous Tissue and Fascia, Left Neck** *See 4 Subcutaneous Tissue and Fascia, Right Neck* **6 Subcutaneous Tissue and Fascia, Chest** Pectoral fascia **7 Subcutaneous Tissue and Fascia, Back** **8 Subcutaneous Tissue and Fascia, Abdomen** **9 Subcutaneous Tissue and Fascia, Buttock** **B Subcutaneous Tissue and Fascia, Perineum** **C Subcutaneous Tissue and Fascia, Pelvic Region** **D Subcutaneous Tissue and Fascia, Right Upper Arm** Axillary fascia Deltoid fascia Infraspinatus fascia Subscapular aponeurosis Supraspinatus fascia **F Subcutaneous Tissue and Fascia, Left Upper Arm** *See D Subcutaneous Tissue and Fascia, Right Upper Arm*	**G Subcutaneous Tissue and Fascia, Right Lower Arm** Antebrachial fascia Bicipital aponeurosis **H Subcutaneous Tissue and Fascia, Left Lower Arm** *See G Subcutaneous Tissue and Fascia, Right Lower Arm* **J Subcutaneous Tissue and Fascia, Right Hand** Palmar fascia (aponeurosis) **K Subcutaneous Tissue and Fascia, Left Hand** *See J Subcutaneous Tissue and Fascia, Right Hand* **L Subcutaneous Tissue and Fascia, Right Upper Leg** Crural fascia Fascia lata Iliac fascia Iliotibial tract (band) **M Subcutaneous Tissue and Fascia, Left Upper Leg** *See L Subcutaneous Tissue and Fascia, Right Upper Leg* **N Subcutaneous Tissue and Fascia, Right Lower Leg** **P Subcutaneous Tissue and Fascia, Left Lower Leg** **Q Subcutaneous Tissue and Fascia, Right Foot** Plantar fascia (aponeurosis) **R Subcutaneous Tissue and Fascia, Left Foot** *See Q Subcutaneous Tissue and Fascia, Right Foot*	**Ø Open** **3 Percutaneous**	**7 Autologous Tissue Substitute** **J Synthetic Substitute** **K Nonautologous Tissue Substitute**	**Z No Qualifier**

Non-OR Procedure   DRG Non-OR Procedure   Valid OR Procedure   HAC Associated Procedure   Combination Only   New/Revised April   New/Revised October

460   ICD-10-PCS 2024

Ø   **Medical and Surgical**
J   **Subcutaneous Tissue and Fascia**
U   **Supplement:**   Definition: Putting in or on biological or synthetic material that physically reinforces and/or augments the function of a portion of a body part
                 Explanation: The biological material is non-living, or is living and from the same individual. The body part may have been previously replaced, and the SUPPLEMENT procedure is performed to physically reinforce and/or augment the function of the replaced body part.

Body Part Character 4		Approach Character 5	Device Character 6	Qualifier Character 7
Ø Subcutaneous Tissue and Fascia, Scalp Galea aponeurotica	**G** Subcutaneous Tissue and Fascia, Right Lower Arm Antebrachial fascia Bicipital aponeurosis	**Ø** Open **3** Percutaneous	**7** Autologous Tissue Substitute **J** Synthetic Substitute **K** Nonautologous Tissue Substitute	**Z** No Qualifier
1 Subcutaneous Tissue and Fascia, Face Chin Masseteric fascia Orbital fascia Submandibular space	**H** Subcutaneous Tissue and Fascia, Left Lower Arm *See G Subcutaneous Tissue and Fascia, Right Lower Arm*			
4 Subcutaneous Tissue and Fascia, Right Neck Deep cervical fascia Pretracheal fascia Prevertebral fascia	**J** Subcutaneous Tissue and Fascia, Right Hand Palmar fascia (aponeurosis)			
5 Subcutaneous Tissue and Fascia, Left Neck *See 4 Subcutaneous Tissue and Fascia, Right Neck*	**K** Subcutaneous Tissue and Fascia, Left Hand *See J Subcutaneous Tissue and Fascia, Right Hand*			
6 Subcutaneous Tissue and Fascia, Chest Pectoral fascia	**L** Subcutaneous Tissue and Fascia, Right Upper Leg Crural fascia Fascia lata Iliac fascia Iliotibial tract (band)			
7 Subcutaneous Tissue and Fascia, Back	**M** Subcutaneous Tissue and Fascia, Left Upper Leg *See L Subcutaneous Tissue and Fascia, Right Upper Leg*			
8 Subcutaneous Tissue and Fascia, Abdomen	**N** Subcutaneous Tissue and Fascia, Right Lower Leg			
9 Subcutaneous Tissue and Fascia, Buttock	**P** Subcutaneous Tissue and Fascia, Left Lower Leg			
B Subcutaneous Tissue and Fascia, Perineum	**Q** Subcutaneous Tissue and Fascia, Right Foot Plantar fascia (aponeurosis)			
C Subcutaneous Tissue and Fascia, Pelvic Region	**R** Subcutaneous Tissue and Fascia, Left Foot *See Q Subcutaneous Tissue and Fascia, Right Foot*			
D Subcutaneous Tissue and Fascia, Right Upper Arm Axillary fascia Deltoid fascia Infraspinatus fascia Subscapular aponeurosis Supraspinatus fascia				
F Subcutaneous Tissue and Fascia, Left Upper Arm *See D Subcutaneous Tissue and Fascia, Right Upper Arm*				

Subcutaneous Tissue and Fascia

Ø   **Medical and Surgical**
J   **Subcutaneous Tissue and Fascia**
W   **Revision**   Definition: Correcting, to the extent possible, a portion of a malfunctioning device or the position of a displaced device
                Explanation: Revision can include correcting a malfunctioning or displaced device by taking out or putting in components of the device such as a screw or pin

Body Part Character 4	Approach Character 5	Device Character 6	Qualifier Character 7
S Subcutaneous Tissue and Fascia, Head and Neck	**Ø** Open **3** Percutaneous	**Ø** Drainage Device **3** Infusion Device **7** Autologous Tissue Substitute **J** Synthetic Substitute **K** Nonautologous Tissue Substitute **N** Tissue Expander **Y** Other Device	**Z** No Qualifier
S Subcutaneous Tissue and Fascia, Head and Neck	**X** External	**Ø** Drainage Device **3** Infusion Device **7** Autologous Tissue Substitute **J** Synthetic Substitute **K** Nonautologous Tissue Substitute **N** Tissue Expander	**Z** No Qualifier
T Subcutaneous Tissue and Fascia, Trunk External oblique aponeurosis Transversalis fascia	**Ø** Open **3** Percutaneous	**Ø** Drainage Device **2** Monitoring Device **3** Infusion Device **7** Autologous Tissue Substitute **F** Subcutaneous Defibrillator Lead **H** Contraceptive Device **J** Synthetic Substitute **K** Nonautologous Tissue Substitute **M** Stimulator Generator **N** Tissue Expander **P** Cardiac Rhythm Related Device **V** Infusion Device, Pump **W** Vascular Access Device, Totally Implantable **X** Vascular Access Device, Tunneled **Y** Other Device	**Z** No Qualifier
T Subcutaneous Tissue and Fascia, Trunk External oblique aponeurosis Transversalis fascia	**X** External	**Ø** Drainage Device **2** Monitoring Device **3** Infusion Device **7** Autologous Tissue Substitute **F** Subcutaneous Defibrillator Lead **H** Contraceptive Device **J** Synthetic Substitute **K** Nonautologous Tissue Substitute **M** Stimulator Generator **N** Tissue Expander **P** Cardiac Rhythm Related Device **V** Infusion Device, Pump **W** Vascular Access Device, Totally Implantable **X** Vascular Access Device, Tunneled	**Z** No Qualifier
V Subcutaneous Tissue and Fascia, Upper Extremity **W** Subcutaneous Tissue and Fascia, Lower Extremity	**Ø** Open **3** Percutaneous	**Ø** Drainage Device **3** Infusion Device **7** Autologous Tissue Substitute **H** Contraceptive Device **J** Synthetic Substitute **K** Nonautologous Tissue Substitute **N** Tissue Expander **V** Infusion Device, Pump **W** Vascular Access Device, Totally Implantable **X** Vascular Access Device, Tunneled **Y** Other Device	**Z** No Qualifier
V Subcutaneous Tissue and Fascia, Upper Extremity **W** Subcutaneous Tissue and Fascia, Lower Extremity	**X** External	**Ø** Drainage Device **3** Infusion Device **7** Autologous Tissue Substitute **H** Contraceptive Device **J** Synthetic Substitute **K** Nonautologous Tissue Substitute **N** Tissue Expander **V** Infusion Device, Pump **W** Vascular Access Device, Totally Implantable **X** Vascular Access Device, Tunneled	**Z** No Qualifier

DRG Non-OR ØJWS[Ø,3][Ø,3,7,J,K,N,Y]Z **DRG Non-OR** ØJWT[Ø,3][Ø,3,7,H,J,K,M,N,V,W,X]Z **DRG Non-OR** ØJWTXMZ **DRG Non-OR** ØJW[V,W][Ø,3][Ø,3,7,H,J,K,N,V,W,X,Y]Z	**Non-OR** ØJWSX[Ø,3,7,J,K,N]Z **Non-OR** ØJWT3YZ **Non-OR** ØJWTX[Ø,2,3,7,F,H,J,K,N,P,V,W,X]Z **Non-OR** ØJW[V,W]X[Ø,3,7,H,J,K,N,V,W,X]Z		**HAC** ØJWT[Ø,3][F,P]Z when reported with SDx K68.11 or T81.4Ø-T81.49, T82.7 with 7th character A

Non-OR Procedure   DRG Non-OR Procedure   Valid OR Procedure   HAC Associated Procedure   Combination Only   New/Revised April   New/Revised October

Ø   **Medical and Surgical**
J   **Subcutaneous Tissue and Fascia**
X   **Transfer**   Definition: Moving, without taking out, all or a portion of a body part to another location to take over the function of all or a portion of a body part

                        Explanation: The body part transferred remains connected to its vascular and nervous supply

Body Part Character 4		Approach Character 5	Device Character 6	Qualifier Character 7
Ø **Subcutaneous Tissue and Fascia, Scalp** Galea aponeurotica	**G** **Subcutaneous Tissue and Fascia, Right Lower Arm** Antebrachial fascia Bicipital aponeurosis	**Ø** Open **3** Percutaneous	**Z** No Device	**B** Skin and Subcutaneous Tissue **C** Skin, Subcutaneous Tissue and Fascia **Z** No Qualifier
1 **Subcutaneous Tissue and Fascia, Face** Chin Masseteric fascia Orbital fascia Submandibular space	**H** **Subcutaneous Tissue and Fascia, Left Lower Arm** *See G Subcutaneous Tissue and Fascia, Right Lower Arm*			
4 **Subcutaneous Tissue and Fascia, Right Neck** Deep cervical fascia Pretracheal fascia Prevertebral fascia	**J** **Subcutaneous Tissue and Fascia, Right Hand** Palmar fascia (aponeurosis)			
5 **Subcutaneous Tissue and Fascia, Left Neck** *See 4 Subcutaneous Tissue and Fascia, Right Neck*	**K** **Subcutaneous Tissue and Fascia, Left Hand** *See J Subcutaneous Tissue and Fascia, Right Hand*			
6 **Subcutaneous Tissue and Fascia, Chest** Pectoral fascia	**L** **Subcutaneous Tissue and Fascia, Right Upper Leg** Crural fascia Fascia lata Iliac fascia Iliotibial tract (band)			
7 **Subcutaneous Tissue and Fascia, Back**	**M** **Subcutaneous Tissue and Fascia, Left Upper Leg** *See L Subcutaneous Tissue and Fascia, Right Upper Leg*			
8 **Subcutaneous Tissue and Fascia, Abdomen**	**N** **Subcutaneous Tissue and Fascia, Right Lower Leg**			
9 **Subcutaneous Tissue and Fascia, Buttock**	**P** **Subcutaneous Tissue and Fascia, Left Lower Leg**			
B **Subcutaneous Tissue and Fascia, Perineum**	**Q** **Subcutaneous Tissue and Fascia, Right Foot** Plantar fascia (aponeurosis)			
C **Subcutaneous Tissue and Fascia, Pelvic Region**	**R** **Subcutaneous Tissue and Fascia, Left Foot** *See Q Subcutaneous Tissue and Fascia, Right Foot*			
D **Subcutaneous Tissue and Fascia, Right Upper Arm** Axillary fascia Deltoid fascia Infraspinatus fascia Subscapular aponeurosis Supraspinatus fascia				
F **Subcutaneous Tissue and Fascia, Left Upper Arm** *See D Subcutaneous Tissue and Fascia, Right Upper Arm*				

Muscles ØK2–ØKX

Character Meanings

This Character Meaning table is provided as a guide to assist the user in the identification of character members that may be found in this section of code tables. It **SHOULD NOT** be used to build a PCS code.

Operation–Character 3	Body Part–Character 4	Approach–Character 5	Device–Character 6	Qualifier–Character 7
2 Change	Ø Head Muscle	Ø Open	Ø Drainage Device	Ø Skin
5 Destruction	1 Facial Muscle	3 Percutaneous	7 Autologous Tissue Substitute	1 Subcutaneous Tissue
8 Division	2 Neck Muscle, Right	4 Percutaneous Endoscopic	J Synthetic Substitute	2 Skin and Subcutaneous Tissue
9 Drainage	3 Neck Muscle, Left	7 Via Natural or Artificial Opening	K Nonautologous Tissue Substitute	5 Latissimus Dorsi Myocutaneous Flap
B Excision	4 Tongue, Palate, Pharynx Muscle	8 Via Natural or Artificial Opening Endoscopic	M Stimulator Lead	6 Transverse Rectus Abdominis Myocutaneous Flap
C Extirpation	5 Shoulder Muscle, Right	X External	Y Other Device	7 Deep Inferior Epigastric Artery Perforator Flap
D Extraction	6 Shoulder Muscle, Left		Z No Device	8 Superficial Inferior Epigastric Artery Flap
H Insertion	7 Upper Arm Muscle, Right			9 Gluteal Artery Perforator Flap
J Inspection	8 Upper Arm Muscle, Left			X Diagnostic
M Reattachment	9 Lower Arm and Wrist Muscle, Right			Z No Qualifier
N Release	B Lower Arm and Wrist Muscle, Left			
P Removal	C Hand Muscle, Right			
Q Repair	D Hand Muscle, Left			
R Replacement	F Trunk Muscle, Right			
S Reposition	G Trunk Muscle, Left			
T Resection	H Thorax Muscle, Right			
U Supplement	J Thorax Muscle, Left			
W Revision	K Abdomen Muscle, Right			
X Transfer	L Abdomen Muscle, Left			
	M Perineum Muscle			
	N Hip Muscle, Right			
	P Hip Muscle, Left			
	Q Upper Leg Muscle, Right			
	R Upper Leg Muscle, Left			
	S Lower Leg Muscle, Right			
	T Lower Leg Muscle, Left			
	V Foot Muscle, Right			
	W Foot Muscle, Left			
	X Upper Muscle			
	Y Lower Muscle			

AHA Coding Clinic for table ØK8
2021, 4Q, 50   Endoscopic division of tongue, palate and pharynx muscle
2020, 2Q, 25   Endoscopic stapling of Zenker's diverticulum

AHA Coding Clinic for table ØKB
2023, 2Q, 30   Excisional debridement and non-excisional debridement at deeper layer same site
2023, 1Q, 32   Zenker's diverticulectomy
2020, 1Q, 27   Delayed reconstruction following mastectomy using gracilis musculocutaneous free flap
2016, 3Q, 20   Excisional debridement of sacrum
2015, 3Q, 3-8   Excisional and nonexcisional debridement

AHA Coding Clinic for table ØKD
2023, 2Q, 30   Excisional debridement and non-excisional debridement at deeper layer same site
2017, 4Q, 41-42   Extraction procedures

AHA Coding Clinic for table ØKH
2020, 4Q, 63   Intercompartmental pressure measurement

AHA Coding Clinic for table ØKN
2017, 2Q, 12   Compartment syndrome and fasciotomy of foot
2017, 2Q, 13   Compartment syndrome and fasciotomy of leg
2015, 2Q, 22   Arthroscopic subacromial decompression
2014, 4Q, 39   Abdominal component release with placement of mesh for hernia repair

AHA Coding Clinic for table ØKQ
2022, 3Q, 13   Repair of prolapsed neovaginal graft
2018, 2Q, 25   Third and fourth degree obstetric lacerations

AHA Coding Clinic for table ØKQ (Continued)
2016, 2Q, 34   Assisted vaginal delivery
2016, 1Q, 7   Obstetrical perineal laceration repair
2014, 4Q, 43   Second degree obstetric perineal laceration
2013, 4Q, 120   Repair of second degree perineum obstetric laceration

AHA Coding Clinic for table ØKS
2022, 3Q, 11   Ulceration and soft tissue redundancy at amputation site due to osteo-integrated implant
2017, 1Q, 41   Manual reduction of hernia

AHA Coding Clinic for table ØKT
2016, 3Q, 30   Resection of malignant neoplasm of infratemporal fossa
2015, 1Q, 38   Abdominoperineal resection with flap closure of the perineum and colostomy

AHA Coding Clinic for table ØKX
2023, 1Q, 34   Repair of Stage 4 pressure ulcer and application of Amniofill®
2022, 3Q, 11   Ulceration and soft tissue redundancy at amputation site due to osteo-integrated implant
2018, 2Q, 18   Transverse rectus abdominis myocutaneous (TRAM) delay
2017, 4Q, 67   New qualifier values - Pedicle flap procedures
2016, 3Q, 30   Resection of femur with interposition arthroplasty
2015, 3Q, 33   Cleft lip repair using Millard rotation advancement
2015, 2Q, 26   Pharyngeal flap to soft palate
2014, 4Q, 41   Abdominoperineal resection (APR) with flap closure of perineum and colostomy
2014, 2Q, 10   Transverse abdominomyocutaneous (TRAM) breast reconstruction
2014, 2Q, 12   Pedicle latissimus myocutaneous flap with placement of breast tissue expanders

Muscles

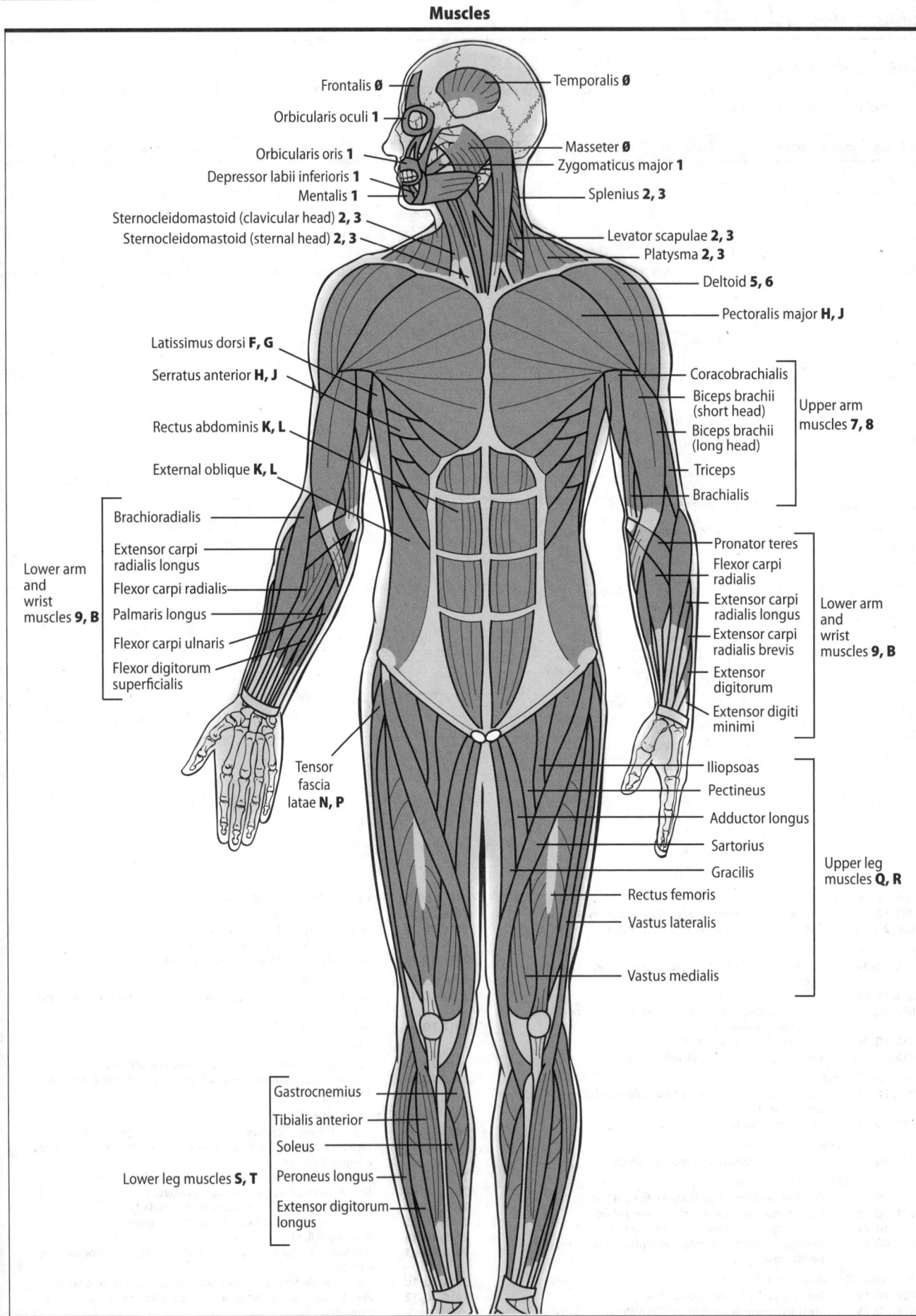

Frontalis **Ø**
Temporalis **Ø**
Orbicularis oculi **1**
Orbicularis oris **1**
Masseter **Ø**
Zygomaticus major **1**
Depressor labii inferioris **1**
Mentalis **1**
Splenius **2, 3**
Sternocleidomastoid (clavicular head) **2, 3**
Sternocleidomastoid (sternal head) **2, 3**
Levator scapulae **2, 3**
Platysma **2, 3**
Deltoid **5, 6**
Pectoralis major **H, J**
Latissimus dorsi **F, G**
Serratus anterior **H, J**
Coracobrachialis
Biceps brachii (short head)
Biceps brachii (long head)
Triceps
Brachialis
Upper arm muscles **7, 8**
Rectus abdominis **K, L**
External oblique **K, L**
Brachioradialis
Extensor carpi radialis longus
Flexor carpi radialis
Palmaris longus
Flexor carpi ulnaris
Flexor digitorum superficialis
Lower arm and wrist muscles **9, B**
Pronator teres
Flexor carpi radialis
Extensor carpi radialis longus
Extensor carpi radialis brevis
Extensor digitorum
Extensor digiti minimi
Lower arm and wrist muscles **9, B**
Tensor fascia latae **N, P**
Iliopsoas
Pectineus
Adductor longus
Sartorius
Gracilis
Rectus femoris
Vastus lateralis
Vastus medialis
Upper leg muscles **Q, R**
Gastrocnemius
Tibialis anterior
Soleus
Peroneus longus
Extensor digitorum longus
Lower leg muscles **S, T**

Ø **Medical and Surgical**
K **Muscles**
2 **Change**   Definition: Taking out or off a device from a body part and putting back an identical or similar device in or on the same body part without cutting or puncturing the skin or a mucous membrane

Explanation: All CHANGE procedures are coded using the approach EXTERNAL

Body Part Character 4	Approach Character 5	Device Character 6	Qualifier Character 7
X Upper Muscle Y Lower Muscle	X External	Ø Drainage Device Y Other Device	Z No Qualifier

Non-OR	All body part, approach, device, and qualifier values

Ø **Medical and Surgical**
K **Muscles**
5 **Destruction**   Definition: Physical eradication of all or a portion of a body part by the direct use of energy, force, or a destructive agent

Explanation: None of the body part is physically taken out

Body Part Character 4			Approach Character 5	Device Character 6	Qualifier Character 7

Ø **Head Muscle**
  Auricularis muscle
  Masseter muscle
  Pterygoid muscle
  Splenius capitis muscle
  Temporalis muscle
  Temporoparietalis muscle
1 **Facial Muscle**
  Buccinator muscle
  Corrugator supercilii muscle
  Depressor anguli oris muscle
  Depressor labii inferioris muscle
  Depressor septi nasi muscle
  Depressor supercilii muscle
  Levator anguli oris muscle
  Levator labii superioris alaeque
    nasi muscle
  Levator labii superioris muscle
  Mentalis muscle
  Nasalis muscle
  Occipitofrontalis muscle
  Orbicularis oris muscle
  Procerus muscle
  Risorius muscle
  Zygomaticus muscle
2 **Neck Muscle, Right**
  Anterior vertebral muscle
  Arytenoid muscle
  Cricothyroid muscle
  Infrahyoid muscle
  Levator scapulae muscle
  Platysma muscle
  Scalene muscle
  Splenius cervicis muscle
  Sternocleidomastoid muscle
  Suprahyoid muscle
  Thyroarytenoid muscle
3 **Neck Muscle, Left**
  See 2 Neck Muscle, Right
4 **Tongue, Palate, Pharynx**
  Muscle
  Chondroglossus muscle
  Genioglossus muscle
  Hyoglossus muscle
  Inferior longitudinal muscle
  Levator veli palatini muscle
  Palatoglossal muscle
  Palatopharyngeal muscle
  Pharyngeal constrictor muscle
  Salpingopharyngeus muscle
  Styloglossus muscle
  Stylopharyngeus muscle
  Superior longitudinal muscle
  Tensor veli palatini muscle
5 **Shoulder Muscle, Right**
  Deltoid muscle
  Infraspinatus muscle
  Subscapularis muscle
  Supraspinatus muscle
  Teres major muscle
  Teres minor muscle
6 **Shoulder Muscle, Left**
  See 5 Shoulder Muscle, Right
	7 **Upper Arm Muscle, Right**
	  Biceps brachii muscle
	  Brachialis muscle
	  Coracobrachialis muscle
	  Triceps brachii muscle
	8 **Upper Arm Muscle, Left**
	  See 7 Upper Arm Muscle, Right
	9 **Lower Arm and Wrist Muscle,**
	  Right
	  Anatomical snuffbox
	  Brachioradialis muscle
	  Extensor carpi radialis muscle
	  Extensor carpi ulnaris muscle
	  Flexor carpi radialis muscle
	  Flexor carpi ulnaris muscle
	  Flexor pollicis longus muscle
	  Palmaris longus muscle
	  Pronator quadratus muscle
	  Pronator teres muscle
	B **Lower Arm and Wrist Muscle,**
	  Left
	  See 9 Lower Arm and Wrist
	    Muscle, Right
	C **Hand Muscle, Right**
	  Hypothenar muscle
	  Palmar interosseous muscle
	  Thenar muscle
	D **Hand Muscle, Left**
	  See C Hand Muscle, Right
	F **Trunk Muscle, Right**
	  Coccygeus muscle
	  Erector spinae muscle
	  Interspinalis muscle
	  Intertransversarius muscle
	  Latissimus dorsi muscle
	  Quadratus lumborum muscle
	  Rhomboid major muscle
	  Rhomboid minor muscle
	  Serratus posterior muscle
	  Transversospinalis muscle
	  Trapezius muscle
	G **Trunk Muscle, Left**
	  See F Trunk Muscle, Right
	H **Thorax Muscle, Right**
	  Intercostal muscle
	  Levatores costarum muscle
	  Pectoralis major muscle
	  Pectoralis minor muscle
	  Serratus anterior muscle
	  Subclavius muscle
	  Subcostal muscle
	  Transverse thoracis muscle
	J **Thorax Muscle, Left**
	  See H Thorax Muscle, Right
	K **Abdomen Muscle, Right**
	  External oblique muscle
	  Internal oblique muscle
	  Pyramidalis muscle
	  Rectus abdominis muscle
	  Transversus abdominis muscle
	L **Abdomen Muscle, Left**
	  See K Abdomen Muscle, Right
		M **Perineum Muscle**
		  Bulbospongiosus muscle
		  Cremaster muscle
		  Deep transverse perineal muscle
		  Ischiocavernosus muscle
		  Levator ani muscle
		  Superficial transverse perineal
		    muscle
		N **Hip Muscle, Right**
		  Gemellus muscle
		  Gluteus maximus muscle
		  Gluteus medius muscle
		  Gluteus minimus muscle
		  Iliacus muscle
		  Obturator muscle
		  Piriformis muscle
		  Psoas muscle
		  Quadratus femoris muscle
		  Tensor fasciae latae muscle
		P **Hip Muscle, Left**
		  See N Hip Muscle, Right
		Q **Upper Leg Muscle, Right**
		  Adductor brevis muscle
		  Adductor longus muscle
		  Adductor magnus muscle
		  Biceps femoris muscle
		  Gracilis muscle
		  Pectineus muscle
		  Quadriceps (femoris)
		  Rectus femoris muscle
		  Sartorius muscle
		  Semimembranosus muscle
		  Semitendinosus muscle
		  Vastus intermedius muscle
		  Vastus lateralis muscle
		  Vastus medialis muscle
		R **Upper Leg Muscle, Left**
		  See Q Upper Leg Muscle, Right
		S **Lower Leg Muscle, Right**
		  Extensor digitorum longus
		    muscle
		  Extensor hallucis longus muscle
		  Fibularis brevis muscle
		  Fibularis longus muscle
		  Flexor digitorum longus muscle
		  Flexor hallucis longus muscle
		  Gastrocnemius muscle
		  Peroneus brevis muscle
		  Peroneus longus muscle
		  Popliteus muscle
		  Soleus muscle
		  Tibialis anterior muscle
		  Tibialis posterior muscle
		T **Lower Leg Muscle, Left**
		  See S Lower Leg Muscle, Right
		V **Foot Muscle, Right**
		  Abductor hallucis muscle
		  Adductor hallucis muscle
		  Extensor digitorum brevis muscle
		  Extensor hallucis brevis muscle
		  Flexor digitorum brevis muscle
		  Flexor hallucis brevis muscle
		  Quadratus plantae muscle
		W **Foot Muscle, Left**
		  See V Foot Muscle, Right
			Ø Open
			3 Percutaneous
			4 Percutaneous
			  Endoscopic
				Z No Device	Z No Qualifier

NC Noncovered Procedure   **LC** Limited Coverage   **QA** Questionable OB Admit   **NT** New Tech Add-on   ⊞ Combination Member   ♂ Male   ♀ Female

ICD-10-PCS 2024   467

ØK2–ØK5

Ø   Medical and Surgical
K   Muscles
8   Division
     Definition: Cutting into a body part, without draining fluids and/or gases from the body part, in order to separate or transect a body part
     Explanation: All or a portion of the body part is separated into two or more portions

Body Part Character 4			Approach Character 5	Device Character 6	Qualifier Character 7

Ø Head Muscle
Auricularis muscle
Masseter muscle
Pterygoid muscle
Splenius capitis muscle
Temporalis muscle
Temporoparietalis muscle
1 Facial Muscle
Buccinator muscle
Corrugator supercilii
  muscle
Depressor anguli oris
  muscle
Depressor labii inferioris
  muscle
Depressor septi nasi muscle
Depressor supercilii muscle
Levator anguli oris muscle
Levator labii superioris
  alaeque nasi muscle
Levator labii superioris
  muscle
Mentalis muscle
Nasalis muscle
Occipitofrontalis muscle
Orbicularis oris muscle
Procerus muscle
Risorius muscle
Zygomaticus muscle
2 Neck Muscle, Right
Anterior vertebral muscle
Arytenoid muscle
Cricothyroid muscle
Infrahyoid muscle
Levator scapulae muscle
Platysma muscle
Scalene muscle
Splenius cervicis muscle
Sternocleidomastoid
  muscle
Suprahyoid muscle
Thyroarytenoid muscle
3 Neck Muscle, Left
See 2 Neck Muscle, Right
Tensor veli palatini muscle
5 Shoulder Muscle, Right
Deltoid muscle
Infraspinatus muscle
Subscapularis muscle
Supraspinatus muscle
Teres major muscle
Teres minor muscle
6 Shoulder Muscle, Left
See 5 Shoulder Muscle, Right
7 Upper Arm Muscle, Right
Biceps brachii muscle
Brachialis muscle
Coracobrachialis muscle
Triceps brachii muscle
8 Upper Arm Muscle, Left
See 7 Upper Arm Muscle,
  Right
	9 Lower Arm and Wrist Muscle,
	  Right
	Anatomical snuffbox
	Brachioradialis muscle
	Extensor carpi radialis muscle
	Extensor carpi ulnaris muscle
	Flexor carpi radialis muscle
	Flexor carpi ulnaris muscle
	Flexor pollicis longus muscle
	Palmaris longus muscle
	Pronator quadratus muscle
	Pronator teres muscle
	B Lower Arm and Wrist Muscle,
	  Left
	See 9 Lower Arm and Wrist
	  Muscle, Right
	C Hand Muscle, Right
	Hypothenar muscle
	Palmar interosseous muscle
	Thenar muscle
	D Hand Muscle, Left
	See C Hand Muscle, Right
	F Trunk Muscle, Right
	Coccygeus muscle
	Erector spinae muscle
	Interspinalis muscle
	Intertransversarius muscle
	Latissimus dorsi muscle
	Quadratus lumborum muscle
	Rhomboid major muscle
	Rhomboid minor muscle
	Serratus posterior muscle
	Transversospinalis muscle
	Trapezius muscle
	G Trunk Muscle, Left
	See F Trunk Muscle, Right
	H Thorax Muscle, Right
	Intercostal muscle
	Levatores costarum muscle
	Pectoralis major muscle
	Pectoralis minor muscle
	Serratus anterior muscle
	Subclavius muscle
	Subcostal muscle
	Transverse thoracis muscle
	J Thorax Muscle, Left
	See H Thorax Muscle, Right
	K Abdomen Muscle, Right
	External oblique muscle
	Internal oblique muscle
	Pyramidalis muscle
	Rectus abdominis muscle
	Transversus abdominis muscle
	L Abdomen Muscle, Left
	See K Abdomen Muscle, Right
	M Perineum Muscle
	Bulbospongiosus muscle
	Cremaster muscle
	Deep transverse perineal muscle
	Ischiocavernosus muscle
	Levator ani muscle
	Superficial transverse perineal
	  muscle
		N Hip Muscle, Right
		Gemellus muscle
		Gluteus maximus muscle
		Gluteus medius muscle
		Gluteus minimus muscle
		Iliacus muscle
		Obturator muscle
		Piriformis muscle
		Psoas muscle
		Quadratus femoris muscle
		Tensor fasciae latae muscle
		P Hip Muscle, Left
		See N Hip Muscle, Right
		Q Upper Leg Muscle, Right
		Adductor brevis muscle
		Adductor longus muscle
		Adductor magnus muscle
		Biceps femoris muscle
		Gracilis muscle
		Pectineus muscle
		Quadriceps (femoris)
		Rectus femoris muscle
		Sartorius muscle
		Semimembranosus muscle
		Semitendinosus muscle
		Vastus intermedius muscle
		Vastus lateralis muscle
		Vastus medialis muscle
		R Upper Leg Muscle, Left
		See Q Upper Leg Muscle, Right
		S Lower Leg Muscle, Right
		Extensor digitorum longus
		  muscle
		Extensor hallucis longus
		  muscle
		Fibularis brevis muscle
		Fibularis longus muscle
		Flexor digitorum longus
		  muscle
		Flexor hallucis longus muscle
		Gastrocnemius muscle
		Peroneus brevis muscle
		Peroneus longus muscle
		Popliteus muscle
		Soleus muscle
		Tibialis anterior muscle
		Tibialis posterior muscle
		T Lower Leg Muscle, Left
		See S Lower Leg Muscle, Right
		V Foot Muscle, Right
		Abductor hallucis muscle
		Adductor hallucis muscle
		Extensor digitorum brevis
		  muscle
		Extensor hallucis brevis
		  muscle
		Flexor digitorum brevis
		  muscle
		Flexor hallucis brevis muscle
		Quadratus plantae muscle
		W Foot Muscle, Left
		See V Foot Muscle, Right
			Ø Open
			3 Percutaneous
			4 Percutaneous
			  Endoscopic
				Z No Device	**Z** No Qualifier

4 Tongue, Palate, Pharynx Muscle
Chondroglossus muscle
Genioglossus muscle
Hyoglossus muscle
Inferior longitudinal muscle
Levator veli palatini muscle
Palatoglossal muscle
Palatopharyngeal muscle
Pharyngeal constrictor muscle
Salpingopharyngeus muscle
Styloglossus muscle
Stylopharyngeus muscle
Superior longitudinal muscle
Tensor veli palatini muscle
			Ø Open
			3 Percutaneous
			4 Percutaneous
			  Endoscopic
			7 Via Natural or
			  Artificial
			  Opening
			8 Via Natural or
			  Artificial
			  Opening
			  Endoscopic
				Z No Device	**Z** No Qualifier

Non-OR Procedure   DRG Non-OR Procedure   Valid OR Procedure   HAC Associated Procedure   Combination Only   New/Revised April   New/Revised October

468   ICD-10-PCS 2024

ØK8–ØK8

Ø   Medical and Surgical
K   Muscles
9   Drainage   Definition: Taking or letting out fluids and/or gases from a body part

Explanation: The qualifier DIAGNOSTIC is used to identify drainage procedures that are biopsies

Body Part Character 4			Approach Character 5	Device Character 6	Qualifier Character 7
Ø Head Muscle Auricularis muscle Masseter muscle Pterygoid muscle Splenius capitis muscle Temporalis muscle Temporoparietalis muscle **1 Facial Muscle** Buccinator muscle Corrugator supercilii muscle Depressor anguli oris muscle Depressor labii inferioris muscle Depressor septi nasi muscle Depressor supercilii muscle Levator anguli oris muscle Levator labii superioris alaeque nasi muscle Levator labii superioris muscle Mentalis muscle Nasalis muscle Occipitofrontalis muscle Orbicularis oris muscle Procerus muscle Risorius muscle Zygomaticus muscle **2 Neck Muscle, Right** Anterior vertebral muscle Arytenoid muscle Cricothyroid muscle Infrahyoid muscle Levator scapulae muscle Platysma muscle Scalene muscle Splenius cervicis muscle Sternocleidomastoid muscle Suprahyoid muscle Thyroarytenoid muscle **3 Neck Muscle, Left** *See 2 Neck Muscle, Right* **4 Tongue, Palate, Pharynx Muscle** Chondroglossus muscle Genioglossus muscle Hyoglossus muscle Inferior longitudinal muscle Levator veli palatini muscle Palatoglossal muscle Palatopharyngeal muscle Pharyngeal constrictor muscle Salpingopharyngeus muscle Styloglossus muscle Stylopharyngeus muscle Superior longitudinal muscle Tensor veli palatini muscle **5 Shoulder Muscle, Right** Deltoid muscle Infraspinatus muscle Subscapularis muscle Supraspinatus muscle Teres major muscle Teres minor muscle **6 Shoulder Muscle, Left** *See 5 Shoulder Muscle, Right*	**7 Upper Arm Muscle, Right** Biceps brachii muscle Brachialis muscle Coracobrachialis muscle Triceps brachii muscle **8 Upper Arm Muscle, Left** *See 7 Upper Arm Muscle, Right* **9 Lower Arm and Wrist Muscle, Right** Anatomical snuffbox Brachioradialis muscle Extensor carpi radialis muscle Extensor carpi ulnaris muscle Flexor carpi radialis muscle Flexor carpi ulnaris muscle Flexor pollicis longus muscle Palmaris longus muscle Pronator quadratus muscle Pronator teres muscle **B Lower Arm and Wrist Muscle, Left** *See 9 Lower Arm and Wrist Muscle, Right* **C Hand Muscle, Right** Hypothenar muscle Palmar interosseous muscle Thenar muscle **D Hand Muscle, Left** *See C Hand Muscle, Right* **F Trunk Muscle, Right** Coccygeus muscle Erector spinae muscle Interspinalis muscle Intertransversarius muscle Latissimus dorsi muscle Quadratus lumborum muscle Rhomboid major muscle Rhomboid minor muscle Serratus posterior muscle Transversospinalis muscle Trapezius muscle **G Trunk Muscle, Left** *See F Trunk Muscle, Right* **H Thorax Muscle, Right** Intercostal muscle Levatores costarum muscle Pectoralis major muscle Pectoralis minor muscle Serratus anterior muscle Subclavius muscle Subcostal muscle Transverse thoracis muscle **J Thorax Muscle, Left** *See H Thorax Muscle, Right* **K Abdomen Muscle, Right** External oblique muscle Internal oblique muscle Pyramidalis muscle Rectus abdominis muscle Transversus abdominis muscle **L Abdomen Muscle, Left** *See K Abdomen Muscle, Right*	**M Perineum Muscle** Bulbospongiosus muscle Cremaster muscle Deep transverse perineal muscle Ischiocavernosus muscle Levator ani muscle Superficial transverse perineal muscle **N Hip Muscle, Right** Gemellus muscle Gluteus maximus muscle Gluteus medius muscle Gluteus minimus muscle Iliacus muscle Obturator muscle Piriformis muscle Psoas muscle Quadratus femoris muscle Tensor fasciae latae muscle **P Hip Muscle, Left** *See N Hip Muscle, Right* **Q Upper Leg Muscle, Right** Adductor brevis muscle Adductor longus muscle Adductor magnus muscle Biceps femoris muscle Gracilis muscle Pectineus muscle Quadriceps (femoris) Rectus femoris muscle Sartorius muscle Semimembranosus muscle Semitendinosus muscle Vastus intermedius muscle Vastus lateralis muscle Vastus medialis muscle **R Upper Leg Muscle, Left** *See Q Upper Leg Muscle, Right* **S Lower Leg Muscle, Right** Extensor digitorum longus muscle Extensor hallucis longus muscle Fibularis brevis muscle Fibularis longus muscle Flexor digitorum longus muscle Flexor hallucis longus muscle Gastrocnemius muscle Peroneus brevis muscle Peroneus longus muscle Popliteus muscle Soleus muscle Tibialis anterior muscle Tibialis posterior muscle **T Lower Leg Muscle, Left** *See S Lower Leg Muscle, Right* **V Foot Muscle, Right** Abductor hallucis muscle Adductor hallucis muscle Extensor digitorum brevis muscle Extensor hallucis brevis muscle Flexor digitorum brevis muscle Flexor hallucis brevis muscle Quadratus plantae muscle **W Foot Muscle, Left** *See V Foot Muscle, Right*	**Ø Open** **3 Percutaneous** **4 Percutaneous Endoscopic**	**Ø Drainage Device**	**Z No Qualifier**

Non-OR   ØK9[Ø,1,2,3,4,5,6,7,8,9,B,C,D,F,G,H,J,K,L,M,N,P,Q,R,S,T,V,W]3ØZ

ØK9 Continued on next page

NC Noncovered Procedure   LC Limited Coverage   QA Questionable OB Admit   NT New Tech Add-on   ✛ Combination Member   ♂ Male   ♀ Female

ICD-10-PCS 2024   469

Muscles

ØK9–ØK9

Ø **Medical and Surgical**   *ØK9 Continued*
K **Muscles**
9 **Drainage**   Definition: Taking or letting out fluids and/or gases from a body part
                     Explanation: The qualifier DIAGNOSTIC is used to identify drainage procedures that are biopsies

Body Part Character 4		Approach Character 5	Device Character 6	Qualifier Character 7
Ø Head Muscle	**7 Upper Arm Muscle, Right**	**Ø Open**	**Z No Device**	**X Diagnostic**
Auricularis muscle	Biceps brachii muscle	**3 Percutaneous**		**Z No Qualifier**
Masseter muscle	Brachialis muscle	**4 Percutaneous**		
Pterygoid muscle	Coracobrachialis muscle	**Endoscopic**		
Splenius capitis muscle	Triceps brachii muscle			
Temporalis muscle	**8 Upper Arm Muscle, Left**			
Temporoparietalis muscle	*See 7 Upper Arm Muscle, Right*			
1 Facial Muscle	**9 Lower Arm and Wrist Muscle, Right**			
Buccinator muscle	Anatomical snuffbox			
Corrugator supercilii muscle	Brachioradialis muscle			
Depressor anguli oris muscle	Extensor carpi radialis muscle			
Depressor labii inferioris muscle	Extensor carpi ulnaris muscle			
Depressor septi nasi muscle	Flexor carpi radialis muscle			
Depressor supercilii muscle	Flexor carpi ulnaris muscle			
Levator anguli oris muscle	Flexor pollicis longus muscle			
Levator labii superioris alaeque nasi muscle	Palmaris longus muscle			
Levator labii superioris muscle	Pronator quadratus muscle			
Mentalis muscle	Pronator teres muscle			
Nasalis muscle	**B Lower Arm and Wrist Muscle, Left**			
Occipitofrontalis muscle	*See 9 Lower Arm and Wrist Muscle, Right*			
Orbicularis oris muscle	**C Hand Muscle, Right**			
Procerus muscle	Hypothenar muscle			
Risorius muscle	Palmar interosseous muscle			
Zygomaticus muscle	Thenar muscle			
2 Neck Muscle, Right	**D Hand Muscle, Left**			
Anterior vertebral muscle	*See C Hand Muscle, Right*			
Arytenoid muscle	**F Trunk Muscle, Right**			
Cricothyroid muscle	Coccygeus muscle			
Infrahyoid muscle	Erector spinae muscle			
Levator scapulae muscle	Interspinalis muscle			
Platysma muscle	Intertransversarius muscle			
Scalene muscle	Latissimus dorsi muscle			
Splenius cervicis muscle	Quadratus lumborum muscle			
Sternocleidomastoid muscle	Rhomboid major muscle			
Suprahyoid muscle	Rhomboid minor muscle			
Thyroarytenoid muscle	Serratus posterior muscle			
3 Neck Muscle, Left	Transversospinalis muscle			
See 2 Neck Muscle, Right	Trapezius muscle			
4 Tongue, Palate, Pharynx Muscle	**G Trunk Muscle, Left**			
Chondroglossus muscle	*See F Trunk Muscle, Right*			
Genioglossus muscle	**H Thorax Muscle, Right**			
Hyoglossus muscle	Intercostal muscle			
Inferior longitudinal muscle	Levatores costarum muscle			
Levator veli palatini muscle	Pectoralis major muscle			
Palatoglossal muscle	Pectoralis minor muscle			
Palatopharyngeal muscle	Serratus anterior muscle			
Pharyngeal constrictor muscle	Subclavius muscle			
Salpingopharyngeus muscle	Subcostal muscle			
Styloglossus muscle	Transverse thoracis muscle			
Stylopharyngeus muscle	**J Thorax Muscle, Left**			
Superior longitudinal muscle	*See H Thorax Muscle, Right*			
Tensor veli palatini muscle	**K Abdomen Muscle, Right**			
5 Shoulder Muscle, Right	External oblique muscle			
Deltoid muscle	Internal oblique muscle			
Infraspinatus muscle	Pyramidalis muscle			
Subscapularis muscle	Rectus abdominis muscle			
Supraspinatus muscle	Transversus abdominis muscle			
Teres major muscle	**L Abdomen Muscle, Left**			
Teres minor muscle	*See K Abdomen Muscle, Right*			
6 Shoulder Muscle, Left				
See 5 Shoulder Muscle, Right				

Middle/Right columns (Body Part continued):

M Perineum Muscle
Bulbospongiosus muscle
Cremaster muscle
Deep transverse perineal muscle
Ischiocavernosus muscle
Levator ani muscle
Superficial transverse perineal muscle

N Hip Muscle, Right
Gemellus muscle
Gluteus maximus muscle
Gluteus medius muscle
Gluteus minimus muscle
Iliacus muscle
Obturator muscle
Piriformis muscle
Psoas muscle
Quadratus femoris muscle
Tensor fasciae latae muscle

P Hip Muscle, Left
See N Hip Muscle, Right

Q Upper Leg Muscle, Right
Adductor brevis muscle
Adductor longus muscle
Adductor magnus muscle
Biceps femoris muscle
Gracilis muscle
Pectineus muscle
Quadriceps (femoris)
Rectus femoris muscle
Sartorius muscle
Semimembranosus muscle
Semitendinosus muscle
Vastus intermedius muscle
Vastus lateralis muscle
Vastus medialis muscle

R Upper Leg Muscle, Left
See Q Upper Leg Muscle, Right

S Lower Leg Muscle, Right
Extensor digitorum longus muscle
Extensor hallucis longus muscle
Fibularis brevis muscle
Fibularis longus muscle
Flexor digitorum longus muscle
Flexor hallucis longus muscle
Gastrocnemius muscle
Peroneus brevis muscle
Peroneus longus muscle
Popliteus muscle
Soleus muscle
Tibialis anterior muscle
Tibialis posterior muscle

T Lower Leg Muscle, Left
See S Lower Leg Muscle, Right

V Foot Muscle, Right
Abductor hallucis muscle
Adductor hallucis muscle
Extensor digitorum brevis muscle
Extensor hallucis brevis muscle
Flexor digitorum brevis muscle
Flexor hallucis brevis muscle
Quadratus plantae muscle

W Foot Muscle, Left
See V Foot Muscle, Right

Non-OR   ØK9[Ø,1,2,3,4,5,6,7,8,9,B,F,G,H,J,K,L,M,N,P,Q,R,S,T,V,W]3ZZ
Non-OR   ØK9[C,D][3,4]ZZ

Non-OR Procedure   DRG Non-OR Procedure   Valid OR Procedure   HAC Associated Procedure   Combination Only   New/Revised April   New/Revised October

470   ICD-10-PCS 2024

Ø   **Medical and Surgical**
K   **Muscles**
B   **Excision**   Definition: Cutting out or off, without replacement, a portion of a body part
                Explanation: The qualifier DIAGNOSTIC is used to identify excision procedures that are biopsies

Body Part Character 4			Approach Character 5	Device Character 6	Qualifier Character 7
Ø Head Muscle	**7 Upper Arm Muscle, Right**	**M Perineum Muscle**	**Ø Open**	**Z No Device**	**X Diagnostic**
Auricularis muscle	Biceps brachii muscle	Bulbospongiosus muscle	**3 Percutaneous**		**Z No Qualifier**
Masseter muscle	Brachialis muscle	Cremaster muscle	**4 Percutaneous**		
Pterygoid muscle	Coracobrachialis muscle	Deep transverse perineal	**Endoscopic**		
Splenius capitis muscle	Triceps brachii muscle	muscle			
Temporalis muscle	**8 Upper Arm Muscle, Left**	Ischiocavernosus muscle			
Temporoparietalis muscle	*See 7 Upper Arm Muscle,*	Levator ani muscle			
1 Facial Muscle	*Right*	Superficial transverse			
Buccinator muscle	**9 Lower Arm and Wrist**	perineal muscle			
Corrugator supercilii	**Muscle, Right**	**N Hip Muscle, Right**			
muscle	Anatomical snuffbox	Gemellus muscle			
Depressor anguli oris	Brachioradialis muscle	Gluteus maximus muscle			
muscle	Extensor carpi radialis	Gluteus medius muscle			
Depressor labii inferioris	muscle	Gluteus minimus muscle			
muscle	Extensor carpi ulnaris	Iliacus muscle			
Depressor septi nasi	muscle	Obturator muscle			
muscle	Flexor carpi radialis	Piriformis muscle			
Depressor supercilii	muscle	Psoas muscle			
muscle	Flexor carpi ulnaris muscle	Quadratus femoris muscle			
Levator anguli oris muscle	Flexor pollicis longus	Tensor fasciae latae			
Levator labii superioris	muscle	muscle			
alaeque nasi muscle	Palmaris longus muscle	**P Hip Muscle, Left**			
Levator labii superioris	Pronator quadratus	*See N Hip Muscle, Right*			
muscle	muscle	**Q Upper Leg Muscle, Right**			
Mentalis muscle	Pronator teres muscle	Adductor brevis muscle			
Nasalis muscle	**B Lower Arm and Wrist**	Adductor longus muscle			
Occipitofrontalis muscle	**Muscle, Left**	Adductor magnus muscle			
Orbicularis oris muscle	*See 9 Lower Arm and Wrist*	Biceps femoris muscle			
Procerus muscle	*Muscle, Right*	Gracilis muscle			
Risorius muscle	**C Hand Muscle, Right**	Pectineus muscle			
Zygomaticus muscle	Hypothenar muscle	Quadriceps (femoris)			
2 Neck Muscle, Right	Palmar interosseous	Rectus femoris muscle			
Anterior vertebral muscle	muscle	Sartorius muscle			
Arytenoid muscle	Thenar muscle	Semimembranosus			
Cricothyroid muscle	**D Hand Muscle, Left**	muscle			
Infrahyoid muscle	*See C Hand Muscle, Right*	Semitendinosus muscle			
Levator scapulae muscle	**F Trunk Muscle, Right**	Vastus intermedius muscle			
Platysma muscle	Coccygeus muscle	Vastus lateralis muscle			
Scalene muscle	Erector spinae muscle	Vastus medialis muscle			
Splenius cervicis muscle	Interspinalis muscle	**R Upper Leg Muscle, Left**			
Sternocleidomastoid	Intertransversarius muscle	*See Q Upper Leg Muscle,*			
muscle	Latissimus dorsi muscle	*Right*			
Suprahyoid muscle	Quadratus lumborum	**S Lower Leg Muscle, Right**			
Thyroarytenoid muscle	muscle	Extensor digitorum longus			
3 Neck Muscle, Left	Rhomboid major muscle	muscle			
See 2 Neck Muscle, Right	Rhomboid minor muscle	Extensor hallucis longus			
4 Tongue, Palate, Pharynx	Serratus posterior muscle	muscle			
Muscle	Transversospinalis muscle	Fibularis brevis muscle			
Chondroglossus muscle	Trapezius muscle	Fibularis longus muscle			
Genioglossus muscle	**G Trunk Muscle, Left**	Flexor digitorum longus			
Hyoglossus muscle	*See F Trunk Muscle, Right*	muscle			
Inferior longitudinal	**H Thorax Muscle; Right**	Flexor hallucis longus			
muscle	Intercostal muscle	muscle			
Levator veli palatini	Levatores costarum	Gastrocnemius muscle			
muscle	muscle	Peroneus brevis muscle			
Palatoglossal muscle	Pectoralis major muscle	Peroneus longus muscle			
Palatopharyngeal muscle	Pectoralis minor muscle	Popliteus muscle			
Pharyngeal constrictor	Serratus anterior muscle	Soleus muscle			
muscle	Subclavius muscle	Tibialis anterior muscle			
Salpingopharyngeus	Subcostal muscle	Tibialis posterior muscle			
muscle	Transverse thoracis	**T Lower Leg Muscle, Left**			
Styloglossus muscle	muscle	*See S Lower Leg Muscle,*			
Stylopharyngeus muscle	**J Thorax Muscle, Left**	*Right*			
Superior longitudinal	*See H Thorax Muscle, Right*	**V Foot Muscle, Right**			
muscle	**K Abdomen Muscle, Right**	Abductor hallucis muscle			
Tensor veli palatini muscle	External oblique muscle	Adductor hallucis muscle			
5 Shoulder Muscle, Right	Internal oblique muscle	Extensor digitorum brevis			
Deltoid muscle	Pyramidalis muscle	muscle			
Infraspinatus muscle	Rectus abdominis muscle	Extensor hallucis brevis			
Subscapularis muscle	Transversus abdominis	muscle			
Supraspinatus muscle	muscle	Flexor digitorum brevis			
Teres major muscle	**L Abdomen Muscle, Left**	muscle			
Teres minor muscle	*See K Abdomen Muscle,*	Flexor hallucis brevis			
6 Shoulder Muscle, Left	*Right*	muscle			
See 5 Shoulder Muscle,		Quadratus plantae muscle			
Right	**W Foot Muscle, Left**				
	See V Foot Muscle, Right				

Non-OR   ØKB[N,P]3Z[X,Z]

NC Noncovered Procedure   LC Limited Coverage   QA Questionable OB Admit   NT New Tech Add-on   ⊞ Combination Member   ♂ Male   ♀ Female

ICD-10-PCS 2024   471

ØKB–ØKB

Muscles

Ø　Medical and Surgical
K　Muscles
C　Extirpation　　Definition: Taking or cutting out solid matter from a body part

Explanation: The solid matter may be an abnormal byproduct of a biological function or a foreign body; it may be imbedded in a body part or in the lumen of a tubular body part. The solid matter may or may not have been previously broken into pieces.

Body Part Character 4			Approach Character 5	Device Character 6	Qualifier Character 7
Ø Head Muscle Auricularis muscle Masseter muscle Pterygoid muscle Splenius capitis muscle Temporalis muscle Temporoparietalis muscle **1 Facial Muscle** Buccinator muscle Corrugator supercilii muscle Depressor anguli oris muscle Depressor labii inferioris muscle Depressor septi nasi muscle Depressor supercilii muscle Levator anguli oris muscle Levator labii superioris alaeque nasi muscle Levator labii superioris muscle Mentalis muscle Nasalis muscle Occipitofrontalis muscle Orbicularis oris muscle Procerus muscle Risorius muscle Zygomaticus muscle **2 Neck Muscle, Right** Anterior vertebral muscle Arytenoid muscle Cricothyroid muscle Infrahyoid muscle Levator scapulae muscle Platysma muscle Scalene muscle Splenius cervicis muscle Sternocleidomastoid muscle Suprahyoid muscle Thyroarytenoid muscle **3 Neck Muscle, Left** *See 2 Neck Muscle, Right* **4 Tongue, Palate, Pharynx Muscle** Chondroglossus muscle Genioglossus muscle Hyoglossus muscle Inferior longitudinal muscle Levator veli palatini muscle Palatoglossal muscle Palatopharyngeal muscle Pharyngeal constrictor muscle Salpingopharyngeus muscle Styloglossus muscle Stylopharyngeus muscle Superior longitudinal muscle Tensor veli palatini muscle **5 Shoulder Muscle, Right** Deltoid muscle Infraspinatus muscle Subscapularis muscle Supraspinatus muscle Teres major muscle Teres minor muscle **6 Shoulder Muscle, Left** *See 5 Shoulder Muscle, Right*	**7 Upper Arm Muscle, Right** Biceps brachii muscle Brachialis muscle Coracobrachialis muscle Triceps brachii muscle **8 Upper Arm Muscle, Left** *See 7 Upper Arm Muscle, Right* **9 Lower Arm and Wrist Muscle, Right** Anatomical snuffbox Brachioradialis muscle Extensor carpi radialis muscle Extensor carpi ulnaris muscle Flexor carpi radialis muscle Flexor carpi ulnaris muscle Flexor pollicis longus muscle Palmaris longus muscle Pronator quadratus muscle Pronator teres muscle **B Lower Arm and Wrist Muscle, Left** *See 9 Lower Arm and Wrist Muscle, Right* **C Hand Muscle, Right** Hypothenar muscle Palmar interosseous muscle Thenar muscle **D Hand Muscle, Left** *See C Hand Muscle, Right* **F Trunk Muscle, Right** Coccygeus muscle Erector spinae muscle Interspinalis muscle Intertransversarius muscle Latissimus dorsi muscle Quadratus lumborum muscle Rhomboid major muscle Rhomboid minor muscle Serratus posterior muscle Transversospinalis muscle Trapezius muscle **G Trunk Muscle, Left** *See F Trunk Muscle, Right* **H Thorax Muscle, Right** Intercostal muscle Levatores costarum muscle Pectoralis major muscle Pectoralis minor muscle Serratus anterior muscle Subclavius muscle Subcostal muscle Transverse thoracis muscle **J Thorax Muscle, Left** *See H Thorax Muscle, Right* **K Abdomen Muscle, Right** External oblique muscle Internal oblique muscle Pyramidalis muscle Rectus abdominis muscle Transversus abdominis muscle **L Abdomen Muscle, Left** *See K Abdomen Muscle, Right*	**M Perineum Muscle** Bulbospongiosus muscle Cremaster muscle Deep transverse perineal muscle Ischiocavernosus muscle Levator ani muscle Superficial transverse perineal muscle **N Hip Muscle, Right** Gemellus muscle Gluteus maximus muscle Gluteus medius muscle Gluteus minimus muscle Iliacus muscle Obturator muscle Piriformis muscle Psoas muscle Quadratus femoris muscle Tensor fasciae latae muscle **P Hip Muscle, Left** *See N Hip Muscle, Right* **Q Upper Leg Muscle, Right** Adductor brevis muscle Adductor longus muscle Adductor magnus muscle Biceps femoris muscle Gracilis muscle Pectineus muscle Quadriceps (femoris) Rectus femoris muscle Sartorius muscle Semimembranosus muscle Semitendinosus muscle Vastus intermedius muscle Vastus lateralis muscle Vastus medialis muscle **R Upper Leg Muscle, Left** *See Q Upper Leg Muscle, Right* **S Lower Leg Muscle, Right** Extensor digitorum longus muscle Extensor hallucis longus muscle Fibularis brevis muscle Fibularis longus muscle Flexor digitorum longus muscle Flexor hallucis longus muscle Gastrocnemius muscle Peroneus brevis muscle Peroneus longus muscle Popliteus muscle Soleus muscle Tibialis anterior muscle Tibialis posterior muscle **T Lower Leg Muscle, Left** *See S Lower Leg Muscle, Right* **V Foot Muscle, Right** Abductor hallucis muscle Adductor hallucis muscle Extensor digitorum brevis muscle Extensor hallucis brevis muscle Flexor digitorum brevis muscle Flexor hallucis brevis muscle Quadratus plantae muscle **W Foot Muscle, Left** *See V Foot Muscle, Right*	**Ø Open** **3 Percutaneous** **4 Percutaneous Endoscopic**	**Z No Device**	**Z No Qualifier**

Ø   **Medical and Surgical**
K   **Muscles**
D   **Extraction**   Definition: Pulling or stripping out or off all or a portion of a body part by the use of force
                       Explanation: The qualifier DIAGNOSTIC is used to identify extraction procedures that are biopsies

Body Part Character 4			Approach Character 5	Device Character 6	Qualifier Character 7
Ø Head Muscle Auricularis muscle Masseter muscle Pterygoid muscle Splenius capitis muscle Temporalis muscle Temporoparietalis muscle **1 Facial Muscle** Buccinator muscle Corrugator supercilii muscle Depressor anguli oris muscle Depressor labii inferioris muscle Depressor septi nasi muscle Depressor supercilii muscle Levator anguli oris muscle Levator labii superioris alaeque nasi muscle Levator labii superioris muscle Mentalis muscle Nasalis muscle Occipitofrontalis muscle Orbicularis oris muscle Procerus muscle Risorius muscle Zygomaticus muscle **2 Neck Muscle, Right** Anterior vertebral muscle Arytenoid muscle Cricothyroid muscle Infrahyoid muscle Levator scapulae muscle Platysma muscle Scalene muscle Splenius cervicis muscle Sternocleidomastoid muscle Suprahyoid muscle Thyroarytenoid muscle **3 Neck Muscle, Left** *See 2 Neck Muscle, Right* **4 Tongue, Palate, Pharynx Muscle** Chondroglossus muscle Genioglossus muscle Hyoglossus muscle Inferior longitudinal muscle Levator veli palatini muscle Palatoglossal muscle Palatopharyngeal muscle Pharyngeal constrictor muscle Salpingopharyngeus muscle Styloglossus muscle Stylopharyngeus muscle Superior longitudinal muscle Tensor veli palatini muscle **5 Shoulder Muscle, Right** Deltoid muscle Infraspinatus muscle Subscapularis muscle Supraspinatus muscle Teres major muscle Teres minor muscle **6 Shoulder Muscle, Left** *See 5 Shoulder Muscle, Right*	**7 Upper Arm Muscle, Right** Biceps brachii muscle Brachialis muscle Coracobrachialis muscle Triceps brachii muscle **8 Upper Arm Muscle, Left** *See 7 Upper Arm Muscle, Right* **9 Lower Arm and Wrist Muscle, Right** Anatomical snuffbox Brachioradialis muscle Extensor carpi radialis muscle Extensor carpi ulnaris muscle Flexor carpi radialis muscle Flexor carpi ulnaris muscle Flexor pollicis longus muscle Palmaris longus muscle Pronator quadratus muscle Pronator teres muscle **B Lower Arm and Wrist Muscle, Left** *See 9 Lower Arm and Wrist Muscle, Right* **C Hand Muscle, Right** Hypothenar muscle Palmar interosseous muscle Thenar muscle **D Hand Muscle, Left** *See C Hand Muscle, Right* **F Trunk Muscle, Right** Coccygeus muscle Erector spinae muscle Interspinalis muscle Intertransversarius muscle Latissimus dorsi muscle Quadratus lumborum muscle Rhomboid major muscle Rhomboid minor muscle Serratus posterior muscle Transversospinalis muscle Trapezius muscle **G Trunk Muscle, Left** *See F Trunk Muscle, Right* **H Thorax Muscle, Right** Intercostal muscle Levatores costarum muscle Pectoralis major muscle Pectoralis minor muscle Serratus anterior muscle Subclavius muscle Subcostal muscle Transverse thoracis muscle **J Thorax Muscle, Left** *See H Thorax Muscle, Right* **K Abdomen Muscle, Right** External oblique muscle Internal oblique muscle Pyramidalis muscle Rectus abdominis muscle Transversus abdominis muscle **L Abdomen Muscle, Left** *See K Abdomen Muscle, Right*	**M Perineum Muscle** Bulbospongiosus muscle Cremaster muscle Deep transverse perineal muscle Ischiocavernosus muscle Levator ani muscle Superficial transverse perineal muscle **N Hip Muscle, Right** Gemellus muscle Gluteus maximus muscle Gluteus medius muscle Gluteus minimus muscle Iliacus muscle Obturator muscle Piriformis muscle Psoas muscle Quadratus femoris muscle Tensor fasciae latae muscle **P Hip Muscle, Left** *See N Hip Muscle, Right* **Q Upper Leg Muscle, Right** Adductor brevis muscle Adductor longus muscle Adductor magnus muscle Biceps femoris muscle Gracilis muscle Pectineus muscle Quadriceps (femoris) Rectus femoris muscle Sartorius muscle Semimembranosus muscle Semitendinosus muscle Vastus intermedius muscle Vastus lateralis muscle Vastus medialis muscle **R Upper Leg Muscle, Left** *See Q Upper Leg Muscle, Right* **S Lower Leg Muscle, Right** Extensor digitorum longus muscle Extensor hallucis longus muscle Fibularis brevis muscle Fibularis longus muscle Flexor digitorum longus muscle Flexor hallucis longus muscle Gastrocnemius muscle Peroneus brevis muscle Peroneus longus muscle Popliteus muscle Soleus muscle Tibialis anterior muscle Tibialis posterior muscle **T Lower Leg Muscle, Left** *See S Lower Leg Muscle, Right* **V Foot Muscle, Right** Abductor hallucis muscle Adductor hallucis muscle Extensor digitorum brevis muscle Extensor hallucis brevis muscle Flexor digitorum brevis muscle Flexor hallucis brevis muscle Quadratus plantae muscle **W Foot Muscle, Left** *See V Foot Muscle, Right*	**Ø Open**	**Z No Device**	**Z No Qualifier**

NC Noncovered Procedure   LC Limited Coverage   QA Questionable OB Admit   NT New Tech Add-on   ✛ Combination Member   ♂ Male   ♀ Female

ICD-10-PCS 2024   473

ØKD–ØKD

Ø   **Medical and Surgical**
K   **Muscles**
H   **Insertion**   Definition: Putting in a nonbiological appliance that monitors, assists, performs, or prevents a physiological function but does not physically take the place of a body part

             Explanation: None

Body Part Character 4	Approach Character 5	Device Character 6	Qualifier Character 7
X Upper Muscle Y Lower Muscle	Ø Open 3 Percutaneous 4 Percutaneous Endoscopic	M Stimulator Lead Y Other Device	Z No Qualifier

Non-OR   ØKH[X,Y][3,4]YZ

Ø   **Medical and Surgical**
K   **Muscles**
J   **Inspection**   Definition: Visually and/or manually exploring a body part

             Explanation: Visual exploration may be performed with or without optical instrumentation. Manual exploration may be performed directly or through intervening body layers.

Body Part Character 4	Approach Character 5	Device Character 6	Qualifier Character 7
X Upper Muscle Y Lower Muscle	Ø Open 3 Percutaneous 4 Percutaneous Endoscopic X External	Z No Device	Z No Qualifier

Non-OR   ØKJ[X,Y][3,X]ZZ

Non-OR Procedure   DRG Non-OR Procedure   Valid OR Procedure   HAC Associated Procedure   Combination Only   New/Revised April   New/Revised October

474   ICD-10-PCS 2024

ØKH–ØKJ

Ø Medical and Surgical
K Muscles
M Reattachment   Definition: Putting back in or on all or a portion of a separated body part to its normal location or other suitable location

Explanation: Vascular circulation and nervous pathways may or may not be reestablished

Body Part Character 4			Approach Character 5	Device Character 6	Qualifier Character 7
Ø Head Muscle Auricularis muscle Masseter muscle Pterygoid muscle Splenius capitis muscle Temporalis muscle Temporoparietalis muscle **1 Facial Muscle** Buccinator muscle Corrugator supercilii muscle Depressor anguli oris muscle Depressor labii inferioris muscle Depressor septi nasi muscle Depressor supercilii muscle Levator anguli oris muscle Levator labii superioris alaeque nasi muscle Levator labii superioris muscle Mentalis muscle Nasalis muscle Occipitofrontalis muscle Orbicularis oris muscle Procerus muscle Risorius muscle Zygomaticus muscle **2 Neck Muscle, Right** Anterior vertebral muscle Arytenoid muscle Cricothyroid muscle Infrahyoid muscle Levator scapulae muscle Platysma muscle Scalene muscle Splenius cervicis muscle Sternocleidomastoid muscle Suprahyoid muscle Thyroarytenoid muscle **3 Neck Muscle, Left** *See 2 Neck Muscle, Right* **4 Tongue, Palate, Pharynx Muscle** Chondroglossus muscle Genioglossus muscle Hyoglossus muscle Inferior longitudinal muscle Levator veli palatini muscle Palatoglossal muscle Palatopharyngeal muscle Pharyngeal constrictor muscle Salpingopharyngeus muscle Styloglossus muscle Stylopharyngeus muscle Superior longitudinal muscle Tensor veli palatini muscle **5 Shoulder Muscle, Right** Deltoid muscle Infraspinatus muscle Subscapularis muscle Supraspinatus muscle Teres major muscle Teres minor muscle **6 Shoulder Muscle, Left** *See 5 Shoulder Muscle, Right*	**7 Upper Arm Muscle, Right** Biceps brachii muscle Brachialis muscle Coracobrachialis muscle Triceps brachii muscle **8 Upper Arm Muscle, Left** *See 7 Upper Arm Muscle, Right* **9 Lower Arm and Wrist Muscle, Right** Anatomical snuffbox Brachioradialis muscle Extensor carpi radialis muscle Extensor carpi ulnaris muscle Flexor carpi radialis muscle Flexor carpi ulnaris muscle Flexor pollicis longus muscle Palmaris longus muscle Pronator quadratus muscle Pronator teres muscle **B Lower Arm and Wrist Muscle, Left** *See 9 Lower Arm and Wrist Muscle, Right* **C Hand Muscle, Right** Hypothenar muscle Palmar interosseous muscle Thenar muscle **D Hand Muscle, Left** *See C Hand Muscle, Right* **F Trunk Muscle, Right** Coccygeus muscle Erector spinae muscle Interspinalis muscle Intertransversarius muscle Latissimus dorsi muscle Quadratus lumborum muscle Rhomboid major muscle Rhomboid minor muscle Serratus posterior muscle Transversospinalis muscle Trapezius muscle **G Trunk Muscle, Left** *See F Trunk Muscle, Right* **H Thorax Muscle, Right** Intercostal muscle Levatores costarum muscle Pectoralis major muscle Pectoralis minor muscle Serratus anterior muscle Subclavius muscle Subcostal muscle Transverse thoracis muscle **J Thorax Muscle, Left** *See H Thorax Muscle, Right* **K Abdomen Muscle, Right** External oblique muscle Internal oblique muscle Pyramidalis muscle Rectus abdominis muscle Transversus abdominis muscle **L Abdomen Muscle, Left** *See K Abdomen Muscle, Right*	**M Perineum Muscle** Bulbospongiosus muscle Cremaster muscle Deep transverse perineal muscle Ischiocavernosus muscle Levator ani muscle Superficial transverse perineal muscle **N Hip Muscle, Right** Gemellus muscle Gluteus maximus muscle Gluteus medius muscle Gluteus minimus muscle Iliacus muscle Obturator muscle Piriformis muscle Psoas muscle Quadratus femoris muscle Tensor fasciae latae muscle **P Hip Muscle, Left** *See N Hip Muscle, Right* **Q Upper Leg Muscle, Right** Adductor brevis muscle Adductor longus muscle Adductor magnus muscle Biceps femoris muscle Gracilis muscle Pectineus muscle Quadriceps (femoris) Rectus femoris muscle Sartorius muscle Semimembranosus muscle Semitendinosus muscle Vastus intermedius muscle Vastus lateralis muscle Vastus medialis muscle **R Upper Leg Muscle, Left** *See Q Upper Leg Muscle, Right* **S Lower Leg Muscle, Right** Extensor digitorum longus muscle Extensor hallucis longus muscle Fibularis brevis muscle Fibularis longus muscle Flexor digitorum longus muscle Flexor hallucis longus muscle Gastrocnemius muscle Peroneus brevis muscle Peroneus longus muscle Popliteus muscle Soleus muscle Tibialis anterior muscle Tibialis posterior muscle **T Lower Leg Muscle, Left** *See S Lower Leg Muscle, Right* **V Foot Muscle, Right** Abductor hallucis muscle Adductor hallucis muscle Extensor digitorum brevis muscle Extensor hallucis brevis muscle Flexor digitorum brevis muscle Flexor hallucis brevis muscle Quadratus plantae muscle **W Foot Muscle, Left** *See V Foot Muscle, Right*	**Ø** Open **4** Percutaneous Endoscopic	**Z** No Device	**Z** No Qualifier

NC Noncovered Procedure   LC Limited Coverage   QA Questionable OB Admit   NT New Tech Add-on   ⊞ Combination Member   ♂ Male   ♀ Female

ICD-10-PCS 2024   475

ØKM–ØKM

Ø   **Medical and Surgical**
K   **Muscles**
N   **Release**   Definition: Freeing a body part from an abnormal physical constraint by cutting or by the use of force
                   Explanation: Some of the restraining tissue may be taken out but none of the body part is taken out

Body Part Character 4			Approach Character 5	Device Character 6	Qualifier Character 7
Ø Head Muscle Auricularis muscle Masseter muscle Pterygoid muscle Splenius capitis muscle Temporalis muscle Temporoparietalis muscle **1 Facial Muscle** Buccinator muscle Corrugator supercilii muscle Depressor anguli oris muscle Depressor labii inferioris muscle Depressor septi nasi muscle Depressor supercilii muscle Levator anguli oris muscle Levator labii superioris alaeque nasi muscle Levator labii superioris muscle Mentalis muscle Nasalis muscle Occipitofrontalis muscle Orbicularis oris muscle Procerus muscle Risorius muscle Zygomaticus muscle **2 Neck Muscle, Right** Anterior vertebral muscle Arytenoid muscle Cricothyroid muscle Infrahyoid muscle Levator scapulae muscle Platysma muscle Scalene muscle Splenius cervicis muscle Sternocleidomastoid muscle Suprahyoid muscle Thyroarytenoid muscle **3 Neck Muscle, Left** *See 2 Neck Muscle, Right* **4 Tongue, Palate, Pharynx Muscle** Chondroglossus muscle Genioglossus muscle Hyoglossus muscle Inferior longitudinal muscle Levator veli palatini muscle Palatoglossal muscle Palatopharyngeal muscle Pharyngeal constrictor muscle Salpingopharyngeus muscle Styloglossus muscle Stylopharyngeus muscle Superior longitudinal muscle Tensor veli palatini muscle **5 Shoulder Muscle, Right** Deltoid muscle Infraspinatus muscle Subscapularis muscle Supraspinatus muscle Teres major muscle Teres minor muscle **6 Shoulder Muscle, Left** *See 5 Shoulder Muscle, Right*	**7 Upper Arm Muscle, Right** Biceps brachii muscle Brachialis muscle Coracobrachialis muscle Triceps brachii muscle **8 Upper Arm Muscle, Left** *See 7 Upper Arm Muscle, Right* **9 Lower Arm and Wrist Muscle, Right** Anatomical snuffbox Brachioradialis muscle Extensor carpi radialis muscle Extensor carpi ulnaris muscle Flexor carpi radialis muscle Flexor carpi ulnaris muscle Flexor pollicis longus muscle Palmaris longus muscle Pronator quadratus muscle Pronator teres muscle **B Lower Arm and Wrist Muscle, Left** *See 9 Lower Arm and Wrist Muscle, Right* **C Hand Muscle, Right** Hypothenar muscle Palmar interosseous muscle Thenar muscle **D Hand Muscle, Left** *See C Hand Muscle, Right* **F Trunk Muscle, Right** Coccygeus muscle Erector spinae muscle Interspinalis muscle Intertransversarius muscle Latissimus dorsi muscle Quadratus lumborum muscle Rhomboid major muscle Rhomboid minor muscle Serratus posterior muscle Transversospinalis muscle Trapezius muscle **G Trunk Muscle, Left** *See F Trunk Muscle, Right* **H Thorax Muscle, Right** Intercostal muscle Levatores costarum muscle Pectoralis major muscle Pectoralis minor muscle Serratus anterior muscle Subclavius muscle Subcostal muscle Transverse thoracis muscle **J Thorax Muscle, Left** *See H Thorax Muscle, Right* **K Abdomen Muscle, Right** External oblique muscle Internal oblique muscle Pyramidalis muscle Rectus abdominis muscle Transversus abdominis muscle **L Abdomen Muscle, Left** *See K Abdomen Muscle, Right*	**M Perineum Muscle** Bulbospongiosus muscle Cremaster muscle Deep transverse perineal muscle Ischiocavernosus muscle Levator ani muscle Superficial transverse perineal muscle **N Hip Muscle, Right** Gemellus muscle Gluteus maximus muscle Gluteus medius muscle Gluteus minimus muscle Iliacus muscle Obturator muscle Piriformis muscle Psoas muscle Quadratus femoris muscle Tensor fasciae latae muscle **P Hip Muscle, Left** *See N Hip Muscle, Right* **Q Upper Leg Muscle, Right** Adductor brevis muscle Adductor longus muscle Adductor magnus muscle Biceps femoris muscle Gracilis muscle Pectineus muscle Quadriceps (femoris) Rectus femoris muscle Sartorius muscle Semimembranosus muscle Semitendinosus muscle Vastus intermedius muscle Vastus lateralis muscle Vastus medialis muscle **R Upper Leg Muscle, Left** *See Q Upper Leg Muscle, Right* **S Lower Leg Muscle, Right** Extensor digitorum longus muscle Extensor hallucis longus muscle Fibularis brevis muscle Fibularis longus muscle Flexor digitorum longus muscle Flexor hallucis longus muscle Gastrocnemius muscle Peroneus brevis muscle Peroneus longus muscle Popliteus muscle Soleus muscle Tibialis anterior muscle Tibialis posterior muscle **T Lower Leg Muscle, Left** *See S Lower Leg Muscle, Right* **V Foot Muscle, Right** Abductor hallucis muscle Adductor hallucis muscle Extensor digitorum brevis muscle Extensor hallucis brevis muscle Flexor digitorum brevis muscle Flexor hallucis brevis muscle Quadratus plantae muscle **W Foot Muscle, Left** *See V Foot Muscle, Right*	**Ø** Open **3** Percutaneous **4** Percutaneous Endoscopic **X** External	**Z** No Device	**Z** No Qualifier

Non-OR   ØKN[Ø,1,2,3,4,5,6,7,8,9,B,C,D,F,G,H,J,K,L,M,N,P,Q,R,S,T,V,W]XZZ

Non-OR Procedure   DRG Non-OR Procedure   Valid OR Procedure   HAC Associated Procedure   Combination Only   New/Revised April   New/Revised October

476   ICD-10-PCS 2024

Ø   Medical and Surgical
K   Muscles
P   Removal   Definition: Taking out or off a device from a body part

Explanation: If a device is taken out and a similar device put in without cutting or puncturing the skin or mucous membrane, the procedure is coded to the root operation CHANGE. Otherwise, the procedure for taking out a device is coded to the root operation REMOVAL.

Body Part Character 4	Approach Character 5	Device Character 6	Qualifier Character 7
X Upper Muscle Y Lower Muscle	Ø Open 3 Percutaneous 4 Percutaneous Endoscopic	Ø Drainage Device 7 Autologous Tissue Substitute J Synthetic Substitute K Nonautologous Tissue Substitute M Stimulator Lead Y Other Device	Z No Qualifier
X Upper Muscle Y Lower Muscle	X External	Ø Drainage Device M Stimulator Lead	Z No Qualifier

Non-OR   ØKP[X,Y][3,4]YZ
Non-OR   ØKP[X,Y]X[Ø,M]Z

NC Noncovered Procedure   LC Limited Coverage   UA Questionable OB Admit   NT New Tech Add-on   ⊞ Combination Member   ♂ Male   ♀ Female

ICD-10-PCS 2024   477

ØKP–ØKP

Ø   Medical and Surgical
K   Muscles
Q   Repair   Definition: Restoring, to the extent possible, a body part to its normal anatomic structure and function

                     Explanation: Used only when the method to accomplish the repair is not one of the other root operations

Body Part Character 4			Approach Character 5	Device Character 6	Qualifier Character 7
Ø Head Muscle Auricularis muscle Masseter muscle Pterygoid muscle Splenius capitis muscle Temporalis muscle Temporoparietalis muscle **1 Facial Muscle** Buccinator muscle Corrugator supercilii muscle Depressor anguli oris muscle Depressor labii inferioris muscle Depressor septi nasi muscle Depressor supercilii muscle Levator anguli oris muscle Levator labii superioris alaeque nasi muscle Levator labii superioris muscle Mentalis muscle Nasalis muscle Occipitofrontalis muscle Orbicularis oris muscle Procerus muscle Risorius muscle Zygomaticus muscle **2 Neck Muscle, Right** Anterior vertebral muscle Arytenoid muscle Cricothyroid muscle Infrahyoid muscle Levator scapulae muscle Platysma muscle Scalene muscle Splenius cervicis muscle Sternocleidomastoid muscle Suprahyoid muscle Thyroarytenoid muscle **3 Neck Muscle, Left** *See 2 Neck Muscle, Right* **4 Tongue, Palate, Pharynx Muscle** Chondroglossus muscle Genioglossus muscle Hyoglossus muscle Inferior longitudinal muscle Levator veli palatini muscle Palatoglossal muscle Palatopharyngeal muscle Pharyngeal constrictor muscle Salpingopharyngeus muscle Styloglossus muscle Stylopharyngeus muscle Superior longitudinal muscle Tensor veli palatini muscle **5 Shoulder Muscle, Right** Deltoid muscle Infraspinatus muscle Subscapularis muscle Supraspinatus muscle Teres major muscle Teres minor muscle **6 Shoulder Muscle, Left** *See 5 Shoulder Muscle, Right*	**7 Upper Arm Muscle, Right** Biceps brachii muscle Brachialis muscle Coracobrachialis muscle Triceps brachii muscle **8 Upper Arm Muscle, Left** *See 7 Upper Arm Muscle, Right* **9 Lower Arm and Wrist Muscle, Right** Anatomical snuffbox Brachioradialis muscle Extensor carpi radialis muscle Extensor carpi ulnaris muscle Flexor carpi radialis muscle Flexor carpi ulnaris muscle Flexor pollicis longus muscle Palmaris longus muscle Pronator quadratus muscle Pronator teres muscle **B Lower Arm and Wrist Muscle, Left** *See 9 Lower Arm and Wrist Muscle, Right* **C Hand Muscle, Right** Hypothenar muscle Palmar interosseous muscle Thenar muscle **D Hand Muscle, Left** *See C Hand Muscle, Right* **F Trunk Muscle, Right** Coccygeus muscle Erector spinae muscle Interspinalis muscle Intertransversarius muscle Latissimus dorsi muscle Quadratus lumborum muscle Rhomboid major muscle Rhomboid minor muscle Serratus posterior muscle Transversospinalis muscle Trapezius muscle **G Trunk Muscle, Left** *See F Trunk Muscle, Right* **H Thorax Muscle, Right** Intercostal muscle Levatores costarum muscle Pectoralis major muscle Pectoralis minor muscle Serratus anterior muscle Subclavius muscle Subcostal muscle Transverse thoracis muscle **J Thorax Muscle, Left** *See H Thorax Muscle, Right* **K Abdomen Muscle, Right** External oblique muscle Internal oblique muscle Pyramidalis muscle Rectus abdominis muscle Transversus abdominis muscle **L Abdomen Muscle, Left** *See K Abdomen Muscle, Right*	**M Perineum Muscle** Bulbospongiosus muscle Cremaster muscle Deep transverse perineal muscle Ischiocavernosus muscle Levator ani muscle Superficial transverse perineal muscle **N Hip Muscle, Right** Gemellus muscle Gluteus maximus muscle Gluteus medius muscle Gluteus minimus muscle Iliacus muscle Obturator muscle Piriformis muscle Psoas muscle Quadratus femoris muscle Tensor fasciae latae muscle **P Hip Muscle, Left** *See N Hip Muscle, Right* **Q Upper Leg Muscle, Right** Adductor brevis muscle Adductor longus muscle Adductor magnus muscle Biceps femoris muscle Gracilis muscle Pectineus muscle Quadriceps (femoris) Rectus femoris muscle Sartorius muscle Semimembranosus muscle Semitendinosus muscle Vastus intermedius muscle Vastus lateralis muscle Vastus medialis muscle **R Upper Leg Muscle, Left** *See Q Upper Leg Muscle, Right* **S Lower Leg Muscle, Right** Extensor digitorum longus muscle Extensor hallucis longus muscle Fibularis brevis muscle Fibularis longus muscle Flexor digitorum longus muscle Flexor hallucis longus muscle Gastrocnemius muscle Peroneus brevis muscle Peroneus longus muscle Popliteus muscle Soleus muscle Tibialis anterior muscle Tibialis posterior muscle **T Lower Leg Muscle, Left** *See S Lower Leg Muscle, Right* **V Foot Muscle, Right** Abductor hallucis muscle Adductor hallucis muscle Extensor digitorum brevis muscle Extensor hallucis brevis muscle Flexor digitorum brevis muscle Flexor hallucis brevis muscle Quadratus plantae muscle **W Foot Muscle, Left** *See V Foot Muscle, Right*	**Ø Open** **3 Percutaneous** **4 Percutaneous Endoscopic**	**Z No Device**	**Z No Qualifier**

Non-OR Procedure   DRG Non-OR Procedure   Valid OR Procedure   HAC Associated Procedure   Combination Only   New/Revised April   New/Revised October

478

ØKQ–ØKQ

ICD-10-PCS 2024

Ø   **Medical and Surgical**
K   **Muscles**
R   **Replacement**   Definition: Putting in or on biological or synthetic material that physically takes the place and/or function of all or a portion of a body part
                Explanation: The body part may have been taken out or replaced, or may be taken out, physically eradicated, or rendered nonfunctional during the REPLACEMENT procedure. A REMOVAL procedure is coded for taking out the device used in a previous replacement procedure.

Body Part Character 4			Approach Character 5	Device Character 6	Qualifier Character 7

Ø   **Head Muscle**
Auricularis muscle
Masseter muscle
Pterygoid muscle
Splenius capitis muscle
Temporalis muscle
Temporoparietalis muscle
1   **Facial Muscle**
Buccinator muscle
Corrugator supercilii
    muscle
Depressor anguli oris
    muscle
Depressor labii inferioris
    muscle
Depressor septi nasi
    muscle
Depressor supercilii
    muscle
Levator anguli oris muscle
Levator labii superioris
    alaeque nasi muscle
Levator labii superioris
    muscle
Mentalis muscle
Nasalis muscle
Occipitofrontalis muscle
Orbicularis oris muscle
Procerus muscle
Risorius muscle
Zygomaticus muscle
2   **Neck Muscle, Right**
Anterior vertebral muscle
Arytenoid muscle
Cricothyroid muscle
Infrahyoid muscle
Levator scapulae muscle
Platysma muscle
Scalene muscle
Splenius cervicis muscle
Sternocleidomastoid
    muscle
Suprahyoid muscle
Thyroarytenoid muscle
3   **Neck Muscle, Left**
See 2 Neck Muscle, Right
4   **Tongue, Palate, Pharynx**
    Muscle
Chondroglossus muscle
Genioglossus muscle
Hyoglossus muscle
Inferior longitudinal
    muscle
Levator veli palatini
    muscle
Palatoglossal muscle
Palatopharyngeal muscle
Pharyngeal constrictor
    muscle
Salpingopharyngeus
    muscle
Styloglossus muscle
Stylopharyngeus muscle
Superior longitudinal
    muscle
Tensor veli palatini muscle
5   **Shoulder Muscle, Right**
Deltoid muscle
Infraspinatus muscle
Subscapularis muscle
Supraspinatus muscle
Teres major muscle
Teres minor muscle
6   **Shoulder Muscle, Left**
See 5 Shoulder Muscle,
    Right
	7 **Upper Arm Muscle, Right**
	Biceps brachii muscle
	Brachialis muscle
	Coracobrachialis muscle
	Triceps brachii muscle
	8 **Upper Arm Muscle, Left**
	See 7 Upper Arm Muscle,
	    Right
	9 **Lower Arm and Wrist**
	    Muscle, Right
	Anatomical snuffbox
	Brachioradialis muscle
	Extensor carpi radialis
	    muscle
	Extensor carpi ulnaris
	    muscle
	Flexor carpi radialis
	    muscle
	Flexor carpi ulnaris muscle
	Flexor pollicis longus
	    muscle
	Palmaris longus muscle
	Pronator quadratus
	    muscle
	Pronator teres muscle
	B **Lower Arm and Wrist**
	    Muscle, Left
	See 9 Lower Arm and Wrist
	    Muscle, Right
	C **Hand Muscle, Right**
	Hypothenar muscle
	Palmar interosseous
	    muscle
	Thenar muscle
	D **Hand Muscle, Left**
	See C Hand Muscle, Right
	F **Trunk Muscle, Right**
	Coccygeus muscle
	Erector spinae muscle
	Interspinalis muscle
	Intertransversarius muscle
	Latissimus dorsi muscle
	Quadratus lumborum
	    muscle
	Rhomboid major muscle
	Rhomboid minor muscle
	Serratus posterior muscle
	Transversospinalis muscle
	Trapezius muscle
	G **Trunk Muscle, Left**
	See F Trunk Muscle, Right
	H **Thorax Muscle, Right**
	Intercostal muscle
	Levatores costarum
	    muscle
	Pectoralis major muscle
	Pectoralis minor muscle
	Serratus anterior muscle
	Subclavius muscle
	Subcostal muscle
	Transverse thoracis
	    muscle
	J **Thorax Muscle, Left**
	See H Thorax Muscle, Right
	K **Abdomen Muscle, Right**
	External oblique muscle
	Internal oblique muscle
	Pyramidalis muscle
	Rectus abdominis muscle
	Transversus abdominis
	    muscle
	L **Abdomen Muscle, Left**
	See K Abdomen Muscle,
	    Right
		M **Perineum Muscle**
		Bulbospongiosus muscle
		Cremaster muscle
		Deep transverse perineal
		    muscle
		Ischiocavernosus muscle
		Levator ani muscle
		Superficial transverse
		    perineal muscle
		N **Hip Muscle, Right**
		Gemellus muscle
		Gluteus maximus muscle
		Gluteus medius muscle
		Gluteus minimus muscle
		Iliacus muscle
		Obturator muscle
		Piriformis muscle
		Psoas muscle
		Quadratus femoris muscle
		Tensor fasciae latae
		    muscle
		P **Hip Muscle, Left**
		See N Hip Muscle, Right
		Q **Upper Leg Muscle, Right**
		Adductor brevis muscle
		Adductor longus muscle
		Adductor magnus muscle
		Biceps femoris muscle
		Gracilis muscle
		Pectineus muscle
		Quadriceps (femoris)
		Rectus femoris muscle
		Sartorius muscle
		Semimembranosus
		    muscle
		Semitendinosus muscle
		Vastus intermedius muscle
		Vastus lateralis muscle
		Vastus medialis muscle
		R **Upper Leg Muscle, Left**
		See Q Upper Leg Muscle,
		    Right
		S **Lower Leg Muscle, Right**
		Extensor digitorum longus
		    muscle
		Extensor hallucis longus
		    muscle
		Fibularis brevis muscle
		Fibularis longus muscle
		Flexor digitorum longus
		    muscle
		Flexor hallucis longus
		    muscle
		Gastrocnemius muscle
		Peroneus brevis muscle
		Peroneus longus muscle
		Popliteus muscle
		Soleus muscle
		Tibialis anterior muscle
		Tibialis posterior muscle
		T **Lower Leg Muscle, Left**
		See S Lower Leg Muscle,
		    Right
		V **Foot Muscle, Right**
		Abductor hallucis muscle
		Adductor hallucis muscle
		Extensor digitorum brevis
		    muscle
		Extensor hallucis brevis
		    muscle
		Flexor digitorum brevis
		    muscle
		Flexor hallucis brevis
		    muscle
		Quadratus plantae muscle
		W **Foot Muscle, Left**
		See V Foot Muscle, Right
			Ø **Open**
			4 **Percutaneous**
			    Endoscopic
				7 **Autologous Tissue**
				    Substitute
				J **Synthetic**
				    Substitute
				K **Nonautologous**
				    Tissue Substitute
					Z **No Qualifier**

NC Noncovered Procedure   **LC** Limited Coverage   **QA** Questionable OB Admit   **NT** New Tech Add-on   ⊞ Combination Member   ♂ Male   ♀ Female

ICD-10-PCS 2024   479

ØKR–ØKR

Ø   Medical and Surgical
K   Muscles
S   Reposition   Definition: Moving to its normal location, or other suitable location, all or a portion of a body part

Explanation: The body part is moved to a new location from an abnormal location, or from a normal location where it is not functioning correctly. The body part may or may not be cut out or off to be moved to the new location.

Body Part Character 4			Approach Character 5	Device Character 6	Qualifier Character 7

Ø Head Muscle
Auricularis muscle
Masseter muscle
Pterygoid muscle
Splenius capitis muscle
Temporalis muscle
Temporoparietalis muscle
1 Facial Muscle
Buccinator muscle
Corrugator supercilii
  muscle
Depressor anguli oris
  muscle
Depressor labii inferioris
  muscle
Depressor septi nasi
  muscle
Depressor supercilii
  muscle
Levator anguli oris muscle
Levator labii superioris
  alaeque nasi muscle
Levator labii superioris
  muscle
Mentalis muscle
Nasalis muscle
Occipitofrontalis muscle
Orbicularis oris muscle
Procerus muscle
Risorius muscle
Zygomaticus muscle
2 Neck Muscle, Right
Anterior vertebral muscle
Arytenoid muscle
Cricothyroid muscle
Infrahyoid muscle
Levator scapulae muscle
Platysma muscle
Scalene muscle
Splenius cervicis muscle
Sternocleidomastoid
  muscle
Suprahyoid muscle
Thyroarytenoid muscle
3 Neck Muscle, Left
See 2 Neck Muscle, Right
**4 Tongue, Palate, Pharynx
  Muscle**
Chondroglossus muscle
Genioglossus muscle
Hyoglossus muscle
Inferior longitudinal
  muscle
Levator veli palatini
  muscle
Palatoglossal muscle
Palatopharyngeal muscle
Pharyngeal constrictor
  muscle
Salpingopharyngeus
  muscle
Styloglossus muscle
Stylopharyngeus muscle
Superior longitudinal
  muscle
Tensor veli palatini muscle
5 Shoulder Muscle, Right
Deltoid muscle
Infraspinatus muscle
Subscapularis muscle
Supraspinatus muscle
Teres major muscle
Teres minor muscle
6 Shoulder Muscle, Left
*See 5 Shoulder Muscle,
  Right*
	7 Upper Arm Muscle, Right
	Biceps brachii muscle
	Brachialis muscle
	Coracobrachialis muscle
	Triceps brachii muscle
	8 Upper Arm Muscle, Left
	*See 7 Upper Arm Muscle,
	  Right*
	**9 Lower Arm and Wrist
	  Muscle, Right**
	Anatomical snuffbox
	Brachioradialis muscle
	Extensor carpi radialis
	  muscle
	Extensor carpi ulnaris
	  muscle
	Flexor carpi radialis
	  muscle
	Flexor carpi ulnaris muscle
	Flexor pollicis longus
	  muscle
	Palmaris longus muscle
	Pronator quadratus
	  muscle
	Pronator teres muscle
	**B Lower Arm and Wrist
	  Muscle, Left**
	*See 9 Lower Arm and Wrist
	  Muscle, Right*
	C Hand Muscle, Right
	Hypothenar muscle
	Palmar interosseous
	  muscle
	Thenar muscle
	D Hand Muscle, Left
	See C Hand Muscle, Right
	F Trunk Muscle, Right
	Coccygeus muscle
	Erector spinae muscle
	Interspinalis muscle
	Intertransversarius muscle
	Latissimus dorsi muscle
	Quadratus lumborum
	  muscle
	Rhomboid major muscle
	Rhomboid minor muscle
	Serratus posterior muscle
	Transversospinalis muscle
	Trapezius muscle
	G Trunk Muscle, Left
	See F Trunk Muscle, Right
	H Thorax Muscle, Right
	Intercostal muscle
	Levatores costarum
	  muscle
	Pectoralis major muscle
	Pectoralis minor muscle
	Serratus anterior muscle
	Subclavius muscle
	Subcostal muscle
	Transverse thoracis
	  muscle
	J Thorax Muscle, Left
	See H Thorax Muscle, Right
	K Abdomen Muscle, Right
	External oblique muscle
	Internal oblique muscle
	Pyramidalis muscle
	Rectus abdominis muscle
	Transversus abdominis
	  muscle
	L Abdomen Muscle, Left
	*See K Abdomen Muscle,
	  Right*
		M Perineum Muscle
		Bulbospongiosus muscle
		Cremaster muscle
		Deep transverse perineal
		  muscle
		Ischiocavernosus muscle
		Levator ani muscle
		Superficial transverse
		  perineal muscle
		N Hip Muscle, Right
		Gemellus muscle
		Gluteus maximus muscle
		Gluteus medius muscle
		Gluteus minimus muscle
		Iliacus muscle
		Obturator muscle
		Piriformis muscle
		Psoas muscle
		Quadratus femoris muscle
		Tensor fasciae latae
		  muscle
		P Hip Muscle, Left
		See N Hip Muscle, Right
		Q Upper Leg Muscle, Right
		Adductor brevis muscle
		Adductor longus muscle
		Adductor magnus muscle
		Biceps femoris muscle
		Gracilis muscle
		Pectineus muscle
		Quadriceps (femoris)
		Rectus femoris muscle
		Sartorius muscle
		Semimembranosus
		  muscle
		Semitendinosus muscle
		Vastus intermedius muscle
		Vastus lateralis muscle
		Vastus medialis muscle
		R Upper Leg Muscle, Left
		*See Q Upper Leg Muscle,
		  Right*
		S Lower Leg Muscle, Right
		Extensor digitorum longus
		  muscle
		Extensor hallucis longus
		  muscle
		Fibularis brevis muscle
		Fibularis longus muscle
		Flexor digitorum longus
		  muscle
		Flexor hallucis longus
		  muscle
		Gastrocnemius muscle
		Peroneus brevis muscle
		Peroneus longus muscle
		Popliteus muscle
		Soleus muscle
		Tibialis anterior muscle
		Tibialis posterior muscle
		T Lower Leg Muscle, Left
		*See S Lower Leg Muscle,
		  Right*
		V Foot Muscle, Right
		Abductor hallucis muscle
		Adductor hallucis muscle
		Extensor digitorum brevis
		  muscle
		Extensor hallucis brevis
		  muscle
		Flexor digitorum brevis
		  muscle
		Flexor hallucis brevis
		  muscle
		Quadratus plantae muscle
		W Foot Muscle, Left
		See V Foot Muscle, Right
			Ø Open
			**4 Percutaneous
			  Endoscopic**
				Z No Device	**Z No Qualifier**

Non-OR Procedure   DRG Non-OR Procedure   Valid OR Procedure   HAC Associated Procedure   Combination Only   New/Revised April   New/Revised October

480   ICD-10-PCS 2024

ØKS–ØKS

Ø   Medical and Surgical
K   Muscles
T   Resection   Definition: Cutting out or off, without replacement, all of a body part
                 Explanation: None

Body Part Character 4			Approach Character 5	Device Character 6	Qualifier Character 7
Ø Head Muscle Auricularis muscle Masseter muscle Pterygoid muscle Splenius capitis muscle Temporalis muscle Temporoparietalis muscle **1 Facial Muscle** Buccinator muscle Corrugator supercilii muscle Depressor anguli oris muscle Depressor labii inferioris muscle Depressor septi nasi muscle Depressor supercilii muscle Levator anguli oris muscle Levator labii superioris alaeque nasi muscle Levator labii superioris muscle Mentalis muscle Nasalis muscle Occipitofrontalis muscle Orbicularis oris muscle Procerus muscle Risorius muscle Zygomaticus muscle **2 Neck Muscle, Right** Anterior vertebral muscle Arytenoid muscle Cricothyroid muscle Infrahyoid muscle Levator scapulae muscle Platysma muscle Scalene muscle Splenius cervicis muscle Sternocleidomastoid muscle Suprahyoid muscle Thyroarytenoid muscle **3 Neck Muscle, Left** *See 2 Neck Muscle, Right* **4 Tongue, Palate, Pharynx Muscle** Chondroglossus muscle Genioglossus muscle Hyoglossus muscle Inferior longitudinal muscle Levator veli palatini muscle Palatoglossal muscle Palatopharyngeal muscle Pharyngeal constrictor muscle Salpingopharyngeus muscle Styloglossus muscle Stylopharyngeus muscle Superior longitudinal muscle Tensor veli palatini muscle **5 Shoulder Muscle, Right** Deltoid muscle Infraspinatus muscle Subscapularis muscle Supraspinatus muscle Teres major muscle Teres minor muscle **6 Shoulder Muscle, Left** *See 5 Shoulder Muscle, Right*	**7 Upper Arm Muscle, Right** Biceps brachii muscle Brachialis muscle Coracobrachialis muscle Triceps brachii muscle **8 Upper Arm Muscle, Left** *See 7 Upper Arm Muscle, Right* **9 Lower Arm and Wrist Muscle, Right** Anatomical snuffbox Brachioradialis muscle Extensor carpi radialis muscle Extensor carpi ulnaris muscle Flexor carpi radialis muscle Flexor carpi ulnaris muscle Flexor pollicis longus muscle Palmaris longus muscle Pronator quadratus muscle Pronator teres muscle **B Lower Arm and Wrist Muscle, Left** *See 9 Lower Arm and Wrist Muscle, Right* **C Hand Muscle, Right** Hypothenar muscle Palmar interosseous muscle Thenar muscle **D Hand Muscle, Left** *See C Hand Muscle, Right* **F Trunk Muscle, Right** Coccygeus muscle Erector spinae muscle Interspinalis muscle Intertransversarius muscle Latissimus dorsi muscle Quadratus lumborum muscle Rhomboid major muscle Rhomboid minor muscle Serratus posterior muscle Transversospinalis muscle Trapezius muscle **G Trunk Muscle, Left** *See F Trunk Muscle, Right* **H Thorax Muscle, Right** ⊞ Intercostal muscle Levatores costarum muscle Pectoralis major muscle Pectoralis minor muscle Serratus anterior muscle Subclavius muscle Subcostal muscle Transverse thoracis muscle **J Thorax Muscle, Left** ⊞ *See H Thorax Muscle, Right* **K Abdomen Muscle, Right** External oblique muscle Internal oblique muscle Pyramidalis muscle Rectus abdominis muscle Transversus abdominis muscle **L Abdomen Muscle, Left** *See K Abdomen Muscle, Right*	**M Perineum Muscle** Bulbospongiosus muscle Cremaster muscle Deep transverse perineal muscle Ischiocavernosus muscle Levator ani muscle Superficial transverse perineal muscle **N Hip Muscle, Right** Gemellus muscle Gluteus maximus muscle Gluteus medius muscle Gluteus minimus muscle Iliacus muscle Obturator muscle Piriformis muscle Psoas muscle Quadratus femoris muscle Tensor fasciae latae muscle **P Hip Muscle, Left** *See N Hip Muscle, Right* **Q Upper Leg Muscle, Right** Adductor brevis muscle Adductor longus muscle Adductor magnus muscle Biceps femoris muscle Gracilis muscle Pectineus muscle Quadriceps (femoris) Rectus femoris muscle Sartorius muscle Semimembranosus muscle Semitendinosus muscle Vastus intermedius muscle Vastus lateralis muscle Vastus medialis muscle **R Upper Leg Muscle, Left** *See Q Upper Leg Muscle, Right* **S Lower Leg Muscle, Right** Extensor digitorum longus muscle Extensor hallucis longus muscle Fibularis brevis muscle Fibularis longus muscle Flexor digitorum longus muscle Flexor hallucis longus muscle Gastrocnemius muscle Peroneus brevis muscle Peroneus longus muscle Popliteus muscle Soleus muscle Tibialis anterior muscle Tibialis posterior muscle **T Lower Leg Muscle, Left** *See S Lower Leg Muscle, Right* **V Foot Muscle, Right** Abductor hallucis muscle Adductor hallucis muscle Extensor digitorum brevis muscle Extensor hallucis brevis muscle Flexor digitorum brevis muscle Flexor hallucis brevis muscle Quadratus plantae muscle **W Foot Muscle, Left** *See V Foot Muscle, Right*	**Ø Open** **4 Percutaneous Endoscopic**	**Z No Device**	**Z No Qualifier**

See Appendix L for Procedure Combinations
⊞   ØKT[H,J]ØZZ

NC Noncovered Procedure   **LC** Limited Coverage   **QA** Questionable OB Admit   **NT** New Tech Add-on   ⊞ Combination Member   ♂ Male   ♀ Female

ICD-10-PCS 2024   **481**

ØKT–ØKT

Ø   **Medical and Surgical**
K   **Muscles**
U   **Supplement**   Definition: Putting in or on biological or synthetic material that physically reinforces and/or augments the function of a portion of a body part

Explanation: The biological material is non-living, or is living and from the same individual. The body part may have been previously replaced, and the SUPPLEMENT procedure is performed to physically reinforce and/or augment the function of the replaced body part.

Body Part Character 4			Approach Character 5	Device Character 6	Qualifier Character 7

Ø Head Muscle
Auricularis muscle
Masseter muscle
Pterygoid muscle
Splenius capitis muscle
Temporalis muscle
Temporoparietalis muscle
1 Facial Muscle
Buccinator muscle
Corrugator supercilii
  muscle
Depressor anguli oris
  muscle
Depressor labii inferioris
  muscle
Depressor septi nasi
  muscle
Depressor supercilii
  muscle
Levator anguli oris muscle
Levator labii superioris
  alaeque nasi muscle
Levator labii superioris
  muscle
Mentalis muscle
Nasalis muscle
Occipitofrontalis muscle
Orbicularis oris muscle
Procerus muscle
Risorius muscle
Zygomaticus muscle
2 Neck Muscle, Right
Anterior vertebral muscle
Arytenoid muscle
Cricothyroid muscle
Infrahyoid muscle
Levator scapulae muscle
Platysma muscle
Scalene muscle
Splenius cervicis muscle
Sternocleidomastoid
  muscle
Suprahyoid muscle
Thyroarytenoid muscle
3 Neck Muscle, Left
See 2 Neck Muscle, Right
4 Tongue, Palate, Pharynx
Muscle
Chondroglossus muscle
Genioglossus muscle
Hyoglossus muscle
Inferior longitudinal
  muscle
Levator veli palatini
  muscle
Palatoglossal muscle
Palatopharyngeal muscle
Pharyngeal constrictor
  muscle
Salpingopharyngeus
  muscle
Styloglossus muscle
Stylopharyngeus muscle
Superior longitudinal
  muscle
Tensor veli palatini muscle
5 Shoulder Muscle, Right
Deltoid muscle
Infraspinatus muscle
Subscapularis muscle
Supraspinatus muscle
Teres major muscle
Teres minor muscle
6 Shoulder Muscle, Left
*See 5 Shoulder Muscle,
  Right*
	7 Upper Arm Muscle, Right
	Biceps brachii muscle
	Brachialis muscle
	Coracobrachialis muscle
	Triceps brachii muscle
	8 Upper Arm Muscle, Left
	*See 7 Upper Arm Muscle,
	  Right*
	9 Lower Arm and Wrist
	Muscle, Right
	Anatomical snuffbox
	Brachioradialis muscle
	Extensor carpi radialis
	  muscle
	Extensor carpi ulnaris
	  muscle
	Flexor carpi radialis
	  muscle
	Flexor carpi ulnaris muscle
	Flexor pollicis longus
	  muscle
	Palmaris longus muscle
	Pronator quadratus
	  muscle
	Pronator teres muscle
	B Lower Arm and Wrist
	Muscle, Left
	*See 9 Lower Arm and Wrist
	  Muscle, Right*
	C Hand Muscle, Right
	Hypothenar muscle
	Palmar interosseous
	  muscle
	Thenar muscle
	D Hand Muscle, Left
	See C Hand Muscle, Left
	F Trunk Muscle, Right
	Coccygeus muscle
	Erector spinae muscle
	Interspinalis muscle
	Intertransversarius muscle
	Latissimus dorsi muscle
	Quadratus lumborum
	  muscle
	Rhomboid major muscle
	Rhomboid minor muscle
	Serratus posterior muscle
	Transversospinalis muscle
	Trapezius muscle
	G Trunk Muscle, Left
	See F Trunk Muscle, Right
	H Thorax Muscle, Right
	Intercostal muscle
	Levatores costarum
	  muscle
	Pectoralis major muscle
	Pectoralis minor muscle
	Serratus anterior muscle
	Subclavius muscle
	Subcostal muscle
	Transverse thoracis
	  muscle
	J Thorax Muscle, Left
	See H Thorax Muscle, Right
	K Abdomen Muscle, Right
	External oblique muscle
	Internal oblique muscle
	Pyramidalis muscle
	Rectus abdominis muscle
	Transversus abdominis
	  muscle
	L Abdomen Muscle, Left
	*See K Abdomen Muscle,
	  Right*
		M Perineum Muscle
		Bulbospongiosus muscle
		Cremaster muscle
		Deep transverse perineal
		  muscle
		Ischiocavernosus muscle
		Levator ani muscle
		Superficial transverse
		  perineal muscle
		N Hip Muscle, Right
		Gemellus muscle
		Gluteus maximus muscle
		Gluteus medius muscle
		Gluteus minimus muscle
		Iliacus muscle
		Obturator muscle
		Piriformis muscle
		Psoas muscle
		Quadratus femoris muscle
		Tensor fasciae latae muscle
		P Hip Muscle, Left
		See N Hip Muscle, Right
		Q Upper Leg Muscle, Right
		Adductor brevis muscle
		Adductor longus muscle
		Adductor magnus muscle
		Biceps femoris muscle
		Gracilis muscle
		Pectineus muscle
		Quadriceps (femoris)
		Rectus femoris muscle
		Sartorius muscle
		Semimembranosus muscle
		Semitendinosus muscle
		Vastus intermedius muscle
		Vastus lateralis muscle
		Vastus medialis muscle
		R Upper Leg Muscle, Left
		*See Q Upper Leg Muscle,
		  Right*
		S Lower Leg Muscle, Right
		Extensor digitorum longus
		  muscle
		Extensor hallucis longus
		  muscle
		Fibularis brevis muscle
		Fibularis longus muscle
		Flexor digitorum longus
		  muscle
		Flexor hallucis longus
		  muscle
		Gastrocnemius muscle
		Peroneus brevis muscle
		Peroneus longus muscle
		Popliteus muscle
		Soleus muscle
		Tibialis anterior muscle
		Tibialis posterior muscle
		T Lower Leg Muscle, Left
		*See S Lower Leg Muscle,
		  Right*
		V Foot Muscle, Right
		Abductor hallucis muscle
		Adductor hallucis muscle
		Extensor digitorum brevis
		  muscle
		Extensor hallucis brevis
		  muscle
		Flexor digitorum brevis
		  muscle
		Flexor hallucis brevis
		  muscle
		Quadratus plantae muscle
		W Foot Muscle, Left
		See V Foot Muscle, Right
			Ø Open
			4 Percutaneous
			  Endoscopic
				7 Autologous Tissue
				  Substitute
				J Synthetic
				  Substitute
				K Nonautologous
				  Tissue Substitute
					Z No Qualifier

Non-OR Procedure   DRG Non-OR Procedure   Valid OR Procedure   HAC Associated Procedure   Combination Only   New/Revised April   New/Revised October

482

ØKU–ØKU

ICD-10-PCS 2024

Ø Medical and Surgical
K Muscles
W Revision   Definition: Correcting, to the extent possible, a portion of a malfunctioning device or the position of a displaced device

Explanation: Revision can include correcting a malfunctioning or displaced device by taking out or putting in components of the device such as a screw or pin

Body Part Character 4	Approach Character 5	Device Character 6	Qualifier Character 7
X Upper Muscle Y Lower Muscle	Ø Open 3 Percutaneous 4 Percutaneous Endoscopic	Ø Drainage Device 7 Autologous Tissue Substitute J Synthetic Substitute K Nonautologous Tissue Substitute M Stimulator Lead Y Other Device	Z No Qualifier
X Upper Muscle Y Lower Muscle	X External	Ø Drainage Device 7 Autologous Tissue Substitute J Synthetic Substitute K Nonautologous Tissue Substitute M Stimulator Lead	Z No Qualifier

Non-OR   ØKW[X,Y][3,4]YZ
Non-OR   ØKW[X,Y]X[Ø,7,J,K,M]Z

NC Noncovered Procedure   **LC** Limited Coverage   **QA** Questionable OB Admit   **NT** New Tech Add-on   ⊞ Combination Member   ♂ Male   ♀ Female

ICD-10-PCS 2024   483

Ø   Medical and Surgical
K   Muscles
X   Transfer   Definition: Moving, without taking out, all or a portion of a body part to another location to take over the function of all or a portion of a body part
               Explanation: The body part transferred remains connected to its vascular and nervous supply

Body Part Character 4			Approach Character 5	Device Character 6	Qualifier Character 7
Ø Head Muscle Auricularis muscle Masseter muscle Pterygoid muscle Splenius capitis muscle Temporalis muscle Temporoparietalis muscle **1 Facial Muscle** Buccinator muscle Corrugator supercilii muscle Depressor anguli oris muscle Depressor labii inferioris muscle Depressor septi nasi muscle Depressor supercilii muscle Levator anguli oris muscle Levator labii superioris alaeque nasi muscle Levator labii superioris muscle Mentalis muscle Nasalis muscle Occipitofrontalis muscle Orbicularis oris muscle Procerus muscle Risorius muscle Zygomaticus muscle **2 Neck Muscle, Right** Anterior vertebral muscle Arytenoid muscle Cricothyroid muscle Infrahyoid muscle Levator scapulae muscle Platysma muscle Scalene muscle Splenius cervicis muscle Sternocleidomastoid muscle Suprahyoid muscle Thyroarytenoid muscle **3 Neck Muscle, Left** *See 2 Neck Muscle, Right* **4 Tongue, Palate, Pharynx Muscle** Chondroglossus muscle Genioglossus muscle Hyoglossus muscle Inferior longitudinal muscle Levator veli palatini muscle Palatoglossal muscle Palatopharyngeal muscle Pharyngeal constrictor muscle Salpingopharyngeus muscle Styloglossus muscle Stylopharyngeus muscle Superior longitudinal muscle Tensor veli palatini muscle **5 Shoulder Muscle, Right** Deltoid muscle Infraspinatus muscle Subscapularis muscle Supraspinatus muscle Teres major muscle Teres minor muscle	**6 Shoulder Muscle, Left** *See 5 Shoulder Muscle, Right* **7 Upper Arm Muscle, Right** Biceps brachii muscle Brachialis muscle Coracobrachialis muscle Triceps brachii muscle **8 Upper Arm Muscle, Left** *See 7 Upper Arm Muscle, Right* **9 Lower Arm and Wrist Muscle, Right** Anatomical snuffbox Brachioradialis muscle Extensor carpi radialis muscle Extensor carpi ulnaris muscle Flexor carpi radialis muscle Flexor carpi ulnaris muscle Flexor pollicis longus muscle Palmaris longus muscle Pronator quadratus muscle Pronator teres muscle **B Lower Arm and Wrist Muscle, Left** *See 9 Lower Arm and Wrist Muscle, Right* **C Hand Muscle, Right** Hypothenar muscle Palmar interosseous muscle Thenar muscle **D Hand Muscle, Left** *See C Hand Muscle, Right* **H Thorax Muscle, Right** Intercostal muscle Levatores costarum muscle Pectoralis major muscle Pectoralis minor muscle Serratus anterior muscle Subclavius muscle Subcostal muscle Transverse thoracis muscle **J Thorax Muscle, Left** *See H Thorax Muscle, Right* **M Perineum Muscle** Bulbospongiosus muscle Cremaster muscle Deep transverse perineal muscle Ischiocavernosus muscle Levator ani muscle Superficial transverse perineal muscle **N Hip Muscle, Right** Gemellus muscle Gluteus maximus muscle Gluteus medius muscle Gluteus minimus muscle Iliacus muscle Obturator muscle Piriformis muscle Psoas muscle Quadratus femoris muscle Tensor fasciae latae muscle	**P Hip Muscle, Left** *See N Hip Muscle, Right* **Q Upper Leg Muscle, Right** Adductor brevis muscle Adductor longus muscle Adductor magnus muscle Biceps femoris muscle Gracilis muscle Pectineus muscle Quadriceps (femoris) Rectus femoris muscle Sartorius muscle Semimembranosus muscle Semitendinosus muscle Vastus intermedius muscle Vastus lateralis muscle Vastus medialis muscle **R Upper Leg Muscle, Left** *See Q Upper Leg Muscle, Right* **S Lower Leg Muscle, Right** Extensor digitorum longus muscle Extensor hallucis longus muscle Fibularis brevis muscle Fibularis longus muscle Flexor digitorum longus muscle Flexor hallucis longus muscle Gastrocnemius muscle Peroneus brevis muscle Peroneus longus muscle Popliteus muscle Soleus muscle Tibialis anterior muscle Tibialis posterior muscle **T Lower Leg Muscle, Left** *See S Lower Leg Muscle, Right* **V Foot Muscle, Right** Abductor hallucis muscle Adductor hallucis muscle Extensor digitorum brevis muscle Extensor hallucis brevis muscle Flexor digitorum brevis muscle Flexor hallucis brevis muscle Quadratus plantae muscle **W Foot Muscle, Left** *See V Foot Muscle, Right*	**Ø Open** **4 Percutaneous Endoscopic**	**Z No Device**	**Ø Skin** **1 Subcutaneous Tissue** **2 Skin and Subcutaneous Tissue** **Z No Qualifier**

ØKX Continued on next page

Non-OR Procedure   DRG Non-OR Procedure   Valid OR Procedure   HAC Associated Procedure   Combination Only   New/Revised April   New/Revised October

484   ICD-10-PCS 2024

Ø   Medical and Surgical
K   Muscles   *ØKX Continued*
X   Transfer   Definition: Moving, without taking out, all or a portion of a body part to another location to take over the function of all or a
                         portion of a body part
                         Explanation: The body part transferred remains connected to its vascular and nervous supply

Body Part Character 4	Approach Character 5	Device Character 6	Qualifier Character 7

F   Trunk Muscle, Right
     Coccygeus muscle
     Erector spinae muscle
     Interspinalis muscle
     Intertransversarius muscle
     Latissimus dorsi muscle
     Quadratus lumborum muscle
     Rhomboid major muscle
     Rhomboid minor muscle
     Serratus posterior muscle
     Transversospinalis muscle
     Trapezius muscle
G   Trunk Muscle, Left
     See F Trunk Muscle, Right
	Ø Open
	4 Percutaneous Endoscopic
		Z No Device	**Ø Skin**
			1 Subcutaneous Tissue
			2 Skin and Subcutaneous Tissue
			5 Latissimus Dorsi Myocutaneous Flap
			7 Deep Inferior Epigastric Artery Perforator Flap
			8 Superficial Inferior Epigastric Artery Flap
			9 Gluteal Artery Perforator Flap
			Z No Qualifier

K   Abdomen Muscle, Right
     External oblique muscle
     Internal oblique muscle
     Pyramidalis muscle
     Rectus abdominis muscle
     Transversus abdominis muscle
L   Abdomen Muscle, Left
     See K Abdomen Muscle, Right
	Ø Open
	4 Percutaneous Endoscopic
		Z No Device	**Ø Skin**
			1 Subcutaneous Tissue
			2 Skin and Subcutaneous Tissue
			6 Transverse Rectus Abdominis Myocutaneous Flap
			Z No Qualifier

NC Noncovered Procedure   **LC** Limited Coverage   **QA** Questionable OB Admit   **NT** New Tech Add-on   ✚ Combination Member   ♂ Male   ♀ Female

ICD-10-PCS 2024   **485**

Tendons ØL2–ØLX

Character Meanings*

This Character Meaning table is provided as a guide to assist the user in the identification of character members that may be found in this section of code tables. It **SHOULD NOT** be used to build a PCS code.

Operation–Character 3	Body Part–Character 4	Approach–Character 5	Device–Character 6	Qualifier–Character 7
2 Change	Ø Head and Neck Tendon	Ø Open	Ø Drainage Device	X Diagnostic
5 Destruction	1 Shoulder Tendon, Right	3 Percutaneous	7 Autologous Tissue Substitute	Z No Qualifier
8 Division	2 Shoulder Tendon, Left	4 Percutaneous Endoscopic	J Synthetic Substitute	
9 Drainage	3 Upper Arm Tendon, Right	X External	K Nonautologous Tissue Substitute	
B Excision	4 Upper Arm Tendon, Left		Y Other Device	
C Extirpation	5 Lower Arm and Wrist Tendon, Right		Z No Device	
D Extraction	6 Lower Arm and Wrist Tendon, Left			
H Insertion	7 Hand Tendon, Right			
J Inspection	8 Hand Tendon, Left			
M Reattachment	9 Trunk Tendon, Right			
N Release	B Trunk Tendon, Left			
P Removal	C Thorax Tendon, Right			
Q Repair	D Thorax Tendon, Left			
R Replacement	F Abdomen Tendon, Right			
S Reposition	G Abdomen Tendon, Left			
T Resection	H Perineum Tendon			
U Supplement	J Hip Tendon, Right			
W Revision	K Hip Tendon, Left			
X Transfer	L Upper Leg Tendon, Right			
	M Upper Leg Tendon, Left			
	N Lower Leg Tendon, Right			
	P Lower Leg Tendon, Left			
	Q Knee Tendon, Right			
	R Knee Tendon, Left			
	S Ankle Tendon, Right			
	T Ankle Tendon, Left			
	V Foot Tendon, Right			
	W Foot Tendon, Left			
	X Upper Tendon			
	Y Lower Tendon			

* Includes synovial membrane.

AHA Coding Clinic for table ØL8
2016, 3Q, 30   Resection of femur with interposition arthroplasty

AHA Coding Clinic for table ØLB
2017, 2Q, 21   Arthroscopic anterior cruciate ligament revision using autograft with anterolateral ligament reconstruction
2015, 3Q, 26   Thumb arthroplasty with resection of trapezium
2014, 3Q, 14   Application of TheraSkin® and excisional debridement
2014, 3Q, 18   Placement of reverse sural fasciocutaneous pedicle flap

AHA Coding Clinic for table ØLD
2017, 4Q, 41   Extraction procedures

AHA Coding Clinic for table ØLQ
2016, 3Q, 32   Rotator cuff repair, tenodesis, decompression, acromioplasty and coracoplasty
2015, 2Q, 11   Repair of patellar and quadriceps tendons with allograft
2013, 3Q, 20   Superior labrum anterior posterior (SLAP) repair and subacromial decompression

AHA Coding Clinic for table ØLS
2016, 3Q, 32   Rotator cuff repair, tenodesis, decompression, acromioplasty and coracoplasty
2015, 3Q, 14   Endoprosthetic replacement of humerus and tendon reattachment

AHA Coding Clinic for table ØLU
2015, 2Q, 11   Repair of patellar and quadriceps tendons with allograft

Foot Tendons

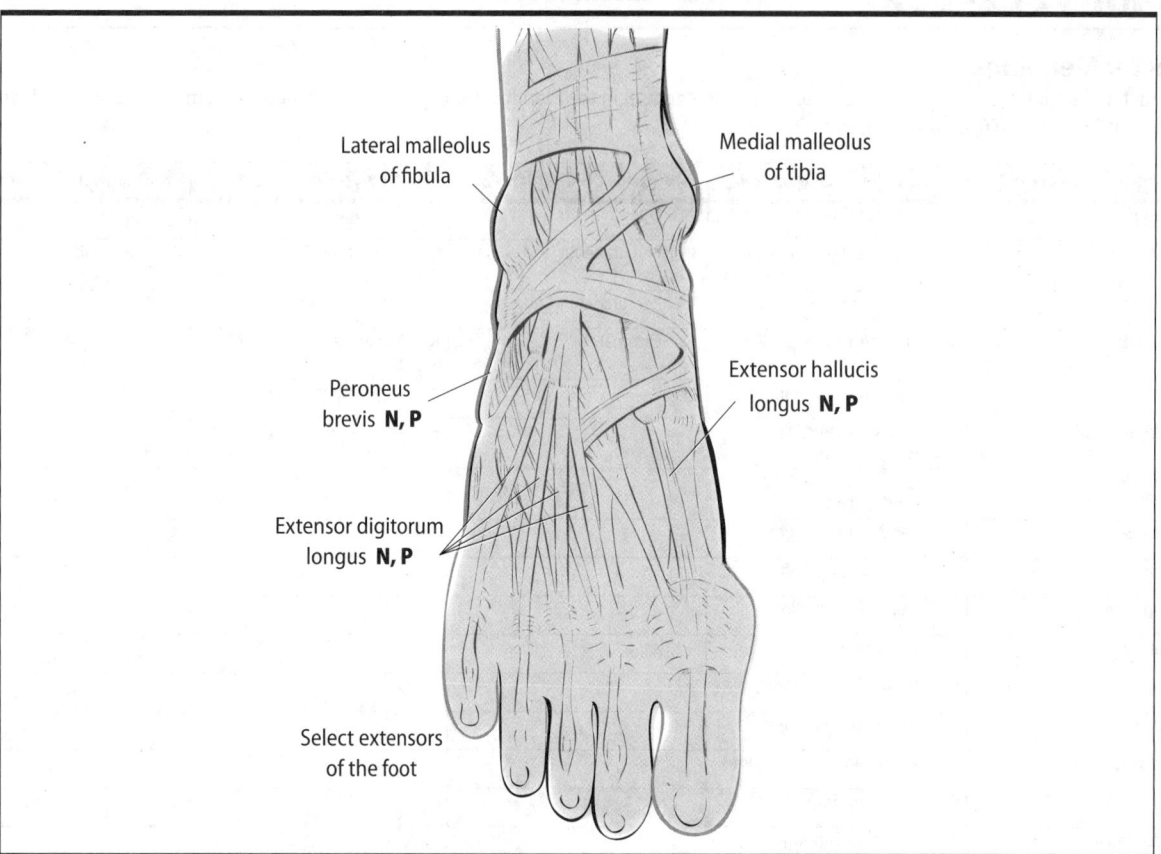

Lateral malleolus
of fibula

Medial malleolus
of tibia

Peroneus
brevis **N, P**

Extensor hallucis
longus **N, P**

Extensor digitorum
longus **N, P**

Select extensors
of the foot

Shoulder Tendons

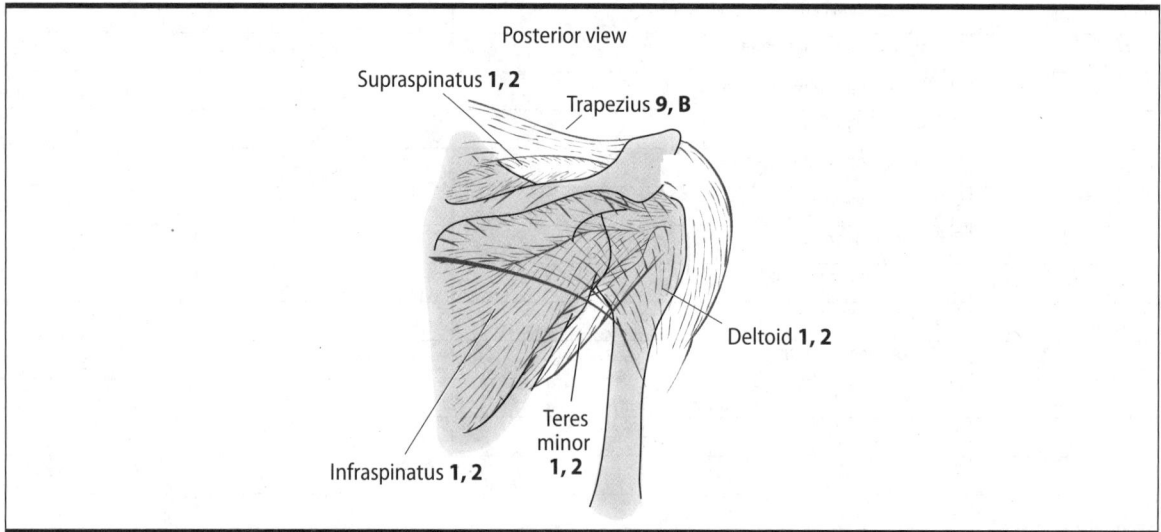

Posterior view

Supraspinatus **1, 2**

Trapezius **9, B**

Deltoid **1, 2**

Teres
minor
1, 2

Infraspinatus **1, 2**

Tendons of Wrist and Hand

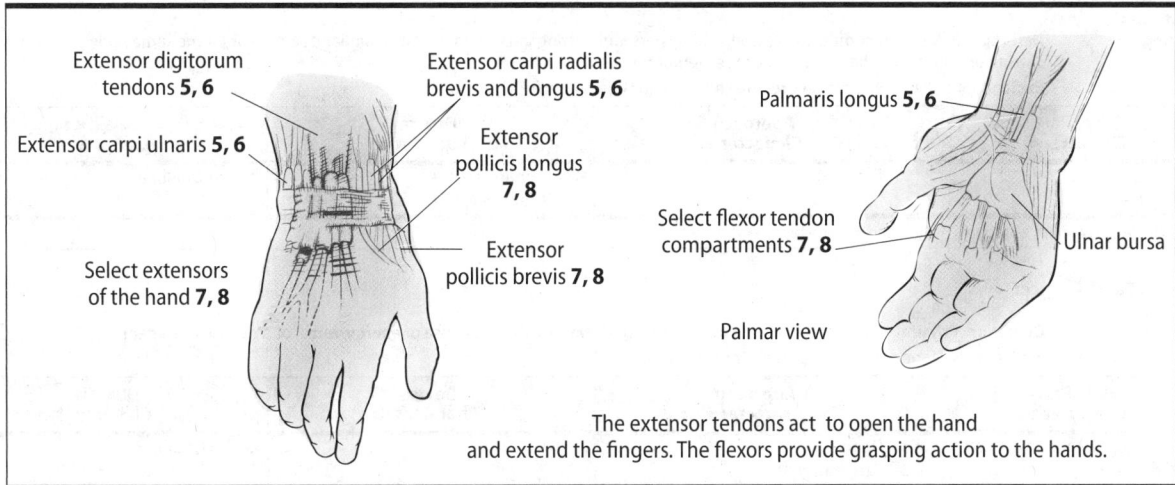

Extensor digitorum tendons **5, 6**

Extensor carpi ulnaris **5, 6**

Extensor carpi radialis brevis and longus **5, 6**

Extensor pollicis longus **7, 8**

Select extensors of the hand **7, 8**

Extensor pollicis brevis **7, 8**

Palmaris longus **5, 6**

Select flexor tendon compartments **7, 8**

Ulnar bursa

Palmar view

The extensor tendons act to open the hand and extend the fingers. The flexors provide grasping action to the hands.

Leg Muscles and Tendons

Head of fibula

Patella

Soleus **N, P**

Anterior tibialis **N, P**

Gastrocnemius **N, P**

Extensor longus **N, P**

Peroneus longus **N, P**

Peroneus brevis **N, P**

Head of femur

Adductor longus **L, M**

Rectus femoris **L, M**

Sartorius **L, M**

Vastus lateralis **L, M**

Patella

Fibula

Ø Medical and Surgical
L Tendons
2 Change

Definition: Taking out or off a device from a body part and putting back an identical or similar device in or on the same body part without cutting or puncturing the skin or a mucous membrane

Explanation: All CHANGE procedures are coded using the approach EXTERNAL

Body Part Character 4	Approach Character 5	Device Character 6	Qualifier Character 7
X Upper Tendon Y Lower Tendon	X External	Ø Drainage Device Y Other Device	Z No Qualifier

Non-OR   All body part, approach, device, and qualifier values

Ø Medical and Surgical
L Tendons
5 Destruction

Definition: Physical eradication of all or a portion of a body part by the direct use of energy, force, or a destructive agent

Explanation: None of the body part is physically taken out

Body Part Character 4	Approach Character 5	Device Character 6	Qualifier Character 7

Ø Head and Neck Tendon
1 Shoulder Tendon, Right
2 Shoulder Tendon, Left
3 Upper Arm Tendon, Right
4 Upper Arm Tendon, Left
5 Lower Arm and Wrist Tendon, Right
6 Lower Arm and Wrist Tendon, Left
7 Hand Tendon, Right
8 Hand Tendon, Left
9 Trunk Tendon, Right
B Trunk Tendon, Left
C Thorax Tendon, Right
D Thorax Tendon, Left
F Abdomen Tendon, Right
G Abdomen Tendon, Left
H Perineum Tendon
J Hip Tendon, Right
K Hip Tendon, Left
L Upper Leg Tendon, Right
M Upper Leg Tendon, Left
N Lower Leg Tendon, Right
   Achilles tendon
P Lower Leg Tendon, Left
   See N Lower Leg Tendon, Right
Q Knee Tendon, Right
   Patellar tendon
R Knee Tendon, Left
   See Q Knee Tendon, Right
S Ankle Tendon, Right
T Ankle Tendon, Left
V Foot Tendon, Right
W Foot Tendon, Left
	Ø Open
	3 Percutaneous
	4 Percutaneous Endoscopic
		Z No Device	Z No Qualifier

Non-OR Procedure   DRG Non-OR Procedure   Valid OR Procedure   HAC Associated Procedure   Combination Only   New/Revised April   New/Revised October

490

ICD-10-PCS 2024

Ø   Medical and Surgical
L   Tendons
8   Division   Definition: Cutting into a body part, without draining fluids and/or gases from the body part, in order to separate or transect a body part
                             Explanation: All or a portion of the body part is separated into two or more portions

Body Part Character 4	Approach Character 5	Device Character 6	Qualifier Character 7

Ø Head and Neck Tendon
1 Shoulder Tendon, Right
2 Shoulder Tendon, Left
3 Upper Arm Tendon, Right
4 Upper Arm Tendon, Left
5 Lower Arm and Wrist Tendon, Right
6 Lower Arm and Wrist Tendon, Left
7 Hand Tendon, Right
8 Hand Tendon, Left
9 Trunk Tendon, Right
B Trunk Tendon, Left
C Thorax Tendon, Right
D Thorax Tendon, Left
F Abdomen Tendon, Right
G Abdomen Tendon, Left
H Perineum Tendon
J Hip Tendon, Right
K Hip Tendon, Left
L Upper Leg Tendon, Right
M Upper Leg Tendon, Left
N Lower Leg Tendon, Right
    Achilles tendon
P Lower Leg Tendon, Left
    See N Lower Leg Tendon, Right
Q Knee Tendon, Right
    Patellar tendon
R Knee Tendon, Left
    See Q Knee Tendon, Right
S Ankle Tendon, Right
T Ankle Tendon, Left
V Foot Tendon, Right
W Foot Tendon, Left
	Ø Open
	3 Percutaneous
	4 Percutaneous Endoscopic
		Z No Device	Z No Qualifier

Ø **Medical and Surgical**
L **Tendons**
9 **Drainage**   Definition: Taking or letting out fluids and/or gases from a body part

Explanation: The qualifier DIAGNOSTIC is used to identify drainage procedures that are biopsies

Body Part Character 4	Approach Character 5	Device Character 6	Qualifier Character 7

Ø Head and Neck Tendon
1 Shoulder Tendon, Right
2 Shoulder Tendon, Left
3 Upper Arm Tendon, Right
4 Upper Arm Tendon, Left
5 Lower Arm and Wrist Tendon, Right
6 Lower Arm and Wrist Tendon, Left
7 Hand Tendon, Right
8 Hand Tendon, Left
9 Trunk Tendon, Right
B Trunk Tendon, Left
C Thorax Tendon, Right
D Thorax Tendon, Left
F Abdomen Tendon, Right
G Abdomen Tendon, Left
H Perineum Tendon
J Hip Tendon, Right
K Hip Tendon, Left
L Upper Leg Tendon, Right
M Upper Leg Tendon, Left
N Lower Leg Tendon, Right
  Achilles tendon
P Lower Leg Tendon, Left
  See N Lower Leg Tendon, Right
Q Knee Tendon, Right
  Patellar tendon
R Knee Tendon, Left
  See Q Knee Tendon, Right
S Ankle Tendon, Right
T Ankle Tendon, Left
V Foot Tendon, Right
W Foot Tendon, Left
	Ø Open
	3 Percutaneous
	4 Percutaneous Endoscopic
		Ø Drainage Device	Z No Qualifier

Ø Head and Neck Tendon
1 Shoulder Tendon, Right
2 Shoulder Tendon, Left
3 Upper Arm Tendon, Right
4 Upper Arm Tendon, Left
5 Lower Arm and Wrist Tendon, Right
6 Lower Arm and Wrist Tendon, Left
7 Hand Tendon, Right
8 Hand Tendon, Left
9 Trunk Tendon, Right
B Trunk Tendon, Left
C Thorax Tendon, Right
D Thorax Tendon, Left
F Abdomen Tendon, Right
G Abdomen Tendon, Left
H Perineum Tendon
J Hip Tendon, Right
K Hip Tendon, Left
L Upper Leg Tendon, Right
M Upper Leg Tendon, Left
N Lower Leg Tendon, Right
  Achilles tendon
P Lower Leg Tendon, Left
  See N Lower Leg Tendon, Right
Q Knee Tendon, Right
  Patellar tendon
R Knee Tendon, Left
  See Q Knee Tendon, Right
S Ankle Tendon, Right
T Ankle Tendon, Left
V Foot Tendon, Right
W Foot Tendon, Left
	Ø Open
	3 Percutaneous
	4 Percutaneous Endoscopic
		Z No Device	X Diagnostic
			Z No Qualifier

Non-OR ØL9[Ø,1,2,3,4,5,6,7,8,9,B,C,D,F,G,H,J,K,L,M,N,P,Q,R,S,T,V,W]3ØZ
Non-OR ØL9[Ø,1,2,3,4,5,6,7,8,9,B,C,D,F,G,H,J,K,L,M,N,P,Q,R,S,T,V,W]3ZZ
Non-OR ØL9[7,8]4ZZ

Ø   **Medical and Surgical**
L   **Tendons**
B   **Excision**   Definition: Cutting out or off, without replacement, a portion of a body part
                  Explanation: The qualifier DIAGNOSTIC is used to identify excision procedures that are biopsies

Body Part Character 4	Approach Character 5	Device Character 6	Qualifier Character 7
Ø Head and Neck Tendon	Ø Open	Z No Device	X Diagnostic
1 Shoulder Tendon, Right	3 Percutaneous		Z No Qualifier
2 Shoulder Tendon, Left	4 Percutaneous Endoscopic		
3 Upper Arm Tendon, Right			
4 Upper Arm Tendon, Left			
5 Lower Arm and Wrist Tendon, Right			
6 Lower Arm and Wrist Tendon, Left			
7 Hand Tendon, Right			
8 Hand Tendon, Left			
9 Trunk Tendon, Right			
B Trunk Tendon, Left			
C Thorax Tendon, Right			
D Thorax Tendon, Left			
F Abdomen Tendon, Right			
G Abdomen Tendon, Left			
H Perineum Tendon			
J Hip Tendon, Right			
K Hip Tendon, Left			
L Upper Leg Tendon, Right			
M Upper Leg Tendon, Left			
N Lower Leg Tendon, Right Achilles tendon			
P Lower Leg Tendon, Left *See N Lower Leg Tendon, Right*			
Q Knee Tendon, Right Patellar tendon			
R Knee Tendon, Left *See Q Knee Tendon, Right*			
S Ankle Tendon, Right			
T Ankle Tendon, Left			
V Foot Tendon, Right			
W Foot Tendon, Left			

NC Noncovered Procedure   **LC** Limited Coverage   **OA** Questionable OB Admit   **NT** New Tech Add-on   ✚ Combination Member   ♂ Male   ♀ Female

ICD-10-PCS 2024   **493**

ØLB–ØLB

Tendons

Ø   **Medical and Surgical**
L   **Tendons**
C   **Extirpation**   Definition: Taking or cutting out solid matter from a body part

Explanation: The solid matter may be an abnormal byproduct of a biological function or a foreign body; it may be imbedded in a body part or in the lumen of a tubular body part. The solid matter may or may not have been previously broken into pieces.

Body Part Character 4	Approach Character 5	Device Character 6	Qualifier Character 7
Ø Head and Neck Tendon	**Ø** Open	**Z** No Device	**Z** No Qualifier
1 Shoulder Tendon, Right	**3** Percutaneous		
2 Shoulder Tendon, Left	**4** Percutaneous Endoscopic		
3 Upper Arm Tendon, Right			
4 Upper Arm Tendon, Left			
5 Lower Arm and Wrist Tendon, Right			
6 Lower Arm and Wrist Tendon, Left			
7 Hand Tendon, Right			
8 Hand Tendon, Left			
9 Trunk Tendon, Right			
B Trunk Tendon, Left			
C Thorax Tendon, Right			
D Thorax Tendon, Left			
F Abdomen Tendon, Right			
G Abdomen Tendon, Left			
H Perineum Tendon			
J Hip Tendon, Right			
K Hip Tendon, Left			
L Upper Leg Tendon, Right			
M Upper Leg Tendon, Left			
N Lower Leg Tendon, Right Achilles tendon			
P Lower Leg Tendon, Left *See N Lower Leg Tendon, Right*			
Q Knee Tendon, Right Patellar tendon			
R Knee Tendon, Left *See Q Knee Tendon, Right*			
S Ankle Tendon, Right			
T Ankle Tendon, Left			
V Foot Tendon, Right			
W Foot Tendon, Left			

Non-OR Procedure   DRG Non-OR Procedure   Valid OR Procedure   HAC Associated Procedure   Combination Only   New/Revised April   New/Revised October

494   ICD-10-PCS 2024

ØLC–ØLC

Ø　Medical and Surgical
L　Tendons
D　Extraction　　Definition: Pulling or stripping out or off all or a portion of a body part by the use of force
　　　　　　　　　Explanation: The qualifier DIAGNOSTIC is used to identify extraction procedures that are biopsies

Body Part Character 4	Approach Character 5	Device Character 6	Qualifier Character 7
Ø Head and Neck Tendon	Ø Open	Z No Device	Z No Qualifier
1 Shoulder Tendon, Right			
2 Shoulder Tendon, Left			
3 Upper Arm Tendon, Right			
4 Upper Arm Tendon, Left			
5 Lower Arm and Wrist Tendon, Right			
6 Lower Arm and Wrist Tendon, Left			
7 Hand Tendon, Right			
8 Hand Tendon, Left			
9 Trunk Tendon, Right			
B Trunk Tendon, Left			
C Thorax Tendon, Right			
D Thorax Tendon, Left			
F Abdomen Tendon, Right			
G Abdomen Tendon, Left			
H Perineum Tendon			
J Hip Tendon, Right			
K Hip Tendon, Left			
L Upper Leg Tendon, Right			
M Upper Leg Tendon, Left			
N Lower Leg Tendon, Right / Achilles tendon			
P Lower Leg Tendon, Left / See N Lower Leg Tendon, Right			
Q Knee Tendon, Right / Patellar tendon			
R Knee Tendon, Left / See Q Knee Tendon, Right			
S Ankle Tendon, Right			
T Ankle Tendon, Left			
V Foot Tendon, Right			
W Foot Tendon, Left			

Ø　Medical and Surgical
L　Tendons
H　Insertion　　Definition: Putting in a nonbiological appliance that monitors, assists, performs, or prevents a physiological function but does not physically take the place of a body part
　　　　　　　　　Explanation: None

Body Part Character 4	Approach Character 5	Device Character 6	Qualifier Character 7
X Upper Tendon	Ø Open	Y Other Device	Z No Qualifier
Y Lower Tendon	3 Percutaneous		
	4 Percutaneous Endoscopic		

Non-OR　ØLH[X,Y][3,4]YZ

Ø　Medical and Surgical
L　Tendons
J　Inspection　　Definition: Visually and/or manually exploring a body part
　　　　　　　　　Explanation: Visual exploration may be performed with or without optical instrumentation. Manual exploration may be performed directly or through intervening body layers.

Body Part Character 4	Approach Character 5	Device Character 6	Qualifier Character 7
X Upper Tendon	Ø Open	Z No Device	Z No Qualifier
Y Lower Tendon	3 Percutaneous		
	4 Percutaneous Endoscopic		
	X External		

Non-OR　ØLJ[X,Y][3,X]ZZ

NC Noncovered Procedure　　LC Limited Coverage　　QA Questionable OB Admit　　NT New Tech Add-on　　⊞ Combination Member　　♂Male　　♀Female
ICD-10-PCS 2024　　　495

ØLD–ØLJ

Ø Medical and Surgical
L Tendons
M Reattachment   Definition: Putting back in or on all or a portion of a separated body part to its normal location or other suitable location

Explanation: Vascular circulation and nervous pathways may or may not be reestablished

Body Part Character 4	Approach Character 5	Device Character 6	Qualifier Character 7

Ø Head and Neck Tendon
1 Shoulder Tendon, Right
2 Shoulder Tendon, Left
3 Upper Arm Tendon, Right
4 Upper Arm Tendon, Left
5 Lower Arm and Wrist Tendon, Right
6 Lower Arm and Wrist Tendon, Left
7 Hand Tendon, Right
8 Hand Tendon, Left
9 Trunk Tendon, Right
B Trunk Tendon, Left
C Thorax Tendon, Right
D Thorax Tendon, Left
F Abdomen Tendon, Right
G Abdomen Tendon, Left
H Perineum Tendon
J Hip Tendon, Right
K Hip Tendon, Left
L Upper Leg Tendon, Right
M Upper Leg Tendon, Left
N Lower Leg Tendon, Right
    Achilles tendon
P Lower Leg Tendon, Left
    See N Lower Leg Tendon, Right
Q Knee Tendon, Right
    Patellar tendon
R Knee Tendon, Left
    See Q Knee Tendon, Right
S Ankle Tendon, Right
T Ankle Tendon, Left
V Foot Tendon, Right
W Foot Tendon, Left
	Ø Open
	4 Percutaneous Endoscopic
		Z No Device	Z No Qualifier

Ø Medical and Surgical
L Tendons
N Release   Definition: Freeing a body part from an abnormal physical constraint by cutting or by the use of force

Explanation: Some of the restraining tissue may be taken out but none of the body part is taken out

Body Part Character 4	Approach Character 5	Device Character 6	Qualifier Character 7

Ø Head and Neck Tendon
1 Shoulder Tendon, Right
2 Shoulder Tendon, Left
3 Upper Arm Tendon, Right
4 Upper Arm Tendon, Left
5 Lower Arm and Wrist Tendon, Right
6 Lower Arm and Wrist Tendon, Left
7 Hand Tendon, Right
8 Hand Tendon, Left
9 Trunk Tendon, Right
B Trunk Tendon, Left
C Thorax Tendon, Right
D Thorax Tendon, Left
F Abdomen Tendon, Right
G Abdomen Tendon, Left
H Perineum Tendon
J Hip Tendon, Right
K Hip Tendon, Left
L Upper Leg Tendon, Right
M Upper Leg Tendon, Left
N Lower Leg Tendon, Right
    Achilles tendon
P Lower Leg Tendon, Left
    See N Lower Leg Tendon, Right
Q Knee Tendon, Right
    Patellar tendon
R Knee Tendon, Left
    See Q Knee Tendon, Right
S Ankle Tendon, Right
T Ankle Tendon, Left
V Foot Tendon, Right
W Foot Tendon, Left
	Ø Open
	3 Percutaneous
	4 Percutaneous Endoscopic
	X External
		Z No Device	Z No Qualifier

Non-OR   ØLN[Ø,1,2,3,4,5,6,7,8,9,B,C,D,F,G,H,J,K,L,M,N,P,Q,R,S,T,V,W]XZZ

Non-OR Procedure   DRG Non-OR Procedure   Valid OR Procedure   HAC Associated Procedure   Combination Only   New/Revised April   New/Revised October

Ø   Medical and Surgical
L   Tendons
P   Removal   Definition: Taking out or off a device from a body part

Explanation: If a device is taken out and a similar device put in without cutting or puncturing the skin or mucous membrane, the procedure is coded to the root operation CHANGE. Otherwise, the procedure for taking out a device is coded to the root operation REMOVAL.

Body Part Character 4	Approach Character 5	Device Character 6	Qualifier Character 7
X Upper Tendon Y Lower Tendon	Ø Open 3 Percutaneous 4 Percutaneous Endoscopic	Ø Drainage Device 7 Autologous Tissue Substitute J Synthetic Substitute K Nonautologous Tissue Substitute Y Other Device	Z No Qualifier
X Upper Tendon Y Lower Tendon	X External	Ø Drainage Device	Z No Qualifier

Non-OR   ØLP[X,Y]3ØZ
Non-OR   ØLP[X,Y][3,4]YZ
Non-OR   ØLP[X,Y]XØZ

Ø   Medical and Surgical
L   Tendons
Q   Repair   Definition: Restoring, to the extent possible, a body part to its normal anatomic structure and function

Explanation: Used only when the method to accomplish the repair is not one of the other root operations

Body Part Character 4	Approach Character 5	Device Character 6	Qualifier Character 7

Ø   Head and Neck Tendon
1   Shoulder Tendon, Right
2   Shoulder Tendon, Left
3   Upper Arm Tendon, Right
4   Upper Arm Tendon, Left
5   Lower Arm and Wrist Tendon, Right
6   Lower Arm and Wrist Tendon, Left
7   Hand Tendon, Right
8   Hand Tendon, Left
9   Trunk Tendon, Right
B   Trunk Tendon, Left
C   Thorax Tendon, Right
D   Thorax Tendon, Left
F   Abdomen Tendon, Right
G   Abdomen Tendon, Left
H   Perineum Tendon
J   Hip Tendon, Right
K   Hip Tendon, Left
L   Upper Leg Tendon, Right
M   Upper Leg Tendon, Left
N   Lower Leg Tendon, Right
     Achilles tendon
P   Lower Leg Tendon, Left
     See N Lower Leg Tendon, Right
Q   Knee Tendon, Right
     Patellar tendon
R   Knee Tendon, Left
     See Q Knee Tendon, Right
S   Ankle Tendon, Right
T   Ankle Tendon, Left
V   Foot Tendon, Right
W   Foot Tendon, Left
	Ø Open
	3 Percutaneous
	4 Percutaneous Endoscopic
		Z No Device	Z No Qualifier

NC Noncovered Procedure   LC Limited Coverage   QA Questionable OB Admit   NT New Tech Add-on   ⊞ Combination Member   ♂ Male   ♀ Female

ICD-10-PCS 2024   497

Ø   **Medical and Surgical**
L   **Tendons**
R   **Replacement**   Definition: Putting in or on biological or synthetic material that physically takes the place and/or function of all or a portion of a body part

                      Explanation: The body part may have been taken out or replaced, or may be taken out, physically eradicated, or rendered nonfunctional during the REPLACEMENT procedure. A REMOVAL procedure is coded for taking out the device used in a previous replacement procedure.

Body Part Character 4	Approach Character 5	Device Character 6	Qualifier Character 7

Ø Head and Neck Tendon
1 Shoulder Tendon, Right
2 Shoulder Tendon, Left
3 Upper Arm Tendon, Right
4 Upper Arm Tendon, Left
5 Lower Arm and Wrist Tendon, Right
6 Lower Arm and Wrist Tendon, Left
7 Hand Tendon, Right
8 Hand Tendon, Left
9 Trunk Tendon, Right
B Trunk Tendon, Left
C Thorax Tendon, Right
D Thorax Tendon, Left
F Abdomen Tendon, Right
G Abdomen Tendon, Left
H Perineum Tendon
J Hip Tendon, Right
K Hip Tendon, Left
L Upper Leg Tendon, Right
M Upper Leg Tendon, Left
N Lower Leg Tendon, Right
    Achilles tendon
P Lower Leg Tendon, Left
    See N Lower Leg Tendon, Right
Q Knee Tendon, Right
    Patellar tendon
R Knee Tendon, Left
    See Q Knee Tendon, Right
S Ankle Tendon, Right
T Ankle Tendon, Left
V Foot Tendon, Right
W Foot Tendon, Left
	Ø Open
	4 Percutaneous Endoscopic
		7 Autologous Tissue Substitute
		J Synthetic Substitute
		K Nonautologous Tissue Substitute
			Z No Qualifier

Ø   **Medical and Surgical**
L   **Tendons**
S   **Reposition**   Definition: Moving to its normal location, or other suitable location, all or a portion of a body part

                      Explanation: The body part is moved to a new location from an abnormal location, or from a normal location where it is not functioning correctly. The body part may or may not be cut out or off to be moved to the new location.

Body Part Character 4	Approach Character 5	Device Character 6	Qualifier Character 7

Ø Head and Neck Tendon
1 Shoulder Tendon, Right
2 Shoulder Tendon, Left
3 Upper Arm Tendon, Right
4 Upper Arm Tendon, Left
5 Lower Arm and Wrist Tendon, Right
6 Lower Arm and Wrist Tendon, Left
7 Hand Tendon, Right
8 Hand Tendon, Left
9 Trunk Tendon, Right
B Trunk Tendon, Left
C Thorax Tendon, Right
D Thorax Tendon, Left
F Abdomen Tendon, Right
G Abdomen Tendon, Left
H Perineum Tendon
J Hip Tendon, Right
K Hip Tendon, Left
L Upper Leg Tendon, Right
M Upper Leg Tendon, Left
N Lower Leg Tendon, Right
    Achilles tendon
P Lower Leg Tendon, Left
    See N Lower Leg Tendon, Right
Q Knee Tendon, Right
    Patellar tendon
R Knee Tendon, Left
    See Q Knee Tendon, Right
S Ankle Tendon, Right
T Ankle Tendon, Left
V Foot Tendon, Right
W Foot Tendon, Left
	Ø Open
	4 Percutaneous Endoscopic
		Z No Device	Z No Qualifier

Non-OR Procedure   DRG Non-OR Procedure   Valid OR Procedure   HAC Associated Procedure   Combination Only   New/Revised April   New/Revised October

Ø **Medical and Surgical**
L **Tendons**
T **Resection**   Definition: Cutting out or off, without replacement, all of a body part
            Explanation: None

Body Part Character 4	Approach Character 5	Device Character 6	Qualifier Character 7
Ø Head and Neck Tendon	Ø Open	Z No Device	Z No Qualifier
1 Shoulder Tendon, Right	4 Percutaneous Endoscopic		
2 Shoulder Tendon, Left			
3 Upper Arm Tendon, Right			
4 Upper Arm Tendon, Left			
5 Lower Arm and Wrist Tendon, Right			
6 Lower Arm and Wrist Tendon, Left			
7 Hand Tendon, Right			
8 Hand Tendon, Left			
9 Trunk Tendon, Right			
B Trunk Tendon, Left			
C Thorax Tendon, Right			
D Thorax Tendon, Left			
F Abdomen Tendon, Right			
G Abdomen Tendon, Left			
H Perineum Tendon			
J Hip Tendon, Right			
K Hip Tendon, Left			
L Upper Leg Tendon, Right			
M Upper Leg Tendon, Left			
N Lower Leg Tendon, Right Achilles tendon			
P Lower Leg Tendon, Left See N Lower Leg Tendon, Right			
Q Knee Tendon, Right Patellar tendon			
R Knee Tendon, Left See Q Knee Tendon, Right			
S Ankle Tendon, Right			
T Ankle Tendon, Left			
V Foot Tendon, Right			
W Foot Tendon, Left			

Ø **Medical and Surgical**
L **Tendons**
U **Supplement**   Definition: Putting in or on biological or synthetic material that physically reinforces and/or augments the function of a portion of a body part
            Explanation: The biological material is non-living, or is living and from the same individual. The body part may have been previously replaced, and the SUPPLEMENT procedure is performed to physically reinforce and/or augment the function of the replaced body part.

Body Part Character 4	Approach Character 5	Device Character 6	Qualifier Character 7
Ø Head and Neck Tendon	Ø Open	7 Autologous Tissue Substitute	Z No Qualifier
1 Shoulder Tendon, Right	4 Percutaneous Endoscopic	J Synthetic Substitute	
2 Shoulder Tendon, Left		K Nonautologous Tissue Substitute	
3 Upper Arm Tendon, Right			
4 Upper Arm Tendon, Left			
5 Lower Arm and Wrist Tendon, Right			
6 Lower Arm and Wrist Tendon, Left			
7 Hand Tendon, Right			
8 Hand Tendon, Left			
9 Trunk Tendon, Right			
B Trunk Tendon, Left			
C Thorax Tendon, Right			
D Thorax Tendon, Left			
F Abdomen Tendon, Right			
G Abdomen Tendon, Left			
H Perineum Tendon			
J Hip Tendon, Right			
K Hip Tendon, Left			
L Upper Leg Tendon, Right			
M Upper Leg Tendon, Left			
N Lower Leg Tendon, Right Achilles tendon			
P Lower Leg Tendon, Left See N Lower Leg Tendon, Right			
Q Knee Tendon, Right Patellar tendon			
R Knee Tendon, Left See Q Knee Tendon, Right			
S Ankle Tendon, Right			
T Ankle Tendon, Left			
V Foot Tendon, Right			
W Foot Tendon, Left			

NC Noncovered Procedure   LC Limited Coverage   QA Questionable OB Admit   NT New Tech Add-on   ⊞ Combination Member   ♂ Male   ♀ Female

ICD-10-PCS 2024   499

Ø Medical and Surgical
L Tendons
W Revision

Definition: Correcting, to the extent possible, a portion of a malfunctioning device or the position of a displaced device

Explanation: Revision can include correcting a malfunctioning or displaced device by taking out or putting in components of the device such as a screw or pin

Body Part Character 4	Approach Character 5	Device Character 6	Qualifier Character 7
X Upper Tendon Y Lower Tendon	Ø Open 3 Percutaneous 4 Percutaneous Endoscopic	Ø Drainage Device 7 Autologous Tissue Substitute J Synthetic Substitute K Nonautologous Tissue Substitute Y Other Device	Z No Qualifier
X Upper Tendon Y Lower Tendon	X External	Ø Drainage Device 7 Autologous Tissue Substitute J Synthetic Substitute K Nonautologous Tissue Substitute	Z No Qualifier

Non-OR   ØLW[X,Y][3,4]YZ
Non-OR   ØLW[X,Y]X[Ø,7,J,K]Z

Ø Medical and Surgical
L Tendons
X Transfer

Definition: Moving, without taking out, all or a portion of a body part to another location to take over the function of all or a portion of a body part

Explanation: The body part transferred remains connected to its vascular and nervous supply

Body Part Character 4	Approach Character 5	Device Character 6	Qualifier Character 7

Ø Head and Neck Tendon
1 Shoulder Tendon, Right
2 Shoulder Tendon, Left
3 Upper Arm Tendon, Right
4 Upper Arm Tendon, Left
5 Lower Arm and Wrist Tendon, Right
6 Lower Arm and Wrist Tendon, Left
7 Hand Tendon, Right
8 Hand Tendon, Left
9 Trunk Tendon, Right
B Trunk Tendon, Left
C Thorax Tendon, Right
D Thorax Tendon, Left
F Abdomen Tendon, Right
G Abdomen Tendon, Left
H Perineum Tendon
J Hip Tendon, Right
K Hip Tendon, Left
L Upper Leg Tendon, Right
M Upper Leg Tendon, Left
N Lower Leg Tendon, Right
   Achilles tendon
P Lower Leg Tendon, Left
   See N Lower Leg Tendon, Right
Q Knee Tendon, Right
   Patellar tendon
R Knee Tendon, Left
   See Q Knee Tendon, Right
S Ankle Tendon, Right
T Ankle Tendon, Left
V Foot Tendon, Right
W Foot Tendon, Left
	Ø Open
	4 Percutaneous Endoscopic
		Z No Device	Z No Qualifier

Non-OR Procedure   DRG Non-OR Procedure   Valid OR Procedure   HAC Associated Procedure   Combination Only   New/Revised April   New/Revised October

500   ICD-10-PCS 2024

ØLW–ØLX

Bursae and Ligaments ØM2–ØMX

Character Meanings*

This Character Meaning table is provided as a guide to assist the user in the identification of character members that may be found in this section of code tables. It **SHOULD NOT** be used to build a PCS code.

Operation–Character 3		Body Part–Character 4		Approach–Character 5		Device–Character 6		Qualifier–Character 7	
2	Change	Ø	Head and Neck Bursa and Ligament	Ø	Open	Ø	Drainage Device	X	Diagnostic
5	Destruction	1	Shoulder Bursa and Ligament, Right	3	Percutaneous	7	Autologous Tissue Substitute	Z	No Qualifier
8	Division	2	Shoulder Bursa and Ligament, Left	4	Percutaneous Endoscopic	J	Synthetic Substitute		
9	Drainage	3	Elbow Bursa and Ligament, Right	X	External	K	Nonautologous Tissue Substitute		
B	Excision	4	Elbow Bursa and Ligament, Left			Y	Other Device		
C	Extirpation	5	Wrist Bursa and Ligament, Right			Z	No Device		
D	Extraction	6	Wrist Bursa and Ligament, Left						
H	Insertion	7	Hand Bursa and Ligament, Right						
J	Inspection	8	Hand Bursa and Ligament, Left						
M	Reattachment	9	Upper Extremity Bursa and Ligament, Right						
N	Release	B	Upper Extremity Bursa and Ligament, Left						
P	Removal	C	Upper Spine Bursa and Ligament						
Q	Repair	D	Lower Spine Bursa and Ligament						
R	Replacement	F	Sternum Bursa and Ligament						
S	Reposition	G	Rib(s) Bursa and Ligament						
T	Resection	H	Abdomen Bursa and Ligament, Right						
U	Supplement	J	Abdomen Bursa and Ligament, Left						
W	Revision	K	Perineum Bursa and Ligament						
X	Transfer	L	Hip Bursa and Ligament, Right						
		M	Hip Bursa and Ligament, Left						
		N	Knee Bursa and Ligament, Right						
		P	Knee Bursa and Ligament, Left						
		Q	Ankle Bursa and Ligament, Right						
		R	Ankle Bursa and Ligament, Left						
		S	Foot Bursa and Ligament, Right						
		T	Foot Bursa and Ligament, Left						
		V	Lower Extremity Bursa and Ligament, Right						
		W	Lower Extremity Bursa and Ligament, Left						
		X	Upper Bursa and Ligament						
		Y	Lower Bursa and Ligament						

* Includes synovial membrane.

AHA Coding Clinic for table ØMB
2018, 3Q, 17   Excisional debridement of periosteum

AHA Coding Clinic for table ØMM
2013, 3Q, 20   Superior labrum anterior posterior (SLAP) repair and subacromial decompression

AHA Coding Clinic for table ØMQ
2014, 3Q, 9   Interspinous ligamentoplasty

AHA Coding Clinic for table ØMT
2017, 2Q, 21   Arthroscopic anterior cruciate ligament revision using autograft with anterolateral ligament reconstruction

AHA Coding Clinic for table ØMU
2017, 2Q, 21   Arthroscopic anterior cruciate ligament revision using autograft with anterolateral ligament reconstruction

Bursae and Ligaments

Shoulder Ligaments

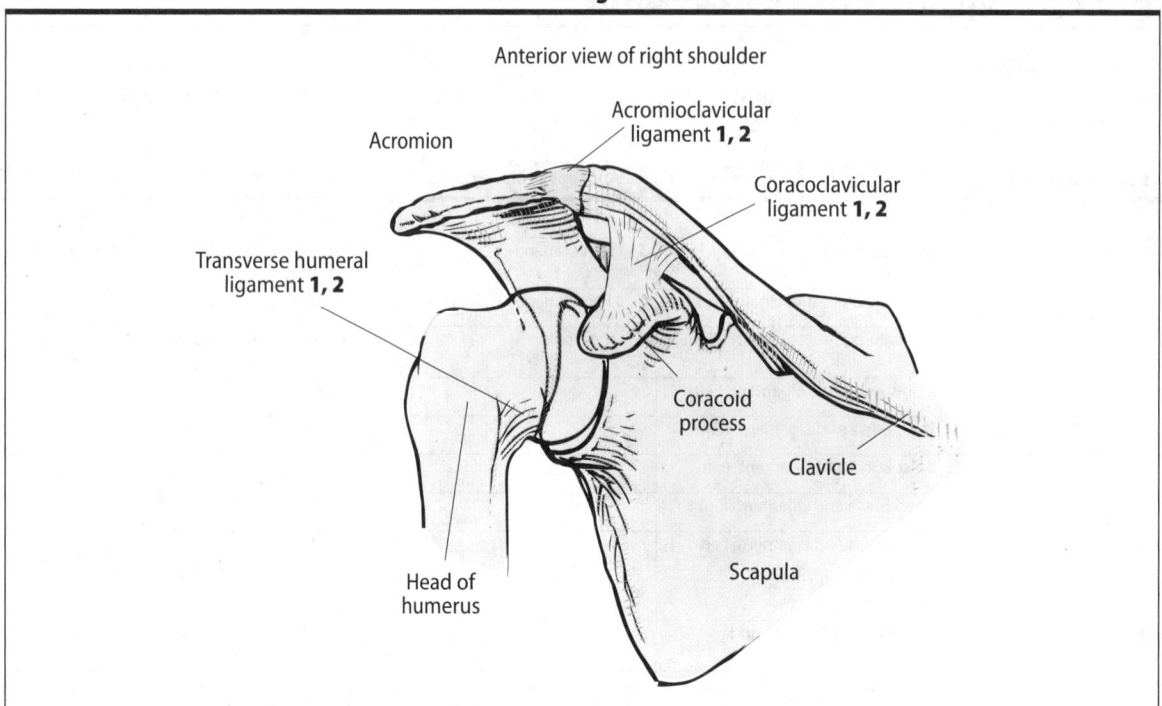

Anterior view of right shoulder

Acromion

Acromioclavicular ligament **1, 2**

Coracoclavicular ligament **1, 2**

Transverse humeral ligament **1, 2**

Coracoid process

Clavicle

Head of humerus

Scapula

Knee Bursae

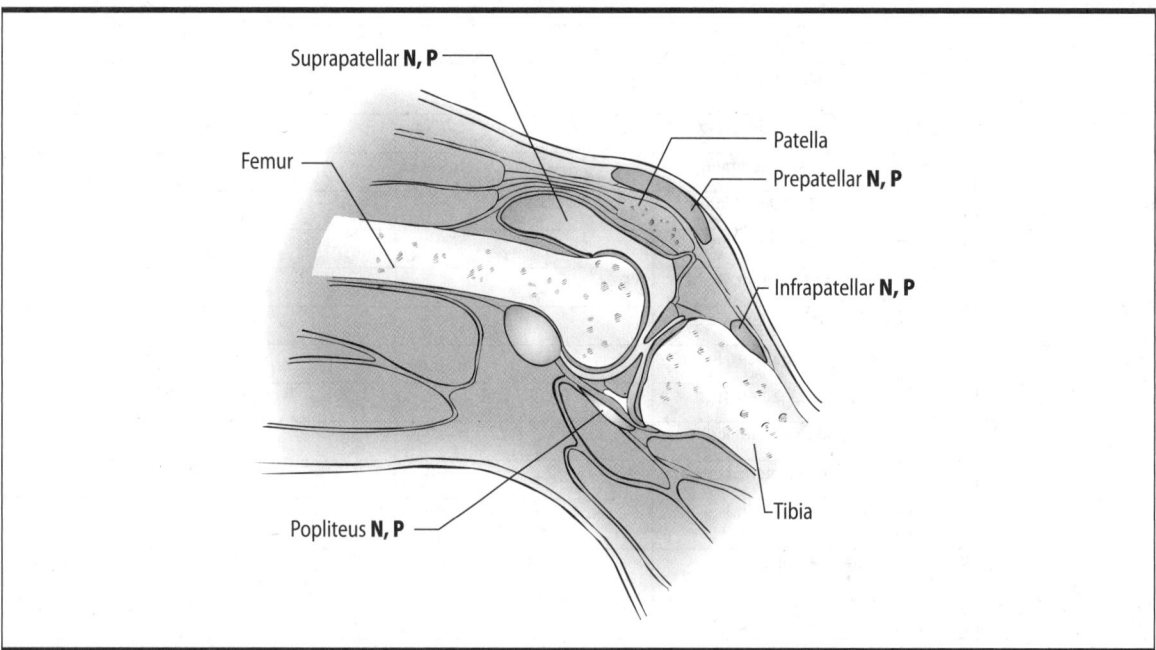

Suprapatellar **N, P**

Femur

Patella

Prepatellar **N, P**

Infrapatellar **N, P**

Popliteus **N, P**

Tibia

Knee Ligaments

Anterior view

Lateral collateral ligament **N, P**

Medial collateral ligament **N, P**

Patella

Posterior cruciate ligament **N, P**
(Behind the Anterior cruciate)

Anterior cruciate ligament **N, P**

Fibula

Tibia

Posterior cruciate
ligament **N, P**

Anterior cruciate ligament **N, P**

Wrist Ligaments

Palmar view

5 4 3 2 1

Flexor carpi
ulnaris **5, 6**

Radial collateral
carpal **5, 6**

Ulnar collateral
carpal **5, 6**

Palmar radiocarpal **5, 6**

Dorsal view

1 2 3 4 5

Radial collateral
carpal **5, 6**

Ulnar collateral
carpal **5, 6**

Dorsal
radiocarpal **5, 6**

Ulnocarpal **5, 6**

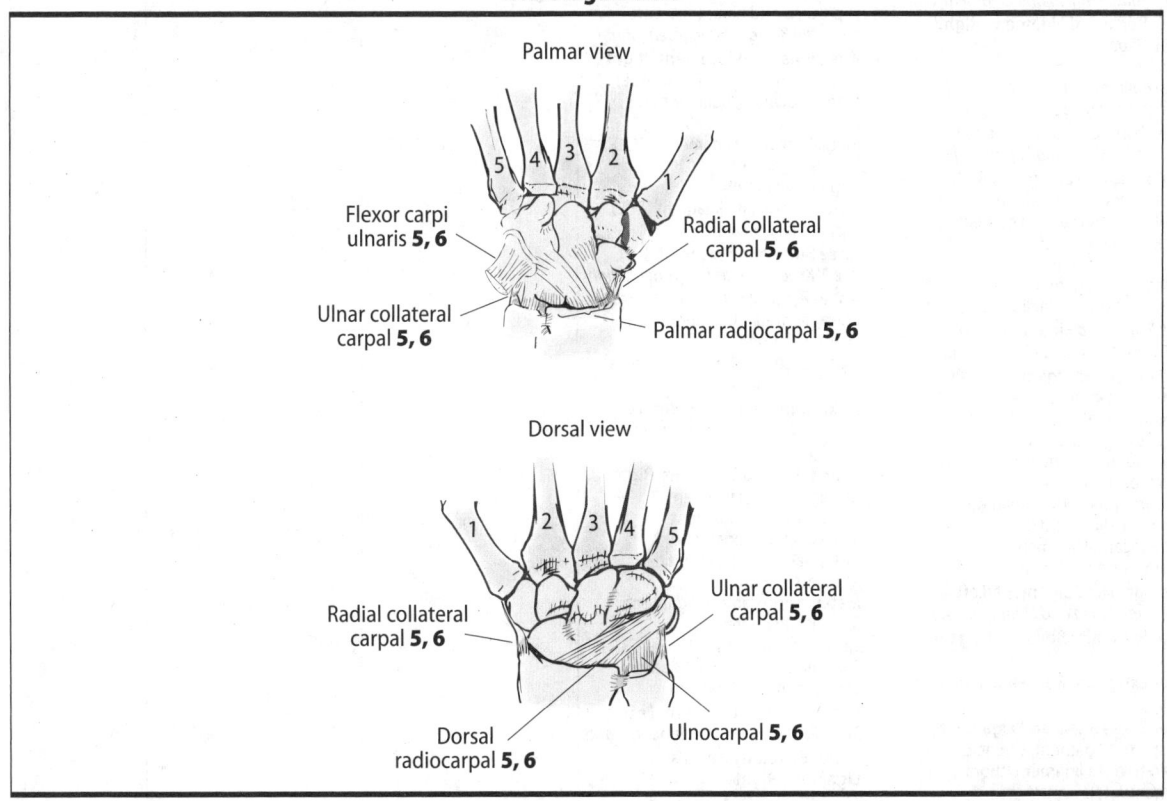

Bursae and Ligaments

Ø **Medical and Surgical**
M **Bursae and Ligaments**
2 **Change**   Definition: Taking out or off a device from a body part and putting back an identical or similar device in or on the same body part without cutting or puncturing the skin or a mucous membrane

Explanation: All CHANGE procedures are coded using the approach EXTERNAL

Body Part Character 4	Approach Character 5	Device Character 6	Qualifier Character 7
X Upper Bursa and Ligament Y Lower Bursa and Ligament	X External	Ø Drainage Device Y Other Device	Z No Qualifier

Non-OR	All body part, approach, device, and qualifier values

Ø **Medical and Surgical**
M **Bursae and Ligaments**
5 **Destruction**   Definition: Physical eradication of all or a portion of a body part by the direct use of energy, force, or a destructive agent

Explanation: None of the body part is physically taken out

Body Part Character 4		Approach Character 5	Device Character 6	Qualifier Character 7
Ø **Head and Neck Bursa and Ligament** Alar ligament of axis Cervical interspinous ligament Cervical intertransverse ligament Cervical ligamentum flavum Interspinous ligament, cervical Intertransverse ligament, cervical Lateral temporomandibular ligament Ligamentum flavum, cervical Sphenomandibular ligament Stylomandibular ligament Transverse ligament of atlas	D **Lower Spine Bursa and Ligament** Iliolumbar ligament Interspinous ligament, lumbar Intertransverse ligament, lumbar Ligamentum flavum, lumbar Sacrococcygeal ligament Sacroiliac ligament Sacrospinous ligament Sacrotuberous ligament Supraspinous ligament	Ø Open 3 Percutaneous 4 Percutaneous Endoscopic	Z No Device	Z No Qualifier
1 **Shoulder Bursa and Ligament, Right** Acromioclavicular ligament Coracoacromial ligament Coracoclavicular ligament Coracohumeral ligament Costoclavicular ligament Glenohumeral ligament Interclavicular ligament Sternoclavicular ligament Subacromial bursa Transverse humeral ligament Transverse scapular ligament	F **Sternum Bursa and Ligament** Costoxiphoid ligament Sternocostal ligament G **Rib(s) Bursa and Ligament** Costotransverse ligament H **Abdomen Bursa and Ligament, Right** J **Abdomen Bursa and Ligament, Left** K **Perineum Bursa and Ligament** L **Hip Bursa and Ligament, Right** Iliofemoral ligament Ischiofemoral ligament Pubofemoral ligament Transverse acetabular ligament Trochanteric bursa			
2 **Shoulder Bursa and Ligament, Left** *See 1 Shoulder Bursa and Ligament, Right* 3 **Elbow Bursa and Ligament, Right** Annular ligament Olecranon bursa Radial collateral ligament Ulnar collateral ligament 4 **Elbow Bursa and Ligament, Left** *See 3 Elbow Bursa and Ligament, Right* 5 **Wrist Bursa and Ligament, Right** Palmar ulnocarpal ligament Radial collateral carpal ligament Radiocarpal ligament Radioulnar ligament Scapholunate ligament Ulnar collateral carpal ligament 6 **Wrist Bursa and Ligament, Left** *See 5 Wrist Bursa and Ligament, Right* 7 **Hand Bursa and Ligament, Right** Carpometacarpal ligament Intercarpal ligament Interphalangeal ligament Lunotriquetral ligament Metacarpal ligament Metacarpophalangeal ligament Pisohamate ligament Pisometacarpal ligament Scaphotrapezium ligament 8 **Hand Bursa and Ligament, Left** *See 7 Hand Bursa and Ligament, Right* 9 **Upper Extremity Bursa and Ligament, Right** B **Upper Extremity Bursa and Ligament, Left** C **Upper Spine Bursa and Ligament** Interspinous ligament, thoracic Intertransverse ligament, thoracic Ligamentum flavum, thoracic Supraspinous ligament	M **Hip Bursa and Ligament, Left** *See L Hip Bursa and Ligament, Right* N **Knee Bursa and Ligament, Right** Anterior cruciate ligament (ACL) Lateral collateral ligament (LCL) Ligament of head of fibula Medial collateral ligament (MCL) Patellar ligament Popliteal ligament Posterior cruciate ligament (PCL) Prepatellar bursa P **Knee Bursa and Ligament, Left** *See N Knee Bursa and Ligament, Right* Q **Ankle Bursa and Ligament, Right** Calcaneofibular ligament Deltoid ligament Ligament of the lateral malleolus Talofibular ligament R **Ankle Bursa and Ligament, Left** *See Q Ankle Bursa and Ligament, Right* S **Foot Bursa and Ligament, Right** Calcaneocuboid ligament Cuneonavicular ligament Intercuneiform ligament Interphalangeal ligament Metatarsal ligament Metatarsophalangeal ligament Subtalar ligament Talocalcaneal ligament Talocalcaneonavicular ligament Tarsometatarsal ligament T **Foot Bursa and Ligament, Left** *See S Foot Bursa and Ligament, Right* V **Lower Extremity Bursa and Ligament, Right** W **Lower Extremity Bursa and Ligament, Left**			

Non-OR Procedure   DRG Non-OR Procedure   Valid OR Procedure   HAC Associated Procedure   Combination Only   New/Revised April   New/Revised October

504   ICD-10-PCS 2024

Bursae and Ligaments

Ø	Medical and Surgical
M	Bursae and Ligaments
8	Division

Definition: Cutting into a body part, without draining fluids and/or gases from the body part, in order to separate or transect a body part

Explanation: All or a portion of the body part is separated into two or more portions

Body Part Character 4		Approach Character 5	Device Character 6	Qualifier Character 7
Ø Head and Neck Bursa and Ligament Alar ligament of axis Cervical interspinous ligament Cervical intertransverse ligament Cervical ligamentum flavum Interspinous ligament, cervical Intertransverse ligament, cervical Lateral temporomandibular ligament Ligamentum flavum, cervical Sphenomandibular ligament Stylomandibular ligament Transverse ligament of atlas	**D Lower Spine Bursa and Ligament** Iliolumbar ligament Interspinous ligament, lumbar Intertransverse ligament, lumbar Ligamentum flavum, lumbar Sacrococcygeal ligament Sacroiliac ligament Sacrospinous ligament Sacrotuberous ligament Supraspinous ligament	**Ø Open** **3 Percutaneous** **4 Percutaneous Endoscopic**	**Z No Device**	**Z No Qualifier**
1 Shoulder Bursa and Ligament, Right Acromioclavicular ligament Coracoacromial ligament Coracoclavicular ligament Coracohumeral ligament Costoclavicular ligament Glenohumeral ligament Interclavicular ligament Sternoclavicular ligament Subacromial bursa Transverse humeral ligament Transverse scapular ligament	**F Sternum Bursa and Ligament** Costoxiphoid ligament Sternocostal ligament **G Rib(s) Bursa and Ligament** Costotransverse ligament **H Abdomen Bursa and Ligament, Right** **J Abdomen Bursa and Ligament, Left** **K Perineum Bursa and Ligament**			
2 Shoulder Bursa and Ligament, Left *See 1 Shoulder Bursa and Ligament, Right*	**L Hip Bursa and Ligament, Right** Iliofemoral ligament Ischiofemoral ligament Pubofemoral ligament Transverse acetabular ligament Trochanteric bursa			
3 Elbow Bursa and Ligament, Right Annular ligament Olecranon bursa Radial collateral ligament Ulnar collateral ligament	**M Hip Bursa and Ligament, Left** *See L Hip Bursa and Ligament, Right*			
4 Elbow Bursa and Ligament, Left *See 3 Elbow Bursa and Ligament, Right*	**N Knee Bursa and Ligament, Right** Anterior cruciate ligament (ACL) Lateral collateral ligament (LCL) Ligament of head of fibula Medial collateral ligament (MCL) Patellar ligament Popliteal ligament Posterior cruciate ligament (PCL) Prepatellar bursa			
5 Wrist Bursa and Ligament, Right Palmar ulnocarpal ligament Radial collateral carpal ligament Radiocarpal ligament Radioulnar ligament Scapholunate ligament Ulnar collateral carpal ligament	**P Knee Bursa and Ligament, Left** *See N Knee Bursa and Ligament, Right*			
6 Wrist Bursa and Ligament, Left *See 5 Wrist Bursa and Ligament, Right*	**Q Ankle Bursa and Ligament, Right** Calcaneofibular ligament Deltoid ligament Ligament of the lateral malleolus Talofibular ligament			
7 Hand Bursa and Ligament, Right Carpometacarpal ligament Intercarpal ligament Interphalangeal ligament Lunotriquetral ligament Metacarpal ligament Metacarpophalangeal ligament Pisohamate ligament Pisometacarpal ligament Scaphotrapezium ligament	**R Ankle Bursa and Ligament, Left** *See Q Ankle Bursa and Ligament, Right*			
8 Hand Bursa and Ligament, Left *See 7 Hand Bursa and Ligament, Right*	**S Foot Bursa and Ligament, Right** Calcaneocuboid ligament Cuneonavicular ligament Intercuneiform ligament Interphalangeal ligament Metatarsal ligament Metatarsophalangeal ligament Subtalar ligament Talocalcaneal ligament Talocalcaneonavicular ligament Tarsometatarsal ligament			
9 Upper Extremity Bursa and Ligament, Right	**T Foot Bursa and Ligament, Left** *See S Foot Bursa and Ligament, Right*			
B Upper Extremity Bursa and Ligament, Left	**V Lower Extremity Bursa and Ligament, Right**			
C Upper Spine Bursa and Ligament Interspinous ligament, thoracic Intertransverse ligament, thoracic Ligamentum flavum, thoracic Supraspinous ligament	**W Lower Extremity Bursa and Ligament, Left**			

NC Noncovered Procedure　　LC Limited Coverage　　QA Questionable OB Admit　　NT New Tech Add-on　　⊞ Combination Member　　♂ Male　　♀ Female

ICD-10-PCS 2024　　　　　　　　　　　　　　　　　　　　　　　　　　　　　　505

Bursae and Ligaments

Ø **Medical and Surgical**
M **Bursae and Ligaments**
9 **Drainage**   Definition: Taking or letting out fluids and/or gases from a body part
                            Explanation: The qualifier DIAGNOSTIC is used to identify drainage procedures that are biopsies

Body Part Character 4		Approach Character 5	Device Character 6	Qualifier Character 7
Ø **Head and Neck Bursa and Ligament** Alar ligament of axis Cervical interspinous ligament Cervical intertransverse ligament Cervical ligamentum flavum Interspinous ligament, cervical Intertransverse ligament, cervical Lateral temporomandibular ligament Ligamentum flavum, cervical Sphenomandibular ligament Stylomandibular ligament Transverse ligament of atlas	**D** **Lower Spine Bursa and Ligament** Iliolumbar ligament Interspinous ligament, lumbar Intertransverse ligament, lumbar Ligamentum flavum, lumbar Sacrococcygeal ligament Sacroiliac ligament Sacrospinous ligament Sacrotuberous ligament Supraspinous ligament	**Ø** Open **3** Percutaneous **4** Percutaneous Endoscopic	**Ø** Drainage Device	**Z** No Qualifier
1 **Shoulder Bursa and Ligament, Right** Acromioclavicular ligament Coracoacromial ligament Coracoclavicular ligament Coracohumeral ligament Costoclavicular ligament Glenohumeral ligament Interclavicular ligament Sternoclavicular ligament Subacromial bursa Transverse humeral ligament Transverse scapular ligament	**F** **Sternum Bursa and Ligament** Costoxiphoid ligament Sternocostal ligament **G** **Rib(s) Bursa and Ligament** Costotransverse ligament **H** **Abdomen Bursa and Ligament, Right** **J** **Abdomen Bursa and Ligament, Left** **K** **Perineum Bursa and Ligament**			
2 **Shoulder Bursa and Ligament, Left** *See* 1 Shoulder Bursa and Ligament, Right	**L** **Hip Bursa and Ligament, Right** Iliofemoral ligament Ischiofemoral ligament Pubofemoral ligament Transverse acetabular ligament Trochanteric bursa			
3 **Elbow Bursa and Ligament, Right** Annular ligament Olecranon bursa Radial collateral ligament Ulnar collateral ligament	**M** **Hip Bursa and Ligament, Left** *See* L Hip Bursa and Ligament, Right			
4 **Elbow Bursa and Ligament, Left** *See* 3 Elbow Bursa and Ligament, Right	**N** **Knee Bursa and Ligament, Right** Anterior cruciate ligament (ACL) Lateral collateral ligament (LCL) Ligament of head of fibula Medial collateral ligament (MCL) Patellar ligament Popliteal ligament Posterior cruciate ligament (PCL) Prepatellar bursa			
5 **Wrist Bursa and Ligament, Right** Palmar ulnocarpal ligament Radial collateral carpal ligament Radiocarpal ligament Radioulnar ligament Scapholunate ligament Ulnar collateral carpal ligament	**P** **Knee Bursa and Ligament, Left** *See* N Knee Bursa and Ligament, Right			
6 **Wrist Bursa and Ligament, Left** *See* 5 Wrist Bursa and Ligament, Right	**Q** **Ankle Bursa and Ligament, Right** Calcaneofibular ligament Deltoid ligament Ligament of the lateral malleolus Talofibular ligament			
7 **Hand Bursa and Ligament, Right** Carpometacarpal ligament Intercarpal ligament Interphalangeal ligament Lunotriquetral ligament Metacarpal ligament Metacarpophalangeal ligament Pisohamate ligament Pisometacarpal ligament Scaphotrapezium ligament	**R** **Ankle Bursa and Ligament, Left** *See* Q Ankle Bursa and Ligament, Right **S** **Foot Bursa and Ligament, Right** Calcaneocuboid ligament Cuneonavicular ligament Intercuneiform ligament Interphalangeal ligament Metatarsal ligament Metatarsophalangeal ligament Subtalar ligament Talocalcaneal ligament Talocalcaneonavicular ligament Tarsometatarsal ligament			
8 **Hand Bursa and Ligament, Left** *See* 7 Hand Bursa and Ligament, Right	**T** **Foot Bursa and Ligament, Left** *See* S Foot Bursa and Ligament, Right			
9 **Upper Extremity Bursa and Ligament, Right** **B** **Upper Extremity Bursa and Ligament, Left**	**V** **Lower Extremity Bursa and Ligament, Right** **W** **Lower Extremity Bursa and Ligament, Left**			
C **Upper Spine Bursa and Ligament** Interspinous ligament, thoracic Intertransverse ligament, thoracic Ligamentum flavum, thoracic Supraspinous ligament				

Non-OR   ØM9[Ø,1,2,3,4,5,6,7,8,9,B,C,D,F,G,H,J,K,L,M,N,P,Q,R,S,T,V,W]3ØZ
Non-OR   ØM9[1,2,3,4,7,8,9,B,C,D,F,G,H,J,K,L,M,V,W]4ØZ

ØM9 Continued on next page

Non-OR Procedure   DRG Non-OR Procedure   Valid OR Procedure   HAC Associated Procedure   Combination Only   New/Revised April   New/Revised October

Ø   Medical and Surgical
M   Bursae and Ligaments
9   Drainage   Definition: Taking or letting out fluids and/or gases from a body part

Explanation: The qualifier DIAGNOSTIC is used to identify drainage procedures that are biopsies

Body Part Character 4		Approach Character 5	Device Character 6	Qualifier Character 7
Ø Head and Neck Bursa and Ligament Alar ligament of axis Cervical interspinous ligament Cervical intertransverse ligament Cervical ligamentum flavum Interspinous ligament, cervical Intertransverse ligament, cervical Lateral temporomandibular ligament Ligamentum flavum, cervical Sphenomandibular ligament Stylomandibular ligament Transverse ligament of atlas	**D Lower Spine Bursa and Ligament** Iliolumbar ligament Interspinous ligament, lumbar Intertransverse ligament, lumbar Ligamentum flavum, lumbar Sacrococcygeal ligament Sacroiliac ligament Sacrospinous ligament Sacrotuberous ligament Supraspinous ligament	**Ø Open** **3 Percutaneous** **4 Percutaneous Endoscopic**	**Z No Device**	**X Diagnostic** **Z No Qualifier**
1 Shoulder Bursa and Ligament, Right Acromioclavicular ligament Coracoacromial ligament Coracoclavicular ligament Coracohumeral ligament Costoclavicular ligament Glenohumeral ligament Interclavicular ligament Sternoclavicular ligament Subacromial bursa Transverse humeral ligament Transverse scapular ligament	**F Sternum Bursa and Ligament** Costoxiphoid ligament Sternocostal ligament **G Rib(s) Bursa and Ligament** Costotransverse ligament **H Abdomen Bursa and Ligament, Right** **J Abdomen Bursa and Ligament, Left** **K Perineum Bursa and Ligament**			
2 Shoulder Bursa and Ligament, Left *See* 1 Shoulder Bursa and Ligament, Right	**L Hip Bursa and Ligament, Right** Iliofemoral ligament Ischiofemoral ligament Pubofemoral ligament Transverse acetabular ligament Trochanteric bursa			
3 Elbow Bursa and Ligament, Right Annular ligament Olecranon bursa Radial collateral ligament Ulnar collateral ligament	**M Hip Bursa and Ligament, Left** *See* L Hip Bursa and Ligament, Right			
4 Elbow Bursa and Ligament, Left *See* 3 Elbow Bursa and Ligament, Right	**N Knee Bursa and Ligament, Right** Anterior cruciate ligament (ACL) Lateral collateral ligament (LCL) Ligament of head of fibula Medial collateral ligament (MCL) Patellar ligament Popliteal ligament Posterior cruciate ligament (PCL) Prepatellar bursa			
5 Wrist Bursa and Ligament, Right Palmar ulnocarpal ligament Radial collateral carpal ligament Radiocarpal ligament Radioulnar ligament Scapholunate ligament Ulnar collateral carpal ligament	**P Knee Bursa and Ligament, Left** *See* N Knee Bursa and Ligament, Right			
6 Wrist Bursa and Ligament, Left *See* 5 Wrist Bursa and Ligament, Right	**Q Ankle Bursa and Ligament, Right** Calcaneofibular ligament Deltoid ligament Ligament of the lateral malleolus Talofibular ligament			
7 Hand Bursa and Ligament, Right Carpometacarpal ligament Intercarpal ligament Interphalangeal ligament Lunotriquetral ligament Metacarpal ligament Metacarpophalangeal ligament Pisohamate ligament Pisometacarpal ligament Scaphotrapezium ligament	**R Ankle Bursa and Ligament, Left** *See* Q Ankle Bursa and Ligament, Right **S Foot Bursa and Ligament, Right** Calcaneocuboid ligament Cuneonavicular ligament Intercuneiform ligament Interphalangeal ligament Metatarsal ligament Metatarsophalangeal ligament Subtalar ligament Talocalcaneal ligament Talocalcaneonavicular ligament Tarsometatarsal ligament			
8 Hand Bursa and Ligament, Left *See* 7 Hand Bursa and Ligament, Right	**T Foot Bursa and Ligament, Left** *See* S Foot Bursa and Ligament, Right			
9 Upper Extremity Bursa and Ligament, Right	**V Lower Extremity Bursa and Ligament, Right**			
B Upper Extremity Bursa and Ligament, Left	**W Lower Extremity Bursa and Ligament, Left**			
C Upper Spine Bursa and Ligament Interspinous ligament, thoracic Intertransverse ligament, thoracic Ligamentum flavum, thoracic Supraspinous ligament				

Non-OR   ØM9[Ø,1,2,3,4,5,6,7,8,C,D,F,G,L,M,N,P,Q,R,S,T][Ø,3,4]ZX
Non-OR   ØM9[Ø,1,2,3,4,5,6,7,8,9,B,C,D,F,G,H,J,K,L,M,N,P,Q,R,S,T,V,W]3ZZ
Non-OR   ØM9[Ø,5,6,7,8,9,B,C,D,F,G,H,J,K,N,P,Q,R,S,T,V,W]4ZZ

NC Noncovered Procedure   LC Limited Coverage   QA Questionable OB Admit   NT New Tech Add-on   ⊞ Combination Member   ♂ Male   ♀ Female

ICD-10-PCS 2024   507

ØM9–ØM9

Bursae and Ligaments

ØMB–ØMB

Ø Medical and Surgical
M Bursae and Ligaments
B Excision   **Definition:** Cutting out or off, without replacement, a portion of a body part

                  Explanation: The qualifier DIAGNOSTIC is used to identify excision procedures that are biopsies

Body Part Character 4		Approach Character 5	Device Character 6	Qualifier Character 7
Ø Head and Neck Bursa and Ligament Alar ligament of axis Cervical interspinous ligament Cervical intertransverse ligament Cervical ligamentum flavum Interspinous ligament, cervical Intertransverse ligament, cervical Lateral temporomandibular ligament Ligamentum flavum, cervical Sphenomandibular ligament Stylomandibular ligament Transverse ligament of atlas	**D Lower Spine Bursa and Ligament** Iliolumbar ligament Interspinous ligament, lumbar Intertransverse ligament, lumbar Ligamentum flavum, lumbar Sacrococcygeal ligament Sacroiliac ligament Sacrospinous ligament Sacrotuberous ligament Supraspinous ligament	**Ø Open** **3 Percutaneous** **4 Percutaneous Endoscopic**	**Z No Device**	**X Diagnostic** **Z No Qualifier**
1 Shoulder Bursa and Ligament, Right Acromioclavicular ligament Coracoacromial ligament Coracoclavicular ligament Coracohumeral ligament Costoclavicular ligament Glenohumeral ligament Interclavicular ligament Sternoclavicular ligament Subacromial bursa Transverse humeral ligament Transverse scapular ligament	**F Sternum Bursa and Ligament** Costoxiphoid ligament Sternocostal ligament **G Rib(s) Bursa and Ligament** Costotransverse ligament **H Abdomen Bursa and Ligament, Right** **J Abdomen Bursa and Ligament, Left** **K Perineum Bursa and Ligament**			
2 Shoulder Bursa and Ligament, Left *See 1 Shoulder Bursa and Ligament, Right*	**L Hip Bursa and Ligament, Right** Iliofemoral ligament Ischiofemoral ligament Pubofemoral ligament Transverse acetabular ligament Trochanteric bursa			
3 Elbow Bursa and Ligament, Right Annular ligament Olecranon bursa Radial collateral ligament Ulnar collateral ligament	**M Hip Bursa and Ligament, Left** *See L Hip Bursa and Ligament, Right*			
4 Elbow Bursa and Ligament, Left *See 3 Elbow Bursa and Ligament, Right*	**N Knee Bursa and Ligament, Right** Anterior cruciate ligament (ACL) Lateral collateral ligament (LCL) Ligament of head of fibula Medial collateral ligament (MCL) Patellar ligament Popliteal ligament Posterior cruciate ligament (PCL) Prepatellar bursa			
5 Wrist Bursa and Ligament, Right Palmar ulnocarpal ligament Radial collateral carpal ligament Radiocarpal ligament Radioulnar ligament Scapholunate ligament Ulnar collateral carpal ligament	**P Knee Bursa and Ligament, Left** *See N Knee Bursa and Ligament, Right*			
6 Wrist Bursa and Ligament, Left *See 5 Wrist Bursa and Ligament, Right*	**Q Ankle Bursa and Ligament, Right** Calcaneofibular ligament Deltoid ligament Ligament of the lateral malleolus Talofibular ligament			
7 Hand Bursa and Ligament, Right Carpometacarpal ligament Intercarpal ligament Interphalangeal ligament Lunotriquetral ligament Metacarpal ligament Metacarpophalangeal ligament Pisohamate ligament Pisometacarpal ligament Scaphotrapezium ligament	**R Ankle Bursa and Ligament, Left** *See Q Ankle Bursa and Ligament, Right* **S Foot Bursa and Ligament, Right** Calcaneocuboid ligament Cuneonavicular ligament Intercuneiform ligament Interphalangeal ligament Metatarsal ligament Metatarsophalangeal ligament Subtalar ligament Talocalcaneal ligament Talocalcaneonavicular ligament Tarsometatarsal ligament			
8 Hand Bursa and Ligament, Left *See 7 Hand Bursa and Ligament, Right*	**T Foot Bursa and Ligament, Left** *See S Foot Bursa and Ligament, Right*			
9 Upper Extremity Bursa and Ligament, Right **B Upper Extremity Bursa and Ligament, Left**	**V Lower Extremity Bursa and Ligament, Right** **W Lower Extremity Bursa and Ligament, Left**			
C Upper Spine Bursa and Ligament Interspinous ligament, thoracic Intertransverse ligament, thoracic Ligamentum flavum, thoracic Supraspinous ligament				

Non-OR   ØMB[Ø,1,2,3,4,5,6,7,8,B,C,D,F,G,L,M,N,P,Q,R,S,T][Ø,3,4]ZX
Non-OR   ØMB94ZX

Non-OR Procedure   DRG Non-OR Procedure   Valid OR Procedure   HAC Associated Procedure   Combination Only   New/Revised April   New/Revised October

Bursae and Ligaments

Ø Medical and Surgical
M Bursae and Ligaments
C Extirpation   Definition: Taking or cutting out solid matter from a body part

Explanation: The solid matter may be an abnormal byproduct of a biological function or a foreign body; it may be imbedded in a body part or in the lumen of a tubular body part. The solid matter may or may not have been previously broken into pieces.

Body Part Character 4		Approach Character 5	Device Character 6	Qualifier Character 7
Ø Head and Neck Bursa and Ligament Alar ligament of axis Cervical interspinous ligament Cervical intertransverse ligament Cervical ligamentum flavum Interspinous ligament, cervical Intertransverse ligament, cervical Lateral temporomandibular ligament Ligamentum flavum, cervical Sphenomandibular ligament Stylomandibular ligament Transverse ligament of atlas **1 Shoulder Bursa and Ligament, Right** Acromioclavicular ligament Coracoacromial ligament Coracoclavicular ligament Coracohumeral ligament Costoclavicular ligament Glenohumeral ligament Interclavicular ligament Sternoclavicular ligament Subacromial bursa Transverse humeral ligament Transverse scapular ligament **2 Shoulder Bursa and Ligament, Left** *See 1 Shoulder Bursa and Ligament, Right* **3 Elbow Bursa and Ligament, Right** Annular ligament Olecranon bursa Radial collateral ligament Ulnar collateral ligament **4 Elbow Bursa and Ligament, Left** *See 3 Elbow Bursa and Ligament, Right* **5 Wrist Bursa and Ligament, Right** Palmar ulnocarpal ligament Radial collateral carpal ligament Radiocarpal ligament Radioulnar ligament Scapholunate ligament Ulnar collateral carpal ligament **6 Wrist Bursa and Ligament, Left** *See 5 Wrist Bursa and Ligament, Right* **7 Hand Bursa and Ligament, Right** Carpometacarpal ligament Intercarpal ligament Interphalangeal ligament Lunotriquetral ligament Metacarpal ligament Metacarpophalangeal ligament Pisohamate ligament Pisometacarpal ligament Scaphotrapezium ligament **8 Hand Bursa and Ligament, Left** *See 7 Hand Bursa and Ligament, Right* **9 Upper Extremity Bursa and Ligament, Right** **B Upper Extremity Bursa and Ligament, Left** **C Upper Spine Bursa and Ligament** Interspinous ligament, thoracic Intertransverse ligament, thoracic Ligamentum flavum, thoracic Supraspinous ligament	**D Lower Spine Bursa and Ligament** Iliolumbar ligament Interspinous ligament, lumbar Intertransverse ligament, lumbar Ligamentum flavum, lumbar Sacrococcygeal ligament Sacroiliac ligament Sacrospinous ligament Sacrotuberous ligament Supraspinous ligament **F Sternum Bursa and Ligament** Costoxiphoid ligament Sternocostal ligament **G Rib(s) Bursa and Ligament** Costotransverse ligament **H Abdomen Bursa and Ligament, Right** **J Abdomen Bursa and Ligament, Left** **K Perineum Bursa and Ligament** **L Hip Bursa and Ligament, Right** Iliofemoral ligament Ischiofemoral ligament Pubofemoral ligament Transverse acetabular ligament Trochanteric bursa **M Hip Bursa and Ligament, Left** *See L Hip Bursa and Ligament, Right* **N Knee Bursa and Ligament, Right** Anterior cruciate ligament (ACL) Lateral collateral ligament (LCL) Ligament of head of fibula Medial collateral ligament (MCL) Patellar ligament Popliteal ligament Posterior cruciate ligament (PCL) Prepatellar bursa **P Knee Bursa and Ligament, Left** *See N Knee Bursa and Ligament, Right* **Q Ankle Bursa and Ligament, Right** Calcaneofibular ligament Deltoid ligament Ligament of the lateral malleolus Talofibular ligament **R Ankle Bursa and Ligament, Left** *See Q Ankle Bursa and Ligament, Right* **S Foot Bursa and Ligament, Right** Calcaneocuboid ligament Cuneonavicular ligament Intercuneiform ligament Interphalangeal ligament Metatarsal ligament Metatarsophalangeal ligament Subtalar ligament Talocalcaneal ligament Talocalcaneonavicular ligament Tarsometatarsal ligament **T Foot Bursa and Ligament, Left** *See S Foot Bursa and Ligament, Right* **V Lower Extremity Bursa and Ligament, Right** **W Lower Extremity Bursa and Ligament, Left**	**Ø Open** **3 Percutaneous** **4 Percutaneous Endoscopic**	**Z No Device**	**Z No Qualifier**

NC Noncovered Procedure   **LC** Limited Coverage   **QA** Questionable OB Admit   **NT** New Tech Add-on   ⊞ Combination Member   ♂ Male   ♀ Female

ICD-10-PCS 2024   509

Bursae and Ligaments

Ø   **Medical and Surgical**
M   **Bursae and Ligaments**
D   **Extraction**   Definition: Pulling or stripping out or off all or a portion of a body part by the use of force
                       Explanation: The qualifier DIAGNOSTIC is used to identify extraction procedures that are biopsies

Body Part Character 4		Approach Character 5	Device Character 6	Qualifier Character 7
Ø Head and Neck Bursa and Ligament Alar ligament of axis Cervical interspinous ligament Cervical intertransverse ligament Cervical ligamentum flavum Interspinous ligament, cervical Intertransverse ligament, cervical Lateral temporomandibular ligament Ligamentum flavum, cervical Sphenomandibular ligament Stylomandibular ligament Transverse ligament of atlas **1 Shoulder Bursa and Ligament, Right** Acromioclavicular ligament Coracoacromial ligament Coracoclavicular ligament Coracohumeral ligament Costoclavicular ligament Glenohumeral ligament Interclavicular ligament Sternoclavicular ligament Subacromial bursa Transverse humeral ligament Transverse scapular ligament **2 Shoulder Bursa and Ligament, Left** *See 1 Shoulder Bursa and Ligament, Right* **3 Elbow Bursa and Ligament, Right** Annular ligament Olecranon bursa Radial collateral ligament Ulnar collateral ligament **4 Elbow Bursa and Ligament, Left** *See 3 Elbow Bursa and Ligament, Right* **5 Wrist Bursa and Ligament, Right** Palmar ulnocarpal ligament Radial collateral carpal ligament Radiocarpal ligament Radioulnar ligament Scapholunate ligament Ulnar collateral carpal ligament **6 Wrist Bursa and Ligament, Left** *See 5 Wrist Bursa and Ligament, Right* **7 Hand Bursa and Ligament, Right** Carpometacarpal ligament Intercarpal ligament Interphalangeal ligament Lunotriquetral ligament Metacarpal ligament Metacarpophalangeal ligament Pisohamate ligament Pisometacarpal ligament Scaphotrapezium ligament **8 Hand Bursa and Ligament, Left** *See 7 Hand Bursa and Ligament, Right* **9 Upper Extremity Bursa and Ligament, Right** **B Upper Extremity Bursa and Ligament, Left** **C Upper Spine Bursa and Ligament** Interspinous ligament, thoracic Intertransverse ligament, thoracic Ligamentum flavum, thoracic Supraspinous ligament	**D Lower Spine Bursa and Ligament** Iliolumbar ligament Interspinous ligament, lumbar Intertransverse ligament, lumbar Ligamentum flavum, lumbar Sacrococcygeal ligament Sacroiliac ligament Sacrospinous ligament Sacrotuberous ligament Supraspinous ligament **F Sternum Bursa and Ligament** Costoxiphoid ligament Sternocostal ligament **G Rib(s) Bursa and Ligament** Costotransverse ligament **H Abdomen Bursa and Ligament, Right** **J Abdomen Bursa and Ligament, Left** **K Perineum Bursa and Ligament** **L Hip Bursa and Ligament, Right** Iliofemoral ligament Ischiofemoral ligament Pubofemoral ligament Transverse acetabular ligament Trochanteric bursa **M Hip Bursa and Ligament, Left** *See L Hip Bursa and Ligament, Right* **N Knee Bursa and Ligament, Right** Anterior cruciate ligament (ACL) Lateral collateral ligament (LCL) Ligament of head of fibula Medial collateral ligament (MCL) Patellar ligament Popliteal ligament Posterior cruciate ligament (PCL) Prepatellar bursa **P Knee Bursa and Ligament, Left** *See N Knee Bursa and Ligament, Right* **Q Ankle Bursa and Ligament, Right** Calcaneofibular ligament Deltoid ligament Ligament of the lateral malleolus Talofibular ligament **R Ankle Bursa and Ligament, Left** *See Q Ankle Bursa and Ligament, Right* **S Foot Bursa and Ligament, Right** Calcaneocuboid ligament Cuneonavicular ligament Intercuneiform ligament Interphalangeal ligament Metatarsal ligament Metatarsophalangeal ligament Subtalar ligament Talocalcaneal ligament Talocalcaneonavicular ligament Tarsometatarsal ligament **T Foot Bursa and Ligament, Left** *See S Foot Bursa and Ligament, Right* **V Lower Extremity Bursa and Ligament, Right** **W Lower Extremity Bursa and Ligament, Left**	**Ø Open** **3 Percutaneous** **4 Percutaneous Endoscopic**	**Z No Device**	**Z No Qualifier**

Ø   **Medical and Surgical**
M   **Bursae and Ligaments**
H   **Insertion**   Definition: Putting in a nonbiological appliance that monitors, assists, performs, or prevents a physiological function but does not physically take the place of a body part
                      Explanation: None

Body Part Character 4	Approach Character 5	Device Character 6	Qualifier Character 7
X Upper Bursa and Ligament Y Lower Bursa and Ligament	Ø Open 3 Percutaneous 4 Percutaneous Endoscopic	Y Other Device	Z No Qualifier

Non-OR   ØMH[X,Y][3,4]YZ

Ø   **Medical and Surgical**
M   **Bursae and Ligaments**
J   **Inspection**   Definition: Visually and/or manually exploring a body part
                      Explanation: Visual exploration may be performed with or without optical instrumentation. Manual exploration may be performed directly or through intervening body layers.

Body Part Character 4	Approach Character 5	Device Character 6	Qualifier Character 7
X Upper Bursa and Ligament Y Lower Bursa and Ligament	Ø Open 3 Percutaneous 4 Percutaneous Endoscopic X External	Z No Device	Z No Qualifier

Non-OR   ØMJ[X,Y][3,X]ZZ

NC Noncovered Procedure   LC Limited Coverage   QA Questionable OB Admit   NT New Tech Add-on   ⊞ Combination Member   ♂ Male   ♀ Female

ICD-10-PCS 2024   511

Ø Medical and Surgical
M Bursae and Ligaments
M Reattachment Definition: Putting back in or on all or a portion of a separated body part to its normal location or other suitable location

Explanation: Vascular circulation and nervous pathways may or may not be reestablished

Body Part Character 4		Approach Character 5	Device Character 6	Qualifier Character 7

Ø Head and Neck Bursa and Ligament
Alar ligament of axis
Cervical interspinous ligament
Cervical intertransverse ligament
Cervical ligamentum flavum
Interspinous ligament, cervical
Intertransverse ligament, cervical
Lateral temporomandibular
   ligament
Ligamentum flavum, cervical
Sphenomandibular ligament
Stylomandibular ligament
Transverse ligament of atlas
	D Lower Spine Bursa and Ligament
	Iliolumbar ligament
	Interspinous ligament, lumbar
	Intertransverse ligament, lumbar
	Ligamentum flavum, lumbar
	Sacrococcygeal ligament
	Sacroiliac ligament
	Sacrospinous ligament
	Sacrotuberous ligament
	Supraspinous ligament
		Ø Open
		4 Percutaneous
		   Endoscopic
			Z No Device	**Z** No Qualifier

1 Shoulder Bursa and Ligament, Right Acromioclavicular ligament Coracoacromial ligament Coracoclavicular ligament Coracohumeral ligament Costoclavicular ligament Glenohumeral ligament Interclavicular ligament Sternoclavicular ligament Subacromial bursa Transverse humeral ligament Transverse scapular ligament	**F Sternum Bursa and Ligament** Costoxiphoid ligament Sternocostal ligament **G Rib(s) Bursa and Ligament** Costotransverse ligament **H Abdomen Bursa and Ligament, Right** **J Abdomen Bursa and Ligament, Left** **K Perineum Bursa and Ligament**			
2 Shoulder Bursa and Ligament, Left *See* 1 Shoulder Bursa and Ligament, Right	**L Hip Bursa and Ligament, Right** Iliofemoral ligament Ischiofemoral ligament Pubofemoral ligament Transverse acetabular ligament Trochanteric bursa			
3 Elbow Bursa and Ligament, Right Annular ligament Olecranon bursa Radial collateral ligament Ulnar collateral ligament	**M Hip Bursa and Ligament, Left** *See* L Hip Bursa and Ligament, Right			
4 Elbow Bursa and Ligament, Left *See* 3 Elbow Bursa and Ligament, Right	**N Knee Bursa and Ligament, Right** Anterior cruciate ligament (ACL) Lateral collateral ligament (LCL) Ligament of head of fibula Medial collateral ligament (MCL) Patellar ligament Popliteal ligament Posterior cruciate ligament (PCL) Prepatellar bursa			
5 Wrist Bursa and Ligament, Right Palmar ulnocarpal ligament Radial collateral carpal ligament Radiocarpal ligament Radioulnar ligament Scapholunate ligament Ulnar collateral carpal ligament	**P Knee Bursa and Ligament, Left** *See* N Knee Bursa and Ligament, Right			
6 Wrist Bursa and Ligament, Left *See* 5 Wrist Bursa and Ligament, Right	**Q Ankle Bursa and Ligament, Right** Calcaneofibular ligament Deltoid ligament Ligament of the lateral malleolus Talofibular ligament			
7 Hand Bursa and Ligament, Right Carpometacarpal ligament Intercarpal ligament Interphalangeal ligament Lunotriquetral ligament Metacarpal ligament Metacarpophalangeal ligament Pisohamate ligament Pisometacarpal ligament Scaphotrapezium ligament	**R Ankle Bursa and Ligament, Left** *See* Q Ankle Bursa and Ligament, Right			
8 Hand Bursa and Ligament, Left *See* 7 Hand Bursa and Ligament, Right	**S Foot Bursa and Ligament, Right** Calcaneocuboid ligament Cuneonavicular ligament Intercuneiform ligament Interphalangeal ligament Metatarsal ligament Metatarsophalangeal ligament Subtalar ligament Talocalcaneal ligament Talocalcaneonavicular ligament Tarsometatarsal ligament			
9 Upper Extremity Bursa and Ligament, Right	**T Foot Bursa and Ligament, Left** *See* S Foot Bursa and Ligament, Right			
B Upper Extremity Bursa and Ligament, Left	**V Lower Extremity Bursa and Ligament, Right**			
C Upper Spine Bursa and Ligament Interspinous ligament, thoracic Intertransverse ligament, thoracic Ligamentum flavum, thoracic Supraspinous ligament	**W Lower Extremity Bursa and Ligament, Left**			

Non-OR Procedure   DRG Non-OR Procedure   Valid OR Procedure   HAC Associated Procedure   Combination Only   New/Revised April   New/Revised October

Bursae and Ligaments

Ø   **Medical and Surgical**
M   **Bursae and Ligaments**
N   **Release**   Definition: Freeing a body part from an abnormal physical constraint by cutting or by the use of force
                   Explanation: Some of the restraining tissue may be taken out but none of the body part is taken out

Body Part Character 4		Approach Character 5	Device Character 6	Qualifier Character 7
Ø **Head and Neck Bursa and Ligament** Alar ligament of axis Cervical interspinous ligament Cervical intertransverse ligament Cervical ligamentum flavum Interspinous ligament, cervical Intertransverse ligament, cervical Lateral temporomandibular ligament Ligamentum flavum, cervical Sphenomandibular ligament Stylomandibular ligament Transverse ligament of atlas **1** **Shoulder Bursa and Ligament, Right** Acromioclavicular ligament Coracoacromial ligament Coracoclavicular ligament Coracohumeral ligament Costoclavicular ligament Glenohumeral ligament Interclavicular ligament Sternoclavicular ligament Subacromial bursa Transverse humeral ligament Transverse scapular ligament **2** **Shoulder Bursa and Ligament, Left** *See 1 Shoulder Bursa and Ligament, Right* **3** **Elbow Bursa and Ligament, Right** Annular ligament Olecranon bursa Radial collateral ligament Ulnar collateral ligament **4** **Elbow Bursa and Ligament, Left** *See 3 Elbow Bursa and Ligament, Right* **5** **Wrist Bursa and Ligament, Right** Palmar ulnocarpal ligament Radial collateral carpal ligament Radiocarpal ligament Radioulnar ligament Scapholunate ligament Ulnar collateral carpal ligament **6** **Wrist Bursa and Ligament, Left** *See 5 Wrist Bursa and Ligament, Right* **7** **Hand Bursa and Ligament, Right** Carpometacarpal ligament Intercarpal ligament Interphalangeal ligament Lunotriquetral ligament Metacarpal ligament Metacarpophalangeal ligament Pisohamate ligament Pisometacarpal ligament Scaphotrapezium ligament **8** **Hand Bursa and Ligament, Left** *See 7 Hand Bursa and Ligament, Right* **9** **Upper Extremity Bursa and Ligament, Right** **B** **Upper Extremity Bursa and Ligament, Left** **C** **Upper Spine Bursa and Ligament** Interspinous ligament, thoracic Intertransverse ligament, thoracic Ligamentum flavum, thoracic Supraspinous ligament	**D** **Lower Spine Bursa and Ligament** Iliolumbar ligament Interspinous ligament, lumbar Intertransverse ligament, lumbar Ligamentum flavum, lumbar Sacrococcygeal ligament Sacroiliac ligament Sacrospinous ligament Sacrotuberous ligament Supraspinous ligament **F** **Sternum Bursa and Ligament** Costoxiphoid ligament Sternocostal ligament **G** **Rib(s) Bursa and Ligament** Costotransverse ligament **H** **Abdomen Bursa and Ligament, Right** **J** **Abdomen Bursa and Ligament, Left** **K** **Perineum Bursa and Ligament** **L** **Hip Bursa and Ligament, Right** Iliofemoral ligament Ischiofemoral ligament Pubofemoral ligament Transverse acetabular ligament Trochanteric bursa **M** **Hip Bursa and Ligament, Left** *See L Hip Bursa and Ligament, Right* **N** **Knee Bursa and Ligament, Right** Anterior cruciate ligament (ACL) Lateral collateral ligament (LCL) Ligament of head of fibula Medial collateral ligament (MCL) Patellar ligament Popliteal ligament Posterior cruciate ligament (PCL) Prepatellar bursa **P** **Knee Bursa and Ligament, Left** *See N Knee Bursa and Ligament, Right* **Q** **Ankle Bursa and Ligament, Right** Calcaneofibular ligament Deltoid ligament Ligament of the lateral malleolus Talofibular ligament **R** **Ankle Bursa and Ligament, Left** *See Q Ankle Bursa and Ligament, Right* **S** **Foot Bursa and Ligament, Right** Calcaneocuboid ligament Cuneonavicular ligament Intercuneiform ligament Interphalangeal ligament Metatarsal ligament Metatarsophalangeal ligament Subtalar ligament Talocalcaneal ligament Talocalcaneonavicular ligament Tarsometatarsal ligament **T** **Foot Bursa and Ligament, Left** *See S Foot Bursa and Ligament, Right* **V** **Lower Extremity Bursa and Ligament, Right** **W** **Lower Extremity Bursa and Ligament, Left**	**Ø** Open **3** Percutaneous **4** Percutaneous Endoscopic **X** External	**Z** No Device	**Z** No Qualifier

Non-OR   ØMN[Ø,1,2,3,4,5,6,7,8,9,B,C,D,F,G,H,J,K,L,M,N,P,Q,R,S,T,V,W]XZZ

Bursae and Ligaments

Ø   Medical and Surgical
M   Bursae and Ligaments
P   Removal   Definition: Taking out or off a device from a body part

Explanation: If a device is taken out and a similar device put in without cutting or puncturing the skin or mucous membrane, the procedure is coded to the root operation CHANGE. Otherwise, the procedure for taking out a device is coded to the root operation REMOVAL.

Body Part Character 4		Approach Character 5		Device Character 6		Qualifier Character 7	
X	Upper Bursa and Ligament	Ø	Open	Ø	Drainage Device	Z	No Qualifier
Y	Lower Bursa and Ligament	3	Percutaneous	7	Autologous Tissue Substitute		
		4	Percutaneous Endoscopic	J	Synthetic Substitute		
				K	Nonautologous Tissue Substitute		
				Y	Other Device		
X	Upper Bursa and Ligament	X	External	Ø	Drainage Device	Z	No Qualifier
Y	Lower Bursa and Ligament						

Non-OR   ØMP[X,Y]3ØZ
Non-OR   ØMP[X,Y][3,4]YZ
Non-OR   ØMP[X,Y]XØZ

Ø　**Medical and Surgical**
M　**Bursae and Ligaments**
Q　**Repair**　　　Definition: Restoring, to the extent possible, a body part to its normal anatomic structure and function
　　　　　　　　　Explanation: Used only when the method to accomplish the repair is not one of the other root operations

Body Part Character 4		Approach Character 5	Device Character 6	Qualifier Character 7
Ø　**Head and Neck Bursa and Ligament** 　　Alar ligament of axis 　　Cervical interspinous ligament 　　Cervical intertransverse ligament 　　Cervical ligamentum flavum 　　Interspinous ligament, cervical 　　Intertransverse ligament, cervical 　　Lateral temporomandibular 　　　ligament 　　Ligamentum flavum, cervical 　　Sphenomandibular ligament 　　Stylomandibular ligament 　　Transverse ligament of atlas 1　**Shoulder Bursa and Ligament, Right** 　　Acromioclavicular ligament 　　Coracoacromial ligament 　　Coracoclavicular ligament 　　Coracohumeral ligament 　　Costoclavicular ligament 　　Glenohumeral ligament 　　Interclavicular ligament 　　Sternoclavicular ligament 　　Subacromial bursa 　　Transverse humeral ligament 　　Transverse scapular ligament 2　**Shoulder Bursa and Ligament, Left** 　　*See 1 Shoulder Bursa and Ligament, Right* 3　**Elbow Bursa and Ligament, Right** 　　Annular ligament 　　Olecranon bursa 　　Radial collateral ligament 　　Ulnar collateral ligament 4　**Elbow Bursa and Ligament, Left** 　　*See 3 Elbow Bursa and Ligament, Right* 5　**Wrist Bursa and Ligament, Right** 　　Palmar ulnocarpal ligament 　　Radial collateral carpal ligament 　　Radiocarpal ligament 　　Radioulnar ligament 　　Scapholunate ligament 　　Ulnar collateral carpal ligament 6　**Wrist Bursa and Ligament, Left** 　　*See 5 Wrist Bursa and Ligament, Right* 7　**Hand Bursa and Ligament, Right** 　　Carpometacarpal ligament 　　Intercarpal ligament 　　Interphalangeal ligament 　　Lunotriquetral ligament 　　Metacarpal ligament 　　Metacarpophalangeal ligament 　　Pisohamate ligament 　　Pisometacarpal ligament 　　Scaphotrapezium ligament 8　**Hand Bursa and Ligament, Left** 　　*See 7 Hand Bursa and Ligament, Right* 9　**Upper Extremity Bursa and Ligament, Right** B　**Upper Extremity Bursa and Ligament, Left** C　**Upper Spine Bursa and Ligament** 　　Interspinous ligament, thoracic 　　Intertransverse ligament, thoracic 　　Ligamentum flavum, thoracic 　　Supraspinous ligament	D　**Lower Spine Bursa and Ligament** 　　Iliolumbar ligament 　　Interspinous ligament, lumbar 　　Intertransverse ligament, lumbar 　　Ligamentum flavum, lumbar 　　Sacrococcygeal ligament 　　Sacroiliac ligament 　　Sacrospinous ligament 　　Sacrotuberous ligament 　　Supraspinous ligament F　**Sternum Bursa and Ligament** 　　Costoxiphoid ligament 　　Sternocostal ligament G　**Rib(s) Bursa and Ligament** 　　Costotransverse ligament H　**Abdomen Bursa and Ligament, Right** J　**Abdomen Bursa and Ligament, Left** K　**Perineum Bursa and Ligament** L　**Hip Bursa and Ligament, Right** 　　Iliofemoral ligament 　　Ischiofemoral ligament 　　Pubofemoral ligament 　　Transverse acetabular ligament 　　Trochanteric bursa M　**Hip Bursa and Ligament, Left** 　　*See L Hip Bursa and Ligament, Right* N　**Knee Bursa and Ligament, Right** 　　Anterior cruciate ligament (ACL) 　　Lateral collateral ligament (LCL) 　　Ligament of head of fibula 　　Medial collateral ligament (MCL) 　　Patellar ligament 　　Popliteal ligament 　　Posterior cruciate ligament (PCL) 　　Prepatellar bursa P　**Knee Bursa and Ligament, Left** 　　*See N Knee Bursa and Ligament, Right* Q　**Ankle Bursa and Ligament, Right** 　　Calcaneofibular ligament 　　Deltoid ligament 　　Ligament of the lateral malleolus 　　Talofibular ligament R　**Ankle Bursa and Ligament, Left** 　　*See Q Ankle Bursa and Ligament, Right* S　**Foot Bursa and Ligament, Right** 　　Calcaneocuboid ligament 　　Cuneonavicular ligament 　　Intercuneiform ligament 　　Interphalangeal ligament 　　Metatarsal ligament 　　Metatarsophalangeal ligament 　　Subtalar ligament 　　Talocalcaneal ligament 　　Talocalcaneonavicular ligament 　　Tarsometatarsal ligament T　**Foot Bursa and Ligament, Left** 　　*See S Foot Bursa and Ligament, Right* V　**Lower Extremity Bursa and Ligament, Right** W　**Lower Extremity Bursa and Ligament, Left**	Ø　Open 3　Percutaneous 4　Percutaneous Endoscopic	Z　No Device	Z　No Qualifier

NC Noncovered Procedure　　**LC** Limited Coverage　　**QA** Questionable OB Admit　　**NT** New Tech Add-on　　✚ Combination Member　　♂ Male　　♀ Female

ICD-10-PCS 2024　　　　　　　　　　　　　　　　　　　　　　　　　　　　　　　　　　　　　515

ØMQ–ØMQ

Bursae and Ligaments

Ø Medical and Surgical
M Bursae and Ligaments
R Replacement   Definition: Putting in or on biological or synthetic material that physically takes the place and/or function of all or a portion of a body part

Explanation: The body part may have been taken out or replaced, or may be taken out, physically eradicated, or rendered nonfunctional during the REPLACEMENT procedure. A REMOVAL procedure is coded for taking out the device used in a previous replacement procedure.

Body Part Character 4		Approach Character 5	Device Character 6	Qualifier Character 7
Ø Head and Neck Bursa and Ligament Alar ligament of axis Cervical interspinous ligament Cervical intertransverse ligament Cervical ligamentum flavum Interspinous ligament, cervical Intertransverse ligament, cervical Lateral temporomandibular ligament Ligamentum flavum, cervical Sphenomandibular ligament Stylomandibular ligament Transverse ligament of atlas **1 Shoulder Bursa and Ligament, Right** Acromioclavicular ligament Coracoacromial ligament Coracoclavicular ligament Coracohumeral ligament Costoclavicular ligament Glenohumeral ligament Interclavicular ligament Sternoclavicular ligament Subacromial bursa Transverse humeral ligament Transverse scapular ligament **2 Shoulder Bursa and Ligament, Left** *See 1 Shoulder Bursa and Ligament, Right* **3 Elbow Bursa and Ligament, Right** Annular ligament Olecranon bursa Radial collateral ligament Ulnar collateral ligament **4 Elbow Bursa and Ligament, Left** *See 3 Elbow Bursa and Ligament, Right* **5 Wrist Bursa and Ligament, Right** Palmar ulnocarpal ligament Radial collateral carpal ligament Radiocarpal ligament Radioulnar ligament Scapholunate ligament Ulnar collateral carpal ligament **6 Wrist Bursa and Ligament, Left** *See 5 Wrist Bursa and Ligament, Right* **7 Hand Bursa and Ligament, Right** Carpometacarpal ligament Intercarpal ligament Interphalangeal ligament Lunotriquetral ligament Metacarpal ligament Metacarpophalangeal ligament Pisohamate ligament Pisometacarpal ligament Scaphotrapezium ligament **8 Hand Bursa and Ligament, Left** *See 7 Hand Bursa and Ligament, Right* **9 Upper Extremity Bursa and Ligament, Right** **B Upper Extremity Bursa and Ligament, Left** **C Upper Spine Bursa and Ligament** Interspinous ligament, thoracic Intertransverse ligament, thoracic Ligamentum flavum, thoracic Supraspinous ligament	**D Lower Spine Bursa and Ligament** Iliolumbar ligament Interspinous ligament, lumbar Intertransverse ligament, lumbar Ligamentum flavum, lumbar Sacrococcygeal ligament Sacroiliac ligament Sacrospinous ligament Sacrotuberous ligament Supraspinous ligament **F Sternum Bursa and Ligament** Costoxiphoid ligament Sternocostal ligament **G Rib(s) Bursa and Ligament** Costotransverse ligament **H Abdomen Bursa and Ligament, Right** **J Abdomen Bursa and Ligament, Left** **K Perineum Bursa and Ligament** **L Hip Bursa and Ligament, Right** Iliofemoral ligament Ischiofemoral ligament Pubofemoral ligament Transverse acetabular ligament Trochanteric bursa **M Hip Bursa and Ligament, Left** *See L Hip Bursa and Ligament, Right* **N Knee Bursa and Ligament, Right** Anterior cruciate ligament (ACL) Lateral collateral ligament (LCL) Ligament of head of fibula Medial collateral ligament (MCL) Patellar ligament Popliteal ligament Posterior cruciate ligament (PCL) Prepatellar bursa **P Knee Bursa and Ligament, Left** *See N Knee Bursa and Ligament, Right* **Q Ankle Bursa and Ligament, Right** Calcaneofibular ligament Deltoid ligament Ligament of the lateral malleolus Talofibular ligament **R Ankle Bursa and Ligament, Left** *See Q Ankle Bursa and Ligament, Right* **S Foot Bursa and Ligament, Right** Calcaneocuboid ligament Cuneonavicular ligament Intercuneiform ligament Interphalangeal ligament Metatarsal ligament Metatarsophalangeal ligament Subtalar ligament Talocalcaneal ligament Talocalcaneonavicular ligament Tarsometatarsal ligament **T Foot Bursa and Ligament, Left** *See S Foot Bursa and Ligament, Right* **V Lower Extremity Bursa and Ligament, Right** **W Lower Extremity Bursa and Ligament, Left**	**Ø Open** **4 Percutaneous Endoscopic**	**7 Autologous Tissue Substitute** **J Synthetic Substitute** **K Nonautologous Tissue Substitute**	**Z No Qualifier**

Non-OR Procedure   DRG Non-OR Procedure   Valid OR Procedure   HAC Associated Procedure   Combination Only   New/Revised April   New/Revised October

516   ICD-10-PCS 2024

Ø Medical and Surgical
M Bursae and Ligaments
S Reposition   Definition: Moving to its normal location, or other suitable location, all or a portion of a body part

                  Explanation: The body part is moved to a new location from an abnormal location, or from a normal location where it is not functioning correctly. The body part may or may not be cut out or off to be moved to the new location.

Body Part Character 4		Approach Character 5	Device Character 6	Qualifier Character 7
Ø Head and Neck Bursa and Ligament Alar ligament of axis Cervical interspinous ligament Cervical intertransverse ligament Cervical ligamentum flavum Interspinous ligament, cervical Intertransverse ligament, cervical Lateral temporomandibular ligament Ligamentum flavum, cervical Sphenomandibular ligament Stylomandibular ligament Transverse ligament of atlas **1 Shoulder Bursa and Ligament, Right** Acromioclavicular ligament Coracoacromial ligament Coracoclavicular ligament Coracohumeral ligament Costoclavicular ligament Glenohumeral ligament Interclavicular ligament Sternoclavicular ligament Subacromial bursa Transverse humeral ligament Transverse scapular ligament **2 Shoulder Bursa and Ligament, Left** *See 1 Shoulder Bursa and Ligament, Right* **3 Elbow Bursa and Ligament, Right** Annular ligament Olecranon bursa Radial collateral ligament Ulnar collateral ligament **4 Elbow Bursa and Ligament, Left** *See 3 Elbow Bursa and Ligament, Right* **5 Wrist Bursa and Ligament, Right** Palmar ulnocarpal ligament Radial collateral carpal ligament Radiocarpal ligament Radioulnar ligament Scapholunate ligament Ulnar collateral carpal ligament **6 Wrist Bursa and Ligament, Left** *See 5 Wrist Bursa and Ligament, Right* **7 Hand Bursa and Ligament, Right** Carpometacarpal ligament Intercarpal ligament Interphalangeal ligament Lunotriquetral ligament Metacarpal ligament Metacarpophalangeal ligament Pisohamate ligament Pisometacarpal ligament Scaphotrapezium ligament **8 Hand Bursa and Ligament, Left** *See 7 Hand Bursa and Ligament, Right* **9 Upper Extremity Bursa and Ligament, Right** **B Upper Extremity Bursa and Ligament, Left** **C Upper Spine Bursa and Ligament** Interspinous ligament, thoracic Intertransverse ligament, thoracic Ligamentum flavum, thoracic Supraspinous ligament	**D Lower Spine Bursa and Ligament** Iliolumbar ligament Interspinous ligament, lumbar Intertransverse ligament, lumbar Ligamentum flavum, lumbar Sacrococcygeal ligament Sacroiliac ligament Sacrospinous ligament Sacrotuberous ligament Supraspinous ligament **F Sternum Bursa and Ligament** Costoxiphoid ligament Sternocostal ligament **G Rib(s) Bursa and Ligament** Costotransverse ligament **H Abdomen Bursa and Ligament, Right** **J Abdomen Bursa and Ligament, Left** **K Perineum Bursa and Ligament** **L Hip Bursa and Ligament, Right** Iliofemoral ligament Ischiofemoral ligament Pubofemoral ligament Transverse acetabular ligament Trochanteric bursa **M Hip Bursa and Ligament, Left** *See L Hip Bursa and Ligament, Right* **N Knee Bursa and Ligament, Right** Anterior cruciate ligament (ACL) Lateral collateral ligament (LCL) Ligament of head of fibula Medial collateral ligament (MCL) Patellar ligament Popliteal ligament Posterior cruciate ligament (PCL) Prepatellar bursa **P Knee Bursa and Ligament, Left** *See N Knee Bursa and Ligament, Right* **Q Ankle Bursa and Ligament, Right** Calcaneofibular ligament Deltoid ligament Ligament of the lateral malleolus Talofibular ligament **R Ankle Bursa and Ligament, Left** *See Q Ankle Bursa and Ligament, Right* **S Foot Bursa and Ligament, Right** Calcaneocuboid ligament Cuneonavicular ligament Intercuneiform ligament Interphalangeal ligament Metatarsal ligament Metatarsophalangeal ligament Subtalar ligament Talocalcaneal ligament Talocalcaneonavicular ligament Tarsometatarsal ligament **T Foot Bursa and Ligament, Left** *See S Foot Bursa and Ligament, Right* **V Lower Extremity Bursa and Ligament, Right** **W Lower Extremity Bursa and Ligament, Left**	**Ø Open** **4 Percutaneous Endoscopic**	**Z No Device**	**Z No Qualifier**

NC Noncovered Procedure   **LC** Limited Coverage   **QA** Questionable OB Admit   **NT** New Tech Add-on   ⊞ Combination Member   ♂ Male   ♀ Female

ICD-10-PCS 2024   517

Bursae and Ligaments

Ø   Medical and Surgical
M   Bursae and Ligaments
T   Resection   Definition: Cutting out or off, without replacement, all of a body part
                Explanation: None

Body Part Character 4		Approach Character 5	Device Character 6	Qualifier Character 7
Ø Head and Neck Bursa and Ligament Alar ligament of axis Cervical interspinous ligament Cervical intertransverse ligament Cervical ligamentum flavum Interspinous ligament, cervical Intertransverse ligament, cervical Lateral temporomandibular ligament Ligamentum flavum, cervical Sphenomandibular ligament Stylomandibular ligament Transverse ligament of atlas **1 Shoulder Bursa and Ligament, Right** Acromioclavicular ligament Coracoacromial ligament Coracoclavicular ligament Coracohumeral ligament Costoclavicular ligament Glenohumeral ligament Interclavicular ligament Sternoclavicular ligament Subacromial bursa Transverse humeral ligament Transverse scapular ligament **2 Shoulder Bursa and Ligament, Left** *See 1 Shoulder Bursa and Ligament, Right* **3 Elbow Bursa and Ligament, Right** Annular ligament Olecranon bursa Radial collateral ligament Ulnar collateral ligament **4 Elbow Bursa and Ligament, Left** *See 3 Elbow Bursa and Ligament, Right* **5 Wrist Bursa and Ligament, Right** Palmar ulnocarpal ligament Radial collateral carpal ligament Radiocarpal ligament Radioulnar ligament Scapholunate ligament Ulnar collateral carpal ligament **6 Wrist Bursa and Ligament, Left** *See 5 Wrist Bursa and Ligament, Right* **7 Hand Bursa and Ligament, Right** Carpometacarpal ligament Intercarpal ligament Interphalangeal ligament Lunotriquetral ligament Metacarpal ligament Metacarpophalangeal ligament Pisohamate ligament Pisometacarpal ligament Scaphotrapezium ligament **8 Hand Bursa and Ligament, Left** *See 7 Hand Bursa and Ligament, Right* **9 Upper Extremity Bursa and Ligament, Right** **B Upper Extremity Bursa and Ligament, Left** **C Upper Spine Bursa and Ligament** Interspinous ligament, thoracic Intertransverse ligament, thoracic Ligamentum flavum, thoracic Supraspinous ligament	**D Lower Spine Bursa and Ligament** Iliolumbar ligament Interspinous ligament, lumbar Intertransverse ligament, lumbar Ligamentum flavum, lumbar Sacrococcygeal ligament Sacroiliac ligament Sacrospinous ligament Sacrotuberous ligament Supraspinous ligament **F Sternum Bursa and Ligament** Costoxiphoid ligament Sternocostal ligament **G Rib(s) Bursa and Ligament** Costotransverse ligament **H Abdomen Bursa and Ligament, Right** **J Abdomen Bursa and Ligament, Left** **K Perineum Bursa and Ligament** **L Hip Bursa and Ligament, Right** Iliofemoral ligament Ischiofemoral ligament Pubofemoral ligament Transverse acetabular ligament Trochanteric bursa **M Hip Bursa and Ligament, Left** *See L Hip Bursa and Ligament, Right* **N Knee Bursa and Ligament, Right** Anterior cruciate ligament (ACL) Lateral collateral ligament (LCL) Ligament of head of fibula Medial collateral ligament (MCL) Patellar ligament Popliteal ligament Posterior cruciate ligament (PCL) Prepatellar bursa **P Knee Bursa and Ligament, Left** *See N Knee Bursa and Ligament, Right* **Q Ankle Bursa and Ligament, Right** Calcaneofibular ligament Deltoid ligament Ligament of the lateral malleolus Talofibular ligament **R Ankle Bursa and Ligament, Left** *See Q Ankle Bursa and Ligament, Right* **S Foot Bursa and Ligament, Right** Calcaneocuboid ligament Cuneonavicular ligament Intercuneiform ligament Interphalangeal ligament Metatarsal ligament Metatarsophalangeal ligament Subtalar ligament Talocalcaneal ligament Talocalcaneonavicular ligament Tarsometatarsal ligament **T Foot Bursa and Ligament, Left** *See S Foot Bursa and Ligament, Right* **V Lower Extremity Bursa and Ligament, Right** **W Lower Extremity Bursa and Ligament, Left**	**Ø Open** **4 Percutaneous Endoscopic**	**Z No Device**	**Z No Qualifier**

Non-OR Procedure   DRG Non-OR Procedure   Valid OR Procedure   HAC Associated Procedure   Combination Only   New/Revised April   New/Revised October

518   ICD-10-PCS 2024

Ø Medical and Surgical
M Bursae and Ligaments
U Supplement Definition: Putting in or on biological or synthetic material that physically reinforces and/or augments the function of a portion of a body part

Explanation: The biological material is non-living, or is living and from the same individual. The body part may have been previously replaced, and the SUPPLEMENT procedure is performed to physically reinforce and/or augment the function of the replaced body part.

Body Part Character 4		Approach Character 5	Device Character 6	Qualifier Character 7
Ø Head and Neck Bursa and Ligament Alar ligament of axis Cervical interspinous ligament Cervical intertransverse ligament Cervical ligamentum flavum Interspinous ligament, cervical Intertransverse ligament, cervical Lateral temporomandibular ligament Ligamentum flavum, cervical Sphenomandibular ligament Stylomandibular ligament Transverse ligament of atlas **1 Shoulder Bursa and Ligament, Right** Acromioclavicular ligament Coracoacromial ligament Coracoclavicular ligament Coracohumeral ligament Costoclavicular ligament Glenohumeral ligament Interclavicular ligament Sternoclavicular ligament Subacromial bursa Transverse humeral ligament Transverse scapular ligament **2 Shoulder Bursa and Ligament, Left** *See 1 Shoulder Bursa and Ligament, Right* **3 Elbow Bursa and Ligament, Right** Annular ligament Olecranon bursa Radial collateral ligament Ulnar collateral ligament **4 Elbow Bursa and Ligament, Left** *See 3 Elbow Bursa and Ligament, Right* **5 Wrist Bursa and Ligament, Right** Palmar ulnocarpal ligament Radial collateral carpal ligament Radiocarpal ligament Radioulnar ligament Scapholunate ligament Ulnar collateral carpal ligament **6 Wrist Bursa and Ligament, Left** *See 5 Wrist Bursa and Ligament, Right* **7 Hand Bursa and Ligament, Right** Carpometacarpal ligament Intercarpal ligament Interphalangeal ligament Lunotriquetral ligament Metacarpal ligament Metacarpophalangeal ligament Pisohamate ligament Pisometacarpal ligament Scaphotrapezium ligament **8 Hand Bursa and Ligament, Left** *See 7 Hand Bursa and Ligament, Right* **9 Upper Extremity Bursa and Ligament, Right** **B Upper Extremity Bursa and Ligament, Left** **C Upper Spine Bursa and Ligament** Interspinous ligament, thoracic Intertransverse ligament, thoracic Ligamentum flavum, thoracic Supraspinous ligament	**D Lower Spine Bursa and Ligament** Iliolumbar ligament Interspinous ligament, lumbar Intertransverse ligament, lumbar Ligamentum flavum, lumbar Sacrococcygeal ligament Sacroiliac ligament Sacrospinous ligament Sacrotuberous ligament Supraspinous ligament **F Sternum Bursa and Ligament** Costoxiphoid ligament Sternocostal ligament **G Rib(s) Bursa and Ligament** Costotransverse ligament **H Abdomen Bursa and Ligament, Right** **J Abdomen Bursa and Ligament, Left** **K Perineum Bursa and Ligament** **L Hip Bursa and Ligament, Right** Iliofemoral ligament Ischiofemoral ligament Pubofemoral ligament Transverse acetabular ligament Trochanteric bursa **M Hip Bursa and Ligament, Left** *See L Hip Bursa and Ligament, Right* **N Knee Bursa and Ligament, Right** Anterior cruciate ligament (ACL) Lateral collateral ligament (LCL) Ligament of head of fibula Medial collateral ligament (MCL) Patellar ligament Popliteal ligament Posterior cruciate ligament (PCL) Prepatellar bursa **P Knee Bursa and Ligament, Left** *See N Knee Bursa and Ligament, Right* **Q Ankle Bursa and Ligament, Right** Calcaneofibular ligament Deltoid ligament Ligament of the lateral malleolus Talofibular ligament **R Ankle Bursa and Ligament, Left** *See Q Ankle Bursa and Ligament, Right* **S Foot Bursa and Ligament, Right** Calcaneocuboid ligament Cuneonavicular ligament Intercuneiform ligament Interphalangeal ligament Metatarsal ligament Metatarsophalangeal ligament Subtalar ligament Talocalcaneal ligament Talocalcaneonavicular ligament Tarsometatarsal ligament **T Foot Bursa and Ligament, Left** *See S Foot Bursa and Ligament, Right* **V Lower Extremity Bursa and Ligament, Right** **W Lower Extremity Bursa and Ligament, Left**	**Ø** Open **4** Percutaneous Endoscopic	**7** Autologous Tissue Substitute **J** Synthetic Substitute **K** Nonautologous Tissue Substitute	**Z** No Qualifier

Bursae and Ligaments

Ø   **Medical and Surgical**
M   **Bursae and Ligaments**
W   **Revision**   Definition: Correcting, to the extent possible, a portion of a malfunctioning device or the position of a displaced device
                  Explanation: Revision can include correcting a malfunctioning or displaced device by taking out or putting in components of the device such as a screw or pin

Body Part Character 4	Approach Character 5	Device Character 6	Qualifier Character 7
X Upper Bursa and Ligament Y Lower Bursa and Ligament	Ø Open 3 Percutaneous 4 Percutaneous Endoscopic	Ø Drainage Device 7 Autologous Tissue Substitute J Synthetic Substitute K Nonautologous Tissue Substitute Y Other Device	Z No Qualifier
X Upper Bursa and Ligament Y Lower Bursa and Ligament	X External	Ø Drainage Device 7 Autologous Tissue Substitute J Synthetic Substitute K Nonautologous Tissue Substitute	Z No Qualifier

Non-OR   ØMW[X,Y][3,4]YZ
Non-OR   ØMW[X,Y]X[Ø,7,J,K]Z

Ø　Medical and Surgical
M　Bursae and Ligaments
X　Transfer　Definition: Moving, without taking out, all or a portion of a body part to another location to take over the function of all or a portion of a body part
　　　　　Explanation: The body part transferred remains connected to its vascular and nervous supply

Body Part Character 4	Approach Character 5	Device Character 6	Qualifier Character 7
Ø　Head and Neck Bursa and Ligament 　Alar ligament of axis 　Cervical interspinous ligament 　Cervical intertransverse ligament 　Cervical ligamentum flavum 　Interspinous ligament, cervical 　Intertransverse ligament, cervical 　Lateral temporomandibular ligament 　Ligamentum flavum, cervical 　Sphenomandibular ligament 　Stylomandibular ligament 　Transverse ligament of atlas **1　Shoulder Bursa and Ligament, Right** 　Acromioclavicular ligament 　Coracoacromial ligament 　Coracoclavicular ligament 　Coracohumeral ligament 　Costoclavicular ligament 　Glenohumeral ligament 　Interclavicular ligament 　Sternoclavicular ligament 　Subacromial bursa 　Transverse humeral ligament 　Transverse scapular ligament **2　Shoulder Bursa and Ligament, Left** 　*See 1 Shoulder Bursa and Ligament, Right* **3　Elbow Bursa and Ligament, Right** 　Annular ligament 　Olecranon bursa 　Radial collateral ligament 　Ulnar collateral ligament **4　Elbow Bursa and Ligament, Left** 　*See 3 Elbow Bursa and Ligament, Right* **5　Wrist Bursa and Ligament, Right** 　Palmar ulnocarpal ligament 　Radial collateral carpal ligament 　Radiocarpal ligament 　Radioulnar ligament 　Scapholunate ligament 　Ulnar collateral carpal ligament **6　Wrist Bursa and Ligament, Left** 　*See 5 Wrist Bursa and Ligament, Right* **7　Hand Bursa and Ligament, Right** 　Carpometacarpal ligament 　Intercarpal ligament 　Interphalangeal ligament 　Lunotriquetral ligament 　Metacarpal ligament 　Metacarpophalangeal ligament 　Pisohamate ligament 　Pisometacarpal ligament 　Scaphotrapezium ligament **8　Hand Bursa and Ligament, Left** 　*See 7 Hand Bursa and Ligament, Right* **9　Upper Extremity Bursa and Ligament, Right** **B　Upper Extremity Bursa and Ligament, Left** **C　Upper Spine Bursa and Ligament** 　Interspinous ligament, thoracic 　Intertransverse ligament, thoracic 　Ligamentum flavum, thoracic 　Supraspinous ligament **D　Lower Spine Bursa and Ligament** 　Iliolumbar ligament 　Interspinous ligament, lumbar 　Intertransverse ligament, lumbar 　Ligamentum flavum, lumbar 　Sacrococcygeal ligament 　Sacroiliac ligament 　Sacrospinous ligament 　Sacrotuberous ligament 　Supraspinous ligament **F　Sternum Bursa and Ligament** 　Costoxiphoid ligament 　Sternocostal ligament **G　Rib(s) Bursa and Ligament** 　Costotransverse ligament **H　Abdomen Bursa and Ligament, Right** **J　Abdomen Bursa and Ligament, Left** **K　Perineum Bursa and Ligament** **L　Hip Bursa and Ligament, Right** 　Iliofemoral ligament 　Ischiofemoral ligament 　Pubofemoral ligament 　Transverse acetabular ligament 　Trochanteric bursa **M　Hip Bursa and Ligament, Left** 　*See L Hip Bursa and Ligament, Right* **N　Knee Bursa and Ligament, Right** 　Anterior cruciate ligament (ACL) 　Lateral collateral ligament (LCL) 　Ligament of head of fibula 　Medial collateral ligament (MCL) 　Patellar ligament 　Popliteal ligament 　Posterior cruciate ligament (PCL) 　Prepatellar bursa **P　Knee Bursa and Ligament, Left** 　*See N Knee Bursa and Ligament, Right* **Q　Ankle Bursa and Ligament, Right** 　Calcaneofibular ligament 　Deltoid ligament 　Ligament of the lateral malleolus 　Talofibular ligament **R　Ankle Bursa and Ligament, Left** 　*See Q Ankle Bursa and Ligament, Right* **S　Foot Bursa and Ligament, Right** 　Calcaneocuboid ligament 　Cuneonavicular ligament 　Intercuneiform ligament 　Interphalangeal ligament 　Metatarsal ligament 　Metatarsophalangeal ligament 　Subtalar ligament 　Talocalcaneal ligament 　Talocalcaneonavicular ligament 　Tarsometatarsal ligament **T　Foot Bursa and Ligament, Left** 　*See S Foot Bursa and Ligament, Right* **V　Lower Extremity Bursa and Ligament, Right** **W　Lower Extremity Bursa and Ligament, Left**	**Ø　Open** **4　Percutaneous Endoscopic**	**Z　No Device**	**Z　No Qualifier**

NC Noncovered Procedure　　**LC** Limited Coverage　　**QA** Questionable OB Admit　　**NT** New Tech Add-on　　⊞ Combination Member　　♂Male　　♀Female

ICD-10-PCS 2024　　　　　　　　　　　　　　　　　　　　　　　　　　　　　　521

Head and Facial Bones ØN2–ØNW

Character Meanings

This Character Meaning table is provided as a guide to assist the user in the identification of character members that may be found in this section of code tables. It **SHOULD NOT** be used to build a PCS code.

Operation–Character 3		Body Part–Character 4		Approach–Character 5		Device–Character 6		Qualifier–Character 7	
2	Change	Ø	Skull	Ø	Open	Ø	Drainage Device	X	Diagnostic
5	Destruction	1	Frontal Bone	3	Percutaneous	3	Infusion Device	Z	No Qualifier
8	Division	3	Parietal Bone, Right	4	Percutaneous Endoscopic	4	Internal Fixation Device		
9	Drainage	4	Parietal Bone, Left	X	External	5	External Fixation Device		
B	Excision	5	Temporal Bone, Right			7	Autologous Tissue Substitute		
C	Extirpation	6	Temporal Bone, Left			J	Synthetic Substitute		
D	Extraction	7	Occipital Bone			K	Nonautologous Tissue Substitute		
H	Insertion	B	Nasal Bone			M	Bone Growth Stimulator		
J	Inspection	C	Sphenoid Bone			N	Neurostimulator Generator		
N	Release	F	Ethmoid Bone, Right			S	Hearing Device		
P	Removal	G	Ethmoid Bone, Left			Y	Other Device		
Q	Repair	H	Lacrimal Bone, Right			Z	No Device		
R	Replacement	J	Lacrimal Bone, Left						
S	Reposition	K	Palatine Bone, Right						
T	Resection	L	Palatine Bone, Left						
U	Supplement	M	Zygomatic Bone, Right						
W	Revision	N	Zygomatic Bone, Left						
		P	Orbit, Right						
		Q	Orbit, Left						
		R	Maxilla						
		T	Mandible, Right						
		V	Mandible, Left						
		W	Facial Bone						
		X	Hyoid Bone						

AHA Coding Clinic for table ØNB

2022, 2Q, 17   Congenital nasal pyriform aperture stenosis and repair
2021, 3Q, 21   Excision of thyroglossal duct cyst
2021, 1Q, 21   Maxillectomy with reconstruction of maxilla
2017, 1Q, 20   Preparatory nasal adhesion repair before definitive cleft palate repair
2015, 3Q, 3-8   Excisional and nonexcisional debridement
2015, 2Q, 12   Orbital exenteration

AHA Coding Clinic for table ØND

2017, 4Q, 41   Extraction procedures

AHA Coding Clinic for table ØNH

2021, 4Q, 51   Insertion of infusion device in skull
2015, 3Q, 13   Nonexcisional debridement of cranial wound with removal and replacement of hardware

AHA Coding Clinic for table ØNP

2023, 1Q, 31   Removal of autologous bone flap due to bone resorption
2022, 4Q, 58-59 Infusion device in head and facial bones
2015, 3Q, 13   Nonexcisional debridement of cranial wound with removal and replacement of hardware

AHA Coding Clinic for table ØNQ

2016, 3Q, 29   Closure of bilateral alveolar clefts

AHA Coding Clinic for table ØNR

2021, 3Q, 29   Repair of superior semicircular canal dehiscence
2021, 1Q, 21   Maxillectomy with reconstruction of maxilla
2017, 3Q, 17   Resection of schwannoma and placement of DuraGen and Lorenz cranial plating system
2017, 3Q, 22   Replacement of native skull bone flap
2017, 1Q, 23   Reconstruction of mandible using titanium and bone
2014, 3Q, 7   Hemi-cranioplasty for repair of cranial defect

AHA Coding Clinic for table ØNS

2022, 1Q, 48   Repair of facial fractures of frontal sinus and orbital roof
2017, 3Q, 22   Replacement of native skull bone flap
2017, 1Q, 20   Preparatory nasal adhesion repair before definitive cleft palate repair
2016, 2Q, 30   Clipping (occlusion) of cerebral artery, decompressive craniectomy and storage of bone flap in abdominal wall
2015, 3Q, 17   Craniosynostosis with cranial vault reconstruction
2015, 3Q, 27   Moyamoya disease and hemispheric pial synangiosis with craniotomy
2014, 3Q, 23   Le Fort I osteotomy
2013, 3Q, 24   Distraction osteogenesis
2013, 3Q, 25   Fracture of frontal bone with repair and coagulation for hemostasis

AHA Coding Clinic for table ØNU

2023, 2Q, 19   Sigmoid sinus dehiscence with mastoidectomy with resurfacing
2021, 3Q, 29   Repair of superior semicircular canal dehiscence
2016, 3Q, 29   Closure of bilateral alveolar clefts
2013, 3Q, 24   Distraction osteogenesis

AHA Coding Clinic for table ØNW

2022, 4Q, 58-59 Infusion device in head and facial bones

Head and Facial Bones

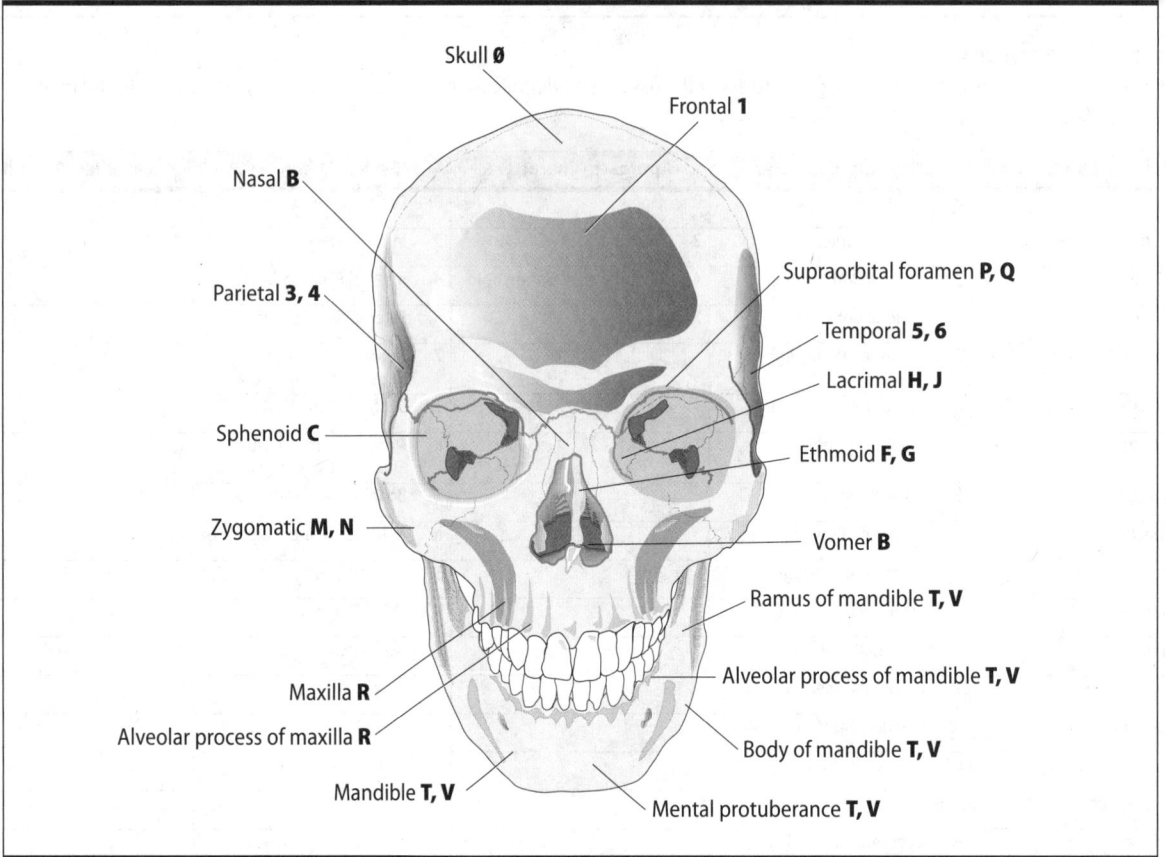

Skull **Ø**

Frontal **1**

Nasal **B**

Supraorbital foramen **P, Q**

Parietal **3, 4**

Temporal **5, 6**

Lacrimal **H, J**

Sphenoid **C**

Ethmoid **F, G**

Zygomatic **M, N**

Vomer **B**

Ramus of mandible **T, V**

Alveolar process of mandible **T, V**

Maxilla **R**

Body of mandible **T, V**

Alveolar process of maxilla **R**

Mandible **T, V**

Mental protuberance **T, V**

Skull Bones

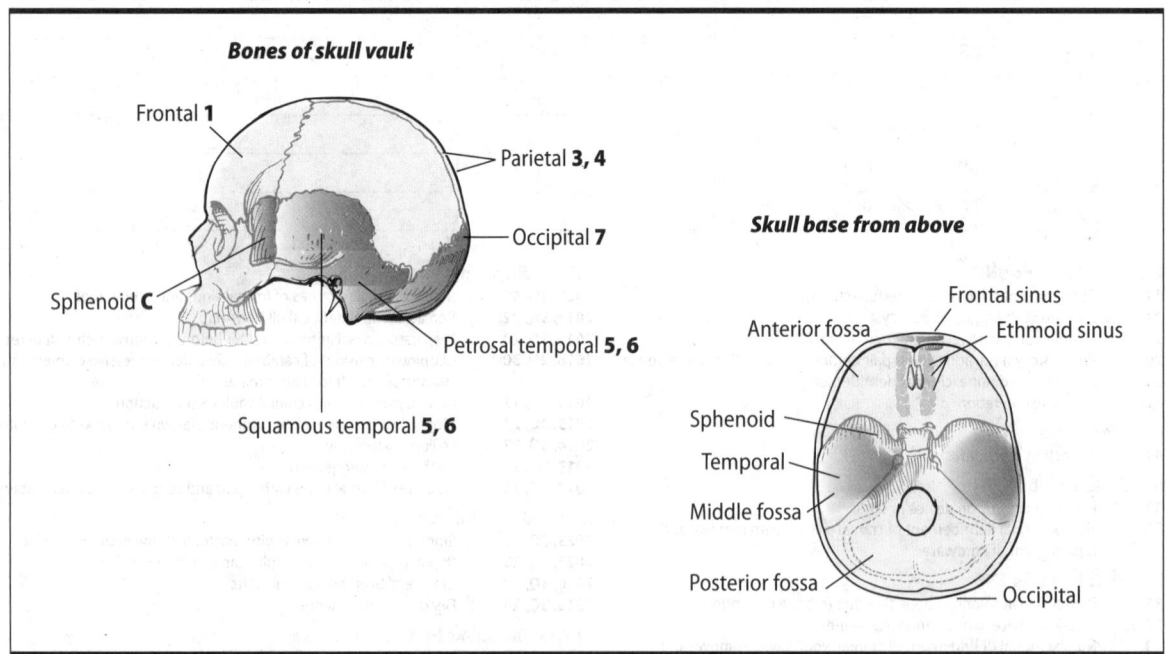

Bones of skull vault

Frontal **1**

Parietal **3, 4**

Occipital **7**

Sphenoid **C**

Petrosal temporal **5, 6**

Squamous temporal **5, 6**

Skull base from above

Frontal sinus

Ethmoid sinus

Anterior fossa

Sphenoid

Temporal

Middle fossa

Posterior fossa

Occipital

Ø   Medical and Surgical
N   Head and Facial Bones
2   Change   Definition: Taking out or off a device from a body part and putting back an identical or similar device in or on the same body part without cutting or puncturing the skin or a mucous membrane
                        Explanation: All CHANGE procedures are coded using the approach EXTERNAL

Body Part Character 4	Approach Character 5	Device Character 6	Qualifier Character 7
Ø Skull B Nasal Bone Vomer of nasal septum W Facial Bone	X External	Ø Drainage Device Y Other Device	Z No Qualifier

| **Non-OR**   All body part, approach, device, and qualifier values |

Ø   Medical and Surgical
N   Head and Facial Bones
5   Destruction   Definition: Physical eradication of all or a portion of a body part by the direct use of energy, force, or a destructive agent
                             Explanation: None of the body part is physically taken out

Body Part Character 4	Approach Character 5	Device Character 6	Qualifier Character 7

Ø   Skull
1   Frontal Bone
     Zygomatic process of frontal bone
3   Parietal Bone, Right
4   Parietal Bone, Left
5   Temporal Bone, Right
     Mastoid process
     Petrous part of temporal bone
     Tympanic part of temporal bone
     Zygomatic process of temporal bone
6   Temporal Bone, Left
     See 5 Temporal Bone, Right
7   Occipital Bone
     Foramen magnum
B   Nasal Bone
     Vomer of nasal septum
C   Sphenoid Bone
     Greater wing
     Lesser wing
     Optic foramen
     Pterygoid process
     Sella turcica
F   Ethmoid Bone, Right
     Cribriform plate
G   Ethmoid Bone, Left
     See F Ethmoid Bone, Right
H   Lacrimal Bone, Right
J   Lacrimal Bone, Left
K   Palatine Bone, Right
L   Palatine Bone, Left
M   Zygomatic Bone, Right
N   Zygomatic Bone, Left
P   Orbit, Right
     Bony orbit
     Orbital portion of ethmoid bone
     Orbital portion of frontal bone
     Orbital portion of lacrimal bone
     Orbital portion of maxilla
     Orbital portion of palatine bone
     Orbital portion of sphenoid bone
     Orbital portion of zygomatic bone
Q   Orbit, Left
     See P Orbit, Right
R   Maxilla
     Alveolar process of maxilla
T   Mandible, Right
     Alveolar process of mandible
     Condyloid process
     Mandibular notch
     Mental foramen
V   Mandible, Left
     See T Mandible, Right
X   Hyoid Bone
	Ø Open
	3 Percutaneous
	4 Percutaneous Endoscopic
		Z No Device	Z No Qualifier

NC Noncovered Procedure   **LC** Limited Coverage   **QA** Questionable OB Admit   **NT** New Tech Add-on   ⊞ Combination Member   ♂ Male   ♀ Female

ICD-10-PCS 2024   ØN2–ØN5   525

Head and Facial Bones

Ø   Medical and Surgical
N   Head and Facial Bones
8   Division   Definition: Cutting into a body part, without draining fluids and/or gases from the body part, in order to separate or transect a body part
                  Explanation: All or a portion of the body part is separated into two or more portions

Body Part Character 4	Approach Character 5	Device Character 6	Qualifier Character 7
Ø Skull	Ø Open	Z No Device	Z No Qualifier
1 Frontal Bone Zygomatic process of frontal bone	3 Percutaneous 4 Percutaneous Endoscopic		
3 Parietal Bone, Right			
4 Parietal Bone, Left			

5   Temporal Bone, Right
     Mastoid process
     Petrous part of temporal bone
     Tympanic part of temporal bone
     Zygomatic process of temporal bone			

6 Temporal Bone, Left *See 5 Temporal Bone, Right*			
7 Occipital Bone Foramen magnum			
B Nasal Bone Vomer of nasal septum			

C   Sphenoid Bone
     Greater wing
     Lesser wing
     Optic foramen
     Pterygoid process
     Sella turcica			

F Ethmoid Bone, Right Cribriform plate			
G Ethmoid Bone, Left *See F Ethmoid Bone, Right*			
H Lacrimal Bone, Right			
J Lacrimal Bone, Left			
K Palatine Bone, Right			
L Palatine Bone, Left			
M Zygomatic Bone, Right			
N Zygomatic Bone, Left			

P   Orbit, Right
     Bony orbit
     Orbital portion of ethmoid bone
     Orbital portion of frontal bone
     Orbital portion of lacrimal bone
     Orbital portion of maxilla
     Orbital portion of palatine bone
     Orbital portion of sphenoid bone
     Orbital portion of zygomatic bone			

Q Orbit, Left *See P Orbit, Right*			
R Maxilla Alveolar process of maxilla			

T   Mandible, Right
     Alveolar process of mandible
     Condyloid process
     Mandibular notch
     Mental foramen			

V Mandible, Left *See T Mandible, Right*			
X Hyoid Bone			

Non-OR   ØN8B[Ø,3,4]ZZ

Ø   Medical and Surgical
N   Head and Facial Bones
9   Drainage   Definition: Taking or letting out fluids and/or gases from a body part
                   Explanation: The qualifier DIAGNOSTIC is used to identify drainage procedures that are biopsies

Body Part Character 4	Approach Character 5	Device Character 6	Qualifier Character 7
Ø Skull	**Ø Open**	**Ø Drainage Device**	**Z No Qualifier**
1 Frontal Bone	**3 Percutaneous**		
Zygomatic process of frontal bone	**4 Percutaneous Endoscopic**		
3 Parietal Bone, Right			
4 Parietal Bone, Left			
5 Temporal Bone, Right			
Mastoid process			
Petrous part of temporal bone			
Tympanic part of temporal bone			
Zygomatic process of temporal bone			
6 Temporal Bone, Left			
See 5 Temporal Bone, Right			
7 Occipital Bone			
Foramen magnum			
B Nasal Bone			
Vomer of nasal septum			
C Sphenoid Bone			
Greater wing			
Lesser wing			
Optic foramen			
Pterygoid process			
Sella turcica			
F Ethmoid Bone, Right			
Cribriform plate			
G Ethmoid Bone, Left			
See F Ethmoid Bone, Right			
H Lacrimal Bone, Right			
J Lacrimal Bone, Left			
K Palatine Bone, Right			
L Palatine Bone, Left			
M Zygomatic Bone, Right			
N Zygomatic Bone, Left			
P Orbit, Right			
Bony orbit			
Orbital portion of ethmoid bone			
Orbital portion of frontal bone			
Orbital portion of lacrimal bone			
Orbital portion of maxilla			
Orbital portion of palatine bone			
Orbital portion of sphenoid bone			
Orbital portion of zygomatic bone			
Q Orbit, Left			
See P Orbit, Right			
R Maxilla			
Alveolar process of maxilla			
T Mandible, Right			
Alveolar process of mandible			
Condyloid process			
Mandibular notch			
Mental foramen			
V Mandible, Left			
See T Mandible, Right			
X Hyoid Bone			

Non-OR ØN9[Ø,1,3,4,5,6,7,C,F,G,H,J,K,L,M,N,P,Q,X]3ØZ
Non-OR ØN9[B,R,T,V][Ø,3,4]ØZ

ØN9 Continued on next page

Ø **Medical and Surgical**
N **Head and Facial Bones**
9 **Drainage**   Definition: Taking or letting out fluids and/or gases from a body part

ØN9 Continued

Explanation: The qualifier DIAGNOSTIC is used to identify drainage procedures that are biopsies

Body Part Character 4	Approach Character 5	Device Character 6	Qualifier Character 7
Ø Skull	**Ø** Open	**Z** No Device	**X** Diagnostic
1 Frontal Bone	**3** Percutaneous		**Z** No Qualifier
Zygomatic process of frontal bone	**4** Percutaneous Endoscopic		
3 Parietal Bone, Right			
4 Parietal Bone, Left			
5 Temporal Bone, Right			
Mastoid process			
Petrous part of temporal bone			
Tympanic part of temporal bone			
Zygomatic process of temporal bone			
6 Temporal Bone, Left			
See 5 Temporal Bone, Right			
7 Occipital Bone			
Foramen magnum			
B Nasal Bone			
Vomer of nasal septum			
C Sphenoid Bone			
Greater wing			
Lesser wing			
Optic foramen			
Pterygoid process			
Sella turcica			
F Ethmoid Bone, Right			
Cribriform plate			
G Ethmoid Bone, Left			
See F Ethmoid Bone, Right			
H Lacrimal Bone, Right			
J Lacrimal Bone, Left			
K Palatine Bone, Right			
L Palatine Bone, Left			
M Zygomatic Bone, Right			
N Zygomatic Bone, Left			
P Orbit, Right			
Bony orbit			
Orbital portion of ethmoid bone			
Orbital portion of frontal bone			
Orbital portion of lacrimal bone			
Orbital portion of maxilla			
Orbital portion of palatine bone			
Orbital portion of sphenoid bone			
Orbital portion of zygomatic bone			
Q Orbit, Left			
See P Orbit, Right			
R Maxilla			
Alveolar process of maxilla			
T Mandible, Right			
Alveolar process of mandible			
Condyloid process			
Mandibular notch			
Mental foramen			
V Mandible, Left			
See T Mandible, Right			
X Hyoid Bone			

Non-OR	ØN9[Ø,1,3,4,5,6,7,C,F,G,H,J,K,L,M,N,P,Q,X]3ZZ
Non-OR	ØN9B[Ø,3,4]Z[X,Z]
Non-OR	ØN9[R,T,V][Ø,3,4]ZZ

Ø **Medical and Surgical**
N **Head and Facial Bones**
B **Excision**　　　　Definition: Cutting out or off, without replacement, a portion of a body part
　　　　　　　　　　　　Explanation: The qualifier DIAGNOSTIC is used to identify excision procedures that are biopsies

Body Part Character 4	Approach Character 5	Device Character 6	Qualifier Character 7
Ø Skull	**Ø** Open	**Z** No Device	**X** Diagnostic
1 Frontal Bone	**3** Percutaneous		**Z** No Qualifier
Zygomatic process of frontal bone	**4** Percutaneous Endoscopic		
3 Parietal Bone, Right			
4 Parietal Bone, Left			
5 Temporal Bone, Right			
Mastoid process			
Petrous part of temporal bone			
Tympanic part of temporal bone			
Zygomatic process of temporal bone			
6 Temporal Bone, Left			
See 5 Temporal Bone, Right			
7 Occipital Bone			
Foramen magnum			
B Nasal Bone			
Vomer of nasal septum			
C Sphenoid Bone			
Greater wing			
Lesser wing			
Optic foramen			
Pterygoid process			
Sella turcica			
F Ethmoid Bone, Right			
Cribriform plate			
G Ethmoid Bone, Left			
See F Ethmoid Bone, Right			
H Lacrimal Bone, Right			
J Lacrimal Bone, Left			
K Palatine Bone, Right			
L Palatine Bone, Left			
M Zygomatic Bone, Right			
N Zygomatic Bone, Left			
P Orbit, Right			
Bony orbit			
Orbital portion of ethmoid bone			
Orbital portion of frontal bone			
Orbital portion of lacrimal bone			
Orbital portion of maxilla			
Orbital portion of palatine bone			
Orbital portion of sphenoid bone			
Orbital portion of zygomatic bone			
Q Orbit, Left			
See P Orbit, Right			
R Maxilla			
Alveolar process of maxilla			
T Mandible, Right			
Alveolar process of mandible			
Condyloid process			
Mandibular notch			
Mental foramen			
V Mandible, Left			
See T Mandible, Right			
X Hyoid Bone			

Non-OR　ØNB[B,R,T,V][Ø,3,4]ZX

NC Noncovered Procedure　　**LC** Limited Coverage　　**QA** Questionable OB Admit　　**NT** New Tech Add-on　　⊞ Combination Member　　♂ Male　　♀ Female

ICD-10-PCS 2024　　　529

ØNB–ØNB

Head and Facial Bones

Ø   **Medical and Surgical**
N   **Head and Facial Bones**
C   **Extirpation**   Definition: Taking or cutting out solid matter from a body part

Explanation: The solid matter may be an abnormal byproduct of a biological function or a foreign body; it may be imbedded in a body part or in the lumen of a tubular body part. The solid matter may or may not have been previously broken into pieces.

Body Part Character 4	Approach Character 5	Device Character 6	Qualifier Character 7

1 **Frontal Bone**
    Zygomatic process of frontal bone
3 **Parietal Bone, Right**
4 **Parietal Bone, Left**
5 **Temporal Bone, Right**
    Mastoid process
    Petrous part of temporal bone
    Tympanic part of temporal bone
    Zygomatic process of temporal bone
6 **Temporal Bone, Left**
    See 5 Temporal Bone, Right
7 **Occipital Bone**
    Foramen magnum
B Nasal Bone
    Vomer of nasal septum
C **Sphenoid Bone**
    Greater wing
    Lesser wing
    Optic foramen
    Pterygoid process
    Sella turcica
F **Ethmoid Bone, Right**
    Cribriform plate
G **Ethmoid Bone, Left**
    See F Ethmoid Bone, Right
H **Lacrimal Bone, Right**
J **Lacrimal Bone, Left**
K **Palatine Bone, Right**
L **Palatine Bone, Left**
M **Zygomatic Bone, Right**
N **Zygomatic Bone, Left**
P **Orbit, Right**
    Bony orbit
    Orbital portion of ethmoid bone
    Orbital portion of frontal bone
    Orbital portion of lacrimal bone
    Orbital portion of maxilla
    Orbital portion of palatine bone
    Orbital portion of sphenoid bone
    Orbital portion of zygomatic bone
Q **Orbit, Left**
    See P Orbit, Right
R Maxilla
    Alveolar process of maxilla
T Mandible, Right
    Alveolar process of mandible
    Condyloid process
    Mandibular notch
    Mental foramen
V Mandible, Left
    See T Mandible, Right
X **Hyoid Bone**
	Ø Open
	3 Percutaneous
	4 Percutaneous Endoscopic
		Z No Device	**Z** No Qualifier

Non-OR   ØNC[B,R,T,V][Ø,3,4]ZZ

Non-OR Procedure   DRG Non-OR Procedure   Valid OR Procedure   HAC Associated Procedure   Combination Only   New/Revised April   New/Revised October

530   ICD-10-PCS 2024

Ø   Medical and Surgical
N   Head and Facial Bones
D   Extraction   Definition: Pulling or stripping out or off all or a portion of a body part by the use of force
                        Explanation: The qualifier DIAGNOSTIC is used to identify extraction procedures that are biopsies

Body Part Character 4	Approach Character 5	Device Character 6	Qualifier Character 7
Ø Skull	**Ø** Open	**Z** No Device	**Z** No Qualifier
1 **Frontal Bone** Zygomatic process of frontal bone			
3 **Parietal Bone, Right**			
4 **Parietal Bone, Left**			

5   **Temporal Bone, Right**
     Mastoid process
     Petrous part of temporal bone
     Tympanic part of temporal bone
     Zygomatic process of temporal bone			

6 **Temporal Bone, Left** *See 5 Temporal Bone, Right*			
7 **Occipital Bone** Foramen magnum			
B **Nasal Bone** Vomer of nasal septum			

C   **Sphenoid Bone**
     Greater wing
     Lesser wing
     Optic foramen
     Pterygoid process
     Sella turcica			

F **Ethmoid Bone, Right** Cribriform plate			
G **Ethmoid Bone, Left** *See F Ethmoid Bone, Right*			
H **Lacrimal Bone, Right**			
J **Lacrimal Bone, Left**			
K **Palatine Bone, Right**			
L **Palatine Bone, Left**			
M **Zygomatic Bone, Right**			
N **Zygomatic Bone, Left**			

P   **Orbit, Right**
     Bony orbit
     Orbital portion of ethmoid bone
     Orbital portion of frontal bone
     Orbital portion of lacrimal bone
     Orbital portion of maxilla
     Orbital portion of palatine bone
     Orbital portion of sphenoid bone
     Orbital portion of zygomatic bone			

Q **Orbit, Left** *See P Orbit, Right*			
R **Maxilla** Alveolar process of maxilla			

T   **Mandible, Right**
     Alveolar process of mandible
     Condyloid process
     Mandibular notch
     Mental foramen			

V **Mandible, Left** *See T Mandible, Right*			
X **Hyoid Bone**			

Head and Facial Bones

Ø   **Medical and Surgical**
N   **Head and Facial Bones**
H   **Insertion**   Definition: Putting in a nonbiological appliance that monitors, assists, performs, or prevents a physiological function but does not physically take the place of a body part

Explanation: None

Body Part Character 4	Approach Character 5	Device Character 6	Qualifier Character 7
Ø Skull ⊞	**Ø** Open	**3** Infusion Device **4** Internal Fixation Device **5** External Fixation Device **M** Bone Growth Stimulator **N** Neurostimulator Generator	**Z** No Qualifier
Ø Skull	**3** Percutaneous **4** Percutaneous Endoscopic	**3** Infusion Device **4** Internal Fixation Device **5** External Fixation Device **M** Bone Growth Stimulator	**Z** No Qualifier

1 Frontal Bone
    Zygomatic process of frontal bone
 3 Parietal Bone, Right
 4 Parietal Bone, Left
 7 Occipital Bone
    Foramen magnum
 C Sphenoid Bone
    Greater wing
    Lesser wing
    Optic foramen
    Pterygoid process
    Sella turcica
 F Ethmoid Bone, Right
    Cribriform plate
 G Ethmoid Bone, Left
    See F Ethmoid Bone, Right
 H Lacrimal Bone, Right
 J Lacrimal Bone, Left
 K Palatine Bone, Right
 L Palatine Bone, Left
 M Zygomatic Bone, Right
 N Zygomatic Bone, Left
 P Orbit, Right
    Bony orbit
    Orbital portion of ethmoid bone
    Orbital portion of frontal bone
    Orbital portion of lacrimal bone
    Orbital portion of maxilla
    Orbital portion of palatine bone
    Orbital portion of sphenoid bone
    Orbital portion of zygomatic bone
 Q Orbit, Left
    See P Orbit, Right
 X Hyoid Bone
	Ø Open
	 3 Percutaneous
	 4 Percutaneous Endoscopic
		4 Internal Fixation Device	**Z** No Qualifier

5 Temporal Bone, Right
    Mastoid process
    Petrous part of temporal bone
    Tympanic part of temporal bone
    Zygomatic process of temporal bone
 6 Temporal Bone, Left
    See 5 Temporal Bone, Right
	Ø Open
	 3 Percutaneous
	 4 Percutaneous Endoscopic
		4 Internal Fixation Device
		 S Hearing Device
			Z No Qualifier

B Nasal Bone Vomer of nasal septum	**Ø** Open **3** Percutaneous **4** Percutaneous Endoscopic	**4** Internal Fixation Device **M** Bone Growth Stimulator	**Z** No Qualifier

R Maxilla
    Alveolar process of maxilla
 T Mandible, Right
    Alveolar process of mandible
    Condyloid process
    Mandibular notch
    Mental foramen
 V Mandible, Left
    See T Mandible, Right
	Ø Open
	 3 Percutaneous
	 4 Percutaneous Endoscopic
		4 Internal Fixation Device
		 5 External Fixation Device
			Z No Qualifier

W Facial Bone	**Ø** Open **3** Percutaneous **4** Percutaneous Endoscopic	**M** Bone Growth Stimulator	**Z** No Qualifier

Non-OR   ØNHØØ5Z
Non-OR   ØNHØ[3,4]5Z
Non-OR   ØNHB[Ø,3,4][4,M]Z

See Appendix L for Procedure Combinations
⊞   ØNHØØNZ

Non-OR Procedure   DRG Non-OR Procedure   Valid OR Procedure   HAC Associated Procedure   Combination Only   New/Revised April   New/Revised October

532   ICD-10-PCS 2024

Ø   Medical and Surgical
N   Head and Facial Bones
J   Inspection   Definition: Visually and/or manually exploring a body part

Explanation: Visual exploration may be performed with or without optical instrumentation. Manual exploration may be performed directly or through intervening body layers.

Body Part Character 4	Approach Character 5	Device Character 6	Qualifier Character 7
Ø Skull B Nasal Bone Vomer of nasal septum W Facial Bone	Ø Open 3 Percutaneous 4 Percutaneous Endoscopic X External	Z No Device	Z No Qualifier

Non-OR   ØNJ[Ø,B,W][3,X]ZZ

Ø   Medical and Surgical
N   Head and Facial Bones
N   Release   Definition: Freeing a body part from an abnormal physical constraint by cutting or by the use of force

Explanation: Some of the restraining tissue may be taken out but none of the body part is taken out

Body Part Character 4	Approach Character 5	Device Character 6	Qualifier Character 7

1   Frontal Bone
     Zygomatic process of frontal bone
3   Parietal Bone, Right
4   Parietal Bone, Left
5   Temporal Bone, Right
     Mastoid process
     Petrous part of temporal bone
     Tympanic part of temporal bone
     Zygomatic process of temporal bone
6   Temporal Bone, Left
     See 5 Temporal Bone, Right
7   Occipital Bone
     Foramen magnum
B   Nasal Bone
     Vomer of nasal septum
C   Sphenoid Bone
     Greater wing
     Lesser wing
     Optic foramen
     Pterygoid process
     Sella turcica
F   Ethmoid Bone, Right
     Cribriform plate
G   Ethmoid Bone, Left
     See F Ethmoid Bone, Right
H   Lacrimal Bone, Right
J   Lacrimal Bone, Left
K   Palatine Bone, Right
L   Palatine Bone, Left
M   Zygomatic Bone, Right
N   Zygomatic Bone, Left
P   Orbit, Right
     Bony orbit
     Orbital portion of ethmoid bone
     Orbital portion of frontal bone
     Orbital portion of lacrimal bone
     Orbital portion of maxilla
     Orbital portion of palatine bone
     Orbital portion of sphenoid bone
     Orbital portion of zygomatic bone
Q   Orbit, Left
     See P Orbit, Right
R   Maxilla
     Alveolar process of maxilla
T   Mandible, Right
     Alveolar process of mandible
     Condyloid process
     Mandibular notch
     Mental foramen
V   Mandible, Left
     See T Mandible, Right
X   Hyoid Bone
	Ø Open
	3 Percutaneous
	4 Percutaneous Endoscopic
		Z No Device	Z No Qualifier

Non-OR   ØNNB[Ø,3,4]ZZ

NC Noncovered Procedure   LC Limited Coverage   QA Questionable OB Admit   NT New Tech Add-on   ⊞ Combination Member   ♂ Male   ♀ Female

ICD-10-PCS 2024   533

Ø Medical and Surgical
N Head and Facial Bones
P Removal   Definition: Taking out or off a device from a body part

Explanation: If a device is taken out and a similar device put in without cutting or puncturing the skin or mucous membrane, the procedure is coded to the root operation CHANGE. Otherwise, the procedure for taking out a device is coded to the root operation REMOVAL.

Body Part Character 4	Approach Character 5	Device Character 6	Qualifier Character 7
Ø Skull	Ø Open	Ø Drainage Device 3 Infusion Device 4 Internal Fixation Device 5 External Fixation Device 7 Autologous Tissue Substitute J Synthetic Substitute K Nonautologous Tissue Substitute M Bone Growth Stimulator N Neurostimulator Generator S Hearing Device	Z No Qualifier
Ø Skull	3 Percutaneous 4 Percutaneous Endoscopic	Ø Drainage Device 3 Infusion Device 4 Internal Fixation Device 5 External Fixation Device 7 Autologous Tissue Substitute J Synthetic Substitute K Nonautologous Tissue Substitute M Bone Growth Stimulator S Hearing Device	Z No Qualifier
Ø Skull	X External	Ø Drainage Device 3 Infusion Device 4 Internal Fixation Device 5 External Fixation Device M Bone Growth Stimulator S Hearing Device	Z No Qualifier
B Nasal Bone Vomer of nasal septum W Facial Bone	Ø Open 3 Percutaneous 4 Percutaneous Endoscopic	Ø Drainage Device 4 Internal Fixation Device 7 Autologous Tissue Substitute J Synthetic Substitute K Nonautologous Tissue Substitute M Bone Growth Stimulator	Z No Qualifier
B Nasal Bone Vomer of nasal septum W Facial Bone	X External	Ø Drainage Device 4 Internal Fixation Device M Bone Growth Stimulator	Z No Qualifier

Non-OR	ØNPØ[3,4]5Z
Non-OR	ØNPØX[Ø,3,5]Z
Non-OR	ØNPB[Ø,3,4][Ø,4,7,J,K,M]Z
Non-OR	ØNPBX[Ø,4,M]Z
Non-OR	ØNPWX[Ø,M]Z

Non-OR Procedure   DRG Non-OR Procedure   Valid OR Procedure   HAC Associated Procedure   Combination Only   New/Revised April   New/Revised October

534   ICD-10-PCS 2024

Ø **Medical and Surgical**
N **Head and Facial Bones**
Q **Repair**　　　　　Definition: Restoring, to the extent possible, a body part to its normal anatomic structure and function
　　　　　　　　　　　　Explanation: Used only when the method to accomplish the repair is not one of the other root operations

Body Part Character 4	Approach Character 5	Device Character 6	Qualifier Character 7
Ø **Skull**	**Ø** Open	**Z** No Device	**Z** No Qualifier
1 **Frontal Bone**	**3** Percutaneous		
Zygomatic process of frontal bone	**4** Percutaneous Endoscopic		
3 **Parietal Bone, Right**	**X** External		
4 **Parietal Bone, Left**			
5 **Temporal Bone, Right**			
Mastoid process			
Petrous part of temporal bone			
Tympanic part of temporal bone			
Zygomatic process of temporal bone			
6 **Temporal Bone, Left**			
See 5 Temporal Bone, Right			
7 **Occipital Bone**			
Foramen magnum			
B **Nasal Bone**			
Vomer of nasal septum			
C **Sphenoid Bone**			
Greater wing			
Lesser wing			
Optic foramen			
Pterygoid process			
Sella turcica			
F **Ethmoid Bone, Right**			
Cribriform plate			
G **Ethmoid Bone, Left**			
See F Ethmoid Bone, Right			
H **Lacrimal Bone, Right**			
J **Lacrimal Bone, Left**			
K **Palatine Bone, Right**			
L **Palatine Bone, Left**			
M **Zygomatic Bone, Right**			
N **Zygomatic Bone, Left**			
P **Orbit, Right**			
Bony orbit			
Orbital portion of ethmoid bone			
Orbital portion of frontal bone			
Orbital portion of lacrimal bone			
Orbital portion of maxilla			
Orbital portion of palatine bone			
Orbital portion of sphenoid bone			
Orbital portion of zygomatic bone			
Q **Orbit, Left**			
See P Orbit, Right			
R **Maxilla**			
Alveolar process of maxilla			
T **Mandible, Right**			
Alveolar process of mandible			
Condyloid process			
Mandibular notch			
Mental foramen			
V **Mandible, Left**			
See T Mandible, Right			
X **Hyoid Bone**			

Non-OR　　ØNQ[Ø,1,3,4,5,6,7,B,C,F,G,H,J,K,L,M,N,P,Q,R,T,V,X]XZZ

NC Noncovered Procedure　　**LC** Limited Coverage　　**QA** Questionable OB Admit　　**NT** New Tech Add-on　　➕ Combination Member　　♂ Male　　♀ Female
ICD-10-PCS 2024　　**535**

ØNQ–ØNQ

Ø Medical and Surgical
N Head and Facial Bones
R Replacement   Definition: Putting in or on biological or synthetic material that physically takes the place and/or function of all or a portion of a body part

Explanation: The body part may have been taken out or replaced, or may be taken out, physically eradicated, or rendered nonfunctional during the REPLACEMENT procedure. A REMOVAL procedure is coded for taking out the device used in a previous replacement procedure.

Body Part Character 4	Approach Character 5	Device Character 6	Qualifier Character 7
Ø Skull	**Ø Open**	**7 Autologous Tissue Substitute**	**Z No Qualifier**
1 Frontal Bone	**3 Percutaneous**	**J Synthetic Substitute**	
Zygomatic process of frontal bone	**4 Percutaneous Endoscopic**	**K Nonautologous Tissue Substitute**	
3 Parietal Bone, Right			
4 Parietal Bone, Left			
5 Temporal Bone, Right			
Mastoid process			
Petrous part of temporal bone			
Tympanic part of temporal bone			
Zygomatic process of temporal bone			
6 Temporal Bone, Left			
See 5 Temporal Bone, Right			
7 Occipital Bone			
Foramen magnum			
B Nasal Bone			
Vomer of nasal septum			
C Sphenoid Bone			
Greater wing			
Lesser wing			
Optic foramen			
Pterygoid process			
Sella turcica			
F Ethmoid Bone, Right			
Cribriform plate			
G Ethmoid Bone, Left			
See F Ethmoid Bone, Right			
H Lacrimal Bone, Right			
J Lacrimal Bone, Left			
K Palatine Bone, Right			
L Palatine Bone, Left			
M Zygomatic Bone, Right			
N Zygomatic Bone, Left			
P Orbit, Right			
Bony orbit			
Orbital portion of ethmoid bone			
Orbital portion of frontal bone			
Orbital portion of lacrimal bone			
Orbital portion of maxilla			
Orbital portion of palatine bone			
Orbital portion of sphenoid bone			
Orbital portion of zygomatic bone			
Q Orbit, Left			
See P Orbit, Right			
R Maxilla			
Alveolar process of maxilla			
T Mandible, Right			
Alveolar process of mandible			
Condyloid process			
Mandibular notch			
Mental foramen			
V Mandible, Left			
See T Mandible, Right			
X Hyoid Bone			

Ø   Medical and Surgical
N   Head and Facial Bones
S   Reposition   Definition: Moving to its normal location, or other suitable location, all or a portion of a body part

                       Explanation: The body part is moved to a new location from an abnormal location, or from a normal location where it is not functioning correctly. The body part may or may not be cut out or off to be moved to the new location.

Body Part Character 4	Approach Character 5	Device Character 6	Qualifier Character 7

Ø Skull
R Maxilla
   Alveolar process of maxilla
T Mandible, Right
   Alveolar process of mandible
   Condyloid process
   Mandibular notch
   Mental foramen
V Mandible, Left
   See T Mandible, Right
	Ø Open
	3 Percutaneous
	4 Percutaneous Endoscopic
		4 Internal Fixation Device
		5 External Fixation Device
		Z No Device
			Z No Qualifier

Ø Skull
R Maxilla
   Alveolar process of maxilla
T Mandible, Right
   Alveolar process of mandible
   Condyloid process
   Mandibular notch
   Mental foramen
V Mandible, Left
   See T Mandible, Right
	X External	**Z** No Device	**Z** No Qualifier

1 Frontal Bone
   Zygomatic process of frontal bone
3 Parietal Bone, Right
4 Parietal Bone, Left
5 Temporal Bone, Right
   Mastoid process
   Petrous part of temporal bone
   Tympanic part of temporal bone
   Zygomatic process of temporal bone
6 Temporal Bone, Left
   See 5 Temporal Bone, Right
7 Occipital Bone
   Foramen magnum
B Nasal Bone
   Vomer of nasal septum
C Sphenoid Bone
   Greater wing
   Lesser wing
   Optic foramen
   Pterygoid process
   Sella turcica
F Ethmoid Bone, Right
   Cribriform plate
G Ethmoid Bone, Left
   See F Ethmoid Bone, Right
H Lacrimal Bone, Right
J Lacrimal Bone, Left
K Palatine Bone, Right
L Palatine Bone, Left
M Zygomatic Bone, Right
N Zygomatic Bone, Left
P Orbit, Right
   Bony orbit
   Orbital portion of ethmoid bone
   Orbital portion of frontal bone
   Orbital portion of lacrimal bone
   Orbital portion of maxilla
   Orbital portion of palatine bone
   Orbital portion of sphenoid bone
   Orbital portion of zygomatic bone
Q Orbit, Left
   See P Orbit, Right
X Hyoid Bone
	Ø Open
	3 Percutaneous
	4 Percutaneous Endoscopic
		4 Internal Fixation Device
		Z No Device
			Z No Qualifier

Non-OR   ØNS[R,T,V][3,4][4,5,Z]Z
Non-OR   ØNS[Ø,R,T,V]XZZ
Non-OR   ØNS[B,C,F,G,H,J,K,L,M,N,P,Q,X][3,4][4,Z]Z

ØNS Continued on next page

NC Noncovered Procedure   LC Limited Coverage   QA Questionable OB Admit   NT New Tech Add-on   ⊞ Combination Member   ♂ Male   ♀ Female

ICD-10-PCS 2024   537

Head and Facial Bones

Ø	Medical and Surgical		*ØNS Continued*
N	Head and Facial Bones		
S	Reposition		

Definition: Moving to its normal location, or other suitable location, all or a portion of a body part

Explanation: The body part is moved to a new location from an abnormal location, or from a normal location where it is not functioning correctly. The body part may or may not be cut out or off to be moved to the new location.

Body Part Character 4	Approach Character 5	Device Character 6	Qualifier Character 7
1 Frontal Bone Zygomatic process of frontal bone **3 Parietal Bone, Right** **4 Parietal Bone, Left** **5 Temporal Bone, Right** Mastoid process Petrous part of temporal bone Tympanic part of temporal bone Zygomatic process of temporal bone **6 Temporal Bone, Left** *See 5 Temporal Bone, Right* **7 Occipital Bone** Foramen magnum **B Nasal Bone** Vomer of nasal septum **C Sphenoid Bone** Greater wing Lesser wing Optic foramen Pterygoid process Sella turcica **F Ethmoid Bone, Right** Cribriform plate **G Ethmoid Bone, Left** *See F Ethmoid Bone, Right* **H Lacrimal Bone, Right** **J Lacrimal Bone, Left** **K Palatine Bone, Right** **L Palatine Bone, Left** **M Zygomatic Bone, Right** **N Zygomatic Bone, Left** **P Orbit, Right** Bony orbit Orbital portion of ethmoid bone Orbital portion of frontal bone Orbital portion of lacrimal bone Orbital portion of maxilla Orbital portion of palatine bone Orbital portion of sphenoid bone Orbital portion of zygomatic bone **Q Orbit, Left** *See P Orbit, Right* **X Hyoid Bone**	**X** External	**Z** No Device	**Z** No Qualifier

Non-OR ØNS[1,3,4,5,6,7,B,C,F,G,H,J,K,L,M,N,P,Q,X]XZZ

Non-OR Procedure   DRG Non-OR Procedure   Valid OR Procedure   HAC Associated Procedure   Combination Only   New/Revised April   New/Revised October

538   ICD-10-PCS 2024

Ø **Medical and Surgical**
N **Head and Facial Bones**
T **Resection** Definition: Cutting out or off, without replacement, all of a body part
Explanation: None

Body Part Character 4	Approach Character 5	Device Character 6	Qualifier Character 7
1 **Frontal Bone** Zygomatic process of frontal bone 3 **Parietal Bone, Right** 4 **Parietal Bone, Left** 5 **Temporal Bone, Right** Mastoid process Petrous part of temporal bone Tympanic part of temporal bone Zygomatic process of temporal bone 6 **Temporal Bone, Left** *See 5 Temporal Bone, Right* 7 **Occipital Bone** Foramen magnum B **Nasal Bone** Vomer of nasal septum C **Sphenoid Bone** Greater wing Lesser wing Optic foramen Pterygoid process Sella turcica F **Ethmoid Bone, Right** Cribriform plate G **Ethmoid Bone, Left** *See F Ethmoid Bone, Right* H **Lacrimal Bone, Right** J **Lacrimal Bone, Left** K **Palatine Bone, Right** L **Palatine Bone, Left** M **Zygomatic Bone, Right** N **Zygomatic Bone, Left** P **Orbit, Right** Bony orbit Orbital portion of ethmoid bone Orbital portion of frontal bone Orbital portion of lacrimal bone Orbital portion of maxilla Orbital portion of palatine bone Orbital portion of sphenoid bone Orbital portion of zygomatic bone Q **Orbit, Left** *See P Orbit, Right* R **Maxilla** Alveolar process of maxilla T **Mandible, Right** Alveolar process of mandible Condyloid process Mandibular notch Mental foramen V **Mandible, Left** *See T Mandible, Right* X **Hyoid Bone**	Ø Open	Z No Device	Z No Qualifier

Head and Facial Bones *(left margin)*

Ø   **Medical and Surgical**
N   **Head and Facial Bones**
U   **Supplement**   Definition: Putting in or on biological or synthetic material that physically reinforces and/or augments the function of a portion of a body part

Explanation: The biological material is non-living, or is living and from the same individual. The body part may have been previously replaced, and the SUPPLEMENT procedure is performed to physically reinforce and/or augment the function of the replaced body part.

Body Part Character 4	Approach Character 5	Device Character 6	Qualifier Character 7
Ø **Skull**	Ø **Open**	7 **Autologous Tissue Substitute**	Z **No Qualifier**
1 **Frontal Bone**	3 **Percutaneous**	J **Synthetic Substitute**	
Zygomatic process of frontal bone	4 **Percutaneous Endoscopic**	K **Nonautologous Tissue Substitute**	
3 **Parietal Bone, Right**			
4 **Parietal Bone, Left**			
5 **Temporal Bone, Right**			
Mastoid process			
Petrous part of temporal bone			
Tympanic part of temporal bone			
Zygomatic process of temporal bone			
6 **Temporal Bone, Left**			
See 5 Temporal Bone, Right			
7 **Occipital Bone**			
Foramen magnum			
B **Nasal Bone**			
Vomer of nasal septum			
C **Sphenoid Bone**			
Greater wing			
Lesser wing			
Optic foramen			
Pterygoid process			
Sella turcica			
F **Ethmoid Bone, Right**			
Cribriform plate			
G **Ethmoid Bone, Left**			
See F Ethmoid Bone, Right			
H **Lacrimal Bone, Right**			
J **Lacrimal Bone, Left**			
K **Palatine Bone, Right**			
L **Palatine Bone, Left**			
M **Zygomatic Bone, Right**			
N **Zygomatic Bone, Left**			
P **Orbit, Right**			
Bony orbit			
Orbital portion of ethmoid bone			
Orbital portion of frontal bone			
Orbital portion of lacrimal bone			
Orbital portion of maxilla			
Orbital portion of palatine bone			
Orbital portion of sphenoid bone			
Orbital portion of zygomatic bone			
Q **Orbit, Left**			
See P Orbit, Right			
R **Maxilla**			
Alveolar process of maxilla			
T **Mandible, Right**			
Alveolar process of mandible			
Condyloid process			
Mandibular notch			
Mental foramen			
V **Mandible, Left**			
See T Mandible, Right			
X **Hyoid Bone**			

Non-OR Procedure   DRG Non-OR Procedure   Valid OR Procedure   HAC Associated Procedure   Combination Only   New/Revised April   New/Revised October

540   ICD-10-PCS 2024

ØNU–ØNU *(left margin)*

Ø   **Medical and Surgical**
N   **Head and Facial Bones**
W   **Revision**   Definition: Correcting, to the extent possible, a portion of a malfunctioning device or the position of a displaced device

                 Explanation: Revision can include correcting a malfunctioning or displaced device by taking out or putting in components of the device such as a screw or pin

Body Part Character 4	Approach Character 5	Device Character 6	Qualifier Character 7
Ø Skull	Ø Open	Ø Drainage Device 3 Infusion Device 4 Internal Fixation Device 5 External Fixation Device 7 Autologous Tissue Substitute J Synthetic Substitute K Nonautologous Tissue Substitute M Bone Growth Stimulator N Neurostimulator Generator S Hearing Device	Z No Qualifier
Ø Skull	3 Percutaneous 4 Percutaneous Endoscopic X External	Ø Drainage Device 3 Infusion Device 4 Internal Fixation Device 5 External Fixation Device 7 Autologous Tissue Substitute J Synthetic Substitute K Nonautologous Tissue Substitute M Bone Growth Stimulator S Hearing Device	Z No Qualifier
B Nasal Bone Vomer of nasal septum W Facial Bone	Ø Open 3 Percutaneous 4 Percutaneous Endoscopic X External	Ø Drainage Device 4 Internal Fixation Device 7 Autologous Tissue Substitute J Synthetic Substitute K Nonautologous Tissue Substitute M Bone Growth Stimulator	Z No Qualifier

Non-OR   ØNWØX[Ø,3,4,5,7,J,K,M,S]Z
Non-OR   ØNWB[Ø,3,4,X][Ø,4,7,J,K,M]Z
Non-OR   ØNWWX[Ø,4,7,J,K,M]Z

Upper Bones ØP2–ØPW

Character Meanings

This Character Meaning table is provided as a guide to assist the user in the identification of character members that may be found in this section of code tables. It **SHOULD NOT** be used to build a PCS code.

Operation–Character 3	Body Part–Character 4	Approach–Character 5	Device–Character 6	Qualifier–Character 7
2 Change	Ø Sternum	Ø Open	Ø Drainage Device OR Internal Fixation Device, Rigid Plate	3 Laser Interstitial Thermal Therapy
5 Destruction	1 Ribs, 1 to 2	3 Percutaneous	3 Spinal Stabilization Device, Vertebral Body Tether	X Diagnostic
8 Division	2 Ribs, 3 or more	4 Percutaneous Endoscopic	4 Internal Fixation Device	Z No Qualifier
9 Drainage	3 Cervical Vertebra	X External	5 External Fixation Device	
B Excision	4 Thoracic Vertebra		6 Internal Fixation Device, Intramedullary	
C Extirpation	5 Scapula, Right		7 Autologous Tissue Substitute OR Internal Fixation Device, Intramedullary Limb Lengthening	
D Extraction	6 Scapula, Left		8 External Fixation Device, Limb Lengthening	
H Insertion	7 Glenoid Cavity, Right		B External Fixation Device, Monoplanar	
J Inspection	8 Glenoid Cavity, Left		C External Fixation Device, Ring	
N Release	9 Clavicle, Right		D External Fixation Device, Hybrid	
P Removal	B Clavicle, Left		J Synthetic Substitute	
Q Repair	C Humeral Head, Right		K Nonautologous Tissue Substitute	
R Replacement	D Humeral Head, Left		M Bone Growth Stimulator	
S Reposition	F Humeral Shaft, Right		Y Other Device	
T Resection	G Humeral Shaft, Left		Z No Device	
U Supplement	H Radius, Right			
W Revision	J Radius, Left			
	K Ulna, Right			
	L Ulna, Left			
	M Carpal, Right			
	N Carpal, Left			
	P Metacarpal, Right			
	Q Metacarpal, Left			
	R Thumb Phalanx, Right			
	S Thumb Phalanx, Left			
	T Finger Phalanx, Right			
	V Finger Phalanx, Left			
	Y Upper Bone			

AHA Coding Clinic for table ØP5
2023, 1Q, 10   Laser interstitial thermal therapy

AHA Coding Clinic for table ØPB
2023, 2Q, 30   Excisional debridement and non-excisional debridement at deeper layer same site
2015, 3Q, 3-8   Excisional and nonexcisional debridement
2015, 2Q, 34   Decompressive laminectomy
2013, 4Q, 109   Separating conjoined twins
2013, 4Q, 116   Spinal decompression
2013, 3Q, 20   Superior labrum anterior posterior (SLAP) repair and subacromial decompression
2012, 4Q, 101   Rib resection with reconstruction of anterior chest wall
2012, 2Q, 19   Multiple decompressive cervical laminectomies

AHA Coding Clinic for table ØPC
2021, 3Q, 15   Curettage of bilateral humeral head and bone graft placement
2019, 3Q, 19   Removal of sternal wire

AHA Coding Clinic for table ØPD
2023, 2Q, 30   Excisional debridement and non-excisional debridement at deeper layer same site
2017, 4Q, 41   Extraction procedures

AHA Coding Clinic for table ØPH
2020, 1Q, 29   Repair of sternal dehiscence using Sternal Talon® device
2019, 4Q, 34   Intramedullary limb lengthening internal fixation device
2019, 2Q, 40   Decompression of spinal cord and placement of instrumentation
2018, 3Q, 26   Anterior vertebral tethering using Dynesys Tethering System
2017, 2Q, 20   Exchange of intramedullary antibiotic impregnated spacer
2016, 4Q, 117   Placement of magnetic growth rods
2014, 4Q, 28   Removal and replacement of displaced growing rods

AHA Coding Clinic for table ØPP
2019, 3Q, 19   Removal of sternal wire
2017, 2Q, 20   Exchange of intramedullary antibiotic impregnated spacer
2016, 4Q, 117   Placement of magnetic growth rods
2014, 4Q, 28   Removal and replacement of displaced growing rods

AHA Coding Clinic for table ØPR
2018, 4Q, 92   Radial head arthroplasty

AHA Coding Clinic for table ØPS
2021, 4Q, 51-52   Vertebral body tethering
2020, 1Q, 33   Spinal fusion without use of bone graft
2018, 3Q, 26   Anterior vertebral tethering using Dynesys Tethering System
2017, 4Q, 53   New and revised body part values - Ribs
2016, 1Q, 21   Elongation derotation flexion casting
2015, 4Q, 33   Ravitch operation
2015, 2Q, 35   Application of tongs to reduce and stabilize cervical fracture
2014, 4Q, 26   Placement of vertical expandable prosthetic titanium rib (VEPTR)
2014, 4Q, 32   Open reduction internal fixation of fracture with debridement
2014, 3Q, 33   Radial fracture treatment with open reduction internal fixation, and release of carpal ligament

AHA Coding Clinic for table ØPT
2015, 3Q, 26   Thumb arthroplasty with resection of trapezium

AHA Coding Clinic for table ØPU
2023, 2Q, 24   Remplissage of subscapularis tendon
2021, 3Q, 15   Curettage of bilateral humeral head and bone graft placement
2015, 2Q, 20   Cervical laminoplasty
2013, 4Q, 109   Separating conjoined twins

AHA Coding Clinic for table ØPW
2014, 4Q, 26   Adjustment of VEPTR lengthening mechanism
2014, 4Q, 27   Bilateral lengthening of growing rods

Upper Bones

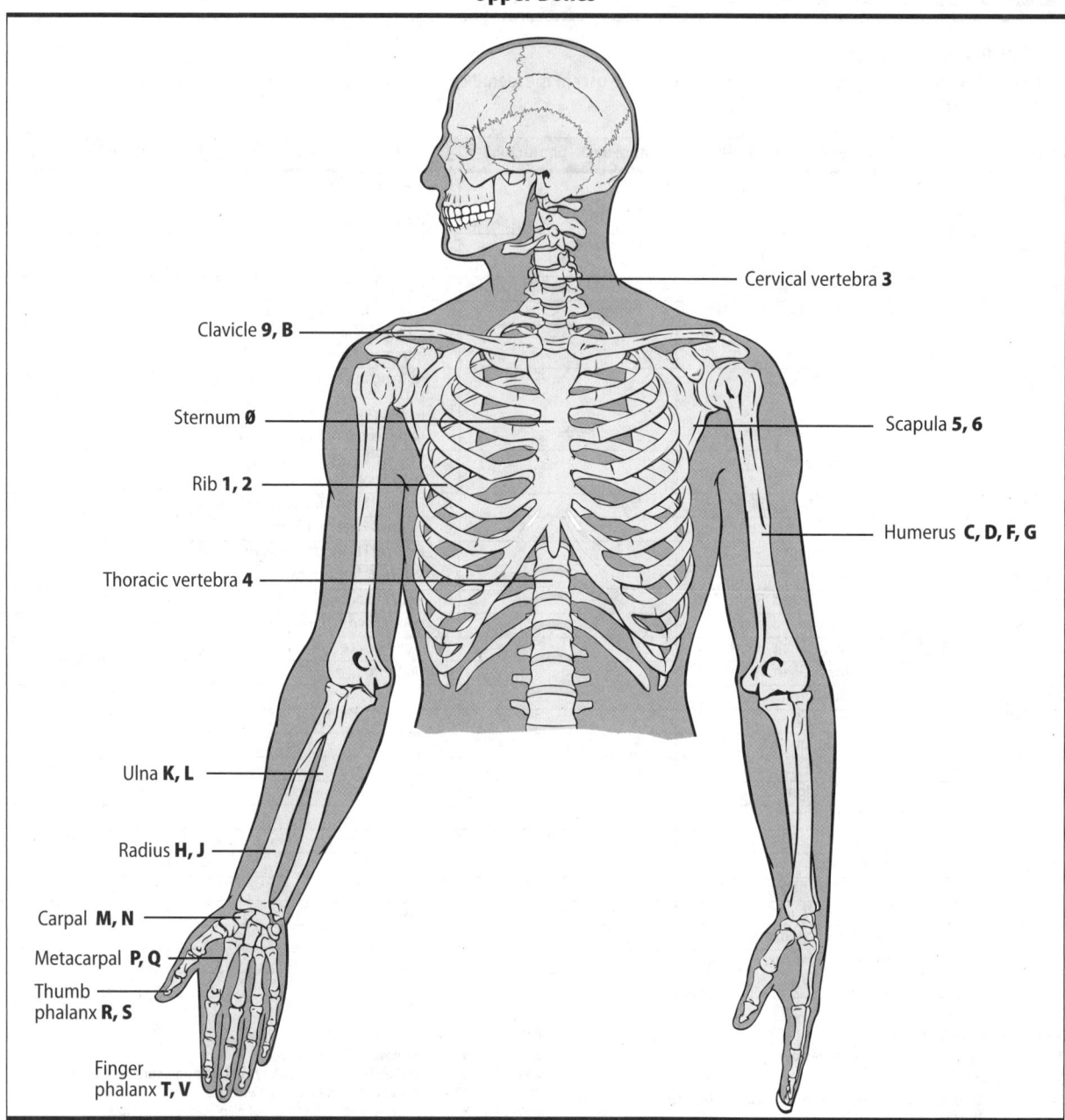

Cervical vertebra **3**

Clavicle **9, B**

Sternum **Ø**

Scapula **5, 6**

Rib **1, 2**

Humerus **C, D, F, G**

Thoracic vertebra **4**

Ulna **K, L**

Radius **H, J**

Carpal **M, N**

Metacarpal **P, Q**

Thumb phalanx **R, S**

Finger phalanx **T, V**

Humerus and Scapula

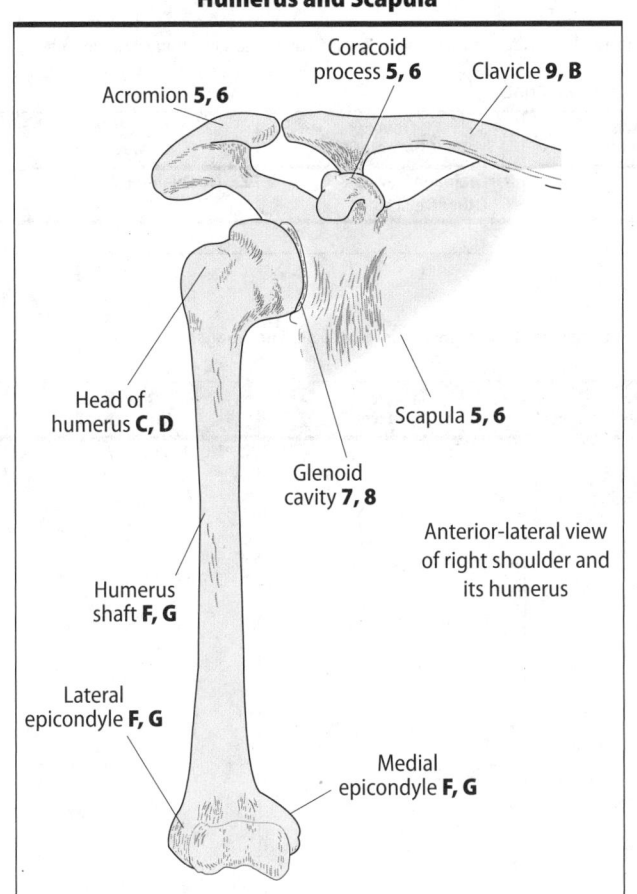

Coracoid process **5, 6**

Acromion **5, 6**

Clavicle **9, B**

Head of humerus **C, D**

Scapula **5, 6**

Glenoid cavity **7, 8**

Anterior-lateral view of right shoulder and its humerus

Humerus shaft **F, G**

Lateral epicondyle **F, G**

Medial epicondyle **F, G**

Radius and Ulna

Olecranon process **K, L**

Radius **H, J**

Coronoid process **K, L**

Ulna **K, L**

Shaft **H, J**

Shaft **K, L**

Radial styloid process **H, J**

Ulnar styloid process **K, L**

Carpal **M, N**

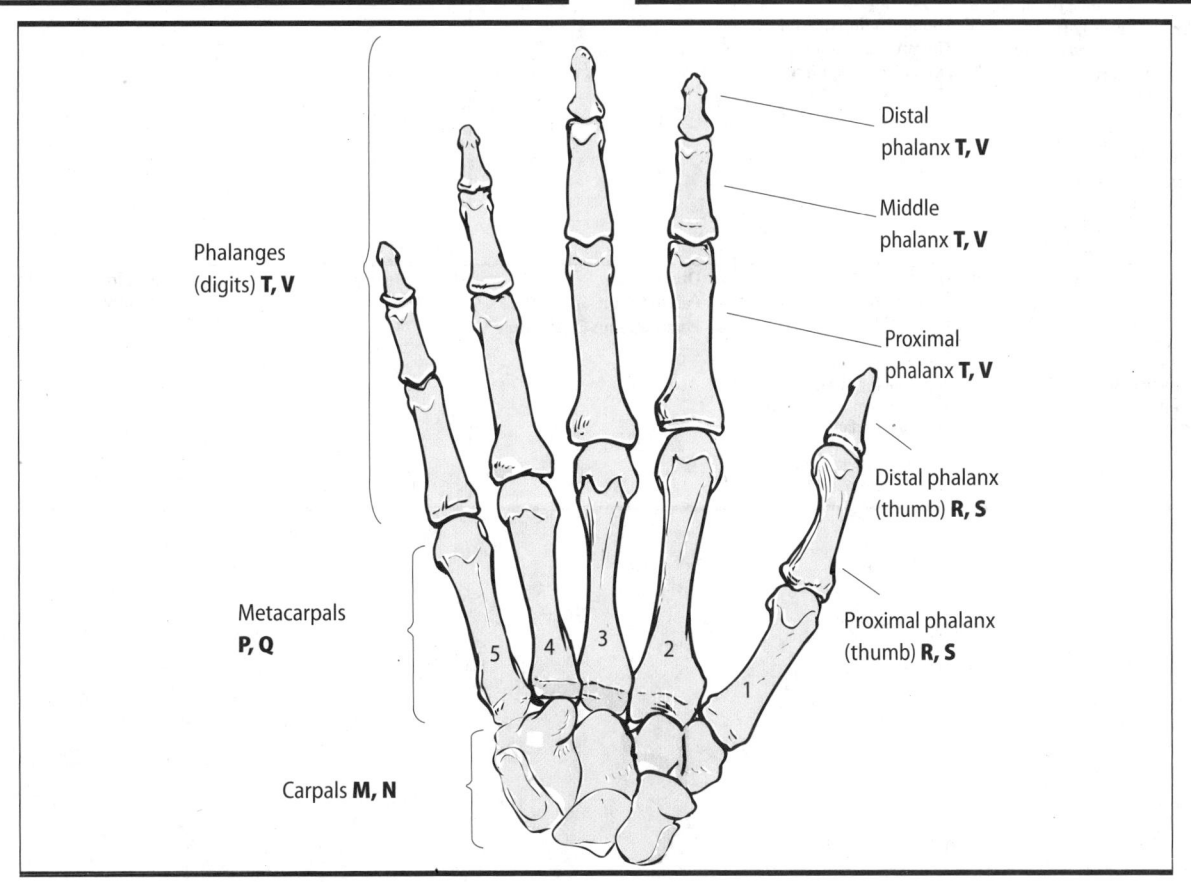

Distal phalanx **T, V**

Middle phalanx **T, V**

Phalanges (digits) **T, V**

Proximal phalanx **T, V**

Distal phalanx (thumb) **R, S**

Metacarpals **P, Q**

Proximal phalanx (thumb) **R, S**

Carpals **M, N**

Ø   **Medical and Surgical**
P   **Upper Bones**
2   **Change**   Definition: Taking out or off a device from a body part and putting back an identical or similar device in or on the same body part without cutting or puncturing the skin or a mucous membrane
                      Explanation: All CHANGE procedures are coded using the approach EXTERNAL

Body Part Character 4	Approach Character 5	Device Character 6	Qualifier Character 7
Y Upper Bone	X External	Ø Drainage Device Y Other Device	Z No Qualifier

Non-OR   All body part, approach, device, and qualifier values

Ø   **Medical and Surgical**
P   **Upper Bones**
5   **Destruction**   Definition: Physical eradication of all or a portion of a body part by the direct use of energy, force, or a destructive agent
                      Explanation: None of the body part is physically taken out

Body Part Character 4	Approach Character 5	Device Character 6	Qualifier Character 7
Ø Sternum Manubrium Suprasternal notch Xiphoid process 1 Ribs, 1 to 2 2 Ribs, 3 or More 5 Scapula, Right Acromion (process) Coracoid process 6 Scapula, Left See 5 Scapula, Right 7 Glenoid Cavity, Right Glenoid fossa (of scapula) 8 Glenoid Cavity, Left See 7 Glenoid Cavity, Right 9 Clavicle, Right B Clavicle, Left C Humeral Head, Right Greater tuberosity Lesser tuberosity Neck of humerus (anatomical)(surgical) D Humeral Head, Left See C Humeral Head, Right F Humeral Shaft, Right Distal humerus Humerus, distal Lateral epicondyle of humerus Medial epicondyle of humerus G Humeral Shaft, Left See F Humeral Shaft, Right H Radius, Right Ulnar notch J Radius, Left See H Radius, Right K Ulna, Right Olecranon process Radial notch L Ulna, Left See K Ulna, Right M Carpal, Right Capitate bone Hamate bone Lunate bone Pisiform bone Scaphoid bone Trapezium bone Trapezoid bone Triquetral bone N Carpal, Left See M Carpal, Right P Metacarpal, Right Q Metacarpal, Left R Thumb Phalanx, Right S Thumb Phalanx, Left T Finger Phalanx, Right V Finger Phalanx, Left	Ø Open 3 Percutaneous 4 Percutaneous Endoscopic	Z No Device	Z No Qualifier
3 Cervical Vertebra Dens Odontoid process Spinous process Transverse foramen Transverse process Vertebral arch Vertebral body Vertebral foramen Vertebral lamina Vertebral pedicle 4 Thoracic Vertebra Spinous process Transverse process Vertebral arch Vertebral body Vertebral foramen Vertebral lamina Vertebral pedicle	Ø Open 3 Percutaneous 4 Percutaneous Endoscopic	Z No Device	3 Laser Interstitial Thermal Therapy Z No Qualifier

0   **Medical and Surgical**
P   **Upper Bones**
8   **Division**   Definition: Cutting into a body part, without draining fluids and/or gases from the body part, in order to separate or transect a body part
                       Explanation: All or a portion of the body part is separated into two or more portions

Body Part Character 4	Approach Character 5	Device Character 6	Qualifier Character 7

0   **Sternum**
    Manubrium
    Suprasternal notch
    Xiphoid process
1   **Ribs, 1 to 2**
2   **Ribs, 3 or More**
3   **Cervical Vertebra**
    Dens
    Odontoid process
    Spinous process
    Transverse foramen
    Transverse process
    Vertebral arch
    Vertebral body
    Vertebral foramen
    Vertebral lamina
    Vertebral pedicle
4   **Thoracic Vertebra**
    Spinous process
    Transverse process
    Vertebral arch
    Vertebral body
    Vertebral foramen
    Vertebral lamina
    Vertebral pedicle
5   **Scapula, Right**
    Acromion (process)
    Coracoid process
6   **Scapula, Left**
    See 5 Scapula, Right
7   **Glenoid Cavity, Right**
    Glenoid fossa (of scapula)
8   **Glenoid Cavity, Left**
    See 7 Glenoid Cavity, Right
9   **Clavicle, Right**
B   **Clavicle, Left**
C   **Humeral Head, Right**
    Greater tuberosity
    Lesser tuberosity
    Neck of humerus (anatomical)(surgical)
D   **Humeral Head, Left**
    See C Humeral Head, Right
F   **Humeral Shaft, Right**
    Distal humerus
    Humerus, distal
    Lateral epicondyle of humerus
    Medial epicondyle of humerus
G   **Humeral Shaft, Left**
    See F Humeral Shaft, Right
H   **Radius, Right**
    Ulnar notch
J   **Radius, Left**
    See H Radius, Right
K   **Ulna, Right**
    Olecranon process
    Radial notch
L   **Ulna, Left**
    See K Ulna, Right
M   **Carpal, Right**
    Capitate bone
    Hamate bone
    Lunate bone
    Pisiform bone
    Scaphoid bone
    Trapezium bone
    Trapezoid bone
    Triquetral bone
N   **Carpal, Left**
    See M Carpal, Right
P   **Metacarpal, Right**
Q   **Metacarpal, Left**
R   **Thumb Phalanx, Right**
S   **Thumb Phalanx, Left**
T   **Finger Phalanx, Right**
V   **Finger Phalanx, Left**
	0 Open
	3 Percutaneous
	4 Percutaneous Endoscopic
		Z No Device	**Z** No Qualifier

NC Noncovered Procedure   **LC** Limited Coverage   **QA** Questionable OB Admit   **NT** New Tech Add-on   ⊞ Combination Member   ♂ Male   ♀ Female

ICD-10-PCS 2024   **547**

0P8–0P8

Upper Bones *(side margin)*

Ø   Medical and Surgical
P   Upper Bones
9   Drainage   Definition: Taking or letting out fluids and/or gases from a body part

Explanation: The qualifier DIAGNOSTIC is used to identify drainage procedures that are biopsies

Body Part Character 4		Approach Character 5	Device Character 6	Qualifier Character 7

Ø   Sternum
    Manubrium
    Suprasternal notch
    Xiphoid process
1   Ribs, 1 to 2
2   Ribs, 3 or More
3   Cervical Vertebra
    Dens
    Odontoid process
    Spinous process
    Transverse foramen
    Transverse process
    Vertebral arch
    Vertebral body
    Vertebral foramen
    Vertebral lamina
    Vertebral pedicle
4   Thoracic Vertebra
    Spinous process
    Transverse process
    Vertebral arch
    Vertebral body
    Vertebral foramen
    Vertebral lamina
    Vertebral pedicle
5   Scapula, Right
    Acromion (process)
    Coracoid process
6   Scapula, Left
    See 5 Scapula, Right
7   Glenoid Cavity, Right
    Glenoid fossa (of scapula)
8   Glenoid Cavity, Left
    See 7 Glenoid Cavity, Right
9   Clavicle, Right
B   Clavicle, Left
C   Humeral Head, Right
    Greater tuberosity
    Lesser tuberosity
    Neck of humerus
      (anatomical)(surgical)
	D Humeral Head, Left
	    See C Humeral Head, Right
	F Humeral Shaft, Right
	    Distal humerus
	    Humerus, distal
	    Lateral epicondyle of
	      humerus
	    Medial epicondyle of
	      humerus
	G Humeral Shaft, Left
	    See F Humeral Shaft, Right
	H Radius, Right
	    Ulnar notch
	J Radius, Left
	    See H Radius, Right
	K Ulna, Right
	    Olecranon process
	    Radial notch
	L Ulna, Left
	    See K Ulna, Right
	M Carpal, Right
	    Capitate bone
	    Hamate bone
	    Lunate bone
	    Pisiform bone
	    Scaphoid bone
	    Trapezium bone
	    Trapezoid bone
	    Triquetral bone
	N Carpal, Left
	    See M Carpal, Right
	P Metacarpal, Right
	Q Metacarpal, Left
	R Thumb Phalanx, Right
	S Thumb Phalanx, Left
	T Finger Phalanx, Right
	V Finger Phalanx, Left
		Ø Open
		3 Percutaneous
		4 Percutaneous Endoscopic
			Ø Drainage Device	Z No Qualifier

Non-OR   ØP9[Ø,1,2,3,4,5,6,7,8,9,B,C,D,F,G,H,J,K,L,M,N,P,Q,R,S,T,V]3ØZ

ØP9 Continued on next page

Ø Medical and Surgical
P Upper Bones
9 Drainage

ØP9 Continued

Definition: Taking or letting out fluids and/or gases from a body part
Explanation: The qualifier DIAGNOSTIC is used to identify drainage procedures that are biopsies

Body Part Character 4		Approach Character 5	Device Character 6	Qualifier Character 7

Ø Sternum
 Manubrium
 Suprasternal notch
 Xiphoid process
 1 Ribs, 1 to 2
 2 Ribs, 3 or More
 3 Cervical Vertebra
 Dens
 Odontoid process
 Spinous process
 Transverse foramen
 Transverse process
 Vertebral arch
 Vertebral body
 Vertebral foramen
 Vertebral lamina
 Vertebral pedicle
 4 Thoracic Vertebra
 Spinous process
 Transverse process
 Vertebral arch
 Vertebral body
 Vertebral foramen
 Vertebral lamina
 Vertebral pedicle
 5 Scapula, Right
 Acromion (process)
 Coracoid process
 6 Scapula, Left
 See 5 Scapula, Right
 7 Glenoid Cavity, Right
 Glenoid fossa (of scapula)
 8 Glenoid Cavity, Left
 See 7 Glenoid Cavity, Right
 9 Clavicle, Right
 B Clavicle, Left
 C Humeral Head, Right
 Greater tuberosity
 Lesser tuberosity
 Neck of humerus
   (anatomical)(surgical)
	D Humeral Head, Left
	 See C Humeral Head, Right
	 F Humeral Shaft, Right
	 Distal humerus
	 Humerus, distal
	 Lateral epicondyle of
	   humerus
	 Medial epicondyle of
	   humerus
	 G Humeral Shaft, Left
	 See F Humeral Shaft, Right
	 H Radius, Right
	 Ulnar notch
	 J Radius, Left
	 See H Radius, Right
	 K Ulna, Right
	 Olecranon process
	 Radial notch
	 L Ulna, Left
	 See K Ulna, Right
	 M Carpal, Right
	 Capitate bone
	 Hamate bone
	 Lunate bone
	 Pisiform bone
	 Scaphoid bone
	 Trapezium bone
	 Trapezoid bone
	 Triquetral bone
	 N Carpal, Left
	 See M Carpal, Right
	 P Metacarpal, Right
	 Q Metacarpal, Left
	 R Thumb Phalanx, Right
	 S Thumb Phalanx, Left
	 T Finger Phalanx, Right
	 V Finger Phalanx, Left
		Ø Open
		 3 Percutaneous
		 4 Percutaneous Endoscopic
			Z No Device	**X Diagnostic**
				 Z No Qualifier

Non-OR   ØP9[Ø,1,2,3,4,5,6,7,8,9,B,C,D,F,G,H,J,K,L,M,N,P,Q,R,S,T,V]3ZZ

NC Noncovered Procedure   LC Limited Coverage   OA Questionable OB Admit   NT New Tech Add-on   ⊞ Combination Member   ♂ Male   ♀ Female

ICD-10-PCS 2024   549

ØP9–ØP9

Upper Bones

Ø Medical and Surgical
P Upper Bones
B Excision   Definition: Cutting out or off, without replacement, a portion of a body part

Explanation: The qualifier DIAGNOSTIC is used to identify excision procedures that are biopsies

Body Part Character 4	Approach Character 5	Device Character 6	Qualifier Character 7
Ø Sternum Manubrium Suprasternal notch Xiphoid process **1 Ribs, 1 to 2** **2 Ribs, 3 or More** **3 Cervical Vertebra** Dens Odontoid process Spinous process Transverse foramen Transverse process Vertebral arch Vertebral body Vertebral foramen Vertebral lamina Vertebral pedicle **4 Thoracic Vertebra** Spinous process Transverse process Vertebral arch Vertebral body Vertebral foramen Vertebral lamina Vertebral pedicle **5 Scapula, Right** Acromion (process) Coracoid process **6 Scapula, Left** *See 5 Scapula, Right* **7 Glenoid Cavity, Right** Glenoid fossa (of scapula) **8 Glenoid Cavity, Left** *See 7 Glenoid Cavity, Right* **9 Clavicle, Right** **B Clavicle, Left** **C Humeral Head, Right** Greater tuberosity Lesser tuberosity Neck of humerus (anatomical)(surgical) **D Humeral Head, Left** *See C Humeral Head, Right* **F Humeral Shaft, Right** Distal humerus Humerus, distal Lateral epicondyle of humerus Medial epicondyle of humerus **G Humeral Shaft, Left** *See F Humeral Shaft, Right* **H Radius, Right** Ulnar notch **J Radius, Left** *See H Radius, Right* **K Ulna, Right** Olecranon process Radial notch **L Ulna, Left** *See K Ulna, Right* **M Carpal, Right** Capitate bone Hamate bone Lunate bone Pisiform bone Scaphoid bone Trapezium bone Trapezoid bone Triquetral bone **N Carpal, Left** *See M Carpal, Right* **P Metacarpal, Right** **Q Metacarpal, Left** **R Thumb Phalanx, Right** **S Thumb Phalanx, Left** **T Finger Phalanx, Right** **V Finger Phalanx, Left**	**Ø Open** **3 Percutaneous** **4 Percutaneous Endoscopic**	**Z No Device**	**X Diagnostic** **Z No Qualifier**

Ø　Medical and Surgical
P　Upper Bones
C　Extirpation　　Definition: Taking or cutting out solid matter from a body part

Explanation: The solid matter may be an abnormal byproduct of a biological function or a foreign body; it may be imbedded in a body part or in the lumen of a tubular body part. The solid matter may or may not have been previously broken into pieces.

Body Part Character 4	Approach Character 5	Device Character 6	Qualifier Character 7
Ø Sternum 　　Manubrium 　　Suprasternal notch 　　Xiphoid process 1 Ribs, 1 to 2 2 Ribs, 3 or More 3 Cervical Vertebra 　　Dens 　　Odontoid process 　　Spinous process 　　Transverse foramen 　　Transverse process 　　Vertebral arch 　　Vertebral body 　　Vertebral foramen 　　Vertebral lamina 　　Vertebral pedicle 4 Thoracic Vertebra 　　Spinous process 　　Transverse process 　　Vertebral arch 　　Vertebral body 　　Vertebral foramen 　　Vertebral lamina 　　Vertebral pedicle 5 Scapula, Right 　　Acromion (process) 　　Coracoid process 6 Scapula, Left 　　*See 5 Scapula, Right* 7 Glenoid Cavity, Right 　　Glenoid fossa (of scapula) 8 Glenoid Cavity, Left 　　*See 7 Glenoid Cavity, Right* 9 Clavicle, Right B Clavicle, Left C Humeral Head, Right 　　Greater tuberosity 　　Lesser tuberosity 　　Neck of humerus (anatomical)(surgical) D Humeral Head, Left 　　*See C Humeral Head, Right* F Humeral Shaft, Right 　　Distal humerus 　　Humerus, distal 　　Lateral epicondyle of humerus 　　Medial epicondyle of humerus G Humeral Shaft, Left 　　*See F Humeral Shaft, Right* H Radius, Right 　　Ulnar notch J Radius, Left 　　*See H Radius, Right* K Ulna, Right 　　Olecranon process 　　Radial notch L Ulna, Left 　　*See K Ulna, Right* M Carpal, Right 　　Capitate bone 　　Hamate bone 　　Lunate bone 　　Pisiform bone 　　Scaphoid bone 　　Trapezium bone 　　Trapezoid bone 　　Triquetral bone N Carpal, Left 　　*See M Carpal, Right* P Metacarpal, Right Q Metacarpal, Left R Thumb Phalanx, Right S Thumb Phalanx, Left T Finger Phalanx, Right V Finger Phalanx, Left	Ø Open 3 Percutaneous 4 Percutaneous Endoscopic	Z No Device	Z No Qualifier

NC Noncovered Procedure　　LC Limited Coverage　　QA Questionable OB Admit　　NT New Tech Add-on　　✛ Combination Member　　♂ Male　　♀ Female

ICD-10-PCS 2024　　　　　　　　　　　　　　　　　　　　　　　　　　　　　　　　　　551

ØPC–ØPC

Upper Bones

Ø   **Medical and Surgical**
P   **Upper Bones**
D   **Extraction**   Definition: Pulling or stripping out or off all or a portion of a body part by the use of force
                        Explanation: The qualifier DIAGNOSTIC is used to identify extraction procedures that are biopsies

Body Part Character 4	Approach Character 5	Device Character 6	Qualifier Character 7
Ø Sternum Manubrium Suprasternal notch Xiphoid process **1 Ribs, 1 to 2** **2 Ribs, 3 or More** **3 Cervical Vertebra** Dens Odontoid process Spinous process Transverse foramen Transverse process Vertebral arch Vertebral body Vertebral foramen Vertebral lamina Vertebral pedicle **4 Thoracic Vertebra** Spinous process Transverse process Vertebral arch Vertebral body Vertebral foramen Vertebral lamina Vertebral pedicle **5 Scapula, Right** Acromion (process) Coracoid process **6 Scapula, Left** *See 5 Scapula, Right* **7 Glenoid Cavity, Right** Glenoid fossa (of scapula) **8 Glenoid Cavity, Left** *See 7 Glenoid Cavity, Right* **9 Clavicle, Right** **B Clavicle, Left** **C Humeral Head, Right** Greater tuberosity Lesser tuberosity Neck of humerus (anatomical)(surgical) **D Humeral Head, Left** *See C Humeral Head, Right* **F Humeral Shaft, Right** Distal humerus Humerus, distal Lateral epicondyle of humerus Medial epicondyle of humerus **G Humeral Shaft, Left** *See F Humeral Shaft, Right* **H Radius, Right** Ulnar notch **J Radius, Left** *See H Radius, Right* **K Ulna, Right** Olecranon process Radial notch **L Ulna, Left** *See K Ulna, Right* **M Carpal, Right** Capitate bone Hamate bone Lunate bone Pisiform bone Scaphoid bone Trapezium bone Trapezoid bone Triquetral bone **N Carpal, Left** *See M Carpal, Right* **P Metacarpal, Right** **Q Metacarpal, Left** **R Thumb Phalanx, Right** **S Thumb Phalanx, Left** **T Finger Phalanx, Right** **V Finger Phalanx, Left**	**Ø Open**	**Z No Device**	**Z No Qualifier**

Ø Medical and Surgical
P Upper Bones
H Insertion

Definition: Putting in a nonbiological appliance that monitors, assists, performs, or prevents a physiological function but does not physically take the place of a body part

Explanation: None

Body Part Character 4		Approach Character 5	Device Character 6	Qualifier Character 7
Ø Sternum Manubrium Suprasternal notch Xiphoid process		**Ø** Open **3** Percutaneous **4** Percutaneous Endoscopic	**Ø** Internal Fixation Device, Rigid Plate **4** Internal Fixation Device	**Z** No Qualifier
1 Ribs, 1 to 2 **2 Ribs, 3 or More** **3 Cervical Vertebra** Dens Odontoid process Spinous process Transverse foramen Transverse process Vertebral arch Vertebral body Vertebral foramen Vertebral lamina Vertebral pedicle **4 Thoracic Vertebra** Spinous process Transverse process Vertebral arch Vertebral body Vertebral foramen Vertebral lamina Vertebral pedicle	**5 Scapula, Right** Acromion (process) Coracoid process **6 Scapula, Left** *See 5 Scapula, Right* **7 Glenoid Cavity, Right** Glenoid fossa (of scapula) **8 Glenoid Cavity, Left** *See 7 Glenoid Cavity, Right* **9 Clavicle, Right** **B Clavicle, Left**	**Ø** Open **3** Percutaneous **4** Percutaneous Endoscopic	**4** Internal Fixation Device	**Z** No Qualifier
C Humeral Head, Right Greater tuberosity Lesser tuberosity Neck of humerus (anatomical)(surgical) **D Humeral Head, Left** *See C Humeral Head, Right*	**H Radius, Right** Ulnar notch **J Radius, Left** *See H Radius, Right* **K Ulna, Right** Olecranon process Radial notch **L Ulna, Left** *See K Ulna, Right*	**Ø** Open **3** Percutaneous **4** Percutaneous Endoscopic	**4** Internal Fixation Device **5** External Fixation Device **6** Internal Fixation Device, Intramedullary **8** External Fixation Device, Limb Lengthening **B** External Fixation Device, Monoplanar **C** External Fixation Device, Ring **D** External Fixation Device, Hybrid	**Z** No Qualifier
F Humeral Shaft, Right Distal humerus Humerus, distal Lateral epicondyle of humerus Medial epicondyle of humerus	**G Humeral Shaft, Left** *See F Humeral Shaft, Right*	**Ø** Open **3** Percutaneous **4** Percutaneous Endoscopic	**4** Internal Fixation Device **5** External Fixation Device **6** Internal Fixation Device, Intramedullary **7** Internal Fixation Device, Intramedullary Limb Lengthening **8** External Fixation Device, Limb Lengthening **B** External Fixation Device, Monoplanar **C** External Fixation Device, Ring **D** External Fixation Device, Hybrid	**Z** No Qualifier
M Carpal, Right Capitate bone Hamate bone Lunate bone Pisiform bone Scaphoid bone Trapezium bone Trapezoid bone Triquetral bone **N Carpal, Left** *See M Carpal, Right*	**P Metacarpal, Right** **Q Metacarpal, Left** **R Thumb Phalanx, Right** **S Thumb Phalanx, Left** **T Finger Phalanx, Right** **V Finger Phalanx, Left**	**Ø** Open **3** Percutaneous **4** Percutaneous Endoscopic	**4** Internal Fixation Device **5** External Fixation Device	**Z** No Qualifier
Y Upper Bone		**Ø** Open **3** Percutaneous **4** Percutaneous Endoscopic	**M** Bone Growth Stimulator	**Z** No Qualifier

Non-OR   ØPH[C,D,H,J,K,L][Ø,3,4]8Z
Non-OR   ØPH[F,G][Ø,3,4]8Z

Ø   **Medical and Surgical**
P   **Upper Bones**
J   **Inspection**   Definition: Visually and/or manually exploring a body part

Explanation: Visual exploration may be performed with or without optical instrumentation. Manual exploration may be performed directly or through intervening body layers.

Body Part Character 4	Approach Character 5	Device Character 6	Qualifier Character 7
Y Upper Bone	Ø Open 3 Percutaneous 4 Percutaneous Endoscopic X External	Z No Device	Z No Qualifier

Non-OR   ØPJY[3,X]ZZ

Ø   **Medical and Surgical**
P   **Upper Bones**
N   **Release**   Definition: Freeing a body part from an abnormal physical constraint by cutting or by the use of force

Explanation: Some of the restraining tissue may be taken out but none of the body part is taken out

Body Part Character 4	Approach Character 5	Device Character 6	Qualifier Character 7

Ø   Sternum
    Manubrium
    Suprasternal notch
    Xiphoid process
1   Ribs, 1 to 2
2   Ribs, 3 or More
3   Cervical Vertebra
    Dens
    Odontoid process
    Spinous process
    Transverse foramen
    Transverse process
    Vertebral arch
    Vertebral body
    Vertebral foramen
    Vertebral lamina
    Vertebral pedicle
4   Thoracic Vertebra
    Spinous process
    Transverse process
    Vertebral arch
    Vertebral body
    Vertebral foramen
    Vertebral lamina
    Vertebral pedicle
5   Scapula, Right
    Acromion (process)
    Coracoid process
6   Scapula, Left
    See 5 Scapula, Right
7   Glenoid Cavity, Right
    Glenoid fossa (of scapula)
8   Glenoid Cavity, Left
    See 7 Glenoid Cavity, Right
9   Clavicle, Right
B   Clavicle, Left
C   Humeral Head, Right
    Greater tuberosity
    Lesser tuberosity
    Neck of humerus
      (anatomical) (surgical)
D   Humeral Head, Left
    See C Humeral Head, Right
	F Humeral Shaft, Right
	    Distal humerus
	    Humerus, distal
	    Lateral epicondyle of
	      humerus
	    Medial epicondyle of
	      humerus
	G Humeral Shaft, Left
	    See F Humeral Shaft, Right
	H Radius, Right
	    Ulnar notch
	J Radius, Left
	    See H Radius, Right
	K Ulna, Right
	    Olecranon process
	    Radial notch
	L Ulna, Left
	    See K Ulna, Right
	M Carpal, Right
	    Capitate bone
	    Hamate bone
	    Lunate bone
	    Pisiform bone
	    Scaphoid bone
	    Trapezium bone
	    Trapezoid bone
	    Triquetral bone
	N Carpal, Left
	    See M Carpal, Right
	P Metacarpal, Right
	Q Metacarpal, Left
	R Thumb Phalanx, Right
	S Thumb Phalanx, Left
	T Finger Phalanx, Right
	V Finger Phalanx, Left
		Ø Open
		3 Percutaneous
		4 Percutaneous Endoscopic
			Z No Device	Z No Qualifier

Non-OR Procedure   DRG Non-OR Procedure   Valid OR Procedure   HAC Associated Procedure   Combination Only   New/Revised April   New/Revised October

554   ICD-10-PCS 2024

ØPJ–ØPN

Ø　Medical and Surgical
P　Upper Bones
P　Removal　　Definition: Taking out or off a device from a body part

Explanation: If a device is taken out and a similar device put in without cutting or puncturing the skin or mucous membrane, the procedure is coded to the root operation CHANGE. Otherwise, the procedure for taking out a device is coded to the root operation REMOVAL.

Body Part Character 4		Approach Character 5	Device Character 6	Qualifier Character 7
Ø Sternum 　Manubrium 　Suprasternal notch 　Xiphoid process **1** Ribs, 1 to 2 **2** Ribs, 3 or More **3** Cervical Vertebra 　Dens 　Odontoid process 　Spinous process 　Transverse foramen 　Transverse process 　Vertebral arch 　Vertebral body 　Vertebral foramen 　Vertebral lamina 　Vertebral pedicle	**4** Thoracic Vertebra 　Spinous process 　Transverse process 　Vertebral arch 　Vertebral body 　Vertebral foramen 　Vertebral lamina 　Vertebral pedicle **5** Scapula, Right 　Acromion (process) 　Coracoid process **6** Scapula, Left 　*See 5 Scapula, Right* **7** Glenoid Cavity, Right 　Glenoid fossa (of scapula) **8** Glenoid Cavity, Left 　*See 7 Glenoid Cavity, Right* **9** Clavicle, Right **B** Clavicle, Left	**Ø** Open **3** Percutaneous **4** Percutaneous Endoscopic	**4** Internal Fixation Device **7** Autologous Tissue Substitute **J** Synthetic Substitute **K** Nonautologous Tissue Substitute	**Z** No Qualifier
Ø Sternum 　Manubrium 　Suprasternal notch 　Xiphoid process **1** Ribs, 1 to 2 **2** Ribs, 3 or More **3** Cervical Vertebra 　Dens 　Odontoid process 　Spinous process 　Transverse foramen 　Transverse process 　Vertebral arch 　Vertebral body 　Vertebral foramen 　Vertebral lamina 　Vertebral pedicle	**4** Thoracic Vertebra 　Spinous process 　Transverse process 　Vertebral arch 　Vertebral body 　Vertebral foramen 　Vertebral lamina 　Vertebral pedicle **5** Scapula, Right 　Acromion (process) 　Coracoid process **6** Scapula, Left 　*See 5 Scapula, Right* **7** Glenoid Cavity, Right 　Glenoid fossa (of scapula) **8** Glenoid Cavity, Left 　*See 7 Glenoid Cavity, Right* **9** Clavicle, Right **B** Clavicle, Left	**X** External	**4** Internal Fixation Device	**Z** No Qualifier
C Humeral Head, Right 　Greater tuberosity 　Lesser tuberosity 　Neck of humerus 　　(anatomical) (surgical) **D** Humeral Head, Left 　*See C Humeral Head, Right* **F** Humeral Shaft, Right 　Distal humerus 　Humerus, distal 　Lateral epicondyle of 　　humerus 　Medial epicondyle of 　　humerus **G** Humeral Shaft, Left 　*See F Humeral Shaft, Right* **H** Radius, Right 　Ulnar notch **J** Radius, Left 　*See H Radius, Right* **K** Ulna, Right 　Olecranon process 　Radial notch	**L** Ulna, Left 　*See K Ulna, Right* **M** Carpal, Right 　Capitate bone 　Hamate bone 　Lunate bone 　Pisiform bone 　Scaphoid bone 　Trapezium bone 　Trapezoid bone 　Triquetral bone **N** Carpal, Left 　*See M Carpal, Right* **P** Metacarpal, Right **Q** Metacarpal, Left **R** Thumb Phalanx, Right **S** Thumb Phalanx, Left **T** Finger Phalanx, Right **V** Finger Phalanx, Left	**Ø** Open **3** Percutaneous **4** Percutaneous Endoscopic	**4** Internal Fixation Device **5** External Fixation Device **7** Autologous Tissue Substitute **J** Synthetic Substitute **K** Nonautologous Tissue Substitute	**Z** No Qualifier

Non-OR　ØPP[Ø,1,2,3,4,5,6,7,8,9,B]X4Z

ØPP Continued on next page

NC Noncovered Procedure　　LC Limited Coverage　　QA Questionable OB Admit　　NT New Tech Add-on　　⊞ Combination Member　　♂Male　　♀Female

ICD-10-PCS 2024　　555

Upper Bones

ØPP Continued

Ø   **Medical and Surgical**
P   **Upper Bones**
P   **Removal**   Definition: Taking out or off a device from a body part

Explanation: If a device is taken out and a similar device put in without cutting or puncturing the skin or mucous membrane, the procedure is coded to the root operation CHANGE. Otherwise, the procedure for taking out a device is coded to the root operation REMOVAL.

Body Part Character 4		Approach Character 5	Device Character 6	Qualifier Character 7

C   **Humeral Head, Right**
    Greater tuberosity
    Lesser tuberosity
    Neck of humerus
      (anatomical) (surgical)
D   **Humeral Head, Left**
    See C Humeral Head, Right
F   **Humeral Shaft, Right**
    Distal humerus
    Humerus, distal
    Lateral epicondyle of
      humerus
    Medial epicondyle of
      humerus
G   **Humeral Shaft, Left**
    See F Humeral Shaft, Right
H   **Radius, Right**
    Ulnar notch
J   **Radius, Left**
    See H Radius, Right
K   **Ulna, Right**
    Olecranon process
Radial notch
	L **Ulna, Left**
	    See K Ulna, Right
	M **Carpal, Right**
	    Capitate bone
	    Hamate bone
	    Lunate bone
	    Pisiform bone
	    Scaphoid bone
	    Trapezium bone
	    Trapezoid bone
	    Triquetral bone
	N **Carpal, Left**
	    See M Carpal, Right
	P **Metacarpal, Right**
	Q **Metacarpal, Left**
	R **Thumb Phalanx, Right**
	S **Thumb Phalanx, Left**
	T **Finger Phalanx, Right**
	V **Finger Phalanx, Left**
		X External	4 **Internal Fixation Device**
			5 **External Fixation Device**
				Z No Qualifier

Y **Upper Bone**		Ø Open 3 Percutaneous 4 Percutaneous Endoscopic X External	Ø **Drainage Device** M **Bone Growth Stimulator**	Z No Qualifier

Non-OR	ØPP[C,D,F,G,H,J,K,L,M,N,P,Q,R,S,T,V]X[4,5]Z
Non-OR	ØPPY3ØZ
Non-OR	ØPPYX[Ø,M]Z

Non-OR Procedure   DRG Non-OR Procedure   Valid OR Procedure   HAC Associated Procedure   Combination Only   New/Revised April   New/Revised October

556   ICD-10-PCS 2024

Ø   **Medical and Surgical**
P   **Upper Bones**
Q   **Repair**   Definition: Restoring, to the extent possible, a body part to its normal anatomic structure and function

                 Explanation: Used only when the method to accomplish the repair is not one of the other root operations

Body Part Character 4		Approach Character 5	Device Character 6	Qualifier Character 7

Ø Sternum
  Manubrium
  Suprasternal notch
  Xiphoid process
1 Ribs, 1 to 2
2 Ribs, 3 or More
3 Cervical Vertebra
  Dens
  Odontoid process
  Spinous process
  Transverse foramen
  Transverse process
  Vertebral arch
  Vertebral body
  Vertebral foramen
  Vertebral lamina
  Vertebral pedicle
4 Thoracic Vertebra
  Spinous process
  Transverse process
  Vertebral arch
  Vertebral body
  Vertebral foramen
  Vertebral lamina
  Vertebral pedicle
5 Scapula, Right
  Acromion (process)
  Coracoid process
6 Scapula, Left
  See 5 Scapula, Right
7 Glenoid Cavity, Right
  Glenoid fossa (of scapula)
8 Glenoid Cavity, Left
  See 7 Glenoid Cavity, Right
9 Clavicle, Right
B Clavicle, Left
C Humeral Head, Right
  Greater tuberosity
  Lesser tuberosity
  Neck of humerus
    (anatomical)(surgical)
D Humeral Head, Left
  See C Humeral Head, Right
	F Humeral Shaft, Right
	  Distal humerus
	  Humerus, distal
	  Lateral epicondyle of
	    humerus
	  Medial epicondyle of
	    humerus
	G Humeral Shaft, Left
	  See F Humeral Shaft, Right
	H Radius, Right
	  Ulnar notch
	J Radius, Left
	  See H Radius, Right
	K Ulna, Right
	  Olecranon process
	  Radial notch
	L Ulna, Left
	  See K Ulna, Right
	M Carpal, Right
	  Capitate bone
	  Hamate bone
	  Lunate bone
	  Pisiform bone
	  Scaphoid bone
	  Trapezium bone
	  Trapezoid bone
	  Triquetral bone
	N Carpal, Left
	  See M Carpal, Right
	P Metacarpal, Right
	Q Metacarpal, Left
	R Thumb Phalanx, Right
	S Thumb Phalanx, Left
	T Finger Phalanx, Right
	V Finger Phalanx, Left
		Ø Open
		3 Percutaneous
		4 Percutaneous Endoscopic
		X External
			Z No Device	**Z No Qualifier**

Non-OR   ØPQ[Ø,1,2,3,4,5,6,7,8,9,B,C,D,F,G,H,J,K,L,M,N,P,Q,R,S,T,V]XZZ

Upper Bones

Ø   **Medical and Surgical**
P   **Upper Bones**
R   **Replacement**   Definition: Putting in or on biological or synthetic material that physically takes the place and/or function of all or a portion of a body part

Explanation: The body part may have been taken out or replaced, or may be taken out, physically eradicated, or rendered nonfunctional during the REPLACEMENT procedure. A REMOVAL procedure is coded for taking out the device used in a previous replacement procedure.

Body Part Character 4		Approach Character 5	Device Character 6	Qualifier Character 7

Ø Sternum
   Manubrium
   Suprasternal notch
   Xiphoid process
1 Ribs, 1 to 2
2 Ribs, 3 or More
3 Cervical Vertebra
   Dens
   Odontoid process
   Spinous process
   Transverse foramen
   Transverse process
   Vertebral arch
   Vertebral body
   Vertebral foramen
   Vertebral lamina
   Vertebral pedicle
4 Thoracic Vertebra
   Spinous process
   Transverse process
   Vertebral arch
   Vertebral body
   Vertebral foramen
   Vertebral lamina
   Vertebral pedicle
5 Scapula, Right
   Acromion (process)
   Coracoid process
6 Scapula, Left
   See 5 Scapula, Right
7 Glenoid Cavity, Right
   Glenoid fossa (of scapula)
8 Glenoid Cavity, Left
   See 7 Glenoid Cavity, Right
9 Clavicle, Right
B Clavicle, Left
C Humeral Head, Right
   Greater tuberosity
   Lesser tuberosity
   Neck of humerus
     (anatomical)(surgical)
D Humeral Head, Left
   See C Humeral Head, Right
	F Humeral Shaft, Right
	   Distal humerus
	   Humerus, distal
	   Lateral epicondyle of
	     humerus
	   Medial epicondyle of
	     humerus
	G Humeral Shaft, Left
	   See F Humeral Shaft, Right
	H Radius, Right
	   Ulnar notch
	J Radius, Left
	   See H Radius, Right
	K Ulna, Right
	   Olecranon process
	   Radial notch
	L Ulna, Left
	   See K Ulna, Right
	M Carpal, Right
	   Capitate bone
	   Hamate bone
	   Lunate bone
	   Pisiform bone
	   Scaphoid bone
	   Trapezium bone
	   Trapezoid bone
	   Triquetral bone
	N Carpal, Left
	   See M Carpal, Right
	P Metacarpal, Right
	Q Metacarpal, Left
	R Thumb Phalanx, Right
	S Thumb Phalanx, Left
	T Finger Phalanx, Right
	V Finger Phalanx, Left
		Ø Open
		3 Percutaneous
		4 Percutaneous Endoscopic
			7 Autologous Tissue
			   Substitute
			J Synthetic Substitute
			K Nonautologous Tissue
			   Substitute
				Z No Qualifier

Non-OR Procedure   DRG Non-OR Procedure   Valid OR Procedure   HAC Associated Procedure   Combination Only   New/Revised April   New/Revised October

558   ICD-10-PCS 2024

Ø   Medical and Surgical
P   Upper Bones
S   Reposition   Definition: Moving to its normal location, or other suitable location, all or a portion of a body part

Explanation: The body part is moved to a new location from an abnormal location, or from a normal location where it is not functioning correctly. The body part may or may not be cut out or off to be moved to the new location.

Body Part Character 4		Approach Character 5	Device Character 6	Qualifier Character 7
Ø Sternum Manubrium Suprasternal notch Xiphoid process		**Ø** Open **3** Percutaneous **4** Percutaneous Endoscopic	**Ø** Internal Fixation Device, Rigid Plate **4** Internal Fixation Device **Z** No Device	**Z** No Qualifier
Ø Sternum Manubrium Suprasternal notch Xiphoid process		**X** External	**Z** No Device	**Z** No Qualifier
1 Ribs, 1 to 2 **2 Ribs, 3 or More** **3 Cervical Vertebra** ⊞ Dens Odontoid process Spinous process Transverse foramen Transverse process Vertebral arch Vertebral body Vertebral foramen Vertebral lamina Vertebral pedicle	**5 Scapula, Right** Acromion (process) Coracoid process **6 Scapula, Left** *See 5 Scapula, Right* **7 Glenoid Cavity, Right** Glenoid fossa (of scapula) **8 Glenoid Cavity, Left** *See 7 Glenoid Cavity, Right* **9 Clavicle, Right** **B Clavicle, Left**	**Ø** Open **3** Percutaneous **4** Percutaneous Endoscopic	**4** Internal Fixation Device **Z** No Device	**Z** No Qualifier
1 Ribs, 1 to 2 **2 Ribs, 3 or More** **3 Cervical Vertebra** Dens Odontoid process Spinous process Transverse foramen Transverse process Vertebral arch Vertebral body Vertebral foramen Vertebral lamina Vertebral pedicle	**5 Scapula, Right** Acromion (process) Coracoid process **6 Scapula, Left** *See 5 Scapula, Right* **7 Glenoid Cavity, Right** Glenoid fossa (of scapula) **8 Glenoid Cavity, Left** *See 7 Glenoid Cavity, Right* **9 Clavicle, Right** **B Clavicle, Left**	**X** External	**Z** No Device	**Z** No Qualifier
4 Thoracic Vertebra Spinous process Transverse process Vertebral arch Vertebral body Vertebral foramen Vertebral lamina Vertebral pedicle		**Ø** Open **4** Percutaneous Endoscopic	**3** Spinal Stabilization Device, Vertebral Body Tether **4** Internal Fixation Device **Z** No Device	**Z** No Qualifier
4 Thoracic Vertebra ⊞ Spinous process Transverse process Vertebral arch Vertebral body Vertebral foramen Vertebral lamina Vertebral pedicle		**3** Percutaneous	**4** Internal Fixation Device **Z** No Device	**Z** No Qualifier
4 Thoracic Vertebra Spinous process Transverse process Vertebral arch Vertebral body Vertebral foramen Vertebral lamina Vertebral pedicle		**X** External	**Z** No Device	**Z** No Qualifier
C Humeral Head, Right Greater tuberosity Lesser tuberosity Neck of humerus (anatomical)(surgical) **D Humeral Head, Left** *See C Humeral Head, Right* **F Humeral Shaft, Right** Distal humerus Humerus, distal Lateral epicondyle of humerus Medial epicondyle of humerus	**G Humeral Shaft, Left** *See F Humeral Shaft, Right* **H Radius, Right** Ulnar notch **J Radius, Left** *See H Radius, Right* **K Ulna, Right** Olecranon process Radial notch **L Ulna, Left** *See K Ulna, Right*	**Ø** Open **3** Percutaneous **4** Percutaneous Endoscopic	**4** Internal Fixation Device **5** External Fixation Device **6** Internal Fixation Device, Intramedullary **B** External Fixation Device, Monoplanar **C** External Fixation Device, Ring **D** External Fixation Device, Hybrid **Z** No Device	**Z** No Qualifier

Non-OR ØPSØ[3,4]ZZ	**Non-OR** ØPS[1,2,3,5,6,7,8,9,B]XZZ	**See Appendix L for Procedure Combinations**
Non-OR ØPSØXZZ	**Non-OR** ØPS4XZZ	⊞ ØPS33ZZ
Non-OR ØPS[1,2,5,6,7,8,9,B][3,4]ZZ	**Non-OR** ØPS[C,D,F,G,H,J,K,L][3,4]ZZ	⊞ ØPS43ZZ

ØPS Continued on next page

NC Noncovered Procedure   LC Limited Coverage   QA Questionable OB Admit   NT New Tech Add-on   ⊞ Combination Member   ♂ Male   ♀ Female

Ø Medical and Surgical
P Upper Bones   *ØPS Continued*
S Reposition Definition: Moving to its normal location, or other suitable location, all or a portion of a body part

Explanation: The body part is moved to a new location from an abnormal location, or from a normal location where it is not functioning correctly. The body part may or may not be cut out or off to be moved to the new location.

Body Part Character 4		Approach Character 5	Device Character 6	Qualifier Character 7

C Humeral Head, Right
   Greater tuberosity
   Lesser tuberosity
   Neck of humerus
      (anatomical)(surgical)
D Humeral Head, Left
   See C Humeral Head, Right
F Humeral Shaft, Right
   Distal humerus
   Humerus, distal
   Lateral epicondyle of humerus
   Medial epicondyle of humerus
	G Humeral Shaft, Left
	   See F Humeral Shaft, Right
	H Radius, Right
	   Ulnar notch
	J Radius, Left
	   See H Radius, Right
	K Ulna, Right
	   Olecranon process
	   Radial notch
	L Ulna, Left
	   See K Ulna, Right
		X External	Z No Device	Z No Qualifier

M Carpal, Right
   Capitate bone
   Hamate bone
   Lunate bone
   Pisiform bone
   Scaphoid bone
   Trapezium bone
   Trapezoid bone
   Triquetral bone
	N Carpal, Left
	   See M Carpal, Right
	P Metacarpal, Right
	Q Metacarpal, Left
	R Thumb Phalanx, Right
	S Thumb Phalanx, Left
	T Finger Phalanx, Right
	V Finger Phalanx, Left
		Ø Open
		3 Percutaneous
		4 Percutaneous Endoscopic
			4 Internal Fixation Device
			5 External Fixation Device
			Z No Device
				Z No Qualifier

M Carpal, Right
   Capitate bone
   Hamate bone
   Lunate bone
   Pisiform bone
   Scaphoid bone
   Trapezium bone
   Trapezoid bone
   Triquetral bone
	N Carpal, Left
	   See M Carpal, Right
	P Metacarpal, Right
	Q Metacarpal, Left
	R Thumb Phalanx, Right
	S Thumb Phalanx, Left
	T Finger Phalanx, Right
	V Finger Phalanx, Left
		X External	Z No Device	Z No Qualifier

Non-OR   ØPS[C,D,F,G,H,J,K,L]XZZ
Non-OR   ØPS[M,N,P,Q,R,S,T,V][3,4]ZZ
Non-OR   ØPS[M,N,P,Q,R,S,T,V]XZZ

Ø Medical and Surgical
P Upper Bones
T Resection Definition: Cutting out or off, without replacement, all of a body part

Explanation: None

Body Part Character 4		Approach Character 5	Device Character 6	Qualifier Character 7

Ø Sternum
   Manubrium
   Suprasternal notch
   Xiphoid process
1 Ribs, 1 to 2
2 Ribs, 3 or More
5 Scapula, Right
   Acromion (process)
   Coracoid process
6 Scapula, Left
   See 5 Scapula, Right
7 Glenoid Cavity, Right
   Glenoid fossa (of scapula)
8 Glenoid Cavity, Left
   See 7 Glenoid Cavity, Right
9 Clavicle, Right
B Clavicle, Left
C Humeral Head, Right
   Greater tuberosity
   Lesser tuberosity
   Neck of humerus
      (anatomical) (surgical)
D Humeral Head, Left
   See C Humeral Head, Right
F Humeral Shaft, Right
   Distal humerus
   Humerus, distal
   Lateral epicondyle of
      humerus
   Medial epicondyle of
      humerus
	G Humeral Shaft, Left
	   See F Humeral Shaft, Right
	H Radius, Right
	   Ulnar notch
	J Radius, Left
	   See H Radius, Right
	K Ulna, Right
	   Olecranon process
	   Radial notch
	L Ulna, Left
	   See K Ulna, Right
	M Carpal, Right
	   Capitate bone
	   Hamate bone
	   Lunate bone
	   Pisiform bone
	   Scaphoid bone
	   Trapezium bone
	   Trapezoid bone
	   Triquetral bone
	N Carpal, Left
	   See M Carpal, Right
	P Metacarpal, Right
	Q Metacarpal, Left
	R Thumb Phalanx, Right
	S Thumb Phalanx, Left
	T Finger Phalanx, Right
	V Finger Phalanx, Left
		Ø Open	Z No Device	Z No Qualifier

Non-OR Procedure   DRG Non-OR Procedure   Valid OR Procedure   HAC Associated Procedure   Combination Only   New/Revised April   New/Revised October

560   ICD-10-PCS 2024

Upper Bones   ØPS–ØPT

Ø   Medical and Surgical
P   Upper Bones
U   Supplement   Definition: Putting in or on biological or synthetic material that physically reinforces and/or augments the function of a portion of a body part

Explanation: The biological material is non-living, or is living and from the same individual. The body part may have been previously replaced, and the SUPPLEMENT procedure is performed to physically reinforce and/or augment the function of the replaced body part.

Body Part Character 4		Approach Character 5	Device Character 6	Qualifier Character 7

Ø Sternum
    Manubrium
    Suprasternal notch
    Xiphoid process
1 Ribs, 1 to 2
2 Ribs, 3 or More
3 Cervical Vertebra ⊞
    Dens
    Odontoid process
    Spinous process
    Transverse foramen
    Transverse process
    Vertebral arch
    Vertebral body
    Vertebral foramen
    Vertebral lamina
    Vertebral pedicle
4 Thoracic Vertebra ⊞
    Spinous process
    Transverse process
    Vertebral arch
    Vertebral body
    Vertebral foramen
    Vertebral lamina
    Vertebral pedicle
5 Scapula, Right
    Acromion (process)
    Coracoid process
6 Scapula, Left
    See 5 Scapula, Right
7 Glenoid Cavity, Right
    Glenoid fossa (of scapula)
8 Glenoid Cavity, Left
    See 7 Glenoid Cavity, Right
9 Clavicle, Right
B Clavicle, Left
C Humeral Head, Right
    Greater tuberosity
    Lesser tuberosity
    Neck of humerus
       (anatomical) (surgical)
	D Humeral Head, Left
	    See C Humeral Head, Right
	F Humeral Shaft, Right
	    Distal humerus
	    Humerus, distal
	    Lateral epicondyle of
	       humerus
	    Medial epicondyle of
	       humerus
	G Humeral Shaft, Left
	    See F Humeral Shaft, Right
	H Radius, Right
	    Ulnar notch
	J Radius, Left
	    See H Radius, Right
	K Ulna, Right
	    Olecranon process
	    Radial notch
	L Ulna, Left
	    See K Ulna, Right
	M Carpal, Right
	    Capitate bone
	    Hamate bone
	    Lunate bone
	    Pisiform bone
	    Scaphoid bone
	    Trapezium bone
	    Trapezoid bone
	    Triquetral bone
	N Carpal, Left
	    See M Carpal, Right
	P Metacarpal, Right
	Q Metacarpal, Left
	R Thumb Phalanx, Right
	S Thumb Phalanx, Left
	T Finger Phalanx, Right
	V Finger Phalanx, Left
		Ø Open
		3 Percutaneous
		4 Percutaneous Endoscopic
			7 Autologous Tissue
			    Substitute
			J Synthetic Substitute
			K Nonautologous Tissue
			    Substitute
				Z No Qualifier

See Appendix L for Procedure Combinations
⊞   ØPU[3,4]3JZ

NC Noncovered Procedure   **LC** Limited Coverage   **QA** Questionable OB Admit   **NT** New Tech Add-on   ⊞ Combination Member   ♂ Male   ♀ Female

ICD-10-PCS 2024   561

ØPU–ØPU

Upper Bones *(left margin)*

Ø   **Medical and Surgical**
P   **Upper Bones**
W   **Revision**   Definition: Correcting, to the extent possible, a portion of a malfunctioning device or the position of a displaced device

Explanation: Revision can include correcting a malfunctioning or displaced device by taking out or putting in components of the device such as a screw or pin

Body Part Character 4		Approach Character 5	Device Character 6	Qualifier Character 7

Ø **Sternum**
  Manubrium
  Suprasternal notch
  Xiphoid process
1 **Ribs, 1 to 2**
2 **Ribs, 3 or More**
3 **Cervical Vertebra**
  Dens
  Odontoid process
  Spinous process
  Transverse foramen
  Transverse process
  Vertebral arch
  Vertebral body
  Vertebral foramen
  Vertebral lamina
  Vertebral pedicle
4 **Thoracic Vertebra**
  Spinous process
  Transverse process
  Vertebral arch
  Vertebral body
  Vertebral foramen
  Vertebral lamina
  Vertebral pedicle
	5 **Scapula, Right**
	  Acromion (process)
	  Coracoid process
	6 **Scapula, Left**
	  See 5 Scapula, Right
	7 **Glenoid Cavity, Right**
	  Glenoid fossa (of scapula)
	8 **Glenoid Cavity, Left**
	  See 7 Glenoid Cavity, Right
	9 **Clavicle, Right**
	B **Clavicle, Left**
		Ø Open
		3 Percutaneous
		4 Percutaneous Endoscopic
		X External
			4 **Internal Fixation Device**
			7 **Autologous Tissue Substitute**
			J **Synthetic Substitute**
			K **Nonautologous Tissue Substitute**
				Z No Qualifier

C **Humeral Head, Right**
  Greater tuberosity
  Lesser tuberosity
  Neck of humerus
    (anatomical)(surgical)
D **Humeral Head, Left**
  See C Humeral Head, Right
F **Humeral Shaft, Right**
  Distal humerus
  Humerus, distal
  Lateral epicondyle of
    humerus
  Medial epicondyle of
    humerus
G **Humeral Shaft, Left**
  See F Humeral Shaft, Right
H **Radius, Right**
  Ulnar notch
J **Radius, Left**
  See H Radius, Right
K **Ulna, Right**
  Olecranon process
  Radial notch
	L **Ulna, Left**
	  See K Ulna, Right
	M **Carpal, Right**
	  Capitate bone
	  Hamate bone
	  Lunate bone
	  Pisiform bone
	  Scaphoid bone
	  Trapezium bone
	  Trapezoid bone
	  Triquetral bone
	N **Carpal, Left**
	  See M Carpal, Right
	P **Metacarpal, Right**
	Q **Metacarpal, Left**
	R **Thumb Phalanx, Right**
	S **Thumb Phalanx, Left**
	T **Finger Phalanx, Right**
	V **Finger Phalanx, Left**
		Ø Open
		3 Percutaneous
		4 Percutaneous Endoscopic
		X External
			4 **Internal Fixation Device**
			5 **External Fixation Device**
			7 **Autologous Tissue Substitute**
			J **Synthetic Substitute**
			K **Nonautologous Tissue Substitute**
				Z No Qualifier

Y **Upper Bone**		Ø Open 3 Percutaneous 4 Percutaneous Endoscopic X External	Ø **Drainage Device** M **Bone Growth Stimulator**	Z No Qualifier

Non-OR   ØPW[Ø,1,2,3,4,5,6,7,8,9,B]X[4,7,J,K]Z
Non-OR   ØPW[C,D,F,G,H,J,K,L,M,N,P,Q,R,S,T,V]X[4,5,7,J,K]Z
Non-OR   ØPWYX[Ø,M]Z

Lower Bones ØQ2–ØQW

Character Meanings

This Character Meaning table is provided as a guide to assist the user in the identification of character members that may be found in this section of code tables. It **SHOULD NOT** be used to build a PCS code.

Operation–Character 3		Body Part–Character 4		Approach–Character 5		Device–Character 6		Qualifier–Character 7	
2	Change	Ø	Lumbar Vertebra	Ø	Open	Ø	Drainage Device	2	Sesamoid Bone(s) 1st Toe
5	Destruction	1	Sacrum	3	Percutaneous	3	Spinal Stabilization Device, Vertebral Body Tether	3	Laser Interstitial Thermal Therapy
8	Division	2	Pelvic Bone, Right	4	Percutaneous Endoscopic	4	Internal Fixation Device	X	Diagnostic
9	Drainage	3	Pelvic Bone, Left	X	External	5	External Fixation Device	Z	No Qualifier
B	Excision	4	Acetabulum, Right			6	Internal Fixation Device, Intramedullary		
C	Extirpation	5	Acetabulum, Left			7	Autologous Tissue Substitute OR Internal Fixation Device, Intramedullary Limb Lengthening		
D	Extraction	6	Upper Femur, Right			8	External Fixation Device, Limb Lengthening		
H	Insertion	7	Upper Femur, Left			B	External Fixation Device, Monoplanar		
J	Inspection	8	Femoral Shaft, Right			C	External Fixation Device, Ring		
N	Release	9	Femoral Shaft, Left			D	External Fixation Device, Hybrid		
P	Removal	B	Lower Femur, Right			J	Synthetic Substitute		
Q	Repair	C	Lower Femur, Left			K	Nonautologous Tissue Substitute		
R	Replacement	D	Patella, Right			M	Bone Growth Stimulator		
S	Reposition	F	Patella, Left			Y	Other Device		
T	Resection	G	Tibia, Right			Z	No Device		
U	Supplement	H	Tibia, Left						
W	Revision	J	Fibula, Right						
		K	Fibula, Left						
		L	Tarsal, Right						
		M	Tarsal, Left						
		N	Metatarsal, Right						
		P	Metatarsal, Left						
		Q	Toe Phalanx, Right						
		R	Toe Phalanx, Left						
		S	Coccyx						
		Y	Lower Bone						

AHA Coding Clinic for table 0Q5

2023, 1Q, 10	Laser interstitial thermal therapy

AHA Coding Clinic for table 0Q8

2018, 1Q, 25	Periacetabular osteotomy for repair of congenital hip dysplasia
2016, 2Q, 31	Periacetabular ostectomy for repair of congenital hip dysplasia

AHA Coding Clinic for table 0Q9

2022, 1Q, 31	Septic arthritis/osteomyelitis of pubic symphysis and aspiration biopsy

AHA Coding Clinic for table 0QB

2023, 2Q, 30	Excisional debridement and non-excisional debridement at deeper layer same site
2021, 4Q, 52-53	Sesamoidectomy of great toe
2021, 2Q, 18	Excision of tibial sesamoid
2020, 2Q, 26	Sacral pressure ulcer with excisional and nonexcisional debridement of same site
2019, 2Q, 19	Cervical spinal fusion, decompression and placement of interfacet stabilization device
2018, 3Q, 17	Excisional debridement of periosteum
2017, 1Q, 23	Reconstruction of mandible using titanium and bone
2016, 3Q, 30	Resection of femur with interposition arthroplasty
2015, 3Q, 3-8	Excisional and nonexcisional debridement
2015, 3Q, 26	Femoral head resection
2015, 2Q, 34	Decompressive laminectomy
2014, 4Q, 25	Femoroacetabular impingement and labral tear with repair
2014, 2Q, 6	Posterior lumbar fusion with discectomy
2013, 4Q, 116	Spinal decompression
2013, 2Q, 39	Ankle fusion, osteotomy, and removal of hardware
2012, 2Q, 19	Multiple decompressive cervical laminectomies

AHA Coding Clinic for table 0QD

2023, 2Q, 30	Excisional debridement and non-excisional debridement at deeper layer same site
2017, 4Q, 41	Extraction procedures

AHA Coding Clinic for table 0QH

2022, 2Q, 19	Limb lengthening surgery
2019, 4Q, 34	Intramedullary limb lengthening internal fixation device
2017, 1Q, 21	Staged scoliosis surgery with iliac fixation and spinal fusion
2016, 3Q, 34	Tibial/fibula epiphysiodesis

AHA Coding Clinic for table 0QP

2023, 1Q, 33	Removal of S2-Alar-Iliac screws
2020, 4Q, 56	Removal of external fixation device
2017, 4Q, 74-75	Magnetic growth rods
2015, 2Q, 6	Planned implant break

AHA Coding Clinic for table 0QQ

2018, 1Q, 15	Pubic symphysis fusion
2014, 3Q, 24	Repair of lipomyelomeningocele and tethered cord

AHA Coding Clinic for table 0QR

2017, 1Q, 22	Total knee replacement and patellar component
2016, 3Q, 30	Resection of femur with interposition arthroplasty

AHA Coding Clinic for table 0QS

2022, 2Q, 19	Limb lengthening surgery
2021, 4Q, 51-52	Vertebral body tethering
2020, 1Q, 33	Spinal fusion without use of bone graft
2019, 3Q, 26	Open reduction with internal fixation and placement of strut allograft
2018, 1Q, 13	Bilateral cuboid osteotomy for repair of congenital talipes equinovarus
2018, 1Q, 25	Periacetabular osteotomy for repair of congenital hip dysplasia
2016, 3Q, 34	Tibial/fibula epiphysiodesis
2014, 4Q, 29	Rotational osteosynthesis
2014, 4Q, 31	Reposition of femur for correction of valgus and recurvatum deformities

AHA Coding Clinic for table 0QT

2017, 1Q, 22	Chopart amputation of foot
2016, 3Q, 30	Resection of femur with interposition arthroplasty
2015, 3Q, 26	Femoral head resection
2014, 4Q, 29	Rotational osteosynthesis

AHA Coding Clinic for table 0QU

2019, 3Q, 26	Open reduction with internal fixation and placement of strut allograft
2019, 2Q, 35	Kiva® kyphoplasty
2015, 3Q, 18	Total hip replacement with acetabular reconstruction
2014, 4Q, 31	Reposition of femur for correction of valgus and recurvatum deformities
2014, 2Q, 12	Percutaneous vertebroplasty using cement
2013, 2Q, 35	Use of bone void filler in grafting

AHA Coding Clinic for table 0QW

2017, 4Q, 74-75	Magnetic growth rods

Lower Bones

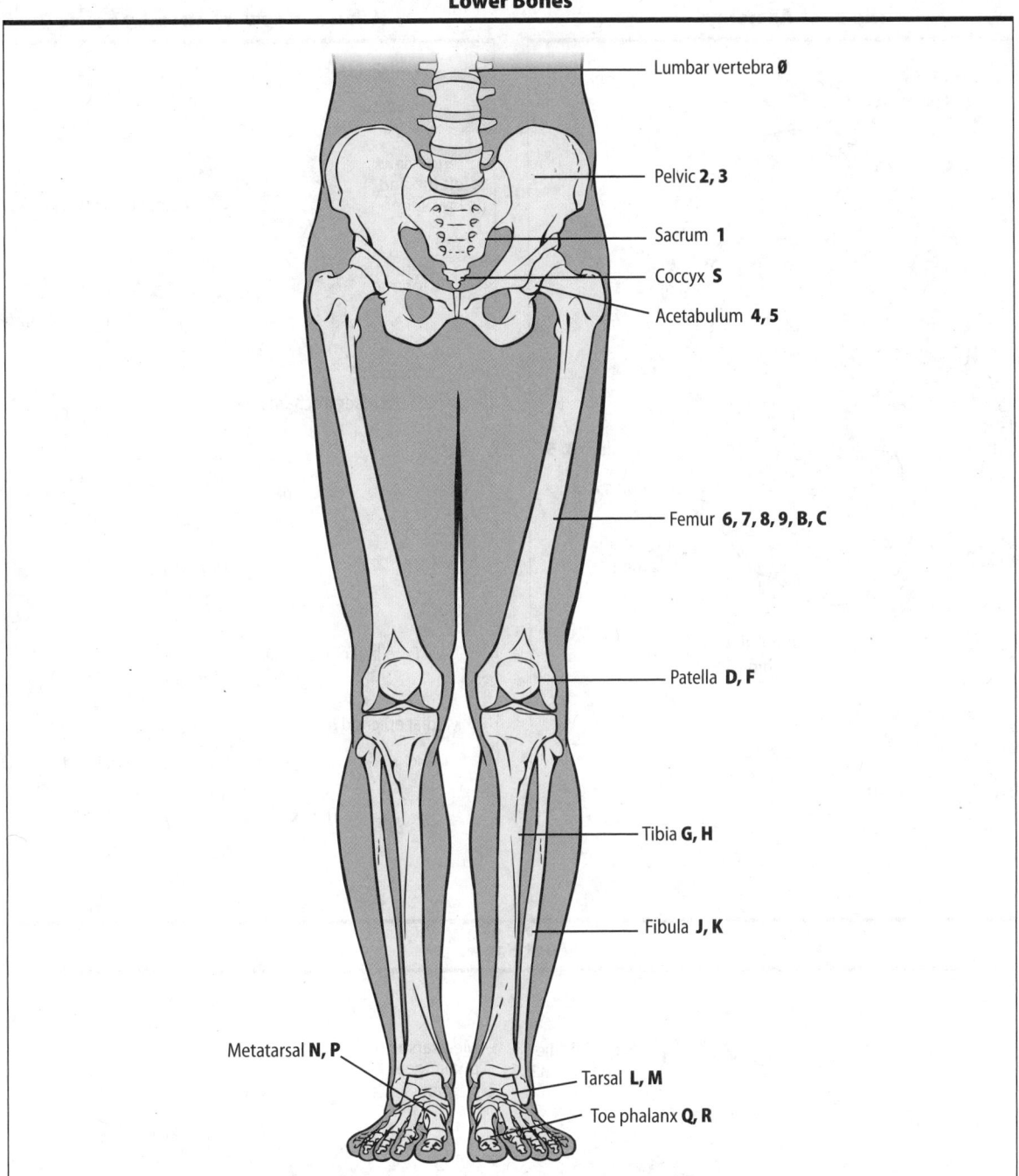

Lumbar vertebra **Ø**

Pelvic **2, 3**

Sacrum **1**

Coccyx **S**

Acetabulum **4, 5**

Femur **6, 7, 8, 9, B, C**

Patella **D, F**

Tibia **G, H**

Fibula **J, K**

Metatarsal **N, P**

Tarsal **L, M**

Toe phalanx **Q, R**

Lower Bones

Hip Bone Anatomy

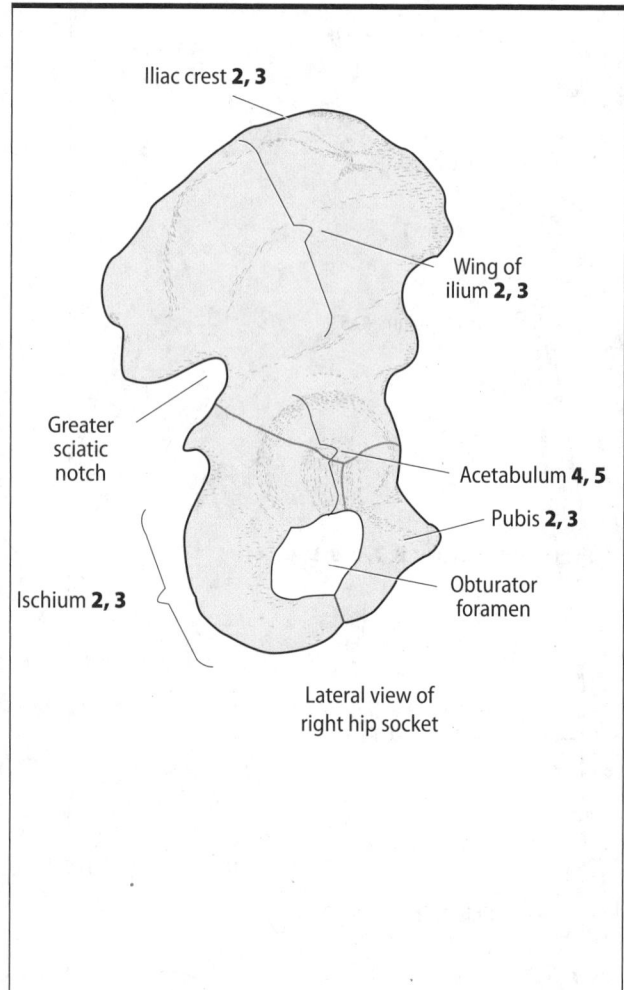

Iliac crest **2, 3**

Wing of ilium **2, 3**

Greater sciatic notch

Acetabulum **4, 5**

Pubis **2, 3**

Obturator foramen

Ischium **2, 3**

Lateral view of right hip socket

Pelvic and Lower Extremity Bones

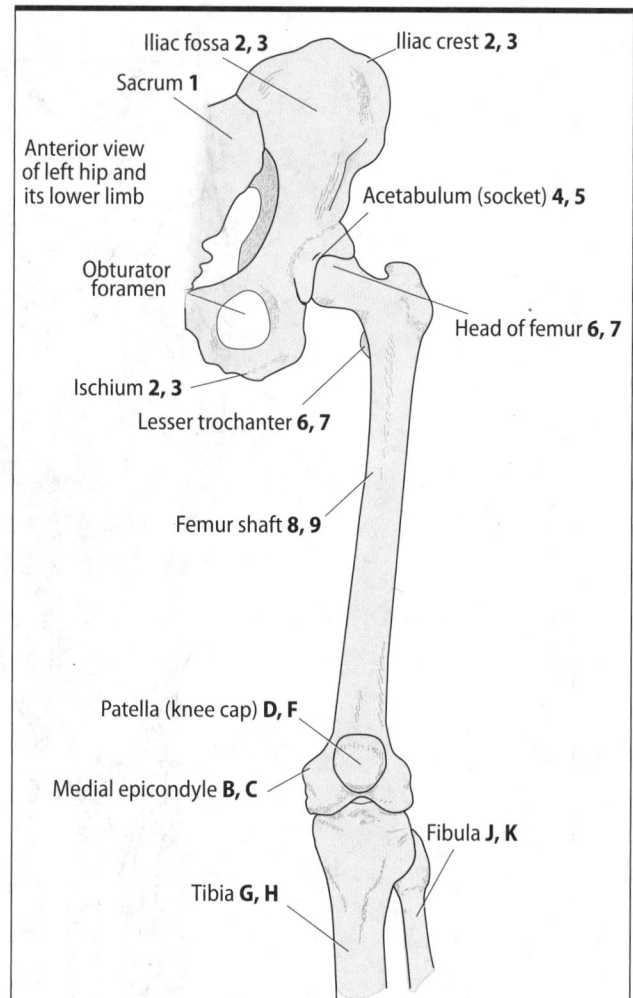

Iliac fossa **2, 3**

Iliac crest **2, 3**

Sacrum **1**

Anterior view of left hip and its lower limb

Acetabulum (socket) **4, 5**

Obturator foramen

Head of femur **6, 7**

Ischium **2, 3**

Lesser trochanter **6, 7**

Femur shaft **8, 9**

Patella (knee cap) **D, F**

Medial epicondyle **B, C**

Fibula **J, K**

Tibia **G, H**

Foot Bones

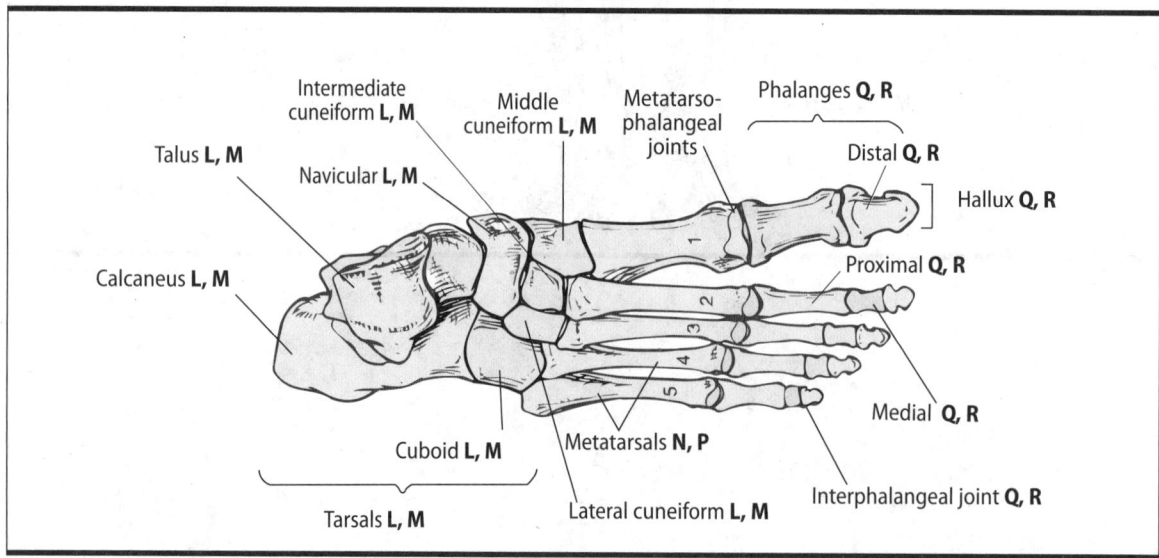

Intermediate cuneiform **L, M**

Middle cuneiform **L, M**

Metatarso-phalangeal joints

Phalanges **Q, R**

Talus **L, M**

Navicular **L, M**

Distal **Q, R**

Calcaneus **L, M**

Hallux **Q, R**

Proximal **Q, R**

Medial **Q, R**

Cuboid **L, M**

Metatarsals **N, P**

Lateral cuneiform **L, M**

Interphalangeal joint **Q, R**

Tarsals **L, M**

0   **Medical and Surgical**
Q   **Lower Bones**
2   **Change**   Definition: Taking out or off a device from a body part and putting back an identical or similar device in or on the same body part without cutting or puncturing the skin or a mucous membrane

                         Explanation: All CHANGE procedures are coded using the approach EXTERNAL

Body Part Character 4		Approach Character 5	Device Character 6	Qualifier Character 7
Y Lower Bone		**X** External	**0** Drainage Device **Y** Other Device	**Z** No Qualifier

Non-OR   All body part, approach, device, and qualifier values

0   **Medical and Surgical**
Q   **Lower Bones**
5   **Destruction**   Definition: Physical eradication of all or a portion of a body part by the direct use of energy, force, or a destructive agent

                         Explanation: None of the body part is physically taken out

Body Part Character 4		Approach Character 5	Device Character 6	Qualifier Character 7

0   Lumbar Vertebra
    Spinous process
    Transverse process
    Vertebral arch
    Vertebral body
    Vertebral foramen
    Vertebral lamina
    Vertebral pedicle
	1 Sacrum	**0** Open
		3 Percutaneous
		4 Percutaneous Endoscopic
			Z No Device	**3** Laser Interstitial Thermal Therapy
				Z No Qualifier

2   Pelvic Bone, Right
    Iliac crest
    Ilium
    Ischium
    Pubis
3   Pelvic Bone, Left
    See 2 Pelvic Bone, Right
4   Acetabulum, Right
5   Acetabulum, Left
6   Upper Femur, Right
    Femoral head
    Greater trochanter
    Lesser trochanter
    Neck of femur
7   Upper Femur, Left
    See 6 Upper Femur, Right
8   Femoral Shaft, Right
    Body of femur
9   Femoral Shaft, Left
    See 8 Femoral Shaft, Right
B   Lower Femur, Right
    Lateral condyle of femur
    Lateral epicondyle of femur
    Medial condyle of femur
    Medial epicondyle of femur
C   Lower Femur, Left
    See B Lower Femur, Right
D   Patella, Right
F   Patella, Left
	G Tibia, Right
	    Lateral condyle of tibia
	    Medial condyle of tibia
	    Medial malleolus
	H Tibia, Left
	    See G Tibia, Right
	J Fibula, Right
	    Body of fibula
	    Head of fibula
	    Lateral malleolus
	K Fibula, Left
	    See J Fibula, Right
	L Tarsal, Right
	    Calcaneus
	    Cuboid bone
	    Intermediate cuneiform
	      bone
	    Lateral cuneiform bone
	    Medial cuneiform bone
	    Navicular bone
	    Talus bone
	M Tarsal, Left
	    See L Tarsal, Right
	N Metatarsal, Right
	    Fibular sesamoid
	    Tibial sesamoid
	P Metatarsal, Left
	    See N Metatarsal, Right
	Q Toe Phalanx, Right
	R Toe Phalanx, Left
	S Coccyx
		0 Open
		3 Percutaneous
		4 Percutaneous Endoscopic
			Z No Device	**Z** No Qualifier

NC Noncovered Procedure   **LC** Limited Coverage   **QA** Questionable OB Admit   **NT** New Tech Add-on   ⊞ Combination Member   ♂ Male   ♀ Female

ICD-10-PCS 2024   567

0Q2–0Q5

Lower Bones

Ø **Medical and Surgical**
Q **Lower Bones**
8 **Division**   Definition: Cutting into a body part, without draining fluids and/or gases from the body part, in order to separate or transect a body part
                        Explanation: All or a portion of the body part is separated into two or more portions

Body Part Character 4	Approach Character 5	Device Character 6	Qualifier Character 7

Ø Lumbar Vertebra
   Spinous process
   Transverse process
   Vertebral arch
   Vertebral body
   Vertebral foramen
   Vertebral lamina
   Vertebral pedicle
1 Sacrum
2 Pelvic Bone, Right
   Iliac crest
   Ilium
   Ischium
   Pubis
3 Pelvic Bone, Left
   See 2 Pelvic Bone, Right
4 Acetabulum, Right
5 Acetabulum, Left
6 Upper Femur, Right
   Femoral head
   Greater trochanter
   Lesser trochanter
   Neck of femur
7 Upper Femur, Left
   See 6 Upper Femur, Right
8 Femoral Shaft, Right
   Body of femur
9 Femoral Shaft, Left
   See 8 Femoral Shaft, Right
B Lower Femur, Right
   Lateral condyle of femur
   Lateral epicondyle of femur
   Medial condyle of femur
   Medial epicondyle of femur
C Lower Femur, Left
   See B Lower Femur, Right
D Patella, Right
F Patella, Left
G Tibia, Right
   Lateral condyle of tibia
   Medial condyle of tibia
   Medial malleolus
H Tibia, Left
   See G Tibia, Right
J Fibula, Right
   Body of fibula
   Head of fibula
   Lateral malleolus
K Fibula, Left
   See J Fibula, Right
L Tarsal, Right
   Calcaneus
   Cuboid bone
   Intermediate cuneiform bone
   Lateral cuneiform bone
   Medial cuneiform bone
   Navicular bone
   Talus bone
M Tarsal, Left
   See L Tarsal, Right
N Metatarsal, Right
   Fibular sesamoid
   Tibial sesamoid
P Metatarsal, Left
   See N Metatarsal, Right
Q Toe Phalanx, Right
R Toe Phalanx, Left
S Coccyx
	Ø Open
	3 Percutaneous
	4 Percutaneous Endoscopic
		Z No Device	Z No Qualifier

Lower Bones

0   **Medical and Surgical**
Q   **Lower Bones**
9   **Drainage**   Definition: Taking or letting out fluids and/or gases from a body part
                      Explanation: The qualifier DIAGNOSTIC is used to identify drainage procedures that are biopsies

Body Part Character 4		Approach Character 5	Device Character 6	Qualifier Character 7

0 Lumbar Vertebra
  Spinous process
  Transverse process
  Vertebral arch
  Vertebral body
  Vertebral foramen
  Vertebral lamina
  Vertebral pedicle
1 Sacrum
2 Pelvic Bone, Right
  Iliac crest
  Ilium
  Ischium
  Pubis
3 Pelvic Bone, Left
  See 2 Pelvic Bone, Right
4 Acetabulum, Right
5 Acetabulum, Left
6 Upper Femur, Right
  Femoral head
  Greater trochanter
  Lesser trochanter
  Neck of femur
7 Upper Femur, Left
  See 6 Upper Femur, Right
8 Femoral Shaft, Right
  Body of femur
9 Femoral Shaft, Left
  See 8 Femoral Shaft, Right
B Lower Femur, Right
  Lateral condyle of femur
  Lateral epicondyle of femur
  Medial condyle of femur
  Medial epicondyle of femur
	C Lower Femur, Left
	  See B Lower Femur, Right
	D Patella, Right
	F Patella, Left
	G Tibia, Right
	  Lateral condyle of tibia
	  Medial condyle of tibia
	  Medial malleolus
	H Tibia, Left
	  See G Tibia, Right
	J Fibula, Right
	  Body of fibula
	  Head of fibula
	  Lateral malleolus
	K Fibula, Left
	  See J Fibula, Right
	L Tarsal, Right
	  Calcaneus
	  Cuboid bone
	  Intermediate cuneiform bone
	  Lateral cuneiform bone
	  Medial cuneiform bone
	  Navicular bone
	  Talus bone
	M Tarsal, Left
	  See L Tarsal, Right
	N Metatarsal, Right
	  Fibular sesamoid
	  Tibial sesamoid
	P Metatarsal, Left
	  See N Metatarsal, Right
	Q Toe Phalanx, Right
	R Toe Phalanx, Left
	S Coccyx
		0 Open
		3 Percutaneous
		4 Percutaneous Endoscopic
			0 Drainage Device	**Z** No Qualifier

0 Lumbar Vertebra
  Spinous process
  Transverse process
  Vertebral arch
  Vertebral body
  Vertebral foramen
  Vertebral lamina
  Vertebral pedicle
1 Sacrum
2 Pelvic Bone, Right
  Iliac crest
  Ilium
  Ischium
  Pubis
3 Pelvic Bone, Left
  See 2 Pelvic Bone, Right
4 Acetabulum, Right
5 Acetabulum, Left
6 Upper Femur, Right
  Femoral head
  Greater trochanter
  Lesser trochanter
  Neck of femur
7 Upper Femur, Left
  See 6 Upper Femur, Right
8 Femoral Shaft, Right
  Body of femur
9 Femoral Shaft, Left
  See 8 Femoral Shaft, Right
B Lower Femur, Right
  Lateral condyle of femur
  Lateral epicondyle of femur
  Medial condyle of femur
  Medial epicondyle of femur
	C Lower Femur, Left
	  See B Lower Femur, Right
	D Patella, Right
	F Patella, Left
	G Tibia, Right
	  Lateral condyle of tibia
	  Medial condyle of tibia
	  Medial malleolus
	H Tibia, Left
	  See G Tibia, Right
	J Fibula, Right
	  Body of fibula
	  Head of fibula
	  Lateral malleolus
	K Fibula, Left
	  See J Fibula, Right
	L Tarsal, Right
	  Calcaneus
	  Cuboid bone
	  Intermediate cuneiform bone
	  Lateral cuneiform bone
	  Medial cuneiform bone
	  Navicular bone
	  Talus bone
	M Tarsal, Left
	  See L Tarsal, Right
	N Metatarsal, Right
	  Fibular sesamoid
	  Tibial sesamoid
	P Metatarsal, Left
	  See N Metatarsal, Right
	Q Toe Phalanx, Right
	R Toe Phalanx, Left
	S Coccyx
		0 Open
		3 Percutaneous
		4 Percutaneous Endoscopic
			Z No Device	**X** Diagnostic
				Z No Qualifier

Non-OR   0Q9[0,1,2,3,4,5,6,7,8,9,B,C,D,F,G,H,J,K,L,M,P,Q,R,S]30Z
Non-OR   0Q9[0,1,2,3,4,5,6,7,8,9,B,C,D,F,G,H,J,K,L,M,P,Q,R,S]3ZZ

NC Noncovered Procedure   **LC** Limited Coverage   **QA** Questionable OB Admit   **NT** New Tech Add-on   ⊞ Combination Member   ♂ Male   ♀ Female

ICD-10-PCS 2024   569

Ø   Medical and Surgical
Q   Lower Bones
B   Excision   Definition: Cutting out or off, without replacement, a portion of a body part

                 Explanation: The qualifier DIAGNOSTIC is used to identify excision procedures that are biopsies

Body Part Character 4	Approach Character 5	Device Character 6	Qualifier Character 7

Ø Lumbar Vertebra
  Spinous process
  Transverse process
  Vertebral arch
  Vertebral body
  Vertebral foramen
  Vertebral lamina
  Vertebral pedicle
1 Sacrum
2 Pelvic Bone, Right
  Iliac crest
  Ilium
  Ischium
  Pubis
3 Pelvic Bone, Left
  See 2 Pelvic Bone, Right
4 Acetabulum, Right
5 Acetabulum, Left
6 Upper Femur, Right
  Femoral head
  Greater trochanter
  Lesser trochanter
  Neck of femur
7 Upper Femur, Left
  See 6 Upper Femur, Right
8 Femoral Shaft, Right
  Body of femur
9 Femoral Shaft, Left
  See 8 Femoral Shaft, Right
B Lower Femur, Right
  Lateral condyle of femur
  Lateral epicondyle of femur
  Medial condyle of femur
  Medial epicondyle of femur
C Lower Femur, Left
  See B Lower Femur, Right
D Patella, Right
F Patella, Left
G Tibia, Right
  Lateral condyle of tibia
  Medial condyle of tibia
  Medial malleolus
H Tibia, Left
  See G Tibia, Right
J Fibula, Right
  Body of fibula
  Head of fibula
  Lateral malleolus
K Fibula, Left
  See J Fibula, Right
L Tarsal, Right
  Calcaneus
  Cuboid bone
  Intermediate cuneiform bone
  Lateral cuneiform bone
  Medial cuneiform bone
  Navicular bone
  Talus bone
M Tarsal, Left
  See L Tarsal, Right
Q Toe Phalanx, Right
R Toe Phalanx, Left
S Coccyx
	Ø Open
	3 Percutaneous
	4 Percutaneous Endoscopic
		Z No Device	**X Diagnostic**
			Z No Qualifier

N Metatarsal, Right
  Fibular sesamoid
  Tibial sesamoid
P Metatarsal, Left
  See N Metatarsal, Right
	Ø Open
	3 Percutaneous
	4 Percutaneous Endoscopic
		Z No Device	**2 Sesamoid Bone(s) 1st Toe**
			X Diagnostic
			Z No Qualifier

Non-OR Procedure   DRG Non-OR Procedure   Valid OR Procedure   HAC Associated Procedure   Combination Only   New/Revised April   New/Revised October

Ø　Medical and Surgical
Q　Lower Bones
C　Extirpation　　Definition: Taking or cutting out solid matter from a body part
　　　　　　　　　　　Explanation: The solid matter may be an abnormal byproduct of a biological function or a foreign body; it may be imbedded in a body part or in the lumen of a tubular body part. The solid matter may or may not have been previously broken into pieces.

Body Part Character 4	Approach Character 5	Device Character 6	Qualifier Character 7
Ø Lumbar Vertebra Spinous process Transverse process Vertebral arch Vertebral body Vertebral foramen Vertebral lamina Vertebral pedicle **1 Sacrum** **2 Pelvic Bone, Right** Iliac crest Ilium Ischium Pubis **3 Pelvic Bone, Left** *See 2 Pelvic Bone, Right* **4 Acetabulum, Right** **5 Acetabulum, Left** **6 Upper Femur, Right** Femoral head Greater trochanter Lesser trochanter Neck of femur **7 Upper Femur, Left** *See 6 Upper Femur, Right* **8 Femoral Shaft, Right** Body of femur **9 Femoral Shaft, Left** *See 8 Femoral Shaft, Right* **B Lower Femur, Right** Lateral condyle of femur Lateral epicondyle of femur Medial condyle of femur Medial epicondyle of femur **C Lower Femur, Left** *See B Lower Femur, Right* **D Patella, Right** **F Patella, Left** **G Tibia, Right** Lateral condyle of tibia Medial condyle of tibia Medial malleolus **H Tibia, Left** *See G Tibia, Right* **J Fibula, Right** Body of fibula Head of fibula Lateral malleolus **K Fibula, Left** *See J Fibula, Right* **L Tarsal, Right** Calcaneus Cuboid bone Intermediate cuneiform bone Lateral cuneiform bone Medial cuneiform bone Navicular bone Talus bone **M Tarsal, Left** *See L Tarsal, Right* **N Metatarsal, Right** Fibular sesamoid Tibial sesamoid **P Metatarsal, Left** *See N Metatarsal, Right* **Q Toe Phalanx, Right** **R Toe Phalanx, Left** **S Coccyx**	**Ø Open** **3 Percutaneous** **4 Percutaneous Endoscopic**	**Z No Device**	**Z No Qualifier**

NC Noncovered Procedure　　**LC** Limited Coverage　　**UA** Questionable OB Admit　　**NT** New Tech Add-on　　⊞ Combination Member　　♂ Male　　♀ Female

ICD-10-PCS 2024　　　571

ØQC–ØQC

Ø Medical and Surgical
Q Lower Bones
D Extraction — Definition: Pulling or stripping out or off all or a portion of a body part by the use of force

Explanation: The qualifier DIAGNOSTIC is used to identify extraction procedures that are biopsies

Body Part Character 4	Approach Character 5	Device Character 6	Qualifier Character 7
Ø Lumbar Vertebra Spinous process Transverse process Vertebral arch Vertebral body Vertebral foramen Vertebral lamina Vertebral pedicle	**Ø Open**	**Z No Device**	**Z No Qualifier**
1 Sacrum			
2 Pelvic Bone, Right Iliac crest Ilium Ischium Pubis			
3 Pelvic Bone, Left *See 2 Pelvic Bone, Right*			
4 Acetabulum, Right			
5 Acetabulum, Left			
6 Upper Femur, Right Femoral head Greater trochanter Lesser trochanter Neck of femur			
7 Upper Femur, Left *See 6 Upper Femur, Right*			
8 Femoral Shaft, Right Body of femur			
9 Femoral Shaft, Left *See 8 Femoral Shaft, Right*			
B Lower Femur, Right Lateral condyle of femur Lateral epicondyle of femur Medial condyle of femur Medial epicondyle of femur			
C Lower Femur, Left *See B Lower Femur, Right*			
D Patella, Right			
F Patella, Left			
G Tibia, Right Lateral condyle of tibia Medial condyle of tibia Medial malleolus			
H Tibia, Left *See G Tibia, Right*			
J Fibula, Right Body of fibula Head of fibula Lateral malleolus			
K Fibula, Left *See J Fibula, Right*			
L Tarsal, Right Calcaneus Cuboid bone Intermediate cuneiform bone Lateral cuneiform bone Medial cuneiform bone Navicular bone Talus bone			
M Tarsal, Left *See L Tarsal, Right*			
N Metatarsal, Right Fibular sesamoid Tibial sesamoid			
P Metatarsal, Left *See N Metatarsal, Right*			
Q Toe Phalanx, Right			
R Toe Phalanx, Left			
S Coccyx			

Ø   **Medical and Surgical**
Q   **Lower Bones**
H   **Insertion**   Definition: Putting in a nonbiological appliance that monitors, assists, performs, or prevents a physiological function but does not physically take the place of a body part

                   Explanation: None

Body Part Character 4		Approach Character 5	Device Character 6	Qualifier Character 7
Ø Lumbar Vertebra Spinous process Transverse process Vertebral arch Vertebral body Vertebral foramen Vertebral lamina Vertebral pedicle **1 Sacrum** **2 Pelvic Bone, Right** Iliac crest Ilium Ischium Pubis **3 Pelvic Bone, Left** *See 2 Pelvic Bone, Right* **4 Acetabulum, Right** **5 Acetabulum, Left**	**D Patella, Right** **F Patella, Left** **L Tarsal, Right** Calcaneus Cuboid bone Intermediate cuneiform bone Lateral cuneiform bone Medial cuneiform bone Navicular bone Talus bone **M Tarsal, Left** *See L Tarsal, Right* **N Metatarsal, Right** Fibular sesamoid Tibial sesamoid **P Metatarsal, Left** *See N Metatarsal, Right* **Q Toe Phalanx, Right** **R Toe Phalanx, Left** **S Coccyx**	**Ø Open** **3 Percutaneous** **4 Percutaneous Endoscopic**	**4 Internal Fixation Device** **5 External Fixation Device**	**Z No Qualifier**
6 Upper Femur, Right Femoral head Greater trochanter Lesser trochanter Neck of femur **7 Upper Femur, Left** *See 6 Upper Femur, Right* **B Lower Femur, Right** Lateral condyle of femur Lateral epicondyle of femur Medial condyle of femur Medial epicondyle of femur	**C Lower Femur, Left** *See B Lower Femur, Right* **J Fibula, Right** Body of fibula Head of fibula Lateral malleolus **K Fibula, Left** *See J Fibula, Right*	**Ø Open** **3 Percutaneous** **4 Percutaneous Endoscopic**	**4 Internal Fixation Device** **5 External Fixation Device** **6 Internal Fixation Device, Intramedullary** **8 External Fixation Device, Limb Lengthening** **B External Fixation Device, Monoplanar** **C External Fixation Device, Ring** **D External Fixation Device, Hybrid**	**Z No Qualifier**
8 Femoral Shaft, Right Body of femur **9 Femoral Shaft, Left** *See 8 Femoral Shaft, Right*	**G Tibia, Right** Lateral condyle of tibia Medial condyle of tibia Medial malleolus **H Tibia, Left** *See G Tibia, Right*	**Ø Open** **3 Percutaneous** **4 Percutaneous Endoscopic**	**4 Internal Fixation Device** **5 External Fixation Device** **6 Internal Fixation Device, Intramedullary** **7 Internal Fixation Device, Intramedullary Limb Lengthening** **8 External Fixation Device, Limb Lengthening** **B External Fixation Device, Monoplanar** **C External Fixation Device, Ring** **D External Fixation Device, Hybrid**	**Z No Qualifier**
Y Lower Bone		**Ø Open** **3 Percutaneous** **4 Percutaneous Endoscopic**	**M Bone Growth Stimulator**	**Z No Qualifier**

Non-OR   ØQH[6,7,B,C,J,K][Ø,3,4]8Z
Non-OR   ØQH[8,9,G,H][Ø,3,4]8Z

Ø   **Medical and Surgical**
Q   **Lower Bones**
J   **Inspection**   Definition: Visually and/or manually exploring a body part

                   Explanation: Visual exploration may be performed with or without optical instrumentation. Manual exploration may be performed directly or through intervening body layers.

Body Part Character 4	Approach Character 5	Device Character 6	Qualifier Character 7
Y Lower Bone	**Ø Open** **3 Percutaneous** **4 Percutaneous Endoscopic** **X External**	**Z No Device**	**Z No Qualifier**

Non-OR   ØQJY[3,X]ZZ

Lower Bones

Ø   Medical and Surgical
Q   Lower Bones
N   Release   Definition: Freeing a body part from an abnormal physical constraint by cutting or by the use of force
                   Explanation: Some of the restraining tissue may be taken out but none of the body part is taken out

Body Part Character 4	Approach Character 5	Device Character 6	Qualifier Character 7

Ø Lumbar Vertebra
  Spinous process
  Transverse process
  Vertebral arch
  Vertebral body
  Vertebral foramen
  Vertebral lamina
  Vertebral pedicle
1 Sacrum
2 Pelvic Bone, Right
  Iliac crest
  Ilium
  Ischium
  Pubis
3 Pelvic Bone, Left
  See 2 Pelvic Bone, Right
4 Acetabulum, Right
5 Acetabulum, Left
6 Upper Femur, Right
  Femoral head
  Greater trochanter
  Lesser trochanter
  Neck of femur
7 Upper Femur, Left
  See 6 Upper Femur, Right
8 Femoral Shaft, Right
  Body of femur
9 Femoral Shaft, Left
  See 8 Femoral Shaft, Right
B Lower Femur, Right
  Lateral condyle of femur
  Lateral epicondyle of femur
  Medial condyle of femur
  Medial epicondyle of femur
C Lower Femur, Left
  See B Lower Femur, Right
D Patella, Right
F Patella, Left
G Tibia, Right
  Lateral condyle of tibia
  Medial condyle of tibia
  Medial malleolus
H Tibia, Left
  See G Tibia, Right
J Fibula, Right
  Body of fibula
  Head of fibula
  Lateral malleolus
K Fibula, Left
  See J Fibula, Right
L Tarsal, Right
  Calcaneus
  Cuboid bone
  Intermediate cuneiform bone
  Lateral cuneiform bone
  Medial cuneiform bone
  Navicular bone
  Talus bone
M Tarsal, Left
  See L Tarsal, Right
N Metatarsal, Right
  Fibular sesamoid
  Tibial sesamoid
P Metatarsal, Left
  See N Metatarsal, Right
Q Toe Phalanx, Right
R Toe Phalanx, Left
S Coccyx
	Ø Open
	3 Percutaneous
	4 Percutaneous Endoscopic
		Z No Device	**Z No Qualifier**

Ø Medical and Surgical
Q Lower Bones
P Removal   Definition: Taking out or off a device from a body part

Explanation: If a device is taken out and a similar device put in without cutting or puncturing the skin or mucous membrane, the procedure is coded to the root operation CHANGE. Otherwise, the procedure for taking out a device is coded to the root operation REMOVAL.

Body Part Character 4		Approach Character 5	Device Character 6	Qualifier Character 7
Ø Lumbar Vertebra Spinous process Transverse process Vertebral arch Vertebral body Vertebral foramen Vertebral lamina Vertebral pedicle **1 Sacrum** **2 Pelvic Bone, Right** Iliac crest Ilium Ischium Pubis **3 Pelvic Bone, Left** *See 2 Pelvic Bone, Right* **4 Acetabulum, Right** **5 Acetabulum, Left** **6 Upper Femur, Right** Femoral head Greater trochanter Lesser trochanter Neck of femur **7 Upper Femur, Left** *See 6 Upper Femur, Right* **8 Femoral Shaft, Right** Body of femur **9 Femoral Shaft, Left** *See 8 Femoral Shaft, Right* **B Lower Femur, Right** Lateral condyle of femur Lateral epicondyle of femur Medial condyle of femur Medial epicondyle of femur	**C Lower Femur, Left** *See B Lower Femur, Right* **D Patella, Right** **F Patella, Left** **G Tibia, Right** Lateral condyle of tibia Medial condyle of tibia Medial malleolus **H Tibia, Left** *See G Tibia, Right* **J Fibula, Right** Body of fibula Head of fibula Lateral malleolus **K Fibula, Left** *See J Fibula, Right* **L Tarsal, Right** Calcaneus Cuboid bone Intermediate cuneiform bone Lateral cuneiform bone Medial cuneiform bone Navicular bone Talus bone **M Tarsal, Left** *See L Tarsal, Right* **N Metatarsal, Right** Fibular sesamoid Tibial sesamoid **P Metatarsal, Left** *See N Metatarsal, Right* **Q Toe Phalanx, Right** **R Toe Phalanx, Left** **S Coccyx**	**Ø Open** **3 Percutaneous** **4 Percutaneous Endoscopic**	**4 Internal Fixation Device** **5 External Fixation Device** **7 Autologous Tissue Substitute** **J Synthetic Substitute** **K Nonautologous Tissue Substitute**	**Z No Qualifier**
Ø Lumbar Vertebra Spinous process Transverse process Vertebral arch Vertebral body Vertebral foramen Vertebral lamina Vertebral pedicle **1 Sacrum** **2 Pelvic Bone, Right** Iliac crest Ilium Ischium Pubis **3 Pelvic Bone, Left** *See 2 Pelvic Bone, Right* **4 Acetabulum, Right** **5 Acetabulum, Left** **6 Upper Femur, Right** Femoral head Greater trochanter Lesser trochanter Neck of femur **7 Upper Femur, Left** *See 6 Upper Femur, Right* **8 Femoral Shaft, Right** Body of femur **9 Femoral Shaft, Left** *See 8 Femoral Shaft, Right* **B Lower Femur, Right** Lateral condyle of femur Lateral epicondyle of femur Medial condyle of femur Medial epicondyle of femur	**C Lower Femur, Left** *See B Lower Femur, Right* **D Patella, Right** **F Patella, Left** **G Tibia, Right** Lateral condyle of tibia Medial condyle of tibia Medial malleolus **H Tibia, Left** *See G Tibia, Right* **J Fibula, Right** Body of fibula Head of fibula Lateral malleolus **K Fibula, Left** *See J Fibula, Right* **L Tarsal, Right** Calcaneus Cuboid bone Intermediate cuneiform bone Lateral cuneiform bone Medial cuneiform bone Navicular bone Talus bone **M Tarsal, Left** *See L Tarsal, Right* **N Metatarsal, Right** Fibular sesamoid Tibial sesamoid **P Metatarsal, Left** *See N Metatarsal, Right* **Q Toe Phalanx, Right** **R Toe Phalanx, Left** **S Coccyx**	**X External**	**4 Internal Fixation Device** **5 External Fixation Device**	**Z No Qualifier**
Y Lower Bone		**Ø Open** **3 Percutaneous** **4 Percutaneous Endoscopic** **X External**	**Ø Drainage Device** **M Bone Growth Stimulator**	**Z No Qualifier**

Non-OR ØQPYX[Ø,M]Z	**Non-OR** ØQPY3ØZ	**Non-OR** ØQP[Ø,1,2,3,4,5,6,7,8,9,B,C,D,F,G,H,J,K,L,M,N,P,Q,R,S]X[4,5]Z	

NC Noncovered Procedure   **LC** Limited Coverage   **QA** Questionable OB Admit   **NT** New Tech Add-on   ⊞ Combination Member   ♂ Male   ♀ Female

ICD-10-PCS 2024   575

ØQP–ØQP

Ø Medical and Surgical
Q Lower Bones
Q Repair Definition: Restoring, to the extent possible, a body part to its normal anatomic structure and function
Explanation: Used only when the method to accomplish the repair is not one of the other root operations

Body Part Character 4	Approach Character 5	Device Character 6	Qualifier Character 7
Ø Lumbar Vertebra Spinous process Transverse process Vertebral arch Vertebral body Vertebral foramen Vertebral lamina Vertebral pedicle **1 Sacrum** **2 Pelvic Bone, Right** Iliac crest Ilium Ischium Pubis **3 Pelvic Bone, Left** See 2 Pelvic Bone, Right **4 Acetabulum, Right** **5 Acetabulum, Left** **6 Upper Femur, Right** Femoral head Greater trochanter Lesser trochanter Neck of femur **7 Upper Femur, Left** See 6 Upper Femur, Right **8 Femoral Shaft, Right** Body of femur **9 Femoral Shaft, Left** See 8 Femoral Shaft, Right **B Lower Femur, Right** Lateral condyle of femur Lateral epicondyle of femur Medial condyle of femur Medial epicondyle of femur **C Lower Femur, Left** See B Lower Femur, Right **D Patella, Right** **F Patella, Left** **G Tibia, Right** Lateral condyle of tibia Medial condyle of tibia Medial malleolus **H Tibia, Left** See G Tibia, Right **J Fibula, Right** Body of fibula Head of fibula Lateral malleolus **K Fibula, Left** See J Fibula, Right **L Tarsal, Right** Calcaneus Cuboid bone Intermediate cuneiform bone Lateral cuneiform bone Medial cuneiform bone Navicular bone Talus bone **M Tarsal, Left** See L Tarsal, Right **N Metatarsal, Right** Fibular sesamoid Tibial sesamoid **P Metatarsal, Left** See N Metatarsal, Right **Q Toe Phalanx, Right** **R Toe Phalanx, Left** **S Coccyx**	**Ø Open** **3 Percutaneous** **4 Percutaneous Endoscopic** **X External**	**Z No Device**	**Z No Qualifier**

Non-OR ØQQ[Ø,1,2,3,4,5,6,7,8,9,B,C,D,F,G,H,J,K,L,M,N,P,Q,R,S]XZZ

Ø   **Medical and Surgical**
Q   **Lower Bones**
R   **Replacement**   Definition: Putting in or on biological or synthetic material that physically takes the place and/or function of all or a portion of a body part

Explanation: The body part may have been taken out or replaced, or may be taken out, physically eradicated, or rendered nonfunctional during the REPLACEMENT procedure. A REMOVAL procedure is coded for taking out the device used in a previous replacement procedure.

Body Part Character 4	Approach Character 5	Device Character 6	Qualifier Character 7

Ø **Lumbar Vertebra**
   Spinous process
   Transverse process
   Vertebral arch
   Vertebral body
   Vertebral foramen
   Vertebral lamina
   Vertebral pedicle
1 **Sacrum**
2 **Pelvic Bone, Right**
   Iliac crest
   Ilium
   Ischium
   Pubis
3 **Pelvic Bone, Left**
   See 2 Pelvic Bone, Right
4 **Acetabulum, Right**
5 **Acetabulum, Left**
6 **Upper Femur, Right**
   Femoral head
   Greater trochanter
   Lesser trochanter
   Neck of femur
7 **Upper Femur, Left**
   See 6 Upper Femur, Right
8 **Femoral Shaft, Right**
   Body of femur
9 **Femoral Shaft, Left**
   See 8 Femoral Shaft, Right
B **Lower Femur, Right**
   Lateral condyle of femur
   Lateral epicondyle of femur
   Medial condyle of femur
   Medial epicondyle of femur
C **Lower Femur, Left**
   See B Lower Femur, Right
D **Patella, Right**
F **Patella, Left**
G **Tibia, Right**
   Lateral condyle of tibia
   Medial condyle of tibia
   Medial malleolus
H **Tibia, Left**
   See G Tibia, Right
J **Fibula, Right**
   Body of fibula
   Head of fibula
   Lateral malleolus
K **Fibula, Left**
   See J Fibula, Right
L **Tarsal, Right**
   Calcaneus
   Cuboid bone
   Intermediate cuneiform bone
   Lateral cuneiform bone
   Medial cuneiform bone
   Navicular bone
   Talus bone
M **Tarsal, Left**
   See L Tarsal, Right
N **Metatarsal, Right**
   Fibular sesamoid
   Tibial sesamoid
P **Metatarsal, Left**
   See N Metatarsal, Right
Q **Toe Phalanx, Right**
R **Toe Phalanx, Left**
S **Coccyx**
	Ø Open
	3 Percutaneous
	4 Percutaneous Endoscopic
		7 Autologous Tissue Substitute
		J Synthetic Substitute
		K Nonautologous Tissue Substitute
			Z No Qualifier

NC Noncovered Procedure   LC Limited Coverage   QA Questionable OB Admit   NT New Tech Add-on   ⊞ Combination Member   ♂ Male   ♀ Female

ICD-10-PCS 2024   **577**

ØQR–ØQR

Lower Bones

Ø   **Medical and Surgical**
Q   **Lower Bones**
S   **Reposition**   Definition: Moving to its normal location, or other suitable location, all or a portion of a body part

Explanation: The body part is moved to a new location from an abnormal location, or from a normal location where it is not functioning correctly. The body part may or may not be cut out or off to be moved to the new location.

Body Part Character 4		Approach Character 5	Device Character 6	Qualifier Character 7

Ø   **Lumbar Vertebra**
    Spinous process
    Transverse process
    Vertebral arch
    Vertebral body
    Vertebral foramen
    Vertebral lamina
    Vertebral pedicle
		Ø Open
		4 Percutaneous Endoscopic
			3 Spinal Stabilization Device,
			    Vertebral Body Tether
			4 Internal Fixation Device
			Z No Device
				Z No Qualifier

Ø   **Lumbar Vertebra**   ⊞
    Spinous process
    Transverse process
    Vertebral arch
    Vertebral body
    Vertebral foramen
    Vertebral lamina
    Vertebral pedicle
		3 Percutaneous	4 Internal Fixation Device
			Z No Device
				Z No Qualifier

Ø   **Lumbar Vertebra**
    Spinous process
    Transverse process
    Vertebral arch
    Vertebral body
    Vertebral foramen
    Vertebral lamina
    Vertebral pedicle
		X External	Z No Device	Z No Qualifier

1 **Sacrum** ⊞ 4 **Acetabulum, Right** 5 **Acetabulum, Left** S **Coccyx** ⊞		Ø Open 3 Percutaneous 4 Percutaneous Endoscopic	4 Internal Fixation Device Z No Device	Z No Qualifier
1 **Sacrum** 4 **Acetabulum, Right** 5 **Acetabulum, Left** S **Coccyx**		X External	Z No Device	Z No Qualifier

2   **Pelvic Bone, Right**
    Iliac crest
    Ilium
    Ischium
    Pubis
3   **Pelvic Bone, Left**
    See 2 Pelvic Bone, Right
D   **Patella, Right**
F   **Patella, Left**
L   **Tarsal, Right**
    Calcaneus
    Cuboid bone
    Intermediate cuneiform
       bone
    Lateral cuneiform bone
    Medial cuneiform bone
    Navicular bone
    Talus bone
	M **Tarsal, Left**
	    See L Tarsal, Right
	Q **Toe Phalanx, Right**
	R **Toe Phalanx, Left**
		Ø Open
		3 Percutaneous
		4 Percutaneous Endoscopic
			4 Internal Fixation Device
			5 External Fixation Device
			Z No Device
				Z No Qualifier

2   **Pelvic Bone, Right**
    Iliac crest
    Ilium
    Ischium
    Pubis
3   **Pelvic Bone, Left**
    See 2 Pelvic Bone, Right
D   **Patella, Right**
F   **Patella, Left**
L   **Tarsal, Right**
    Calcaneus
    Cuboid bone
    Intermediate cuneiform
       bone
    Lateral cuneiform bone
    Medial cuneiform bone
    Navicular bone
    Talus bone
	M **Tarsal, Left**
	    See L Tarsal, Right
	Q **Toe Phalanx, Right**
	R **Toe Phalanx, Left**
		X External	Z No Device	Z No Qualifier

Non-OR	ØQSØXZZ	See Appendix L for Procedure Combinations
Non-OR	ØQS[4,5][3,4]ZZ	⊞ ØQSØ3ZZ
Non-OR	ØQS[1,4,5,S]XZZ	⊞ ØQS[1,S]3ZZ
Non-OR	ØQS[2,3,D,F,L,M,Q,R][3,4]ZZ	
Non-OR	ØQS[2,3,D,F,L,M,Q,R]XZZ	

ØQS Continued on next page

Non-OR Procedure   DRG Non-OR Procedure   Valid OR Procedure   HAC Associated Procedure   Combination Only   New/Revised April   New/Revised October

578   ICD-10-PCS 2024

Ø Medical and Surgical
Q Lower Bones
S Reposition

ØQS Continued

Definition: Moving to its normal location, or other suitable location, all or a portion of a body part

Explanation: The body part is moved to a new location from an abnormal location, or from a normal location where it is not functioning correctly. The body part may or may not be cut out or off to be moved to the new location.

Body Part Character 4	Approach Character 5	Device Character 6	Qualifier Character 7

6 Upper Femur, Right
 Femoral head
 Greater trochanter
 Lesser trochanter
 Neck of femur
7 Upper Femur, Left
 See 6 Upper Femur, Right
8 Femoral Shaft, Right
 Body of femur
9 Femoral Shaft, Left
 See 8 Femoral Shaft, Right
B Lower Femur, Right
 Lateral condyle of femur
 Lateral epicondyle of femur
 Medial condyle of femur
 Medial epicondyle of femur
C Lower Femur, Left
 See B Lower Femur, Right
G Tibia, Right
 Lateral condyle of tibia
 Medial condyle of tibia
 Medial malleolus
H Tibia, Left
 See G Tibia, Right
J Fibula, Right
 Body of fibula
 Head of fibula
 Lateral malleolus
K Fibula, Left
 See J Fibula, Right
	Ø Open
	3 Percutaneous
	4 Percutaneous Endoscopic
		4 Internal Fixation Device
		5 External Fixation Device
		6 Internal Fixation Device,
		  Intramedullary
		B External Fixation Device,
		  Monoplanar
		C External Fixation Device, Ring
		D External Fixation Device, Hybrid
		Z No Device
			Z No Qualifier

6 Upper Femur, Right Femoral head Greater trochanter Lesser trochanter Neck of femur **7 Upper Femur, Left** *See 6 Upper Femur, Right* **8 Femoral Shaft, Right** Body of femur **9 Femoral Shaft, Left** *See 8 Femoral Shaft, Right* **B Lower Femur, Right** Lateral condyle of femur Lateral epicondyle of femur Medial condyle of femur Medial epicondyle of femur **C Lower Femur, Left** *See B Lower Femur, Right* **G Tibia, Right** Lateral condyle of tibia Medial condyle of tibia Medial malleolus **H Tibia, Left** *See G Tibia, Right* **J Fibula, Right** Body of fibula Head of fibula Lateral malleolus **K Fibula, Left** *See J Fibula, Right*	**X** External	**Z** No Device	**Z** No Qualifier
N Metatarsal, Right Fibular sesamoid Tibial sesamoid **P Metatarsal, Left** *See N Metatarsal, Right*	**Ø** Open **3** Percutaneous **4** Percutaneous Endoscopic	**4** Internal Fixation Device **5** External Fixation Device **Z** No Device	**2** Sesamoid Bone(s) 1st Toe **Z** No Qualifier
N Metatarsal, Right Fibular sesamoid Tibial sesamoid **P Metatarsal, Left** *See N Metatarsal, Right*	**X** External	**Z** No Device	**2** Sesamoid Bone(s) 1st Toe **Z** No Qualifier

Non-OR ØQS[6,7,8,9,B,C,G,H,J,K][3,4]ZZ
Non-OR ØQS[6,7,8,9,B,C,G,H,J,K]XZZ
Non-OR ØQS[N,P][3,4]Z[2,Z]
Non-OR ØQS[N,P]XZ[2,Z]

NC Noncovered Procedure **LC** Limited Coverage **QA** Questionable OB Admit **NT** New Tech Add-on ⊞ Combination Member ♂ Male ♀ Female

ICD-10-PCS 2024   579

Ø Medical and Surgical
Q Lower Bones
T Resection

Definition: Cutting out or off, without replacement, all of a body part
Explanation: None

Body Part Character 4		Approach Character 5	Device Character 6	Qualifier Character 7
2 Pelvic Bone, Right Iliac crest Ilium Ischium Pubis	**F Patella, Left** **G Tibia, Right** Lateral condyle of tibia Medial condyle of tibia Medial malleolus	**Ø Open**	**Z No Device**	**Z No Qualifier**
3 Pelvic Bone, Left *See 2 Pelvic Bone, Right*	**H Tibia, Left** *See G Tibia, Right*			
4 Acetabulum, Right	**J Fibula, Right** Body of fibula			
5 Acetabulum, Left	Head of fibula Lateral malleolus			
6 Upper Femur, Right Femoral head Greater trochanter Lesser trochanter Neck of femur	**K Fibula, Left** *See J Fibula, Right* **L Tarsal, Right** Calcaneus Cuboid bone			
7 Upper Femur, Left *See 6 Upper Femur, Right*	Intermediate cuneiform bone Lateral cuneiform bone Medial cuneiform bone			
8 Femoral Shaft, Right Body of femur	Navicular bone Talus bone			
9 Femoral Shaft, Left *See 8 Femoral Shaft, Right*	**M Tarsal, Left** *See L Tarsal, Right*			

B Lower Femur, Right
Lateral condyle of femur
Lateral epicondyle of
  femur
Medial condyle of femur
Medial epicondyle of
  femur
	N Metatarsal, Right
	Fibular sesamoid
	Tibial sesamoid
	P Metatarsal, Left
	See N Metatarsal, Right			

C Lower Femur, Left *See B Lower Femur, Right*	**Q Toe Phalanx, Right** **R Toe Phalanx, Left**			
D Patella, Right	**S Coccyx**			

Ø Medical and Surgical
Q Lower Bones
U Supplement

Definition: Putting in or on biological or synthetic material that physically reinforces and/or augments the function of a portion of a body part
Explanation: The biological material is non-living, or is living and from the same individual. The body part may have been previously replaced, and the SUPPLEMENT procedure is performed to physically reinforce and/or augment the function of the replaced body part.

Body Part Character 4		Approach Character 5	Device Character 6	Qualifier Character 7
Ø Lumbar Vertebra ⊞ Spinous process Transverse process Vertebral arch Vertebral body Vertebral foramen Vertebral lamina Vertebral pedicle	**C Lower Femur, Left** *See B Lower Femur, Right* **D Patella, Right** **F Patella, Left** **G Tibia, Right** Lateral condyle of tibia Medial condyle of tibia Medial malleolus	**Ø Open** **3 Percutaneous** **4 Percutaneous Endoscopic**	**7 Autologous Tissue Substitute** **J Synthetic Substitute** **K Nonautologous Tissue Substitute**	**Z No Qualifier**
1 Sacrum ⊞	**H Tibia, Left** *See G Tibia, Right*			
2 Pelvic Bone, Right Iliac crest Ilium Ischium Pubis	**J Fibula, Right** Body of fibula Head of fibula Lateral malleolus			
3 Pelvic Bone, Left *See 2 Pelvic Bone, Right*	**K Fibula, Left** *See J Fibula, Right*			
4 Acetabulum, Right	**L Tarsal, Right** Calcaneus Cuboid bone			
5 Acetabulum, Left	Intermediate cuneiform bone			
6 Upper Femur, Right Femoral head Greater trochanter Lesser trochanter Neck of femur	Lateral cuneiform bone Medial cuneiform bone Navicular bone Talus bone			
7 Upper Femur, Left *See 6 Upper Femur, Right*	**M Tarsal, Left** *See L Tarsal, Right*			
8 Femoral Shaft, Right Body of femur	**N Metatarsal, Right** Fibular sesamoid Tibial sesamoid			
9 Femoral Shaft, Left *See 8 Femoral Shaft, Right*	**P Metatarsal, Left** *See N Metatarsal, Right*			
B Lower Femur, Right Lateral condyle of femur Lateral epicondyle of femur Medial condyle of femur Medial epicondyle of femur	**Q Toe Phalanx, Right** **R Toe Phalanx, Left** **S Coccyx** ⊞			

See Appendix L for Procedure Combinations
⊞   ØQU[Ø,1,S]3JZ

Non-OR Procedure   DRG Non-OR Procedure   Valid OR Procedure   HAC Associated Procedure   Combination Only   New/Revised April   New/Revised October

580   ICD-10-PCS 2024

0   Medical and Surgical
Q   Lower Bones
W   Revision   Definition: Correcting, to the extent possible, a portion of a malfunctioning device or the position of a displaced device

Explanation: Revision can include correcting a malfunctioning or displaced device by taking out or putting in components of the device such as a screw or pin

Body Part Character 4	Approach Character 5	Device Character 6	Qualifier Character 7
0 Lumbar Vertebra Spinous process Transverse process Vertebral arch Vertebral body Vertebral foramen Vertebral lamina Vertebral pedicle **1** Sacrum **4** Acetabulum, Right **5** Acetabulum, Left **S** Coccyx	**0** Open **3** Percutaneous **4** Percutaneous Endoscopic **X** External	**4** Internal Fixation Device **7** Autologous Tissue Substitute **J** Synthetic Substitute **K** Nonautologous Tissue Substitute	**Z** No Qualifier
2 Pelvic Bone, Right Iliac crest Ilium Ischium Pubis **3** Pelvic Bone, Left *See 2 Pelvic Bone, Right* **6** Upper Femur, Right Femoral head Greater trochanter Lesser trochanter Neck of femur **7** Upper Femur, Left *See 6 Upper Femur, Right* **8** Femoral Shaft, Right Body of femur **9** Femoral Shaft, Left *See 8 Femoral Shaft, Right* **B** Lower Femur, Right Lateral condyle of femur Lateral epicondyle of femur Medial condyle of femur Medial epicondyle of femur **C** Lower Femur, Left *See B Lower Femur, Right* **D** Patella, Right **F** Patella, Left **G** Tibia, Right Lateral condyle of tibia Medial condyle of tibia Medial malleolus **H** Tibia, Left *See G Tibia, Right* **J** Fibula, Right Body of fibula Head of fibula Lateral malleolus **K** Fibula, Left *See J Fibula, Right* **L** Tarsal, Right Calcaneus Cuboid bone Intermediate cuneiform bone Lateral cuneiform bone Medial cuneiform bone Navicular bone Talus bone **M** Tarsal, Left *See L Tarsal, Right* **N** Metatarsal, Right Fibular sesamoid Tibial sesamoid **P** Metatarsal, Left *See N Metatarsal, Right* **Q** Toe Phalanx, Right **R** Toe Phalanx, Left	**0** Open **3** Percutaneous **4** Percutaneous Endoscopic **X** External	**4** Internal Fixation Device **5** External Fixation Device **7** Autologous Tissue Substitute **J** Synthetic Substitute **K** Nonautologous Tissue Substitute	**Z** No Qualifier
Y Lower Bone	**0** Open **3** Percutaneous **4** Percutaneous Endoscopic **X** External	**0** Drainage Device **M** Bone Growth Stimulator	**Z** No Qualifier

Non-OR   0QW[0,1,4,5,S]X[4,7,J,K]Z
Non-OR   0QW[2,3,6,7,8,9,B,C,D,F,G,H,J,K,L,M,N,P,Q,R]X[4,5,7,J,K]Z
Non-OR   0QWYX[0,M]Z

🆖 Noncovered Procedure   🆑 Limited Coverage   🆀 Questionable OB Admit   🆕 New Tech Add-on   ⊞ Combination Member   ♂ Male   ♀ Female

ICD-10-PCS 2024   581

0QW–0QW

Upper Joints ØR2–ØRW

Character Meanings*

This Character Meaning table is provided as a guide to assist the user in the identification of character members that may be found in this section of code tables. It **SHOULD NOT** be used to build a PCS code.

Operation–Character 3	Body Part–Character 4	Approach–Character 5	Device–Character 6	Qualifier–Character 7
2 Change	Ø Occipital-cervical Joint	Ø Open	Ø Drainage Device OR Synthetic Substitute, Reverse Ball and Socket	Ø Anterior Approach, Anterior Column
5 Destruction	1 Cervical Vertebral Joint	3 Percutaneous	3 Infusion Device OR Internal Fixation Device, Sustained Compression	1 Posterior Approach, Posterior Column
9 Drainage	2 Cervical Vertebral Joint, 2 or more	4 Percutaneous Endoscopic	4 Internal Fixation Device	6 Humeral Surface
B Excision	3 Cervical Vertebral Disc	X External	5 External Fixation Device	7 Glenoid Surface
C Extirpation	4 Cervicothoracic Vertebral Joint		7 Autologous Tissue Substitute	J Posterior Approach, Anterior Column
G Fusion	5 Cervicothoracic Vertebral Disc		8 Spacer	X Diagnostic
H Insertion	6 Thoracic Vertebral Joint		A Interbody Fusion Device	Z No Qualifier
J Inspection	7 Thoracic Vertebral Joint, 2 to 7		B Spinal Stabilization Device, Interspinous Process	
N Release	8 Thoracic Vertebral Joint, 8 or more		C Spinal Stabilization Device, Pedicle-Based	
P Removal	9 Thoracic Vertebral Disc		D Spinal Stabilization Device, Facet Replacement	
Q Repair	A Thoracolumbar Vertebral Joint		J Synthetic Substitute	
R Replacement	B Thoracolumbar Vertebral Disc		K Nonautologous Tissue Substitute	
S Reposition	C Temporomandibular Joint, Right		Y Other Device	
T Resection	D Temporomandibular Joint, Left		Z No Device	
U Supplement	E Sternoclavicular Joint, Right			
W Revision	F Sternoclavicular Joint, Left			
	G Acromioclavicular Joint, Right			
	H Acromioclavicular Joint, Left			
	J Shoulder Joint, Right			
	K Shoulder Joint, Left			
	L Elbow Joint, Right			
	M Elbow Joint, Left			
	N Wrist Joint, Right			
	P Wrist Joint, Left			
	Q Carpal Joint, Right			
	R Carpal Joint, Left			
	S Carpometacarpal Joint, Right			
	T Carpometacarpal Joint, Left			
	U Metacarpophalangeal Joint, Right			
	V Metacarpophalangeal Joint, Left			
	W Finger Phalangeal Joint, Right			
	X Finger Phalangeal Joint, Left			
	Y Upper Joint			

* Includes synovial membrane.

AHA Coding Clinic for table ØRB

2019, 3Q, 26	Acromioclavicular joint reconstruction using allograft

AHA Coding Clinic for table ØRG

2023, 2Q, 25	Spinal fusion using allograft bone graft and bone marrow aspirate
2022, 3Q, 21	Breakage of intervertebral cage during surgery
2021, 4Q, 67	Posterior dynamic distraction
2021, 1Q, 18	Placement of interspinous distraction device (spacer) for decompression
2021, 1Q, 53	Official guidelines for coding and reporting for interbody fusion device B3.10c
2020, 4Q, 56-58	Intramedullary sustained compression joint fusion
2020, 2Q, 27	Spinal fusion with NuVasive® VersaTie®
2020, 1Q, 33	Spinal fusion without use of bone graft
2019, 3Q, 28	Use of VERTE-STACK™ implant with fusion
2019, 3Q, 35	Fusion procedures of the spine (guideline B3.10c)
2019, 2Q, 19	Cervical spinal fusion, decompression and placement of interfacet stabilization device
2019, 1Q, 30	Spinal fusion performed at same level as decompressive laminectomy
2018, 4Q, 43	Joint fusion device value
2018, 1Q, 22	Spinal fusion procedures without bone graft
2017, 4Q, 62	Added and revised device values - Nerve substitutes
2017, 4Q, 76	Radiolucent porous interbody fusion device
2017, 2Q, 23	Decompression of spinal cord and placement of instrumentation
2014, 3Q, 30	Spinal fusion and fixation instrumentation
2014, 2Q, 7	Anterior cervical thoracic fusion with total discectomy
2013, 1Q, 21-23	Spinal fusion of thoracic and lumbar vertebrae
2013, 1Q, 29	Cervical and thoracic spinal fusion

AHA Coding Clinic for table ØRH

2021, 1Q, 18	Placement of interspinous distraction device (spacer) for decompression
2019, 2Q, 40	Decompression of spinal cord and placement of instrumentation
2018, 3Q, 26	Anterior vertebral tethering using Dynesys Tethering System
2017, 2Q, 23	Decompression of spinal cord and placement of instrumentation
2016, 3Q, 32	Rotator cuff repair, tenodesis, decompression, acromioplasty and coracoplasty

AHA Coding Clinic for table ØRN

2019, 1Q, 30	Spinal fusion performed at same level as decompressive laminectomy
2016, 3Q, 32	Rotator cuff repair, tenodesis, decompression, acromioplasty and coracoplasty
2015, 2Q, 22	Arthroscopic subacromial decompression
2015, 2Q, 23	Arthroscopic release of shoulder joint

AHA Coding Clinic for table ØRP

2022, 3Q, 21	Breakage of intervertebral cage during surgery
2021, 4Q, 53	Shoulder hemiarthroplasty
2017, 4Q, 107	Total ankle replacement versus revision

AHA Coding Clinic for table ØRQ

2016, 1Q, 30	Thermal capsulorrhaphy of shoulder

AHA Coding Clinic for table ØRR

2018, 4Q, 92	Radial head arthroplasty
2017, 4Q, 107	Total ankle replacement versus revision
2015, 3Q, 14	Endoprosthetic replacement of humerus and tendon reattachment
2015, 1Q, 27	Reverse total shoulder arthroplasty

AHA Coding Clinic for table ØRS

2019, 3Q, 26	Acromioclavicular joint reconstruction using allograft
2018, 3Q, 26	Anterior vertebral tethering using Dynesys Tethering System
2015, 2Q, 35	Application of tongs to reduce and stabilize cervical fracture
2014, 4Q, 32	Open reduction internal fixation of fracture with debridement
2014, 3Q, 33	Radial fracture treatment with open reduction internal fixation, and release of carpal ligament
2013, 2Q, 39	Application of cervical tongs for reduction of cervical fracture

AHA Coding Clinic for table ØRT

2019, 3Q, 26	Acromioclavicular joint reconstruction using allograft
2014, 2Q, 7	Anterior cervical thoracic fusion with total discectomy

AHA Coding Clinic for table ØRU

2019, 3Q, 26	Acromioclavicular joint reconstruction using allograft
2015, 3Q, 26	Thumb arthroplasty with resection of trapezium

AHA Coding Clinic for table ØRW

2021, 4Q, 53	Shoulder hemiarthroplasty
2017, 4Q, 107	Total ankle replacement versus revision

Upper Joints

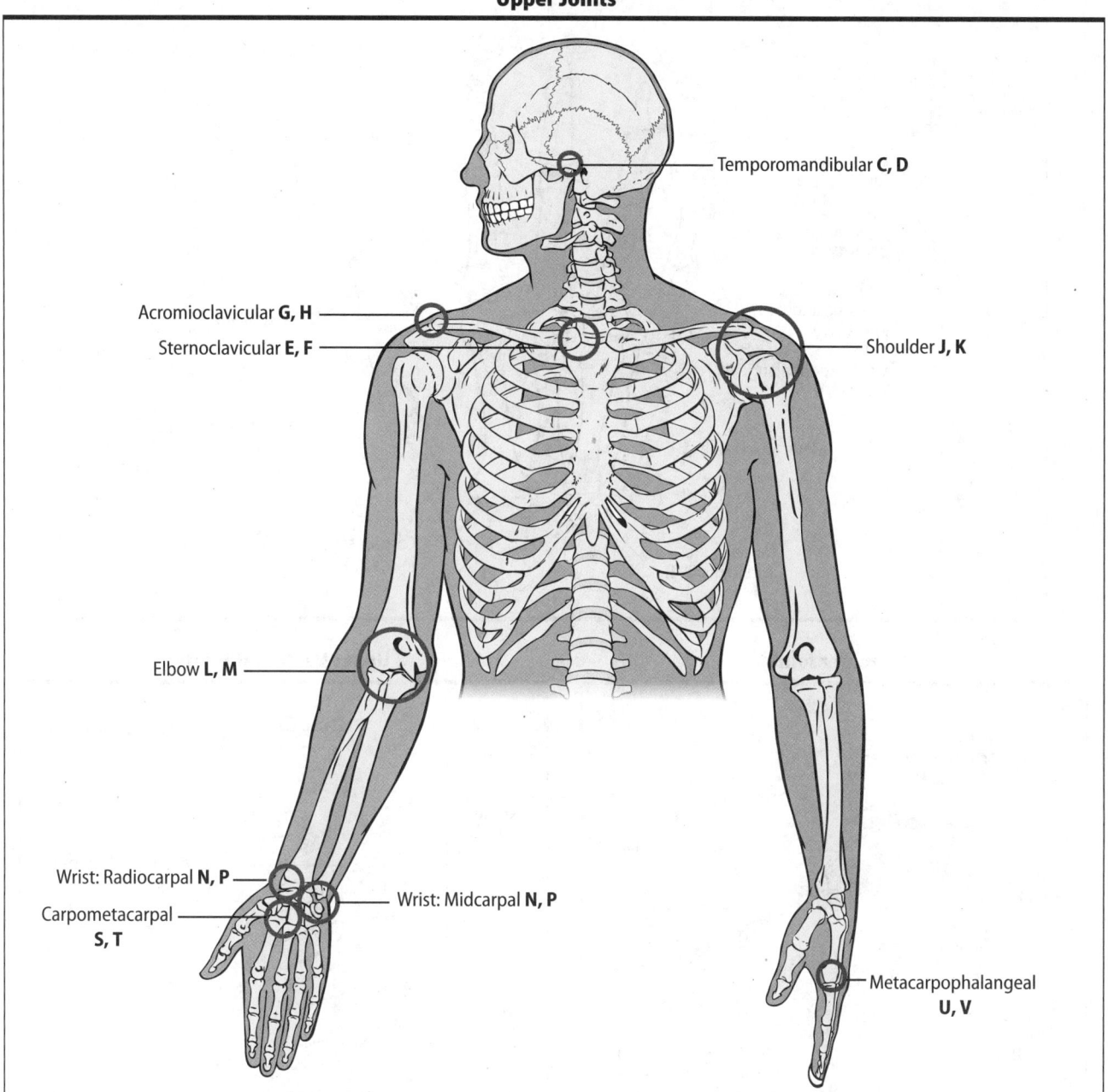

Temporomandibular **C, D**

Acromioclavicular **G, H**

Sternoclavicular **E, F**

Shoulder **J, K**

Elbow **L, M**

Wrist: Radiocarpal **N, P**

Wrist: Midcarpal **N, P**

Carpometacarpal
S, T

Metacarpophalangeal
U, V

Hand Joints

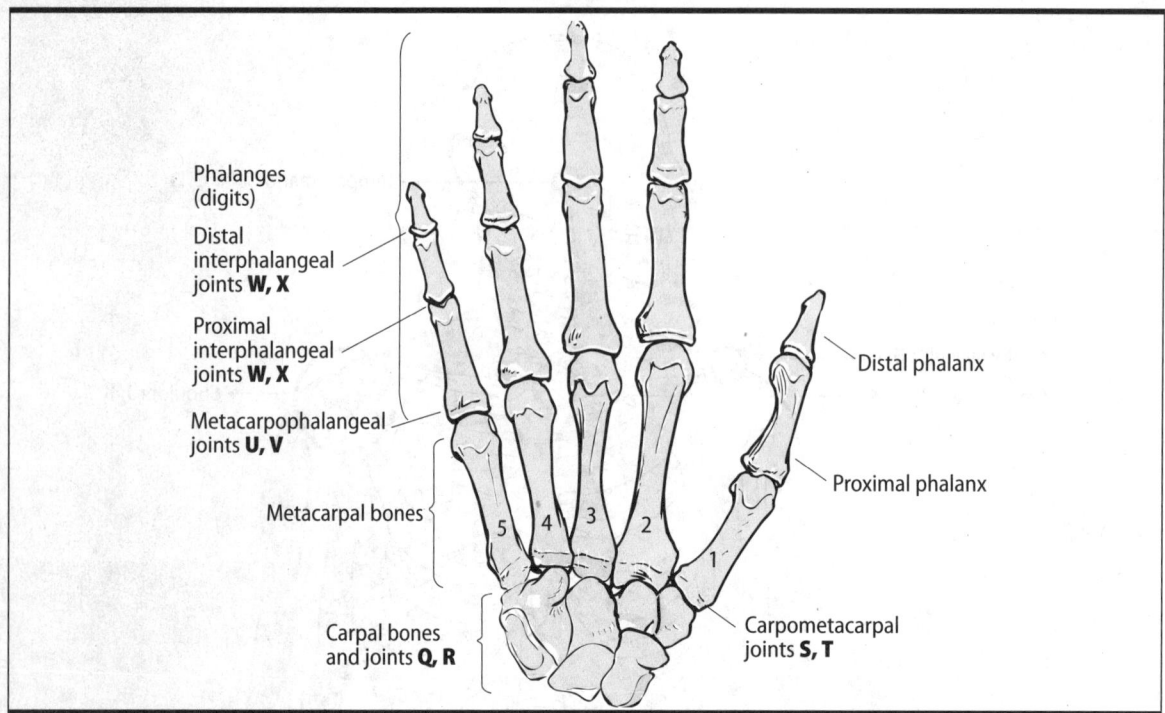

Phalanges (digits)

Distal interphalangeal joints **W, X**

Proximal interphalangeal joints **W, X**

Metacarpophalangeal joints **U, V**

Metacarpal bones

Carpal bones and joints **Q, R**

Distal phalanx

Proximal phalanx

Carpometacarpal joints **S, T**

Shoulder Joints

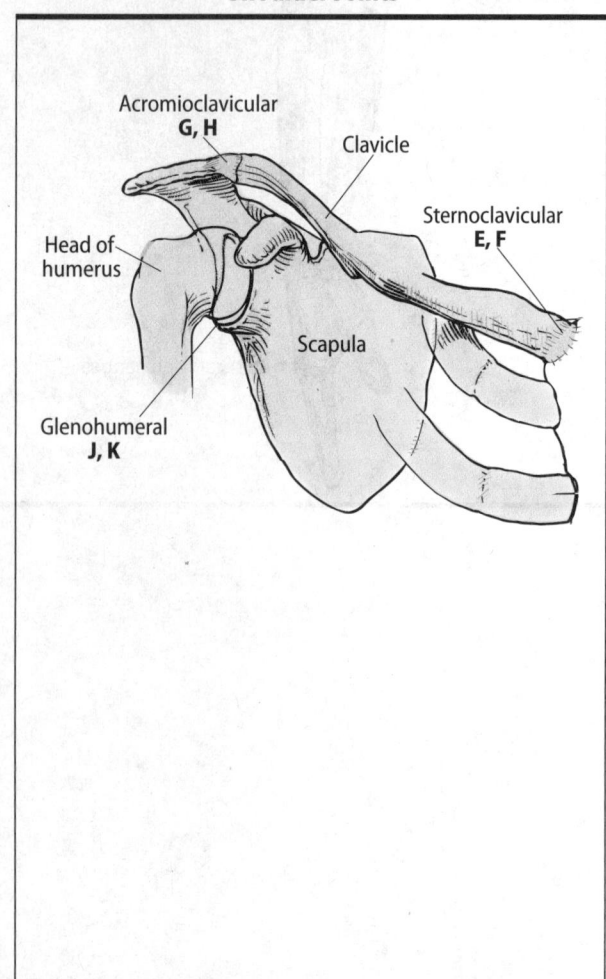

Acromioclavicular **G, H**

Clavicle

Head of humerus

Sternoclavicular **E, F**

Scapula

Glenohumeral **J, K**

Upper Vertebral Joints

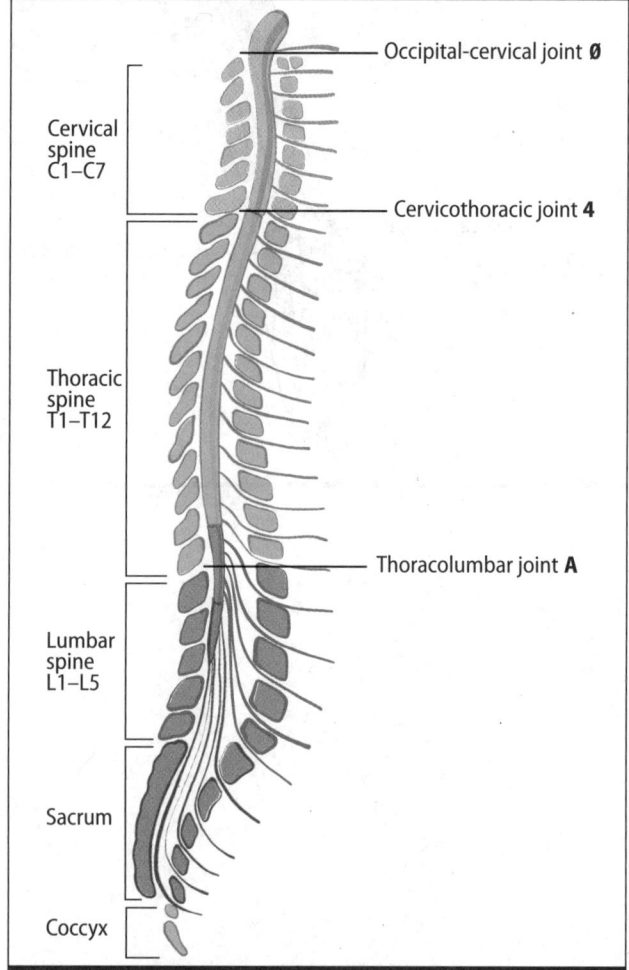

Occipital-cervical joint **Ø**

Cervical spine C1–C7

Cervicothoracic joint **4**

Thoracic spine T1–T12

Thoracolumbar joint **A**

Lumbar spine L1–L5

Sacrum

Coccyx

0   **Medical and Surgical**
R   **Upper Joints**
2   **Change**   Definition: Taking out or off a device from a body part and putting back an identical or similar device in or on the same body part without cutting or puncturing the skin or a mucous membrane
                       Explanation: All CHANGE procedures are coded using the approach EXTERNAL

Body Part Character 4	Approach Character 5	Device Character 6	Qualifier Character 7
Y Upper Joint	**X** External	**0** Drainage Device **Y** Other Device	**Z** No Qualifier

> **Non-OR**   All body part, approach, device, and qualifier values

0   **Medical and Surgical**
R   **Upper Joints**
5   **Destruction**   Definition: Physical eradication of all or a portion of a body part by the direct use of energy, force, or a destructive agent
                       Explanation: None of the body part is physically taken out

Body Part Character 4	Approach Character 5	Device Character 6	Qualifier Character 7

0   Occipital-cervical Joint
1   Cervical Vertebral Joint
     Atlantoaxial joint
     Cervical facet joint
3   Cervical Vertebral Disc
4   Cervicothoracic Vertebral Joint
     Cervicothoracic facet joint
5   Cervicothoracic Vertebral Disc
6   Thoracic Vertebral Joint
     Costotransverse joint
     Costovertebral joint
     Thoracic facet joint
9   Thoracic Vertebral Disc
A   Thoracolumbar Vertebral Joint
     Thoracolumbar facet joint
B   Thoracolumbar Vertebral Disc
C   Temporomandibular Joint, Right
D   Temporomandibular Joint, Left
E   Sternoclavicular Joint, Right
F   Sternoclavicular Joint, Left
G   Acromioclavicular Joint, Right
H   Acromioclavicular Joint, Left
J   Shoulder Joint, Right
     Glenohumeral joint
     Glenoid ligament (labrum)
K   Shoulder Joint, Left
     See J Shoulder Joint, Right
L   Elbow Joint, Right
     Distal humerus, involving joint
     Humeroradial joint
     Humeroulnar joint
     Proximal radioulnar joint
M   Elbow Joint, Left
     See L Elbow Joint, Right
N   Wrist Joint, Right
     Distal radioulnar joint
     Radiocarpal joint
P   Wrist Joint, Left
     See N Wrist Joint, Right
Q   Carpal Joint, Right
     Intercarpal joint
     Midcarpal joint
R   Carpal Joint, Left
     See Q Carpal Joint, Right
S   Carpometacarpal Joint, Right
T   Carpometacarpal Joint, Left
U   Metacarpophalangeal Joint, Right
V   Metacarpophalangeal Joint, Left
W   Finger Phalangeal Joint, Right
     Interphalangeal (IP) joint
X   Finger Phalangeal Joint, Left
     See W Finger Phalangeal Joint, Right
	0 Open
	3 Percutaneous
	4 Percutaneous Endoscopic
		Z No Device	**Z** No Qualifier

> **Non-OR**   0R5[3,5,9,B][3,4]ZZ

Upper Joints

0   **Medical and Surgical**
R   **Upper Joints**
9   **Drainage**   Definition: Taking or letting out fluids and/or gases from a body part

Explanation: The qualifier DIAGNOSTIC is used to identify drainage procedures that are biopsies

Body Part Character 4		Approach Character 5	Device Character 6	Qualifier Character 7

0 Occipital-cervical Joint
1 Cervical Vertebral Joint
  Atlantoaxial joint
  Cervical facet joint
3 Cervical Vertebral Disc
4 Cervicothoracic Vertebral Joint
  Cervicothoracic facet joint
5 Cervicothoracic Vertebral Disc
6 Thoracic Vertebral Joint
  Costotransverse joint
  Costovertebral joint
  Thoracic facet joint
9 Thoracic Vertebral Disc
A Thoracolumbar Vertebral Joint
  Thoracolumbar facet joint
B Thoracolumbar Vertebral Disc
C Temporomandibular Joint, Right
D Temporomandibular Joint, Left
E Sternoclavicular Joint, Right
F Sternoclavicular Joint, Left
G Acromioclavicular Joint, Right
H Acromioclavicular Joint, Left
J Shoulder Joint, Right
  Glenohumeral joint
  Glenoid ligament (labrum)
K Shoulder Joint, Left
  See J Shoulder Joint, Right
	L Elbow Joint, Right
	  Distal humerus, involving joint
	  Humeroradial joint
	  Humeroulnar joint
	  Proximal radioulnar joint
	M Elbow Joint, Left
	  See L Elbow Joint, Right
	N Wrist Joint, Right
	  Distal radioulnar joint
	  Radiocarpal joint
	P Wrist Joint, Left
	  See N Wrist Joint, Right
	Q Carpal Joint, Right
	  Intercarpal joint
	  Midcarpal joint
	R Carpal Joint, Left
	  See Q Carpal Joint, Right
	S Carpometacarpal Joint, Right
	T Carpometacarpal Joint, Left
	U Metacarpophalangeal Joint, Right
	V Metacarpophalangeal Joint, Left
	W Finger Phalangeal Joint, Right
	  Interphalangeal (IP) joint
	X Finger Phalangeal Joint, Left
	  See W Finger Phalangeal Joint, Right
		0 Open
		3 Percutaneous
		4 Percutaneous Endoscopic
			0 Drainage Device	**Z** No Qualifier

0 Occipital-cervical Joint
1 Cervical Vertebral Joint
  Atlantoaxial joint
  Cervical facet joint
3 Cervical Vertebral Disc
4 Cervicothoracic Vertebral Joint
  Cervicothoracic facet joint
5 Cervicothoracic Vertebral Disc
6 Thoracic Vertebral Joint
  Costotransverse joint
  Costovertebral joint
  Thoracic facet joint
9 Thoracic Vertebral Disc
A Thoracolumbar Vertebral Joint
  Thoracolumbar facet joint
B Thoracolumbar Vertebral Disc
C Temporomandibular Joint, Right
D Temporomandibular Joint, Left
E Sternoclavicular Joint, Right
F Sternoclavicular Joint, Left
G Acromioclavicular Joint, Right
H Acromioclavicular Joint, Left
J Shoulder Joint, Right
  Glenohumeral joint
  Glenoid ligament (labrum)
K Shoulder Joint, Left
  See J Shoulder Joint, Right
	L Elbow Joint, Right
	  Distal humerus, involving joint
	  Humeroradial joint
	  Humeroulnar joint
	  Proximal radioulnar joint
	M Elbow Joint, Left
	  See L Elbow Joint, Right
	N Wrist Joint, Right
	  Distal radioulnar joint
	  Radiocarpal joint
	P Wrist Joint, Left
	  See N Wrist Joint, Right
	Q Carpal Joint, Right
	  Intercarpal joint
	  Midcarpal joint
	R Carpal Joint, Left
	  See Q Carpal Joint, Right
	S Carpometacarpal Joint, Right
	T Carpometacarpal Joint, Left
	U Metacarpophalangeal Joint, Right
	V Metacarpophalangeal Joint, Left
	W Finger Phalangeal Joint, Right
	  Interphalangeal (IP) joint
	X Finger Phalangeal Joint, Left
	  See W Finger Phalangeal Joint, Right
		0 Open
		3 Percutaneous
		4 Percutaneous Endoscopic
			Z No Device	**X** Diagnostic
				Z No Qualifier

Non-OR	0R9[0,1,3,4,5,6,9,A,B,E,F,G,H,J,K,L,M,N,P,Q,R,S,T,U,V,W,X][3,4]0Z
Non-OR	0R9[C,D]30Z
Non-OR	0R9[0,1,3,4,5,6,9,A,B,E,F,G,H,J,K,L,M,N,P,Q,R,S,T,U,V,W,X][0,3,4]ZX
Non-OR	0R9[0,1,3,4,5,6,9,A,B,E,F,G,H,J,K,L,M,N,P,Q,R,S,T,U,V,W,X][3,4]ZZ
Non-OR	0R9[C,D]3ZZ

Non-OR Procedure   DRG Non-OR Procedure   Valid OR Procedure   HAC Associated Procedure   Combination Only   New/Revised April   New/Revised October

Ø **Medical and Surgical**
R **Upper Joints**
B **Excision**　　　　Definition: Cutting out or off, without replacement, a portion of a body part
　　　　　　　　　　Explanation: The qualifier DIAGNOSTIC is used to identify excision procedures that are biopsies

Body Part Character 4	Approach Character 5	Device Character 6	Qualifier Character 7
Ø Occipital-cervical Joint **1** Cervical Vertebral Joint 　　Atlantoaxial joint 　　Cervical facet joint **3** Cervical Vertebral Disc **4** Cervicothoracic Vertebral Joint 　　Cervicothoracic facet joint **5** Cervicothoracic Vertebral Disc **6** Thoracic Vertebral Joint 　　Costotransverse joint 　　Costovertebral joint 　　Thoracic facet joint **9** Thoracic Vertebral Disc **A** Thoracolumbar Vertebral Joint 　　Thoracolumbar facet joint **B** Thoracolumbar Vertebral Disc **C** Temporomandibular Joint, Right **D** Temporomandibular Joint, Left **E** Sternoclavicular Joint, Right **F** Sternoclavicular Joint, Left **G** Acromioclavicular Joint, Right **H** Acromioclavicular Joint, Left **J** Shoulder Joint, Right 　　Glenohumeral joint 　　Glenoid ligament (labrum) **K** Shoulder Joint, Left 　　*See J Shoulder Joint, Right* **L** Elbow Joint, Right 　　Distal humerus, involving joint 　　Humeroradial joint 　　Humeroulnar joint 　　Proximal radioulnar joint **M** Elbow Joint, Left 　　*See L Elbow Joint, Right* **N** Wrist Joint, Right 　　Distal radioulnar joint 　　Radiocarpal joint **P** Wrist Joint, Left 　　*See N Wrist Joint, Right* **Q** Carpal Joint, Right 　　Intercarpal joint 　　Midcarpal joint **R** Carpal Joint, Left 　　*See Q Carpal Joint, Right* **S** Carpometacarpal Joint, Right **T** Carpometacarpal Joint, Left **U** Metacarpophalangeal Joint, Right **V** Metacarpophalangeal Joint, Left **W** Finger Phalangeal Joint, Right 　　Interphalangeal (IP) joint **X** Finger Phalangeal Joint, Left 　　*See W Finger Phalangeal Joint, Right*	**Ø** Open **3** Percutaneous **4** Percutaneous Endoscopic	**Z** No Device	**X** Diagnostic **Z** No Qualifier

Non-OR　　ØRB[Ø,1,3,4,5,6,9,A,B,E,F,G,H,J,K,L,M,N,P,Q,R,S,T,U,V,W,X][Ø,3,4]ZX

NC Noncovered Procedure　LC Limited Coverage　QA Questionable OB Admit　NT New Tech Add-on　⊞ Combination Member　♂Male　♀Female

ICD-10-PCS 2024　　　　　　　　　　　　　　　　　　　　　　　　　　　　　　　　　　　　　**589**

Upper Joints

Ø   **Medical and Surgical**
R   **Upper Joints**
C   **Extirpation**   Definition: Taking or cutting out solid matter from a body part

Explanation: The solid matter may be an abnormal byproduct of a biological function or a foreign body; it may be imbedded in a body part or in the lumen of a tubular body part. The solid matter may or may not have been previously broken into pieces.

Body Part Character 4	Approach Character 5	Device Character 6	Qualifier Character 7
Ø **Occipital-cervical Joint**	**Ø** Open	**Z** No Device	**Z** No Qualifier

1   **Cervical Vertebral Joint**
    Atlantoaxial joint
    Cervical facet joint
	3 Percutaneous
	4 Percutaneous Endoscopic		

3 **Cervical Vertebral Disc**			
4 **Cervicothoracic Vertebral Joint** Cervicothoracic facet joint			
5 **Cervicothoracic Vertebral Disc**			

6   **Thoracic Vertebral Joint**
    Costotransverse joint
    Costovertebral joint
    Thoracic facet joint			

9 **Thoracic Vertebral Disc**			
A **Thoracolumbar Vertebral Joint** Thoracolumbar facet joint			
B **Thoracolumbar Vertebral Disc**			
C **Temporomandibular Joint, Right**			
D **Temporomandibular Joint, Left**			
E **Sternoclavicular Joint, Right**			
F **Sternoclavicular Joint, Left**			
G **Acromioclavicular Joint, Right**			
H **Acromioclavicular Joint, Left**			

J   **Shoulder Joint, Right**
    Glenohumeral joint
    Glenoid ligament (labrum)			

K **Shoulder Joint, Left** *See J Shoulder Joint, Right*			

L   **Elbow Joint, Right**
    Distal humerus, involving joint
    Humeroradial joint
    Humeroulnar joint
    Proximal radioulnar joint			

M **Elbow Joint, Left** *See L Elbow Joint, Right*			

N   **Wrist Joint, Right**
    Distal radioulnar joint
    Radiocarpal joint			

P **Wrist Joint, Left** *See N Wrist Joint, Right*			

Q   **Carpal Joint, Right**
    Intercarpal joint
    Midcarpal joint			

R **Carpal Joint, Left** *See Q Carpal Joint, Right*			
S **Carpometacarpal Joint, Right**			
T **Carpometacarpal Joint, Left**			
U **Metacarpophalangeal Joint, Right**			
V **Metacarpophalangeal Joint, Left**			
W **Finger Phalangeal Joint, Right** Interphalangeal (IP) joint			
X **Finger Phalangeal Joint, Left** *See W Finger Phalangeal Joint, Right*			

Ø Medical and Surgical
R Upper Joints
G Fusion   Definition: Joining together portions of an articular body part rendering the articular body part immobile
              Explanation: The body part is joined together by fixation device, bone graft, or other means

Body Part Character 4	Approach Character 5	Device Character 6	Qualifier Character 7
Ø Occipital-cervical Joint **1 Cervical Vertebral Joint** Atlantoaxial joint Cervical facet joint **2 Cervical Vertebral Joints, 2 or more** Cervical facet joint **4 Cervicothoracic Vertebral Joint** Cervicothoracic facet joint **6 Thoracic Vertebral Joint** Costotransverse joint Costovertebral joint Thoracic facet joint **7 Thoracic Vertebral Joints, 2 to 7** ⊞ **8 Thoracic Vertebral Joints, 8 or more** **A Thoracolumbar Vertebral Joint** Thoracolumbar facet joint	**Ø Open** **3 Percutaneous** **4 Percutaneous Endoscopic**	**7 Autologous Tissue Substitute** **J Synthetic Substitute** **K Nonautologous Tissue Substitute**	**Ø Anterior Approach, Anterior Column** **1 Posterior Approach, Posterior Column** **J Posterior Approach, Anterior Column**
Ø Occipital-cervical Joint **1 Cervical Vertebral Joint** Atlantoaxial joint Cervical facet joint **2 Cervical Vertebral Joints, 2 or more** Cervical facet joint **4 Cervicothoracic Vertebral Joint** Cervicothoracic facet joint **6 Thoracic Vertebral Joint** Costotransverse joint Costovertebral joint Thoracic facet joint **7 Thoracic Vertebral Joints, 2 to 7** ⊞ **8 Thoracic Vertebral Joints, 8 or more** **A Thoracolumbar Vertebral Joint** Thoracolumbar facet joint	**Ø Open** **3 Percutaneous** **4 Percutaneous Endoscopic**	**A Interbody Fusion Device**	**Ø Anterior Approach, Anterior Column** **J Posterior Approach, Anterior Column**
C Temporomandibular Joint, Right **D Temporomandibular Joint, Left** **E Sternoclavicular Joint, Right** **F Sternoclavicular Joint, Left** **G Acromioclavicular Joint, Right** **H Acromioclavicular Joint, Left** **J Shoulder Joint, Right** Glenohumeral joint Glenoid ligament (labrum) **K Shoulder Joint, Left** *See J Shoulder Joint, Right*	**Ø Open** **3 Percutaneous** **4 Percutaneous Endoscopic**	**4 Internal Fixation Device** **7 Autologous Tissue Substitute** **J Synthetic Substitute** **K Nonautologous Tissue Substitute**	**Z No Qualifier**
L Elbow Joint, Right Distal humerus, involving joint Humeroradial joint Humeroulnar joint Proximal radioulnar joint **M Elbow Joint, Left** *See L Elbow Joint, Right* **N Wrist Joint, Right** Distal radioulnar joint Radiocarpal joint **P Wrist Joint, Left** *See N Wrist Joint, Right* **Q Carpal Joint, Right** Intercarpal joint Midcarpal joint **R Carpal Joint, Left** *See Q Carpal Joint, Right* **S Carpometacarpal Joint, Right** **T Carpometacarpal Joint, Left** **U Metacarpophalangeal Joint, Right** **V Metacarpophalangeal Joint, Left** **W Finger Phalangeal Joint, Right** Interphalangeal (IP) joint **X Finger Phalangeal Joint, Left** *See W Finger Phalangeal Joint, Right*	**Ø Open** **3 Percutaneous** **4 Percutaneous Endoscopic**	**3 Internal Fixation Device, Sustained Compression** **4 Internal Fixation Device** **5 External Fixation Device** **7 Autologous Tissue Substitute** **J Synthetic Substitute** **K Nonautologous Tissue Substitute**	**Z No Qualifier**

HAC   ØRG[Ø,1,2,4,6,7,8,A][Ø,3,4][7,J,K][Ø,1,J] when reported with SDx K68.11 or
          T81.4Ø–T81.49, T84.6Ø-T84.619, T84.63-T84.7 with 7th character A
HAC   ØRG[Ø,1,2,4,6,7,8,A][Ø,3,4]A[Ø,J] when reported with SDx K68.11 or T81.4Ø–T81.49,
          T84.6Ø-T84.619, T84.63-T84.7 with 7th character A
HAC   ØRG[E,F,G,H,J,K][Ø,3,4][4,7,J,K]Z when reported with SDx K68.11 or T81.4Ø–T81.49,
          T84.6Ø-T84.619, T84.63-T84.7 with 7th character A
HAC   ØRG[L,M][Ø,3,4][3,4,5,7,J,K]Z when reported with SDx K68.11 or T81.4Ø–T81.49,
          T84.6Ø-T84.619, T84.63-T84.7 with 7th character A

See Appendix L for Procedure Combinations
⊞   ØRG7[Ø,3,4][7,J,K][Ø,1,J]
⊞   ØRG7[Ø,3,4]A[Ø,J]

🆖 Noncovered Procedure   🆑 Limited Coverage   🆗 Questionable OB Admit   🆕 New Tech Add-on   ⊞ Combination Member   ♂ Male   ♀ Female

ICD-10-PCS 2024   591

Ø   Medical and Surgical
R   Upper Joints
H   Insertion

Definition: Putting in a nonbiological appliance that monitors, assists, performs, or prevents a physiological function but does not physically take the place of a body part

Explanation: None

Body Part Character 4	Approach Character 5	Device Character 6	Qualifier Character 7

Ø Occipital-cervical Joint
1 Cervical Vertebral Joint
  Atlantoaxial joint
  Cervical facet joint
4 Cervicothoracic Vertebral Joint
  Cervicothoracic facet joint
6 Thoracic Vertebral Joint
  Costotransverse joint
  Costovertebral joint
  Thoracic facet joint
A Thoracolumbar Vertebral Joint
  Thoracolumbar facet joint
	Ø Open
	3 Percutaneous
	4 Percutaneous Endoscopic
		3 Infusion Device
		4 Internal Fixation Device
		8 Spacer
		B Spinal Stabilization Device, Interspinous Process
		C Spinal Stabilization Device, Pedicle-Based
		D Spinal Stabilization Device, Facet Replacement
			Z No Qualifier

3 Cervical Vertebral Disc 5 Cervicothoracic Vertebral Disc 9 Thoracic Vertebral Disc B Thoracolumbar Vertebral Disc	Ø Open 3 Percutaneous 4 Percutaneous Endoscopic	3 Infusion Device	Z No Qualifier

C Temporomandibular Joint, Right
D Temporomandibular Joint, Left
E Sternoclavicular Joint, Right
F Sternoclavicular Joint, Left
G Acromioclavicular Joint, Right
H Acromioclavicular Joint, Left
J Shoulder Joint, Right
  Glenohumeral joint
  Glenoid ligament (labrum)
K Shoulder Joint, Left
  See J Shoulder Joint, Right
	Ø Open
	3 Percutaneous
	4 Percutaneous Endoscopic
		3 Infusion Device
		4 Internal Fixation Device
		8 Spacer
			Z No Qualifier

L Elbow Joint, Right
  Distal humerus, involving joint
  Humeroradial joint
  Humeroulnar joint
  Proximal radioulnar joint
M Elbow Joint, Left
  See L Elbow Joint, Right
N Wrist Joint, Right
  Distal radioulnar joint
  Radiocarpal joint
P Wrist Joint, Left
  See N Wrist Joint, Right
Q Carpal Joint, Right
  Intercarpal joint
  Midcarpal joint
R Carpal Joint, Left
  See Q Carpal Joint, Right
S Carpometacarpal Joint, Right
T Carpometacarpal Joint, Left
U Metacarpophalangeal Joint, Right
V Metacarpophalangeal Joint, Left
W Finger Phalangeal Joint, Right
  Interphalangeal (IP) joint
X Finger Phalangeal Joint, Left
  See W Finger Phalangeal Joint, Right
	Ø Open
	3 Percutaneous
	4 Percutaneous Endoscopic
		3 Infusion Device
		4 Internal Fixation Device
		5 External Fixation Device
		8 Spacer
			Z No Qualifier

Non-OR ØRH[Ø,1,4,6,A][Ø,3,4][3,8]Z
Non-OR ØRH[3,5,9,B][Ø,3,4]3Z
Non-OR ØRH[C,D][Ø,4]8Z
Non-OR ØRH[C,D]3[3,8]Z
Non-OR ØRH[E,F,G,H][Ø,3,4][3,8]Z
Non-OR ØRH[J,K][Ø,3,4]3Z
Non-OR ØRH[J,K]38Z
Non-OR ØRH[L,M,N,P,Q,R,S,T,U,V,W,X][Ø,3,4][3,8]Z

Ø   Medical and Surgical
R   Upper Joints
J   Inspection   Definition: Visually and/or manually exploring a body part

Explanation: Visual exploration may be performed with or without optical instrumentation. Manual exploration may be performed directly or through intervening body layers.

Body Part Character 4	Approach Character 5	Device Character 6	Qualifier Character 7
Ø Occipital-cervical Joint **1** Cervical Vertebral Joint 　Atlantoaxial joint 　Cervical facet joint **3** Cervical Vertebral Disc **4** Cervicothoracic Vertebral Joint 　Cervicothoracic facet joint **5** Cervicothoracic Vertebral Disc **6** Thoracic Vertebral Joint 　Costotransverse joint 　Costovertebral joint 　Thoracic facet joint **9** Thoracic Vertebral Disc **A** Thoracolumbar Vertebral Joint 　Thoracolumbar facet joint **B** Thoracolumbar Vertebral Disc **C** Temporomandibular Joint, Right **D** Temporomandibular Joint, Left **E** Sternoclavicular Joint, Right **F** Sternoclavicular Joint, Left **G** Acromioclavicular Joint, Right **H** Acromioclavicular Joint, Left **J** Shoulder Joint, Right 　Glenohumeral joint 　Glenoid ligament (labrum) **K** Shoulder Joint, Left 　*See J Shoulder Joint, Right* **L** Elbow Joint, Right 　Distal humerus, involving joint 　Humeroradial joint 　Humeroulnar joint 　Proximal radioulnar joint **M** Elbow Joint, Left 　*See L Elbow Joint, Right* **N** Wrist Joint, Right 　Distal radioulnar joint 　Radiocarpal joint **P** Wrist Joint, Left 　*See N Wrist Joint, Right* **Q** Carpal Joint, Right 　Intercarpal joint 　Midcarpal joint **R** Carpal Joint, Left 　*See Q Carpal Joint, Right* **S** Carpometacarpal Joint, Right **T** Carpometacarpal Joint, Left **U** Metacarpophalangeal Joint, Right **V** Metacarpophalangeal Joint, Left **W** Finger Phalangeal Joint, Right 　Interphalangeal (IP) joint **X** Finger Phalangeal Joint, Left 　*See W Finger Phalangeal Joint, Right*	**Ø** Open **3** Percutaneous **4** Percutaneous Endoscopic **X** External	**Z** No Device	**Z** No Qualifier

Non-OR　ØRJ[Ø,1,3,4,5,6,9,A,B,C,D,E,F,G,H,J,K,L,M,N,P,Q,R,S,T,U,V,W,X][3,X]ZZ

NC Noncovered Procedure　　**LC** Limited Coverage　　**QA** Questionable OB Admit　　**NT** New Tech Add-on　　⊞ Combination Member　　♂ Male　　♀ Female

ICD-10-PCS 2024　　　　　　　　　　　　　　　　　　　　　　　　　　　　　　　　　　　　　　593

ØRJ–ØRJ

Ø Medical and Surgical
R Upper Joints
N Release

Definition: Freeing a body part from an abnormal physical constraint by cutting or by the use of force
Explanation: Some of the restraining tissue may be taken out but none of the body part is taken out

Body Part Character 4	Approach Character 5	Device Character 6	Qualifier Character 7
Ø Occipital-cervical Joint	Ø Open	Z No Device	Z No Qualifier
1 Cervical Vertebral Joint	3 Percutaneous		
Atlantoaxial joint	4 Percutaneous Endoscopic		
Cervical facet joint	X External		
3 Cervical Vertebral Disc			
4 Cervicothoracic Vertebral Joint			
Cervicothoracic facet joint			
5 Cervicothoracic Vertebral Disc			
6 Thoracic Vertebral Joint			
Costotransverse joint			
Costovertebral joint			
Thoracic facet joint			
9 Thoracic Vertebral Disc			
A Thoracolumbar Vertebral Joint			
Thoracolumbar facet joint			
B Thoracolumbar Vertebral Disc			
C Temporomandibular Joint, Right			
D Temporomandibular Joint, Left			
E Sternoclavicular Joint, Right			
F Sternoclavicular Joint, Left			
G Acromioclavicular Joint, Right			
H Acromioclavicular Joint, Left			
J Shoulder Joint, Right			
Glenohumeral joint			
Glenoid ligament (labrum)			
K Shoulder Joint, Left			
See J Shoulder Joint, Right			
L Elbow Joint, Right			
Distal humerus, involving joint			
Humeroradial joint			
Humeroulnar joint			
Proximal radioulnar joint			
M Elbow Joint, Left			
See L Elbow Joint, Right			
N Wrist Joint, Right			
Distal radioulnar joint			
Radiocarpal joint			
P Wrist Joint, Left			
See N Wrist Joint, Right			
Q Carpal Joint, Right			
Intercarpal joint			
Midcarpal joint			
R Carpal Joint, Left			
See Q Carpal Joint, Right			
S Carpometacarpal Joint, Right			
T Carpometacarpal Joint, Left			
U Metacarpophalangeal Joint, Right			
V Metacarpophalangeal Joint, Left			
W Finger Phalangeal Joint, Right			
Interphalangeal (IP) joint			
X Finger Phalangeal Joint, Left			
See W Finger Phalangeal Joint, Right			

Non-OR   ØRN[Ø,1,3,4,5,6,9,A,B,C,D,E,F,G,H,J,K,L,M,N,P,Q,R,S,T,U,V,W,X]XZZ

Non-OR Procedure   DRG Non-OR Procedure   Valid OR Procedure   HAC Associated Procedure   Combination Only   New/Revised April   New/Revised October

594   ICD-10-PCS 2024

Ø   Medical and Surgical
R   Upper Joints
P   Removal   Definition: Taking out or off a device from a body part

Explanation: If a device is taken out and a similar device put in without cutting or puncturing the skin or mucous membrane, the procedure is coded to the root operation CHANGE. Otherwise, the procedure for taking out the device is coded to the root operation REMOVAL.

Body Part Character 4	Approach Character 5	Device Character 6	Qualifier Character 7

Ø Occipital-cervical Joint
1 Cervical Vertebral Joint
   Atlantoaxial joint
   Cervical facet joint
4 Cervicothoracic Vertebral Joint
   Cervicothoracic facet joint
6 Thoracic Vertebral Joint
   Costotransverse joint
   Costovertebral joint
   Thoracic facet joint
A Thoracolumbar Vertebral Joint
   Thoracolumbar facet joint
	Ø Open
	3 Percutaneous
	4 Percutaneous Endoscopic
		Ø Drainage Device
		3 Infusion Device
		4 Internal Fixation Device
		7 Autologous Tissue Substitute
		8 Spacer
		A Interbody Fusion Device
		J Synthetic Substitute
		K Nonautologous Tissue Substitute
			Z No Qualifier

Ø Occipital-cervical Joint
1 Cervical Vertebral Joint
   Atlantoaxial joint
   Cervical facet joint
4 Cervicothoracic Vertebral Joint
   Cervicothoracic facet joint
6 Thoracic Vertebral Joint
   Costotransverse joint
   Costovertebral joint
   Thoracic facet joint
A Thoracolumbar Vertebral Joint
   Thoracolumbar facet joint
	X External	Ø Drainage Device
		3 Infusion Device
		4 Internal Fixation Device
			Z No Qualifier

3 Cervical Vertebral Disc 5 Cervicothoracic Vertebral Disc 9 Thoracic Vertebral Disc B Thoracolumbar Vertebral Disc	Ø Open 3 Percutaneous 4 Percutaneous Endoscopic	Ø Drainage Device 3 Infusion Device 7 Autologous Tissue Substitute J Synthetic Substitute K Nonautologous Tissue Substitute	Z No Qualifier
3 Cervical Vertebral Disc 5 Cervicothoracic Vertebral Disc 9 Thoracic Vertebral Disc B Thoracolumbar Vertebral Disc	X External	Ø Drainage Device 3 Infusion Device	Z No Qualifier
C Temporomandibular Joint, Right D Temporomandibular Joint, Left E Sternoclavicular Joint, Right F Sternoclavicular Joint, Left G Acromioclavicular Joint, Right H Acromioclavicular Joint, Left	Ø Open 3 Percutaneous 4 Percutaneous Endoscopic	Ø Drainage Device 3 Infusion Device 4 Internal Fixation Device 7 Autologous Tissue Substitute 8 Spacer J Synthetic Substitute K Nonautologous Tissue Substitute	Z No Qualifier
C Temporomandibular Joint, Right D Temporomandibular Joint, Left E Sternoclavicular Joint, Right F Sternoclavicular Joint, Left G Acromioclavicular Joint, Right H Acromioclavicular Joint, Left	X External	Ø Drainage Device 3 Infusion Device 4 Internal Fixation Device	Z No Qualifier

J Shoulder Joint, Right
   Glenohumeral joint
   Glenoid ligament (labrum)
K Shoulder Joint, Left
   See J Shoulder Joint, Right
	Ø Open
	3 Percutaneous
	4 Percutaneous Endoscopic
		Ø Drainage Device
		3 Infusion Device
		4 Internal Fixation Device
		7 Autologous Tissue Substitute
		8 Spacer
		K Nonautologous Tissue Substitute
			Z No Qualifier

J Shoulder Joint, Right
   Glenohumeral joint
   Glenoid ligament (labrum)
K Shoulder Joint, Left
   See J Shoulder Joint, Right
	Ø Open
	3 Percutaneous
	4 Percutaneous Endoscopic
		J Synthetic Substitute	6 Humeral Surface
			7 Glenoid Surface
			Z No Qualifier

J Shoulder Joint, Right
   Glenohumeral joint
   Glenoid ligament (labrum)
K Shoulder Joint, Left
   See J Shoulder Joint, Right
	X External	Ø Drainage Device
		3 Infusion Device
		4 Internal Fixation Device
			Z No Qualifier

Non-OR ØRP[Ø,1,4,6,A]3[Ø,3,8]Z	Non-OR ØRP[C,D,E,F,G,H][Ø,4]8Z
Non-OR ØRP[Ø,1,4,6,A][Ø,4]8Z	Non-OR ØRP[C,D]X[Ø,3]Z
Non-OR ØRP[Ø,1,4,6,A]X[Ø,3,4]Z	Non-OR ØRP[E,F,G,H,J,K]X[Ø,3,4]Z
Non-OR ØRP[3,5,9,B]3[Ø,3]Z	Non-OR ØRP[J,K]3[Ø,3,8]Z
Non-OR ØRP[3,5,9,B]X[Ø,3]Z	Non-OR ØRP[J,K]X[Ø,3,4]Z
Non-OR ØRP[C,D,E,F,G,H]3[Ø,3,8]Z	

ØRP Continued on next page

NC Noncovered Procedure   LC Limited Coverage   OA Questionable OB Admit   NT New Tech Add-on   ⊞ Combination Member   ♂ Male   ♀ Female

ICD-10-PCS 2024   595

ØRP–ØRP

Upper Joints

Ø   **Medical and Surgical**
R   **Upper Joints**
P   **Removal**   Definition: Taking out or off a device from a body part

ØRP Continued

Explanation: If a device is taken out and a similar device put in without cutting or puncturing the skin or mucous membrane, the procedure is coded to the root operation CHANGE. Otherwise, the procedure for taking out the device is coded to the root operation REMOVAL.

Body Part Character 4	Approach Character 5	Device Character 6	Qualifier Character 7
L Elbow Joint, Right Distal humerus, involving joint Humeroradial joint Humeroulnar joint Proximal radioulnar joint **M** Elbow Joint, Left *See L Elbow Joint, Right* **N** Wrist Joint, Right Distal radioulnar joint Radiocarpal joint **P** Wrist Joint, Left *See N Wrist Joint, Right* **Q** Carpal Joint, Right Intercarpal joint Midcarpal joint **R** Carpal Joint, Left *See Q Carpal Joint, Right* **S** Carpometacarpal Joint, Right **T** Carpometacarpal Joint, Left **U** Metacarpophalangeal Joint, Right **V** Metacarpophalangeal Joint, Left **W** Finger Phalangeal Joint, Right Interphalangeal (IP) joint **X** Finger Phalangeal Joint, Left *See W Finger Phalangeal Joint, Right*	**Ø** Open **3** Percutaneous **4** Percutaneous Endoscopic	**Ø** Drainage Device **3** Infusion Device **4** Internal Fixation Device **5** External Fixation Device **7** Autologous Tissue Substitute **8** Spacer **J** Synthetic Substitute **K** Nonautologous Tissue Substitute	**Z** No Qualifier
L Elbow Joint, Right Distal humerus, involving joint Humeroradial joint Humeroulnar joint Proximal radioulnar joint **M** Elbow Joint, Left *See L Elbow Joint, Right* **N** Wrist Joint, Right Distal radioulnar joint Radiocarpal joint **P** Wrist Joint, Left *See N Wrist Joint, Right* **Q** Carpal Joint, Right Intercarpal joint Midcarpal joint **R** Carpal Joint, Left *See Q Carpal Joint, Right* **S** Carpometacarpal Joint, Right **T** Carpometacarpal Joint, Left **U** Metacarpophalangeal Joint, Right **V** Metacarpophalangeal Joint, Left **W** Finger Phalangeal Joint, Right Interphalangeal (IP) joint **X** Finger Phalangeal Joint, Left *See W Finger Phalangeal Joint, Right*	**X** External	**Ø** Drainage Device **3** Infusion Device **4** Internal Fixation Device **5** External Fixation Device	**Z** No Qualifier

Non-OR   ØRP[L,M,N,P,Q,R,S,T,U,V,W,X]3[Ø,3,8]Z
Non-OR   ØRP[L,M,N,P,Q,R,S,T,U,V,W,X][Ø,4]8Z
Non-OR   ØRP[L,M,N,P,Q,R,S,T,U,V,W,X]X[Ø,3,4,5]Z

Ø   Medical and Surgical
R   Upper Joints
Q   Repair

Definition: Restoring, to the extent possible, a body part to its normal anatomic structure and function

Explanation: Used only when the method to accomplish the repair is not one of the other root operations

Body Part Character 4	Approach Character 5	Device Character 6	Qualifier Character 7

Ø Occipital-cervical Joint
1 Cervical Vertebral Joint
   Atlantoaxial joint
   Cervical facet joint
3 Cervical Vertebral Disc
4 Cervicothoracic Vertebral Joint
   Cervicothoracic facet joint
5 Cervicothoracic Vertebral Disc
6 Thoracic Vertebral Joint
   Costotransverse joint
   Costovertebral joint
   Thoracic facet joint
9 Thoracic Vertebral Disc
A Thoracolumbar Vertebral Joint
   Thoracolumbar facet joint
B Thoracolumbar Vertebral Disc
C Temporomandibular Joint, Right
D Temporomandibular Joint, Left
E Sternoclavicular Joint, Right
F Sternoclavicular Joint, Left
G Acromioclavicular Joint, Right
H Acromioclavicular Joint, Left
J Shoulder Joint, Right
   Glenohumeral joint
   Glenoid ligament (labrum)
K Shoulder Joint, Left
   See J Shoulder Joint, Right
L Elbow Joint, Right
   Distal humerus, involving joint
   Humeroradial joint
   Humeroulnar joint
   Proximal radioulnar joint
M Elbow Joint, Left
   See L Elbow Joint, Right
N Wrist Joint, Right
   Distal radioulnar joint
   Radiocarpal joint
P Wrist Joint, Left
   See N Wrist Joint, Right
Q Carpal Joint, Right
   Intercarpal joint
   Midcarpal joint
R Carpal Joint, Left
   See Q Carpal Joint, Right
S Carpometacarpal Joint, Right
T Carpometacarpal Joint, Left
U Metacarpophalangeal Joint, Right
V Metacarpophalangeal Joint, Left
W Finger Phalangeal Joint, Right
   Interphalangeal (IP) joint
X Finger Phalangeal Joint, Left
   See W Finger Phalangeal Joint, Right
	Ø Open
	3 Percutaneous
	4 Percutaneous Endoscopic
	X External
		Z No Device	**Z No Qualifier**

Non-OR   ØRQ[Ø,1,3,4,5,6,9,A,B,C,D,E,F,G,H,J,K,L,M,N,P,Q,R,S,T,U,V,W,X]XZZ

HAC   ØRQ[E,F,G,H,J,K,L,M][Ø,3,4]ZZ when reported with SDx K68.11 or T81.40–T81.49, T84.60-T84.619, T84.63-T84.7 with 7th character A

Ø Medical and Surgical
R Upper Joints
R Replacement   Definition: Putting in or on biological or synthetic material that physically takes the place and/or function of all or a portion of a body part

Explanation: The body part may have been taken out or replaced, or may be taken out, physically eradicated, or rendered nonfunctional during the REPLACEMENT procedure. A REMOVAL procedure is coded for taking out the device used in a previous replacement procedure.

Body Part Character 4	Approach Character 5	Device Character 6	Qualifier Character 7

Ø Occipital-cervical Joint
1 Cervical Vertebral Joint
   Atlantoaxial joint
   Cervical facet joint
3 Cervical Vertebral Disc
4 Cervicothoracic Vertebral Joint
   Cervicothoracic facet joint
5 Cervicothoracic Vertebral Disc
6 Thoracic Vertebral Joint
   Costotransverse joint
   Costovertebral joint
   Thoracic facet joint
9 Thoracic Vertebral Disc
A Thoracolumbar Vertebral Joint
   Thoracolumbar facet joint
B Thoracolumbar Vertebral Disc
C Temporomandibular Joint, Right
D Temporomandibular Joint, Left
E Sternoclavicular Joint, Right
F Sternoclavicular Joint, Left
G Acromioclavicular Joint, Right
H Acromioclavicular Joint, Left
L Elbow Joint, Right
   Distal humerus, involving joint
   Humeroradial joint
   Humeroulnar joint
   Proximal radioulnar joint
M Elbow Joint, Left
   See L Elbow Joint, Right
N Wrist Joint, Right
   Distal radioulnar joint
   Radiocarpal joint
P Wrist Joint, Left
   See N Wrist Joint, Right
Q Carpal Joint, Right
   Intercarpal joint
   Midcarpal joint
R Carpal Joint, Left
   See Q Carpal Joint, Right
S Carpometacarpal Joint, Right
T Carpometacarpal Joint, Left
U Metacarpophalangeal Joint, Right
V Metacarpophalangeal Joint, Left
W Finger Phalangeal Joint, Right
   Interphalangeal (IP) joint
X Finger Phalangeal Joint, Left
   See W Finger Phalangeal Joint, Right
	Ø Open	**7 Autologous Tissue Substitute**
		J Synthetic Substitute
		K Nonautologous Tissue Substitute
			Z No Qualifier

J Shoulder Joint, Right
   Glenohumeral joint
   Glenoid ligament (labrum)
K Shoulder Joint, Left
   See J Shoulder Joint, Right
	Ø Open	**Ø Synthetic Substitute, Reverse Ball and Socket**
		7 Autologous Tissue Substitute
		K Nonautologous Tissue Substitute
			Z No Qualifier

J Shoulder Joint, Right
   Glenohumeral joint
   Glenoid ligament (labrum)
K Shoulder Joint, Left
   See J Shoulder Joint, Right
	Ø Open	**J Synthetic Substitute**	**6 Humeral Surface**
			7 Glenoid Surface
			Z No Qualifier

Non-OR Procedure   DRG Non-OR Procedure   Valid OR Procedure   HAC Associated Procedure   Combination Only   New/Revised April   New/Revised October

598   ICD-10-PCS 2024

ØRR–ØRR

Ø   **Medical and Surgical**
R   **Upper Joints**
S   **Reposition**

Definition: Moving to its normal location, or other suitable location, all or a portion of a body part
Explanation: The body part is moved to a new location from an abnormal location, or from a normal location where it is not functioning correctly. The body part may or may not be cut out or off to be moved to the new location.

Body Part Character 4	Approach Character 5	Device Character 6	Qualifier Character 7

Ø Occipital-cervical Joint
1 Cervical Vertebral Joint
   Atlantoaxial joint
   Cervical facet joint
4 Cervicothoracic Vertebral Joint
   Cervicothoracic facet joint
6 Thoracic Vertebral Joint
   Costotransverse joint
   Costovertebral joint
   Thoracic facet joint
A Thoracolumbar Vertebral Joint
   Thoracolumbar facet joint
C Temporomandibular Joint, Right
D Temporomandibular Joint, Left
E Sternoclavicular Joint, Right
F Sternoclavicular Joint, Left
G Acromioclavicular Joint, Right
H Acromioclavicular Joint, Left
J Shoulder Joint, Right
   Glenohumeral joint
   Glenoid ligament (labrum)
K Shoulder Joint, Left
   See J Shoulder Joint, Right
	Ø Open
	3 Percutaneous
	4 Percutaneous Endoscopic
	X External
		4 Internal Fixation Device
		Z No Device
			Z No Qualifier

L Elbow Joint, Right
   Distal humerus, involving joint
   Humeroradial joint
   Humeroulnar joint
   Proximal radioulnar joint
M Elbow Joint, Left
   See L Elbow Joint, Right
N Wrist Joint, Right
   Distal radioulnar joint
   Radiocarpal joint
P Wrist Joint, Left
   See N Wrist Joint, Right
Q Carpal Joint, Right
   Intercarpal joint
   Midcarpal joint
R Carpal Joint, Left
   See Q Carpal Joint, Right
S Carpometacarpal Joint, Right
T Carpometacarpal Joint, Left
U Metacarpophalangeal Joint, Right
V Metacarpophalangeal Joint, Left
W Finger Phalangeal Joint, Right
   Interphalangeal (IP) joint
X Finger Phalangeal Joint, Left
   See W Finger Phalangeal Joint, Right
	Ø Open
	3 Percutaneous
	4 Percutaneous Endoscopic
	X External
		4 Internal Fixation Device
		5 External Fixation Device
		Z No Device
			Z No Qualifier

Non-OR   ØRS[Ø,1,4,6,A,C,D,E,F,G,H,J,K][3,4,X][4,Z]Z
Non-OR   ØRS[L,M,N,P,Q,R,S,T,U,V,W,X][3,4,X][4,5,Z]Z

NC Noncovered Procedure   LC Limited Coverage   QA Questionable OB Admit   NT New Tech Add-on   ⊞ Combination Member   ♂ Male   ♀ Female
ICD-10-PCS 2024   599

ØRS–ØRS

Upper Joints

ØRT–ØRT

Ø Medical and Surgical
R Upper Joints
T Resection   Definition: Cutting out or off, without replacement, all of a body part
                Explanation: None

Body Part Character 4	Approach Character 5	Device Character 6	Qualifier Character 7

3 Cervical Vertebral Disc
4 Cervicothoracic Vertebral Joint
    Cervicothoracic facet joint
5 Cervicothoracic Vertebral Disc
9 Thoracic Vertebral Disc
B Thoracolumbar Vertebral Disc
C Temporomandibular Joint, Right
D Temporomandibular Joint, Left
E Sternoclavicular Joint, Right
F Sternoclavicular Joint, Left
G Acromioclavicular Joint, Right
H Acromioclavicular Joint, Left
J Shoulder Joint, Right
    Glenohumeral joint
    Glenoid ligament (labrum)
K Shoulder Joint, Left
    See J Shoulder Joint, Right
L Elbow Joint, Right
    Distal humerus, involving joint
    Humeroradial joint
    Humeroulnar joint
    Proximal radioulnar joint
M Elbow Joint, Left
    See L Elbow Joint, Right
N Wrist Joint, Right
    Distal radioulnar joint
    Radiocarpal joint
P Wrist Joint, Left
    See N Wrist Joint, Right
Q Carpal Joint, Right
    Intercarpal joint
    Midcarpal joint
R Carpal Joint, Left
    See Q Carpal Joint, Right
S Carpometacarpal Joint, Right
T Carpometacarpal Joint, Left
U Metacarpophalangeal Joint, Right
V Metacarpophalangeal Joint, Left
W Finger Phalangeal Joint, Right
    Interphalangeal (IP) joint
X Finger Phalangeal Joint, Left
    See W Finger Phalangeal Joint, Right
	Ø Open	**Z** No Device	**Z** No Qualifier

Upper Joints *(side tab)*

Ø   Medical and Surgical
R   Upper Joints
U   Supplement   Definition: Putting in or on biological or synthetic material that physically reinforces and/or augments the function of a portion of a body part

Explanation: The biological material is non-living, or is living and from the same individual. The body part may have been previously replaced, and the SUPPLEMENT procedure is performed to physically reinforce and/or augment the function of the replaced body part.

Body Part Character 4	Approach Character 5	Device Character 6	Qualifier Character 7
Ø Occipital-cervical Joint	**Ø Open**	**7 Autologous Tissue**	**Z No Qualifier**
1 Cervical Vertebral Joint	**3 Percutaneous**	**Substitute**	
Atlantoaxial joint	**4 Percutaneous Endoscopic**	**J Synthetic Substitute**	
Cervical facet joint		**K Nonautologous Tissue**	
3 Cervical Vertebral Disc		**Substitute**	
4 Cervicothoracic Vertebral Joint			
Cervicothoracic facet joint			
5 Cervicothoracic Vertebral Disc			
6 Thoracic Vertebral Joint			
Costotransverse joint			
Costovertebral joint			
Thoracic facet joint			
9 Thoracic Vertebral Disc			
A Thoracolumbar Vertebral Joint			
Thoracolumbar facet joint			
B Thoracolumbar Vertebral Disc			
C Temporomandibular Joint, Right			
D Temporomandibular Joint, Left			
E Sternoclavicular Joint, Right			
F Sternoclavicular Joint, Left			
G Acromioclavicular Joint, Right			
H Acromioclavicular Joint, Left			
J Shoulder Joint, Right			
Glenohumeral joint			
Glenoid ligament (labrum)			
K Shoulder Joint, Left			
See J Shoulder Joint, Right			
L Elbow Joint, Right			
Distal humerus, involving joint			
Humeroradial joint			
Humeroulnar joint			
Proximal radioulnar joint			
M Elbow Joint, Left			
See L Elbow Joint, Right			
N Wrist Joint, Right			
Distal radioulnar joint			
Radiocarpal joint			
P Wrist Joint, Left			
See N Wrist Joint, Right			
Q Carpal Joint, Right			
Intercarpal joint			
Midcarpal joint			
R Carpal Joint, Left			
See Q Carpal Joint, Right			
S Carpometacarpal Joint, Right			
T Carpometacarpal Joint, Left			
U Metacarpophalangeal Joint, Right			
V Metacarpophalangeal Joint, Left			
W Finger Phalangeal Joint, Right			
Interphalangeal (IP) joint			
X Finger Phalangeal Joint, Left			
See W Finger Phalangeal Joint, Right			

HAC   ØRU[E,F,G,H,J,K,L,M][Ø,3,4][7,J,K]Z when reported with SDx K68.11 or T81.4Ø–T81.49, T84.6Ø-T84.619, T84.63-T84.7 with 7th character A

NC Noncovered Procedure   LC Limited Coverage   QA Questionable OB Admit   NT New Tech Add-on   ⊞ Combination Member   ♂ Male   ♀ Female

ICD-10-PCS 2024   601

ØRU–ØRU *(side tab)*

Ø   **Medical and Surgical**
R   **Upper Joints**
W   **Revision**   Definition: Correcting, to the extent possible, a portion of a malfunctioning device or the position of a displaced device

Explanation: Revision can include correcting a malfunctioning or displaced device by taking out or putting in components of the device such as a screw or pin

Body Part Character 4	Approach Character 5	Device Character 6	Qualifier Character 7

Ø Occipital-cervical Joint
1 Cervical Vertebral Joint
   Atlantoaxial joint
   Cervical facet joint
4 Cervicothoracic Vertebral Joint
   Cervicothoracic facet joint
6 Thoracic Vertebral Joint
   Costotransverse joint
   Costovertebral joint
   Thoracic facet joint
A Thoracolumbar Vertebral Joint
   Thoracolumbar facet joint
	Ø Open
	3 Percutaneous
	4 Percutaneous Endoscopic
	X External
		Ø Drainage Device
		3 Infusion Device
		4 Internal Fixation Device
		7 Autologous Tissue Substitute
		8 Spacer
		A Interbody Fusion Device
		J Synthetic Substitute
		K Nonautologous Tissue Substitute
			Z No Qualifier

3 Cervical Vertebral Disc 5 Cervicothoracic Vertebral Disc 9 Thoracic Vertebral Disc B Thoracolumbar Vertebral Disc	Ø Open 3 Percutaneous 4 Percutaneous Endoscopic X External	Ø Drainage Device 3 Infusion Device 7 Autologous Tissue Substitute J Synthetic Substitute K Nonautologous Tissue Substitute	Z No Qualifier
C Temporomandibular Joint, Right D Temporomandibular Joint, Left E Sternoclavicular Joint, Right F Sternoclavicular Joint, Left G Acromioclavicular Joint, Right H Acromioclavicular Joint, Left	Ø Open 3 Percutaneous 4 Percutaneous Endoscopic X External	Ø Drainage Device 3 Infusion Device 4 Internal Fixation Device 7 Autologous Tissue Substitute 8 Spacer J Synthetic Substitute K Nonautologous Tissue Substitute	Z No Qualifier

J Shoulder Joint, Right
   Glenohumeral joint
   Glenoid ligament (labrum)
K Shoulder Joint, Left
   See J Shoulder Joint, Right
	Ø Open
	3 Percutaneous
	4 Percutaneous Endoscopic
	X External
		Ø Drainage Device
		3 Infusion Device
		4 Internal Fixation Device
		7 Autologous Tissue Substitute
		8 Spacer
		J Synthetic Substitute
		K Nonautologous Tissue Substitute
			Z No Qualifier

J Shoulder Joint, Right
   Glenohumeral joint
   Glenoid ligament (labrum)
K Shoulder Joint, Left
   See J Shoulder Joint, Right
	Ø Open
	3 Percutaneous
	4 Percutaneous Endoscopic
	X External
		J Synthetic Substitute	6 Humeral Surface
			7 Glenoid Surface
			Z No Qualifier

L Elbow Joint, Right
   Distal humerus, involving joint
   Humeroradial joint
   Humeroulnar joint
   Proximal radioulnar joint
M Elbow Joint, Left
   See L Elbow Joint, Right
N Wrist Joint, Right
   Distal radioulnar joint
   Radiocarpal joint
P Wrist Joint, Left
   See N Wrist Joint, Right
Q Carpal Joint, Right
   Intercarpal joint
   Midcarpal joint
R Carpal Joint, Left
   See Q Carpal Joint, Right
S Carpometacarpal Joint, Right
T Carpometacarpal Joint, Left
U Metacarpophalangeal Joint, Right
V Metacarpophalangeal Joint, Left
W Finger Phalangeal Joint, Right
   Interphalangeal (IP) joint
X Finger Phalangeal Joint, Left
   See W Finger Phalangeal Joint, Right
	Ø Open
	3 Percutaneous
	4 Percutaneous Endoscopic
	X External
		Ø Drainage Device
		3 Infusion Device
		4 Internal Fixation Device
		5 External Fixation Device
		7 Autologous Tissue Substitute
		8 Spacer
		J Synthetic Substitute
		K Nonautologous Tissue Substitute
			Z No Qualifier

Non-OR	ØRW[Ø,1,4,6,A]X[Ø,3,4,7,8,A,J,K]Z
Non-OR	ØRW[3,5,9,B]X[Ø,3,7,J,K]Z
Non-OR	ØRW[C,D,E,F,G,H]X[Ø,3,4,7,8,J,K]Z
Non-OR	ØRW[J,K]X[Ø,3,4,7,8,J,K]Z
Non-OR	ØRW[J,K]XJ[6,7,Z]
Non-OR	ØRW[L,M,N,P,Q,R,S,T,U,V,W,X]X[Ø,3,4,5,7,8,J,K]Z

Non-OR Procedure   DRG Non-OR Procedure   Valid OR Procedure   HAC Associated Procedure   Combination Only   New/Revised April   New/Revised October

602   ICD-10-PCS 2024

Lower Joints ØS2–ØSW

Character Meanings*

This Character Meaning table is provided as a guide to assist the user in the identification of character members that may be found in this section of code tables. It **SHOULD NOT** be used to build a PCS code.

Operation–Character 3		Body Part–Character 4		Approach–Character 5		Device–Character 6		Qualifier–Character 7	
2	Change	Ø	Lumbar Vertebral Joint	Ø	Open	Ø	Drainage Device OR Synthetic Substitute, Polyethylene	Ø	Anterior Approach, Anterior Column
5	Destruction	1	Lumbar Vertebral Joint, 2 or more	3	Percutaneous	1	Synthetic Substitute, Metal	1	Posterior Approach, Posterior Column
9	Drainage	2	Lumbar Vertebral Disc	4	Percutaneous Endoscopic	2	Synthetic Substitute, Metal on Polyethylene	9	Cemented
B	Excision	3	Lumbosacral Joint	X	External	3	Infusion Device OR Internal Fixation Device, Sustained Compression OR Synthetic Substitute, Ceramic	A	Uncemented
C	Extirpation	4	Lumbosacral Disc			4	Internal Fixation Device OR Synthetic Substitute, Ceramic on Polyethylene	C	Patellar Surface
G	Fusion	5	Sacrococcygeal Joint			5	External Fixation Device	J	Posterior Approach, Anterior Column
H	Insertion	6	Coccygeal Joint			6	Synthetic Substitute, Oxidized Zirconium on Polyethylene	X	Diagnostic
J	Inspection	7	Sacroiliac Joint, Right			7	Autologous Tissue Substitute	Z	No Qualifier
N	Release	8	Sacroiliac Joint, Left			8	Spacer		
P	Removal	9	Hip Joint, Right			9	Liner		
Q	Repair	A	Hip Joint, Acetabular Surface, Right			A	Interbody Fusion Device		
R	Replacement	B	Hip Joint, Left			B	Resurfacing Device OR Spinal Stabilization Device, Interspinous Process		
S	Reposition	C	Knee Joint, Right			C	Spinal Stabilization Device, Pedicle-Based		
T	Resection	D	Knee Joint, Left			D	Spinal Stabilization Device, Facet Replacement		
U	Supplement	E	Hip Joint, Acetabular Surface, Left			E	Articulating Spacer		
W	Revision	F	Ankle Joint, Right			J	Synthetic Substitute		
		G	Ankle Joint, Left			K	Nonautologous Tissue Substitute		
		H	Tarsal Joint, Right			L	Synthetic Substitute, Unicondylar Medial		
		J	Tarsal Joint, Left			M	Synthetic Substitute, Unicondylar Lateral		
		K	Tarsometatarsal Joint, Right			N	Synthetic Substitute, Patellofemoral		
		L	Tarsometatarsal Joint, Left			Y	Other Device		
		M	Metatarsal-Phalangeal Joint, Right			Z	No Device		
		N	Metatarsal-Phalangeal Joint, Left						
		P	Toe Phalangeal Joint, Right						
		Q	Toe Phalangeal Joint, Left						
		R	Hip Joint, Femoral Surface, Right						
		S	Hip Joint, Femoral Surface, Left						
		T	Knee Joint, Femoral Surface, Right						
		U	Knee Joint, Femoral Surface, Left						
		V	Knee Joint, Tibial Surface, Right						
		W	Knee Joint, Tibial Surface, Left						
		Y	Lower Joint						

* Includes synovial membrane.

AHA Coding Clinic for table ØS9

| 2018, 2Q, 17 | Arthroscopic drainage of knee and nonexcisional debridement |
| 2017, 1Q, 50 | Dry aspiration of ankle joint |

AHA Coding Clinic for table ØSB

2017, 4Q, 76	Radiolucent porous interbody fusion device
2016, 2Q, 16	Decompressive laminectomy/foraminotomy and lumbar discectomy
2016, 1Q, 20	Metatarsophalangeal joint resection arthroplasty
2015, 1Q, 34	Arthroscopic meniscectomy with debridement and abrasion chondroplasty
2014, 2Q, 6	Posterior lumbar fusion with discectomy

AHA Coding Clinic for table ØSG

2023, 2Q, 25	Spinal fusion using allograft bone graft and bone marrow aspirate
2022, 3Q, 21	Breakage of intervertebral cage during surgery
2022, 2Q, 23	Sacroiliac joint fusion
2021, 4Q, 67	Posterior dynamic distraction
2021, 3Q, 24	Mid-foot fusion with bone graft
2021, 3Q, 25	Placement of X-Spine Axle Cage
2021, 1Q, 18	Placement of interspinous distraction device (spacer) for decompression
2021, 1Q, 53	Official guidelines for coding and reporting for interbody fusion device B3.10c
2020, 4Q, 56-58	Intramedullary sustained compression joint fusion
2020, 2Q, 27	Spinal fusion with NuVasive® VersaTie®
2020, 1Q, 33	Spinal fusion without use of bone graft
2019, 3Q, 35	Fusion procedures of the spine (guideline B3.10c)
2019, 1Q, 30	Spinal fusion performed at same level as decompressive laminectomy
2018, 4Q, 43	Joint fusion device value
2018, 1Q, 22	Spinal fusion procedures without bone graft
2017, 4Q, 76	Radiolucent porous interbody fusion device
2017, 2Q, 23	Decompression of spinal cord and placement of instrumentation
2014, 3Q, 30	Spinal fusion and fixation instrumentation
2014, 3Q, 36	Lumbar interbody fusion of two vertebral levels
2014, 2Q, 6	Posterior lumbar fusion with discectomy
2013, 3Q, 25	360-degree spinal fusion
2013, 2Q, 39	Ankle fusion, osteotomy, and removal of hardware
2013, 1Q, 21-23	Spinal fusion of thoracic and lumbar vertebrae

AHA Coding Clinic for table ØSH

2021, 3Q, 25	Placement of X-Spine Axle Cage
2021, 1Q, 18	Placement of interspinous distraction device (spacer) for decompression
2017, 2Q, 23	Decompression of spinal cord and placement of instrumentation

AHA Coding Clinic for table ØSJ

| 2017, 1Q, 50 | Dry aspiration of ankle joint |

AHA Coding Clinic for table ØSN

| 2020, 2Q, 26 | Arthroscopic manipulation and nonexcisional debridement of knee joint |
| 2019, 1Q, 30 | Spinal fusion performed at same level as decompressive laminectomy |

AHA Coding Clinic for table ØSP

2022, 3Q, 21	Breakage of intervertebral cage during surgery
2021, 3Q, 25	Revision total knee arthroplasty
2021, 1Q, 17	Revision of ankle arthroplasty with placement of tibial insert
2018, 4Q, 43	Articulating spacer for hip and knee joint
2018, 2Q, 16	Exchange of tibial polyethylene component with stabilizing insert (tibial tray)
2017, 4Q, 107	Total ankle replacement versus revision
2016, 4Q, 110-112	Removal and revision of hip and knee devices
2015, 2Q, 18	Total knee revision
2015, 2Q, 19	Revision of femoral head and acetabular liner
2013, 2Q, 39	Ankle fusion, osteotomy, and removal of hardware

AHA Coding Clinic for table ØSQ

| 2014, 4Q, 25 | Femoroacetabular impingement and labral tear with repair |

AHA Coding Clinic for table ØSR

2022, 1Q, 39	Provisional total hip arthroplasty
2021, 3Q, 25	Revision total knee arthroplasty
2021, 1Q, 17	Revision of ankle arthroplasty with placement of tibial insert
2020, 3Q, 33	Total hip arthroplasty using dual mobility components
2018, 4Q, 43	Articulating spacer for hip and knee joint
2018, 2Q, 16	Exchange of tibial polyethylene component with stabilizing insert (tibial tray)
2017, 4Q, 38-39	Oxidized zirconium on polyethylene bearing surface
2017, 4Q, 107	Total ankle replacement versus revision
2017, 1Q, 22	Total knee replacement and patellar component
2016, 4Q, 110-111	Partial (unicondylar) knee replacement
2016, 4Q, 111-112	Removal and revision of hip and knee devices
2016, 3Q, 35	Use of cemented versus uncemented qualifier for joint replacement
2015, 3Q, 18	Total hip replacement with acetabular reconstruction
2015, 2Q, 18	Total knee revision
2015, 2Q, 19	Revision of femoral head and acetabular liner

AHA Coding Clinic for table ØSS

2022, 3Q, 27	Ankle and tarsal joint distraction
2022, 2Q, 22	Ankle distraction procedure
2016, 2Q, 31	Periacetabular ostectomy for repair of congenital hip dysplasia

AHA Coding Clinic for table ØST

| 2016, 1Q, 20 | Metatarsophalangeal joint resection arthroplasty |
| 2014, 4Q, 29 | Rotational osteosynthesis |

AHA Coding Clinic for table ØSU

2022, 1Q, 47	Matrix-induced autologous chondrocyte implantation
2021, 1Q, 17	Revision of ankle arthroplasty with placement of tibial insert
2018, 2Q, 16	Exchange of tibial polyethylene component with stabilizing insert (tibial tray)
2016, 4Q, 111	Removal and revision of hip and knee devices
2015, 2Q, 19	Revision of femoral head and acetabular liner

AHA Coding Clinic for table ØSW

2017, 4Q, 107	Total ankle replacement versus revision
2016, 4Q, 110-112	Removal and revision of hip and knee devices
2015, 2Q, 18	Total knee revision
2015, 2Q, 19	Revision of femoral head and acetabular liner

Lower Joints

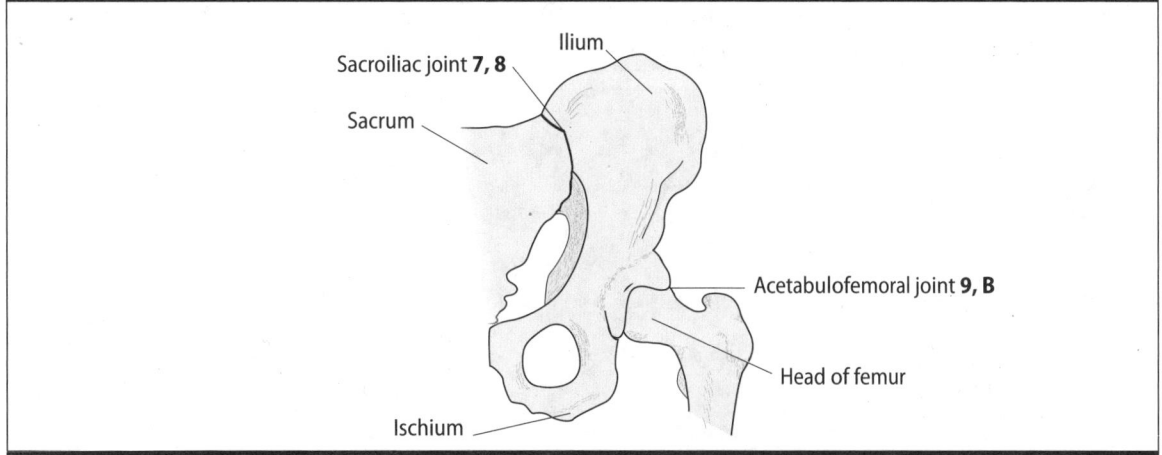

Sacroiliac **7, 8**

Lumbosacral **3**

Sacrococcygeal joint **5**

Hip **9, B**

Knee **C, D**

Ankle **F, G**

(Transverse) tarsal **H, J**

Metatarsal-phalangeal **M, N**

Hip Joint

Sacroiliac joint **7, 8**

Ilium

Sacrum

Acetabulofemoral joint **9, B**

Head of femur

Ischium

Knee Joint

Anterior view

Patella

Medial meniscus cartilage

Lateral meniscus cartilage

Lateral view

Femur

Synovial cavity

Patella

Tibia

Foot Joints

Phalanges

Metatarso-phalangeal joints **M, N**

Tarsal joints **H, J**

Tarsometatarsal joints **K, L**

Distal interphalangeal joint **P, Q**

Proximal interphalangeal joint **P, Q**

Tarsals

Metatarsals

0   **Medical and Surgical**
S   **Lower Joints**
2   **Change**   Definition: Taking out or off a device from a body part and putting back an identical or similar device in or on the same body part without cutting or puncturing the skin or a mucous membrane

                      Explanation: All CHANGE procedures are coded using the approach EXTERNAL

Body Part Character 4	Approach Character 5	Device Character 6	Qualifier Character 7
Y Lower Joint	X External	0 Drainage Device Y Other Device	Z No Qualifier

     Non-OR   All body part, approach, device, and qualifier values

---

0   **Medical and Surgical**
S   **Lower Joints**
5   **Destruction**   Definition: Physical eradication of all or a portion of a body part by the direct use of energy, force, or a destructive agent

                      Explanation: None of the body part is physically taken out

Body Part Character 4	Approach Character 5	Device Character 6	Qualifier Character 7

0   Lumbar Vertebral Joint
     Lumbar facet joint
2   Lumbar Vertebral Disc
3   Lumbosacral Joint
     Lumbosacral facet joint
4   Lumbosacral Disc
5   Sacrococcygeal Joint
     Sacrococcygeal symphysis
6   Coccygeal Joint
7   Sacroiliac Joint, Right
8   Sacroiliac Joint, Left
9   Hip Joint, Right
     Acetabulofemoral joint
B   Hip Joint, Left
     See 9 Hip Joint, Right
C   Knee Joint, Right
     Femoropatellar joint
     Femorotibial joint
     Lateral meniscus
     Medial meniscus
     Patellofemoral joint
     Tibiofemoral joint
D   Knee Joint, Left
     See C Knee Joint, Right
F   Ankle Joint, Right
     Inferior tibiofibular joint
     Talocrural joint
G   Ankle Joint, Left
     See F Ankle Joint, Right
H   Tarsal Joint, Right
     Calcaneocuboid joint
     Cuboideonavicular joint
     Cuneonavicular joint
     Intercuneiform joint
     Subtalar (talocalcaneal) joint
     Talocalcaneal (subtalar) joint
     Talocalcaneonavicular joint
J   Tarsal Joint, Left
     See H Tarsal Joint, Right
K   Tarsometatarsal Joint, Right
L   Tarsometatarsal Joint, Left
M   Metatarsal-Phalangeal Joint, Right
     Metatarsophalangeal (MTP) joint
N   Metatarsal-Phalangeal Joint, Left
     See M Metatarsal-Phalangeal Joint, Right
P   Toe Phalangeal Joint, Right
     Interphalangeal (IP) joint
Q   Toe Phalangeal Joint, Left
     See P Toe Phalangeal Joint, Right
	0 Open
	3 Percutaneous
	4 Percutaneous Endoscopic
		Z No Device	Z No Qualifier

NC Noncovered Procedure   **LC** Limited Coverage   **QA** Questionable OB Admit   **NT** New Tech Add-on   ⊞ Combination Member   ♂ Male   ♀ Female

ICD-10-PCS 2024   607

0S2–0S5

Ø Medical and Surgical
S Lower Joints
9 Drainage   Definition: Taking or letting out fluids and/or gases from a body part
Explanation: The qualifier DIAGNOSTIC is used to identify drainage procedures that are biopsies

Body Part Character 4		Approach Character 5	Device Character 6	Qualifier Character 7
Ø Lumbar Vertebral Joint Lumbar facet joint 2 Lumbar Vertebral Disc 3 Lumbosacral Joint Lumbosacral facet joint 4 Lumbosacral Disc 5 Sacrococcygeal Joint Sacrococcygeal symphysis 6 Coccygeal Joint 7 Sacroiliac Joint, Right 8 Sacroiliac Joint, Left 9 Hip Joint, Right Acetabulofemoral joint B Hip Joint, Left *See 9 Hip Joint, Right* C Knee Joint, Right Femoropatellar joint Femorotibial joint Lateral meniscus Medial meniscus Patellofemoral joint Tibiofemoral joint D Knee Joint, Left *See C Knee Joint, Right* F Ankle Joint, Right Inferior tibiofibular joint Talocrural joint G Ankle Joint, Left *See F Ankle Joint, Right*	H Tarsal Joint, Right Calcaneocuboid joint Cuboideonavicular joint Cuneonavicular joint Intercuneiform joint Subtalar (talocalcaneal) joint Talocalcaneal (subtalar) joint Talocalcaneonavicular joint J Tarsal Joint, Left *See H Tarsal Joint, Right* K Tarsometatarsal Joint, Right L Tarsometatarsal Joint, Left M Metatarsal-Phalangeal Joint, Right Metatarsophalangeal (MTP) joint N Metatarsal-Phalangeal Joint, Left *See M Metatarsal-Phalangeal Joint, Right* P Toe Phalangeal Joint, Right Interphalangeal (IP) joint Q Toe Phalangeal Joint, Left *See P Toe Phalangeal Joint, Right*	Ø Open 3 Percutaneous 4 Percutaneous Endoscopic	Ø Drainage Device	Z No Qualifier
Ø Lumbar Vertebral Joint Lumbar facet joint 2 Lumbar Vertebral Disc 3 Lumbosacral Joint Lumbosacral facet joint 4 Lumbosacral Disc 5 Sacrococcygeal Joint Sacrococcygeal symphysis 6 Coccygeal Joint 7 Sacroiliac Joint, Right 8 Sacroiliac Joint, Left 9 Hip Joint, Right Acetabulofemoral joint B Hip Joint, Left *See 9 Hip Joint, Right* C Knee Joint, Right Femoropatellar joint Femorotibial joint Lateral meniscus Medial meniscus Patellofemoral joint Tibiofemoral joint D Knee Joint, Left *See C Knee Joint, Right* F Ankle Joint, Right Inferior tibiofibular joint Talocrural joint G Ankle Joint, Left *See F Ankle Joint, Right*	H Tarsal Joint, Right Calcaneocuboid joint Cuboideonavicular joint Cuneonavicular joint Intercuneiform joint Subtalar (talocalcaneal) joint Talocalcaneal (subtalar) joint Talocalcaneonavicular joint J Tarsal Joint, Left *See H Tarsal Joint, Right* K Tarsometatarsal Joint, Right L Tarsometatarsal Joint, Left M Metatarsal-Phalangeal Joint, Right Metatarsophalangeal (MTP) joint N Metatarsal-Phalangeal Joint, Left *See M Metatarsal-Phalangeal Joint, Right* P Toe Phalangeal Joint, Right Interphalangeal (IP) joint Q Toe Phalangeal Joint, Left *See P Toe Phalangeal Joint, Right*	Ø Open 3 Percutaneous 4 Percutaneous Endoscopic	Z No Device	X Diagnostic Z No Qualifier

Non-OR   ØS9[Ø,2,3,4,5,6,7,8,9,B,C,D,F,G,H,J,K,L,M,N,P,Q][3,4]ØZ
Non-OR   ØS9[Ø,2,3,4,5,6,7,8,9,B,C,D,F,G,H,J,K,L,M,N,P,Q][Ø,3,4]ZX
Non-OR   ØS9[Ø,2,3,4,5,6,7,8,9,B,C,D,F,G,H,J,K,L,M,N,P,Q][3,4]ZZ

Non-OR Procedure   DRG Non-OR Procedure   Valid OR Procedure   HAC Associated Procedure   Combination Only   New/Revised April   New/Revised October
608   ICD-10-PCS 2024

ØS9–ØS9

Ø   Medical and Surgical
S   Lower Joints
B   Excision   Definition: Cutting out or off, without replacement, a portion of a body part
                     Explanation: The qualifier DIAGNOSTIC is used to identify excision procedures that are biopsies

Body Part Character 4	Approach Character 5	Device Character 6	Qualifier Character 7
Ø Lumbar Vertebral Joint Lumbar facet joint **2 Lumbar Vertebral Disc** **3 Lumbosacral Joint** Lumbosacral facet joint **4 Lumbosacral Disc** **5 Sacrococcygeal Joint** Sacrococcygeal symphysis **6 Coccygeal Joint** **7 Sacroiliac Joint, Right** **8 Sacroiliac Joint, Left** **9 Hip Joint, Right** Acetabulofemoral joint **B Hip Joint, Left** *See 9 Hip Joint, Right* **C Knee Joint, Right** Femoropatellar joint Femorotibial joint Lateral meniscus Medial meniscus Patellofemoral joint Tibiofemoral joint **D Knee Joint, Left** *See C Knee Joint, Right* **F Ankle Joint, Right** Inferior tibiofibular joint Talocrural joint **G Ankle Joint, Left** *See F Ankle Joint, Right* **H Tarsal Joint, Right** Calcaneocuboid joint Cuboideonavicular joint Cuneonavicular joint Intercuneiform joint Subtalar (talocalcaneal) joint Talocalcaneal (subtalar) joint Talocalcaneonavicular joint **J Tarsal Joint, Left** *See H Tarsal Joint, Right* **K Tarsometatarsal Joint, Right** **L Tarsometatarsal Joint, Left** **M Metatarsal-Phalangeal Joint, Right** Metatarsophalangeal (MTP) joint **N Metatarsal-Phalangeal Joint, Left** *See M Metatarsal-Phalangeal Joint, Right* **P Toe Phalangeal Joint, Right** Interphalangeal (IP) joint **Q Toe Phalangeal Joint, Left** *See P Toe Phalangeal Joint, Right*	**Ø** Open **3** Percutaneous **4** Percutaneous Endoscopic	**Z** No Device	**X** Diagnostic **Z** No Qualifier

Non-OR   ØSB[Ø,2,3,4,5,6,7,8,9,B,C,D,F,G,H,J,K,L,M,N,P,Q][Ø,3,4]ZX

Lower Joints *(left margin)*

Ø   **Medical and Surgical**
S   **Lower Joints**
C   **Extirpation**   Definition: Taking or cutting out solid matter from a body part

Explanation: The solid matter may be an abnormal byproduct of a biological function or a foreign body; it may be imbedded in a body part or in the lumen of a tubular body part. The solid matter may or may not have been previously broken into pieces.

Body Part Character 4	Approach Character 5	Device Character 6	Qualifier Character 7

Ø Lumbar Vertebral Joint
  Lumbar facet joint
2 Lumbar Vertebral Disc
3 Lumbosacral Joint
  Lumbosacral facet joint
4 Lumbosacral Disc
5 Sacrococcygeal Joint
  Sacrococcygeal symphysis
6 Coccygeal Joint
7 Sacroiliac Joint, Right
8 Sacroiliac Joint, Left
9 Hip Joint, Right
  Acetabulofemoral joint
B Hip Joint, Left
  See 9 Hip Joint, Right
C Knee Joint, Right
  Femoropatellar joint
  Femorotibial joint
  Lateral meniscus
  Medial meniscus
  Patellofemoral joint
  Tibiofemoral joint
D Knee Joint, Left
  See C Knee Joint, Right
F Ankle Joint, Right
  Inferior tibiofibular joint
  Talocrural joint
G Ankle Joint, Left
  See F Ankle Joint, Right
H Tarsal Joint, Right
  Calcaneocuboid joint
  Cuboideonavicular joint
  Cuneonavicular joint
  Intercuneiform joint
  Subtalar (talocalcaneal) joint
  Talocalcaneal (subtalar) joint
  Talocalcaneonavicular joint
J Tarsal Joint, Left
  See H Tarsal Joint, Right
K Tarsometatarsal Joint, Right
L Tarsometatarsal Joint, Left
M Metatarsal-Phalangeal Joint, Right
  Metatarsophalangeal (MTP) joint
N Metatarsal-Phalangeal Joint, Left
  See M Metatarsal-Phalangeal Joint, Right
P Toe Phalangeal Joint, Right
  Interphalangeal (IP) joint
Q Toe Phalangeal Joint, Left
  See P Toe Phalangeal Joint, Right
	Ø Open
	3 Percutaneous
	4 Percutaneous Endoscopic
		Z No Device	Z No Qualifier

Ø Medical and Surgical
S Lower Joints
G Fusion   Definition: Joining together portions of an articular body part rendering the articular body part immobile
                     Explanation: The body part is joined together by fixation device, bone graft, or other means

Body Part Character 4	Approach Character 5	Device Character 6	Qualifier Character 7
Ø Lumbar Vertebral Joint Lumbar facet joint **1 Lumbar Vertebral Joints, 2 or more** ⊞ **3 Lumbosacral Joint** Lumbosacral facet joint	**Ø** Open **3** Percutaneous **4** Percutaneous Endoscopic	**7** Autologous Tissue Substitute **J** Synthetic Substitute **K** Nonautologous Tissue Substitute	**Ø** Anterior Approach, Anterior Column **1** Posterior Approach, Posterior Column **J** Posterior Approach, Anterior Column
Ø Lumbar Vertebral Joint Lumbar facet joint **1 Lumbar Vertebral Joints, 2 or more** ⊞ **3 Lumbosacral Joint** Lumbosacral facet joint	**Ø** Open **3** Percutaneous **4** Percutaneous Endoscopic	**A** Interbody Fusion Device	**Ø** Anterior Approach, Anterior Column **J** Posterior Approach, Anterior Column
5 Sacrococcygeal Joint Sacrococcygeal symphysis **6 Coccygeal Joint** **7 Sacroiliac Joint, Right** **8 Sacroiliac Joint, Left**	**Ø** Open **3** Percutaneous **4** Percutaneous Endoscopic	**4** Internal Fixation Device **7** Autologous Tissue Substitute **J** Synthetic Substitute **K** Nonautologous Tissue Substitute	**Z** No Qualifier
9 Hip Joint, Right Acetabulofemoral joint **B Hip Joint, Left** *See 9 Hip Joint, Right* **C Knee Joint, Right** Femoropatellar joint Femorotibial joint Lateral meniscus Medial meniscus Patellofemoral joint Tibiofemoral joint **D Knee Joint, Left** *See C Knee Joint, Right* **F Ankle Joint, Right** Inferior tibiofibular joint Talocrural joint **G Ankle Joint, Left** *See F Ankle Joint, Right* **H Tarsal Joint, Right** Calcaneocuboid joint Cuboideonavicular joint Cuneonavicular joint Intercuneiform joint Subtalar (talocalcaneal) joint Talocalcaneal (subtalar) joint Talocalcaneonavicular joint **J Tarsal Joint, Left** *See H Tarsal Joint, Right* **K Tarsometatarsal Joint, Right** **L Tarsometatarsal Joint, Left** **M Metatarsal-Phalangeal Joint, Right** Metatarsophalangeal (MTP) joint **N Metatarsal-Phalangeal Joint, Left** *See M Metatarsal-Phalangeal Joint, Right* **P Toe Phalangeal Joint, Right** Interphalangeal (IP) joint **Q Toe Phalangeal Joint, Left** *See P Toe Phalangeal Joint, Right*	**Ø** Open **3** Percutaneous **4** Percutaneous Endoscopic	**3** Internal Fixation Device, Sustained Compression **4** Internal Fixation Device **5** External Fixation Device **7** Autologous Tissue Substitute **J** Synthetic Substitute **K** Nonautologous Tissue Substitute	**Z** No Qualifier

HAC   ØSG[Ø,1,3][Ø,3,4][7,J,K][Ø,1,J] when reported with SDx K68.11 or T81.4Ø–T81.49, T84.6Ø-T84.619, T84.63-T84.7 with 7th character A
HAC   ØSG[Ø,1,3][Ø,3,4]A[Ø,J] when reported with SDx K68.11 or T81.4Ø–T81.49, T84.6Ø-T84.619, T84.63-T84.7 with 7th character A
HAC   ØSG[7,8][Ø,3,4][4,7,J,K]Z when reported with SDx K68.11 or T81.4Ø–T81.49, T84.6Ø-T84.619, T84.63-T84.7 with 7th character A

See Appendix L for Procedure Combinations
⊞   ØSG1[Ø,3,4][7,J,K][Ø,1,J]
⊞   ØSG1[Ø,3,4]A[Ø,J]

Lower Joints

Ø	Medical and Surgical	
S	Lower Joints	
H	Insertion	Definition: Putting in a nonbiological appliance that monitors, assists, performs, or prevents a physiological function but does not physically take the place of a body part
		Explanation: None

Body Part Character 4	Approach Character 5	Device Character 6	Qualifier Character 7

Ø Lumbar Vertebral Joint
   Lumbar facet joint
3 Lumbosacral Joint
   Lumbosacral facet joint
	Ø Open
	3 Percutaneous
	4 Percutaneous Endoscopic
		3 Infusion Device
		4 Internal Fixation Device
		8 Spacer
		B Spinal Stabilization Device,
		   Interspinous Process
		C Spinal Stabilization Device,
		   Pedicle-Based
		D Spinal Stabilization Device, Facet
		   Replacement
			Z No Qualifier

2 Lumbar Vertebral Disc 4 Lumbosacral Disc	Ø Open 3 Percutaneous 4 Percutaneous Endoscopic	3 Infusion Device 8 Spacer	Z No Qualifier
5 Sacrococcygeal Joint Sacrococcygeal symphysis 6 Coccygeal Joint 7 Sacroiliac Joint, Right 8 Sacroiliac Joint, Left	Ø Open 3 Percutaneous 4 Percutaneous Endoscopic	3 Infusion Device 4 Internal Fixation Device 8 Spacer	Z No Qualifier

9 Hip Joint, Right
   Acetabulofemoral joint
B Hip Joint, Left
   See 9 Hip Joint, Right
C Knee Joint, Right
   Femoropatellar joint
   Femorotibial joint
   Lateral meniscus
   Medial meniscus
   Patellofemoral joint
   Tibiofemoral joint
D Knee Joint, Left
   See C Knee Joint, Right
F Ankle Joint, Right
   Inferior tibiofibular joint
   Talocrural joint
G Ankle Joint, Left
   See F Ankle Joint, Right
H Tarsal Joint, Right
   Calcaneocuboid joint
   Cuboideonavicular joint
   Cuneonavicular joint
   Intercuneiform joint
   Subtalar (talocalcaneal) joint
   Talocalcaneal (subtalar) joint
   Talocalcaneonavicular joint
J Tarsal Joint, Left
   See H Tarsal Joint, Right
K Tarsometatarsal Joint, Right
L Tarsometatarsal Joint, Left
M Metatarsal-Phalangeal Joint, Right
   Metatarsophalangeal (MTP) joint
N Metatarsal-Phalangeal Joint, Left
   See M Metatarsal-Phalangeal Joint, Right
P Toe Phalangeal Joint, Right
   Interphalangeal (IP) joint
Q Toe Phalangeal Joint, Left
   See P Toe Phalangeal Joint, Right
	Ø Open
	3 Percutaneous
	4 Percutaneous Endoscopic
		3 Infusion Device
		4 Internal Fixation Device
		5 External Fixation Device
		8 Spacer
			Z No Qualifier

Non-OR	ØSH[Ø,3][Ø,3,4][3,8]Z
Non-OR	ØSH[2,4][Ø,3,4][3,8]Z
Non-OR	ØSH[5,6,7,8][Ø,3,4][3,8]Z
Non-OR	ØSH[9,B,C,D][Ø,3,4]3Z
Non-OR	ØSH[9,B,C,D][3,4]8Z
Non-OR	ØSH[F,G,H,J,K,L,M,N,P,Q][Ø,3,4][3,8]Z

Non-OR Procedure   DRG Non-OR Procedure   Valid OR Procedure   HAC Associated Procedure   Combination Only   New/Revised April   New/Revised October

612   ICD-10-PCS 2024

Ø　Medical and Surgical
S　Lower Joints
J　Inspection　　Definition: Visually and/or manually exploring a body part

Explanation: Visual exploration may be performed with or without optical instrumentation. Manual exploration may be performed directly or through intervening body layers.

Body Part Character 4		Approach Character 5	Device Character 6	Qualifier Character 7
Ø　Lumbar Vertebral Joint 　　Lumbar facet joint 2　Lumbar Vertebral Disc 3　Lumbosacral Joint 　　Lumbosacral facet joint 4　Lumbosacral Disc 5　Sacrococcygeal Joint 　　Sacrococcygeal symphysis 6　Coccygeal Joint 7　Sacroiliac Joint, Right 8　Sacroiliac Joint, Left 9　Hip Joint, Right 　　Acetabulofemoral joint B　Hip Joint, Left 　　*See* 9 Hip Joint, Right C　Knee Joint, Right 　　Femoropatellar joint 　　Femorotibial joint 　　Lateral meniscus 　　Medial meniscus 　　Patellofemoral joint 　　Tibiofemoral joint D　Knee Joint, Left 　　*See* C Knee Joint, Right F　Ankle Joint, Right 　　Inferior tibiofibular joint 　　Talocrural joint G　Ankle Joint, Left 　　*See* F Ankle Joint, Right	H　Tarsal Joint, Right 　　Calcaneocuboid joint 　　Cuboideonavicular joint 　　Cuneonavicular joint 　　Intercuneiform joint 　　Subtalar (talocalcaneal) joint 　　Talocalcaneal (subtalar) joint 　　Talocalcaneonavicular joint J　Tarsal Joint, Left 　　*See* H Tarsal Joint, Right K　Tarsometatarsal Joint, 　　Right L　Tarsometatarsal Joint, Left M　Metatarsal-Phalangeal 　　Joint, Right 　　Metatarsophalangeal (MTP) 　　joint N　Metatarsal-Phalangeal 　　Joint, Left 　　*See* M Metatarsal-Phalangeal 　　Joint, Right P　Toe Phalangeal Joint, Right 　　Interphalangeal (IP) joint Q　Toe Phalangeal Joint, Left 　　*See* P Toe Phalangeal Joint, 　　Right	Ø　Open 3　Percutaneous 4　Percutaneous Endoscopic X　External	Z　No Device	Z　No Qualifier

Non-OR　ØSJ[Ø,2,3,4,5,6,7,8,9,B,C,D,F,G,H,J,K,L,M,N,P,Q][3,X]ZZ

Ø　Medical and Surgical
S　Lower Joints
N　Release　　Definition: Freeing a body part from an abnormal physical constraint by cutting or by the use of force

Explanation: Some of the restraining tissue may be taken out but none of the body part is taken out

Body Part Character 4		Approach Character 5	Device Character 6	Qualifier Character 7
Ø　Lumbar Vertebral Joint 　　Lumbar facet joint 2　Lumbar Vertebral Disc 3　Lumbosacral Joint 　　Lumbosacral facet joint 4　Lumbosacral Disc 5　Sacrococcygeal Joint 　　Sacrococcygeal symphysis 6　Coccygeal Joint 7　Sacroiliac Joint, Right 8　Sacroiliac Joint, Left 9　Hip Joint, Right 　　Acetabulofemoral joint B　Hip Joint, Left 　　*See* 9 Hip Joint, Right C　Knee Joint, Right 　　Femoropatellar joint 　　Femorotibial joint 　　Lateral meniscus 　　Medial meniscus 　　Patellofemoral joint 　　Tibiofemoral joint D　Knee Joint, Left 　　*See* C Knee Joint, Right F　Ankle Joint, Right 　　Inferior tibiofibular joint 　　Talocrural joint G　Ankle Joint, Left 　　*See* F Ankle Joint, Right	H　Tarsal Joint, Right 　　Calcaneocuboid joint 　　Cuboideonavicular joint 　　Cuneonavicular joint 　　Intercuneiform joint 　　Subtalar (talocalcaneal) joint 　　Talocalcaneal (subtalar) joint 　　Talocalcaneonavicular joint J　Tarsal Joint, Left 　　*See* H Tarsal Joint, Right K　Tarsometatarsal Joint, 　　Right L　Tarsometatarsal Joint, Left M　Metatarsal-Phalangeal 　　Joint, Right 　　Metatarsophalangeal (MTP) 　　joint N　Metatarsal-Phalangeal 　　Joint, Left 　　*See* M Metatarsal-Phalangeal 　　Joint, Right P　Toe Phalangeal Joint, Right 　　Interphalangeal (IP) joint Q　Toe Phalangeal Joint, Left 　　*See* P Toe Phalangeal Joint, 　　Right	Ø　Open 3　Percutaneous 4　Percutaneous Endoscopic X　External	Z　No Device	Z　No Qualifier

Non-OR　ØSN[Ø,2,3,4,5,6,7,8,9,B,C,D,F,G,H,J,K,L,M,N,P,Q]XZZ

NC Noncovered Procedure　　**LC** Limited Coverage　　**QA** Questionable OB Admit　　**NT** New Tech Add-on　　⊞ Combination Member　　♂ Male　　♀ Female

ICD-10-PCS 2024　　　613

ØSJ–ØSN

Lower Joints

Ø Medical and Surgical
S Lower Joints
P Removal   Definition: Taking out or off a device from a body part

Explanation: If a device is taken out and a similar device put in without cutting or puncturing the skin or mucous membrane, the procedure is coded to the root operation CHANGE. Otherwise, the procedure for taking out the device is coded to the root operation REMOVAL.

Body Part Character 4	Approach Character 5	Device Character 6	Qualifier Character 7
Ø Lumbar Vertebral Joint Lumbar facet joint 3 Lumbosacral Joint Lumbosacral facet joint	Ø Open 3 Percutaneous 4 Percutaneous Endoscopic	Ø Drainage Device 3 Infusion Device 4 Internal Fixation Device 7 Autologous Tissue Substitute 8 Spacer A Interbody Fusion Device J Synthetic Substitute K Nonautologous Tissue Substitute	Z No Qualifier
Ø Lumbar Vertebral Joint Lumbar facet joint 3 Lumbosacral Joint Lumbosacral facet joint	X External	Ø Drainage Device 3 Infusion Device 4 Internal Fixation Device	Z No Qualifier
2 Lumbar Vertebral Disc 4 Lumbosacral Disc	Ø Open 3 Percutaneous 4 Percutaneous Endoscopic	Ø Drainage Device 3 Infusion Device 7 Autologous Tissue Substitute J Synthetic Substitute K Nonautologous Tissue Substitute	Z No Qualifier
2 Lumbar Vertebral Disc 4 Lumbosacral Disc	X External	Ø Drainage Device 3 Infusion Device	Z No Qualifier
5 Sacrococcygeal Joint Sacrococcygeal symphysis 6 Coccygeal Joint 7 Sacroiliac Joint, Right 8 Sacroiliac Joint, Left	Ø Open 3 Percutaneous 4 Percutaneous Endoscopic	Ø Drainage Device 3 Infusion Device 4 Internal Fixation Device 7 Autologous Tissue Substitute 8 Spacer J Synthetic Substitute K Nonautologous Tissue Substitute	Z No Qualifier
5 Sacrococcygeal Joint Sacrococcygeal symphysis 6 Coccygeal Joint 7 Sacroiliac Joint, Right 8 Sacroiliac Joint, Left	X External	Ø Drainage Device 3 Infusion Device 4 Internal Fixation Device	Z No Qualifier
9 Hip Joint, Right ⊞ Acetabulofemoral joint B Hip Joint, Left ⊞ See 9 Hip Joint, Right	Ø Open	Ø Drainage Device 3 Infusion Device 4 Internal Fixation Device 5 External Fixation Device 7 Autologous Tissue Substitute 8 Spacer 9 Liner B Resurfacing Device E Articulating Spacer J Synthetic Substitute K Nonautologous Tissue Substitute	Z No Qualifier
9 Hip Joint, Right ⊞ Acetabulofemoral joint B Hip Joint, Left ⊞ See 9 Hip Joint, Right	3 Percutaneous 4 Percutaneous Endoscopic	Ø Drainage Device 3 Infusion Device 4 Internal Fixation Device 5 External Fixation Device 7 Autologous Tissue Substitute 8 Spacer J Synthetic Substitute K Nonautologous Tissue Substitute	Z No Qualifier
9 Hip Joint, Right Acetabulofemoral joint B Hip Joint, Left See 9 Hip Joint, Right	X External	Ø Drainage Device 3 Infusion Device 4 Internal Fixation Device 5 External Fixation Device	Z No Qualifier

Non-OR	ØSP[Ø,3][Ø,3,4]8Z	
Non-OR	ØSP[Ø,3]3[Ø,3]Z	
Non-OR	ØSP[Ø,3]X[Ø,3,4]Z	
Non-OR	ØSP[2,4]3[Ø,3]Z	
Non-OR	ØSP[2,4]X[Ø,3]Z	
Non-OR	ØSP[5,6,7,8][Ø,3,4]8Z	
Non-OR	ØSP[5,6,7,8]3[Ø,3]Z	
Non-OR	ØSP[5,6,7,8]X[Ø,3,4]Z	
Non-OR	ØSP[9,B]3[Ø,3,8]Z	
Non-OR	ØSP[9,B]X[Ø,3,4,5]Z	

See Appendix L for Procedure Combinations
Combo-only   ØSP[9,B]48Z
⊞   ØSP[9,B]Ø[8,9,B,E,J]Z
⊞   ØSP[9,B]4JZ

ØSP Continued on next page

Non-OR Procedure   DRG Non-OR Procedure   Valid OR Procedure   HAC Associated Procedure   Combination Only   New/Revised April   New/Revised October

Ø   Medical and Surgical
S   Lower Joints
P   Removal   Definition: Taking out or off a device from a body part

ØSP Continued

Explanation: If a device is taken out and a similar device put in without cutting or puncturing the skin or mucous membrane, the procedure is coded to the root operation CHANGE. Otherwise, the procedure for taking out the device is coded to the root operation REMOVAL.

Body Part Character 4	Approach Character 5	Device Character 6	Qualifier Character 7

A Hip Joint, Acetabular Surface, Right ⊞
E Hip Joint, Acetabular Surface, Left ⊞
R Hip Joint, Femoral Surface, Right ⊞
S Hip Joint, Femoral Surface, Left ⊞
T Knee Joint, Femoral Surface, Right ⊞
    Femoropatellar joint
    Patellofemoral joint
U Knee Joint, Femoral Surface, Left ⊞
    See T Knee Joint, Femoral Surface, Right
V Knee Joint, Tibial Surface, Right ⊞
    Femorotibial joint
    Tibiofemoral joint
W Knee Joint, Tibial Surface, Left ⊞
    See V Knee Joint, Tibial Surface, Right
	Ø Open
	3 Percutaneous
	4 Percutaneous Endoscopic
		J Synthetic Substitute	Z No Qualifier

C Knee Joint, Right ⊞
    Femoropatellar joint
    Femorotibial joint
    Lateral meniscus
    Medial meniscus
    Patellofemoral joint
    Tibiofemoral joint
D Knee Joint, Left ⊞
    See C Knee Joint, Right
	Ø Open	Ø Drainage Device
		3 Infusion Device
		4 Internal Fixation Device
		5 External Fixation Device
		7 Autologous Tissue Substitute
		8 Spacer
		9 Liner
		E Articulating Spacer
		K Nonautologous Tissue Substitute
		L Synthetic Substitute, Unicondylar Medial
		M Synthetic Substitute, Unicondylar Lateral
		N Synthetic Substitute, Patellofemoral
			Z No Qualifier

C Knee Joint, Right ⊞
    Femoropatellar joint
    Femorotibial joint
    Lateral meniscus
    Medial meniscus
    Patellofemoral joint
    Tibiofemoral joint
D Knee Joint, Left ⊞
    See C Knee Joint, Right
	Ø Open	J Synthetic Substitute	C Patellar Surface
			Z No Qualifier

C Knee Joint, Right ⊞
    Femoropatellar joint
    Femorotibial joint
    Lateral meniscus
    Medial meniscus
    Patellofemoral joint
    Tibiofemoral joint
D Knee Joint, Left ⊞
    See C Knee Joint, Right
	3 Percutaneous
	4 Percutaneous Endoscopic
		Ø Drainage Device
		3 Infusion Device
		4 Internal Fixation Device
		5 External Fixation Device
		7 Autologous Tissue Substitute
		8 Spacer
		K Nonautologous Tissue Substitute
		L Synthetic Substitute, Unicondylar Medial
		M Synthetic Substitute, Unicondylar Lateral
		N Synthetic Substitute, Patellofemoral
			Z No Qualifier

C Knee Joint, Right ⊞
    Femoropatellar joint
    Femorotibial joint
    Lateral meniscus
    Medial meniscus
    Patellofemoral joint
    Tibiofemoral joint
D Knee Joint, Left ⊞
    See C Knee Joint, Right
	3 Percutaneous
	4 Percutaneous Endoscopic
		J Synthetic Substitute	C Patellar Surface
			Z No Qualifier

Non-OR   ØSP[C,D]3[Ø,3]Z

See Appendix L for Procedure Combinations
Combo-only   ØSP[C,D][3,4]8Z
⊞   ØSP[A,E,R,S,T,U,V,W][Ø,4]JZ
⊞   ØSP[C,D]Ø[8,9,E,L,M,N]Z
⊞   ØSP[C,D]ØJ[C,Z]
⊞   ØSP[C,D]4[L,M,N]Z
⊞   ØSP[C,D]4J[C,Z]

ØSP Continued on next page

NC Noncovered Procedure   **LC** Limited Coverage   **QA** Questionable OB Admit   **NT** New Tech Add-on   ⊞ Combination Member   ♂ Male   ♀ Female

ICD-10-PCS 2024   615

ØSP–ØSP

Ø Medical and Surgical *ØSP Continued*
S Lower Joints
P Removal Definition: Taking out or off a device from a body part

Explanation: If a device is taken out and a similar device put in without cutting or puncturing the skin or mucous membrane, the procedure is coded to the root operation CHANGE. Otherwise, the procedure for taking out the device is coded to the root operation REMOVAL.

Body Part Character 4	Approach Character 5	Device Character 6	Qualifier Character 7
C Knee Joint, Right Femoropatellar joint Femorotibial joint Lateral meniscus Medial meniscus Patellofemoral joint Tibiofemoral joint **D** Knee Joint, Left *See C Knee Joint, Right*	**X** External	**Ø** Drainage Device **3** Infusion Device **4** Internal Fixation Device **5** External Fixation Device	**Z** No Qualifier
F Ankle Joint, Right Inferior tibiofibular joint Talocrural joint **G** Ankle Joint, Left *See F Ankle Joint, Right* **H** Tarsal Joint, Right Calcaneocuboid joint Cuboideonavicular joint Cuneonavicular joint Intercuneiform joint Subtalar (talocalcaneal) joint Talocalcaneal (subtalar) joint Talocalcaneonavicular joint **J** Tarsal Joint, Left *See H Tarsal Joint, Right* **K** Tarsometatarsal Joint, Right **L** Tarsometatarsal Joint, Left **M** Metatarsal-Phalangeal Joint, Right Metatarsophalangeal (MTP) joint **N** Metatarsal-Phalangeal Joint, Left *See M Metatarsal-Phalangeal Joint, Right* **P** Toe Phalangeal Joint, Right Interphalangeal (IP) joint **Q** Toe Phalangeal Joint, Left *See P Toe Phalangeal Joint, Right*	**Ø** Open **3** Percutaneous **4** Percutaneous Endoscopic	**Ø** Drainage Device **3** Infusion Device **4** Internal Fixation Device **5** External Fixation Device **7** Autologous Tissue Substitute **8** Spacer **J** Synthetic Substitute **K** Nonautologous Tissue Substitute	**Z** No Qualifier
F Ankle Joint, Right Inferior tibiofibular joint Talocrural joint **G** Ankle Joint, Left *See F Ankle Joint, Right* **H** Tarsal Joint, Right Calcaneocuboid joint Cuboideonavicular joint Cuneonavicular joint Intercuneiform joint Subtalar (talocalcaneal) joint Talocalcaneal (subtalar) joint Talocalcaneonavicular joint **J** Tarsal Joint, Left *See H Tarsal Joint, Right* **K** Tarsometatarsal Joint, Right **L** Tarsometatarsal Joint, Left **M** Metatarsal-Phalangeal Joint, Right Metatarsophalangeal (MTP) joint **N** Metatarsal-Phalangeal Joint, Left *See M Metatarsal-Phalangeal Joint, Right* **P** Toe Phalangeal Joint, Right Interphalangeal (IP) joint **Q** Toe Phalangeal Joint, Left *See P Toe Phalangeal Joint, Right*	**X** External	**Ø** Drainage Device **3** Infusion Device **4** Internal Fixation Device **5** External Fixation Device	**Z** No Qualifier

Non-OR ØSP[C,D]X[Ø,3,4,5]Z
Non-OR ØSP[F,G,H,J,K,L,M,N,P,Q]3[Ø,3,8]Z
Non-OR ØSP[F,G,H,J,K,L,M,N,P,Q][Ø,4]8Z
Non-OR ØSP[F,G,H,J,K,L,M,N,P,Q]X[Ø,3,4,5]Z

Ø   Medical and Surgical
S   Lower Joints
Q   Repair   Definition: Restoring, to the extent possible, a body part to its normal anatomic structure and function
                          Explanation: Used only when the method to accomplish the repair is not one of the other root operations

Body Part Character 4	Approach Character 5	Device Character 6	Qualifier Character 7
Ø Lumbar Vertebral Joint Lumbar facet joint **2 Lumbar Vertebral Disc** **3 Lumbosacral Joint** Lumbosacral facet joint **4 Lumbosacral Disc** **5 Sacrococcygeal Joint** Sacrococcygeal symphysis **6 Coccygeal Joint** **7 Sacroiliac Joint, Right** **8 Sacroiliac Joint, Left** **9 Hip Joint, Right** Acetabulofemoral joint **B Hip Joint, Left** *See 9 Hip Joint, Right* **C Knee Joint, Right** Femoropatellar joint Femorotibial joint Lateral meniscus Medial meniscus Patellofemoral joint Tibiofemoral joint **D Knee Joint, Left** *See C Knee Joint, Right* **F Ankle Joint, Right** Inferior tibiofibular joint Talocrural joint **G Ankle Joint, Left** *See F Ankle Joint, Right* **H Tarsal Joint, Right** Calcaneocuboid joint Cuboideonavicular joint Cuneonavicular joint Intercuneiform joint Subtalar (talocalcaneal) joint Talocalcaneal (subtalar) joint Talocalcaneonavicular joint **J Tarsal Joint, Left** *See H Tarsal Joint, Right* **K Tarsometatarsal Joint, Right** **L Tarsometatarsal Joint, Left** **M Metatarsal-Phalangeal Joint, Right** Metatarsophalangeal (MTP) joint **N Metatarsal-Phalangeal Joint, Left** *See M Metatarsal-Phalangeal Joint, Right* **P Toe Phalangeal Joint, Right** Interphalangeal (IP) joint **Q Toe Phalangeal Joint, Left** *See P Toe Phalangeal Joint, Right*	**Ø Open** **3 Percutaneous** **4 Percutaneous Endoscopic** **X External**	**Z No Device**	**Z No Qualifier**

Non-OR   ØSQ[Ø,2,3,4,5,6,7,8,9,B,C,D,F,G,H,J,K,L,M,N,P,Q]XZZ

Lower Joints (side tab)

Ø **Medical and Surgical**
S **Lower Joints**
R **Replacement** Definition: Putting in or on biological or synthetic material that physically takes the place and/or function of all or a portion of a body part

Explanation: The body part may have been taken out or replaced, or may be taken out, physically eradicated, or rendered nonfunctional during the REPLACEMENT procedure. A REMOVAL procedure is coded for taking out the device used in a previous replacement procedure.

Body Part Character 4	Approach Character 5	Device Character 6	Qualifier Character 7

Ø Lumbar Vertebral Joint
  Lumbar facet joint
2 Lumbar Vertebral Disc NC
3 Lumbosacral Joint
  Lumbosacral facet joint
4 Lumbosacral Disc NC
5 Sacrococcygeal Joint
  Sacrococcygeal symphysis
6 Coccygeal Joint
7 Sacroiliac Joint, Right
8 Sacroiliac Joint, Left
H Tarsal Joint, Right
  Calcaneocuboid joint
  Cuboideonavicular joint
  Cuneonavicular joint
  Intercuneiform joint
  Subtalar (talocalcaneal) joint
  Talocalcaneal (subtalar) joint
  Talocalcaneonavicular joint
J Tarsal Joint, Left
  See H Tarsal Joint, Right
K Tarsometatarsal Joint, Right
L Tarsometatarsal Joint, Left
M Metatarsal-Phalangeal Joint, Right
  Metatarsophalangeal (MTP) joint
N Metatarsal-Phalangeal Joint, Left
  See M Metatarsal-Phalangeal Joint, Right
P Toe Phalangeal Joint, Right
  Interphalangeal (IP) joint
Q Toe Phalangeal Joint, Left
  See P Toe Phalangeal Joint, Right
	Ø Open	7 Autologous Tissue Substitute
		J Synthetic Substitute
		K Nonautologous Tissue Substitute
			Z No Qualifier

9 Hip Joint, Right ⊞
  Acetabulofemoral joint
B Hip Joint, Left ⊞
  See 9 Hip Joint, Right
	Ø Open	1 Synthetic Substitute, Metal
		2 Synthetic Substitute, Metal on Polyethylene
		3 Synthetic Substitute, Ceramic
		4 Synthetic Substitute, Ceramic on Polyethylene
		6 Synthetic Substitute, Oxidized Zirconium on Polyethylene
		J Synthetic Substitute
			9 Cemented
			A Uncemented
			Z No Qualifier

9 Hip Joint, Right ⊞
  Acetabulofemoral joint
B Hip Joint, Left ⊞
  See 9 Hip Joint, Right
	Ø Open	7 Autologous Tissue Substitute
		E Articulating Spacer
		K Nonautologous Tissue Substitute
			Z No Qualifier

A Hip Joint, Acetabular Surface, Right ⊞ E Hip Joint, Acetabular Surface, Left ⊞	Ø Open	Ø Synthetic Substitute, Polyethylene 1 Synthetic Substitute, Metal 3 Synthetic Substitute, Ceramic J Synthetic Substitute	9 Cemented A Uncemented Z No Qualifier
A Hip Joint, Acetabular Surface, Right E Hip Joint, Acetabular Surface, Left	Ø Open	7 Autologous Tissue Substitute K Nonautologous Tissue Substitute	Z No Qualifier

HAC ØSR[9,B]Ø[1,2,3,4,6,J][9,A,Z] when reported with SDx of I26.Ø2-I26.Ø9, I26.92-I26.99, or I82.4Ø1-I82.4Z9
HAC ØSR[9,B]Ø[7,E,K]Z when reported with SDx of I26.Ø2-I26.Ø9, I26.92-I26.99, or I82.4Ø1-I82.4Z9
HAC ØSR[A,E]Ø[Ø,1,3,J][9,A,Z] when reported with SDx of I26.Ø2-I26.Ø9, I26.92-I26.99, or I82.4Ø1-I82.4Z9
HAC ØSR[A,E]Ø[7,K]Z when reported with SDx of I26.Ø2-I26.Ø9, I26.92-I26.99, or I82.4Ø1-I82.4Z9
NC ØSR[2,4]ØJZ when beneficiary age is over 6Ø

See Appendix L for Procedure Combinations
⊞ ØSR[9,B]Ø[1,2,3,4,6,J][9,A,Z]
⊞ ØSR[9,B]ØEZ
⊞ ØSR[A,E]Ø[Ø,1,3,J][9,A,Z]

ØSR Continued on next page

Non-OR Procedure   DRG Non-OR Procedure   Valid OR Procedure   HAC Associated Procedure   Combination Only   New/Revised April   New/Revised October

Ø   **Medical and Surgical**
S   **Lower Joints**
R   **Replacement**

ØSR Continued

Definition: Putting in or on biological or synthetic material that physically takes the place and/or function of all or a portion of a body part

Explanation: The body part may have been taken out or replaced, or may be taken out, physically eradicated, or rendered nonfunctional during the REPLACEMENT procedure. A REMOVAL procedure is coded for taking out the device used in a previous replacement procedure.

Body Part Character 4	Approach Character 5	Device Character 6	Qualifier Character 7
C Knee Joint, Right ⊞ Femoropatellar joint Femorotibial joint Lateral meniscus Medial meniscus Patellofemoral joint Tibiofemoral joint **D Knee Joint, Left** ⊞ *See C Knee Joint, Right*	Ø Open	6 Synthetic Substitute, Oxidized Zirconium on Polyethylene J Synthetic Substitute L Synthetic Substitute, Unicondylar Medial M Synthetic Substitute, Unicondylar Lateral N Synthetic Substitute, Patellofemoral	9 Cemented A Uncemented Z No Qualifier
C Knee Joint, Right ⊞ Femoropatellar joint Femorotibial joint Lateral meniscus Medial meniscus Patellofemoral joint Tibiofemoral joint **D Knee Joint, Left** ⊞ *See C Knee Joint, Right*	Ø Open	7 Autologous Tissue Substitute E Articulating Spacer K Nonautologous Tissue Substitute	Z No Qualifier
F Ankle Joint, Right Inferior tibiofibular joint Talocrural joint **G Ankle Joint, Left** *See F Ankle Joint, Right* **T Knee Joint, Femoral Surface, Right** Femoropatellar joint Patellofemoral joint **U Knee Joint, Femoral Surface, Left** *See T Knee Joint, Femoral Surface, Right* **V Knee Joint, Tibial Surface, Right** Femorotibial joint Tibiofemoral joint **W Knee Joint, Tibial Surface, Left** *See V Knee Joint, Tibial Surface, Right*	Ø Open	7 Autologous Tissue Substitute K Nonautologous Tissue Substitute	Z No Qualifier
F Ankle Joint, Right Inferior tibiofibular joint Talocrural joint **G Ankle Joint, Left** *See F Ankle Joint, Right* **T Knee Joint, Femoral Surface, Right** ⊞ Femoropatellar joint Patellofemoral joint **U Knee Joint, Femoral Surface, Left** ⊞ *See T Knee Joint, Femoral Surface, Right* **V Knee Joint, Tibial Surface, Right** ⊞ Femorotibial joint Tibiofemoral joint **W Knee Joint, Tibial Surface, Left** ⊞ *See V Knee Joint, Tibial Surface, Right*	Ø Open	J Synthetic Substitute	9 Cemented A Uncemented Z No Qualifier
R Hip Joint, Femoral Surface, Right ⊞ **S Hip Joint, Femoral Surface, Left** ⊞	Ø Open	1 Synthetic Substitute, Metal 3 Synthetic Substitute, Ceramic J Synthetic Substitute	9 Cemented A Uncemented Z No Qualifier
R Hip Joint, Femoral Surface, Right **S Hip Joint, Femoral Surface, Left**	Ø Open	7 Autologous Tissue Substitute K Nonautologous Tissue Substitute	Z No Qualifier

HAC   ØSR[C,D]Ø[6,J,L,M,N][9,A,Z] when reported with SDx of I26.Ø2-I26.Ø9, I26.92-I26.99 or I82.4Ø1-I82.4Z9

HAC   ØSR[C,D]Ø[7,E,K]Z when reported with SDx of I26.Ø2-I26.Ø9, I26.92-I26.99 or I82.4Ø1-I82.4Z9

HAC   ØSR[T,U,V,W]Ø[7,K]Z when reported with SDx of I26.Ø2-I26.Ø9, I26.92-I26.99 or I82.4Ø1-I82.4Z9

HAC   ØSR[T,U,V,W]ØJ[9,A,Z] when reported with SDx of I26.Ø2-I26.Ø9, I26.92-I26.99 or I82.4Ø1-I82.4Z9

HAC   ØSR[R,S]Ø[1,3,J][9,A,Z] when reported with SDx of I26.Ø2-I26.Ø9, I26.92-I26.99, or I82.4Ø1-I82.4Z9

HAC   ØSR[R,S]Ø[7,K]Z when reported with SDx of I26.Ø2-I26.Ø9, I26.92-I26.99, or I82.4Ø1-I82.4Z9

See Appendix L for Procedure Combinations
⊞ ØSR[C,D]Ø[6,J,L,M,N][9,A,Z]
⊞ ØSR[C,D]ØEZ
⊞ ØSR[T,U,V,W]ØJ[9,A,Z]
⊞ ØSR[R,S]Ø[1,3,J][9,A,Z]

NC Noncovered Procedure   **LC** Limited Coverage   **QA** Questionable OB Admit   **NT** New Tech Add-on   ⊞ Combination Member   ♂ Male   ♀ Female

Ø **Medical and Surgical**
S **Lower Joints**
S **Reposition** Definition: Moving to its normal location, or other suitable location, all or a portion of a body part

Explanation: The body part is moved to a new location from an abnormal location, or from a normal location where it is not functioning correctly. The body part may or may not be cut out or off to be moved to the new location.

Body Part Character 4	Approach Character 5	Device Character 6	Qualifier Character 7
Ø **Lumbar Vertebral Joint** Lumbar facet joint **3** **Lumbosacral Joint** Lumbosacral facet joint **5** **Sacrococcygeal Joint** Sacrococcygeal symphysis **6** **Coccygeal Joint** **7** **Sacroiliac Joint, Right** **8** **Sacroiliac Joint, Left**	**Ø** Open **3** Percutaneous **4** Percutaneous Endoscopic **X** External	**4** Internal Fixation Device **Z** No Device	**Z** No Qualifier
9 Hip Joint, Right Acetabulofemoral joint **B** Hip Joint, Left *See 9 Hip Joint, Right* **C** Knee Joint, Right Femoropatellar joint Femorotibial joint Lateral meniscus Medial meniscus Patellofemoral joint Tibiofemoral joint **D** Knee Joint, Left *See C Knee Joint, Right* **F** Ankle Joint, Right Inferior tibiofibular joint Talocrural joint **G** Ankle Joint, Left *See F Ankle Joint, Right* **H** Tarsal Joint, Right Calcaneocuboid joint Cuboideonavicular joint Cuneonavicular joint Intercuneiform joint Subtalar (talocalcaneal) joint Talocalcaneal (subtalar) joint Talocalcaneonavicular joint **J** Tarsal Joint, Left *See H Tarsal Joint, Right* **K** Tarsometatarsal Joint, Right **L** Tarsometatarsal Joint, Left **M** Metatarsal-Phalangeal Joint, Right Metatarsophalangeal (MTP) joint **N** Metatarsal-Phalangeal Joint, Left *See M Metatarsal-Phalangeal Joint, Right* **P** Toe Phalangeal Joint, Right Interphalangeal (IP) joint **Q** Toe Phalangeal Joint, Left *See P Toe Phalangeal Joint, Right*	**Ø** Open **3** Percutaneous **4** Percutaneous Endoscopic **X** External	**4** Internal Fixation Device **5** External Fixation Device **Z** No Device	**Z** No Qualifier

Non-OR	ØSS[Ø,3,5,6,][3,4,X][4,Z]Z
Non-OR	ØSS[7,8]3ZZ
Non-OR	ØSS[7,8][4,X][4,Z]Z
Non-OR	ØSS[9,B]3ZZ
Non-OR	ØSS[9,B][3,4,X]5Z
Non-OR	ØSS[9,B][4,X][4,Z]Z
Non-OR	ØSS[C,D,F,G,H,J,K,L,M,N,P,Q][3,4,X][4,5,Z]Z

Non-OR Procedure   DRG Non-OR Procedure   Valid OR Procedure   HAC Associated Procedure   Combination Only   New/Revised April   New/Revised October

620

ICD-10-PCS 2024

Ø   Medical and Surgical
S   Lower Joints
T   Resection   Definition: Cutting out or off, without replacement, all of a body part
                 Explanation: None

Body Part Character 4	Approach Character 5	Device Character 6	Qualifier Character 7

2   Lumbar Vertebral Disc
4   Lumbosacral Disc
5   Sacrococcygeal Joint
     Sacrococcygeal symphysis
6   Coccygeal Joint
7   Sacroiliac Joint, Right
8   Sacroiliac Joint, Left
9   Hip Joint, Right
     Acetabulofemoral joint
B   Hip Joint, Left
     See 9 Hip Joint, Right
C   Knee Joint, Right
     Femoropatellar joint
     Femorotibial joint
     Lateral meniscus
     Medial meniscus
     Patellofemoral joint
     Tibiofemoral joint
D   Knee Joint, Left
     See C Knee Joint, Right
F   Ankle Joint, Right
     Inferior tibiofibular joint
     Talocrural joint
G   Ankle Joint, Left
     See F Ankle Joint, Right
H   Tarsal Joint, Right
     Calcaneocuboid joint
     Cuboideonavicular joint
     Cuneonavicular joint
     Intercuneiform joint
     Subtalar (talocalcaneal) joint
     Talocalcaneal (subtalar) joint
     Talocalcaneonavicular joint
J   Tarsal Joint, Left
     See H Tarsal Joint, Right
K   Tarsometatarsal Joint, Right
L   Tarsometatarsal Joint, Left
M   Metatarsal-Phalangeal Joint, Right
     Metatarsophalangeal (MTP) joint
N   Metatarsal-Phalangeal Joint, Left
     See M Metatarsal-Phalangeal Joint, Right
P   Toe Phalangeal Joint, Right
     Interphalangeal (IP) joint
Q   Toe Phalangeal Joint, Left
     See P Toe Phalangeal Joint, Right
	Ø Open	**Z** No Device	**Z** No Qualifier

NC Noncovered Procedure   **LC** Limited Coverage   **QA** Questionable OB Admit   **NT** New Tech Add-on   ⊞ Combination Member   ♂ Male   ♀ Female

ICD-10-PCS 2024   621

ØST–ØST

Ø   **Medical and Surgical**
S   **Lower Joints**
U   **Supplement**   Definition: Putting in or on biological or synthetic material that physically reinforces and/or augments the function of a portion of a body part

Explanation: The biological material is non-living, or is living and from the same individual. The body part may have been previously replaced, and the SUPPLEMENT procedure is performed to physically reinforce and/or augment the function of the replaced body part.

Body Part Character 4		Approach Character 5	Device Character 6	Qualifier Character 7
Ø	**Lumbar Vertebral Joint** Lumbar facet joint	**Ø** Open **3** Percutaneous **4** Percutaneous Endoscopic	**7** Autologous Tissue Substitute **J** Synthetic Substitute **K** Nonautologous Tissue Substitute	**Z** No Qualifier
2	**Lumbar Vertebral Disc**			
3	**Lumbosacral Joint** Lumbosacral facet joint			
4	**Lumbosacral Disc**			
5	**Sacrococcygeal Joint** Sacrococcygeal symphysis			
6	**Coccygeal Joint**			
7	**Sacroiliac Joint, Right**			
8	**Sacroiliac Joint, Left**			
F	**Ankle Joint, Right** Inferior tibiofibular joint Talocrural joint			
G	**Ankle Joint, Left** *See F Ankle Joint, Right*			
H	**Tarsal Joint, Right** Calcaneocuboid joint Cuboideonavicular joint Cuneonavicular joint Intercuneiform joint Subtalar (talocalcaneal) joint Talocalcaneal (subtalar) joint Talocalcaneonavicular joint			
J	**Tarsal Joint, Left** *See H Tarsal Joint, Right*			
K	**Tarsometatarsal Joint, Right**			
L	**Tarsometatarsal Joint, Left**			
M	**Metatarsal-Phalangeal Joint, Right** Metatarsophalangeal (MTP) joint			
N	**Metatarsal-Phalangeal Joint, Left** *See M Metatarsal-Phalangeal Joint, Right*			
P	**Toe Phalangeal Joint, Right** Interphalangeal (IP) joint			
Q	**Toe Phalangeal Joint, Left** *See P Toe Phalangeal Joint, Right*			
9	**Hip Joint, Right** ⊞ Acetabulofemoral joint	**Ø** Open	**7** Autologous Tissue Substitute **9** Liner **B** Resurfacing Device **J** Synthetic Substitute **K** Nonautologous Tissue Substitute	**Z** No Qualifier
B	**Hip Joint, Left** ⊞ *See 9 Hip Joint, Right*			
9	**Hip Joint, Right** Acetabulofemoral joint	**3** Percutaneous **4** Percutaneous Endoscopic	**7** Autologous Tissue Substitute **J** Synthetic Substitute **K** Nonautologous Tissue Substitute	**Z** No Qualifier
B	**Hip Joint, Left** *See 9 Hip Joint, Right*			
A	**Hip Joint, Acetabular Surface, Right** ⊞	**Ø** Open	**9** Liner **B** Resurfacing Device	**Z** No Qualifier
E	**Hip Joint, Acetabular Surface, Left** ⊞			
R	**Hip Joint, Femoral Surface, Right** ⊞			
S	**Hip Joint, Femoral Surface, Left** ⊞			
C	**Knee Joint, Right** Femoropatellar joint Femorotibial joint Lateral meniscus Medial meniscus Patellofemoral joint Tibiofemoral joint	**Ø** Open	**7** Autologous Tissue Substitute **J** Synthetic Substitute **K** Nonautologous Tissue Substitute	**Z** No Qualifier
D	**Knee Joint, Left** *See C Knee Joint, Right*			
C	**Knee Joint, Right** Femoropatellar joint Femorotibial joint Lateral meniscus Medial meniscus Patellofemoral joint Tibiofemoral joint	**Ø** Open	**9** Liner	**C** Patellar Surface **Z** No Qualifier
D	**Knee Joint, Left** *See C Knee Joint, Right*			

HAC	ØSU[9,B]ØBZ when reported with SDx of I26.Ø2-I26.Ø9, I26.92-I26.99, or I82.4Ø1-I82.4Z9	**See Appendix L for Procedure Combinations**	
		⊞ ØSU[9,B]Ø9Z	
HAC	ØSU[A,E,R,S]ØBZ when reported with SDx of I26.Ø2-I26.Ø9, I26.92-I26.99, or I82.4Ø1-I82.4Z9	⊞ ØSU[A,E,R,S]Ø9Z	

ØSU Continued on next page

Non-OR Procedure   DRG Non-OR Procedure   Valid OR Procedure   HAC Associated Procedure   Combination Only   New/Revised April   New/Revised October

Ø   Medical and Surgical
S   Lower Joints
U   Supplement

ØSU Continued

Definition: Putting in or on biological or synthetic material that physically reinforces and/or augments the function of a portion of a body part
Explanation: The biological material is non-living, or is living and from the same individual. The body part may have been previously replaced, and the SUPPLEMENT procedure is performed to physically reinforce and/or augment the function of the replaced body part.

Body Part Character 4	Approach Character 5	Device Character 6	Qualifier Character 7
C Knee Joint, Right Femoropatellar joint Femorotibial joint Lateral meniscus Medial meniscus Patellofemoral joint Tibiofemoral joint **D Knee Joint, Left** *See C Knee Joint, Right*	**3** Percutaneous **4** Percutaneous Endoscopic	**7** Autologous Tissue Substitute **J** Synthetic Substitute **K** Nonautologous Tissue Substitute	**Z** No Qualifier
T Knee Joint, Femoral Surface, Right Femoropatellar joint Patellofemoral joint **U Knee Joint, Femoral Surface, Left** *See T Knee Joint, Femoral Surface, Right* **V Knee Joint, Tibial Surface, Right** ⊞ Femorotibial joint Tibiofemoral joint **W Knee Joint, Tibial Surface, Left** ⊞ *See V Knee Joint, Tibial Surface, Right*	**Ø** Open	**9** Liner	**Z** No Qualifier

See Appendix L for Procedure Combinations
⊞   ØSU[V,W]Ø9Z

NC Noncovered Procedure   **LC** Limited Coverage   **QA** Questionable OB Admit   **NT** New Tech Add-on   ⊞ Combination Member   ♂ Male   ♀ Female

ICD-10-PCS 2024   **623**

ØSU–ØSU

Lower Joints

Ø   Medical and Surgical
S   Lower Joints
W   Revision   Definition: Correcting, to the extent possible, a portion of a malfunctioning device or the position of a displaced device

Explanation: Revision can include correcting a malfunctioning or displaced device by taking out or putting in components of the device such as a screw or pin

Body Part Character 4	Approach Character 5	Device Character 6	Qualifier Character 7
Ø Lumbar Vertebral Joint Lumbar facet joint 3 Lumbosacral Joint Lumbosacral facet joint	Ø Open 3 Percutaneous 4 Percutaneous Endoscopic X External	Ø Drainage Device 3 Infusion Device 4 Internal Fixation Device 7 Autologous Tissue Substitute 8 Spacer A Interbody Fusion Device J Synthetic Substitute K Nonautologous Tissue Substitute	Z No Qualifier
2 Lumbar Vertebral Disc 4 Lumbosacral Disc	Ø Open 3 Percutaneous 4 Percutaneous Endoscopic X External	Ø Drainage Device 3 Infusion Device 7 Autologous Tissue Substitute J Synthetic Substitute K Nonautologous Tissue Substitute	Z No Qualifier
5 Sacrococcygeal Joint Sacrococcygeal symphysis 6 Coccygeal Joint 7 Sacroiliac Joint, Right 8 Sacroiliac Joint, Left	Ø Open 3 Percutaneous 4 Percutaneous Endoscopic X External	Ø Drainage Device 3 Infusion Device 4 Internal Fixation Device 7 Autologous Tissue Substitute 8 Spacer J Synthetic Substitute K Nonautologous Tissue Substitute	Z No Qualifier
9 Hip Joint, Right Acetabulofemoral joint B Hip Joint, Left *See 9 Hip Joint, Right*	Ø Open	Ø Drainage Device 3 Infusion Device 4 Internal Fixation Device 5 External Fixation Device 7 Autologous Tissue Substitute 8 Spacer 9 Liner B Resurfacing Device J Synthetic Substitute K Nonautologous Tissue Substitute	Z No Qualifier
9 Hip Joint, Right Acetabulofemoral joint B Hip Joint, Left *See 9 Hip Joint, Right*	3 Percutaneous 4 Percutaneous Endoscopic X External	Ø Drainage Device 3 Infusion Device 4 Internal Fixation Device 5 External Fixation Device 7 Autologous Tissue Substitute 8 Spacer J Synthetic Substitute K Nonautologous Tissue Substitute	Z No Qualifier

A Hip Joint, Acetabular Surface, Right
E Hip Joint, Acetabular Surface, Left
R Hip Joint, Femoral Surface, Right
S Hip Joint, Femoral Surface, Left
T Knee Joint, Femoral Surface, Right
Femoropatellar joint
Patellofemoral joint
U Knee Joint, Femoral Surface, Left
   See T Knee Joint, Femoral Surface, Right
V Knee Joint, Tibial Surface, Right
Femorotibial joint
Tibiofemoral joint
W Knee Joint, Tibial Surface, Left
   See V Knee Joint, Tibial Surface, Right
	Ø Open
	3 Percutaneous
	4 Percutaneous Endoscopic
	X External
		J Synthetic Substitute	Z No Qualifier

C Knee Joint, Right Femoropatellar joint Femorotibial joint Lateral meniscus Medial meniscus Patellofemoral joint Tibiofemoral joint D Knee Joint, Left *See C Knee Joint, Right*	Ø Open	Ø Drainage Device 3 Infusion Device 4 Internal Fixation Device 5 External Fixation Device 7 Autologous Tissue Substitute 8 Spacer 9 Liner K Nonautologous Tissue Substitute	Z No Qualifier

Non-OR	ØSW[Ø,3]X[Ø,3,4,7,8,A,J,K]Z
Non-OR	ØSW[2,4]X[Ø,3,7,J,K]Z
Non-OR	ØSW[5,6,7,8]X[Ø,3,4,7,8,J,K]Z
Non-OR	ØSW[9,B]X[Ø,3,4,5,7,8,J,K]Z
Non-OR	ØSW[A,E,R,S,T,U,V,W]XJZ

ØSW Continued on next page

Non-OR Procedure   DRG Non-OR Procedure   Valid OR Procedure   HAC Associated Procedure   Combination Only   New/Revised April   New/Revised October

624   ICD-10-PCS 2024

Ø Medical and Surgical
S Lower Joints
W Revision   Definition: Correcting, to the extent possible, a portion of a malfunctioning device or the position of a displaced device

ØSW Continued

Explanation: Revision can include correcting a malfunctioning or displaced device by taking out or putting in components of the device such as a screw or pin

Body Part Character 4	Approach Character 5	Device Character 6	Qualifier Character 7

C Knee Joint, Right
  Femoropatellar joint
  Femorotibial joint
  Lateral meniscus
  Medial meniscus
  Patellofemoral joint
  Tibiofemoral joint
D Knee Joint, Left
  See C Knee Joint, Right
	Ø Open	**J** Synthetic Substitute	**C** Patellar Surface
			Z No Qualifier

C Knee Joint, Right
  Femoropatellar joint
  Femorotibial joint
  Lateral meniscus
  Medial meniscus
  Patellofemoral joint
  Tibiofemoral joint
D Knee Joint, Left
  See C Knee Joint, Right
	3 Percutaneous
	4 Percutaneous Endoscopic
	X External
		Ø Drainage Device
		3 Infusion Device
		4 Internal Fixation Device
		5 External Fixation Device
		7 Autologous Tissue Substitute
		8 Spacer
		K Nonautologous Tissue Substitute
			Z No Qualifier

C Knee Joint, Right
  Femoropatellar joint
  Femorotibial joint
  Lateral meniscus
  Medial meniscus
  Patellofemoral joint
  Tibiofemoral joint
D Knee Joint, Left
  See C Knee Joint, Right
	3 Percutaneous
	4 Percutaneous Endoscopic
	X External
		J Synthetic Substitute	**C** Patellar Surface
			Z No Qualifier

F Ankle Joint, Right
  Inferior tibiofibular joint
  Talocrural joint
G Ankle Joint, Left
  See F Ankle Joint, Right
H Tarsal Joint, Right
  Calcaneocuboid joint
  Cuboideonavicular joint
  Cuneonavicular joint
  Intercuneiform joint
  Subtalar (talocalcaneal) joint
  Talocalcaneal (subtalar) joint
  Talocalcaneonavicular joint
J Tarsal Joint, Left
  See H Tarsal Joint, Right
K Tarsometatarsal Joint, Right
L Tarsometatarsal Joint, Left
M Metatarsal-Phalangeal Joint, Right
  Metatarsophalangeal (MTP) joint
N Metatarsal-Phalangeal Joint, Left
  See M Metatarsal-Phalangeal Joint, Right
P Toe Phalangeal Joint, Right
  Interphalangeal (IP) joint
Q Toe Phalangeal Joint, Left
  See P Toe Phalangeal Joint, Right
	Ø Open
	3 Percutaneous
	4 Percutaneous Endoscopic
	X External
		Ø Drainage Device
		3 Infusion Device
		4 Internal Fixation Device
		5 External Fixation Device
		7 Autologous Tissue Substitute
		8 Spacer
		J Synthetic Substitute
		K Nonautologous Tissue Substitute
			Z No Qualifier

Non-OR   ØSW[C,D]X[Ø,3,4,5,7,8,K]Z
Non-OR   ØSW[C,D]XJ[C,Z]
Non-OR   ØSW[F,G,H,J,K,L,M,N,P,Q]X[Ø,3,4,5,7,8,J,K]Z

NC Noncovered Procedure   LC Limited Coverage   QA Questionable OB Admit   NT New Tech Add-on   ⊞ Combination Member   ♂ Male   ♀ Female

ICD-10-PCS 2024   625

Urinary System ØT1–ØTY

Character Meanings

This Character Meaning table is provided as a guide to assist the user in the identification of character members that may be found in this section of code tables. It **SHOULD NOT** be used to build a PCS code.

Operation–Character 3	Body Part–Character 4	Approach–Character 5	Device–Character 6	Qualifier–Character 7
1 Bypass	Ø Kidney, Right	Ø Open	Ø Drainage Device	Ø Allogeneic
2 Change	1 Kidney, Left	3 Percutaneous	1 Radioactive Element	1 Syngeneic
5 Destruction	2 Kidneys, Bilateral	4 Percutaneous Endoscopic	2 Monitoring Device	2 Zooplastic
7 Dilation	3 Kidney Pelvis, Right	7 Via Natural or Artificial Opening	3 Infusion Device	3 Kidney Pelvis, Right
8 Division	4 Kidney Pelvis, Left	8 Via Natural or Artificial Opening Endoscopic	7 Autologous Tissue Substitute	4 Kidney Pelvis, Left
9 Drainage	5 Kidney	X External	C Extraluminal Device	6 Ureter, Right
B Excision	6 Ureter, Right		D Intraluminal Device	7 Ureter, Left
C Extirpation	7 Ureter, Left		J Synthetic Substitute	8 Colon
D Extraction	8 Ureters, Bilateral		K Nonautologous Tissue Substitute	9 Colocutaneous
F Fragmentation	9 Ureter		L Artificial Sphincter	A Ileum
H Insertion	B Bladder		M Stimulator Lead	B Bladder
J Inspection	C Bladder Neck		Y Other Device	C Ileocutaneous
L Occlusion	D Urethra		Z No Device	D Cutaneous
M Reattachment				X Diagnostic
N Release				Z No Qualifier
P Removal				
Q Repair				
R Replacement				
S Reposition				
T Resection				
U Supplement				
V Restriction				
W Revision				
Y Transplantation				

AHA Coding Clinic for table ØT1
2017, 3Q, 20	Creation of Indiana pouch
2017, 3Q, 21	Augmentation cystoplasty with Indiana pouch and continent urinary diversion
2017, 1Q, 37	Perineal urethrostomy
2015, 3Q, 34	Redo urinary diversion surgery via left ureteral reimplantation

AHA Coding Clinic for table ØT7
2019, 2Q, 16	Reimplantation of ureters with insertion of tubes
2017, 4Q, 111	Exchange of ureteral stent
2016, 2Q, 27	Exchange of ureteral stents
2015, 2Q, 8	Urinary calculi fragmentation and evacuation
2013, 4Q, 123	Urolift® procedure

AHA Coding Clinic for table ØT9
2017, 3Q, 19	Ureteral stent placement for urinary leakage
2017, 3Q, 20	Creation of Indiana pouch
2017, 3Q, 21	Augmentation cystoplasty with Indiana pouch and continent urinary diversion

AHA Coding Clinic for table ØTB
2016, 1Q, 19	Biopsy of neobladder malignancy
2015, 3Q, 34	Excision of Mitrofanoff polyp
2014, 2Q, 8	Ileoscopy with excision of polyp of Ileal loop urinary diversion

AHA Coding Clinic for table ØTC
2019, 3Q, 4	Evacuation of clots from bladder dome
2016, 3Q, 23	Ureteral stone migrating into bladder
2015, 2Q, 7	Urinary calculi fragmentation and evacuation
2015, 2Q, 8	Urinary calculi fragmentation and evacuation
2013, 4Q, 122	Laser lithotripsy with removal of fragments

AHA Coding Clinic for table ØTF
2015, 2Q, 7	Urinary calculi fragmentation and evacuation
2013, 4Q, 122	Extracorporeal shock wave lithotripsy
2013, 4Q, 122	Laser lithotripsy with removal of fragments

AHA Coding Clinic for table ØTH
2020, 4Q, 43-44	Insertion of radioactive element
2019, 2Q, 16	Reimplantation of ureters with insertion of tubes

AHA Coding Clinic for table ØTP
2017, 4Q, 111	Exchange of ureteral stent
2016, 2Q, 27	Exchange of ureteral stents

AHA Coding Clinic for table ØTQ
2018, 2Q, 27	Dismembered pyeloplasty
2017, 1Q, 37	Perineal urethrostomy

AHA Coding Clinic for table ØTR
2017, 3Q, 20	Creation of Indiana pouch

AHA Coding Clinic for table ØTS
2019, 1Q, 29	Young-Dees-Leadbetter bladder neck reconstruction
2018, 2Q, 27	Dismembered pyeloplasty
2017, 1Q, 36	Dismembered pyeloplasty
2016, 1Q, 15	Pubovaginal sling placement

AHA Coding Clinic for table ØTT
2014, 3Q, 16	Hand-assisted laparoscopy nephroureterectomy

AHA Coding Clinic for table ØTU
2019, 1Q, 29	Young-Dees-Leadbetter bladder neck reconstruction
2017, 3Q, 21	Augmentation cystoplasty with Indiana pouch and continent urinary diversion

AHA Coding Clinic for table ØTV
2015, 2Q, 11	Cystourethroscopic Deflux® injection

AHA Coding Clinic for table ØTY
2023, 2Q, 32	Preparation of donor organ before transplantation

Urinary System

- Inferior vena cava
- Aorta
- Right kidney **Ø**
- Left kidney **1**
- Left ureter **7**
- Right ureter **6**
- Urinary bladder **B**
- Ureteral orifice **6, 7, 8, 9**
- Bladder neck **C**
- Urethra **D**
- Urogenital diaphragm

Kidney

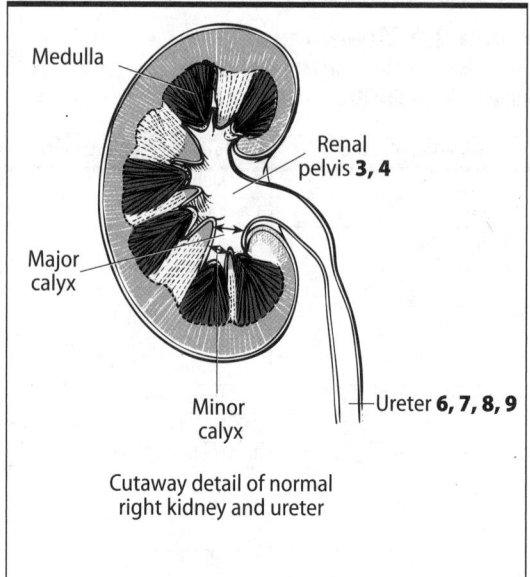

- Medulla
- Renal pelvis **3, 4**
- Major calyx
- Minor calyx
- Ureter **6, 7, 8, 9**

Cutaway detail of normal right kidney and ureter

Bladder

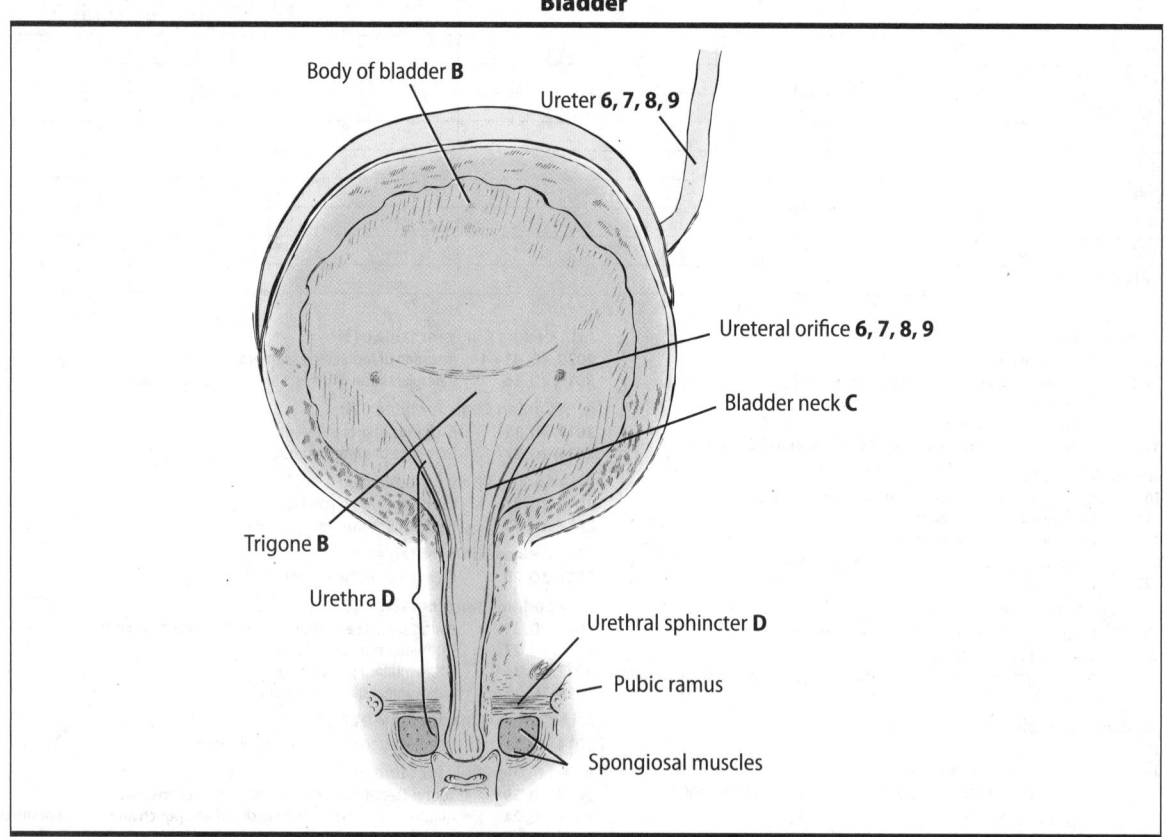

- Body of bladder **B**
- Ureter **6, 7, 8, 9**
- Ureteral orifice **6, 7, 8, 9**
- Bladder neck **C**
- Trigone **B**
- Urethra **D**
- Urethral sphincter **D**
- Pubic ramus
- Spongiosal muscles

Ø   Medical and Surgical
T   Urinary System
1   Bypass   Definition: Altering the route of passage of the contents of a tubular body part

Explanation: Rerouting contents of a body part to a downstream area of the normal route, to a similar route and body part, or to an abnormal route and dissimilar body part. Includes one or more anastomoses, with or without the use of a device.

Body Part Character 4	Approach Character 5	Device Character 6	Qualifier Character 7

3   Kidney Pelvis, Right
     Ureteropelvic junction (UPJ)
 4   Kidney Pelvis, Left
     See 3 Kidney Pelvis, Right
	Ø Open
	 4 Percutaneous Endoscopic
		7 Autologous Tissue Substitute
		 J Synthetic Substitute
		 K Nonautologous Tissue Substitute
		 Z No Device
			3 Kidney Pelvis, Right
			 4 Kidney Pelvis, Left
			 6 Ureter, Right
			 7 Ureter, Left
			 8 Colon
			 9 Colocutaneous
			 A Ileum
			 B Bladder
			 C Ileocutaneous
			 D Cutaneous

3   Kidney Pelvis, Right
     Ureteropelvic junction (UPJ)
 4   Kidney Pelvis, Left
     See 3 Kidney Pelvis, Right
	3 Percutaneous	**J** Synthetic Substitute	**D** Cutaneous

6   Ureter, Right
     Ureteral orifice
     Ureterovesical orifice
 7   Ureter, Left
     See 6 Ureter, Right
 8   Ureters, Bilateral
     See 6 Ureter, Right
	Ø Open
	 4 Percutaneous Endoscopic
		7 Autologous Tissue Substitute
		 J Synthetic Substitute
		 K Nonautologous Tissue Substitute
		 Z No Device
			6 Ureter, Right
			 7 Ureter, Left
			 8 Colon
			 9 Colocutaneous
			 A Ileum
			 B Bladder
			 C Ileocutaneous
			 D Cutaneous

6   Ureter, Right
     Ureteral orifice
     Ureterovesical orifice
 7   Ureter, Left
     See 6 Ureter, Right
 8   Ureters, Bilateral
     See 6 Ureter, Right
	3 Percutaneous	**J** Synthetic Substitute	**D** Cutaneous

B Bladder Trigone of bladder	**Ø** Open **4** Percutaneous Endoscopic	**7** Autologous Tissue Substitute **J** Synthetic Substitute **K** Nonautologous Tissue Substitute **Z** No Device	**9** Colocutaneous **C** Ileocutaneous **D** Cutaneous
B Bladder Trigone of bladder	**3** Percutaneous	**J** Synthetic Substitute	**D** Cutaneous

Ø   Medical and Surgical
T   Urinary System
2   Change   Definition: Taking out or off a device from a body part and putting back an identical or similar device in or on the same body part without cutting or puncturing the skin or a mucous membrane

Explanation: All CHANGE procedures are coded using the approach EXTERNAL

Body Part Character 4	Approach Character 5	Device Character 6	Qualifier Character 7

5   Kidney
     Renal calyx
     Renal capsule
     Renal cortex
     Renal segment
 9   Ureter
     Ureteral orifice
     Ureterovesical orifice
 B   Bladder
     Trigone of bladder
 D   Urethra
     Bulbourethral (Cowper's) gland
     Cowper's (bulbourethral) gland
     External urethral sphincter
     Internal urethral sphincter
     Membranous urethra
     Penile urethra
     Prostatic urethra
	X External	**Ø** Drainage Device
		 Y Other Device
			Z No Qualifier

Non-OR   All body part, approach, device, and qualifier values

NC Noncovered Procedure   **LC** Limited Coverage   **QA** Questionable OB Admit   **NT** New Tech Add-on   ⊞ Combination Member   ♂ Male   ♀ Female

ICD-10-PCS 2024   629

ØT1–ØT2

Urinary System (side tab)

Ø Medical and Surgical
T Urinary System
5 Destruction

Definition: Physical eradication of all or a portion of a body part by the direct use of energy, force, or a destructive agent

Explanation: None of the body part is physically taken out

Body Part Character 4	Approach Character 5	Device Character 6	Qualifier Character 7
Ø Kidney, Right Renal calyx Renal capsule Renal cortex Renal segment 1 Kidney, Left *See Ø Kidney, Right* 3 Kidney Pelvis, Right Ureteropelvic junction (UPJ) 4 Kidney Pelvis, Left *See 3 Kidney Pelvis, Right* 6 Ureter, Right Ureteral orifice Ureterovesical orifice 7 Ureter, Left *See 6 Ureter, Right* B Bladder Trigone of bladder C Bladder Neck	Ø Open 3 Percutaneous 4 Percutaneous Endoscopic 7 Via Natural or Artificial Opening 8 Via Natural or Artificial Opening Endoscopic	Z No Device	Z No Qualifier
D Urethra Bulbourethral (Cowper's) gland Cowper's (bulbourethral) gland External urethral sphincter Internal urethral sphincter Membranous urethra Penile urethra Prostatic urethra	Ø Open 3 Percutaneous 4 Percutaneous Endoscopic 7 Via Natural or Artificial Opening 8 Via Natural or Artificial Opening Endoscopic X External	Z No Device	Z No Qualifier

Non-OR   ØT5D[Ø,3,4,7,8,X]ZZ

Ø Medical and Surgical
T Urinary System
7 Dilation

Definition: Expanding an orifice or the lumen of a tubular body part

Explanation: The orifice can be a natural orifice or an artificially created orifice. Accomplished by stretching a tubular body part using intraluminal pressure or by cutting part of the orifice or wall of the tubular body part.

Body Part Character 4	Approach Character 5	Device Character 6	Qualifier Character 7
3 Kidney Pelvis, Right Ureteropelvic junction (UPJ) 4 Kidney Pelvis, Left *See 3 Kidney Pelvis, Right* 6 Ureter, Right Ureteral orifice Ureterovesical orifice 7 Ureter, Left *See 6 Ureter, Right* 8 Ureters, Bilateral *See 6 Ureter, Right* B Bladder Trigone of bladder C Bladder Neck D Urethra Bulbourethral (Cowper's) gland Cowper's (bulbourethral) gland External urethral sphincter Internal urethral sphincter Membranous urethra Penile urethra Prostatic urethra	Ø Open 3 Percutaneous 4 Percutaneous Endoscopic 7 Via Natural or Artificial Opening 8 Via Natural or Artificial Opening Endoscopic	D Intraluminal Device Z No Device	Z No Qualifier

Non-OR   ØT7[6,7,8][Ø,3,4,7]DZ
Non-OR   ØT7[6,7,8]7ZZ
Non-OR   ØT788ZZ
Non-OR   ØT7B7[D,Z]Z
Non-OR   ØT7C[Ø,3,4]ZZ
Non-OR   ØT7[C,D][Ø,3,4]DZ
Non-OR   ØT7[C,D][7,8][D,Z]Z

Ø Medical and Surgical
T Urinary System
8 Division

Definition: Cutting into a body part, without draining fluids and/or gases from the body part, in order to separate or transect a body part

Explanation: All or a portion of the body part is separated into two or more portions

Body Part Character 4	Approach Character 5	Device Character 6	Qualifier Character 7
2 Kidneys, Bilateral Renal calyx Renal capsule Renal cortex Renal segment C Bladder Neck	Ø Open 3 Percutaneous 4 Percutaneous Endoscopic	Z No Device	Z No Qualifier

Non-OR Procedure   DRG Non-OR Procedure   Valid OR Procedure   HAC Associated Procedure   Combination Only   New/Revised April   New/Revised October

Ø **Medical and Surgical**
T **Urinary System**
9 **Drainage** Definition: Taking or letting out fluids and/or gases from a body part
Explanation: The qualifier DIAGNOSTIC is used to identify drainage procedures that are biopsies

Body Part Character 4	Approach Character 5	Device Character 6	Qualifier Character 7
Ø Kidney, Right Renal calyx Renal capsule Renal cortex Renal segment **1** Kidney, Left *See Ø Kidney, Right* **3** Kidney Pelvis, Right Ureteropelvic junction (UPJ) **4** Kidney Pelvis, Left *See 3 Kidney Pelvis, Right* **6** Ureter, Right Ureteral orifice Ureterovesical orifice **7** Ureter, Left *See 6 Ureter, Right* **8** Ureters, Bilateral *See 6 Ureter, Right* **B** Bladder Trigone of bladder **C** Bladder Neck	**Ø** Open **3** Percutaneous **4** Percutaneous Endoscopic **7** Via Natural or Artificial Opening **8** Via Natural or Artificial Opening Endoscopic	**Ø** Drainage Device	**Z** No Qualifier
Ø Kidney, Right Renal calyx Renal capsule Renal cortex Renal segment **1** Kidney, Left *See Ø Kidney, Right* **3** Kidney Pelvis, Right Ureteropelvic junction (UPJ) **4** Kidney Pelvis, Left *See 3 Kidney Pelvis, Right* **6** Ureter, Right Ureteral orifice Ureterovesical orifice **7** Ureter, Left *See 6 Ureter, Right* **8** Ureters, Bilateral *See 6 Ureter, Right* **B** Bladder Trigone of bladder **C** Bladder Neck	**Ø** Open **3** Percutaneous **4** Percutaneous Endoscopic **7** Via Natural or Artificial Opening **8** Via Natural or Artificial Opening Endoscopic	**Z** No Device	**X** Diagnostic **Z** No Qualifier
D Urethra Bulbourethral (Cowper's) gland Cowper's (bulbourethral) gland External urethral sphincter Internal urethral sphincter Membranous urethra Penile urethra Prostatic urethra	**Ø** Open **3** Percutaneous **4** Percutaneous Endoscopic **7** Via Natural or Artificial Opening **8** Via Natural or Artificial Opening Endoscopic **X** External	**Ø** Drainage Device	**Z** No Qualifier
D Urethra Bulbourethral (Cowper's) gland Cowper's (bulbourethral) gland External urethral sphincter Internal urethral sphincter Membranous urethra Penile urethra Prostatic urethra	**Ø** Open **3** Percutaneous **4** Percutaneous Endoscopic **7** Via Natural or Artificial Opening **8** Via Natural or Artificial Opening Endoscopic **X** External	**Z** No Device	**X** Diagnostic **Z** No Qualifier

Non-OR	ØT9[Ø,1,3,4]3ØZ
Non-OR	ØT9[6,7,8][Ø,3,4,7,8]ØZ
Non-OR	ØT9[B,C][3,4,7,8]ØZ
Non-OR	ØT9[Ø,1,3,4,6,7,8][3,4,7,8]ZX
Non-OR	ØT9[Ø,1,3,4][3,4]ZZ
Non-OR	ØT9[6,7,8]3ZZ
Non-OR	ØT9[B,C][3,4,7,8]ZZ
Non-OR	ØT9D3ØZ
Non-OR	ØT9D[Ø,3,4,7,8,X]ZX
Non-OR	ØT9D3ZZ

NC Noncovered Procedure **LC** Limited Coverage **QA** Questionable OB Admit **NT** New Tech Add-on ⊞ Combination Member ♂ Male ♀ Female
ICD-10-PCS 2024 631

ØT9–ØT9

Urinary System

Ø	Medical and Surgical
T	Urinary System
B	Excision Definition: Cutting out or off, without replacement, a portion of a body part

Explanation: The qualifier DIAGNOSTIC is used to identify excision procedures that are biopsies

Body Part Character 4	Approach Character 5	Device Character 6	Qualifier Character 7

Ø **Kidney, Right**
   Renal calyx
   Renal capsule
   Renal cortex
   Renal segment
1 **Kidney, Left**
   See Ø Kidney, Right
3 **Kidney Pelvis, Right**
   Ureteropelvic junction (UPJ)
4 **Kidney Pelvis, Left**
   See 3 Kidney Pelvis, Right
6 **Ureter, Right**
   Ureteral orifice
   Ureterovesical orifice
7 **Ureter, Left**
   See 6 Ureter, Right
B **Bladder**
   Trigone of bladder
C **Bladder Neck**
	Ø Open
	3 Percutaneous
	4 Percutaneous Endoscopic
	7 Via Natural or Artificial Opening
	8 Via Natural or Artificial Opening Endoscopic
		Z No Device	X Diagnostic
			Z No Qualifier

D **Urethra**
   Bulbourethral (Cowper's) gland
   Cowper's (bulbourethral) gland
   External urethral sphincter
   Internal urethral sphincter
   Membranous urethra
   Penile urethra
   Prostatic urethra
	Ø Open
	3 Percutaneous
	4 Percutaneous Endoscopic
	7 Via Natural or Artificial Opening
	8 Via Natural or Artificial Opening Endoscopic
	X External
		Z No Device	X Diagnostic
			Z No Qualifier

Non-OR   ØTB[Ø,1,3,4,6,7][3,4,7,8]ZX
Non-OR   ØTBD[Ø,3,4,7,8,X]ZX

Ø	Medical and Surgical
T	Urinary System
C	Extirpation Definition: Taking or cutting out solid matter from a body part

Explanation: The solid matter may be an abnormal byproduct of a biological function or a foreign body; it may be imbedded in a body part or in the lumen of a tubular body part. The solid matter may or may not have been previously broken into pieces.

Body Part Character 4	Approach Character 5	Device Character 6	Qualifier Character 7

Ø **Kidney, Right**
   Renal calyx
   Renal capsule
   Renal cortex
   Renal segment
1 **Kidney, Left**
   See Ø Kidney, Right
3 **Kidney Pelvis, Right**
   Ureteropelvic junction (UPJ)
4 **Kidney Pelvis, Left**
   See 3 Kidney Pelvis, Right
6 **Ureter, Right**
   Ureteral orifice
   Ureterovesical orifice
7 **Ureter, Left**
   See 6 Ureter, Right
B **Bladder**
   Trigone of bladder
C **Bladder Neck**
	Ø Open
	3 Percutaneous
	4 Percutaneous Endoscopic
	7 Via Natural or Artificial Opening
	8 Via Natural or Artificial Opening Endoscopic
		Z No Device	Z No Qualifier

D **Urethra**
   Bulbourethral (Cowper's) gland
   Cowper's (bulbourethral) gland
   External urethral sphincter
   Internal urethral sphincter
   Membranous urethra
   Penile urethra
   Prostatic urethra
	Ø Open
	3 Percutaneous
	4 Percutaneous Endoscopic
	7 Via Natural or Artificial Opening
	8 Via Natural or Artificial Opening Endoscopic
	X External
		Z No Device	Z No Qualifier

Non-OR   ØTC[Ø,1,3,4,6,7]8ZZ
Non-OR   ØTC[B,C][7,8]ZZ
Non-OR   ØTCD[7,8,X]ZZ

Non-OR Procedure   DRG Non-OR Procedure   Valid OR Procedure   HAC Associated Procedure   Combination Only   New/Revised April   New/Revised October

632   ICD-10-PCS 2024

Ø   **Medical and Surgical**
T   **Urinary System**
D   **Extraction**   Definition: Pulling or stripping out or off all or a portion of a body part by the use of force

                     Explanation: The qualifier DIAGNOSTIC is used to identify extraction procedures that are biopsies

Body Part Character 4	Approach Character 5	Device Character 6	Qualifier Character 7

Ø   **Kidney, Right**
    Renal calyx
    Renal capsule
    Renal cortex
    Renal segment
1   **Kidney, Left**
    See Ø Kidney, Right
	Ø Open
	3 Percutaneous
	4 Percutaneous Endoscopic
		Z No Device	**Z** No Qualifier

Ø   **Medical and Surgical**
T   **Urinary System**
F   **Fragmentation**   Definition: Breaking solid matter in a body part into pieces

                     Explanation: Physical force (e.g., manual, ultrasonic) applied directly or indirectly is used to break the solid matter into pieces. The solid matter may be an abnormal byproduct of a biological function or a foreign body. The pieces of solid matter are not taken out.

Body Part Character 4	Approach Character 5	Device Character 6	Qualifier Character 7

3   **Kidney Pelvis, Right**
    Ureteropelvic junction (UPJ)
4   **Kidney Pelvis, Left**
    See 3 Kidney Pelvis, Right
6   **Ureter, Right**
    Ureteral orifice
    Ureterovesical orifice
7   **Ureter, Left**
    See 6 Ureter, Right
B   **Bladder**
    Trigone of bladder
C   **Bladder Neck**
D   **Urethra**   `NC`
    Bulbourethral (Cowper's) gland
    Cowper's (bulbourethral) gland
    External urethral sphincter
    Internal urethral sphincter
    Membranous urethra
    Penile urethra
    Prostatic urethra
	Ø Open
	3 Percutaneous
	4 Percutaneous Endoscopic
	7 Via Natural or Artificial Opening
	8 Via Natural or Artificial Opening Endoscopic
	X External
		Z No Device	**Z** No Qualifier

Non-OR   ØTF[3,4][Ø,7,8]ZZ
Non-OR   ØTF[6,7,B,C,D][Ø,3,4,7,8]ZZ
Non-OR   ØTF[3,4,6,7,B,C,D]XZZ
`NC`   ØTFDXZZ

NC Noncovered Procedure   **LC** Limited Coverage   **QA** Questionable OB Admit   **NT** New Tech Add-on   ⊞ Combination Member   ♂ Male   ♀ Female

ICD-10-PCS 2024   633

Ø   **Medical and Surgical**
T   **Urinary System**
H   **Insertion**   Definition: Putting in a nonbiological appliance that monitors, assists, performs, or prevents a physiological function but does not physically take the place of a body part

                         Explanation: None

Body Part Character 4	Approach Character 5	Device Character 6	Qualifier Character 7

5   Kidney
    Renal calyx
    Renal capsule
    Renal cortex
    Renal segment
	Ø Open
	3 Percutaneous
	4 Percutaneous Endoscopic
	7 Via Natural or Artificial Opening
	8 Via Natural or Artificial Opening Endoscopic
		1 Radioactive Element
		2 Monitoring Device
		3 Infusion Device
		Y Other Device
			Z No Qualifier

9   Ureter
    Ureteral orifice
    Ureterovesical orifice
	Ø Open
	3 Percutaneous
	4 Percutaneous Endoscopic
	7 Via Natural or Artificial Opening
	8 Via Natural or Artificial Opening Endoscopic
		1 Radioactive Element
		2 Monitoring Device
		3 Infusion Device
		M Stimulator Lead
		Y Other Device
			Z No Qualifier

B Bladder ^{NC} Trigone of bladder	**Ø** Open **3** Percutaneous **4** Percutaneous Endoscopic **7** Via Natural or Artificial Opening **8** Via Natural or Artificial Opening Endoscopic	**1** Radioactive Element **2** Monitoring Device **3** Infusion Device **L** Artificial Sphincter **M** Stimulator Lead **Y** Other Device	**Z** No Qualifier
C Bladder Neck	**Ø** Open **3** Percutaneous **4** Percutaneous Endoscopic **7** Via Natural or Artificial Opening **8** Via Natural or Artificial Opening Endoscopic	**L** Artificial Sphincter	**Z** No Qualifier

D   Urethra
    Bulbourethral (Cowper's) gland
    Cowper's (bulbourethral) gland
    External urethral sphincter
    Internal urethral sphincter
    Membranous urethra
    Penile urethra
    Prostatic urethra
	Ø Open
	3 Percutaneous
	4 Percutaneous Endoscopic
	7 Via Natural or Artificial Opening
	8 Via Natural or Artificial Opening Endoscopic
		1 Radioactive Element
		2 Monitoring Device
		3 Infusion Device
		L Artificial Sphincter
		Y Other Device
			Z No Qualifier

D   Urethra
    Bulbourethral (Cowper's) gland
    Cowper's (bulbourethral) gland
    External urethral sphincter
    Internal urethral sphincter
    Membranous urethra
    Penile urethra
    Prostatic urethra
	X External	**2** Monitoring Device
		3 Infusion Device
		L Artificial Sphincter
			Z No Qualifier

Non-OR ØTH5Ø3Z	**Non-OR** ØTHB3[1,3,Y]Z
Non-OR ØTH53[1,3,Y]Z	**Non-OR** ØTHB4[3,Y]Z
Non-OR ØTH54[3,Y]Z	**Non-OR** ØTHB7[1,2,3,Y]Z
Non-OR ØTH57[1,2,3,Y]Z	**Non-OR** ØTHB8[2,3]Z
Non-OR ØTH58[2,3]Z	**Non-OR** ØTHD03Z
Non-OR ØTH9Ø3Z	**Non-OR** ØTHD3[1,3,Y]Z
Non-OR ØTH93[1,3,Y]Z	**Non-OR** ØTHD4[3,Y]Z
Non-OR ØTH94[3,Y]Z	**Non-OR** ØTHD7[1,2,3,Y]Z
Non-OR ØTH97[1,2,3,Y]Z	**Non-OR** ØTHD8[2,3,Y]Z
Non-OR ØTH98[2,3]Z	**Non-OR** ØTHDX3Z
Non-OR ØTHBØ3Z	^{NC} ØTHB[Ø,3,4,7,8]MZ

Non-OR Procedure   DRG Non-OR Procedure   Valid OR Procedure   HAC Associated Procedure   Combination Only   New/Revised April   New/Revised October

634   ICD-10-PCS 2024

ØTH–ØTH

Ø　**Medical and Surgical**
T　**Urinary System**
J　**Inspection**　　　Definition: Visually and/or manually exploring a body part

Explanation: Visual exploration may be performed with or without optical instrumentation. Manual exploration may be performed directly or through intervening body layers.

Body Part Character 4	Approach Character 5	Device Character 6	Qualifier Character 7
5 Kidney Renal calyx Renal capsule Renal cortex Renal segment **9** Ureter Ureteral orifice Ureterovesical orifice **B** Bladder Trigone of bladder **D** Urethra Bulbourethral (Cowper's) gland Cowper's (bulbourethral) gland External urethral sphincter Internal urethral sphincter Membranous urethra Penile urethra Prostatic urethra	**Ø** Open **3** Percutaneous **4** Percutaneous Endoscopic **7** Via Natural or Artificial Opening **8** Via Natural or Artificial Opening Endoscopic **X** External	**Z** No Device	**Z** No Qualifier

Non-OR　ØTJ[5,9,D][3,4,7,8,X]ZZ
Non-OR　ØTJB[3,7,8,X]ZZ

Ø　**Medical and Surgical**
T　**Urinary System**
L　**Occlusion**　　　Definition: Completely closing an orifice or the lumen of a tubular body part

Explanation: The orifice can be a natural orifice or an artificially created orifice

Body Part Character 4	Approach Character 5	Device Character 6	Qualifier Character 7
3 Kidney Pelvis, Right Ureteropelvic junction (UPJ) **4** Kidney Pelvis, Left *See 3 Kidney Pelvis, Right* **6** Ureter, Right Ureteral orifice Ureterovesical orifice **7** Ureter, Left *See 6 Ureter, Right* **B** Bladder Trigone of bladder **C** Bladder Neck	**Ø** Open **3** Percutaneous **4** Percutaneous Endoscopic	**C** Extraluminal Device **D** Intraluminal Device **Z** No Device	**Z** No Qualifier
3 Kidney Pelvis, Right Ureteropelvic junction (UPJ) **4** Kidney Pelvis, Left *See 3 Kidney Pelvis, Right* **6** Ureter, Right Ureteral orifice Ureterovesical orifice **7** Ureter, Left *See 6 Ureter, Right* **B** Bladder Trigone of bladder **C** Bladder Neck	**7** Via Natural or Artificial Opening **8** Via Natural or Artificial Opening Endoscopic	**D** Intraluminal Device **Z** No Device	**Z** No Qualifier
D Urethra Bulbourethral (Cowper's) gland Cowper's (bulbourethral) gland External urethral sphincter Internal urethral sphincter Membranous urethra Penile urethra Prostatic urethra	**Ø** Open **3** Percutaneous **4** Percutaneous Endoscopic **X** External	**C** Extraluminal Device **D** Intraluminal Device **Z** No Device	**Z** No Qualifier
D Urethra Bulbourethral (Cowper's) gland Cowper's (bulbourethral) gland External urethral sphincter Internal urethral sphincter Membranous urethra Penile urethra Prostatic urethra	**7** Via Natural or Artificial Opening **8** Via Natural or Artificial Opening Endoscopic	**D** Intraluminal Device **Z** No Device	**Z** No Qualifier

NC Noncovered Procedure　LC Limited Coverage　QA Questionable OB Admit　NT New Tech Add-on　⊞ Combination Member　♂Male　♀Female

ICD-10-PCS 2024　　　　　　　　　　　　　　　　　　　　　　　　　　　　　　　　　　　　635

Urinary System

Ø   **Medical and Surgical**
T   **Urinary System**
M   **Reattachment**   Definition: Putting back in or on all or a portion of a separated body part to its normal location or other suitable location

                       Explanation: Vascular circulation and nervous pathways may or may not be reestablished

Body Part Character 4	Approach Character 5	Device Character 6	Qualifier Character 7
Ø Kidney, Right Renal calyx Renal capsule Renal cortex Renal segment **1 Kidney, Left** *See Ø Kidney, Right* **2 Kidneys, Bilateral** *See Ø Kidney, Right* **3 Kidney Pelvis, Right** Ureteropelvic junction (UPJ) **4 Kidney Pelvis, Left** *See 3 Kidney Pelvis, Right* **6 Ureter, Right** Ureteral orifice Ureterovesical orifice **7 Ureter, Left** *See 6 Ureter, Right* **8 Ureters, Bilateral** *See 6 Ureter, Right* **B Bladder** Trigone of bladder **C Bladder Neck** **D Urethra** Bulbourethral (Cowper's) gland Cowper's (bulbourethral) gland External urethral sphincter Internal urethral sphincter Membranous urethra Penile urethra Prostatic urethra	**Ø** Open **4** Percutaneous Endoscopic	**Z** No Device	**Z** No Qualifier

Ø   **Medical and Surgical**
T   **Urinary System**
N   **Release**   Definition: Freeing a body part from an abnormal physical constraint by cutting or by the use of force

                Explanation: Some of the restraining tissue may be taken out but none of the body part is taken out

Body Part Character 4	Approach Character 5	Device Character 6	Qualifier Character 7
Ø Kidney, Right Renal calyx Renal capsule Renal cortex Renal segment **1 Kidney, Left** *See Ø Kidney, Right* **3 Kidney Pelvis, Right** Ureteropelvic junction (UPJ) **4 Kidney Pelvis, Left** *See 3 Kidney Pelvis, Right* **6 Ureter, Right** Ureteral orifice Ureterovesical orifice **7 Ureter, Left** *See 6 Ureter, Right* **B Bladder** Trigone of bladder **C Bladder Neck**	**Ø** Open **3** Percutaneous **4** Percutaneous Endoscopic **7** Via Natural or Artificial Opening **8** Via Natural or Artificial Opening Endoscopic	**Z** No Device	**Z** No Qualifier
D Urethra Bulbourethral (Cowper's) gland Cowper's (bulbourethral) gland External urethral sphincter Internal urethral sphincter Membranous urethra Penile urethra Prostatic urethra	**Ø** Open **3** Percutaneous **4** Percutaneous Endoscopic **7** Via Natural or Artificial Opening **8** Via Natural or Artificial Opening Endoscopic **X** External	**Z** No Device	**Z** No Qualifier

Non-OR Procedure   DRG Non-OR Procedure   Valid OR Procedure   HAC Associated Procedure   Combination Only   New/Revised April   New/Revised October

636   ICD-10-PCS 2024

Ø Medical and Surgical
T Urinary System
P Removal   Definition: Taking out or off a device from a body part

Explanation: If a device is taken out and a similar device put in without cutting or puncturing the skin or mucous membrane, the procedure is coded to the root operation CHANGE. Otherwise, the procedure for taking out the device is coded to the root operation REMOVAL.

Body Part Character 4	Approach Character 5	Device Character 6	Qualifier Character 7
5 Kidney Renal calyx Renal capsule Renal cortex Renal segment	Ø Open 3 Percutaneous 4 Percutaneous Endoscopic 7 Via Natural or Artificial Opening 8 Via Natural or Artificial Opening Endoscopic	Ø Drainage Device 2 Monitoring Device 3 Infusion Device 7 Autologous Tissue Substitute C Extraluminal Device D Intraluminal Device J Synthetic Substitute K Nonautologous Tissue Substitute Y Other Device	Z No Qualifier
5 Kidney Renal calyx Renal capsule Renal cortex Renal segment	X External	Ø Drainage Device 2 Monitoring Device 3 Infusion Device D Intraluminal Device	Z No Qualifier
9 Ureter Ureteral orifice Ureterovesical orifice	Ø Open 3 Percutaneous 4 Percutaneous Endoscopic 7 Via Natural or Artificial Opening 8 Via Natural or Artificial Opening Endoscopic	Ø Drainage Device 2 Monitoring Device 3 Infusion Device 7 Autologous Tissue Substitute C Extraluminal Device D Intraluminal Device J Synthetic Substitute K Nonautologous Tissue Substitute M Stimulator Lead Y Other Device	Z No Qualifier
9 Ureter Ureteral orifice Ureterovesical orifice	X External	Ø Drainage Device 2 Monitoring Device 3 Infusion Device D Intraluminal Device M Stimulator Lead	Z No Qualifier
B Bladder [NC] Trigone of bladder	Ø Open 3 Percutaneous 4 Percutaneous Endoscopic 7 Via Natural or Artificial Opening 8 Via Natural or Artificial Opening Endoscopic	Ø Drainage Device 2 Monitoring Device 3 Infusion Device 7 Autologous Tissue Substitute C Extraluminal Device D Intraluminal Device J Synthetic Substitute K Nonautologous Tissue Substitute L Artificial Sphincter M Stimulator Lead Y Other Device	Z No Qualifier
B Bladder Trigone of bladder	X External	Ø Drainage Device 2 Monitoring Device 3 Infusion Device D Intraluminal Device L Artificial Sphincter M Stimulator Lead	Z No Qualifier
D Urethra Bulbourethral (Cowper's) gland Cowper's (bulbourethral) gland External urethral sphincter Internal urethral sphincter Membranous urethra Penile urethra Prostatic urethra	Ø Open 3 Percutaneous 4 Percutaneous Endoscopic 7 Via Natural or Artificial Opening 8 Via Natural or Artificial Opening Endoscopic	Ø Drainage Device 2 Monitoring Device 3 Infusion Device 7 Autologous Tissue Substitute C Extraluminal Device D Intraluminal Device J Synthetic Substitute K Nonautologous Tissue Substitute L Artificial Sphincter Y Other Device	Z No Qualifier
D Urethra Bulbourethral (Cowper's) gland Cowper's (bulbourethral) gland External urethral sphincter Internal urethral sphincter Membranous urethra Penile urethra Prostatic urethra	X External	Ø Drainage Device 2 Monitoring Device 3 Infusion Device D Intraluminal Device L Artificial Sphincter	Z No Qualifier

Non-OR ØTP5[3,4,7]YZ	**Non-OR** ØTP9[7,8][Ø,2,3,D]Z	**Non-OR** ØTPB[7,8][Ø,2,3,D]Z	**Non-OR** ØTPD[7,8][Ø,2,3,D,Y]Z
Non-OR ØTP5[7,8][Ø,2,3,D]Z	**Non-OR** ØTP9X[Ø,2,3,D]Z	**Non-OR** ØTPBX[Ø,2,3,D,L]Z	**Non-OR** ØTPDX[Ø,2,3,D]Z
Non-OR ØTP5X[Ø,2,3,D]Z	**Non-OR** ØTPB[3,4,7]YZ	**Non-OR** ØTPD[3,4]YZ	[NC] ØTPB[Ø,3,4,7,8]MZ
Non-OR ØTP9[3,4,7]YZ			

[NC] Noncovered Procedure   [LC] Limited Coverage   [QA] Questionable OB Admit   [NT] New Tech Add-on   ⊞ Combination Member   ♂ Male   ♀ Female

Urinary System

ØTQ–ØTR

Ø	**Medical and Surgical**		
T	**Urinary System**		
Q	**Repair**	Definition: Restoring, to the extent possible, a body part to its normal anatomic structure and function	
		Explanation: Used only when the method to accomplish the repair is not one of the other root operations	

Body Part Character 4	Approach Character 5	Device Character 6	Qualifier Character 7

Ø **Kidney, Right**
  Renal calyx
  Renal capsule
  Renal cortex
  Renal segment
1 **Kidney, Left**
  See Ø Kidney, Right
3 **Kidney Pelvis, Right**
  Ureteropelvic junction (UPJ)
4 **Kidney Pelvis, Left**
  See 3 Kidney Pelvis, Right
6 **Ureter, Right**
  Ureteral orifice
  Ureterovesical orifice
7 **Ureter, Left**
  See 6 Ureter, Right
B **Bladder** ⊞
  Trigone of bladder
C **Bladder Neck**
	Ø Open
	3 Percutaneous
	4 Percutaneous Endoscopic
	7 Via Natural or Artificial Opening
	8 Via Natural or Artificial Opening Endoscopic
		Z No Device	Z No Qualifier

D **Urethra**
  Bulbourethral (Cowper's) gland
  Cowper's (bulbourethral) gland
  External urethral sphincter
  Internal urethral sphincter
  Membranous urethra
  Penile urethra
  Prostatic urethra
	Ø Open
	3 Percutaneous
	4 Percutaneous Endoscopic
	7 Via Natural or Artificial Opening
	8 Via Natural or Artificial Opening Endoscopic
	X External
		Z No Device	Z No Qualifier

See Appendix L for Procedure Combinations
  ⊞   ØTQB[Ø,3,4]ZZ

Ø	**Medical and Surgical**		
T	**Urinary System**		
R	**Replacement**	Definition: Putting in or on biological or synthetic material that physically takes the place and/or function of all or a portion of a body part	
		Explanation: The body part may have been taken out or replaced, or may be taken out, physically eradicated, or rendered nonfunctional during the REPLACEMENT procedure. A REMOVAL procedure is coded for taking out the device used in a previous replacement procedure.	

Body Part Character 4	Approach Character 5	Device Character 6	Qualifier Character 7

3 **Kidney Pelvis, Right**
  Ureteropelvic junction (UPJ)
4 **Kidney Pelvis, Left**
  See 3 Kidney Pelvis, Right
6 **Ureter, Right**
  Ureteral orifice
  Ureterovesical orifice
7 **Ureter, Left**
  See 6 Ureter, Right
B **Bladder**
  Trigone of bladder
C **Bladder Neck**
	Ø Open
	4 Percutaneous Endoscopic
	7 Via Natural or Artificial Opening
	8 Via Natural or Artificial Opening Endoscopic
		7 Autologous Tissue Substitute
		J Synthetic Substitute
		K Nonautologous Tissue Substitute
			Z No Qualifier

D **Urethra**
  Bulbourethral (Cowper's) gland
  Cowper's (bulbourethral) gland
  External urethral sphincter
  Internal urethral sphincter
  Membranous urethra
  Penile urethra
  Prostatic urethra
	Ø Open
	4 Percutaneous Endoscopic
	7 Via Natural or Artificial Opening
	8 Via Natural or Artificial Opening Endoscopic
	X External
		7 Autologous Tissue Substitute
		J Synthetic Substitute
		K Nonautologous Tissue Substitute
			Z No Qualifier

Non-OR Procedure   DRG Non-OR Procedure   Valid OR Procedure   HAC Associated Procedure   Combination Only   New/Revised April   New/Revised October

638   ICD-10-PCS 2024

Urinary System

Ø   Medical and Surgical
T   Urinary System
S   Reposition   Definition: Moving to its normal location, or other suitable location, all or a portion of a body part

Explanation: The body part is moved to a new location from an abnormal location, or from a normal location where it is not functioning correctly. The body part may or may not be cut out or off to be moved to the new location.

Body Part Character 4	Approach Character 5	Device Character 6	Qualifier Character 7

Ø   Kidney, Right
    Renal calyx
    Renal capsule
    Renal cortex
    Renal segment
1   Kidney, Left
    See Ø Kidney, Right
2   Kidneys, Bilateral
    See Ø Kidney, Right
3   Kidney Pelvis, Right
    Ureteropelvic junction (UPJ)
4   Kidney Pelvis, Left
    See 3 Kidney Pelvis, Right
6   Ureter, Right
    Ureteral orifice
    Ureterovesical orifice
7   Ureter, Left
    See 6 Ureter, Right
8   Ureters, Bilateral
    See 6 Ureter, Right
B   Bladder
    Trigone of bladder
C   Bladder Neck
D   Urethra
    Bulbourethral (Cowper's) gland
    Cowper's (bulbourethral) gland
    External urethral sphincter
    Internal urethral sphincter
    Membranous urethra
    Penile urethra
    Prostatic urethra
	Ø Open
	4 Percutaneous Endoscopic
		Z No Device	Z No Qualifier

Ø   Medical and Surgical
T   Urinary System
T   Resection   Definition: Cutting out or off, without replacement, all of a body part

Explanation: None

Body Part Character 4	Approach Character 5	Device Character 6	Qualifier Character 7

Ø   Kidney, Right
    Renal calyx
    Renal capsule
    Renal cortex
    Renal segment
1   Kidney, Left
    See Ø Kidney, Right
2   Kidneys, Bilateral
    See Ø Kidney, Right
	Ø Open
	4 Percutaneous Endoscopic
		Z No Device	Z No Qualifier

3   Kidney Pelvis, Right
    Ureteropelvic junction (UPJ)
4   Kidney Pelvis, Left
    See 3 Kidney Pelvis, Right
6   Ureter, Right
    Ureteral orifice
    Ureterovesical orifice
7   Ureter, Left
    See 6 Ureter, Right
B   Bladder ⊞
    Trigone of bladder
C   Bladder Neck
D   Urethra
    Bulbourethral (Cowper's) gland
    Cowper's (bulbourethral) gland
    External urethral sphincter
    Internal urethral sphincter
    Membranous urethra
    Penile urethra
    Prostatic urethra
	Ø Open
	4 Percutaneous Endoscopic
	7 Via Natural or Artificial Opening
	8 Via Natural or Artificial Opening Endoscopic
		Z No Device	Z No Qualifier

Non-OR   ØTTD[4,7,8]ZZ

See Appendix L for Procedure Combinations
    Combo-only   ØTTDØZZ
           ⊞   ØTTBØZZ

NC Noncovered Procedure   **LC** Limited Coverage   **QA** Questionable OB Admit   **NT** New Tech Add-on   ⊞ Combination Member   ♂ Male   ♀ Female

ICD-10-PCS 2024   639

Ø   Medical and Surgical
T   Urinary System
U   Supplement   Definition: Putting in or on biological or synthetic material that physically reinforces and/or augments the function of a portion of a body part

Explanation: The biological material is non-living, or is living and from the same individual. The body part may have been previously replaced, and the SUPPLEMENT procedure is performed to physically reinforce and/or augment the function of the replaced body part.

Body Part Character 4	Approach Character 5	Device Character 6	Qualifier Character 7

3 **Kidney Pelvis, Right**
   Ureteropelvic junction (UPJ)
4 **Kidney Pelvis, Left**
   See 3 Kidney Pelvis, Right
6 **Ureter, Right**
   Ureteral orifice
   Ureterovesical orifice
7 **Ureter, Left**
   See 6 Ureter, Right
B **Bladder**
   Trigone of bladder
C **Bladder Neck**
	Ø **Open**
	4 **Percutaneous Endoscopic**
	7 **Via Natural or Artificial Opening**
	8 **Via Natural or Artificial Opening
	   Endoscopic**
		7 **Autologous Tissue Substitute**
		J **Synthetic Substitute**
		K **Nonautologous Tissue Substitute**
			Z **No Qualifier**

D **Urethra**
   Bulbourethral (Cowper's) gland
   Cowper's (bulbourethral) gland
   External urethral sphincter
   Internal urethral sphincter
   Membranous urethra
   Penile urethra
   Prostatic urethra
	Ø **Open**
	4 **Percutaneous Endoscopic**
	7 **Via Natural or Artificial Opening**
	8 **Via Natural or Artificial Opening
	   Endoscopic**
	X **External**
		7 **Autologous Tissue Substitute**
		J **Synthetic Substitute**
		K **Nonautologous Tissue Substitute**
			Z **No Qualifier**

Ø   Medical and Surgical
T   Urinary System
V   Restriction   Definition: Partially closing an orifice or the lumen of a tubular body part

Explanation: The orifice can be a natural orifice or an artificially created orifice

Body Part Character 4	Approach Character 5	Device Character 6	Qualifier Character 7

3 **Kidney Pelvis, Right**
   Ureteropelvic junction (UPJ)
4 **Kidney Pelvis, Left**
   See 3 Kidney Pelvis, Right
6 **Ureter, Right**
   Ureteral orifice
   Ureterovesical orifice
7 **Ureter, Left**
   See 6 Ureter, Right
B **Bladder**
   Trigone of bladder
C **Bladder Neck**
	Ø **Open**
	3 **Percutaneous**
	4 **Percutaneous Endoscopic**
		C **Extraluminal Device**
		D **Intraluminal Device**
		Z **No Device**
			Z **No Qualifier**

3 **Kidney Pelvis, Right**
   Ureteropelvic junction (UPJ)
4 **Kidney Pelvis, Left**
   See 3 Kidney Pelvis, Right
6 **Ureter, Right**
   Ureteral orifice
   Ureterovesical orifice
7 **Ureter, Left**
   See 6 Ureter, Right
B **Bladder**
   Trigone of bladder
C **Bladder Neck**
	7 **Via Natural or Artificial Opening**
	8 **Via Natural or Artificial Opening
	   Endoscopic**
		D **Intraluminal Device**
		Z **No Device**
			Z **No Qualifier**

D **Urethra**
   Bulbourethral (Cowper's) gland
   Cowper's (bulbourethral) gland
   External urethral sphincter
   Internal urethral sphincter
   Membranous urethra
   Penile urethra
   Prostatic urethra
	Ø **Open**
	3 **Percutaneous**
	4 **Percutaneous Endoscopic**
		C **Extraluminal Device**
		D **Intraluminal Device**
		Z **No Device**
			Z **No Qualifier**

D **Urethra**
   Bulbourethral (Cowper's) gland
   Cowper's (bulbourethral) gland
   External urethral sphincter
   Internal urethral sphincter
   Membranous urethra
   Penile urethra
   Prostatic urethra
	7 **Via Natural or Artificial Opening**
	8 **Via Natural or Artificial Opening
	   Endoscopic**
		D **Intraluminal Device**
		Z **No Device**
			Z **No Qualifier**

D **Urethra**
   Bulbourethral (Cowper's) gland
   Cowper's (bulbourethral) gland
   External urethral sphincter
   Internal urethral sphincter
   Membranous urethra
   Penile urethra
   Prostatic urethra
	X **External**	Z **No Device**	Z **No Qualifier**

Non-OR Procedure   DRG Non-OR Procedure   Valid OR Procedure   HAC Associated Procedure   Combination Only   New/Revised April   New/Revised October

640   ICD-10-PCS 2024

ØTU–ØTV

Ø Medical and Surgical
T Urinary System
W Revision
Definition: Correcting, to the extent possible, a portion of a malfunctioning device or the position of a displaced device
Explanation: Revision can include correcting a malfunctioning or displaced device by taking out or putting in components of the device such as a screw or pin

Body Part Character 4	Approach Character 5	Device Character 6	Qualifier Character 7
5 Kidney Renal calyx Renal capsule Renal cortex Renal segment	Ø Open 3 Percutaneous 4 Percutaneous Endoscopic 7 Via Natural or Artificial Opening 8 Via Natural or Artificial Opening Endoscopic	Ø Drainage Device 2 Monitoring Device 3 Infusion Device 7 Autologous Tissue Substitute C Extraluminal Device D Intraluminal Device J Synthetic Substitute K Nonautologous Tissue Substitute Y Other Device	Z No Qualifier
5 Kidney Renal calyx Renal capsule Renal cortex Renal segment	X External	Ø Drainage Device 2 Monitoring Device 3 Infusion Device 7 Autologous Tissue Substitute C Extraluminal Device D Intraluminal Device J Synthetic Substitute K Nonautologous Tissue Substitute	Z No Qualifier
9 Ureter Ureteral orifice Ureterovesical orifice	Ø Open 3 Percutaneous 4 Percutaneous Endoscopic 7 Via Natural or Artificial Opening 8 Via Natural or Artificial Opening Endoscopic	Ø Drainage Device 2 Monitoring Device 3 Infusion Device 7 Autologous Tissue Substitute C Extraluminal Device D Intraluminal Device J Synthetic Substitute K Nonautologous Tissue Substitute M Stimulator Lead Y Other Device	Z No Qualifier
9 Ureter Ureteral orifice Ureterovesical orifice	X External	Ø Drainage Device 2 Monitoring Device 3 Infusion Device 7 Autologous Tissue Substitute C Extraluminal Device D Intraluminal Device J Synthetic Substitute K Nonautologous Tissue Substitute M Stimulator Lead	Z No Qualifier
B Bladder Trigone of bladder	Ø Open 3 Percutaneous 4 Percutaneous Endoscopic 7 Via Natural or Artificial Opening 8 Via Natural or Artificial Opening Endoscopic	Ø Drainage Device 2 Monitoring Device 3 Infusion Device 7 Autologous Tissue Substitute C Extraluminal Device D Intraluminal Device J Synthetic Substitute K Nonautologous Tissue Substitute L Artificial Sphincter M Stimulator Lead Y Other Device	Z No Qualifier
B Bladder Trigone of bladder	X External	Ø Drainage Device 2 Monitoring Device 3 Infusion Device 7 Autologous Tissue Substitute C Extraluminal Device D Intraluminal Device J Synthetic Substitute K Nonautologous Tissue Substitute L Artificial Sphincter M Stimulator Lead	Z No Qualifier

Non-OR ØTW5[3,4,7]YZ
Non-OR ØTW5X[Ø,2,3,7,C,D,J,K]Z
Non-OR ØTW9[3,4,7]YZ

Non-OR ØTW9X[Ø,2,3,7,C,D,J,K,M]Z
Non-OR ØTWB[3,4,7]YZ
Non-OR ØTWBX[Ø,2,3,7,C,D,J,K,L,M]Z

ØTW Continued on next page

NC Noncovered Procedure   LC Limited Coverage   QA Questionable OB Admit   NT New Tech Add-on   ⊞ Combination Member   ♂ Male   ♀ Female
ICD-10-PCS 2024   641

ØTW–ØTW

Ø **Medical and Surgical**
T **Urinary System**
W **Revision** — Definition: Correcting, to the extent possible, a portion of a malfunctioning device or the position of a displaced device

ØTW Continued

Explanation: Revision can include correcting a malfunctioning or displaced device by taking out or putting in components of the device such as a screw or pin

Body Part Character 4	Approach Character 5	Device Character 6	Qualifier Character 7
D Urethra Bulbourethral (Cowper's) gland Cowper's (bulbourethral) gland External urethral sphincter Internal urethral sphincter Membranous urethra Penile urethra Prostatic urethra	**Ø** Open **3** Percutaneous **4** Percutaneous Endoscopic **7** Via Natural or Artificial Opening **8** Via Natural or Artificial Opening Endoscopic	**Ø** Drainage Device **2** Monitoring Device **3** Infusion Device **7** Autologous Tissue Substitute **C** Extraluminal Device **D** Intraluminal Device **J** Synthetic Substitute **K** Nonautologous Tissue Substitute **L** Artificial Sphincter **Y** Other Device	**Z** No Qualifier
D Urethra Bulbourethral (Cowper's) gland Cowper's (bulbourethral) gland External urethral sphincter Internal urethral sphincter Membranous urethra Penile urethra Prostatic urethra	**X** External	**Ø** Drainage Device **2** Monitoring Device **3** Infusion Device **7** Autologous Tissue Substitute **C** Extraluminal Device **D** Intraluminal Device **J** Synthetic Substitute **K** Nonautologous Tissue Substitute **L** Artificial Sphincter	**Z** No Qualifier

Non-OR   ØTWD[3,4,7,8]YZ
Non-OR   ØTWDX[Ø,2,3,7,C,D,J,K,L]Z

Ø **Medical and Surgical**
T **Urinary System**
Y **Transplantation** — Definition: Putting in or on all or a portion of a living body part taken from another individual or animal to physically take the place and/or function of all or a portion of a similar body part

Explanation: The native body part may or may not be taken out, and the transplanted body part may take over all or a portion of its function

Body Part Character 4	Approach Character 5	Device Character 6	Qualifier Character 7
Ø Kidney, Right `LC` ⊞ Renal calyx Renal capsule Renal cortex Renal segment **1** Kidney, Left `LC` ⊞ *See Ø Kidney, Right*	**Ø** Open	**Z** No Device	**Ø** Allogeneic **1** Syngeneic **2** Zooplastic

`LC`   ØTY[Ø,1]ØZ[Ø,1,2]

See Appendix L for Procedure Combinations
⊞   ØTY[Ø,1]ØZ[Ø,1,2]

Non-OR Procedure   DRG Non-OR Procedure   Valid OR Procedure   HAC Associated Procedure   Combination Only   New/Revised April   New/Revised October

642

ICD-10-PCS 2024

Female Reproductive System ØU1–ØUY

Character Meanings

This Character Meaning table is provided as a guide to assist the user in the identification of character members that may be found in this section of code tables. It **SHOULD NOT** be used to build a PCS code.

Operation–Character 3		Body Part–Character 4		Approach–Character 5		Device–Character 6		Qualifier–Character 7	
1	Bypass	Ø	Ovary, Right	Ø	Open	Ø	Drainage Device	Ø	Allogeneic
2	Change	1	Ovary, Left	3	Percutaneous	1	Radioactive Element	1	Syngeneic
5	Destruction	2	Ovaries, Bilateral	4	Percutaneous Endoscopic	3	Infusion Device	2	Zooplastic
7	Dilation	3	Ovary	7	Via Natural or Artificial Opening	7	Autologous Tissue Substitute	5	Fallopian Tube, Right
8	Division	4	Uterine Supporting Structure	8	Via Natural or Artificial Opening Endoscopic	C	Extraluminal Device	6	Fallopian Tube, Left
9	Drainage	5	Fallopian Tube, Right	F	Via Natural or Artificial Opening With Percutaneous Endoscopic Assistance	D	Intraluminal Device	9	Uterus
B	Excision	6	Fallopian Tube, Left	X	External	G	Intraluminal Device, Pessary	L	Supracervical
C	Extirpation	7	Fallopian Tubes, Bilateral			H	Contraceptive Device	X	Diagnostic
D	Extraction	8	Fallopian Tube			J	Synthetic Substitute	Z	No Qualifier
F	Fragmentation	9	Uterus			K	Nonautologous Tissue Substitute		
H	Insertion	B	Endometrium			Y	Other Device		
J	Inspection	C	Cervix			Z	No Device		
L	Occlusion	D	Uterus and Cervix						
M	Reattachment	F	Cul-de-sac						
N	Release	G	Vagina						
P	Removal	H	Vagina and Cul-de-sac						
Q	Repair	J	Clitoris						
S	Reposition	K	Hymen						
T	Resection	L	Vestibular Gland						
U	Supplement	M	Vulva						
V	Restriction	N	Ova						
W	Revision								
Y	Transplantation								

AHA Coding Clinic for table ØU5
2015, 3Q, 31   Tubal ligation for sterilization

AHA Coding Clinic for table ØU7
2020, 2Q, 30   Duhrssen cervical incision

AHA Coding Clinic for table ØU9
2016, 4Q, 58   Longitudinal vaginal septum

AHA Coding Clinic for table ØUB
2018, 1Q, 23   Tubal ligation procedure
2015, 3Q, 31   Laparoscopic partial salpingectomy for ectopic pregnancy
2015, 3Q, 31   Tubal ligation for sterilization
2014, 4Q, 16   Excision of multiple uterine fibroids
2014, 3Q, 12   Excision of skin tag from labia majora

AHA Coding Clinic for table ØUC
2015, 3Q, 30   Removal of cervical cerclage
2013, 2Q, 38   Evacuation of clot post-partum

AHA Coding Clinic for table ØUH
2020, 4Q, 43-44   Insertion of radioactive element
2018, 1Q, 25   Intrauterine brachytherapy & placement of tandems & ovoids
2013, 2Q, 34   Placement of intrauterine device via open approach

AHA Coding Clinic for table ØUJ
2015, 1Q, 33   Robotic-assisted laparoscopic hysterectomy converted to open procedure

AHA Coding Clinic for table ØUL
2018, 1Q, 23   Tubal ligation procedure
2015, 3Q, 31   Tubal ligation for sterilization

AHA Coding Clinic for table ØUP
2022, 3Q, 13   Repair of prolapsed neovaginal graft

AHA Coding Clinic for table ØUQ
2020, 4Q, 59-60   Extraction of ectopic products of conception
2014, 4Q, 18   Obstetrical periurethral laceration
2013, 4Q, 120   Repair of clitoral obstetric laceration

AHA Coding Clinic for table ØUS
2016, 1Q, 9   Anteversion of retroverted pregnant uterus

AHA Coding Clinic for table ØUT
2022, 1Q, 21   Gravid hysterectomy due to placenta increta
2017, 4Q, 68   New qualifier values - Supracervical hysterectomy
2015, 1Q, 33   Robotic-assisted laparoscopic hysterectomy converted to open procedure
2013, 3Q, 28   Total hysterectomy
2013, 1Q, 24   Excision versus Resection of remaining ovarian remnant following previous excision

AHA Coding Clinic for table ØUV
2015, 3Q, 30   Insertion of cervical cerclage

AHA Coding Clinic for table ØUY
2023, 2Q, 32   Preparation of donor organ before transplantation
2018, 4Q, 40   Uterus transplant

Female Reproductive System

Female Internal/External Structures

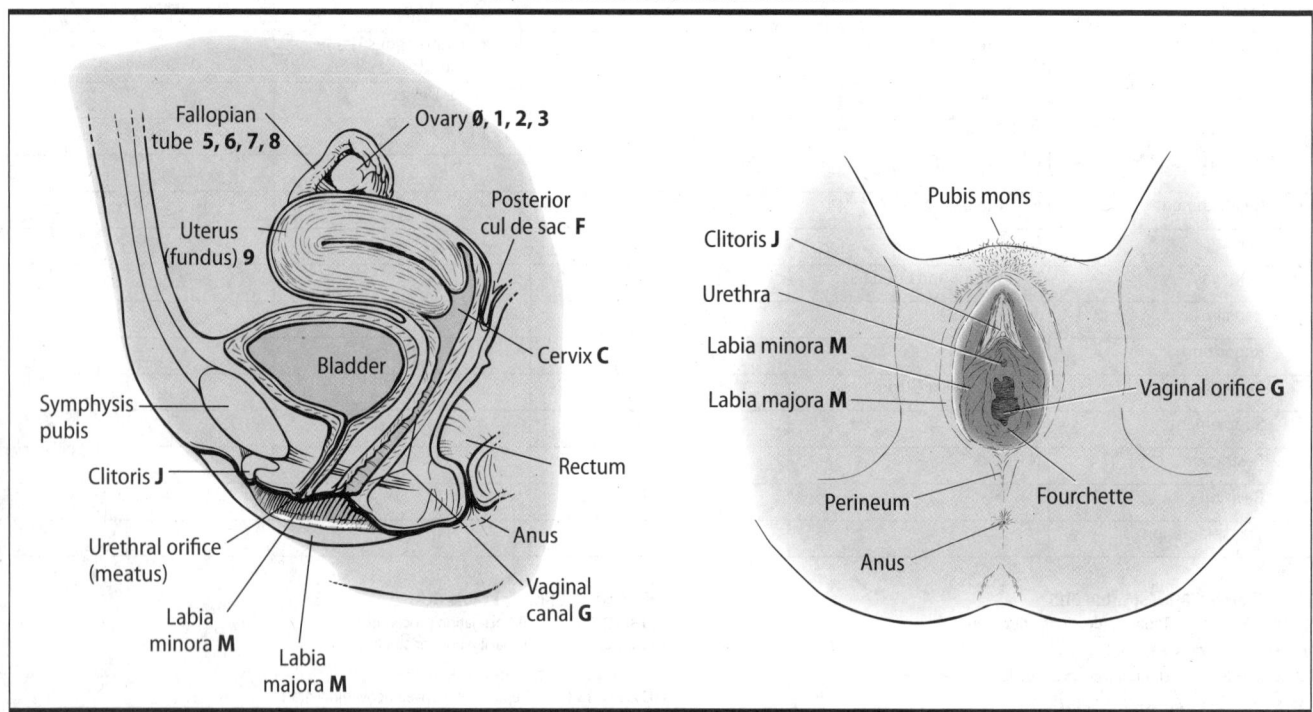

Ø   Medical and Surgical
U   Female Reproductive System
1   Bypass   Definition: Altering the route of passage of the contents of a tubular body part

Explanation: Rerouting contents of a body part to a downstream area of the normal route, to a similar route and body part, or to an abnormal route and dissimilar body part. Includes one or more anastomoses, with or without the use of a device.

Body Part Character 4	Approach Character 5	Device Character 6	Qualifier Character 7

5 Fallopian Tube, Right ♀
    Oviduct
    Salpinx
    Uterine tube
6 Fallopian Tube, Left ♀
    See 5 Fallopian Tube, Right
	Ø Open
	4 Percutaneous Endoscopic
		7 Autologous Tissue Substitute
		J Synthetic Substitute
		K Nonautologous Tissue Substitute
		Z No Device
			5 Fallopian Tube, Right
			6 Fallopian Tube, Left
			9 Uterus

♀   All body part, approach, device, and qualifier values

Ø   Medical and Surgical
U   Female Reproductive System
2   Change   Definition: Taking out or off a device from a body part and putting back an identical or similar device in or on the same body part without cutting or puncturing the skin or a mucous membrane

Explanation: All CHANGE procedures are coded using the approach EXTERNAL

Body Part Character 4	Approach Character 5	Device Character 6	Qualifier Character 7

3 Ovary ♀
8 Fallopian Tube ♀
M Vulva ♀
    Labia majora
    Labia minora
	X External	Ø Drainage Device
		Y Other Device
			Z No Qualifier

D Uterus and Cervix ♀	X External	Ø Drainage Device H Contraceptive Device Y Other Device	Z No Qualifier
H Vagina and Cul-de-sac ♀	X External	Ø Drainage Device G Intraluminal Device, Pessary Y Other Device	Z No Qualifier

Non-OR   All body part, approach, device, and qualifier values   ♀   All body part, approach, device, and qualifier values

Female Reproductive System

Ø   Medical and Surgical
U   Female Reproductive System
5   Destruction   Definition: Physical eradication of all or a portion of a body part by the direct use of energy, force, or a destructive agent
                      Explanation: None of the body part is physically taken out

Body Part Character 4	Approach Character 5	Device Character 6	Qualifier Character 7

Ø Ovary, Right ♀
1 Ovary, Left ♀
2 Ovaries, Bilateral ♀
4 Uterine Supporting Structure ♀
   Broad ligament
   Infundibulopelvic ligament
   Ovarian ligament
   Round ligament of uterus
	Ø Open
	3 Percutaneous
	4 Percutaneous Endoscopic
	8 Via Natural or Artificial Opening Endoscopic
		Z No Device	Z No Qualifier

5 Fallopian Tube, Right ♀
   Oviduct
   Salpinx
   Uterine tube
6 Fallopian Tube, Left ♀
   See 5 Fallopian Tube, Right
7 Fallopian Tubes, Bilateral **NC** ♀
9 Uterus ♀
   Fundus uteri
   Myometrium
   Perimetrium
   Uterine cornu
B Endometrium ♀
C Cervix ♀
F Cul-de-sac ♀
	Ø Open
	3 Percutaneous
	4 Percutaneous Endoscopic
	7 Via Natural or Artificial Opening
	8 Via Natural or Artificial Opening Endoscopic
		Z No Device	Z No Qualifier

G Vagina ♀ K Hymen ♀	Ø Open 3 Percutaneous 4 Percutaneous Endoscopic 7 Via Natural or Artificial Opening 8 Via Natural or Artificial Opening Endoscopic X External	Z No Device	Z No Qualifier

J Clitoris ♀
L Vestibular Gland ♀
   Bartholin's (greater vestibular) gland
   Greater vestibular (Bartholin's) gland
   Paraurethral (Skene's) gland
   Skene's (paraurethral) gland
M Vulva ♀
   Labia majora
   Labia minora
	Ø Open
	X External
		Z No Device	Z No Qualifier

NC   ØU57[Ø,3,4,7,8]ZZ with principal or secondary diagnosis of Z3Ø.2   ♀   All body part, approach, device, and qualifier values

Ø   Medical and Surgical
U   Female Reproductive System
7   Dilation   Definition: Expanding an orifice or the lumen of a tubular body part

Explanation: The orifice can be a natural orifice or an artificially created orifice. Accomplished by stretching a tubular body part using intraluminal pressure or by cutting part of the orifice or wall of the tubular body part.

Body Part Character 4	Approach Character 5	Device Character 6	Qualifier Character 7
5 Fallopian Tube, Right ♀ Oviduct Salpinx Uterine tube **6 Fallopian Tube, Left** ♀ *See 5 Fallopian Tube, Right* **7 Fallopian Tubes, Bilateral** ♀ **9 Uterus** ♀ Fundus uteri Myometrium Perimetrium Uterine cornu **C Cervix** ♀ **G Vagina** ♀	**Ø** Open **3** Percutaneous **4** Percutaneous Endoscopic **7** Via Natural or Artificial Opening **8** Via Natural or Artificial Opening Endoscopic	**D** Intraluminal Device **Z** No Device	**Z** No Qualifier
K Hymen ♀	**Ø** Open **3** Percutaneous **4** Percutaneous Endoscopic **7** Via Natural or Artificial Opening **8** Via Natural or Artificial Opening Endoscopic **X** External	**D** Intraluminal Device **Z** No Device	**Z** No Qualifier

Non-OR	ØU7C[Ø,3,4,7,8][D,Z]Z	♀	All body part, approach, device, and qualifier values
Non-OR	ØU7G[7,8][D,Z]Z		

Ø   Medical and Surgical
U   Female Reproductive System
8   Division   Definition: Cutting into a body part, without draining fluids and/or gases from the body part, in order to separate or transect a body part

Explanation: All or a portion of the body part is separated into two or more portions

Body Part Character 4	Approach Character 5	Device Character 6	Qualifier Character 7
Ø Ovary, Right ♀ **1 Ovary, Left** ♀ **2 Ovaries, Bilateral** ♀ **4 Uterine Supporting Structure** ♀ Broad ligament Infundibulopelvic ligament Ovarian ligament Round ligament of uterus	**Ø** Open **3** Percutaneous **4** Percutaneous Endoscopic	**Z** No Device	**Z** No Qualifier
K Hymen ♀	**7** Via Natural or Artificial Opening **8** Via Natural or Artificial Opening Endoscopic **X** External	**Z** No Device	**Z** No Qualifier

Non-OR	ØU8K[7,8,X]ZZ	♀	All body part, approach, device, and qualifier values

---

NC Noncovered Procedure   LC Limited Coverage   QA Questionable OB Admit   NT New Tech Add-on   ⊞ Combination Member   ♂ Male   ♀ Female

Female Reproductive System

Ø   **Medical and Surgical**
U   **Female Reproductive System**
9   **Drainage**   Definition: Taking or letting out fluids and/or gases from a body part
                    Explanation: The qualifier DIAGNOSTIC is used to identify drainage procedures that are biopsies

Body Part Character 4	Approach Character 5	Device Character 6	Qualifier Character 7
Ø Ovary, Right ♀ 1 Ovary, Left ♀ 2 Ovaries, Bilateral ♀	Ø Open 3 Percutaneous 4 Percutaneous Endoscopic 8 Via Natural or Artificial Opening Endoscopic	Ø Drainage Device	Z No Qualifier
Ø Ovary, Right ♀ 1 Ovary, Left ♀ 2 Ovaries, Bilateral ♀	Ø Open 3 Percutaneous 4 Percutaneous Endoscopic 8 Via Natural or Artificial Opening Endoscopic	Z No Device	X Diagnostic Z No Qualifier
Ø Ovary, Right ♀ 1 Ovary, Left ♀ 2 Ovaries, Bilateral ♀	X External	Z No Device	Z No Qualifier

4 Uterine Supporting Structure ♀
   Broad ligament
   Infundibulopelvic ligament
   Ovarian ligament
   Round ligament of uterus
	Ø Open
	3 Percutaneous
	4 Percutaneous Endoscopic
	8 Via Natural or Artificial Opening Endoscopic
		Ø Drainage Device	Z No Qualifier

4 Uterine Supporting Structure ♀
   Broad ligament
   Infundibulopelvic ligament
   Ovarian ligament
   Round ligament of uterus
	Ø Open
	3 Percutaneous
	4 Percutaneous Endoscopic
	8 Via Natural or Artificial Opening Endoscopic
		Z No Device	X Diagnostic
			Z No Qualifier

5 Fallopian Tube, Right ♀
   Oviduct
   Salpinx
   Uterine tube
6 Fallopian Tube, Left ♀
   See 5 Fallopian Tube, Right
7 Fallopian Tubes, Bilateral ♀
9 Uterus ♀
   Fundus uteri
   Myometrium
   Perimetrium
   Uterine cornu
C Cervix ♀
F Cul-de-sac ♀
	Ø Open
	3 Percutaneous
	4 Percutaneous Endoscopic
	7 Via Natural or Artificial Opening
	8 Via Natural or Artificial Opening Endoscopic
		Ø Drainage Device	Z No Qualifier

5 Fallopian Tube, Right ♀
   Oviduct
   Salpinx
   Uterine tube
6 Fallopian Tube, Left ♀
   See 5 Fallopian Tube, Right
7 Fallopian Tubes, Bilateral ♀
9 Uterus ♀
   Fundus uteri
   Myometrium
   Perimetrium
   Uterine cornu
C Cervix ♀
F Cul-de-sac ♀
	Ø Open
	3 Percutaneous
	4 Percutaneous Endoscopic
	7 Via Natural or Artificial Opening
	8 Via Natural or Artificial Opening Endoscopic
		Z No Device	X Diagnostic
			Z No Qualifier

Non-OR ØU9[Ø,1,2][3,8]ØZ		**Non-OR** ØU9[5,6,7,9,C]3ØZ	
Non-OR ØU9[Ø,1,2][3,8]ZZ		**Non-OR** ØU9F[3,4]ØZ	
Non-OR ØU9[Ø,1,2]8ZX		**Non-OR** ØU9[5,6,7][3,4,7,8]ZZ	
Non-OR ØU94[3,8]ØZ		**Non-OR** ØU9[9,C]3ZZ	
Non-OR ØU94[3,8]ZZ		**Non-OR** ØU9F[3,4]ZZ	
Non-OR ØU948ZX		♀ All body part, approach, device, and qualifier values	

ØU9 Continued on next page

Non-OR Procedure   DRG Non-OR Procedure   Valid OR Procedure   HAC Associated Procedure   Combination Only   New/Revised April   New/Revised October

0U9 Continued

0   **Medical and Surgical**
U   **Female Reproductive System**
9   **Drainage**   Definition: Taking or letting out fluids and/or gases from a body part
                   Explanation: The qualifier DIAGNOSTIC is used to identify drainage procedures that are biopsies

Body Part Character 4	Approach Character 5	Device Character 6	Qualifier Character 7
G Vagina ♀ **K** Hymen ♀	**0** Open **3** Percutaneous **4** Percutaneous Endoscopic **7** Via Natural or Artificial Opening **8** Via Natural or Artificial Opening Endoscopic **X** External	**0** Drainage Device	**Z** No Qualifier
G Vagina ♀ **K** Hymen ♀	**0** Open **3** Percutaneous **4** Percutaneous Endoscopic **7** Via Natural or Artificial Opening **8** Via Natural or Artificial Opening Endoscopic **X** External	**Z** No Device	**X** Diagnostic **Z** No Qualifier

J Clitoris ♀
L Vestibular Gland ♀
   Bartholin's (greater vestibular) gland
   Greater vestibular (Bartholin's) gland
   Paraurethral (Skene's) gland
   Skene's (paraurethral) gland
M Vulva ♀
   Labia majora
   Labia minora
	0 Open
	X External
		0 Drainage Device	**Z** No Qualifier

J Clitoris ♀
L Vestibular Gland ♀
   Bartholin's (greater vestibular) gland
   Greater vestibular (Bartholin's) gland
   Paraurethral (Skene's) gland
   Skene's (paraurethral) gland
M Vulva ♀
   Labia majora
   Labia minora
	0 Open
	X External
		Z No Device	**X** Diagnostic
			Z No Qualifier

Non-OR 0U9G30Z		**Non-OR** 0U9L[0,X]0Z	
Non-OR 0U9K[0,3,4,7,8,X]0Z		**Non-OR** 0U9L[0,X]Z[X,Z]	
Non-OR 0U9G3ZZ		♀ All body part, approach, device, and qualifier values	
Non-OR 0U9K[0,3,4,7,8,X]ZZ			

NC Noncovered Procedure   **LC** Limited Coverage   **QA** Questionable OB Admit   **NT** New Tech Add-on   ⊞ Combination Member   ♂ Male   ♀ Female

ICD-10-PCS 2024   **649**

Female Reproductive System

Ø   Medical and Surgical
U   Female Reproductive System
B   Excision   Definition: Cutting out or off, without replacement, a portion of a body part
                Explanation: The qualifier DIAGNOSTIC is used to identify excision procedures that are biopsies

Body Part Character 4	Approach Character 5	Device Character 6	Qualifier Character 7

Ø Ovary, Right ♀
1 Ovary, Left ♀
2 Ovaries, Bilateral ♀
4 Uterine Supporting Structure ♀
    Broad ligament
    Infundibulopelvic ligament
    Ovarian ligament
    Round ligament of uterus
5 Fallopian Tube, Right ♀
    Oviduct
    Salpinx
    Uterine tube
6 Fallopian Tube, Left ♀
    See 5 Fallopian Tube, Right
7 Fallopian Tubes, Bilateral ♀
9 Uterus ♀
    Fundus uteri
    Myometrium
    Perimetrium
    Uterine cornu
C Cervix ♀
F Cul-de-sac ♀
	Ø Open
	3 Percutaneous
	4 Percutaneous Endoscopic
	7 Via Natural or Artificial Opening
	8 Via Natural or Artificial Opening
	    Endoscopic
		Z No Device	**X** Diagnostic
			Z No Qualifier

G Vagina ♀ **K** Hymen ♀	**Ø** Open **3** Percutaneous **4** Percutaneous Endoscopic **7** Via Natural or Artificial Opening **8** Via Natural or Artificial Opening Endoscopic **X** External	**Z** No Device	**X** Diagnostic **Z** No Qualifier

J Clitoris ♀
L Vestibular Gland ♀
    Bartholin's (greater vestibular) gland
    Greater vestibular (Bartholin's) gland
    Paraurethral (Skene's) gland
    Skene's (paraurethral) gland
M Vulva ♀
    Labia majora
    Labia minora
	Ø Open
	X External
		Z No Device	**X** Diagnostic
			Z No Qualifier

♀   All body part, approach, device, and qualifier values

Non-OR Procedure   DRG Non-OR Procedure   Valid OR Procedure   HAC Associated Procedure   Combination Only   New/Revised April   New/Revised October

650   ICD-10-PCS 2024

Female Reproductive System

Ø	Medical and Surgical
U	Female Reproductive System
C	Extirpation Definition: Taking or cutting out solid matter from a body part

Explanation: The solid matter may be an abnormal byproduct of a biological function or a foreign body; it may be imbedded in a body part or in the lumen of a tubular body part. The solid matter may or may not have been previously broken into pieces.

Body Part Character 4		Approach Character 5	Device Character 6	Qualifier Character 7

Ø Ovary, Right ♀
1 Ovary, Left ♀
2 Ovaries, Bilateral ♀
4 Uterine Supporting Structure ♀
   Broad ligament
   Infundibulopelvic ligament
   Ovarian ligament
   Round ligament of uterus
		Ø Open
		3 Percutaneous
		4 Percutaneous Endoscopic
		8 Via Natural or Artificial Opening
		   Endoscopic
			Z No Device	**Z** No Qualifier

5 Fallopian Tube, Right ♀
   Oviduct
   Salpinx
   Uterine tube
6 Fallopian Tube, Left ♀
   See 5 Fallopian Tube, Right
7 Fallopian Tubes, Bilateral ♀
9 Uterus ♀
   Fundus uteri
   Myometrium
   Perimetrium
   Uterine cornu
B Endometrium ♀
C Cervix ♀
F Cul-de-sac ♀
		Ø Open
		3 Percutaneous
		4 Percutaneous Endoscopic
		7 Via Natural or Artificial Opening
		8 Via Natural or Artificial Opening
		   Endoscopic
			Z No Device	**Z** No Qualifier

G Vagina ♀ **K** Hymen ♀		**Ø** Open **3** Percutaneous **4** Percutaneous Endoscopic **7** Via Natural or Artificial Opening **8** Via Natural or Artificial Opening Endoscopic **X** External	**Z** No Device	**Z** No Qualifier

J Clitoris ♀
L Vestibular Gland ♀
   Bartholin's (greater vestibular) gland
   Greater vestibular (Bartholin's) gland
   Paraurethral (Skene's) gland
   Skene's (paraurethral) gland
M Vulva ♀
   Labia majora
   Labia minora
		Ø Open
		X External
			Z No Device	**Z** No Qualifier

Non-OR	ØUC9[7,8]ZZ	**Non-OR**	ØUCMXZZ
Non-OR	ØUCG[7,8,X]ZZ	♀	All body part, approach, device, and qualifier values
Non-OR	ØUCK[Ø,3,4,7,8,X]ZZ		

Ø	Medical and Surgical
U	Female Reproductive System
D	Extraction Definition: Pulling or stripping out or off all or a portion of a body part by the use of force

Explanation: The qualifier DIAGNOSTIC is used to identify extraction procedures that are biopsies

Body Part Character 4		Approach Character 5	Device Character 6	Qualifier Character 7
B Endometrium ♀		**7** Via Natural or Artificial Opening **8** Via Natural or Artificial Opening Endoscopic	**Z** No Device	**X** Diagnostic **Z** No Qualifier
N Ova ♀		**Ø** Open **3** Percutaneous **4** Percutaneous Endoscopic	**Z** No Device	**Z** No Qualifier

♀	All body part, approach, device, and qualifier values

NC Noncovered Procedure   **LC** Limited Coverage   **QA** Questionable OB Admit   **NT** New Tech Add-on   ⊞ Combination Member   ♂ Male   ♀ Female

ICD-10-PCS 2024   651

Female Reproductive System

ØUC–ØUD

Female Reproductive System (side tab)

Ø   **Medical and Surgical**
U   **Female Reproductive System**
F   **Fragmentation**   Definition: Breaking solid matter in a body part into pieces

Explanation: Physical force (e.g., manual, ultrasonic) applied directly or indirectly is used to break the solid matter into pieces. The solid matter may be an abnormal byproduct of a biological function or a foreign body. The pieces of solid matter are not taken out.

Body Part Character 4	Approach Character 5	Device Character 6	Qualifier Character 7

5   Fallopian Tube, Right   NC ♀
    Oviduct
    Salpinx
    Uterine tube
6   Fallopian Tube, Left   NC ♀
    See 5 Fallopian Tube, Right
7   Fallopian Tubes, Bilateral   NC ♀
9   Uterus   NC ♀
    Fundus uteri
    Myometrium
    Perimetrium
    Uterine cornu
	Ø Open
	3 Percutaneous
	4 Percutaneous Endoscopic
	7 Via Natural or Artificial Opening
	8 Via Natural or Artificial Opening
	    Endoscopic
	X External
		Z No Device	Z No Qualifier

Non-OR	ØUF[5,6,7,9]XZZ
NC	ØUF[5,6,7,9]XZZ

♀   All body part, approach, device, and qualifier values

Ø   **Medical and Surgical**
U   **Female Reproductive System**
H   **Insertion**   Definition: Putting in a nonbiological appliance that monitors, assists, performs, or prevents a physiological function but does not physically take the place of a body part

Explanation: None

Body Part Character 4	Approach Character 5	Device Character 6	Qualifier Character 7
3 Ovary ♀	Ø Open 3 Percutaneous 4 Percutaneous Endoscopic	1 Radioactive Element 3 Infusion Device Y Other Device	Z No Qualifier
3 Ovary ♀	7 Via Natural or Artificial Opening 8 Via Natural or Artificial Opening Endoscopic	1 Radioactive Element Y Other Device	Z No Qualifier
8 Fallopian Tube ♀ D Uterus and Cervix ♀ H Vagina and Cul-de-sac ♀	Ø Open 3 Percutaneous 4 Percutaneous Endoscopic 7 Via Natural or Artificial Opening 8 Via Natural or Artificial Opening Endoscopic	3 Infusion Device Y Other Device	Z No Qualifier

9   Uterus   ♀
    Fundus uteri
    Myometrium
    Perimetrium
    Uterine cornu
	Ø Open
	7 Via Natural or Artificial Opening
	8 Via Natural or Artificial Opening
	    Endoscopic
		1 Radioactive Element
		H Contraceptive Device
			Z No Qualifier

C Cervix ♀	Ø Open 3 Percutaneous 4 Percutaneous Endoscopic	1 Radioactive Element	Z No Qualifier
C Cervix ♀	7 Via Natural or Artificial Opening 8 Via Natural or Artificial Opening Endoscopic	1 Radioactive Element H Contraceptive Device	Z No Qualifier
F Cul-de-sac ♀	7 Via Natural or Artificial Opening 8 Via Natural or Artificial Opening Endoscopic	G Intraluminal Device, Pessary	Z No Qualifier
G Vagina ♀	Ø Open 3 Percutaneous 4 Percutaneous Endoscopic X External	1 Radioactive Element	Z No Qualifier
G Vagina ♀	7 Via Natural or Artificial Opening 8 Via Natural or Artificial Opening Endoscopic	1 Radioactive Element G Intraluminal Device, Pessary	Z No Qualifier

Non-OR	ØUH3[Ø,4][3,Y]Z		Non-OR	ØUH9[Ø,7,8][1,H]Z
Non-OR	ØUH33[1,3,Y]Z		Non-OR	ØUHC[7,8]HZ
Non-OR	ØUH3[7,8][1,Y]Z		Non-OR	ØUHF[7,8]HZ
Non-OR	ØUH[8,D][Ø,3,4,7,8][3,Y]Z		Non-OR	ØUHG[7,8]HZ
Non-OR	ØUHH[3,4]YZ		♀	All body part, approach, device, and qualifier values
Non-OR	ØUHH[7,8][3,Y]Z			

Non-OR Procedure   DRG Non-OR Procedure   Valid OR Procedure   HAC Associated Procedure   Combination Only   New/Revised April   New/Revised October

Ø   **Medical and Surgical**
U   **Female Reproductive System**
J   **Inspection**   Definition: Visually and/or manually exploring a body part

                   Explanation: Visual exploration may be performed with or without optical instrumentation. Manual exploration may be performed directly or through intervening body layers.

Body Part Character 4		Approach Character 5	Device Character 6	Qualifier Character 7
3 Ovary	♀	Ø Open 3 Percutaneous 4 Percutaneous Endoscopic 8 Via Natural or Artificial Opening Endoscopic X External	Z No Device	Z No Qualifier
8 Fallopian Tube D Uterus and Cervix H Vagina and Cul-de-sac	♀ ♀ ♀	Ø Open 3 Percutaneous 4 Percutaneous Endoscopic 7 Via Natural or Artificial Opening 8 Via Natural or Artificial Opening Endoscopic X External	Z No Device	Z No Qualifier

M   Vulva
     Labia majora
     Labia minora
	♀	Ø Open
		X External
			Z No Device	Z No Qualifier

Non-OR   ØUJ3[3,8,X]ZZ
Non-OR   ØUJ[8,D,H][3,7,8,X]ZZ

Non-OR   ØUJMXZZ
♀   All body part, approach, device, and qualifier values

Ø   **Medical and Surgical**
U   **Female Reproductive System**
L   **Occlusion**   Definition: Completely closing an orifice or the lumen of a tubular body part

                   Explanation: The orifice can be a natural orifice or an artificially created orifice

Body Part Character 4		Approach Character 5	Device Character 6	Qualifier Character 7

5   Fallopian Tube, Right
     Oviduct
     Salpinx
     Uterine tube
6   Fallopian Tube, Left
     See 5 Fallopian Tube, Right
7   Fallopian Tubes, Bilateral NC
	♀
	
	♀
	
	♀
		Ø Open
		3 Percutaneous
		4 Percutaneous Endoscopic
			C Extraluminal Device
			D Intraluminal Device
			Z No Device
				Z No Qualifier

5   Fallopian Tube, Right
     Oviduct
     Salpinx
     Uterine tube
6   Fallopian Tube, Left
     See 5 Fallopian Tube, Right
7   Fallopian Tubes, Bilateral NC
	♀
	
	♀
	
	♀
		7 Via Natural or Artificial Opening
		8 Via Natural or Artificial Opening Endoscopic
			D Intraluminal Device
			Z No Device
				Z No Qualifier

F Cul-de-sac G Vagina	♀ ♀	7 Via Natural or Artificial Opening 8 Via Natural or Artificial Opening Endoscopic	D Intraluminal Device Z No Device	Z No Qualifier

NC   ØUL7[Ø,3,4][C,D,Z]Z with principal or secondary diagnosis of Z30.2
NC   ØUL7[7,8][D,Z]Z with principal or secondary diagnosis of Z30.2

♀   All body part, approach, device, and qualifier values

Female Reproductive System

Ø Medical and Surgical
U Female Reproductive System
M Reattachment　　Definition: Putting back in or on all or a portion of a separated body part to its normal location or other suitable location
　　　　　　　　　　　Explanation: Vascular circulation and nervous pathways may or may not be reestablished

Body Part Character 4	Approach Character 5	Device Character 6	Qualifier Character 7
Ø Ovary, Right ♀ **1** Ovary, Left ♀ **2** Ovaries, Bilateral ♀ **4** Uterine Supporting Structure ♀ 　　Broad ligament 　　Infundibulopelvic ligament 　　Ovarian ligament 　　Round ligament of uterus **5** Fallopian Tube, Right ♀ 　　Oviduct 　　Salpinx 　　Uterine tube **6** Fallopian Tube, Left ♀ 　　See 5 Fallopian Tube, Right **7** Fallopian Tubes, Bilateral ♀ **9** Uterus ♀ 　　Fundus uteri 　　Myometrium 　　Perimetrium 　　Uterine cornu **C** Cervix ♀ **F** Cul-de-sac ♀ **G** Vagina ♀	**Ø** Open **4** Percutaneous Endoscopic	**Z** No Device	**Z** No Qualifier
J Clitoris ♀ **M** Vulva ♀ 　　Labia majora 　　Labia minora	**X** External	**Z** No Device	**Z** No Qualifier
K Hymen ♀	**Ø** Open **4** Percutaneous Endoscopic **X** External	**Z** No Device	**Z** No Qualifier

♀　　All body part, approach, device, and qualifier values

Ø   **Medical and Surgical**
U   **Female Reproductive System**
N   **Release**   Definition: Freeing a body part from an abnormal physical constraint by cutting or by the use of force
                   Explanation: Some of the restraining tissue may be taken out but none of the body part is taken out

Body Part Character 4		Approach Character 5	Device Character 6	Qualifier Character 7

Ø Ovary, Right
1 Ovary, Left
2 Ovaries, Bilateral
4 Uterine Supporting Structure
    Broad ligament
    Infundibulopelvic ligament
    Ovarian ligament
    Round ligament of uterus
	♀
	♀
	♀
	♀
		Ø Open
		3 Percutaneous
		4 Percutaneous Endoscopic
		8 Via Natural or Artificial Opening
		    Endoscopic
			Z No Device	**Z** No Qualifier

5 Fallopian Tube, Right
    Oviduct
    Salpinx
    Uterine tube
6 Fallopian Tube, Left
    See 5 Fallopian Tube, Right
7 Fallopian Tubes, Bilateral
9 Uterus
    Fundus uteri
    Myometrium
    Perimetrium
    Uterine cornu
C Cervix
F Cul-de-sac
	♀
	
	♀
	♀
	
	♀
	♀
		Ø Open
		3 Percutaneous
		4 Percutaneous Endoscopic
		7 Via Natural or Artificial Opening
		8 Via Natural or Artificial Opening
		    Endoscopic
			Z No Device	**Z** No Qualifier

G Vagina **K** Hymen	♀ ♀	**Ø** Open **3** Percutaneous **4** Percutaneous Endoscopic **7** Via Natural or Artificial Opening **8** Via Natural or Artificial Opening Endoscopic **X** External	**Z** No Device	**Z** No Qualifier

J Clitoris
L Vestibular Gland
    Bartholin's (greater vestibular) gland
    Greater vestibular (Bartholin's) gland
    Paraurethral (Skene's) gland
    Skene's (paraurethral) gland
M Vulva
    Labia majora
    Labia minora
	♀
	♀
	
	♀
		Ø Open
		X External
			Z No Device	**Z** No Qualifier

     ♀   All body part, approach, device, and qualifier values

NC Noncovered Procedure   **LC** Limited Coverage   **QA** Questionable OB Admit   **NT** New Tech Add-on   ✛ Combination Member   ♂ Male   ♀ Female

ICD-10-PCS 2024   **655**

Ø **Medical and Surgical**
U **Female Reproductive System**
P **Removal** — Definition: Taking out or off a device from a body part

Explanation: If a device is taken out and a similar device put in without cutting or puncturing the skin or mucous membrane, the procedure is coded to the root operation CHANGE. Otherwise, the procedure for taking out the device is coded to the root operation REMOVAL.

Body Part Character 4	Approach Character 5	Device Character 6	Qualifier Character 7
3 Ovary ♀	Ø Open 3 Percutaneous 4 Percutaneous Endoscopic	Ø Drainage Device 3 Infusion Device Y Other Device	Z No Qualifier
3 Ovary ♀	7 Via Natural or Artificial Opening 8 Via Natural or Artificial Opening Endoscopic	Y Other Device	Z No Qualifier
3 Ovary ♀	X External	Ø Drainage Device 3 Infusion Device	Z No Qualifier
8 Fallopian Tube ♀	Ø Open 3 Percutaneous 4 Percutaneous Endoscopic 7 Via Natural or Artificial Opening 8 Via Natural or Artificial Opening Endoscopic	Ø Drainage Device 3 Infusion Device 7 Autologous Tissue Substitute C Extraluminal Device D Intraluminal Device J Synthetic Substitute K Nonautologous Tissue Substitute Y Other Device	Z No Qualifier
8 Fallopian Tube ♀	X External	Ø Drainage Device 3 Infusion Device D Intraluminal Device	Z No Qualifier
D Uterus and Cervix ♀	Ø Open 3 Percutaneous 4 Percutaneous Endoscopic 7 Via Natural or Artificial Opening 8 Via Natural or Artificial Opening Endoscopic	Ø Drainage Device 1 Radioactive Element 3 Infusion Device 7 Autologous Tissue Substitute C Extraluminal Device D Intraluminal Device H Contraceptive Device J Synthetic Substitute K Nonautologous Tissue Substitute Y Other Device	Z No Qualifier
D Uterus and Cervix ♀	X External	Ø Drainage Device 3 Infusion Device D Intraluminal Device H Contraceptive Device	Z No Qualifier
H Vagina and Cul-de-sac ♀	Ø Open 3 Percutaneous 4 Percutaneous Endoscopic 7 Via Natural or Artificial Opening 8 Via Natural or Artificial Opening Endoscopic	Ø Drainage Device 1 Radioactive Element 3 Infusion Device 7 Autologous Tissue Substitute D Intraluminal Device J Synthetic Substitute K Nonautologous Tissue Substitute Y Other Device	Z No Qualifier
H Vagina and Cul-de-sac ♀	X External	Ø Drainage Device 1 Radioactive Element 3 Infusion Device D Intraluminal Device	Z No Qualifier
M Vulva Labia majora Labia minora ♀	Ø Open	Ø Drainage Device 7 Autologous Tissue Substitute J Synthetic Substitute K Nonautologous Tissue Substitute	Z No Qualifier
M Vulva Labia majora Labia minora ♀	X External	Ø Drainage Device	Z No Qualifier

Non-OR ØUP3[3,4]YZ		**Non-OR** ØUPD[7,8][Ø,3,C,D,H,Y]Z	
Non-OR ØUP3[7,8]YZ		**Non-OR** ØUPDX[Ø,3,D,H]Z	
Non-OR ØUP3X[Ø,3]Z		**Non-OR** ØUPH[3,4]YZ	
Non-OR ØUP8[3,4]YZ		**Non-OR** ØUPH[7,8][Ø,3,D,Y]Z	
Non-OR ØUP8[7,8][Ø,3,D,Y]Z		**Non-OR** ØUPHX[Ø,1,3,D]Z	
Non-OR ØUP8X[Ø,3,D]Z		**Non-OR** ØUPMXØZ	
Non-OR ØUPD[3,4][C,Y]Z		♀ All body part, approach, device, and qualifier values	

Ø   **Medical and Surgical**
U   **Female Reproductive System**
Q   **Repair**   Definition: Restoring, to the extent possible, a body part to its normal anatomic structure and function

Explanation: Used only when the method to accomplish the repair is not one of the other root operations

Body Part Character 4	Approach Character 5	Device Character 6	Qualifier Character 7

Ø Ovary, Right ♀
 1 Ovary, Left ♀
 2 Ovaries, Bilateral ♀
 4 Uterine Supporting Structure ♀
    Broad ligament
    Infundibulopelvic ligament
    Ovarian ligament
    Round ligament of uterus
	Ø Open
	 3 Percutaneous
	 4 Percutaneous Endoscopic
	 8 Via Natural or Artificial Opening Endoscopic
		Z No Device	Z No Qualifier

5 Fallopian Tube, Right ♀
    Oviduct
    Salpinx
    Uterine tube
 6 Fallopian Tube, Left ♀
    See 5 Fallopian Tube, Right
 7 Fallopian Tubes, Bilateral ♀
 9 Uterus ♀
    Fundus uteri
    Myometrium
    Perimetrium
    Uterine cornu
 C Cervix ♀
 F Cul-de-sac ♀
	Ø Open
	 3 Percutaneous
	 4 Percutaneous Endoscopic
	 7 Via Natural or Artificial Opening
	 8 Via Natural or Artificial Opening Endoscopic
		Z No Device	Z No Qualifier

G Vagina ♀ K Hymen ♀	Ø Open 3 Percutaneous 4 Percutaneous Endoscopic 7 Via Natural or Artificial Opening 8 Via Natural or Artificial Opening Endoscopic X External	Z No Device	Z No Qualifier

J Clitoris ♀
 L Vestibular Gland ♀
    Bartholin's (greater vestibular) gland
    Greater vestibular (Bartholin's) gland
    Paraurethral (Skene's) gland
    Skene's (paraurethral) gland
 M Vulva ♀
    Labia majora
    Labia minora
	Ø Open
	 X External
		Z No Device	Z No Qualifier

Non-OR   ØUQG[7,X]ZZ
Non-OR   ØUQKXZZ

Non-OR   ØUQMXZZ
♀   All body part, approach, device, and qualifier values

Ø   **Medical and Surgical**
U   **Female Reproductive System**
S   **Reposition**   Definition: Moving to its normal location, or other suitable location, all or a portion of a body part

Explanation: The body part is moved to a new location from an abnormal location, or from a normal location where it is not functioning correctly. The body part may or may not be cut out or off to be moved to the new location.

Body Part Character 4	Approach Character 5	Device Character 6	Qualifier Character 7

Ø Ovary, Right ♀
 1 Ovary, Left ♀
 2 Ovaries, Bilateral ♀
 4 Uterine Supporting Structure ♀
    Broad ligament
    Infundibulopelvic ligament
    Ovarian ligament
    Round ligament of uterus
 5 Fallopian Tube, Right ♀
    Oviduct
    Salpinx
    Uterine tube
 6 Fallopian Tube, Left ♀
    See 5 Fallopian Tube, Right
 7 Fallopian Tubes, Bilateral ♀
 C Cervix ♀
 F Cul-de-sac ♀
	Ø Open
	 4 Percutaneous Endoscopic
	 8 Via Natural or Artificial Opening Endoscopic
		Z No Device	Z No Qualifier

9 Uterus ♀
    Fundus uteri
    Myometrium
    Perimetrium
    Uterine cornu
 G Vagina ♀
	Ø Open
	 4 Percutaneous Endoscopic
	 7 Via Natural or Artificial Opening
	 8 Via Natural or Artificial Opening Endoscopic
	 X External
		Z No Device	Z No Qualifier

Non-OR   ØUS9XZZ   ♀   All body part, approach, device, and qualifier values

NC Noncovered Procedure   LC Limited Coverage   QA Questionable OB Admit   NT New Tech Add-on   ⊞ Combination Member   ♂ Male   ♀ Female

ICD-10-PCS 2024   657

ØUQ–ØUS

Female Reproductive System

Ø   **Medical and Surgical**
U   **Female Reproductive System**
T   **Resection**   Definition: Cutting out or off, without replacement, all of a body part
                            Explanation: None

Body Part Character 4	Approach Character 5	Device Character 6	Qualifier Character 7

Ø Ovary, Right ♀
1 Ovary, Left ♀
2 Ovaries, Bilateral ⊞♀
5 Fallopian Tube, Right ♀
   Oviduct
   Salpinx
   Uterine tube
6 Fallopian Tube, Left ♀
   See 5 Fallopian Tube, Right
7 Fallopian Tubes, Bilateral ⊞♀
	Ø Open
	4 Percutaneous Endoscopic
	7 Via Natural or Artificial Opening
	8 Via Natural or Artificial Opening Endoscopic
	F Via Natural or Artificial Opening With Percutaneous Endoscopic Assistance
		Z No Device	Z No Qualifier

4 Uterine Supporting Structure ⊞♀
   Broad ligament
   Infundibulopelvic ligament
   Ovarian ligament
   Round ligament of uterus
C Cervix ⊞♀
F Cul-de-sac ♀
G Vagina ⊞♀
	Ø Open
	4 Percutaneous Endoscopic
	7 Via Natural or Artificial Opening
	8 Via Natural or Artificial Opening Endoscopic
		Z No Device	Z No Qualifier

9 Uterus ⊞♀
   Fundus uteri
   Myometrium
   Perimetrium
   Uterine cornu
	Ø Open
	4 Percutaneous Endoscopic
	7 Via Natural or Artificial Opening
	8 Via Natural or Artificial Opening Endoscopic
	F Via Natural or Artificial Opening With Percutaneous Endoscopic Assistance
		Z No Device	L Supracervical
			Z No Qualifier

J Clitoris ♀
L Vestibular Gland ♀
   Bartholin's (greater vestibular) gland
   Greater vestibular (Bartholin's) gland
   Paraurethral (Skene's) gland
   Skene's (paraurethral) gland
M Vulva ⊞♀
   Labia majora
   Labia minora
	Ø Open
	X External
		Z No Device	Z No Qualifier

K Hymen ♀	Ø Open 4 Percutaneous Endoscopic 7 Via Natural or Artificial Opening 8 Via Natural or Artificial Opening Endoscopic X External	Z No Device	Z No Device

♀   All body part, approach, device, and qualifier values

See Appendix L for Procedure Combinations
⊞   ØUT[2,7]ØZZ
⊞   ØUT[4,C][Ø,4,7,8]ZZ
⊞   ØUTGØZZ
⊞   ØUT9[Ø,4,7,8,F]ZZ
⊞   ØUTM[Ø,X]ZZ

Ø   **Medical and Surgical**
U   **Female Reproductive System**
U   **Supplement**   Definition: Putting in or on biological or synthetic material that physically reinforces and/or augments the function of a portion of a body part

Explanation: The biological material is non-living, or is living and from the same individual. The body part may have been previously replaced, and the SUPPLEMENT procedure is performed to physically reinforce and/or augment the function of the replaced body part.

Body Part Character 4		Approach Character 5	Device Character 6	Qualifier Character 7

4 Uterine Supporting Structure ♀
  Broad ligament
  Infundibulopelvic ligament
  Ovarian ligament
  Round ligament of uterus
		Ø Open
		4 Percutaneous Endoscopic
			7 Autologous Tissue Substitute
			J Synthetic Substitute
			K Nonautologous Tissue Substitute
				Z No Qualifier

5 Fallopian Tube, Right ♀
  Oviduct
  Salpinx
  Uterine tube
6 Fallopian Tube, Left ♀
  See 5 Fallopian Tube, Right
7 Fallopian Tubes, Bilateral ♀
F Cul-de-sac ♀
		Ø Open
		4 Percutaneous Endoscopic
		7 Via Natural or Artificial Opening
		8 Via Natural or Artificial Opening Endoscopic
			7 Autologous Tissue Substitute
			J Synthetic Substitute
			K Nonautologous Tissue Substitute
				Z No Qualifier

G Vagina ♀ **K** Hymen ♀		**Ø** Open **4** Percutaneous Endoscopic **7** Via Natural or Artificial Opening **8** Via Natural or Artificial Opening Endoscopic **X** External	**7** Autologous Tissue Substitute **J** Synthetic Substitute **K** Nonautologous Tissue Substitute	**Z** No Qualifier

J Clitoris ♀
M Vulva ♀
  Labia majora
  Labia minora
		Ø Open
		X External
			7 Autologous Tissue Substitute
			J Synthetic Substitute
			K Nonautologous Tissue Substitute
				Z No Qualifier

  ♀   All body part, approach, device, and qualifier values

Ø   **Medical and Surgical**
U   **Female Reproductive System**
V   **Restriction**   Definition: Partially closing an orifice or the lumen of a tubular body part

Explanation: The orifice can be a natural orifice or an artificially created orifice

Body Part Character 4		Approach Character 5	Device Character 6	Qualifier Character 7
C Cervix ♀		**Ø** Open **3** Percutaneous **4** Percutaneous Endoscopic	**C** Extraluminal Device **D** Intraluminal Device **Z** No Device	**Z** No Qualifier
C Cervix ♀		**7** Via Natural or Artificial Opening **8** Via Natural or Artificial Opening Endoscopic	**D** Intraluminal Device **Z** No Device	**Z** No Qualifier

  ♀   All body part, approach, device, and qualifier values

NC Noncovered Procedure   **LC** Limited Coverage   **OA** Questionable OB Admit   **NT** New Tech Add-on   ⊞ Combination Member   ♂ Male   ♀ Female

ICD-10-PCS 2024   659

ØUU–ØUV

Female Reproductive System

Ø   **Medical and Surgical**
U   **Female Reproductive System**
W   **Revision**   Definition: Correcting, to the extent possible, a portion of a malfunctioning device or the position of a displaced device
                     Explanation: Revision can include correcting a malfunctioning or displaced device by taking out or putting in components of the device such as a screw or pin

Body Part Character 4	Approach Character 5	Device Character 6	Qualifier Character 7
3 Ovary ♀	Ø Open 3 Percutaneous 4 Percutaneous Endoscopic	Ø Drainage Device 3 Infusion Device Y Other Device	Z No Qualifier
3 Ovary ♀	7 Via Natural or Artificial Opening 8 Via Natural or Artificial Opening Endoscopic	Y Other Device	Z No Qualifier
3 Ovary ♀	X External	Ø Drainage Device 3 Infusion Device	Z No Qualifier
8 Fallopian Tube ♀	Ø Open 3 Percutaneous 4 Percutaneous Endoscopic 7 Via Natural or Artificial Opening 8 Via Natural or Artificial Opening Endoscopic	Ø Drainage Device 3 Infusion Device 7 Autologous Tissue Substitute C Extraluminal Device D Intraluminal Device J Synthetic Substitute K Nonautologous Tissue Substitute Y Other Device	Z No Qualifier
8 Fallopian Tube ♀	X External	Ø Drainage Device 3 Infusion Device 7 Autologous Tissue Substitute C Extraluminal Device D Intraluminal Device J Synthetic Substitute K Nonautologous Tissue Substitute	Z No Qualifier
D Uterus and Cervix ♀	Ø Open 3 Percutaneous 4 Percutaneous Endoscopic 7 Via Natural or Artificial Opening 8 Via Natural or Artificial Opening Endoscopic	Ø Drainage Device 1 Radioactive Element 3 Infusion Device 7 Autologous Tissue Substitute C Extraluminal Device D Intraluminal Device H Contraceptive Device J Synthetic Substitute K Nonautologous Tissue Substitute Y Other Device	Z No Qualifier
D Uterus and Cervix ♀	X External	Ø Drainage Device 3 Infusion Device 7 Autologous Tissue Substitute C Extraluminal Device D Intraluminal Device H Contraceptive Device J Synthetic Substitute K Nonautologous Tissue Substitute	Z No Qualifier
H Vagina and Cul-de-sac ♀	Ø Open 3 Percutaneous 4 Percutaneous Endoscopic 7 Via Natural or Artificial Opening 8 Via Natural or Artificial Opening Endoscopic	Ø Drainage Device 1 Radioactive Element 3 Infusion Device 7 Autologous Tissue Substitute D Intraluminal Device J Synthetic Substitute K Nonautologous Tissue Substitute Y Other Device	Z No Qualifier
H Vagina and Cul-de-sac ♀	X External	Ø Drainage Device 3 Infusion Device 7 Autologous Tissue Substitute D Intraluminal Device J Synthetic Substitute K Nonautologous Tissue Substitute	Z No Qualifier

M Vulva ♀
    Labia majora
    Labia minora
	Ø Open
	X External
		Ø Drainage Device
		7 Autologous Tissue Substitute
		J Synthetic Substitute
		K Nonautologous Tissue Substitute
			Z No Qualifier

Non-OR ØUW3[3,4]YZ	**Non-OR** ØUWDX[Ø,3,7,C,D,H,J,K]Z
Non-OR ØUW3[7,8]YZ	**Non-OR** ØUWH[3,4,7,8]YZ
Non-OR ØUW3X[Ø,3]Z	**Non-OR** ØUWHX[Ø,3,7,D,J,K]Z
Non-OR ØUW8[3,4,7,8]YZ	**Non-OR** ØUWMX[Ø,7,J,K]Z
Non-OR ØUW8X[Ø,3,7,C,D,J,K]Z	♀ All body part, approach, device, and qualifier values
Non-OR ØUWD[3,4,7,8]YZ	

Non-OR Procedure   DRG Non-OR Procedure   Valid OR Procedure   HAC Associated Procedure   Combination Only   New/Revised April   New/Revised October

Ø   **Medical and Surgical**
U   **Female Reproductive System**
Y   **Transplantation**   Definition: Putting in or on all or a portion of a living body part taken from another individual or animal to physically take the place and/or function of all or a portion of a similar body part

         Explanation: The native body part may or may not be taken out, and the transplanted body part may take over all or a portion of its function

Body Part Character 4		Approach Character 5	Device Character 6	Qualifier Character 7
Ø Ovary, Right ♀ 1 Ovary, Left ♀ 9 Uterus ♀		Ø Open	Z No Device	Ø Allogeneic 1 Syngeneic 2 Zooplastic
♀ All body part, approach, device, and qualifier values				

NC Noncovered Procedure   LC Limited Coverage   QA Questionable OB Admit   NT New Tech Add-on   ⊞ Combination Member   ♂ Male   ♀ Female

ICD-10-PCS 2024   **661**

Male Reproductive System ØV1–ØVY

Character Meanings

This Character Meaning table is provided as a guide to assist the user in the identification of character members that may be found in this section of code tables. It **SHOULD NOT** be used to build a PCS code.

Operation–Character 3		Body Part–Character 4		Approach–Character 5		Device–Character 6		Qualifier–Character 7	
1	Bypass	Ø	Prostate	Ø	Open	Ø	Drainage Device	Ø	Allogeneic
2	Change	1	Seminal Vesicle, Right	3	Percutaneous	1	Radioactive Element	1	Syngeneic
5	Destruction	2	Seminal Vesicle, Left	4	Percutaneous Endoscopic	3	Infusion Device	2	Zooplastic
7	Dilation	3	Seminal Vesicles, Bilateral	7	Via Natural or Artificial Opening	7	Autologous Tissue Substitute	3	Laser Interstitial Thermal Therapy
9	Drainage	4	Prostate and Seminal Vesicles	8	Via Natural or Artificial Opening Endoscopic	C	Extraluminal Device	D	Urethra
B	Excision	5	Scrotum	X	External	D	Intraluminal Device	J	Epididymis, Right
C	Extirpation	6	Tunica Vaginalis, Right			J	Synthetic Substitute	K	Epididymis, Left
H	Insertion	7	Tunica Vaginalis, Left			K	Nonautologous Tissue Substitute	N	Vas Deferens, Right
J	Inspection	8	Scrotum and Tunica Vaginalis			Y	Other Device	P	Vas Deferens, Left
L	Occlusion	9	Testis, Right			Z	No Device	S	Penis
M	Reattachment	B	Testis, Left					X	Diagnostic
N	Release	C	Testes, Bilateral					Z	No Qualifier
P	Removal	D	Testis						
Q	Repair	F	Spermatic Cord, Right						
R	Replacement	G	Spermatic Cord, Left						
S	Reposition	H	Spermatic Cords, Bilateral						
T	Resection	J	Epididymis, Right						
U	Supplement	K	Epididymis, Left						
W	Revision	L	Epididymis, Bilateral						
X	Transfer	M	Epididymis and Spermatic Cord						
Y	Transplantation	N	Vas Deferens, Right						
		P	Vas Deferens, Left						
		Q	Vas Deferens, Bilateral						
		R	Vas Deferens						
		S	Penis						
		T	Prepuce						

AHA Coding Clinic for table ØV1
2018, 3Q, 12   Al-Ghorab distal penile shunt surgery

AHA Coding Clinic for table ØV5
2022, 4Q, 53-54   Laser interstitial thermal therapy

AHA Coding Clinic for table ØV9
2018, 3Q, 12   Al-Ghorab distal penile shunt surgery

AHA Coding Clinic for table ØVB
2020, 1Q, 31   Repair of buried penis
2019, 3Q, 18   Radical prostatectomy and lymph node dissection with biopsy of neurovascular bundle
2016, 1Q, 23   Transurethral resection of ejaculatory ducts
2014, 4Q, 33   Radical prostatectomy

AHA Coding Clinic for table ØVH
2020, 4Q, 43-44   Insertion of radioactive element

AHA Coding Clinic for table ØVP
2016, 2Q, 28   Removal of multi-component inflatable penile prosthesis with placement of new malleable device

AHA Coding Clinic for table ØVQ
2018, 3Q, 12   Al-Ghorab distal penile shunt surgery

AHA Coding Clinic for table ØVT
2020, 4Q, 99   Robotic-assisted prostatectomy with extension of incision for specimen removal
2019, 3Q, 18   Radical prostatectomy and lymph node dissection with biopsy of neurovascular bundle
2014, 4Q, 33   Radical prostatectomy

AHA Coding Clinic for table ØVU
2020, 1Q, 31   Repair of buried penis
2016, 2Q, 28   Removal of multi-component inflatable penile prosthesis with placement of new malleable device
2015, 3Q, 25   Placement of inflatable penile prosthesis

AHA Coding Clinic for table ØVX
2018, 4Q, 40   Transfer of prepuce

AHA Coding Clinic for table ØVY
2023, 2Q, 32   Preparation of donor organ before transplantation
2020, 4Q, 58   Male reproductive organ transplant

Male Reproductive System

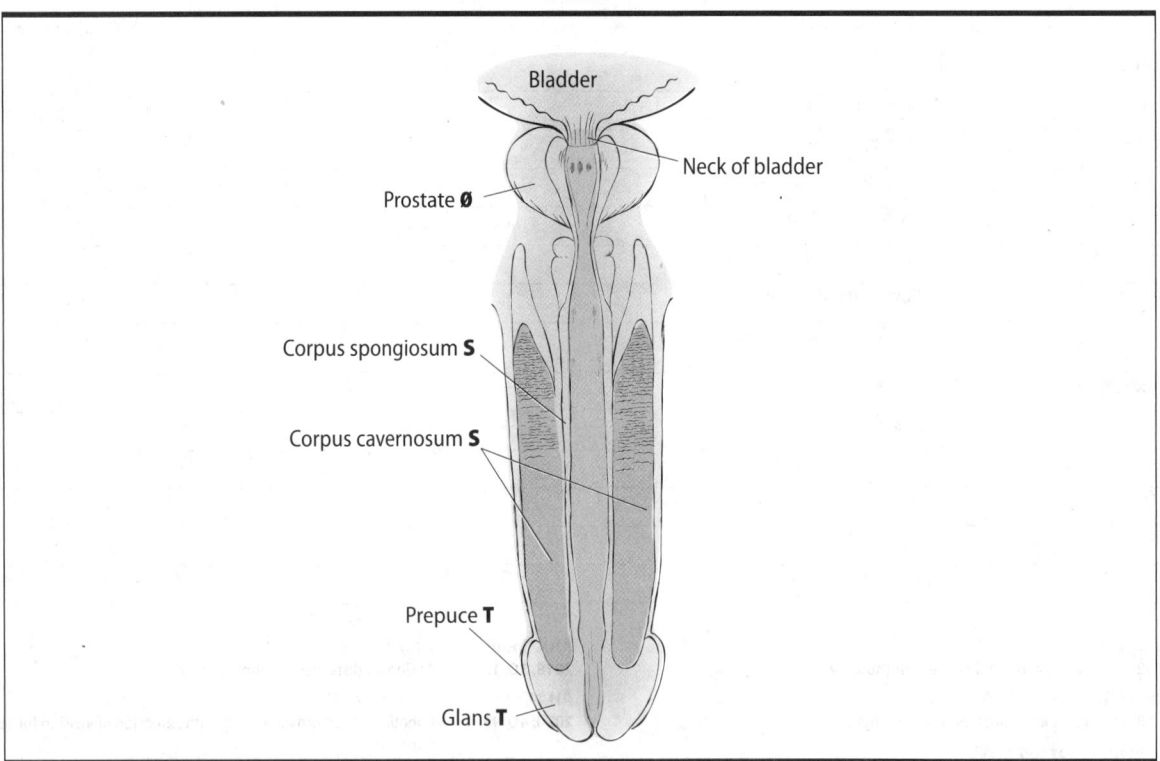

Penis

Ø　Medical and Surgical
V　Male Reproductive System
1　Bypass　　Definition: Altering the route of passage of the contents of a tubular body part

Explanation: Rerouting contents of a body part to a downstream area of the normal route, to a similar route and body part, or to an abnormal route and dissimilar body part. Includes one or more anastomoses, with or without the use of a device.

Body Part Character 4	Approach Character 5	Device Character 6	Qualifier Character 7
N　Vas Deferens, Right　♂ 　　Ductus deferens 　　Ejaculatory duct P　Vas Deferens, Left　♂ 　　*See N Vas Deferens, Right* Q　Vas Deferens, Bilateral　♂ 　　*See N Vas Deferens, Right*	Ø　Open 4　Percutaneous Endoscopic	7　Autologous Tissue Substitute J　Synthetic Substitute K　Nonautologous Tissue Substitute Z　No Device	J　Epididymis, Right K　Epididymis, Left N　Vas Deferens, Right P　Vas Deferens, Left

♂　All body part, approach, device, and qualifier values

Ø　Medical and Surgical
V　Male Reproductive System
2　Change　　Definition: Taking out or off a device from a body part and putting back an identical or similar device in or on the same body part without cutting or puncturing the skin or a mucous membrane

Explanation: All CHANGE procedures are coded using the approach EXTERNAL

Body Part Character 4	Approach Character 5	Device Character 6	Qualifier Character 7
4　Prostate and Seminal Vesicles　♂ 8　Scrotum and Tunica Vaginalis　♂ D　Testis　♂ M　Epididymis and Spermatic Cord　♂ R　Vas Deferens　♂ 　　Ductus deferens 　　Ejaculatory duct S　Penis　♂ 　　Corpus cavernosum 　　Corpus spongiosum	X　External	Ø　Drainage Device Y　Other Device	Z　No Qualifier

Non-OR　All body part, approach, device, and qualifier values　　♂　All body part, approach, device, and qualifier values

Ø　Medical and Surgical
V　Male Reproductive System
5　Destruction　　Definition: Physical eradication of all or a portion of a body part by the direct use of energy, force, or a destructive agent

Explanation: None of the body part is physically taken out

Body Part Character 4	Approach Character 5	Device Character 6	Qualifier Character 7
Ø　Prostate　♂	Ø　Open 3　Percutaneous 4　Percutaneous Endoscopic	Z　No Device	3　Laser Interstitial Thermal Therapy Z　No Qualifier
Ø　Prostate　♂	7　Via Natural or Artificial Opening 8　Via Natural or Artificial Opening 　　Endoscopic	Z　No Device	Z　No Qualifier
1　Seminal Vesicle, Right　♂ 2　Seminal Vesicle, Left　♂ 3　Seminal Vesicles, Bilateral　♂ 6　Tunica Vaginalis, Right　♂ 7　Tunica Vaginalis, Left　♂ 9　Testis, Right　♂ B　Testis, Left　♂ C　Testes, Bilateral　♂	Ø　Open 3　Percutaneous 4　Percutaneous Endoscopic	Z　No Device	Z　No Qualifier
5　Scrotum　♂ S　Penis　♂ 　　Corpus cavernosum 　　Corpus spongiosum T　Prepuce　♂ 　　Foreskin 　　Glans penis	Ø　Open 3　Percutaneous 4　Percutaneous Endoscopic X　External	Z　No Device	Z　No Qualifier
F　Spermatic Cord, Right　♂ G　Spermatic Cord, Left　♂ H　Spermatic Cords, Bilateral　♂ J　Epididymis, Right　♂ K　Epididymis, Left　♂ L　Epididymis, Bilateral　♂ N　Vas Deferens, Right　NC ♂ 　　Ductus deferens 　　Ejaculatory duct P　Vas Deferens, Left　NC ♂ 　　*See N Vas Deferens, Right* Q　Vas Deferens, Bilateral　NC ♂ 　　*See N Vas Deferens, Right*	Ø　Open 3　Percutaneous 4　Percutaneous Endoscopic 8　Via Natural or Artificial Opening 　　Endoscopic	Z　No Device	Z　No Qualifier

Non-OR　ØV55[Ø,3,4,X]ZZ
Non-OR　ØV5[N,P,Q][Ø,3,4,8]ZZ
NC　ØV5[N,P,Q][Ø,3,4]ZZ with principal or secondary diagnosis of Z3Ø.2
♂　All body part, approach, device, and qualifier values

NC Noncovered Procedure　　LC Limited Coverage　　OA Questionable OB Admit　　NT New Tech Add-on　　⊞ Combination Member　　♂ Male　　♀ Female

Male Reproductive System *(left margin)*

Ø Medical and Surgical
V Male Reproductive System
7 Dilation   Definition: Expanding an orifice or the lumen of a tubular body part

Explanation: The orifice can be a natural orifice or an artificially created orifice. Accomplished by stretching a tubular body part using intraluminal pressure or by cutting part of the orifice or wall of the tubular body part.

Body Part Character 4	Approach Character 5	Device Character 6	Qualifier Character 7

N Vas Deferens, Right ♂
   Ductus deferens
   Ejaculatory duct
P Vas Deferens, Left ♂
   See N Vas Deferens, Right
Q Vas Deferens, Bilateral ♂
   See N Vas Deferens, Right
	Ø Open
	3 Percutaneous
	4 Percutaneous Endoscopic
		D Intraluminal Device
		Z No Device
			Z No Qualifier

♂   All body part, approach, device, and qualifier values

Ø Medical and Surgical
V Male Reproductive System
9 Drainage   Definition: Taking or letting out fluids and/or gases from a body part

Explanation: The qualifier DIAGNOSTIC is used to identify drainage procedures that are biopsies

Body Part Character 4	Approach Character 5	Device Character 6	Qualifier Character 7
Ø Prostate ♂	Ø Open 3 Percutaneous 4 Percutaneous Endoscopic 7 Via Natural or Artificial Opening 8 Via Natural or Artificial Opening Endoscopic	Ø Drainage Device	Z No Qualifier
Ø Prostate ♂	Ø Open 3 Percutaneous 4 Percutaneous Endoscopic 7 Via Natural or Artificial Opening 8 Via Natural or Artificial Opening Endoscopic	Z No Device	X Diagnostic Z No Qualifier

1 Seminal Vesicle, Right ♂
2 Seminal Vesicle, Left ♂
3 Seminal Vesicles, Bilateral ♂
6 Tunica Vaginalis, Right ♂
7 Tunica Vaginalis, Left ♂
9 Testis, Right ♂
B Testis, Left ♂
C Testes, Bilateral ♂
F Spermatic Cord, Right ♂
G Spermatic Cord, Left ♂
H Spermatic Cords, Bilateral ♂
J Epididymis, Right ♂
K Epididymis, Left ♂
L Epididymis, Bilateral ♂
N Vas Deferens, Right ♂
   Ductus deferens
   Ejaculatory duct
P Vas Deferens, Left ♂
   See N Vas Deferens, Right
Q Vas Deferens, Bilateral ♂
   See N Vas Deferens, Right
	Ø Open
	3 Percutaneous
	4 Percutaneous Endoscopic
		Ø Drainage Device	Z No Qualifier

Non-OR ØV9Ø[3,4]ØZ		**Non-OR** ØV9[6,7,F,G,H,N,P,Q][Ø,3,4]ØZ	
Non-OR ØV9Ø[3,4]Z[X,Z]		**Non-OR** ØV9[J,K,L]3ØZ	
Non-OR ØV9Ø[7,8]ZX		♂ All body part, approach, device, and qualifier values	
Non-OR ØV9[1,2,3,9,B,C][3,4]ØZ			

ØV9 Continued on next page

Non-OR Procedure   DRG Non-OR Procedure   Valid OR Procedure   HAC Associated Procedure   Combination Only   New/Revised April   New/Revised October

666   ICD-10-PCS 2024

Ø Medical and Surgical
V Male Reproductive System
9 Drainage Definition: Taking or letting out fluids and/or gases from a body part

ØV9 Continued

Explanation: The qualifier DIAGNOSTIC is used to identify drainage procedures that are biopsies

Body Part Character 4		Approach Character 5	Device Character 6	Qualifier Character 7
1 Seminal Vesicle, Right ♂		Ø Open	Z No Device	X Diagnostic
2 Seminal Vesicle, Left ♂		3 Percutaneous		Z No Qualifier
3 Seminal Vesicles, Bilateral ♂		4 Percutaneous Endoscopic		
6 Tunica Vaginalis, Right ♂				
7 Tunica Vaginalis, Left ♂				
9 Testis, Right ♂				
B Testis, Left ♂				
C Testes, Bilateral ♂				
F Spermatic Cord, Right ♂				
G Spermatic Cord, Left ♂				
H Spermatic Cords, Bilateral ♂				
J Epididymis, Right ♂				
K Epididymis, Left ♂				
L Epididymis, Bilateral ♂				
N Vas Deferens, Right ♂				
Ductus deferens				
Ejaculatory duct				
P Vas Deferens, Left ♂				
See N Vas Deferens, Right				
Q Vas Deferens, Bilateral ♂				
See N Vas Deferens, Right				
5 Scrotum ♂		Ø Open	Ø Drainage Device	Z No Qualifier
S Penis ♂		3 Percutaneous		
Corpus cavernosum		4 Percutaneous Endoscopic		
Corpus spongiosum		X External		
T Prepuce ♂				
Foreskin				
Glans penis				
5 Scrotum ♂		Ø Open	Z No Device	X Diagnostic
S Penis ♂		3 Percutaneous		Z No Qualifier
Corpus cavernosum		4 Percutaneous Endoscopic		
Corpus spongiosum		X External		
T Prepuce ♂				
Foreskin				
Glans penis				

Non-OR	ØV9[1,2,3,9,B,C][3,4]Z[X,Z]	**Non-OR**	ØV9[S,T]3ØZ
Non-OR	ØV9[6,7,F,G,H,J,K,L,N,P,Q][Ø,3,4]ZX	**Non-OR**	ØV95ØZX
Non-OR	ØV9[6,7,F,G,H,N,P,Q][Ø,3,4]ZZ	**Non-OR**	ØV95[3,4,X]Z[X,Z]
Non-OR	ØV9[J,K,L]3ZZ	**Non-OR**	ØV9[S,T]3ZZ
Non-OR	ØV95[Ø,3,4,X]ØZ	♂	All body part, approach, device, and qualifier values

Male Reproductive System

Ø   **Medical and Surgical**
V   **Male Reproductive System**
B   **Excision**   Definition: Cutting out or off, without replacement, a portion of a body part
       Explanation: The qualifier DIAGNOSTIC is used to identify excision procedures that are biopsies

Body Part Character 4	Approach Character 5	Device Character 6	Qualifier Character 7
Ø Prostate ♂	Ø Open 3 Percutaneous 4 Percutaneous Endoscopic 7 Via Natural or Artificial Opening 8 Via Natural or Artificial Opening Endoscopic	Z No Device	X Diagnostic Z No Qualifier
1 Seminal Vesicle, Right ♂ 2 Seminal Vesicle, Left ♂ 3 Seminal Vesicles, Bilateral ♂ 6 Tunica Vaginalis, Right ♂ 7 Tunica Vaginalis, Left ♂ 9 Testis, Right ♂ B Testis, Left ♂ C Testes, Bilateral ♂	Ø Open 3 Percutaneous 4 Percutaneous Endoscopic	Z No Device	X Diagnostic Z No Qualifier

5 Scrotum ♂
S Penis ♂
  Corpus cavernosum
  Corpus spongiosum
T Prepuce ♂
  Foreskin
  Glans penis
	Ø Open
	3 Percutaneous
	4 Percutaneous Endoscopic
	X External
		Z No Device	X Diagnostic
			Z No Qualifier

F Spermatic Cord, Right ♂
G Spermatic Cord, Left ♂
H Spermatic Cords, Bilateral ♂
J Epididymis, Right ♂
K Epididymis, Left ♂
L Epididymis, Bilateral ♂
N Vas Deferens, Right NC ♂
  Ductus deferens
  Ejaculatory duct
P Vas Deferens, Left NC ♂
  See N Vas Deferens, Right
Q Vas Deferens, Bilateral NC ♂
  See N Vas Deferens, Right
	Ø Open
	3 Percutaneous
	4 Percutaneous Endoscopic
	8 Via Natural or Artificial Opening Endoscopic
		Z No Device	X Diagnostic
			Z No Qualifier

Non-OR ØVBØ[3,4,7,8]ZX
Non-OR ØVB[1,2,3,9,B,C][3,4]ZX
Non-OR ØVB[6,7][Ø,3,4]ZX
Non-OR ØVB5ØZX
Non-OR ØVB5[3,4,X]Z[X,Z]

Non-OR ØVB[F,G,H,J,K,L][Ø,3,4,8]ZX
Non-OR ØVB[N,P,Q][Ø,3,4,8]Z[X,Z]
NC ØVB[N,P,Q][Ø,3,4]ZZ with principal or secondary diagnosis of Z3Ø.2
♂ All body part, approach, device, and qualifier values

Ø　Medical and Surgical
V　Male Reproductive System
C　Extirpation　　Definition: Taking or cutting out solid matter from a body part

Explanation: The solid matter may be an abnormal byproduct of a biological function or a foreign body; it may be imbedded in a body part or in the lumen of a tubular body part. The solid matter may or may not have been previously broken into pieces.

Body Part Character 4	Approach Character 5	Device Character 6	Qualifier Character 7
Ø　Prostate　♂	Ø　Open 3　Percutaneous 4　Percutaneous Endoscopic 7　Via Natural or Artificial Opening 8　Via Natural or Artificial Opening Endoscopic	Z　No Device	Z　No Qualifier
1　Seminal Vesicle, Right　♂ 2　Seminal Vesicle, Left　♂ 3　Seminal Vesicles, Bilateral　♂ 6　Tunica Vaginalis, Right　♂ 7　Tunica Vaginalis, Left　♂ 9　Testis, Right　♂ B　Testis, Left　♂ C　Testes, Bilateral　♂ F　Spermatic Cord, Right　♂ G　Spermatic Cord, Left　♂ H　Spermatic Cords, Bilateral　♂ J　Epididymis, Right　♂ K　Epididymis, Left　♂ L　Epididymis, Bilateral　♂ N　Vas Deferens, Right　♂ 　　Ductus deferens 　　Ejaculatory duct P　Vas Deferens, Left　♂ 　　*See N Vas Deferens, Right* Q　Vas Deferens, Bilateral　♂ 　　*See N Vas Deferens, Right*	Ø　Open 3　Percutaneous 4　Percutaneous Endoscopic	Z　No Device	Z　No Qualifier
5　Scrotum　♂ S　Penis　♂ 　　Corpus cavernosum 　　Corpus spongiosum T　Prepuce　♂ 　　Foreskin 　　Glans penis	Ø　Open 3　Percutaneous 4　Percutaneous Endoscopic X　External	Z　No Device	Z　No Qualifier

Non-OR　ØVC[6,7,N,P,Q][Ø,3,4]ZZ
Non-OR　ØVC5[3,4,X]ZZ

Non-OR　ØVCSXZZ
♂　All body part, approach, device, and qualifier values

Male Reproductive System *(side tab)*

Ø   **Medical and Surgical**
V   **Male Reproductive System**
H   **Insertion**   Definition: Putting in a nonbiological appliance that monitors, assists, performs, or prevents a physiological function but does not physically take the place of a body part

                       Explanation: None

Body Part Character 4		Approach Character 5	Device Character 6	Qualifier Character 7
Ø Prostate ♂		Ø Open 3 Percutaneous 4 Percutaneous Endoscopic 7 Via Natural or Artificial Opening 8 Via Natural or Artificial Opening Endoscopic	1 Radioactive Element	Z No Qualifier

4 Prostate and Seminal Vesicles ♂
8 Scrotum and Tunica Vaginalis ♂
M Epididymis and Spermatic Cord ♂
R Vas Deferens ♂
    Ductus deferens
    Ejaculatory duct
		Ø Open
		3 Percutaneous
		4 Percutaneous Endoscopic
		7 Via Natural or Artificial Opening
		8 Via Natural or Artificial Opening Endoscopic
			3 Infusion Device
			Y Other Device
				Z No Qualifier

D Testis ♂		Ø Open 3 Percutaneous 4 Percutaneous Endoscopic 7 Via Natural or Artificial Opening 8 Via Natural or Artificial Opening Endoscopic	1 Radioactive Element 3 Infusion Device Y Other Device	Z No Qualifier

S Penis ♂
    Corpus cavernosum
    Corpus spongiosum
		Ø Open
		3 Percutaneous
		4 Percutaneous Endoscopic
			3 Infusion Device
			Y Other Device
				Z No Qualifier

S Penis ♂
    Corpus cavernosum
    Corpus spongiosum
		7 Via Natural or Artificial Opening
		8 Via Natural or Artificial Opening Endoscopic
			Y Other Device	Z No Qualifier

S Penis ♂
    Corpus cavernosum
    Corpus spongiosum
		X External	3 Infusion Device	Z No Qualifier

Non-OR   ØVH[4,8,M,R][Ø,3,4,7,8][3,Y]Z
Non-OR   ØVHD[Ø,3,4,7,8][1,3,Y]Z
Non-OR   ØVHS[Ø,3,4][3,Y]Z
Non-OR   ØVHS[7,8]YZ

Non-OR   ØVHSX3Z
♂   All body part, approach, device, and qualifier values

Ø   **Medical and Surgical**
V   **Male Reproductive System**
J   **Inspection**   Definition: Visually and/or manually exploring a body part

                       Explanation: Visual exploration may be performed with or without optical instrumentation. Manual exploration may be performed directly or through intervening body layers.

Body Part Character 4		Approach Character 5	Device Character 6	Qualifier Character 7

4 Prostate and Seminal Vesicles ♂
8 Scrotum and Tunica Vaginalis ♂
D Testis ♂
M Epididymis and Spermatic Cord ♂
R Vas Deferens ♂
    Ductus deferens
    Ejaculatory duct
S Penis ♂
    Corpus cavernosum
    Corpus spongiosum
		Ø Open
		3 Percutaneous
		4 Percutaneous Endoscopic
		X External
			Z No Device	Z No Qualifier

Non-OR   ØVJ[4,D,M,R][3,X]ZZ
Non-OR   ØVJ8[Ø,3,4,X]ZZ
Non-OR   ØVJS[3,4,X]ZZ

♂   All body part, approach, device, and qualifier values

Non-OR Procedure   DRG Non-OR Procedure   Valid OR Procedure   HAC Associated Procedure   Combination Only   New/Revised April   New/Revised October

670   ICD-10-PCS 2024

Ø   **Medical and Surgical**
V   **Male Reproductive System**
L   **Occlusion**   Definition: Completely closing an orifice or the lumen of a tubular body part
                 Explanation: The orifice can be a natural orifice or an artificially created orifice

Body Part Character 4	Approach Character 5	Device Character 6	Qualifier Character 7

F Spermatic Cord, Right NC ♂
G Spermatic Cord, Left NC ♂
H Spermatic Cords, Bilateral NC ♂
N Vas Deferens, Right NC ♂
   Ductus deferens
   Ejaculatory duct
P Vas Deferens, Left NC ♂
   See N Vas Deferens, Right
Q Vas Deferens, Bilateral NC ♂
   See N Vas Deferens, Right
	Ø Open
	3 Percutaneous
	4 Percutaneous Endoscopic
	8 Via Natural or Artificial Opening Endoscopic
		C Extraluminal Device
		D Intraluminal Device
		Z No Device
			Z No Qualifier

Non-OR   ØVL[F,G,H][Ø,3,4,8][C,D,Z]Z
Non-OR   ØVL[N,P,Q][Ø,3,4,8][C,Z]Z

NC ØVL[F,G,H][Ø,3,4][C,D,Z]Z with principal or secondary diagnosis of Z3Ø.2
NC ØVL[N,P,Q][Ø,3,4][C,Z]Z with principal or secondary diagnosis of Z3Ø.2
♂ All body part, approach, device, and qualifier values

Ø   **Medical and Surgical**
V   **Male Reproductive System**
M   **Reattachment**   Definition: Putting back in or on all or a portion of a separated body part to its normal location or other suitable location
                 Explanation: Vascular circulation and nervous pathways may or may not be reestablished

Body Part Character 4	Approach Character 5	Device Character 6	Qualifier Character 7

5 Scrotum ♂
S Penis ♂
   Corpus cavernosum
   Corpus spongiosum
	X External	Z No Device	Z No Qualifier

6 Tunica Vaginalis, Right ♂ 7 Tunica Vaginalis, Left ♂ 9 Testis, Right ♂ B Testis, Left ♂ C Testes, Bilateral ♂ F Spermatic Cord, Right ♂ G Spermatic Cord, Left ♂ H Spermatic Cords, Bilateral ♂	Ø Open 4 Percutaneous Endoscopic	Z No Device	Z No Qualifier

♂ All body part, approach, device, and qualifier values

Male Reproductive System

Ø　Medical and Surgical
V　Male Reproductive System
N　Release　　Definition: Freeing a body part from an abnormal physical constraint by cutting or by the use of force
　　　　　　　　　Explanation: Some of the restraining tissue may be taken out but none of the body part is taken out

Body Part Character 4	Approach Character 5	Device Character 6	Qualifier Character 7
Ø Prostate ♂	Ø Open 3 Percutaneous 4 Percutaneous Endoscopic 7 Via Natural or Artificial Opening 8 Via Natural or Artificial Opening Endoscopic	Z No Device	Z No Qualifier
1 Seminal Vesicle, Right ♂ 2 Seminal Vesicle, Left ♂ 3 Seminal Vesicles, Bilateral ♂ 6 Tunica Vaginalis, Right ♂ 7 Tunica Vaginalis, Left ♂ 9 Testis, Right ♂ B Testis, Left ♂ C Testes, Bilateral ♂	Ø Open 3 Percutaneous 4 Percutaneous Endoscopic	Z No Device	Z No Qualifier
5 Scrotum ♂ S Penis ♂ 　　Corpus cavernosum 　　Corpus spongiosum T Prepuce ♂ 　　Foreskin 　　Glans penis	Ø Open 3 Percutaneous 4 Percutaneous Endoscopic X External	Z No Device	Z No Qualifier
F Spermatic Cord, Right ♂ G Spermatic Cord, Left ♂ H Spermatic Cords, Bilateral ♂ J Epididymis, Right ♂ K Epididymis, Left ♂ L Epididymis, Bilateral ♂ N Vas Deferens, Right ♂ 　　Ductus deferens 　　Ejaculatory duct P Vas Deferens, Left ♂ 　　*See N Vas Deferens, Right* Q Vas Deferens, Bilateral ♂ 　　*See N Vas Deferens, Right*	Ø Open 3 Percutaneous 4 Percutaneous Endoscopic 8 Via Natural or Artificial Opening Endoscopic	Z No Device	Z No Qualifier

Non-OR　ØVN[9,B,C][Ø,3,4]ZZ　　　　　　　　　　　　♂　All body part, approach, device, and qualifier values
Non-OR　ØVNT[Ø,3,4,X]ZZ

Ø   **Medical and Surgical**
V   **Male Reproductive System**
P   **Removal**   Definition: Taking out or off a device from a body part

Explanation: If a device is taken out and a similar device put in without cutting or puncturing the skin or mucous membrane, the procedure is coded to the root operation CHANGE. Otherwise, the procedure for taking out the device is coded to the root operation REMOVAL.

Body Part Character 4	Approach Character 5	Device Character 6	Qualifier Character 7
4 Prostate and Seminal Vesicles ♂	Ø Open 3 Percutaneous 4 Percutaneous Endoscopic 7 Via Natural or Artificial Opening 8 Via Natural or Artificial Opening Endoscopic	Ø Drainage Device 1 Radioactive Element 3 Infusion Device 7 Autologous Tissue Substitute J Synthetic Substitute K Nonautologous Tissue Substitute Y Other Device	Z No Qualifier
4 Prostate and Seminal Vesicles ♂	X External	Ø Drainage Device 1 Radioactive Element 3 Infusion Device	Z No Qualifier

8   Scrotum and Tunica Vaginalis ♂
D   Testis ♂
S   Penis ♂
     Corpus cavernosum
     Corpus spongiosum
	Ø Open
	3 Percutaneous
	4 Percutaneous Endoscopic
	7 Via Natural or Artificial Opening
	8 Via Natural or Artificial Opening Endoscopic
		Ø Drainage Device
		3 Infusion Device
		7 Autologous Tissue Substitute
		J Synthetic Substitute
		K Nonautologous Tissue Substitute
		Y Other Device
			Z No Qualifier

8   Scrotum and Tunica Vaginalis ♂
D   Testis ♂
S   Penis ♂
     Corpus cavernosum
     Corpus spongiosum
	X External	Ø Drainage Device
		3 Infusion Device
			Z No Qualifier

M Epididymis and Spermatic Cord ♂	Ø Open 3 Percutaneous 4 Percutaneous Endoscopic 7 Via Natural or Artificial Opening 8 Via Natural or Artificial Opening Endoscopic	Ø Drainage Device 3 Infusion Device 7 Autologous Tissue Substitute C Extraluminal Device J Synthetic Substitute K Nonautologous Tissue Substitute Y Other Device	Z No Qualifier
M Epididymis and Spermatic Cord ♂	X External	Ø Drainage Device 3 Infusion Device	Z No Qualifier

R   Vas Deferens ♂
     Ductus deferens
     Ejaculatory duct
	Ø Open
	3 Percutaneous
	4 Percutaneous Endoscopic
	7 Via Natural or Artificial Opening
	8 Via Natural or Artificial Opening Endoscopic
		Ø Drainage Device
		3 Infusion Device
		7 Autologous Tissue Substitute
		C Extraluminal Device
		D Intraluminal Device
		J Synthetic Substitute
		K Nonautologous Tissue Substitute
		Y Other Device
			Z No Qualifier

R   Vas Deferens ♂
     Ductus deferens
     Ejaculatory duct
	X External	Ø Drainage Device
		3 Infusion Device
		D Intraluminal Device
			Z No Qualifier

Non-OR	ØVP4[3,4]YZ	Non-OR	ØVPM[3,4]YZ
Non-OR	ØVP4[7,8][Ø,3,Y]Z	Non-OR	ØVPM[7,8][Ø,3,Y]Z
Non-OR	ØVP4X[Ø,1,3]Z	Non-OR	ØVPMX[Ø,3]Z
Non-OR	ØVP8[Ø,3,4,7,8][Ø,3,7,J,K,Y]Z	Non-OR	ØVPR[Ø,3,4][Ø,3,7,C,J,K,Y]Z
Non-OR	ØVP[D,S][3,4]YZ	Non-OR	ØVPR[7,8][Ø,3,7,C,D,J,K,Y]Z
Non-OR	ØVP[D,S][7,8][Ø,3,Y]Z	Non-OR	ØVPRX[Ø,3,D]Z
Non-OR	ØVP[8,D,S]X[Ø,3]Z	♂	All body part, approach, device, and qualifier values

NC Noncovered Procedure   LC Limited Coverage   QA Questionable OB Admit   NT New Tech Add-on   ⊞ Combination Member   ♂ Male   ♀ Female

ICD-10-PCS 2024   673

ØVP–ØVP

Ø Medical and Surgical
V Male Reproductive System
Q Repair   Definition: Restoring, to the extent possible, a body part to its normal anatomic structure and function

Explanation: Used only when the method to accomplish the repair is not one of the other root operations

Body Part Character 4	Approach Character 5	Device Character 6	Qualifier Character 7
Ø Prostate ♂	Ø Open 3 Percutaneous 4 Percutaneous Endoscopic 7 Via Natural or Artificial Opening 8 Via Natural or Artificial Opening Endoscopic	Z No Device	Z No Qualifier
1 Seminal Vesicle, Right ♂ 2 Seminal Vesicle, Left ♂ 3 Seminal Vesicles, Bilateral ♂ 6 Tunica Vaginalis, Right ♂ 7 Tunica Vaginalis, Left ♂ 9 Testis, Right ♂ B Testis, Left ♂ C Testes, Bilateral ♂	Ø Open 3 Percutaneous 4 Percutaneous Endoscopic	Z No Device	Z No Qualifier

5 Scrotum ♂
S Penis ♂
  Corpus cavernosum
  Corpus spongiosum
T Prepuce ♂
  Foreskin
  Glans penis
	Ø Open
	3 Percutaneous
	4 Percutaneous Endoscopic
	X External
		Z No Device	Z No Qualifier

F Spermatic Cord, Right ♂
G Spermatic Cord, Left ♂
H Spermatic Cords, Bilateral ♂
J Epididymis, Right ♂
K Epididymis, Left ♂
L Epididymis, Bilateral ♂
N Vas Deferens, Right ♂
  Ductus deferens
  Ejaculatory duct
P Vas Deferens, Left ♂
  See N Vas Deferens, Right
Q Vas Deferens, Bilateral ♂
  See N Vas Deferens, Right
	Ø Open
	3 Percutaneous
	4 Percutaneous Endoscopic
	8 Via Natural or Artificial Opening Endoscopic
		Z No Device	Z No Qualifier

Non-OR   ØVQ[6,7][Ø,3,4]ZZ
Non-OR   ØVQ5[Ø,3,4,X]ZZ
♂   All body part, approach, device, and qualifier values

Ø Medical and Surgical
V Male Reproductive System
R Replacement   Definition: Putting in or on biological or synthetic material that physically takes the place and/or function of all or a portion of a body part

Explanation: The body part may have been taken out or replaced, or may be taken out, physically eradicated, or rendered nonfunctional during the REPLACEMENT procedure. A REMOVAL procedure is coded for taking out the device used in a previous replacement procedure.

Body Part Character 4	Approach Character 5	Device Character 6	Qualifier Character 7
9 Testis, Right ♂ B Testis, Left ♂ C Testes, Bilateral ♂	Ø Open	J Synthetic Substitute	Z No Qualifier

♂   All body part, approach, device, and qualifier values

Ø Medical and Surgical
V Male Reproductive System
S Reposition   Definition: Moving to its normal location, or other suitable location, all or a portion of a body part

Explanation: The body part is moved to a new location from an abnormal location, or from a normal location where it is not functioning correctly. The body part may or may not be cut out or off to be moved to the new location.

Body Part Character 4	Approach Character 5	Device Character 6	Qualifier Character 7
9 Testis, Right ♂ B Testis, Left ♂ C Testes, Bilateral ♂ F Spermatic Cord, Right ♂ G Spermatic Cord, Left ♂ H Spermatic Cords, Bilateral ♂	Ø Open 3 Percutaneous 4 Percutaneous Endoscopic 8 Via Natural or Artificial Opening Endoscopic	Z No Device	Z No Qualifier

♂   All body part, approach, device, and qualifier values

Ø   **Medical and Surgical**
V   **Male Reproductive System**
T   **Resection**   Definition: Cutting out or off, without replacement, all of a body part
                 Explanation: None

Body Part Character 4	Approach Character 5	Device Character 6	Qualifier Character 7
Ø Prostate ⊞ ♂	**Ø** Open **4** Percutaneous Endoscopic **7** Via Natural or Artificial Opening **8** Via Natural or Artificial Opening Endoscopic	**Z** No Device	**Z** No Qualifier

1   Seminal Vesicle, Right   ♂
2   Seminal Vesicle, Left   ♂
3   Seminal Vesicles, Bilateral   ⊞ ♂
6   Tunica Vaginalis, Right   ♂
7   Tunica Vaginalis, Left   ♂
9   Testis, Right   ♂
B   Testis, Left   ♂
C   Testes, Bilateral   ♂
F   Spermatic Cord, Right   ♂
G   Spermatic Cord, Left   ♂
H   Spermatic Cords, Bilateral   ♂
J   Epididymis, Right   ♂
K   Epididymis, Left   ♂
L   Epididymis, Bilateral   ♂
N   Vas Deferens, Right   NC ♂
      Ductus deferens
      Ejaculatory duct
P   Vas Deferens, Left   NC ♂
      See N Vas Deferens, Right
Q   Vas Deferens, Bilateral   NC ♂
      See N Vas Deferens, Right
	Ø Open
	4 Percutaneous Endoscopic
		Z No Device	**Z** No Qualifier

5   Scrotum   ♂
S   Penis   ♂
      Corpus cavernosum
      Corpus spongiosum
T   Prepuce   ♂
      Foreskin
      Glans penis
	Ø Open
	4 Percutaneous Endoscopic
	X External
		Z No Device	**Z** No Qualifier

Non-OR ØVT[N,P,Q][Ø,4]ZZ		**See Appendix L for Procedure Combinations**
Non-OR ØVT[5,T][Ø,4,X]ZZ		⊞ ØVTØ[Ø,4,7,8]ZZ
NC ØVT[N,P,Q][Ø,4]ZZ with principal or secondary diagnosis of Z3Ø.2		⊞ ØVT3[Ø,4]ZZ
♂ All body part, approach, device, and qualifier values		

NC Noncovered Procedure   **LC** Limited Coverage   **QA** Questionable OB Admit   **NT** New Tech Add-on   ⊞ Combination Member   ♂ Male   ♀ Female

ICD-10-PCS 2024   **675**

Male Reproductive System

Ø   **Medical and Surgical**
V   **Male Reproductive System**
U   **Supplement**   Definition: Putting in or on biological or synthetic material that physically reinforces and/or augments the function of a portion of a body part
                       Explanation: The biological material is non-living, or is living and from the same individual. The body part may have been previously replaced, and the SUPPLEMENT procedure is performed to physically reinforce and/or augment the function of the replaced body part.

Body Part Character 4	Approach Character 5	Device Character 6	Qualifier Character 7

1 Seminal Vesicle, Right ♂
2 Seminal Vesicle, Left ♂
3 Seminal Vesicles, Bilateral ♂
6 Tunica Vaginalis, Right ♂
7 Tunica Vaginalis, Left ♂
F Spermatic Cord, Right ♂
G Spermatic Cord, Left ♂
H Spermatic Cords, Bilateral ♂
J Epididymis, Right ♂
K Epididymis, Left ♂
L Epididymis, Bilateral ♂
N Vas Deferens, Right ♂
    Ductus deferens
    Ejaculatory duct
P Vas Deferens, Left ♂
    See N Vas Deferens, Right
Q Vas Deferens, Bilateral ♂
    See N Vas Deferens, Right
	Ø Open
	4 Percutaneous Endoscopic
	8 Via Natural or Artificial Opening
	    Endoscopic
		7 Autologous Tissue Substitute
		J Synthetic Substitute
		K Nonautologous Tissue Substitute
			Z No Qualifier

5 Scrotum ♂
S Penis ♂
    Corpus cavernosum
    Corpus spongiosum
T Prepuce ♂
    Foreskin
    Glans penis
	Ø Open
	4 Percutaneous Endoscopic
	X External
		7 Autologous Tissue Substitute
		J Synthetic Substitute
		K Nonautologous Tissue Substitute
			Z No Qualifier

9 Testis, Right ♂ B Testis, Left ♂ C Testes, Bilateral ♂	Ø Open	7 Autologous Tissue Substitute J Synthetic Substitute K Nonautologous Tissue Substitute	Z No Qualifier

Non-OR   ØVUSX[7,J,K]Z   ♂   All body part, approach, device, and qualifier values

Non-OR Procedure   DRG Non-OR Procedure   Valid OR Procedure   HAC Associated Procedure   Combination Only   New/Revised April   New/Revised October

Ø   Medical and Surgical
V   Male Reproductive System
W   Revision   Definition: Correcting, to the extent possible, a portion of a malfunctioning device or the position of a displaced device
                 Explanation: Revision can include correcting a malfunctioning or displaced device by taking out or putting in components of the device such as a screw or pin

Body Part Character 4	Approach Character 5	Device Character 6	Qualifier Character 7

4 Prostate and Seminal Vesicles ♂
8 Scrotum and Tunica Vaginalis ♂
D Testis ♂
S Penis ♂
   Corpus cavernosum
   Corpus spongiosum
	Ø Open
	3 Percutaneous
	4 Percutaneous Endoscopic
	7 Via Natural or Artificial Opening
	8 Via Natural or Artificial Opening Endoscopic
		Ø Drainage Device
		3 Infusion Device
		7 Autologous Tissue Substitute
		J Synthetic Substitute
		K Nonautologous Tissue Substitute
		Y Other Device
			Z No Qualifier

4 Prostate and Seminal Vesicles ♂
8 Scrotum and Tunica Vaginalis ♂
D Testis ♂
S Penis ♂
   Corpus cavernosum
   Corpus spongiosum
	X External	Ø Drainage Device
		3 Infusion Device
		7 Autologous Tissue Substitute
		J Synthetic Substitute
		K Nonautologous Tissue Substitute
			Z No Qualifier

M Epididymis and Spermatic Cord ♂	Ø Open 3 Percutaneous 4 Percutaneous Endoscopic 7 Via Natural or Artificial Opening 8 Via Natural or Artificial Opening Endoscopic	Ø Drainage Device 3 Infusion Device 7 Autologous Tissue Substitute C Extraluminal Device J Synthetic Substitute K Nonautologous Tissue Substitute Y Other Device	Z No Qualifier
M Epididymis and Spermatic Cord ♂	X External	Ø Drainage Device 3 Infusion Device 7 Autologous Tissue Substitute C Extraluminal Device J Synthetic Substitute K Nonautologous Tissue Substitute	Z No Qualifier

R Vas Deferens ♂
   Ductus deferens
   Ejaculatory duct
	Ø Open
	3 Percutaneous
	4 Percutaneous Endoscopic
	7 Via Natural or Artificial Opening
	8 Via Natural or Artificial Opening Endoscopic
		Ø Drainage Device
		3 Infusion Device
		7 Autologous Tissue Substitute
		C Extraluminal Device
		D Intraluminal Device
		J Synthetic Substitute
		K Nonautologous Tissue Substitute
		Y Other Device
			Z No Qualifier

R Vas Deferens ♂
   Ductus deferens
   Ejaculatory duct
	X External	Ø Drainage Device
		3 Infusion Device
		7 Autologous Tissue Substitute
		C Extraluminal Device
		D Intraluminal Device
		J Synthetic Substitute
		K Nonautologous Tissue Substitute
			Z No Qualifier

Non-OR	ØVW[4,D,S][3,4,7,8]YZ	Non-OR	ØVWMX[Ø,3,7,C,J,K]Z
Non-OR	ØVW8[Ø,3,4,7,8][Ø,3,7,J,K,Y]Z	Non-OR	ØVWR[Ø,3,4,7,8][Ø,3,7,C,D,J,K,Y]Z
Non-OR	ØVW[4,8,D,S]X[Ø,3,7,J,K]Z	Non-OR	ØVWRX[Ø,3,7,C,D,J,K]Z
Non-OR	ØVWM[3,4,7,8]YZ	♂	All body part, approach, device, and qualifier values

NC Noncovered Procedure   LC Limited Coverage   QA Questionable OB Admit   NT New Tech Add-on   ⊞ Combination Member   ♂ Male   ♀ Female

ICD-10-PCS 2024   677

Male Reproductive System

Ø   **Medical and Surgical**
V   **Male Reproductive System**
X   **Transfer**   Definition: Moving, without taking out, all or a portion of a body part to another location to take over the function of all or a portion of a body part

Explanation: The body part transferred remains connected to its vascular and nervous supply

Body Part Character 4	Approach Character 5	Device Character 6	Qualifier Character 7

T   Prepuce
     Foreskin
     Glans penis
	Ø Open
	X External
		Z No Device	D Urethra
			S Penis

Ø   **Medical and Surgical**
V   **Male Reproductive System**
Y   **Transplantation**   Definition: Putting in or on all or a portion of a living body part taken from another individual or animal to physically take the place and/or function of all or a portion of a similar body part

Explanation: The native body part may or may not be taken out, and the transplanted body part may take over all or a portion of its function

Body Part Character 4	Approach Character 5	Device Character 6	Qualifier Character 7

5   Scrotum   ♂
S   Penis   ♂
     Corpus cavernosum
     Corpus spongiosum
	Ø Open	Z No Device	Ø Allogeneic
			1 Syngeneic
			2 Zooplastic

♂   All body part, approach, device, and qualifier values

Anatomical Regions, General ØWØ–ØWY

Character Meanings

This Character Meaning table is provided as a guide to assist the user in the identification of character members that may be found in this section of code tables. It **SHOULD NOT** be used to build a PCS code.

Operation–Character 3	Body Region–Character 4	Approach–Character 5	Device–Character 6	Qualifier–Character 7
Ø Alteration	Ø Head	Ø Open	Ø Drainage Device	Ø Vagina OR Allogeneic
1 Bypass	1 Cranial Cavity	3 Percutaneous	1 Radioactive Element	1 Penis OR Syngeneic
2 Change	2 Face	4 Percutaneous Endoscopic	3 Infusion Device	2 Stoma
3 Control	3 Oral Cavity and Throat	7 Via Natural or Artificial Opening	7 Autologous Tissue Substitute	4 Cutaneous
4 Creation	4 Upper Jaw	8 Via Natural or Artificial Opening Endoscopic	G Defibrillator Lead	6 Bladder
8 Division	5 Lower Jaw	X External	J Synthetic Substitute	9 Pleural Cavity, Right
9 Drainage	6 Neck		K Nonautologous Tissue Substitute	B Pleural Cavity, Left
B Excision	8 Chest Wall		Y Other Device	G Peritoneal Cavity
C Extirpation	9 Pleural Cavity, Right		Z No Device	J Pelvic Cavity
F Fragmentation	B Pleural Cavity, Left			W Upper Vein
H Insertion	C Mediastinum			X Diagnostic
J Inspection	D Pericardial Cavity			Y Lower Vein
M Reattachment	F Abdominal Wall			Z No Qualifier
P Removal	G Peritoneal Cavity			
Q Repair	H Retroperitoneum			
U Supplement	J Pelvic Cavity			
W Revision	K Upper Back			
Y Transplantation	L Lower Back			
	M Perineum, Male			
	N Perineum, Female			
	P Gastrointestinal Tract			
	Q Respiratory Tract			
	R Genitourinary Tract			

AHA Coding Clinic for table ØWØ
2015, 1Q, 31   Bilateral browpexy

AHA Coding Clinic for table ØW1
2020, 4Q, 55   Insertion of subcutaneous pump system for ascites drainage
2018, 4Q, 41-42 Anatomical regions bypass qualifiers
2015, 2Q, 36   Insertion of infusion device into peritoneal cavity
2013, 4Q, 126-127 Creation of percutaneous cutaneoperitoneal fistula

AHA Coding Clinic for table ØW3
2023, 2Q, 26   Control of bleeding with Hemospray®
2021, 3Q, 26   Cavoatrial junction tear with repair and relief of cardiac tamponade
2019, 3Q, 4   Evacuation of subdural hematoma and control of bleeding artery
2018, 4Q, 38   Control of epistaxis
2018, 1Q, 19   Argon plasma coagulation of duodenal arteriovenous malformation
2018, 1Q, 19   Control of epistaxis via silver nitrate cauterization
2017, 4Q, 57-58 Added approach values - Transorifice esophageal vein banding
2017, 4Q, 105   Control of gastrointestinal bleeding
2017, 4Q, 106   Control of bleeding of external naris using suture
2017, 4Q, 106   Nasal packing for epistaxis
2016, 4Q, 99-100 Root operation Control
2014, 4Q, 44   Bakri balloon for control of postpartum hemorrhage
2013, 3Q, 23   Control of intraoperative bleeding

AHA Coding Clinic for table ØW4
2019, 4Q, 30   Transfer large intestine to vagina
2016, 4Q, 101   Root operation Creation

AHA Coding Clinic for table ØW9
2022, 4Q, 59-60 Drainage of the parapharyngeal space and retropharyngeal space
2021, 3Q, 17   Incision and drainage of retropharyngeal space abscess
2021, 3Q, 21   Drainage of midline neck abscess
2021, 3Q, 26   Cavoatrial junction tear with repair and relief of cardiac tamponade
2020, 4Q, 56   Transvaginal drainage of pelvis
2017, 3Q, 12   Therapeutic and diagnostic paracentesis
2017, 2Q, 16   Incision and drainage of floor of mouth

AHA Coding Clinic for table ØWB
2021, 3Q, 21   Excision of thyroglossal duct cyst
2019, 1Q, 27   Excision of pelvic sidewall mass
2017, 2Q, 16   Excision of floor of mouth
2016, 1Q, 21   Excision of urachal mass
2013, 4Q, 119   Excision of inclusion cyst of perineum

AHA Coding Clinic for table ØWC
2022, 1Q, 42   Removal of fat necrosis from retroperitoneum and space of Retzius
2019, 4Q, 35   Extirpation of jaw
2017, 2Q, 16   Excision of floor of mouth

AHA Coding Clinic for table ØWH
2021, 2Q, 14   Peritoneal dialysis catheter placement
2019, 4Q, 43   Unidirectional source brachytherapy
2018, 1Q, 25   Intrauterine brachytherapy & placement of tandems & ovoids
2017, 4Q, 104   Intrauterine brachytherapy & placement of tandems & ovoids
2016, 2Q, 14   Insertion of peritoneal totally implantable venous access device
2015, 2Q, 36   Insertion of infusion device into peritoneal cavity

AHA Coding Clinic for table ØWJ
2022, 3Q, 19   Aortic cross-clamping and exploratory thoracotomy
2021, 2Q, 19   Electromagnetic stealth guided ventriculoperitoneal shunt insertion with endoscopy
2019, 1Q, 3-8   Whipple procedure
2019, 1Q, 25   Laparoscopic appendectomy converted to open procedure
2018, 3Q, 29   Decommissioning of left ventricular assist device with exploration of mediastinum
2016, 4Q, 58   Longitudinal vaginal septum
2013, 2Q, 36   Insertion of ventriculoperitoneal shunt with laparoscopic assistance

AHA Coding Clinic for table ØWP
2021, 2Q, 14   Removal of peritoneal dialysis catheter

AHA Coding Clinic for table ØWQ
2017, 4Q, 106   Control of bleeding of external naris using suture
2017, 3Q, 8   Removal of silo and closure of gastroschisis
2016, 3Q, 3-7   Stoma creation & takedown procedures
2014, 4Q, 38   Abdominoplasty and abdominal wall plication for hernia repair
2014, 3Q, 28   Ileostomy takedown and parastomal hernia repair

AHA Coding Clinic for table ØWU
2017, 3Q, 8   First stage of gastroschisis repair with silo placement
2016, 3Q, 40   Omentoplasty
2015, 2Q, 29   Placement of Ioban™ antimicrobial drape over surgical wound
2014, 4Q, 39   Abdominal component release with placement of mesh for hernia repair
2012, 4Q, 101   Rib resection with reconstruction of anterior chest wall

AHA Coding Clinic for table ØWW
2015, 2Q, 9   Revision of ventriculoperitoneal (VP) shunt

AHA Coding Clinic for table ØWY
2016, 4Q, 112-113 Transplantation

Anatomical Regions, General

Ø   **Medical and Surgical**
W   **Anatomical Regions, General**
Ø   **Alteration**   Definition: Modifying the anatomic structure of a body part without affecting the function of the body part

                        Explanation: Principal purpose is to improve appearance

Body Part Character 4	Approach Character 5	Device Character 6	Qualifier Character 7

Ø Head
2 Face
4 Upper Jaw
5 Lower Jaw
6 Neck
   Parapharyngeal space
   Retropharyngeal space
8 Chest Wall
F Abdominal Wall
K Upper Back
L Lower Back
M Perineum, Male   ♂
N Perineum, Female   ♀
	Ø Open
	3 Percutaneous
	4 Percutaneous Endoscopic
		7 Autologous Tissue Substitute
		J Synthetic Substitute
		K Nonautologous Tissue Substitute
		Z No Device
			Z No Qualifier

    ♂   ØWØM[Ø,3,4][7,J,K,Z]Z
    ♀   ØWØN[Ø,3,4][7,J,K,Z]Z

Ø   **Medical and Surgical**
W   **Anatomical Regions, General**
1   **Bypass**   Definition: Altering the route of passage of the contents of a tubular body part

                        Explanation: Rerouting contents of a body part to a downstream area of the normal route, to a similar route and body part, or to an abnormal route and dissimilar body part. Includes one or more anastomoses, with or without the use of a device.

Body Part Character 4	Approach Character 5	Device Character 6	Qualifier Character 7
1 Cranial Cavity	Ø Open	J Synthetic Substitute	9 Pleural Cavity, Right B Pleural Cavity, Left G Peritoneal Cavity J Pelvic Cavity

9 Pleural Cavity, Right
B Pleural Cavity, Left
J Pelvic Cavity
   Retropubic space
   Space of Retzius
	Ø Open
	3 Percutaneous
	4 Percutaneous Endoscopic
		J Synthetic Substitute	4 Cutaneous
			9 Pleural Cavity, Right
			B Pleural Cavity, Left
			G Peritoneal Cavity
			J Pelvic Cavity
			W Upper Vein
			Y Lower Vein

G Peritoneal Cavity Abdominal cavity	Ø Open 3 Percutaneous 4 Percutaneous Endoscopic	J Synthetic Substitute	4 Cutaneous 6 Bladder 9 Pleural Cavity, Right B Pleural Cavity, Left G Peritoneal Cavity J Pelvic Cavity W Upper Vein Y Lower Vein

    Non-OR   ØW1[9,B][Ø,3,4]J[4,G,W,Y]
    Non-OR   ØW1J[Ø,3,4]J[4,W,Y]
    Non-OR   ØW1G[Ø,3,4]J[9,B,G,J]

Non-OR Procedure   DRG Non-OR Procedure   Valid OR Procedure   HAC Associated Procedure   Combination Only   New/Revised April   New/Revised October

680   ICD-10-PCS 2024

ØWØ–ØW1

Ø   Medical and Surgical
W Anatomical Regions, General
2   Change   Definition: Taking out or off a device from a body part and putting back an identical or similar device in or on the same body part without cutting or puncturing the skin or a mucous membrane
               Explanation: All CHANGE procedures are coded using the approach EXTERNAL

Body Part Character 4	Approach Character 5	Device Character 6	Qualifier Character 7

Ø Head
1 Cranial Cavity
2 Face
4 Upper Jaw
5 Lower Jaw
6 Neck
     Parapharyngeal space
     Retropharyngeal space
8 Chest Wall
9 Pleural Cavity, Right
B Pleural Cavity, Left
C Mediastinum
     Mediastinal cavity
     Mediastinal space
D Pericardial Cavity
F Abdominal Wall
G Peritoneal Cavity
     Abdominal cavity
H Retroperitoneum
     Retroperitoneal cavity
     Retroperitoneal space
J Pelvic Cavity
     Retropubic space
     Space of Retzius
K Upper Back
L Lower Back
M Perineum, Male   ♂
N Perineum, Female   ♀
	X External	Ø Drainage Device
		Y Other Device
			Z No Qualifier

Non-OR	All body part, approach, device, and qualifier values	♂ ♀	ØW2MX[Ø,Y]Z ØW2NX[Ø,Y]Z

NC Noncovered Procedure   **LC** Limited Coverage   **QA** Questionable OB Admit   **NT** New Tech Add-on   ⊞ Combination Member   ♂ Male   ♀ Female

ICD-10-PCS 2024   **681**

Ø   Medical and Surgical
W   Anatomical Regions, General
3   Control   Definition: Stopping, or attempting to stop, postprocedural or other acute bleeding

                Explanation: None

Body Part Character 4	Approach Character 5	Device Character 6	Qualifier Character 7

Ø Head
1 Cranial Cavity
2 Face
4 Upper Jaw
5 Lower Jaw
6 Neck
   Parapharyngeal space
   Retropharyngeal space
8 Chest Wall
9 Pleural Cavity, Right
B Pleural Cavity, Left
C Mediastinum
   Mediastinal cavity
   Mediastinal space
D Pericardial Cavity
F Abdominal Wall
G Peritoneal Cavity
   Abdominal cavity
H Retroperitoneum
   Retroperitoneal cavity
   Retroperitoneal space
J Pelvic Cavity
   Retropubic space
   Space of Retzius
K Upper Back
L Lower Back
M Perineum, Male ♂
N Perineum, Female ♀
	Ø Open
	3 Percutaneous
	4 Percutaneous Endoscopic
		Z No Device	Z No Qualifier

3 Oral Cavity and Throat	Ø Open 3 Percutaneous 4 Percutaneous Endoscopic 7 Via Natural or Artificial Opening 8 Via Natural or Artificial Opening Endoscopic X External	Z No Device	Z No Qualifier
P Gastrointestinal Tract Q Respiratory Tract R Genitourinary Tract	Ø Open 3 Percutaneous 4 Percutaneous Endoscopic 7 Via Natural or Artificial Opening 8 Via Natural or Artificial Opening Endoscopic	Z No Device	Z No Qualifier

Non-OR   ØW3P8ZZ

                                         ♂   ØW3M[Ø,3,4]ZZ
                                         ♀   ØW3N[Ø,3,4]ZZ

Ø   Medical and Surgical
W   Anatomical Regions, General
4   Creation   Definition: Putting in or on biological or synthetic material to form a new body part that to the extent possible replicates the anatomic structure or function of an absent body part

                Explanation: Used for gender reassignment surgery and corrective procedures in individuals with congenital anomalies

Body Part Character 4	Approach Character 5	Device Character 6	Qualifier Character 7
M Perineum, Male ♂	Ø Open	7 Autologous Tissue Substitute J Synthetic Substitute K Nonautologous Tissue Substitute	Ø Vagina
N Perineum, Female ♀	Ø Open	7 Autologous Tissue Substitute J Synthetic Substitute K Nonautologous Tissue Substitute	1 Penis

♂   ØW4MØ[7,J,K]Ø
♀   ØW4NØ[7,J,K]1

Ø   Medical and Surgical
W   Anatomical Regions, General
8   Division   Definition: Cutting into a body part, without draining fluids and/or gases from the body part, in order to separate or transect a body part

                Explanation: All or a portion of the body part is separated into two or more portions

Body Part Character 4	Approach Character 5	Device Character 6	Qualifier Character 7
N Perineum, Female ♀	X External	Z No Device	Z No Qualifier

Non-OR   ØW8NXZZ   ♀   ØW8NXZZ

Non-OR Procedure   DRG Non-OR Procedure   Valid OR Procedure   HAC Associated Procedure   Combination Only   New/Revised April   New/Revised October

Ø   **Medical and Surgical**
W   **Anatomical Regions, General**
9   **Drainage**   Definition: Taking or letting out fluids and/or gases from a body part

                           Explanation: The qualifier DIAGNOSTIC is used to identify drainage procedures that are biopsies

Body Part Character 4	Approach Character 5	Device Character 6	Qualifier Character 7

Ø **Head**
1 **Cranial Cavity**
2 **Face**
3 **Oral Cavity and Throat**
4 **Upper Jaw**
5 **Lower Jaw**
8 **Chest Wall**
9 **Pleural Cavity, Right**
B **Pleural Cavity, Left**
C **Mediastinum**
    Mediastinal cavity
    Mediastinal space
D **Pericardial Cavity**
F **Abdominal Wall**
G **Peritoneal Cavity**
    Abdominal cavity
H **Retroperitoneum**
    Retroperitoneal cavity
    Retroperitoneal space
K **Upper Back**
L **Lower Back**
M **Perineum, Male**   ♂
N **Perineum, Female**   ♀
	Ø Open
	3 Percutaneous
	4 Percutaneous Endoscopic
		Ø Drainage Device	**Z** No Qualifier

Ø **Head**
1 **Cranial Cavity**
2 **Face**
3 **Oral Cavity and Throat**
4 **Upper Jaw**
5 **Lower Jaw**
8 **Chest Wall**
9 **Pleural Cavity, Right**
B **Pleural Cavity, Left**
C **Mediastinum**
    Mediastinal cavity
    Mediastinal space
D **Pericardial Cavity**
F **Abdominal Wall**
G **Peritoneal Cavity**
    Abdominal cavity
H **Retroperitoneum**
    Retroperitoneal cavity
    Retroperitoneal space
K **Upper Back**
L **Lower Back**
M **Perineum, Male**   ♂
N **Perineum, Female**   ♀
	Ø Open
	3 Percutaneous
	4 Percutaneous Endoscopic
		Z No Device	**X** Diagnostic
			Z No Qualifier

6 **Neck**
    Parapharyngeal space
    Retropharyngeal space
J **Pelvic Cavity**
    Retropubic space
    Space of Retzius
	Ø Open
	3 Percutaneous
	4 Percutaneous Endoscopic
	7 Via Natural or Artificial Opening
	8 Via Natural or Artificial Opening
	    Endoscopic
		Ø Drainage Device	**Z** No Qualifier

6 **Neck**
    Parapharyngeal space
    Retropharyngeal space
J **Pelvic Cavity**
    Retropubic space
    Space of Retzius
	Ø Open
	3 Percutaneous
	4 Percutaneous Endoscopic
	7 Via Natural or Artificial Opening
	8 Via Natural or Artificial Opening
	    Endoscopic
		Z No Device	**X** Diagnostic
			Z No Qualifier

Non-OR	ØW9[Ø,8,9,B,K,L,M]ØØZ	♂	ØW9M[Ø,3,4]ØZ
Non-OR	ØW9[Ø,1,2,3,4,5,8,9,B,C,D,F,G,H,K,L,M,N]3ØZ	♂	ØW9M[Ø,3,4]Z[X,Z]
Non-OR	ØW9[Ø,1,8,F,K,L,M]4ØZ	♀	ØW9N[Ø,3,4]ØZ
Non-OR	ØW9[Ø,2,3,4,5,8,9,B,K,L,M,N]ØZX	♀	ØW9N[Ø,3]Z[X,Z]
Non-OR	ØW9[Ø,1,2,3,4,5,8,9,B,C,D,G,K,L,M,N]3ZX	♀	ØW9N4ZZ
Non-OR	ØW9[Ø,1,2,3,4,5,8,C,K,L,M,N]4ZX		
Non-OR	ØW9[Ø,8,9,B,K,L,M]ØZZ		
Non-OR	ØW9[Ø,1,2,3,4,5,8,9,B,C,D,F,G,H,K,L,M,N]3ZZ		
Non-OR	ØW9[Ø,1,8,F,K,L,M]4ZZ		
Non-OR	ØW9[6,J][3,7,8]ØZ		
Non-OR	ØW96[Ø,4]ZX		
Non-OR	ØW9[6,J][3,7,8]Z[X,Z]		

Anatomical Regions, General

Ø   **Medical and Surgical**
W   **Anatomical Regions, General**
B   **Excision**   Definition: Cutting out or off, without replacement, a portion of a body part

                Explanation: The qualifier DIAGNOSTIC is used to identify excision procedures that are biopsies

Body Part Character 4	Approach Character 5	Device Character 6	Qualifier Character 7
Ø Head 2 Face 3 Oral Cavity and Throat 4 Upper Jaw 5 Lower Jaw 8 Chest Wall K Upper Back L Lower Back M Perineum, Male ♂ N Perineum, Female ♀	Ø Open 3 Percutaneous 4 Percutaneous Endoscopic X External	Z No Device	X Diagnostic Z No Qualifier

6 Neck
   Parapharyngeal space
   Retropharyngeal space
F Abdominal Wall
	Ø Open
	3 Percutaneous
	4 Percutaneous Endoscopic
		Z No Device	X Diagnostic
			Z No Qualifier

6 Neck
   Parapharyngeal space
   Retropharyngeal space
F Abdominal Wall
	X External	Z No Device	2 Stoma
			X Diagnostic
			Z No Qualifier

C Mediastinum
   Mediastinal cavity
   Mediastinal space
H Retroperitoneum
   Retroperitoneal cavity
   Retroperitoneal space
	Ø Open
	3 Percutaneous
	4 Percutaneous Endoscopic
		Z No Device	X Diagnostic
			Z No Qualifier

Non-OR	ØWB[Ø,2,4,5,8,K,L,M][Ø,3,4,X]ZX	♂	ØWBM[Ø,3,4,X]Z[X,Z]
Non-OR	ØWB6[Ø,3,4]ZX	♀	ØWBN[Ø,3,4,X]Z[X,Z]
Non-OR	ØWB6XZX		
Non-OR	ØWBH[3,4]ZX		

Ø   **Medical and Surgical**
W   **Anatomical Regions, General**
C   **Extirpation**   Definition: Taking or cutting out solid matter from a body part

                Explanation: The solid matter may be an abnormal byproduct of a biological function or a foreign body; it may be imbedded in a body part or in the lumen of a tubular body part. The solid matter may or may not have been previously broken into pieces.

Body Part Character 4	Approach Character 5	Device Character 6	Qualifier Character 7

1 Cranial Cavity
3 Oral Cavity and Throat
9 Pleural Cavity, Right
B Pleural Cavity, Left
C Mediastinum
   Mediastinal cavity
   Mediastinal space
D Pericardial Cavity
G Peritoneal Cavity
   Abdominal cavity
H Retroperitoneum
   Retroperitoneal cavity
   Retroperitoneal space
J Pelvic Cavity
   Retropubic space
   Space of Retzius
	Ø Open
	3 Percutaneous
	4 Percutaneous Endoscopic
	X External
		Z No Device	Z No Qualifier

4 Upper Jaw 5 Lower Jaw	Ø Open 3 Percutaneous 4 Percutaneous Endoscopic	Z No Device	Z No Qualifier
P Gastrointestinal Tract Q Respiratory Tract R Genitourinary Tract	Ø Open 3 Percutaneous 4 Percutaneous Endoscopic 7 Via Natural or Artificial Opening 8 Via Natural or Artificial Opening Endoscopic X External	Z No Device	Z No Qualifier

Non-OR	ØWC[1,3]XZZ
Non-OR	ØWC[9,B][Ø,3,4,X]ZZ
Non-OR	ØWC[C,D,G,H,J]XZZ
Non-OR	ØWC[4,5]3ZZ
Non-OR	ØWC[P,R][7,8,X]ZZ
Non-OR	ØWCQ[Ø,3,4,X]ZZ

Non-OR Procedure   DRG Non-OR Procedure   Valid OR Procedure   HAC Associated Procedure   Combination Only   New/Revised April   New/Revised October

Ø   **Medical and Surgical**
W   **Anatomical Regions, General**
F   **Fragmentation**   Definition: Breaking solid matter in a body part into pieces

                 Explanation: Physical force (e.g., manual, ultrasonic) applied directly or indirectly is used to break the solid matter into pieces. The solid matter may be an abnormal byproduct of a biological function or a foreign body. The pieces of solid matter are not taken out.

Body Part Character 4	Approach Character 5	Device Character 6	Qualifier Character 7

1   Cranial Cavity   NC
3   Oral Cavity and Throat   NC
9   Pleural Cavity, Right   NC
B   Pleural Cavity, Left   NC
C   Mediastinum   NC
     Mediastinal cavity
     Mediastinal space
D   Pericardial Cavity
G   Peritoneal Cavity   NC
     Abdominal cavity
J   Pelvic Cavity   NC
     Retropubic space
     Space of Retzius
	Ø Open
	3 Percutaneous
	4 Percutaneous Endoscopic
	X External
		Z No Device	Z No Qualifier

P Gastrointestinal Tract NC Q Respiratory Tract NC R Genitourinary Tract	Ø Open 3 Percutaneous 4 Percutaneous Endoscopic 7 Via Natural or Artificial Opening 8 Via Natural or Artificial Opening Endoscopic X External	Z No Device	Z No Qualifier

Non-OR ØWF[1,3,9,B,C,G]XZZ	**Non-OR** ØWFQXZZ	NC ØWF[1,3,9,B,C,G,J]XZZ	
Non-OR ØWFJ[Ø,3,4,X]ZZ	**Non-OR** ØWFR[Ø,3,4,7,8,X]ZZ	NC ØWF[P,Q]XZZ	
Non-OR ØWFP[Ø,3,4,7,8,X]ZZ			

NC Noncovered Procedure   LC Limited Coverage   QA Questionable OB Admit   NT New Tech Add-on   ⊞ Combination Member   ♂ Male   ♀ Female

ICD-10-PCS 2024   **685**

Ø Medical and Surgical
W Anatomical Regions, General
H Insertion   Definition: Putting in a nonbiological appliance that monitors, assists, performs, or prevents a physiological function but does not physically take the place of a body part
              Explanation: None

Body Part Character 4	Approach Character 5	Device Character 6	Qualifier Character 7

Ø Head
1 Cranial Cavity
2 Face
3 Oral Cavity and Throat
4 Upper Jaw
5 Lower Jaw
6 Neck
   Parapharyngeal space
   Retropharyngeal space
8 Chest Wall
9 Pleural Cavity, Right
B Pleural Cavity, Left
D Pericardial Cavity
F Abdominal Wall
G Peritoneal Cavity
   Abdominal cavity
H Retroperitoneum
   Retroperitoneal cavity
   Retroperitoneal space
J Pelvic Cavity
   Retropubic space
   Space of Retzius
K Upper Back
L Lower Back
M Perineum, Male
N Perineum, Female ♀
	Ø Open
	3 Percutaneous
	4 Percutaneous Endoscopic
		1 Radioactive Element
		3 Infusion Device
		Y Other Device
			Z No Qualifier

C Mediastinum
   Mediastinal cavity
   Mediastinal space
	Ø Open
	3 Percutaneous
	4 Percutaneous Endoscopic
		1 Radioactive Element
		3 Infusion Device
		G Defibrillator Lead
		Y Other Device
			Z No Qualifier

P Gastrointestinal Tract Q Respiratory Tract R Genitourinary Tract	Ø Open 3 Percutaneous 4 Percutaneous Endoscopic 7 Via Natural or Artificial Opening 8 Via Natural or Artificial Opening Endoscopic	1 Radioactive Element 3 Infusion Device Y Other Device	Z No Qualifier

DRG Non-OR	ØWH[Ø,2,4,5,6,K,L,M][Ø,3,4][3,Y]Z	
Non-OR	ØWH1[Ø,3,4]3Z	
Non-OR	ØWH[8,9,B][Ø,3,4][3,Y]Z	
Non-OR	ØWHPØYZ	

Non-OR	ØWHP[3,4,7,8][3,Y]Z
Non-OR	ØWHQ[Ø,7,8][3,Y]Z
Non-OR	ØWHR[Ø,3,4,7,8][3,Y]Z
♀	ØWHN[Ø,3,4][3,Y]Z

Ø   **Medical and Surgical**
W   **Anatomical Regions, General**
J   **Inspection**   Definition: Visually and/or manually exploring a body part

Explanation: Visual exploration may be performed with or without optical instrumentation. Manual exploration may be performed directly or through intervening body layers.

Body Part Character 4	Approach Character 5	Device Character 6	Qualifier Character 7

Ø Head
2 Face
3 Oral Cavity and Throat
4 Upper Jaw
5 Lower Jaw
6 Neck
   Parapharyngeal space
   Retropharyngeal space
8 Chest Wall
F Abdominal Wall
K Upper Back
L Lower Back
M Perineum, Male   ♂
N Perineum, Female   ♀
	Ø Open
	3 Percutaneous
	4 Percutaneous Endoscopic
	X External
		Z No Device	**Z** No Qualifier

1 Cranial Cavity
9 Pleural Cavity, Right
B Pleural Cavity, Left
C Mediastinum
   Mediastinal cavity
   Mediastinal space
D Pericardial Cavity
G Peritoneal Cavity
   Abdominal cavity
H Retroperitoneum
   Retroperitoneal cavity
   Retroperitoneal space
J Pelvic Cavity
   Retropubic space
   Space of Retzius
	Ø Open
	3 Percutaneous
	4 Percutaneous Endoscopic
		Z No Device	**Z** No Qualifier

P Gastrointestinal Tract **Q** Respiratory Tract **R** Genitourinary Tract	**Ø** Open **3** Percutaneous **4** Percutaneous Endoscopic **7** Via Natural or Artificial Opening **8** Via Natural or Artificial Opening Endoscopic	**Z** No Device	**Z** No Qualifier

DRG Non-OR	ØWJ[Ø,2,4,5,K,L]ØZZ	♂	ØWJM[Ø,3,4,X]ZZ
DRG Non-OR	ØWJM[Ø,4]ZZ	♀	ØWJN[Ø,3,4,X]ZZ
Non-OR	ØWJ3ØZZ		
Non-OR	ØWJ[Ø,2,3,4,5,6,8,F,K,L,M,N][3,X]ZZ		
Non-OR	ØWJ[Ø,2,3,4,5,K,L]4ZZ		
Non-OR	ØWJDØZZ		
Non-OR	ØWJ[1,9,B,C,D,G,H,J]3ZZ		
Non-OR	ØWJ[P,Q,R][3,7,8]ZZ		

Ø   **Medical and Surgical**
W   **Anatomical Regions, General**
M   **Reattachment**   Definition: Putting back in or on all or a portion of a separated body part to its normal location or other suitable location

Explanation: Vascular circulation and nervous pathways may or may not be reestablished

Body Part Character 4	Approach Character 5	Device Character 6	Qualifier Character 7

2 Face
4 Upper Jaw
5 Lower Jaw
6 Neck
   Parapharyngeal space
   Retropharyngeal space
8 Chest Wall
F Abdominal Wall
K Upper Back
L Lower Back
M Perineum, Male   ♂
N Perineum, Female   ♀
	Ø Open	**Z** No Device	**Z** No Qualifier

♂	ØWMMØZZ
♀	ØWMNØZZ

Anatomical Regions, General

Ø **Medical and Surgical**
W **Anatomical Regions, General**
P **Removal**   Definition: Taking out or off a device from a body part

       Explanation: If a device is taken out and a similar device put in without cutting or puncturing the skin or mucous membrane, the procedure is coded to the root operation CHANGE. Otherwise, the procedure for taking out the device is coded to the root operation REMOVAL.

Body Part Character 4	Approach Character 5	Device Character 6	Qualifier Character 7

Ø Head
2 Face
4 Upper Jaw
5 Lower Jaw
6 Neck
  Parapharyngeal space
  Retropharyngeal space
8 Chest Wall
F Abdominal Wall
K Upper Back
L Lower Back
M Perineum, Male ♂
N Perineum, Female ♀
	Ø Open
	3 Percutaneous
	4 Percutaneous Endoscopic
	X External
		Ø Drainage Device
		1 Radioactive Element
		3 Infusion Device
		7 Autologous Tissue Substitute
		J Synthetic Substitute
		K Nonautologous Tissue Substitute
		Y Other Device
			Z No Qualifier

1 Cranial Cavity
9 Pleural Cavity, Right
B Pleural Cavity, Left
G Peritoneal Cavity
  Abdominal cavity
J Pelvic Cavity
  Retropubic space
  Space of Retzius
	Ø Open
	3 Percutaneous
	4 Percutaneous Endoscopic
		Ø Drainage Device
		1 Radioactive Element
		3 Infusion Device
		J Synthetic Substitute
		Y Other Device
			Z No Qualifier

1 Cranial Cavity
9 Pleural Cavity, Right
B Pleural Cavity, Left
G Peritoneal Cavity
  Abdominal cavity
J Pelvic Cavity
  Retropubic space
  Space of Retzius
	X External	Ø Drainage Device
		1 Radioactive Element
		3 Infusion Device
			Z No Qualifier

C Mediastinum
  Mediastinal cavity
  Mediastinal space
	Ø Open
	3 Percutaneous
	4 Percutaneous Endoscopic
	X External
		Ø Drainage Device
		1 Radioactive Element
		3 Infusion Device
		7 Autologous Tissue Substitute
		G Defibrillator Lead
		J Synthetic Substitute
		K Nonautologous Tissue Substitute
		Y Other Device
			Z No Qualifier

D Pericardial Cavity
H Retroperitoneum
  Retroperitoneal cavity
  Retroperitoneal space
	Ø Open
	3 Percutaneous
	4 Percutaneous Endoscopic
		Ø Drainage Device
		1 Radioactive Element
		3 Infusion Device
		Y Other Device
			Z No Qualifier

D Pericardial Cavity
H Retroperitoneum
  Retroperitoneal cavity
  Retroperitoneal space
	X External	Ø Drainage Device
		1 Radioactive Element
		3 Infusion Device
			Z No Qualifier

P Gastrointestinal Tract Q Respiratory Tract R Genitourinary Tract	Ø Open 3 Percutaneous 4 Percutaneous Endoscopic 7 Via Natural or Artificial Opening 8 Via Natural or Artificial Opening Endoscopic X External	1 Radioactive Element 3 Infusion Device Y Other Device	Z No Qualifier

Non-OR	ØWP[Ø,2,4,5,6,8][Ø,3,4,X][Ø,1,3,7,J,K,Y]Z
Non-OR	ØWPFX[Ø,1,3,7,J,K,Y]Z
Non-OR	ØWP[K,L][Ø,3,4,X][Ø,1,3,7,J,K,Y]Z
Non-OR	ØWPM[Ø,3,4][Ø,1,3,J,Y]Z
Non-OR	ØWPMX[Ø,1,3,Y]Z
Non-OR	ØWPNX[Ø,1,3,7,J,K,Y]Z
Non-OR	ØWP1[Ø,3,4]3Z
Non-OR	ØWP[9,B,J][Ø,3,4][Ø,1,3,J,Y]Z
Non-OR	ØWP[1,9,B,G,J]X[Ø,1,3]Z
Non-OR	ØWPCX[Ø,1,3,7,J,K,Y]Z
Non-OR	ØWP[D,H]X[Ø,1,3]Z
Non-OR	ØWPP[3,4,7,8,X][1,3,Y]Z
Non-OR	ØWPQ73Z
Non-OR	ØWPQ8[3,Y]Z
Non-OR	ØWPQ[Ø,X][1,3,Y]Z
Non-OR	ØWPR[Ø,3,4,7,8,X][1,3,Y]Z

♂ ØWPM[Ø,3,4,X][Ø,1,3,7,J,K,Y]Z
♀ ØWPN[Ø,3,4,X][Ø,1,3,7,J,K,Y]Z

Non-OR Procedure   DRG Non-OR Procedure   Valid OR Procedure   HAC Associated Procedure   Combination Only   New/Revised April   New/Revised October

688   ICD-10-PCS 2024

Ø **Medical and Surgical**
W **Anatomical Regions, General**
Q **Repair**   Definition: Restoring, to the extent possible, a body part to its normal anatomic structure and function

                         Explanation: Used only when the method to accomplish the repair is not one of the other root operations

Body Part Character 4	Approach Character 5	Device Character 6	Qualifier Character 7
Ø Head 2 Face 3 Oral Cavity and Throat 4 Upper Jaw 5 Lower Jaw 8 Chest Wall K Upper Back L Lower Back M Perineum, Male ♂ N Perineum, Female ♀	Ø Open 3 Percutaneous 4 Percutaneous Endoscopic X External	Z No Device	Z No Qualifier

6 Neck
   Parapharyngeal space
   Retropharyngeal space
F Abdominal Wall
	Ø Open
	3 Percutaneous
	4 Percutaneous Endoscopic
		Z No Device	Z No Qualifier

6 Neck
   Parapharyngeal space
   Retropharyngeal space
F Abdominal Wall ✛
	X External	Z No Device	2 Stoma
			Z No Qualifier

C Mediastinum
   Mediastinal cavity
   Mediastinal space
	Ø Open
	3 Percutaneous
	4 Percutaneous Endoscopic
		Z No Device	Z No Qualifier

Non-OR   ØWQNXZZ
♂   ØWQM[Ø,3,4,X]ZZ
♀   ØWQN[Ø,3,4,X]ZZ

See Appendix L for Procedure Combinations
✛   ØWQFXZ[2,Z]

Ø **Medical and Surgical**
W **Anatomical Regions, General**
U **Supplement**   Definition: Putting in or on biological or synthetic material that physically reinforces and/or augments the function of a portion of a body part

                         Explanation: The biological material is non-living, or is living and from the same individual. The body part may have been previously replaced, and the SUPPLEMENT procedure is performed to physically reinforce and/or augment the function of the replaced body part.

Body Part Character 4	Approach Character 5	Device Character 6	Qualifier Character 7

Ø Head
2 Face
4 Upper Jaw
5 Lower Jaw
6 Neck
   Parapharyngeal space
   Retropharyngeal space
8 Chest Wall
C Mediastinum
   Mediastinal cavity
   Mediastinal space
F Abdominal Wall
K Upper Back
L Lower Back
M Perineum, Male ♂
N Perineum, Female ♀
	Ø Open
	4 Percutaneous Endoscopic
		7 Autologous Tissue Substitute
		J Synthetic Substitute
		K Nonautologous Tissue Substitute
			Z No Qualifier

♂   ØWUM[Ø,4][7,J,K]Z
♀   ØWUN[Ø,4][7,J,K]Z

NC Noncovered Procedure   **LC** Limited Coverage   **QA** Questionable OB Admit   **NT** New Tech Add-on   ✛ Combination Member   ♂ Male   ♀ Female

ICD-10-PCS 2024   **689**

Ø   **Medical and Surgical**
W   **Anatomical Regions, General**
W   **Revision**   Definition: Correcting, to the extent possible, a portion of a malfunctioning device or the position of a displaced device
                       Explanation: Revision can include correcting a malfunctioning or displaced device by taking out or putting in components of the device such as a screw or pin

Body Part Character 4	Approach Character 5	Device Character 6	Qualifier Character 7

Ø Head
2 Face
4 Upper Jaw
5 Lower Jaw
6 Neck
   Parapharyngeal space
   Retropharyngeal space
8 Chest Wall
F Abdominal Wall
K Upper Back
L Lower Back
M Perineum, Male ♂
N Perineum, Female ♀
	Ø Open
	3 Percutaneous
	4 Percutaneous Endoscopic
	X External
		Ø Drainage Device
		1 Radioactive Element
		3 Infusion Device
		7 Autologous Tissue Substitute
		J Synthetic Substitute
		K Nonautologous Tissue Substitute
		Y Other Device
			Z No Qualifier

1 Cranial Cavity
9 Pleural Cavity, Right
B Pleural Cavity, Left
G Peritoneal Cavity
   Abdominal cavity
J Pelvic Cavity
   Retropubic space
   Space of Retzius
	Ø Open
	3 Percutaneous
	4 Percutaneous Endoscopic
	X External
		Ø Drainage Device
		1 Radioactive Element
		3 Infusion Device
		J Synthetic Substitute
		Y Other Device
			Z No Qualifier

C Mediastinum
   Mediastinal cavity
   Mediastinal space
	Ø Open
	3 Percutaneous
	4 Percutaneous Endoscopic
	X External
		Ø Drainage Device
		1 Radioactive Element
		3 Infusion Device
		7 Autologous Tissue Substitute
		G Defibrillator Lead
		J Synthetic Substitute
		K Nonautologous Tissue Substitute
		Y Other Device
			Z No Qualifier

D Pericardial Cavity
H Retroperitoneum
   Retroperitoneal cavity
   Retroperitoneal space
	Ø Open
	3 Percutaneous
	4 Percutaneous Endoscopic
	X External
		Ø Drainage Device
		1 Radioactive Element
		3 Infusion Device
		Y Other Device
			Z No Qualifier

P Gastrointestinal Tract Q Respiratory Tract R Genitourinary Tract	Ø Open 3 Percutaneous 4 Percutaneous Endoscopic 7 Via Natural or Artificial Opening 8 Via Natural or Artificial Opening Endoscopic X External	1 Radioactive Element 3 Infusion Device Y Other Device	Z No Qualifier

DRG Non-OR   ØWW[Ø,2,4,5,6,K,L][Ø,3,4][Ø,1,3,7,J,K,Y]Z
DRG Non-OR   ØWWM[Ø,3,4][Ø,1,3,J,Y]Z
Non-OR   ØWW[Ø,2,4,5,6,F,K,L,M,N]X[Ø,1,3,7,J,K,Y]Z
Non-OR   ØWW8[Ø,3,4,X][Ø,1,3,7,J,K,Y]Z
Non-OR   ØWW[1,G,J]X[Ø,1,3,J,Y]Z
Non-OR   ØWW[9,B][Ø,3,4,X][Ø,1,3,J,Y]Z
Non-OR   ØWWCX[Ø,1,3,7,J,K,Y]Z
Non-OR   ØWW[D,H]X[Ø,1,3,Y]Z
Non-OR   ØWWP[3,4,7,8,X][1,3,Y]Z
Non-OR   ØWWQ[Ø,X][1,3,Y]Z
Non-OR   ØWWR[Ø,3,4,7,8,X][1,3,Y]Z

♂   ØWWM[Ø,3,4,X][Ø,1,3,7,J,K,Y]Z
♀   ØWWN[Ø,3,4,X][Ø,1,3,7,K,Y]Z

Ø   **Medical and Surgical**
W   **Anatomical Regions, General**
Y   **Transplantation**   Definition: Putting in or on all or a portion of a living body part taken from another individual or animal to physically take the place and/or function of all or a portion of a similar body part
                       Explanation: The native body part may or may not be taken out, and the transplanted body part may take over all or a portion of its function

Body Part Character 4	Approach Character 5	Device Character 6	Qualifier Character 7
2 Face	Ø Open	Z No Device	Ø Allogeneic 1 Syngeneic

Anatomical Regions, Upper Extremities ØXØ–ØXY

Character Meanings

This Character Meaning table is provided as a guide to assist the user in the identification of character members that may be found in this section of code tables. It **SHOULD NOT** be used to build a PCS code.

Operation–Character 3		Body Part–Character 4		Approach–Character 5		Device–Character 6		Qualifier–Character 7	
Ø	Alteration	Ø	Forequarter, Right	Ø	Open	Ø	Drainage Device	Ø	Allogeneic OR Complete
2	Change	1	Forequarter, Left	3	Percutaneous	1	Radioactive Element	1	High OR Syngeneic
3	Control	2	Shoulder Region, Right	4	Percutaneous Endoscopic	3	Infusion Device	2	Mid
6	Detachment	3	Shoulder Region, Left	X	External	7	Autologous Tissue Substitute	3	Low
9	Drainage	4	Axilla, Right			J	Synthetic Substitute	4	Complete 1st Ray
B	Excision	5	Axilla, Left			K	Nonautologous Tissue Substitute	5	Complete 2nd Ray
H	Insertion	6	Upper Extremity, Right			Y	Other Device	6	Complete 3rd Ray
J	Inspection	7	Upper Extremity, Left			Z	No Device	7	Complete 4th Ray
M	Reattachment	8	Upper Arm, Right					8	Complete 5th Ray
P	Removal	9	Upper Arm, Left					9	Partial 1st Ray
Q	Repair	B	Elbow Region, Right					B	Partial 2nd Ray
R	Replacement	C	Elbow Region, Left					C	Partial 3rd Ray
U	Supplement	D	Lower Arm, Right					D	Partial 4th Ray
W	Revision	F	Lower Arm, Left					F	Partial 5th Ray
X	Transfer	G	Wrist Region, Right					L	Thumb, Right
Y	Transplantation	H	Wrist Region, Left					M	Thumb, Left
		J	Hand, Right					N	Toe, Right
		K	Hand, Left					P	Toe, Left
		L	Thumb, Right					X	Diagnostic
		M	Thumb, Left					Z	No Qualifier
		N	Index Finger, Right						
		P	Index Finger, Left						
		Q	Middle Finger, Right						
		R	Middle Finger, Left						
		S	Ring Finger, Right						
		T	Ring Finger, Left						
		V	Little Finger, Right						
		W	Little Finger, Left						

AHA Coding Clinic for table ØX3

2016, 4Q, 99	Root operation Control
2015, 1Q, 35	Evacuation of hematoma for control of postprocedural bleeding
2013, 3Q, 23	Control of intraoperative bleeding

AHA Coding Clinic for table ØX6

2017, 2Q, 3-4	Qualifiers for the root operation detachment
2017, 2Q, 18	Removal of polydactyl digits
2017, 1Q, 52	Further distal phalangeal amputation
2016, 3Q, 33	Traumatic amputation of fingers with further revision amputation

AHA Coding Clinic for table ØXH

2017, 2Q, 20	Exchange of intramedullary antibiotic impregnated spacer

AHA Coding Clinic for table ØXP

2017, 2Q, 20	Exchange of intramedullary antibiotic impregnated spacer

AHA Coding Clinic for table ØXY

2016, 4Q, 112-113	Transplantation

Detachment Qualifier Descriptions

Qualifier Definition	Upper Arm	Lower Arm
1 **High:** Amputation at the proximal portion of the shaft of the:	Humerus	Radius/Ulna
2 **Mid:** Amputation at the middle portion of the shaft of the:	Humerus	Radius/Ulna
3 **Low:** Amputation at the distal portion of the shaft of the:	Humerus	Radius/Ulna

Qualifier Definition	Hand
0 **Complete 1st through 5th Rays** Ray: digit of hand or foot with corresponding metacarpus or metatarsus	Through carpo-metacarpal joint, **Wrist**
4 **Complete 1st Ray**	Through carpo-metacarpal joint, **Thumb**
5 **Complete 2nd Ray**	Through carpo-metacarpal joint, **Index Finger**
6 **Complete 3rd Ray**	Through carpo-metacarpal joint, **Middle Finger**
7 **Complete 4th Ray**	Through carpo-metacarpal joint, **Ring Finger**
8 **Complete 5th Ray**	Through carpo-metacarpal joint, **Little Finger**
9 **Partial 1st Ray**	Anywhere along shaft or head of metacarpal bone, **Thumb**
B **Partial 2nd Ray**	Anywhere along shaft or head of metacarpal bone, **Index Finger**
C **Partial 3rd Ray**	Anywhere along shaft or head of metacarpal bone, **Middle Finger**
D **Partial 4th Ray**	Anywhere along shaft or head of metacarpal bone, **Ring Finger**
F **Partial 5th Ray**	Anywhere along shaft or head of metacarpal bone, **Little Finger**

Qualifier Definition	Thumb/Finger
0 Complete	At the metacarpophalangeal joint
1 High	Anywhere along the proximal phalanx
2 Mid	Through the proximal interphalangeal joint or anywhere along the middle phalanx
3 Low	Through the distal interphalangeal joint or anywhere along the distal phalanx

Ø   **Medical and Surgical**
X   **Anatomical Regions, Upper Extremities**
Ø   **Alteration**   Definition: Modifying the anatomic structure of a body part without affecting the function of the body part
                 Explanation: Principal purpose is to improve appearance

Body Part Character 4	Approach Character 5	Device Character 6	Qualifier Character 7
2 Shoulder Region, Right 3 Shoulder Region, Left 4 Axilla, Right 5 Axilla, Left 6 Upper Extremity, Right 7 Upper Extremity, Left 8 Upper Arm, Right 9 Upper Arm, Left B Elbow Region, Right C Elbow Region, Left D Lower Arm, Right F Lower Arm, Left G Wrist Region, Right H Wrist Region, Left	Ø Open 3 Percutaneous 4 Percutaneous Endoscopic	7 Autologous Tissue Substitute J Synthetic Substitute K Nonautologous Tissue Substitute Z No Device	Z No Qualifier

Ø   **Medical and Surgical**
X   **Anatomical Regions, Upper Extremities**
2   **Change**   Definition: Taking out or off a device from a body part and putting back an identical or similar device in or on the same body part without cutting or puncturing the skin or a mucous membrane
                 Explanation: All CHANGE procedures are coded using the approach EXTERNAL

Body Part Character 4	Approach Character 5	Device Character 6	Qualifier Character 7
6 Upper Extremity, Right 7 Upper Extremity, Left	X External	Ø Drainage Device Y Other Device	Z No Qualifier

Non-OR   All body part, approach, device, and qualifier values

Ø   **Medical and Surgical**
X   **Anatomical Regions, Upper Extremities**
3   **Control**   Definition: Stopping, or attempting to stop, postprocedural or other acute bleeding
                 Explanation: None

Body Part Character 4	Approach Character 5	Device Character 6	Qualifier Character 7
2 Shoulder Region, Right 3 Shoulder Region, Left 4 Axilla, Right 5 Axilla, Left 6 Upper Extremity, Right 7 Upper Extremity, Left 8 Upper Arm, Right 9 Upper Arm, Left B Elbow Region, Right C Elbow Region, Left D Lower Arm, Right F Lower Arm, Left G Wrist Region, Right H Wrist Region, Left J Hand, Right K Hand, Left	Ø Open 3 Percutaneous 4 Percutaneous Endoscopic	Z No Device	Z No Qualifier

NC Noncovered Procedure   LC Limited Coverage   QA Questionable OB Admit   COM New Tech Add-on   ⊞ Combination Member   ♂ Male   ♀ Female

ICD-10-PCS 2024   693

Ø　Medical and Surgical
X　Anatomical Regions, Upper Extremities
6　Detachment　　Definition: Cutting off all or a portion of the upper or lower extremities

Explanation: The body part value is the site of the detachment, with a qualifier if applicable to further specify the level where the extremity was detached

Body Part Character 4	Approach Character 5	Device Character 6	Qualifier Character 7
Ø　Forequarter, Right 1　Forequarter, Left 2　Shoulder Region, Right 3　Shoulder Region, Left B　Elbow Region, Right C　Elbow Region, Left	Ø　Open	Z　No Device	Z　No Qualifier
8　Upper Arm, Right 9　Upper Arm, Left D　Lower Arm, Right F　Lower Arm, Left	Ø　Open	Z　No Device	1　High 2　Mid 3　Low
J　Hand, Right K　Hand, Left	Ø　Open	Z　No Device	Ø　Complete 4　Complete 1st Ray 5　Complete 2nd Ray 6　Complete 3rd Ray 7　Complete 4th Ray 8　Complete 5th Ray 9　Partial 1st Ray B　Partial 2nd Ray C　Partial 3rd Ray D　Partial 4th Ray F　Partial 5th Ray
L　Thumb, Right M　Thumb, Left N　Index Finger, Right P　Index Finger, Left Q　Middle Finger, Right R　Middle Finger, Left S　Ring Finger, Right T　Ring Finger, Left V　Little Finger, Right W　Little Finger, Left	Ø　Open	Z　No Device	Ø　Complete 1　High 2　Mid 3　Low

Ø Medical and Surgical
X Anatomical Regions, Upper Extremities
9 Drainage　　　Definition: Taking or letting out fluids and/or gases from a body part
　　　　　Explanation: The qualifier DIAGNOSTIC is used to identify drainage procedures that are biopsies

Body Part Character 4	Approach Character 5	Device Character 6	Qualifier Character 7
2 Shoulder Region, Right 3 Shoulder Region, Left 4 Axilla, Right 5 Axilla, Left 6 Upper Extremity, Right 7 Upper Extremity, Left 8 Upper Arm, Right 9 Upper Arm, Left B Elbow Region, Right C Elbow Region, Left D Lower Arm, Right F Lower Arm, Left G Wrist Region, Right H Wrist Region, Left J Hand, Right K Hand, Left	Ø Open 3 Percutaneous 4 Percutaneous Endoscopic	Ø Drainage Device	Z No Qualifier
2 Shoulder Region, Right 3 Shoulder Region, Left 4 Axilla, Right 5 Axilla, Left 6 Upper Extremity, Right 7 Upper Extremity, Left 8 Upper Arm, Right 9 Upper Arm, Left B Elbow Region, Right C Elbow Region, Left D Lower Arm, Right F Lower Arm, Left G Wrist Region, Right H Wrist Region, Left J Hand, Right K Hand, Left	Ø Open 3 Percutaneous 4 Percutaneous Endoscopic	Z No Device	X Diagnostic Z No Qualifier

Non-OR　All body part, approach, device, and qualifier values

Ø Medical and Surgical
X Anatomical Regions, Upper Extremities
B Excision　　　Definition: Cutting out or off, without replacement, a portion of a body part
　　　　　Explanation: The qualifier DIAGNOSTIC is used to identify excision procedures that are biopsies

Body Part Character 4	Approach Character 5	Device Character 6	Qualifier Character 7
2 Shoulder Region, Right 3 Shoulder Region, Left 4 Axilla, Right 5 Axilla, Left 6 Upper Extremity, Right 7 Upper Extremity, Left 8 Upper Arm, Right 9 Upper Arm, Left B Elbow Region, Right C Elbow Region, Left D Lower Arm, Right F Lower Arm, Left G Wrist Region, Right H Wrist Region, Left J Hand, Right K Hand, Left	Ø Open 3 Percutaneous 4 Percutaneous Endoscopic	Z No Device	X Diagnostic Z No Qualifier

Non-OR　ØXB[2,3,4,5,6,7,8,9,B,C,D,F,G,H,J,K][Ø,3,4]ZX

Anatomical Regions, Upper Extremities (left margin)

Ø Medical and Surgical
X Anatomical Regions, Upper Extremities
H Insertion   Definition: Putting in a nonbiological appliance that monitors, assists, performs, or prevents a physiological function but does not physically take the place of a body part

Explanation: None

Body Part Character 4	Approach Character 5	Device Character 6	Qualifier Character 7
2 Shoulder Region, Right	Ø Open	1 Radioactive Element	Z No Qualifier
3 Shoulder Region, Left	3 Percutaneous	3 Infusion Device	
4 Axilla, Right	4 Percutaneous Endoscopic	Y Other Device	
5 Axilla, Left			
6 Upper Extremity, Right			
7 Upper Extremity, Left			
8 Upper Arm, Right			
9 Upper Arm, Left			
B Elbow Region, Right			
C Elbow Region, Left			
D Lower Arm, Right			
F Lower Arm, Left			
G Wrist Region, Right			
H Wrist Region, Left			
J Hand, Right			
K Hand, Left			

DRG Non-OR   ØXH[2,3,4,5,6,7,8,9,B,C,D,F,G,H,J,K][Ø,3,4][3,Y]Z

Ø Medical and Surgical
X Anatomical Regions, Upper Extremities
J Inspection   Definition: Visually and/or manually exploring a body part

Explanation: Visual exploration may be performed with or without optical instrumentation. Manual exploration may be performed directly or through intervening body layers.

Body Part Character 4	Approach Character 5	Device Character 6	Qualifier Character 7
2 Shoulder Region, Right	Ø Open	Z No Device	Z No Qualifier
3 Shoulder Region, Left	3 Percutaneous		
4 Axilla, Right	4 Percutaneous Endoscopic		
5 Axilla, Left	X External		
6 Upper Extremity, Right			
7 Upper Extremity, Left			
8 Upper Arm, Right			
9 Upper Arm, Left			
B Elbow Region, Right			
C Elbow Region, Left			
D Lower Arm, Right			
F Lower Arm, Left			
G Wrist Region, Right			
H Wrist Region, Left			
J Hand, Right			
K Hand, Left			

DRG Non-OR   ØXJ[2,3,4,5,6,7,8,9,B,C,D,F,G,H,J,K]ØZZ
Non-OR   ØXJ[2,3,4,5,6,7,8,9,B,C,D,F,G,H][3,4,X]ZZ
Non-OR   ØXJ[J,K][3,X]ZZ

Ø   **Medical and Surgical**
X   **Anatomical Regions, Upper Extremities**
M   **Reattachment**   Definition: Putting back in or on all or a portion of a separated body part to its normal location or other suitable location

                 Explanation: Vascular circulation and nervous pathways may or may not be reestablished

Body Part Character 4	Approach Character 5	Device Character 6	Qualifier Character 7
Ø Forequarter, Right	Ø Open	Z No Device	Z No Qualifier
1 Forequarter, Left			
2 Shoulder Region, Right			
3 Shoulder Region, Left			
4 Axilla, Right			
5 Axilla, Left			
6 Upper Extremity, Right			
7 Upper Extremity, Left			
8 Upper Arm, Right			
9 Upper Arm, Left			
B Elbow Region, Right			
C Elbow Region, Left			
D Lower Arm, Right			
F Lower Arm, Left			
G Wrist Region, Right			
H Wrist Region, Left			
J Hand, Right			
K Hand, Left			
L Thumb, Right			
M Thumb, Left			
N Index Finger, Right			
P Index Finger, Left			
Q Middle Finger, Right			
R Middle Finger, Left			
S Ring Finger, Right			
T Ring Finger, Left			
V Little Finger, Right			
W Little Finger, Left			

Ø   **Medical and Surgical**
X   **Anatomical Regions, Upper Extremities**
P   **Removal**   Definition: Taking out or off a device from a body part

                 Explanation: If a device is taken out and a similar device put in without cutting or puncturing the skin or mucous membrane, the procedure is coded to the root operation CHANGE. Otherwise, the procedure for taking out the device is coded to the root operation REMOVAL.

Body Part Character 4	Approach Character 5	Device Character 6	Qualifier Character 7
6 Upper Extremity, Right	Ø Open	Ø Drainage Device	Z No Qualifier
7 Upper Extremity, Left	3 Percutaneous	1 Radioactive Element	
	4 Percutaneous Endoscopic	3 Infusion Device	
	X External	7 Autologous Tissue Substitute	
		J Synthetic Substitute	
		K Nonautologous Tissue Substitute	
		Y Other Device	

Non-OR   All body part, approach, device, and qualifier values

NC Noncovered Procedure   **LC** Limited Coverage   **QA** Questionable OB Admit   **COM** New Tech Add-on   ⊞ Combination Member   ♂ Male   ♀ Female

ICD-10-PCS 2024   **697**

Ø Medical and Surgical
X Anatomical Regions, Upper Extremities
Q Repair   Definition: Restoring, to the extent possible, a body part to its normal anatomic structure and function
                 Explanation: Used only when the method to accomplish the repair is not one of the other root operations

Body Part Character 4	Approach Character 5	Device Character 6	Qualifier Character 7
2 Shoulder Region, Right	Ø Open	Z No Device	Z No Qualifier
3 Shoulder Region, Left	3 Percutaneous		
4 Axilla, Right	4 Percutaneous Endoscopic		
5 Axilla, Left	X External		
6 Upper Extremity, Right			
7 Upper Extremity, Left			
8 Upper Arm, Right			
9 Upper Arm, Left			
B Elbow Region, Right			
C Elbow Region, Left			
D Lower Arm, Right			
F Lower Arm, Left			
G Wrist Region, Right			
H Wrist Region, Left			
J Hand, Right			
K Hand, Left			
L Thumb, Right			
M Thumb, Left			
N Index Finger, Right			
P Index Finger, Left			
Q Middle Finger, Right			
R Middle Finger, Left			
S Ring Finger, Right			
T Ring Finger, Left			
V Little Finger, Right			
W Little Finger, Left			

Ø Medical and Surgical
X Anatomical Regions, Upper Extremities
R Replacement   Definition: Putting in or on biological or synthetic material that physically takes the place and/or function of all or a portion of a body part
                      Explanation: The body part may have been taken out or replaced, or may be taken out, physically eradicated, or rendered nonfunctional during the REPLACEMENT procedure. A REMOVAL procedure is coded for taking out the device used in a previous replacement procedure.

Body Part Character 4	Approach Character 5	Device Character 6	Qualifier Character 7
L Thumb, Right	Ø Open	7 Autologous Tissue Substitute	N Toe, Right
M Thumb, Left	4 Percutaneous Endoscopic		P Toe, Left

Ø   **Medical and Surgical**
X   **Anatomical Regions, Upper Extremities**
U   **Supplement**   Definition: Putting in or on biological or synthetic material that physically reinforces and/or augments the function of a portion of a body part
           Explanation: The biological material is non-living, or is living and from the same individual. The body part may have been previously replaced, and the SUPPLEMENT procedure is performed to physically reinforce and/or augment the function of the replaced body part.

Body Part Character 4	Approach Character 5	Device Character 6	Qualifier Character 7
2 Shoulder Region, Right	Ø Open	7 Autologous Tissue Substitute	Z No Qualifier
3 Shoulder Region, Left	4 Percutaneous Endoscopic	J Synthetic Substitute	
4 Axilla, Right		K Nonautologous Tissue Substitute	
5 Axilla, Left			
6 Upper Extremity, Right			
7 Upper Extremity, Left			
8 Upper Arm, Right			
9 Upper Arm, Left			
B Elbow Region, Right			
C Elbow Region, Left			
D Lower Arm, Right			
F Lower Arm, Left			
G Wrist Region, Right			
H Wrist Region, Left			
J Hand, Right			
K Hand, Left			
L Thumb, Right			
M Thumb, Left			
N Index Finger, Right			
P Index Finger, Left			
Q Middle Finger, Right			
R Middle Finger, Left			
S Ring Finger, Right			
T Ring Finger, Left			
V Little Finger, Right			
W Little Finger, Left			

Anatomical Regions, Upper Extremities

ØXU–ØXU

NC Noncovered Procedure   LC Limited Coverage   QA Questionable OB Admit   COM New Tech Add-on   ⊞ Combination Member   ♂ Male   ♀ Female

ICD-10-PCS 2024   **699**

Ø Medical and Surgical
X Anatomical Regions, Upper Extremities
W Revision   Definition: Correcting, to the extent possible, a portion of a malfunctioning device or the position of a displaced device

Explanation: Revision can include correcting a malfunctioning or displaced device by taking out or putting in components of the device such as a screw or pin

Body Part Character 4	Approach Character 5	Device Character 6	Qualifier Character 7
6 Upper Extremity, Right 7 Upper Extremity, Left	Ø Open 3 Percutaneous 4 Percutaneous Endoscopic X External	Ø Drainage Device 3 Infusion Device 7 Autologous Tissue Substitute J Synthetic Substitute K Nonautologous Tissue Substitute Y Other Device	Z No Qualifier

DRG Non-OR   ØXW[6,7][Ø,3,4][Ø,3,7,J,K,Y]Z
Non-OR   ØXW[6,7]X[Ø,3,7,J,K,Y]Z

Ø Medical and Surgical
X Anatomical Regions, Upper Extremities
X Transfer   Definition: Moving, without taking out, all or a portion of a body part to another location to take over the function of all or a portion of a body part

Explanation: The body part transferred remains connected to its vascular and nervous supply

Body Part Character 4	Approach Character 5	Device Character 6	Qualifier Character 7
N Index Finger, Right	Ø Open	Z No Device	L Thumb, Right
P Index Finger, Left	Ø Open	Z No Device	M Thumb, Left

Ø Medical and Surgical
X Anatomical Regions, Upper Extremities
Y Transplantation   Definition: Putting in or on all or a portion of a living body part taken from another individual or animal to physically take the place and/or function of all or a portion of a similar body part

Explanation: The native body part may or may not be taken out, and the transplanted body part may take over all or a portion of its function

Body Part Character 4	Approach Character 5	Device Character 6	Qualifier Character 7
J Hand, Right K Hand, Left	Ø Open	Z No Device	Ø Allogeneic 1 Syngeneic

Anatomical Regions, Lower Extremities ØYØ–ØYW

Character Meanings

This Character Meaning table is provided as a guide to assist the user in the identification of character members that may be found in this section of code tables. It **SHOULD NOT** be used to build a PCS code.

Operation–Character 3		Body Part–Character 4		Approach–Character 5		Device–Character 6		Qualifier–Character 7	
Ø	Alteration	Ø	Buttock, Right	Ø	Open	Ø	Drainage Device	Ø	Complete
2	Change	1	Buttock, Left	3	Percutaneous	1	Radioactive Element	1	High
3	Control	2	Hindquarter, Right	4	Percutaneous Endoscopic	3	Infusion Device	2	Mid
6	Detachment	3	Hindquarter, Left	X	External	7	Autologous Tissue Substitute	3	Low
9	Drainage	4	Hindquarter, Bilateral			J	Synthetic Substitute	4	Complete 1st Ray
B	Excision	5	Inguinal Region, Right			K	Nonautologous Tissue Substitute	5	Complete 2nd Ray
H	Insertion	6	Inguinal Region, Left			Y	Other Device	6	Complete 3rd Ray
J	Inspection	7	Femoral Region, Right			Z	No Device	7	Complete 4th Ray
M	Reattachment	8	Femoral Region, Left					8	Complete 5th Ray
P	Removal	9	Lower Extremity, Right					9	Partial 1st Ray
Q	Repair	A	Inguinal Region, Bilateral					B	Partial 2nd Ray
U	Supplement	B	Lower Extremity, Left					C	Partial 3rd Ray
W	Revision	C	Upper Leg, Right					D	Partial 4th Ray
		D	Upper Leg, Left					F	Partial 5th Ray
		E	Femoral Region, Bilateral					X	Diagnostic
		F	Knee Region, Right					Z	No Qualifier
		G	Knee Region, Left						
		H	Lower Leg, Right						
		J	Lower Leg, Left						
		K	Ankle Region, Right						
		L	Ankle Region, Left						
		M	Foot, Right						
		N	Foot, Left						
		P	1st Toe, Right						
		Q	1st Toe, Left						
		R	2nd Toe, Right						
		S	2nd Toe, Left						
		T	3rd Toe, Right						
		U	3rd Toe, Left						
		V	4th Toe, Right						
		W	4th Toe, Left						
		X	5th Toe, Right						
		Y	5th Toe, Left						

AHA Coding Clinic for table ØY3

| 2016, 4Q, 99 | Root operation Control |
| 2013, 3Q, 23 | Control of intraoperative bleeding |

AHA Coding Clinic for table ØY6

2019, 2Q, 17	Cryoamputation of lower leg
2017, 2Q, 3-4	Qualifiers for the root operation detachment
2017, 1Q, 22	Chopart amputation of foot
2015, 2Q, 28	Partial amputation of hallux at interphalangeal Joint
2015, 1Q, 28	Mid-foot amputation

AHA Coding Clinic for table ØY9

| 2015, 1Q, 22 | Incision and drainage of abscess of femoropopliteal bypass site |
| 2015, 1Q, 22 | Incision and drainage of groin abscess |

AHA Coding Clinic for table ØYH

| 2023, 1Q, 27 | Bilateral traumatic amputation with Stage 1 placement of OPRA device |
| 2023, 1Q, 29 | Stage 2 placement of OPRA device |

AHA Coding Clinic for table ØYW

| 2023, 1Q, 29 | Stage 2 placement of OPRA device |

Detachment Qualifier Descriptions

Qualifier Definition	Upper Leg	Lower Leg
1 **High:** Amputation at the proximal portion of the shaft of the:	Femur	Tibia/Fibula
2 **Mid:** Amputation at the middle portion of the shaft of the:	Femur	Tibia/Fibula
3 **Low:** Amputation at the distal portion of the shaft of the:	Femur	Tibia/Fibula

Qualifier Definition	Foot
0 Complete 1st through 5th Rays Ray: digit of hand or foot with corresponding metacarpus or metatarsus	Through tarso-metatarsal Joint, **Ankle**
4 Complete 1st Ray	Through tarso-metatarsal joint, **Great Toe**
5 Complete 2nd Ray	Through tarso-metatarsal joint, **2nd Toe**
6 Complete 3rd Ray	Through tarso-metatarsal joint, **3rd Toe**
7 Complete 4th Ray	Through tarso-metatarsal joint, **4th Toe**
8 Complete 5th Ray	Through tarso-metatarsal joint, **Little Toe**
9 Partial 1st Ray	Anywhere along shaft or head of metatarsal bone, **Great Toe**
B Partial 2nd Ray	Anywhere along shaft or head of metatarsal bone, **2nd Toe**
C Partial 3rd Ray	Anywhere along shaft or head of metatarsal bone, **3rd Toe**
D Partial 4th Ray	Anywhere along shaft or head of metatarsal bone, **4th Toe**
F Partial 5th Ray	Anywhere along shaft or head of metatarsal bone, **Little Toe**

Qualifier Definition	Toe
0 Complete	At the metatarsal-phalangeal joint
1 High	Anywhere along the proximal phalanx
2 Mid	Through the proximal interphalangeal joint or anywhere along the middle phalanx
3 Low	Through the distal interphalangeal joint or anywhere along the distal phalanx

Ø   **Medical and Surgical**
Y   **Anatomical Regions, Lower Extremities**
Ø   **Alteration**   Definition: Modifying the anatomic structure of a body part without affecting the function of the body part
                   Explanation: Principal purpose is to improve appearance

Body Part Character 4	Approach Character 5	Device Character 6	Qualifier Character 7
Ø Buttock, Right 1 Buttock, Left 9 Lower Extremity, Right B Lower Extremity, Left C Upper Leg, Right D Upper Leg, Left F Knee Region, Right G Knee Region, Left H Lower Leg, Right J Lower Leg, Left K Ankle Region, Right L Ankle Region, Left	Ø Open 3 Percutaneous 4 Percutaneous Endoscopic	7 Autologous Tissue Substitute J Synthetic Substitute K Nonautologous Tissue Substitute Z No Device	Z No Qualifier

Ø   **Medical and Surgical**
Y   **Anatomical Regions, Lower Extremities**
2   **Change**   Definition: Taking out or off a device from a body part and putting back an identical or similar device in or on the same body part without
                   cutting or puncturing the skin or a mucous membrane
                   Explanation: All CHANGE procedures are coded using the approach EXTERNAL

Body Part Character 4	Approach Character 5	Device Character 6	Qualifier Character 7
9 Lower Extremity, Right B Lower Extremity, Left	X External	Ø Drainage Device Y Other Device	Z No Qualifier

     Non-OR   All body part, approach, device, and qualifier values

Ø   **Medical and Surgical**
Y   **Anatomical Regions, Lower Extremities**
3   **Control**   Definition: Stopping, or attempting to stop, postprocedural or other acute bleeding
                   Explanation: None

Body Part Character 4	Approach Character 5	Device Character 6	Qualifier Character 7

Ø   Buttock, Right
1   Buttock, Left
5   Inguinal Region, Right
     Inguinal canal
     Inguinal triangle
6   Inguinal Region, Left
     See 5 Inguinal Region, Right
7   Femoral Region, Right
8   Femoral Region, Left
9   Lower Extremity, Right
B   Lower Extremity, Left
C   Upper Leg, Right
D   Upper Leg, Left
F   Knee Region, Right
G   Knee Region, Left
H   Lower Leg, Right
J   Lower Leg, Left
K   Ankle Region, Right
L   Ankle Region, Left
M   Foot, Right
N   Foot, Left
	Ø Open
	3 Percutaneous
	4 Percutaneous Endoscopic
		Z No Device	Z No Qualifier

NC Noncovered Procedure   LC Limited Coverage   QA Questionable OB Admit   COM New Tech Add-on   ⊞ Combination Member   ♂ Male   ♀ Female

ICD-10-PCS 2024   **703**

Ø Medical and Surgical
Y Anatomical Regions, Lower Extremities
6 Detachment   Definition: Cutting off all or a portion of the upper or lower extremities
                Explanation: The body part value is the site of the detachment, with a qualifier if applicable to further specify the level where the extremity was detached

Body Part Character 4	Approach Character 5	Device Character 6	Qualifier Character 7
2 Hindquarter, Right 3 Hindquarter, Left 4 Hindquarter, Bilateral 7 Femoral Region, Right 8 Femoral Region, Left F Knee Region, Right G Knee Region, Left	Ø Open	Z No Device	Z No Qualifier
C Upper Leg, Right D Upper Leg, Left H Lower Leg, Right J Lower Leg, Left	Ø Open	Z No Device	1 High 2 Mid 3 Low
M Foot, Right N Foot, Left	Ø Open	Z No Device	Ø Complete 4 Complete 1st Ray 5 Complete 2nd Ray 6 Complete 3rd Ray 7 Complete 4th Ray 8 Complete 5th Ray 9 Partial 1st Ray B Partial 2nd Ray C Partial 3rd Ray D Partial 4th Ray F Partial 5th Ray

P 1st Toe, Right
  Hallux
Q 1st Toe, Left
  See 1st Toe, Right
R 2nd Toe, Right
S 2nd Toe, Left
T 3rd Toe, Right
U 3rd Toe, Left
V 4th Toe, Right
W 4th Toe, Left
X 5th Toe, Right
Y 5th Toe, Left
	Ø Open	Z No Device	Ø Complete
			1 High
			2 Mid
			3 Low

Ø   **Medical and Surgical**
Y   **Anatomical Regions, Lower Extremities**
9   **Drainage**   Definition: Taking or letting out fluids and/or gases from a body part
                           Explanation: The qualifier DIAGNOSTIC is used to identify drainage procedures that are biopsies

Body Part Character 4	Approach Character 5	Device Character 6	Qualifier Character 7

Ø Buttock, Right
1 Buttock, Left
5 Inguinal Region, Right
    Inguinal canal
    Inguinal triangle
6 Inguinal Region, Left
    See 5 Inguinal Region, Right
7 Femoral Region, Right
8 Femoral Region, Left
9 Lower Extremity, Right
B Lower Extremity, Left
C Upper Leg, Right
D Upper Leg, Left
F Knee Region, Right
G Knee Region, Left
H Lower Leg, Right
J Lower Leg, Left
K Ankle Region, Right
L Ankle Region, Left
M Foot, Right
N Foot, Left
	Ø Open
	3 Percutaneous
	4 Percutaneous Endoscopic
		Ø Drainage Device	**Z** No Qualifier

Ø Buttock, Right
1 Buttock, Left
5 Inguinal Region, Right
    Inguinal canal
    Inguinal triangle
6 Inguinal Region, Left
    See 5 Inguinal Region, Right
7 Femoral Region, Right
8 Femoral Region, Left
9 Lower Extremity, Right
B Lower Extremity, Left
C Upper Leg, Right
D Upper Leg, Left
F Knee Region, Right
G Knee Region, Left
H Lower Leg, Right
J Lower Leg, Left
K Ankle Region, Right
L Ankle Region, Left
M Foot, Right
N Foot, Left
	Ø Open
	3 Percutaneous
	4 Percutaneous Endoscopic
		Z No Device	**X** Diagnostic
			Z No Qualifier

Non-OR   ØY9[Ø,1,7,8,9,B,C,D,F,G,H,J,K,L,M,N][Ø,3,4]ØZ
Non-OR   ØY9[5,6]3ØZ
Non-OR   ØY9[Ø,1,7,8,9,B,C,D,F,G,H,J,K,L,M,N][Ø,3,4]Z[X,Z]
Non-OR   ØY9[5,6]3ZZ

Anatomical Regions, Lower Extremities

Ø   **Medical and Surgical**
Y   **Anatomical Regions, Lower Extremities**
B   **Excision**   Definition: Cutting out or off, without replacement, a portion of a body part

                  Explanation: The qualifier DIAGNOSTIC is used to identify excision procedures that are biopsies

Body Part Character 4	Approach Character 5	Device Character 6	Qualifier Character 7

Ø Buttock, Right
1 Buttock, Left
5 Inguinal Region, Right
   Inguinal canal
   Inguinal triangle
6 Inguinal Region, Left
   See 5 Inguinal Region, Right
7 Femoral Region, Right
8 Femoral Region, Left
9 Lower Extremity, Right
B Lower Extremity, Left
C Upper Leg, Right
D Upper Leg, Left
F Knee Region, Right
G Knee Region, Left
H Lower Leg, Right
J Lower Leg, Left
K Ankle Region, Right
L Ankle Region, Left
M Foot, Right
N Foot, Left
	Ø Open
	3 Percutaneous
	4 Percutaneous Endoscopic
		Z No Device	X Diagnostic
			Z No Qualifier

Non-OR   ØYB[Ø,1,9,B,C,D,F,G,H,J,K,L,M,N][Ø,3,4]ZX

Ø   **Medical and Surgical**
Y   **Anatomical Regions, Lower Extremities**
H   **Insertion**   Definition: Putting in a nonbiological appliance that monitors, assists, performs, or prevents a physiological function but does not physically take the place of a body part

                  Explanation: None

Body Part Character 4	Approach Character 5	Device Character 6	Qualifier Character 7

Ø Buttock, Right
1 Buttock, Left
5 Inguinal Region, Right
   Inguinal canal
   Inguinal triangle
6 Inguinal Region, Left
   See 5 Inguinal Region, Right
7 Femoral Region, Right
8 Femoral Region, Left
9 Lower Extremity, Right
B Lower Extremity, Left
C Upper Leg, Right
D Upper Leg, Left
F Knee Region, Right
G Knee Region, Left
H Lower Leg, Right
J Lower Leg, Left
K Ankle Region, Right
L Ankle Region, Left
M Foot, Right
N Foot, Left
	Ø Open
	3 Percutaneous
	4 Percutaneous Endoscopic
		1 Radioactive Element
		3 Infusion Device
		Y Other Device
			Z No Qualifier

DRG Non-OR   ØYH[Ø,1,5,6,7,8,9,B,C,D,F,G,H,J,K,L,M,N][Ø,3,4][3,Y]Z

Non-OR Procedure   DRG Non-OR Procedure   Valid OR Procedure   HAC Associated Procedure   Combination Only   New/Revised April   New/Revised October

706   ICD-10-PCS 2024

Ø   Medical and Surgical
Y   Anatomical Regions, Lower Extremities
J   Inspection   Definition: Visually and/or manually exploring a body part

                     Explanation: Visual exploration may be performed with or without optical instrumentation. Manual exploration may be performed directly or through intervening body layers.

Body Part Character 4	Approach Character 5	Device Character 6	Qualifier Character 7
Ø Buttock, Right	**Ø** Open	**Z** No Device	**Z** No Qualifier
1 Buttock, Left	**3** Percutaneous		
5 Inguinal Region, Right	**4** Percutaneous Endoscopic		
Inguinal canal	**X** External		
Inguinal triangle			
6 Inguinal Region, Left			
See 5 Inguinal Region, Right			
7 Femoral Region, Right			
8 Femoral Region, Left			
9 Lower Extremity, Right			
A Inguinal Region, Bilateral			
See 5 Inguinal Region, Right			
B Lower Extremity, Left			
C Upper Leg, Right			
D Upper Leg, Left			
E Femoral Region, Bilateral			
F Knee Region, Right			
G Knee Region, Left			
H Lower Leg, Right			
J Lower Leg, Left			
K Ankle Region, Right			
L Ankle Region, Left			
M Foot, Right			
N Foot, Left			

DRG Non-OR	ØYJ[Ø,1,8,9,B,C,D,E,F,G,H,J,K,L,M,N]ØZZ
Non-OR	ØYJ[Ø,1,9,B,C,D,F,G,H,J,K,L,M,N][3,4,X]ZZ
Non-OR	ØYJ[5,6,7,8,A,E][3,X]ZZ

Anatomical Regions, Lower Extremities *(left margin)*

Ø **Medical and Surgical**
Y **Anatomical Regions, Lower Extremities**
M **Reattachment** Definition: Putting back in or on all or a portion of a separated body part to its normal location or other suitable location
Explanation: Vascular circulation and nervous pathways may or may not be reestablished

Body Part Character 4	Approach Character 5	Device Character 6	Qualifier Character 7
Ø Buttock, Right	Ø Open	Z No Device	Z No Qualifier
1 Buttock, Left			
2 Hindquarter, Right			
3 Hindquarter, Left			
4 Hindquarter, Bilateral			

5 Inguinal Region, Right
  Inguinal canal
  Inguinal triangle			

6 Inguinal Region, Left *See 5 Inguinal Region, Right*			
7 Femoral Region, Right			
8 Femoral Region, Left			
9 Lower Extremity, Right			
B Lower Extremity, Left			
C Upper Leg, Right			
D Upper Leg, Left			
F Knee Region, Right			
G Knee Region, Left			
H Lower Leg, Right			
J Lower Leg, Left			
K Ankle Region, Right			
L Ankle Region, Left			
M Foot, Right			
N Foot, Left			
P 1st Toe, Right Hallux			
Q 1st Toe, Left *See 1st Toe, Right*			
R 2nd Toe, Right			
S 2nd Toe, Left			
T 3rd Toe, Right			
U 3rd Toe, Left			
V 4th Toe, Right			
W 4th Toe, Left			
X 5th Toe, Right			
Y 5th Toe, Left			

Ø **Medical and Surgical**
Y **Anatomical Regions, Lower Extremities**
P **Removal** Definition: Taking out or off a device from a body part
Explanation: If a device is taken out and a similar device put in without cutting or puncturing the skin or mucous membrane, the procedure is coded to the root operation CHANGE. Otherwise, the procedure for taking out the device is coded to the root operation REMOVAL.

Body Part Character 4	Approach Character 5	Device Character 6	Qualifier Character 7
9 Lower Extremity, Right	Ø Open	Ø Drainage Device	Z No Qualifier
B Lower Extremity, Left	3 Percutaneous	1 Radioactive Element	
	4 Percutaneous Endoscopic	3 Infusion Device	
	X External	7 Autologous Tissue Substitute	
		J Synthetic Substitute	
		K Nonautologous Tissue Substitute	
		Y Other Device	

Non-OR All body part, approach, device, and qualifier values

Ø   **Medical and Surgical**
Y   **Anatomical Regions, Lower Extremities**
Q   **Repair**   Definition: Restoring, to the extent possible, a body part to its normal anatomic structure and function

                             Explanation: Used only when the method to accomplish the repair is not one of the other root operations

Body Part Character 4	Approach Character 5	Device Character 6	Qualifier Character 7
Ø Buttock, Right	**Ø** Open	**Z** No Device	**Z** No Qualifier
1 Buttock, Left	**3** Percutaneous		
5 Inguinal Region, Right	**4** Percutaneous Endoscopic		
Inguinal canal	**X** External		
Inguinal triangle			
6 Inguinal Region, Left			
See 5 Inguinal Region, Right			
7 Femoral Region, Right			
8 Femoral Region, Left			
9 Lower Extremity, Right			
A Inguinal Region, Bilateral			
See 5 Inguinal Region, Right			
B Lower Extremity, Left			
C Upper Leg, Right			
D Upper Leg, Left			
E Femoral Region, Bilateral			
F Knee Region, Right			
G Knee Region, Left			
H Lower Leg, Right			
J Lower Leg, Left			
K Ankle Region, Right			
L Ankle Region, Left			
M Foot, Right			
N Foot, Left			
P 1st Toe, Right			
Hallux			
Q 1st Toe, Left			
See 1st Toe, Right			
R 2nd Toe, Right			
S 2nd Toe, Left			
T 3rd Toe, Right			
U 3rd Toe, Left			
V 4th Toe, Right			
W 4th Toe, Left			
X 5th Toe, Right			
Y 5th Toe, Left			

Non-OR   ØYQ[5,6,7,8,A,E]XZZ

NC Noncovered Procedure   **LC** Limited Coverage   **QA** Questionable OB Admit   **COM** New Tech Add-on   ⊞ Combination Member   ♂ Male   ♀ Female

ICD-10-PCS 2024   **709**

Ø   Medical and Surgical
Y   Anatomical Regions, Lower Extremities
U   Supplement   Definition: Putting in or on biological or synthetic material that physically reinforces and/or augments the function of a portion of a body part
                    Explanation: The biological material is non-living, or is living and from the same individual. The body part may have been previously replaced, and the SUPPLEMENT procedure is performed to physically reinforce and/or augment the function of the replaced body part.

Body Part Character 4	Approach Character 5	Device Character 6	Qualifier Character 7

Ø   Buttock, Right
1   Buttock, Left
5   Inguinal Region, Right
     Inguinal canal
     Inguinal triangle
6   Inguinal Region, Left
     See 5 Inguinal Region, Right
7   Femoral Region, Right
8   Femoral Region, Left
9   Lower Extremity, Right
A   Inguinal Region, Bilateral
     See 5 Inguinal Region, Right
B   Lower Extremity, Left
C   Upper Leg, Right
D   Upper Leg, Left
E   Femoral Region, Bilateral
F   Knee Region, Right
G   Knee Region, Left
H   Lower Leg, Right
J   Lower Leg, Left
K   Ankle Region, Right
L   Ankle Region, Left
M   Foot, Right
N   Foot, Left
P   1st Toe, Right
     Hallux
Q   1st Toe, Left
     See 1st Toe, Right
R   2nd Toe, Right
S   2nd Toe, Left
T   3rd Toe, Right
U   3rd Toe, Left
V   4th Toe, Right
W   4th Toe, Left
X   5th Toe, Right
Y   5th Toe, Left
	Ø Open
	4 Percutaneous Endoscopic
		7 Autologous Tissue Substitute
		J Synthetic Substitute
		K Nonautologous Tissue Substitute
			Z No Qualifier

Ø   Medical and Surgical
Y   Anatomical Regions, Lower Extremities
W   Revision   Definition: Correcting, to the extent possible, a portion of a malfunctioning device or the position of a displaced device
                Explanation: Revision can include correcting a malfunctioning or displaced device by taking out or putting in components of the device such as a screw or pin

Body Part Character 4	Approach Character 5	Device Character 6	Qualifier Character 7
9 Lower Extremity, Right B Lower Extremity, Left	Ø Open 3 Percutaneous 4 Percutaneous Endoscopic X External	Ø Drainage Device 3 Infusion Device 7 Autologous Tissue Substitute J Synthetic Substitute K Nonautologous Tissue Substitute Y Other Device	Z No Qualifier

DRG Non-OR   ØYW[9,B][Ø,3,4][Ø,3,7,J,K,Y]Z
Non-OR   ØYW[9,B]X[Ø,3,7,J,K,Y]Z

Obstetrics 1Ø2–1ØY

Character Meanings

This Character Meaning table is provided as a guide to assist the user in the identification of character members that may be found in this section of code tables. It **SHOULD NOT** be used to build a PCS code.

Ø: Pregnancy

Operation–Character 3		Body Part–Character 4		Approach–Character 5		Device–Character 6		Qualifier–Character 7	
2	Change	Ø	Products of Conception	Ø	Open	3	Monitoring Electrode	Ø	High
9	Drainage	1	Products of Conception, Retained	3	Percutaneous	Y	Other Device	1	Low
A	Abortion	2	Products of Conception, Ectopic	4	Percutaneous Endoscopic	Z	No Device	2	Extraperitoneal
D	Extraction			7	Via Natural or Artificial Opening			3	Low Forceps
E	Delivery			8	Via Natural or Artificial Opening Endoscopic			4	Mid Forceps
H	Insertion			X	External			5	High Forceps
J	Inspection							6	Vacuum
P	Removal							7	Internal Version
Q	Repair							8	Other
S	Reposition							9	Fetal Blood OR Manual
T	Resection							A	Fetal Cerebrospinal Fluid
Y	Transplantation							B	Fetal Fluid, Other
								C	Amniotic Fluid, Therapeutic
								D	Fluid, Other
								E	Nervous System
								F	Cardiovascular System
								G	Lymphatics & Hemic
								H	Eye
								J	Ear, Nose & Sinus
								K	Respiratory System
								L	Mouth & Throat
								M	Gastrointestinal System
								N	Hepatobiliary & Pancreas
								P	Endocrine System
								Q	Skin
								R	Musculoskeletal System
								S	Urinary System
								T	Female Reproductive System
								U	Amniotic Fluid, Diagnostic
								V	Male Reproductive System
								W	Laminaria
								X	Abortifacient
								Y	Other Body System
								Z	No Qualifier

AHA Coding Clinic for table 1Ø9

| 2014, 3Q, 12 | Fetoscopic laser photocoagulation and laser microseptostomy for twin-twin transfusion syndrome |
| 2014, 2Q, 9 | Pitocin administration to augment labor |

AHA Coding Clinic for table 1ØA

| 2022, 1Q, 21 | Gravid hysterectomy due to placenta increta |
| 2022, 1Q, 41 | Intrauterine Cook balloon placement for ectopic pregnancy |

AHA Coding Clinic for table 1ØD

2022, 1Q, 19	Spontaneous abortion with retained placenta of Twin B
2021, 1Q, 52	Removal of ectopic pregnancy via laparotomy
2020, 4Q, 59-60	Extraction of ectopic products of conception
2018, 4Q, 49-51	Revised qualifier values for root operation "extraction" (cesarean delivery)
2018, 2Q, 17	High transverse cesarean section
2016, 1Q, 9	Vaginal delivery assisted by vacuum and low forceps extraction
2014, 4Q, 43	Cesarean delivery assisted by vacuum extraction
2014, 4Q, 43	Vacuum dilation and curettage for blighted ovum

AHA Coding Clinic for table 1ØE

2017, 3Q, 5	Delivery of placenta
2016, 2Q, 34	Assisted vaginal delivery
2014, 4Q, 17	RH (D) alloimmunization (sensitization)
2014, 2Q, 9	Pitocin administration to augment labor

AHA Coding Clinic for table 1ØH

| 2013, 2Q, 36 | Intrauterine pressure monitor |

AHA Coding Clinic for table 1ØQ

| 2021, 2Q, 21 | Ex Utero intrapartum treatment procedure |
| 2014, 3Q, 12 | Fetoscopic laser photocoagulation and laser microseptostomy for twin-twin transfusion syndrome |

AHA Coding Clinic for table 1ØT

| 2020, 3Q, 47 | Removal of ectopic cornual pregnancy |
| 2015, 3Q, 31 | Laparoscopic partial salpingectomy for ectopic pregnancy |

1   Obstetrics
Ø   Pregnancy
2   Change   Definition: Taking out or off a device from a body part and putting back an identical or similar device in or on the same body part without cutting or puncturing the skin or a mucous membrane
Explanation: None

Body Part Character 4		Approach Character 5	Device Character 6	Qualifier Character 7
Ø Products of Conception ♀	7	Via Natural or Artificial Opening	3 Monitoring Electrode Y Other Device	Z No Qualifier

Non-OR   All body part, approach, device, and qualifier values
♀   All body part, approach, device, and qualifier values

1   Obstetrics
Ø   Pregnancy
9   Drainage   Definition: Taking or letting out fluids and/or gases from a body part
Explanation: None

Body Part Character 4		Approach Character 5	Device Character 6	Qualifier Character 7
Ø Products of Conception ♀	Ø 3 4 7 8	Open Percutaneous Percutaneous Endoscopic Via Natural or Artificial Opening Via Natural or Artificial Opening Endoscopic	Z No Device	9 Fetal Blood A Fetal Cerebrospinal Fluid B Fetal Fluid, Other C Amniotic Fluid, Therapeutic D Fluid, Other U Amniotic Fluid, Diagnostic

Non-OR   All body part, approach, device, and qualifier values
♀   All body part, approach, device, and qualifier values

1   Obstetrics
Ø   Pregnancy
A   Abortion   Definition: Artificially terminating a pregnancy
Explanation: None

Body Part Character 4		Approach Character 5	Device Character 6	Qualifier Character 7
Ø Products of Conception ♀	Ø 3 4 8	Open Percutaneous Percutaneous Endoscopic Via Natural or Artificial Opening Endoscopic	Z No Device	Z No Qualifier
Ø Products of Conception ♀	7	Via Natural or Artificial Opening	Z No Device	6 Vacuum W Laminaria X Abortifacient Z No Qualifier

Non-OR   1ØA07Z[6,W,X]
♀   All body part, approach, device, and qualifier values

1   Obstetrics
Ø   Pregnancy
D   Extraction   Definition: Pulling or stripping out or off all or a portion of a body part by the use of force
Explanation: None

Body Part Character 4		Approach Character 5	Device Character 6	Qualifier Character 7
Ø Products of Conception QA ♀	Ø	Open	Z No Device	Ø High 1 Low 2 Extraperitoneal
Ø Products of Conception QA ♀	7	Via Natural or Artificial Opening	Z No Device	3 Low Forceps 4 Mid Forceps 5 High Forceps 6 Vacuum 7 Internal Version 8 Other
1 Products of Conception, Retained ♀	7 8	Via Natural or Artificial Opening Via Natural or Artificial Opening Endoscopic	Z No Device	9 Manual Z No Qualifier
2 Products of Conception, Ectopic ♀	Ø 4 7 8	Open Percutaneous Endoscopic Via Natural or Artificial Opening Via Natural or Artificial Opening Endoscopic	Z No Device	Z No Qualifier

DRG Non-OR   1ØDØ7Z[3,4,5,6,7,8]
QA   1ØDØØZ[Ø,1,2] except when a corresponding SDX of Z37.Ø-Z37.9 is also reported
QA   1ØDØ7Z[3,4,5,7] except when a corresponding SDX of Z37.Ø-Z37.9 is also reported
♀   All body part, approach, device, and qualifier values

Non-OR Procedure   DRG Non-OR Procedure   Valid OR Procedure   HAC Associated Procedure   Combination Only   New/Revised April   New/Revised October

712   ICD-10-PCS 2024

1Ø2–1ØD

1   Obstetrics
Ø   Pregnancy
E   Delivery   Definition: Assisting the passage of the products of conception from the genital canal

          Explanation: None

Body Part Character 4	Approach Character 5	Device Character 6	Qualifier Character 7
Ø Products of Conception **QA** ♀	X External	Z No Device	Z No Qualifier

DRG Non-OR   10EØXZZ
QA   10EØXZZ except when a corresponding SDX of Z37.Ø-Z37.9 is also reported
♀   All body part, approach, device, and qualifier values

1   Obstetrics
Ø   Pregnancy
H   Insertion   Definition: Putting in a nonbiological appliance that monitors, assists, performs, or prevents a physiological function but does not physically take the place of a body part

          Explanation: None

Body Part Character 4	Approach Character 5	Device Character 6	Qualifier Character 7
Ø Products of Conception ♀	Ø Open 7 Via Natural or Artificial Opening	3 Monitoring Electrode Y Other Device	Z No Qualifier

Non-OR   All body part, approach, device, and qualifier values
♀   All body part, approach, device, and qualifier values

1   Obstetrics
Ø   Pregnancy
J   Inspection   Definition: Visually and/or manually exploring a body part

          Explanation: Visual exploration may be performed with or without optical instrumentation. Manual exploration may be performed directly or through intervening body layers.

Body Part Character 4	Approach Character 5	Device Character 6	Qualifier Character 7

Ø   Products of Conception   ♀
1   Products of Conception,
     Retained   ♀
2   Products of Conception, Ectopic   ♀
	Ø Open
	3 Percutaneous
	4 Percutaneous Endoscopic
	7 Via Natural or Artificial Opening
	8 Via Natural or Artificial Opening
	     Endoscopic
	X External
		Z No Device	Z No Qualifier

Non-OR   All body part, approach, device, and qualifier values
♀   All body part, approach, device, and qualifier values

1   Obstetrics
Ø   Pregnancy
P   Removal   Definition: Taking out or off a device from a body part, region or orifice

          Explanation: If a device is taken out and a similar device put in without cutting or puncturing the skin or mucous membrane, the procedure is coded to the root operation CHANGE. Otherwise, the procedure for taking out a device is coded to the root operation REMOVAL.

Body Part Character 4	Approach Character 5	Device Character 6	Qualifier Character 7
Ø Products of Conception ♀	Ø Open 7 Via Natural or Artificial Opening	3 Monitoring Electrode Y Other Device	Z No Qualifier

Non-OR   All body part, approach, device, and qualifier values
♀   All body part, approach, device, and qualifier values

1   Obstetrics
Ø   Pregnancy
Q   Repair   Definition: Restoring, to the extent possible, a body part to its normal anatomic structure and function

          Explanation: Used only when the method to accomplish the repair is not one of the other root operations

Body Part Character 4	Approach Character 5	Device Character 6	Qualifier Character 7
Ø Products of Conception ♀	Ø Open 3 Percutaneous 4 Percutaneous Endoscopic 7 Via Natural or Artificial Opening 8 Via Natural or Artificial Opening Endoscopic	Y Other Device Z No Device	E Nervous System F Cardiovascular System G Lymphatics and Hemic H Eye J Ear, Nose and Sinus K Respiratory System L Mouth and Throat M Gastrointestinal System N Hepatobiliary and Pancreas P Endocrine System Q Skin R Musculoskeletal System S Urinary System T Female Reproductive System V Male Reproductive System Y Other Body System

Non-OR   All body part, approach, device, and qualifier values
♀   All body part, approach, device, and qualifier values

NC Noncovered Procedure   **LC** Limited Coverage   **QA** Questionable OB Admit   **NT** New Tech Add-on   ✚ Combination Member   ♂ Male   ♀ Female

1   Obstetrics
0   Pregnancy
S   Reposition

Definition: Moving to its normal location, or other suitable location, all or a portion of a body part

Explanation: The body part is moved to a new location from an abnormal location, or from a normal location where it is not functioning correctly. The body part may or may not be cut out or off to be moved to the new location.

Body Part Character 4	Approach Character 5	Device Character 6	Qualifier Character 7
0 Products of Conception ♀	7 Via Natural or Artificial Opening X External	Z No Device	Z No Qualifier
2 Products of Conception, Ectopic ♀	0 Open 3 Percutaneous 4 Percutaneous Endoscopic 7 Via Natural or Artificial Opening 8 Via Natural or Artificial Opening Endoscopic	Z No Device	Z No Qualifier

Non-OR   10S0[7,X]ZZ
♀   All body part, approach, device, and qualifier values

---

1   Obstetrics
0   Pregnancy
T   Resection

Definition: Cutting out or off, without replacement, all of a body part

Explanation: None

Body Part Character 4	Approach Character 5	Device Character 6	Qualifier Character 7
2 Products of Conception, Ectopic ♀	0 Open 3 Percutaneous 4 Percutaneous Endoscopic 7 Via Natural or Artificial Opening 8 Via Natural or Artificial Opening Endoscopic	Z No Device	Z No Qualifier

♀   All body part, approach, device, and qualifier values

---

1   Obstetrics
0   Pregnancy
Y   Transplantation

Definition: Putting in or on all or a portion of a living body part taken from another individual or animal to physically take the place and/or function of all or a portion of a similar body part

Explanation: The native body part may or may not be taken out, and the transplanted body part may take over all or a portion of its function

Body Part Character 4	Approach Character 5	Device Character 6	Qualifier Character 7
0 Products of Conception ♀	3 Percutaneous 4 Percutaneous Endoscopic 7 Via Natural or Artificial Opening	Z No Device	E Nervous System F Cardiovascular System G Lymphatics and Hemic H Eye J Ear, Nose and Sinus K Respiratory System L Mouth and Throat M Gastrointestinal System N Hepatobiliary and Pancreas P Endocrine System Q Skin R Musculoskeletal System S Urinary System T Female Reproductive System V Male Reproductive System Y Other Body System

Non-OR   All body part, approach, device, and qualifier values
♀   All body part, approach, device, and qualifier values

Non-OR Procedure   DRG Non-OR Procedure   Valid OR Procedure   HAC Associated Procedure   Combination Only   New/Revised April   New/Revised October

Placement 2WØ–2Y5

AHA Coding Clinic for table 2W6

2015, 2Q, 35   Application of tongs to reduce and stabilize cervical fracture
2013, 2Q, 39   Application of cervical tongs for reduction of cervical fracture

AHA Coding Clinic for table 2Y4

2018, 4Q, 38   Control of epistaxis
2017, 4Q, 106   Nasal packing for epistaxis

2   Placement
W   Anatomical Regions
Ø   Change   Definition: Taking out or off a device from a body part and putting back an identical or similar device in or on the same body part without cutting or puncturing the skin or a mucous membrane

Body Region Character 4	Approach Character 5	Device Character 6	Qualifier Character 7
Ø Head 2 Neck 3 Abdominal Wall 4 Chest Wall 5 Back 6 Inguinal Region, Right 7 Inguinal Region, Left 8 Upper Extremity, Right 9 Upper Extremity, Left A Upper Arm, Right B Upper Arm, Left C Lower Arm, Right D Lower Arm, Left E Hand, Right F Hand, Left G Thumb, Right H Thumb, Left J Finger, Right K Finger, Left L Lower Extremity, Right M Lower Extremity, Left N Upper Leg, Right P Upper Leg, Left Q Lower Leg, Right R Lower Leg, Left S Foot, Right T Foot, Left U Toe, Right V Toe, Left	X External	Ø Traction Apparatus 1 Splint 2 Cast 3 Brace 4 Bandage 5 Packing Material 6 Pressure Dressing 7 Intermittent Pressure Device Y Other Device	Z No Qualifier
1 Face	X External	Ø Traction Apparatus 1 Splint 2 Cast 3 Brace 4 Bandage 5 Packing Material 6 Pressure Dressing 7 Intermittent Pressure Device 9 Wire Y Other Device	Z No Qualifier

NC Noncovered Procedure   **LC** Limited Coverage   **QA** Questionable OB Admit   **NT** New Tech Add-on   ⊞ Combination Member   ♂ Male   ♀ Female

ICD-10-PCS 2024   715

2　**Placement**
W　**Anatomical Regions**
1　**Compression**　　Definition: Putting pressure on a body region

Body Region Character 4	Approach Character 5	Device Character 6	Qualifier Character 7
Ø Head 1 Face 2 Neck 3 Abdominal Wall 4 Chest Wall 5 Back 6 Inguinal Region, Right 7 Inguinal Region, Left 8 Upper Extremity, Right 9 Upper Extremity, Left A Upper Arm, Right B Upper Arm, Left C Lower Arm, Right D Lower Arm, Left E Hand, Right F Hand, Left G Thumb, Right H Thumb, Left J Finger, Right K Finger, Left L Lower Extremity, Right M Lower Extremity, Left N Upper Leg, Right P Upper Leg, Left Q Lower Leg, Right R Lower Leg, Left S Foot, Right T Foot, Left U Toe, Right V Toe, Left	X External	6 Pressure Dressing 7 Intermittent Pressure Device	Z No Qualifier

2　**Placement**
W　**Anatomical Regions**
2　**Dressing**　　Definition: Putting material on a body region for protection

Body Region Character 4	Approach Character 5	Device Character 6	Qualifier Character 7
Ø Head 1 Face 2 Neck 3 Abdominal Wall 4 Chest Wall 5 Back 6 Inguinal Region, Right 7 Inguinal Region, Left 8 Upper Extremity, Right 9 Upper Extremity, Left A Upper Arm, Right B Upper Arm, Left C Lower Arm, Right D Lower Arm, Left E Hand, Right F Hand, Left G Thumb, Right H Thumb, Left J Finger, Right K Finger, Left L Lower Extremity, Right M Lower Extremity, Left N Upper Leg, Right P Upper Leg, Left Q Lower Leg, Right R Lower Leg, Left S Foot, Right T Foot, Left U Toe, Right V Toe, Left	X External	4 Bandage	Z No Qualifier

Non-OR Procedure　　DRG Non-OR Procedure　　Valid OR Procedure　　HAC Associated Procedure　　Combination Only　　New/Revised April　　New/Revised October

716　　　　　　　　　　　　　　　　　　　　　　　　　　　　　　　　　　　　　ICD-10-PCS 2024

2   Placement
W   Anatomical Regions
3   Immobilization   Definition: Limiting or preventing motion of a body region

Body Region Character 4	Approach Character 5	Device Character 6	Qualifier Character 7
Ø Head **2** Neck **3** Abdominal Wall **4** Chest Wall **5** Back **6** Inguinal Region, Right **7** Inguinal Region, Left **8** Upper Extremity, Right **9** Upper Extremity, Left **A** Upper Arm, Right **B** Upper Arm, Left **C** Lower Arm, Right **D** Lower Arm, Left **E** Hand, Right **F** Hand, Left **G** Thumb, Right **H** Thumb, Left **J** Finger, Right **K** Finger, Left **L** Lower Extremity, Right **M** Lower Extremity, Left **N** Upper Leg, Right **P** Upper Leg, Left **Q** Lower Leg, Right **R** Lower Leg, Left **S** Foot, Right **T** Foot, Left **U** Toe, Right **V** Toe, Left	**X** External	**1** Splint **2** Cast **3** Brace **Y** Other Device	**Z** No Qualifier
1 Face	**X** External	**1** Splint **2** Cast **3** Brace **9** Wire **Y** Other Device	**Z** No Qualifier

2   Placement
W   Anatomical Regions
4   Packing   Definition: Putting material in a body region or orifice

Body Region Character 4	Approach Character 5	Device Character 6	Qualifier Character 7
Ø Head **1** Face **2** Neck **3** Abdominal Wall **4** Chest Wall **5** Back **6** Inguinal Region, Right **7** Inguinal Region, Left **8** Upper Extremity, Right **9** Upper Extremity, Left **A** Upper Arm, Right **B** Upper Arm, Left **C** Lower Arm, Right **D** Lower Arm, Left **E** Hand, Right **F** Hand, Left **G** Thumb, Right **H** Thumb, Left **J** Finger, Right **K** Finger, Left **L** Lower Extremity, Right **M** Lower Extremity, Left **N** Upper Leg, Right **P** Upper Leg, Left **Q** Lower Leg, Right **R** Lower Leg, Left **S** Foot, Right **T** Foot, Left **U** Toe, Right **V** Toe, Left	**X** External	**5** Packing Material	**Z** No Qualifier

NC Noncovered Procedure   **LC** Limited Coverage   **QA** Questionable OB Admit   **NT** New Tech Add-on   ⊞ Combination Member   ♂ Male   ♀ Female

ICD-10-PCS 2024   717

2W3–2W4

Placement

2   **Placement**
W   **Anatomical Regions**
5   **Removal**   Definition: Taking out or off a device from a body part

Body Region Character 4	Approach Character 5	Device Character 6	Qualifier Character 7
Ø Head 2 Neck 3 Abdominal Wall 4 Chest Wall 5 Back 6 Inguinal Region, Right 7 Inguinal Region, Left 8 Upper Extremity, Right 9 Upper Extremity, Left A Upper Arm, Right B Upper Arm, Left C Lower Arm, Right D Lower Arm, Left E Hand, Right F Hand, Left G Thumb, Right H Thumb, Left J Finger, Right K Finger, Left L Lower Extremity, Right M Lower Extremity, Left N Upper Leg, Right P Upper Leg, Left Q Lower Leg, Right R Lower Leg, Left S Foot, Right T Foot, Left U Toe, Right V Toe, Left	X External	Ø Traction Apparatus 1 Splint 2 Cast 3 Brace 4 Bandage 5 Packing Material 6 Pressure Dressing 7 Intermittent Pressure Device Y Other Device	Z No Qualifier
1 Face	X External	Ø Traction Apparatus 1 Splint 2 Cast 3 Brace 4 Bandage 5 Packing Material 6 Pressure Dressing 7 Intermittent Pressure Device 9 Wire Y Other Device	Z No Qualifier

Non-OR Procedure   DRG Non-OR Procedure   Valid OR Procedure   HAC Associated Procedure   Combination Only   New/Revised April   New/Revised October

718   ICD-10-PCS 2024

2   **Placement**
W   **Anatomical Regions**
6   **Traction**   Definition: Exerting a pulling force on a body region in a distal direction

Body Region Character 4	Approach Character 5	Device Character 6	Qualifier Character 7
Ø Head 1 Face 2 Neck 3 Abdominal Wall 4 Chest Wall 5 Back 6 Inguinal Region, Right 7 Inguinal Region, Left 8 Upper Extremity, Right 9 Upper Extremity, Left A Upper Arm, Right B Upper Arm, Left C Lower Arm, Right D Lower Arm, Left E Hand, Right F Hand, Left G Thumb, Right H Thumb, Left J Finger, Right K Finger, Left L Lower Extremity, Right M Lower Extremity, Left N Upper Leg, Right P Upper Leg, Left Q Lower Leg, Right R Lower Leg, Left S Foot, Right T Foot, Left U Toe, Right V Toe, Left	X External	Ø Traction Apparatus Z No Device	Z No Qualifier

2   **Placement**
Y   **Anatomical Orifices**
Ø   **Change**   Definition: Taking out or off a device from a body part and putting back an identical or similar device in or on the same body part without cutting or puncturing the skin or a mucous membrane

Body Region Character 4	Approach Character 5	Device Character 6	Qualifier Character 7
Ø Mouth and Pharynx 1 Nasal 2 Ear 3 Anorectal 4 Female Genital Tract ♀ 5 Urethra	X External	5 Packing Material	Z No Qualifier

♀   2YØ4X5Z

2   **Placement**
Y   **Anatomical Orifices**
4   **Packing**   Definition: Putting material in a body region or orifice

Body Region Character 4	Approach Character 5	Device Character 6	Qualifier Character 7
Ø Mouth and Pharynx 1 Nasal 2 Ear 3 Anorectal 4 Female Genital Tract ♀ 5 Urethra	X External	5 Packing Material	Z No Qualifier

♀   2Y44X5Z

2   **Placement**
Y   **Anatomical Orifices**
5   **Removal**   Definition: Taking out or off a device from a body part

Body Region Character 4	Approach Character 5	Device Character 6	Qualifier Character 7
Ø Mouth and Pharynx 1 Nasal 2 Ear 3 Anorectal 4 Female Genital Tract ♀ 5 Urethra	X External	5 Packing Material	Z No Qualifier

♀   2Y54X5Z

NC Noncovered Procedure   LC Limited Coverage   QA Questionable OB Admit   NT New Tech Add-on   ⊞ Combination Member   ♂ Male   ♀ Female

ICD-10-PCS 2024   **719**

2W6–2Y5

Administration 3Ø2–3E1

AHA Coding Clinic for table 3Ø2

2023, 1Q, 10-11	Intraosseous administration of blood products
2021, 4Q, 54	Nonautologous pathogen reduced cryoprecipitated fibrinogen complex
2020, 4Q, 60-61	Transfusion stem cell progenitor cells
2019, 4Q, 35	Transfusion of blood products
2019, 4Q, 36	T-cell depleted hematopoietic stem cells for transplantation
2016, 4Q, 113	Bone marrow and stem cell transfusion (Transplantation)

AHA Coding Clinic for table 3EØ

2023, 2Q, 33	Testing of premature rupture of membranes via indigo carmine injection
2022, 4Q, 60-61	Introduction of other therapeutic monoclonal antibody
2022, 4Q, 61	Introduction of bone-substitute material
2022, 3Q, 26	Tumor-infiltrating lymphocyte therapy
2022, 1Q, 8	Other monoclonal antibody
2021, 4Q, 54-55	Antineoplastic monoclonal antibody
2021, 4Q, 110	New/revised frequently asked questions regarding ICD-10-CM/PCS coding for COVID-19
2021, 1Q, 49	Frequently asked questions regarding ICD-10-CM and ICD-10-PCS coding for COVID-19
2020, 4Q, 49-50	Intravascular ultrasound assisted thrombolysis
2020, 4Q, 95	Frequently asked questions regarding ICD-10-PCS coding for COVID-19
2020, 3Q, 17-21	New procedure codes for introduction or infusion of therapeutics
2019, 4Q, 36-37	Hyperthermic antineoplastic chemotherapy
2018, 3Q, 7	Coronary brachytherapy with angioplasty
2018, 1Q, 8	Placement of bone morphogenetic protein & spinal fusion surgery
2017, 2Q, 14	Infusion of tPA into pleural cavity
2017, 1Q, 37	Injection of glue into enteric fistula tract
2016, 4Q, 113-114	Substances applied to cranial cavity and brain
2016, 3Q, 29	Closure of bilateral alveolar clefts
2016, 1Q, 20	Metatarsophalangeal joint resection arthroplasty

AHA Coding Clinic for table 3EØ (Continued)

2015, 3Q, 24	Esophagogastroduodenoscopy with epinephrine injection for control of bleeding
2015, 3Q, 29	Placement of adhesion barrier
2015, 2Q, 29	Insertion of nasogastric tube for drainage and feeding
2015, 2Q, 31	Thoracoscopic talc pleurodesis
2015, 1Q, 31	Intrathecal chemotherapy
2015, 1Q, 38	Chemoembolization of the hepatic artery
2014, 4Q, 16	Administration of RH (D) immunoglobulin
2014, 4Q, 17	RH (D) alloimmunization (sensitization)
2014, 4Q, 19	Ultrasound accelerated thrombolysis
2014, 4Q, 34	Resection of brain malignancy with implantation of chemotherapeutic wafer
2014, 4Q, 38	Placement of saline and Seprafilm solution into abdominal cavity
2014, 3Q, 26	Coil embolization of·gastroduodenal artery with chemoembolization of hepatic artery
2014, 2Q, 8	Medical induction of labor with Cervidil tampon insertion
2014, 2Q, 10	Prophylactic Neulasta injection for infection prevention
2013, 4Q, 124	Administration of tPA for stroke treatment prior to transfer
2013, 1Q, 27	Injection of sclerosing agent into an esophageal varix

AHA Coding Clinic for table 3E1

2021, 4Q, 55	Laparoscopic irrigation of peritoneal cavity
2019, 4Q, 38	Irrigation of joint using irrigating substance
2017, 3Q, 14	Bronchoscopy with suctioning and washings for removal of mucus plug

NC Noncovered Procedure   LC Limited Coverage   QA Questionable OB Admit   NT New Tech Add-on   ✚ Combination Member   ♂ Male   ♀ Female

ICD-10-PCS 2024   721

3   Administration
0   Circulatory
2   Transfusion   Definition: Putting in blood or blood products

Body System/Region Character 4		Approach Character 5	Substance Character 6	Qualifier Character 7
3 Peripheral Vein NC 4 Central Vein NC		3 Percutaneous	A Stem Cells, Embryonic	Z No Qualifier
3 Peripheral Vein 4 Central Vein		3 Percutaneous	C Hematopoietic Stem/Progenitor Cells, Genetically Modified	0 Autologous

3   Peripheral Vein
4   Central Vein
		3 Percutaneous	D Pathogen Reduced NT
			    Cryoprecipitated Fibrinogen
			    Complex
				1 Nonautologous

3 Peripheral Vein NC 4 Central Vein NC		3 Percutaneous	G Bone Marrow X Stem Cells, Cord Blood Y Stem Cells, Hematopoietic	0 Autologous 2 Allogeneic, Related 3 Allogeneic, Unrelated 4 Allogeneic, Unspecified
3 Peripheral Vein 4 Central Vein		3 Percutaneous	H Whole Blood J Serum Albumin K Frozen Plasma L Fresh Plasma M Plasma Cryoprecipitate N Red Blood Cells P Frozen Red Cells Q White Cells R Platelets S Globulin T Fibrinogen V Antihemophilic Factors W Factor IX	0 Autologous 1 Nonautologous
3 Peripheral Vein 4 Central Vein		3 Percutaneous	U Stem Cells, T-cell Depleted Hematopoietic	2 Allogeneic, Related 3 Allogeneic, Unrelated 4 Allogeneic, Unspecified
7 Products of Conception, ♀ Circulatory		3 Percutaneous 7 Via Natural or Artificial Opening	H Whole Blood J Serum Albumin K Frozen Plasma L Fresh Plasma M Plasma Cryoprecipitate N Red Blood Cells P Frozen Red Cells Q White Cells R Platelets S Globulin T Fibrinogen V Antihemophilic Factors W Factor IX	1 Nonautologous
8 Vein		3 Percutaneous	B 4-Factor Prothrombin Complex Concentrate	1 Nonautologous
A Bone Marrow		3 Percutaneous	H Whole Blood J Serum Albumin K Frozen Plasma L Fresh Plasma N Red Blood Cells P Frozen Red Cells R Platelets	0 Autologous 1 Nonautologous

DRG Non-OR	302[3,4]3AZ
DRG Non-OR	302[3,4]3C0
DRG Non-OR	302[3,4]3[G,X,Y][0,2,3,4]
DRG Non-OR	302[3,4]3U[2,3,4]

NC   302[3,4]3AZ Only when reported with PDx or SDx of C91.00, C92.00, C92.10, C92.11, C92.40, C92.50, C92.60, C92.A0, C93.00, C94.00, C95.00

NC   302[3,4]3[G,Y]0 Only when reported with PDx or SDx of C91.00, C92.00, C92.10, C92.11, C92.40, C92.50, C92.60, C92.A0, C93.00, C94.00, C95.00

NT   302[3,4]3D1 for Intercept® (PRCFC) in combination with dx code D62, D65, D68.2, D68.4, or D68.9

♀   3027[3,7][H,J,K,L,M,N,P,Q,R,S,T,V,W]1

3   Administration
C   Indwelling Device
1   Irrigation   Definition: Putting in or on a cleansing substance

Body System/Region Character 4	Approach Character 5	Substance Character 6	Qualifier Character 7
Z None	X External	8 Irrigating Substance	Z No Qualifier

Non-OR Procedure   DRG Non-OR Procedure   Valid OR Procedure   HAC Associated Procedure   Combination Only   New/Revised April   New/Revised October

722   ICD-10-PCS 2024

302–3C1

3   Administration
E   Physiological Systems and Anatomical Regions
0   Introduction   Definition: Putting in or on a therapeutic, diagnostic, nutritional, physiological, or prophylactic substance except blood or blood products

Body System/Region Character 4	Approach Character 5	Substance Character 6	Qualifier Character 7
0 Skin and Mucous Membranes	X External	0 Antineoplastic	5 Other Antineoplastic M Monoclonal Antibody
0 Skin and Mucous Membranes	X External	2 Anti-infective	8 Oxazolidinones 9 Other Anti-infective
0 Skin and Mucous Membranes	X External	3 Anti-inflammatory 4 Serum, Toxoid and Vaccine B Anesthetic Agent K Other Diagnostic Substance M Pigment N Analgesics, Hypnotics, Sedatives T Destructive Agent	Z No Qualifier
0 Skin and Mucous Membranes	X External	G Other Therapeutic Substance	C Other Substance
1 Subcutaneous Tissue	0 Open	2 Anti-infective	A Anti-Infective Envelope
1 Subcutaneous Tissue	3 Percutaneous	0 Antineoplastic	5 Other Antineoplastic M Monoclonal Antibody
1 Subcutaneous Tissue	3 Percutaneous	2 Anti-infective	8 Oxazolidinones 9 Other Anti-infective A Anti-Infective Envelope
1 Subcutaneous Tissue	3 Percutaneous	3 Anti-inflammatory 6 Nutritional Substance 7 Electrolytic and Water Balance Substance B Anesthetic Agent H Radioactive Substance K Other Diagnostic Substance N Analgesics, Hypnotics, Sedatives T Destructive Agent	Z No Qualifier
1 Subcutaneous Tissue	3 Percutaneous	4 Serum, Toxoid and Vaccine	0 Influenza Vaccine Z No Qualifier
1 Subcutaneous Tissue	3 Percutaneous	G Other Therapeutic Substance	C Other Substance
1 Subcutaneous Tissue	3 Percutaneous	V Hormone	G Insulin J Other Hormone
2 Muscle	3 Percutaneous	0 Antineoplastic	5 Other Antineoplastic M Monoclonal Antibody
2 Muscle	3 Percutaneous	2 Anti-infective	8 Oxazolidinones 9 Other Anti-infective
2 Muscle	3 Percutaneous	3 Anti-inflammatory 6 Nutritional Substance 7 Electrolytic and Water Balance Substance B Anesthetic Agent H Radioactive Substance K Other Diagnostic Substance N Analgesics, Hypnotics, Sedatives T Destructive Agent	Z No Qualifier
2 Muscle	3 Percutaneous	4 Serum, Toxoid and Vaccine	0 Influenza Vaccine Z No Qualifier
2 Muscle	3 Percutaneous	G Other Therapeutic Substance	C Other Substance
3 Peripheral Vein	0 Open	0 Antineoplastic	2 High-dose Interleukin-2 3 Low-dose Interleukin-2 5 Other Antineoplastic M Monoclonal Antibody P Clofarabine
3 Peripheral Vein	0 Open	1 Thrombolytic	6 Recombinant Human- activated Protein C 7 Other Thrombolytic
3 Peripheral Vein	0 Open	2 Anti-infective	8 Oxazolidinones 9 Other Anti-infective

DRG Non-OR   3E03002
DRG Non-OR   3E03017

3E0 Continued on next page

NC Noncovered Procedure   LC Limited Coverage   QA Questionable OB Admit   NT New Tech Add-on   ⊞ Combination Member   ♂ Male   ♀ Female

ICD-10-PCS 2024   723

Administration

3   **Administration**
E   **Physiological Systems and Anatomical Regions**
Ø   **Introduction**   Definition: Putting in or on a therapeutic, diagnostic, nutritional, physiological, or prophylactic substance except blood or blood products

3EØ Continued

Body System/Region Character 4	Approach Character 5	Substance Character 6	Qualifier Character 7
3 Peripheral Vein	Ø Open	3 Anti-inflammatory 4 Serum, Toxoid and Vaccine 6 Nutritional Substance 7 Electrolytic and Water Balance Substance F Intracirculatory Anesthetic H Radioactive Substance K Other Diagnostic Substance N Analgesics, Hypnotics, Sedatives P Platelet Inhibitor R Antiarrhythmic T Destructive Agent X Vasopressor	Z No Qualifier
3 Peripheral Vein	Ø Open	G Other Therapeutic Substance	C Other Substance N Blood Brain Barrier Disruption
3 Peripheral Vein	Ø Open	U Pancreatic Islet Cells	Ø Autologous 1 Nonautologous
3 Peripheral Vein	Ø Open	V Hormone	G Insulin H Human B-type Natriuretic Peptide J Other Hormone
3 Peripheral Vein	Ø Open	W Immunotherapeutic	K Immunostimulator L Immunosuppressive
3 Peripheral Vein	3 Percutaneous	Ø Antineoplastic	2 High-dose Interleukin-2 3 Low-dose Interleukin-2 5 Other Antineoplastic M Monoclonal Antibody P Clofarabine
3 Peripheral Vein	3 Percutaneous	1 Thrombolytic	6 Recombinant Human- activated Protein C 7 Other Thrombolytic
3 Peripheral Vein	3 Percutaneous	2 Anti-infective	8 Oxazolidinones 9 Other Anti-infective
3 Peripheral Vein	3 Percutaneous	3 Anti-inflammatory 4 Serum, Toxoid and Vaccine 6 Nutritional Substance 7 Electrolytic and Water Balance Substance F Intracirculatory Anesthetic H Radioactive Substance K Other Diagnostic Substance N Analgesics, Hypnotics, Sedatives P Platelet Inhibitor R Antiarrhythmic T Destructive Agent X Vasopressor	Z No Qualifier
3 Peripheral Vein	3 Percutaneous	G Other Therapeutic Substance	C Other Substance N Blood Brain Barrier Disruption Q Glucarpidase R Other Therapeutic Monoclonal Antibody
3 Peripheral Vein	3 Percutaneous	U Pancreatic Islet Cells	Ø Autologous 1 Nonautologous
3 Peripheral Vein	3 Percutaneous	V Hormone	G Insulin H Human B-type Natriuretic Peptide J Other Hormone
3 Peripheral Vein	3 Percutaneous	W Immunotherapeutic	K Immunostimulator L Immunosuppressive
4 Central Vein	Ø Open	Ø Antineoplastic	2 High-dose Interleukin-2 3 Low-dose Interleukin-2 5 Other Antineoplastic M Monoclonal Antibody P Clofarabine
4 Central Vein	Ø Open	1 Thrombolytic	6 Recombinant Human- activated Protein C 7 Other Thrombolytic

Valid OR 3EØ3ØTZ		**DRG Non-OR** 3EØ33U[Ø,1]	
DRG Non-OR 3EØ3ØU[Ø,1]		**DRG Non-OR** 3EØ4ØØ2	
DRG Non-OR 3EØ33Ø2		**DRG Non-OR** 3EØ4Ø17	
DRG Non-OR 3EØ3317			

3EØ Continued on next page

Non-OR Procedure   DRG Non-OR Procedure   Valid OR Procedure   HAC Associated Procedure   Combination Only   New/Revised April   New/Revised October

724   ICD-10-PCS 2024

3   **Administration**
E   **Physiological Systems and Anatomical Regions**
Ø   **Introduction**   Definition: Putting in or on a therapeutic, diagnostic, nutritional, physiological, or prophylactic substance except blood or blood products

3EØ Continued

Body System/Region Character 4	Approach Character 5	Substance Character 6	Qualifier Character 7
4 Central Vein	Ø Open	2 Anti-infective	8 Oxazolidinones 9 Other Anti-infective
4 Central Vein	Ø Open	3 Anti-inflammatory 4 Serum, Toxoid and Vaccine 6 Nutritional Substance 7 Electrolytic and Water Balance Substance F Intracirculatory Anesthetic H Radioactive Substance K Other Diagnostic Substance N Analgesics, Hypnotics, Sedatives P Platelet Inhibitor R Antiarrhythmic T Destructive Agent X Vasopressor	Z No Qualifier
4 Central Vein	Ø Open	G Other Therapeutic Substance	C Other Substance N Blood Brain Barrier Disruption
4 Central Vein	Ø Open	V Hormone	G Insulin H Human B-type Natriuretic Peptide J Other Hormone
4 Central Vein	Ø Open	W Immunotherapeutic	K Immunostimulator L Immunosuppressive
4 Central Vein	3 Percutaneous	Ø Antineoplastic	2 High-dose Interleukin-2 3 Low-dose Interleukin-2 5 Other Antineoplastic M Monoclonal Antibody P Clofarabine
4 Central Vein	3 Percutaneous	1 Thrombolytic	6 Recombinant Human- activated Protein C 7 Other Thrombolytic
4 Central Vein	3 Percutaneous	2 Anti-infective	8 Oxazolidinones 9 Other Anti-infective
4 Central Vein	3 Percutaneous	3 Anti-inflammatory 4 Serum, Toxoid and Vaccine 6 Nutritional Substance 7 Electrolytic and Water Balance Substance F Intracirculatory Anesthetic H Radioactive Substance K Other Diagnostic Substance N Analgesics, Hypnotics, Sedatives P Platelet Inhibitor R Antiarrhythmic T Destructive Agent X Vasopressor	Z No Qualifier
4 Central Vein	3 Percutaneous	G Other Therapeutic Substance	C Other Substance N Blood Brain Barrier Disruption Q Glucarpidase R Other Therapeutic Monoclonal Antibody
4 Central Vein	3 Percutaneous	V Hormone	G Insulin H Human B-type Natriuretic Peptide J Other Hormone
4 Central Vein	3 Percutaneous	W Immunotherapeutic	K Immunostimulator L Immunosuppressive
5 Peripheral Artery 6 Central Artery	Ø Open 3 Percutaneous	Ø Antineoplastic	2 High-dose Interleukin-2 3 Low-dose Interleukin-2 5 Other Antineoplastic M Monoclonal Antibody P Clofarabine
5 Peripheral Artery 6 Central Artery	Ø Open 3 Percutaneous	1 Thrombolytic	6 Recombinant Human- activated Protein C 7 Other Thrombolytic
5 Peripheral Artery 6 Central Artery	Ø Open 3 Percutaneous	2 Anti-infective	8 Oxazolidinones 9 Other Anti-infective

Valid OR   3E04ØTZ
DRG Non-OR   3E04302
DRG Non-OR   3E04317
DRG Non-OR   3E0[5,6][Ø,3]Ø2
DRG Non-OR   3E0[5,6][Ø,3]17

3EØ Continued on next page

NC Noncovered Procedure   LC Limited Coverage   QA Questionable OB Admit   NT New Tech Add-on   ⊞ Combination Member   ♂ Male   ♀ Female

Administration (left margin, vertical)

3   **Administration**
E   **Physiological Systems and Anatomical Regions**   *3E0 Continued*
0   **Introduction**   Definition: Putting in or on a therapeutic, diagnostic, nutritional, physiological, or prophylactic substance except blood or blood products

Body System/Region Character 4	Approach Character 5	Substance Character 6	Qualifier Character 7
5 Peripheral Artery 6 Central Artery	0 Open 3 Percutaneous	3 Anti-inflammatory 4 Serum, Toxoid and Vaccine 6 Nutritional Substance 7 Electrolytic and Water Balance Substance F Intracirculatory Anesthetic H Radioactive Substance K Other Diagnostic Substance N Analgesics, Hypnotics, Sedatives P Platelet Inhibitor R Antiarrhythmic T Destructive Agent X Vasopressor	Z No Qualifier
5 Peripheral Artery 6 Central Artery	0 Open 3 Percutaneous	G Other Therapeutic Substance	C Other Substance N Blood Brain Barrier Disruption
5 Peripheral Artery 6 Central Artery	0 Open 3 Percutaneous	V Hormone	G Insulin H Human B-type Natriuretic Peptide J Other Hormone
5 Peripheral Artery 6 Central Artery	0 Open 3 Percutaneous	W Immunotherapeutic	K Immunostimulator L Immunosuppressive
7 Coronary Artery 8 Heart	0 Open 3 Percutaneous	1 Thrombolytic	6 Recombinant Human- activated Protein C 7 Other Thrombolytic
7 Coronary Artery 8 Heart	0 Open 3 Percutaneous	G Other Therapeutic Substance	C Other Substance
7 Coronary Artery 8 Heart	0 Open 3 Percutaneous	K Other Diagnostic Substance P Platelet Inhibitor	Z No Qualifier
7 Coronary Artery 8 Heart	4 Percutaneous Endoscopic	G Other Therapeutic Substance	C Other Substance
9 Nose	3 Percutaneous 7 Via Natural or Artificial Opening X External	0 Antineoplastic	5 Other Antineoplastic M Monoclonal Antibody
9 Nose	3 Percutaneous 7 Via Natural or Artificial Opening X External	2 Anti-infective	8 Oxazolidinones 9 Other Anti-infective
9 Nose	3 Percutaneous 7 Via Natural or Artificial Opening X External	3 Anti-inflammatory 4 Serum, Toxoid and Vaccine B Anesthetic Agent H Radioactive Substance K Other Diagnostic Substance N Analgesics, Hypnotics, Sedatives T Destructive Agent	Z No Qualifier
9 Nose	3 Percutaneous 7 Via Natural or Artificial Opening X External	G Other Therapeutic Substance	C Other Substance
A Bone Marrow	3 Percutaneous	0 Antineoplastic	5 Other Antineoplastic M Monoclonal Antibody
A Bone Marrow	3 Percutaneous	G Other Therapeutic Substance	C Other Substance
B Ear	3 Percutaneous 7 Via Natural or Artificial Opening X External	0 Antineoplastic	4 Liquid Brachytherapy Radioisotope 5 Other Antineoplastic M Monoclonal Antibody
B Ear	3 Percutaneous 7 Via Natural or Artificial Opening X External	2 Anti-infective	8 Oxazolidinones 9 Other Anti-infective
B Ear	3 Percutaneous 7 Via Natural or Artificial Opening X External	3 Anti-inflammatory B Anesthetic Agent H Radioactive Substance K Other Diagnostic Substance N Analgesics, Hypnotics, Sedatives T Destructive Agent	Z No Qualifier
B Ear	3 Percutaneous 7 Via Natural or Artificial Opening X External	G Other Therapeutic Substance	C Other Substance

DRG Non-OR   3E08[0,3]17

3E0 Continued on next page

Non-OR Procedure   DRG Non-OR Procedure   Valid OR Procedure   HAC Associated Procedure   Combination Only   New/Revised April   New/Revised October

3 Administration
E Physiological Systems and Anatomical Regions

3E0 Continued

0 Introduction   Definition: Putting in or on a therapeutic, diagnostic, nutritional, physiological, or prophylactic substance except blood or blood products

Body System/Region Character 4	Approach Character 5	Substance Character 6	Qualifier Character 7
C Eye	**3** Percutaneous **7** Via Natural or Artificial Opening **X** External	**0** Antineoplastic	**4** Liquid Brachytherapy Radioisotope **5** Other Antineoplastic **M** Monoclonal Antibody
C Eye	**3** Percutaneous **7** Via Natural or Artificial Opening **X** External	**2** Anti-infective	**8** Oxazolidinones **9** Other Anti-infective
C Eye	**3** Percutaneous **7** Via Natural or Artificial Opening **X** External	**3** Anti-inflammatory **B** Anesthetic Agent **H** Radioactive Substance **K** Other Diagnostic Substance **M** Pigment **N** Analgesics, Hypnotics, Sedatives **T** Destructive Agent	**Z** No Qualifier
C Eye	**3** Percutaneous **7** Via Natural or Artificial Opening **X** External	**G** Other Therapeutic Substance	**C** Other Substance
C Eye	**3** Percutaneous **7** Via Natural or Artificial Opening **X** External	**S** Gas	**F** Other Gas
D Mouth and Pharynx	**3** Percutaneous **7** Via Natural or Artificial Opening **X** External	**0** Antineoplastic	**4** Liquid Brachytherapy Radioisotope **5** Other Antineoplastic **M** Monoclonal Antibody
D Mouth and Pharynx	**3** Percutaneous **7** Via Natural or Artificial Opening **X** External	**2** Anti-infective	**8** Oxazolidinones **9** Other Anti-infective
D Mouth and Pharynx	**3** Percutaneous **7** Via Natural or Artificial Opening **X** External	**3** Anti-inflammatory **4** Serum, Toxoid and Vaccine **6** Nutritional Substance **7** Electrolytic and Water Balance Substance **B** Anesthetic Agent **H** Radioactive Substance **K** Other Diagnostic Substance **N** Analgesics, Hypnotics, Sedatives **R** Antiarrhythmic **T** Destructive Agent	**Z** No Qualifier
D Mouth and Pharynx	**3** Percutaneous **7** Via Natural or Artificial Opening **X** External	**G** Other Therapeutic Substance	**C** Other Substance
E Products of Conception ♀ **G** Upper GI **H** Lower GI **K** Genitourinary Tract **N** Male Reproductive ♂	**3** Percutaneous **7** Via Natural or Artificial Opening **8** Via Natural or Artificial Opening Endoscopic	**0** Antineoplastic	**4** Liquid Brachytherapy Radioisotope **5** Other Antineoplastic **M** Monoclonal Antibody
E Products of Conception ♀ **G** Upper GI **H** Lower GI **K** Genitourinary Tract **N** Male Reproductive ♂	**3** Percutaneous **7** Via Natural or Artificial Opening **8** Via Natural or Artificial Opening Endoscopic	**2** Anti-infective	**8** Oxazolidinones **9** Other Anti-infective
E Products of Conception ♀ **G** Upper GI **H** Lower GI **K** Genitourinary Tract **N** Male Reproductive ♂	**3** Percutaneous **7** Via Natural or Artificial Opening **8** Via Natural or Artificial Opening Endoscopic	**3** Anti-inflammatory **6** Nutritional Substance **7** Electrolytic and Water Balance Substance **B** Anesthetic Agent **H** Radioactive Substance **K** Other Diagnostic Substance **N** Analgesics, Hypnotics, Sedatives **T** Destructive Agent	**Z** No Qualifier
E Products of Conception ♀ **G** Upper GI **H** Lower GI **K** Genitourinary Tract **N** Male Reproductive ♂	**3** Percutaneous **7** Via Natural or Artificial Opening **8** Via Natural or Artificial Opening Endoscopic	**G** Other Therapeutic Substance	**C** Other Substance

♂   All approach, substance, and qualifier values for body system/region (character 4) with this icon
♀   All approach, substance, and qualifier values for body system/region (character 4) with this icon

3E0 Continued on next page

Administration

3   Administration   *3E0 Continued*
E   Physiological Systems and Anatomical Regions
0   Introduction   Definition: Putting in or on a therapeutic, diagnostic, nutritional, physiological, or prophylactic substance except blood or blood products

Body System/Region Character 4	Approach Character 5	Substance Character 6	Qualifier Character 7
E Products of Conception ♀ G Upper GI H Lower GI K Genitourinary Tract N Male Reproductive ♂	3 Percutaneous 7 Via Natural or Artificial Opening 8 Via Natural or Artificial Opening Endoscopic	S Gas	F Other Gas
E Products of Conception ♀ G Upper GI H Lower GI K Genitourinary Tract N Male Reproductive ♂	4 Percutaneous Endoscopic	G Other Therapeutic Substance	C Other Substance
F Respiratory Tract	3 Percutaneous 7 Via Natural or Artificial Opening 8 Via Natural or Artificial Opening Endoscopic	0 Antineoplastic	4 Liquid Brachytherapy Radioisotope 5 Other Antineoplastic M Monoclonal Antibody
F Respiratory Tract	3 Percutaneous 7 Via Natural or Artificial Opening 8 Via Natural or Artificial Opening Endoscopic	2 Anti-infective	8 Oxazolidinones 9 Other Anti-infective
F Respiratory Tract	3 Percutaneous 7 Via Natural or Artificial Opening 8 Via Natural or Artificial Opening Endoscopic	3 Anti-inflammatory 6 Nutritional Substance 7 Electrolytic and Water Balance Substance B Anesthetic Agent H Radioactive Substance K Other Diagnostic Substance N Analgesics, Hypnotics, Sedatives T Destructive Agent	Z No Qualifier
F Respiratory Tract	3 Percutaneous 7 Via Natural or Artificial Opening 8 Via Natural or Artificial Opening Endoscopic	G Other Therapeutic Substance	C Other Substance
F Respiratory Tract	3 Percutaneous 7 Via Natural or Artificial Opening 8 Via Natural or Artificial Opening Endoscopic	S Gas	D Nitric Oxide F Other Gas
F Respiratory Tract	4 Percutaneous Endoscopic	G Other Therapeutic Substance	C Other Substance
J Biliary and Pancreatic Tract	3 Percutaneous 7 Via Natural or Artificial Opening 8 Via Natural or Artificial Opening Endoscopic	0 Antineoplastic	4 Liquid Brachytherapy Radioisotope 5 Other Antineoplastic M Monoclonal Antibody
J Biliary and Pancreatic Tract	3 Percutaneous 7 Via Natural or Artificial Opening 8 Via Natural or Artificial Opening Endoscopic	2 Anti-infective	8 Oxazolidinones 9 Other Anti-infective
J Biliary and Pancreatic Tract	3 Percutaneous 7 Via Natural or Artificial Opening 8 Via Natural or Artificial Opening Endoscopic	3 Anti-inflammatory 6 Nutritional Substance 7 Electrolytic and Water Balance Substance B Anesthetic Agent H Radioactive Substance K Other Diagnostic Substance N Analgesics, Hypnotics, Sedatives T Destructive Agent	Z No Qualifier
J Biliary and Pancreatic Tract	3 Percutaneous 7 Via Natural or Artificial Opening 8 Via Natural or Artificial Opening Endoscopic	G Other Therapeutic Substance	C Other Substance
J Biliary and Pancreatic Tract	3 Percutaneous 7 Via Natural or Artificial Opening 8 Via Natural or Artificial Opening Endoscopic	S Gas	F Other Gas

♂   All approach, substance, and qualifier values for body system/region (character 4) with this icon
♀   All approach, substance, and qualifier values for body system/region (character 4) with this icon

3E0 Continued on next page

Non-OR Procedure   DRG Non-OR Procedure   Valid OR Procedure   HAC Associated Procedure   Combination Only   New/Revised April   New/Revised October

3　**Administration**　　　　　　　　　　　　　　　　　　　　　　　　　　　**3E0 Continued**
E　**Physiological Systems and Anatomical Regions**
0　**Introduction**　　Definition: Putting in or on a therapeutic, diagnostic, nutritional, physiological, or prophylactic substance except blood or blood products

Body System/Region Character 4		Approach Character 5	Substance Character 6	Qualifier Character 7
J	Biliary and Pancreatic Tract	3 Percutaneous 7 Via Natural or Artificial Opening 8 Via Natural or Artificial Opening Endoscopic	U Pancreatic Islet Cells	0 Autologous 1 Nonautologous
J	Biliary and Pancreatic Tract	4 Percutaneous Endoscopic	G Other Therapeutic Substance	C Other Substance
L	Pleural Cavity	0 Open	5 Adhesion Barrier	Z No Qualifier
L	Pleural Cavity	3 Percutaneous	0 Antineoplastic	4 Liquid Brachytherapy Radioisotope 5 Other Antineoplastic M Monoclonal Antibody
L	Pleural Cavity	3 Percutaneous	2 Anti-infective	8 Oxazolidinones 9 Other Anti-infective
L	Pleural Cavity	3 Percutaneous	3 Anti-inflammatory 5 Adhesion Barrier 6 Nutritional Substance 7 Electrolytic and Water Balance Substance B Anesthetic Agent H Radioactive Substance K Other Diagnostic Substance N Analgesics, Hypnotics, Sedatives T Destructive Agent	Z No Qualifier
L	Pleural Cavity	3 Percutaneous	G Other Therapeutic Substance	C Other Substance
L	Pleural Cavity	3 Percutaneous	S Gas	F Other Gas
L	Pleural Cavity	4 Percutaneous Endoscopic	5 Adhesion Barrier	Z No Qualifier
L	Pleural Cavity	4 Percutaneous Endoscopic	G Other Therapeutic Substance	C Other Substance
L	Pleural Cavity	7 Via Natural or Artificial Opening	0 Antineoplastic	4 Liquid Brachytherapy Radioisotope 5 Other Antineoplastic M Monoclonal Antibody
L	Pleural Cavity	7 Via Natural or Artificial Opening	S Gas	F Other Gas
M	Peritoneal Cavity	0 Open	5 Adhesion Barrier	Z No Qualifier
M	Peritoneal Cavity	3 Percutaneous	0 Antineoplastic	4 Liquid Brachytherapy Radioisotope 5 Other Antineoplastic M Monoclonal Antibody Y Hyperthermic
M	Peritoneal Cavity	3 Percutaneous	2 Anti-infective	8 Oxazolidinones 9 Other Anti-infective
M	Peritoneal Cavity	3 Percutaneous	3 Anti-inflammatory 5 Adhesion Barrier 6 Nutritional Substance 7 Electrolytic and Water Balance Substance B Anesthetic Agent H Radioactive Substance K Other Diagnostic Substance N Analgesics, Hypnotics, Sedatives T Destructive Agent	Z No Qualifier
M	Peritoneal Cavity	3 Percutaneous	G Other Therapeutic Substance	C Other Substance
M	Peritoneal Cavity	3 Percutaneous	S Gas	F Other Gas
M	Peritoneal Cavity	4 Percutaneous Endoscopic	5 Adhesion Barrier	Z No Qualifier
M	Peritoneal Cavity	4 Percutaneous Endoscopic	G Other Therapeutic Substance	C Other Substance
M	Peritoneal Cavity	7 Via Natural or Artificial Opening	0 Antineoplastic	4 Liquid Brachytherapy Radioisotope 5 Other Antineoplastic M Monoclonal Antibody
M	Peritoneal Cavity	7 Via Natural or Artificial Opening	S Gas	F Other Gas
P	Female Reproductive ♀	0 Open	5 Adhesion Barrier	Z No Qualifier
P	Female Reproductive ♀	3 Percutaneous	0 Antineoplastic	4 Liquid Brachytherapy Radioisotope 5 Other Antineoplastic M Monoclonal Antibody
P	Female Reproductive ♀	3 Percutaneous	2 Anti-infective	8 Oxazolidinones 9 Other Anti-infective

Valid OR　　3E0L4GC
DRG Non-OR　3E0J[3,7,8]U[0,1]
♀　　　　All approach, substance, and qualifier values for body system/region (character 4) with this icon

3E0 Continued on next page

Administration

3   **Administration**
E   **Physiological Systems and Anatomical Regions**
Ø   **Introduction**   Definition: Putting in or on a therapeutic, diagnostic, nutritional, physiological, or prophylactic substance except blood or blood products

3EØ Continued

Body System/Region Character 4	Approach Character 5	Substance Character 6	Qualifier Character 7
P Female Reproductive ♀	3 Percutaneous	3 Anti-inflammatory 5 Adhesion Barrier 6 Nutritional Substance 7 Electrolytic and Water Balance Substance B Anesthetic Agent H Radioactive Substance K Other Diagnostic Substance L Sperm N Analgesics, Hypnotics, Sedatives T Destructive Agent V Hormone	Z No Qualifier
P Female Reproductive ♀	3 Percutaneous	G Other Therapeutic Substance	C Other Substance
P Female Reproductive ♀	3 Percutaneous	Q Fertilized Ovum	Ø Autologous 1 Nonautologous
P Female Reproductive ♀	3 Percutaneous	S Gas	F Other Gas
P Female Reproductive ♀	4 Percutaneous Endoscopic	5 Adhesion Barrier	Z No Qualifier
P Female Reproductive ♀	4 Percutaneous Endoscopic	G Other Therapeutic Substance	C Other Substance
P Female Reproductive ♀	7 Via Natural or Artificial Opening	Ø Antineoplastic	4 Liquid Brachytherapy Radioisotope 5 Other Antineoplastic M Monoclonal Antibody
P Female Reproductive ♀	7 Via Natural or Artificial Opening	2 Anti-infective	8 Oxazolidinones 9 Other Anti-infective
P Female Reproductive ♀	7 Via Natural or Artificial Opening	3 Anti-inflammatory 6 Nutritional Substance 7 Electrolytic and Water Balance Substance B Anesthetic Agent H Radioactive Substance K Other Diagnostic Substance L Sperm N Analgesics, Hypnotics, Sedatives T Destructive Agent V Hormone	Z No Qualifier
P Female Reproductive ♀	7 Via Natural or Artificial Opening	G Other Therapeutic Substance	C Other Substance
P Female Reproductive ♀	7 Via Natural or Artificial Opening	Q Fertilized Ovum	Ø Autologous 1 Nonautologous
P Female Reproductive ♀	7 Via Natural or Artificial Opening	S Gas	F Other Gas
P Female Reproductive ♀	8 Via Natural or Artificial Opening Endoscopic	Ø Antineoplastic	4 Liquid Brachytherapy Radioisotope 5 Other Antineoplastic M Monoclonal Antibody
P Female Reproductive ♀	8 Via Natural or Artificial Opening Endoscopic	2 Anti-infective	8 Oxazolidinones 9 Other Anit-infective

P Female Reproductive ♀	8 Via Natural or Artificial Opening
	    Endoscopic
		3 Anti-inflammatory
		6 Nutritional Substance
		7 Electrolytic and Water Balance
		    Substance
		B Anesthetic Agent
		H Radioactive Substance
		K Other Diagnostic Substance
		N Analgesics, Hypnotics, Sedatives
		T Destructive Agent
			Z No Qualifier

P Female Reproductive ♀	8 Via Natural or Artificial Opening Endoscopic	G Other Therapeutic Substance	C Other Substance
P Female Reproductive ♀	8 Via Natural or Artificial Opening Endoscopic	S Gas	F Other Gas
Q Cranial Cavity and Brain	Ø Open 3 Percutaneous	Ø Antineoplastic	4 Liquid Brachytherapy Radioisotope 5 Other Antineoplastic M Monoclonal Antibody
Q Cranial Cavity and Brain	Ø Open 3 Percutaneous	2 Anti-infective	8 Oxazolidinones 9 Other Anti-infective

Valid OR   3EØP3Q[Ø,1]
Valid OR   3EØP7Q[Ø,1]
DRG Non-OR   3EØQ[Ø,3]Ø5
♀   All approach, substance, and qualifier values for body system/region (character 4) with this icon

3EØ Continued on next page

Non-OR Procedure   DRG Non-OR Procedure   Valid OR Procedure   HAC Associated Procedure   Combination Only   New/Revised April   New/Revised October

730   ICD-10-PCS 2024

3   **Administration**

E   **Physiological Systems and Anatomical Regions**

Ø   **Introduction**   Definition: Putting in or on a therapeutic, diagnostic, nutritional, physiological, or prophylactic substance except blood or blood products

3EØ Continued

Body System/Region Character 4	Approach Character 5	Substance Character 6	Qualifier Character 7
Q Cranial Cavity and Brain	Ø Open 3 Percutaneous	3 Anti-inflammatory 6 Nutritional Substance 7 Electrolytic and Water Balance Substance A Stem Cells, Embryonic B Anesthetic Agent H Radioactive Substance K Other Diagnostic Substance N Analgesics, Hypnotics, Sedatives T Destructive Agent	Z No Qualifier
Q Cranial Cavity and Brain	Ø Open 3 Percutaneous	E Stem Cells, Somatic	Ø Autologous 1 Nonautologous
Q Cranial Cavity and Brain	Ø Open 3 Percutaneous	G Other Therapeutic Substance	C Other Substance
Q Cranial Cavity and Brain	Ø Open 3 Percutaneous	S Gas	F Other Gas
Q Cranial Cavity and Brain	7 Via Natural or Artificial Opening	Ø Antineoplastic	4 Liquid Brachytherapy Radioisotope 5 Other Antineoplastic M Monoclonal Antibody
Q Cranial Cavity and Brain	7 Via Natural or Artificial Opening	S Gas	F Other Gas
R Spinal Canal	Ø Open	A Stem Cells, Embryonic	Z No Qualifier
R Spinal Canal	Ø Open	E Stem Cells, Somatic	Ø Autologous 1 Nonautologous
R Spinal Canal	3 Percutaneous	Ø Antineoplastic	2 High-dose Interleukin-2 3 Low-dose Interleukin-2 4 Liquid Brachytherapy Radioisotope 5 Other Antineoplastic M Monoclonal Antibody
R Spinal Canal	3 Percutaneous	2 Anti-infective	8 Oxazolidinones 9 Other Anti-infective
R Spinal Canal	3 Percutaneous	3 Anti-inflammatory 6 Nutritional Substance 7 Electrolytic and Water Balance Substance A Stem Cells, Embryonic B Anesthetic Agent H Radioactive Substance K Other Diagnostic Substance N Analgesics, Hypnotics, Sedatives T Destructive Agent	Z No Qualifier
R Spinal Canal	3 Percutaneous	E Stem Cells, Somatic	Ø Autologous 1 Nonautologous
R Spinal Canal	3 Percutaneous	G Other Therapeutic Substance	C Other Substance
R Spinal Canal	3 Percutaneous	S Gas	F Other Gas
R Spinal Canal	7 Via Natural or Artificial Opening	S Gas	F Other Gas
S Epidural Space	3 Percutaneous	Ø Antineoplastic	2 High-dose Interleukin-2 3 Low-dose Interleukin-2 4 Liquid Brachytherapy Radioisotope 5 Other Antineoplastic M Monoclonal Antibody
S Epidural Space	3 Percutaneous	2 Anti-infective	8 Oxazolidinones 9 Other Anti-infective
S Epidural Space	3 Percutaneous	3 Anti-inflammatory 6 Nutritional Substance 7 Electrolytic and Water Balance Substance B Anesthetic Agent H Radioactive Substance K Other Diagnostic Substance N Analgesics, Hypnotics, Sedatives T Destructive Agent	Z No Qualifier

DRG Non-OR	3EØQ7Ø5
DRG Non-OR	3EØR3Ø2
DRG Non-OR	3EØS3Ø2

3EØ Continued on next page

NC Noncovered Procedure   **LC** Limited Coverage   **QA** Questionable OB Admit   **NT** New Tech Add-on   ⊞ Combination Member   ♂ Male   ♀ Female

ICD-10-PCS 2024   731

3EØ–3EØ

Administration *(left margin)*

3   Administration
E   Physiological Systems and Anatomical Regions
Ø   Introduction   Definition: Putting in or on a therapeutic, diagnostic, nutritional, physiological, or prophylactic substance except blood or blood products

3EØ Continued

Body System/Region Character 4		Approach Character 5		Substance Character 6		Qualifier Character 7	
S	Epidural Space	3	Percutaneous	G	Other Therapeutic Substance	C	Other Substance
S	Epidural Space	3	Percutaneous	S	Gas	F	Other Gas
S	Epidural Space	7	Via Natural or Artificial Opening	S	Gas	F	Other Gas
T X	Peripheral Nerves and Plexi Cranial Nerves	3	Percutaneous	3 B T	Anti-inflammatory Anesthetic Agent Destructive Agent	Z	No Qualifier
T X	Peripheral Nerves and Plexi Cranial Nerves	3	Percutaneous	G	Other Therapeutic Substance	C	Other Substance
U	Joints	Ø	Open	2	Anti-infective	8 9	Oxazolidinones Other Anti-infective
U	Joints	Ø	Open	G	Other Therapeutic Substance	B	Recombinant Bone Morphogenetic Protein
U	Joints	3	Percutaneous	Ø	Antineoplastic	4 5 M	Liquid Brachytherapy Radioisotope Other Antineoplastic Monoclonal Antibody
U	Joints	3	Percutaneous	2	Anti-infective	8 9	Oxazolidinones Other Anti-infective
U	Joints	3	Percutaneous	3 6 7 B H K N T	Anti-inflammatory Nutritional Substance Electrolytic and Water Balance Substance Anesthetic Agent Radioactive Substance Other Diagnostic Substance Analgesics, Hypnotics, Sedatives Destructive Agent	Z	No Qualifier
U	Joints	3	Percutaneous	G	Other Therapeutic Substance	B C	Recombinant Bone Morphogenetic Protein Other Substance
U	Joints	3	Percutaneous	S	Gas	F	Other Gas
U	Joints	4	Percutaneous Endoscopic	G	Other Therapeutic Substance	C	Other Substance
V	Bones	Ø	Open	G	Other Therapeutic Substance	B C	Recombinant Bone Morphogenetic Protein Other Substance
V	Bones	3	Percutaneous	Ø	Antineoplastic	5 M	Other Antineoplastic Monoclonal Antibody
V	Bones	3	Percutaneous	2	Anti-infective	8 9	Oxazolidinones Other Anti-infective
V	Bones	3	Percutaneous	3 6 7 B H K N T	Anti-inflammatory Nutritional Substance Electrolytic and Water Balance Substance Anesthetic Agent Radioactive Substance Other Diagnostic Substance Analgesics, Hypnotics, Sedatives Destructive Agent	Z	No Qualifier
V	Bones	3	Percutaneous	G	Other Therapeutic Substance	B C	Recombinant Bone Morphogenetic Protein Other Substance
V	Bones	4	Percutaneous Endoscopic	G	Other Therapeutic Substance	C	Other Substance
W	Lymphatics	3	Percutaneous	Ø	Antineoplastic	5 M	Other Antineoplastic Monoclonal Antibody
W	Lymphatics	3	Percutaneous	2	Anti-infective	8 9	Oxazolidinones Other Anti-infective
W	Lymphatics	3	Percutaneous	3 6 7 B H K N T	Anti-inflammatory Nutritional Substance Electrolytic and Water Balance Substance Anesthetic Agent Radioactive Substance Other Diagnostic Substance Analgesics, Hypnotics, Sedatives Destructive Agent	Z	No Qualifier
W	Lymphatics	3	Percutaneous	G	Other Therapeutic Substance	C	Other Substance

3EØ Continued on next page

3E0 Continued

3   **Administration**
E   **Physiological Systems and Anatomical Regions**
0   **Introduction**   Definition: Putting in or on a therapeutic, diagnostic, nutritional, physiological, or prophylactic substance except blood or blood products

Body System/Region Character 4	Approach Character 5	Substance Character 6	Qualifier Character 7
Y Pericardial Cavity	**3** Percutaneous	**0** Antineoplastic	**4** Liquid Brachytherapy Radioisotope **5** Other Antineoplastic **M** Monoclonal Antibody
Y Pericardial Cavity	**3** Percutaneous	**2** Anti-infective	**8** Oxazolidinones **9** Other Anti-infective
Y Pericardial Cavity	**3** Percutaneous	**3** Anti-inflammatory **6** Nutritional Substance **7** Electrolytic and Water Balance Substance **B** Anesthetic Agent **H** Radioactive Substance **K** Other Diagnostic Substance **N** Analgesics, Hypnotics, Sedatives **T** Destructive Agent	**Z** No Qualifier
Y Pericardial Cavity	**3** Percutaneous	**G** Other Therapeutic Substance	**C** Other Substance
Y Pericardial Cavity	**3** Percutaneous	**S** Gas	**F** Other Gas
Y Pericardial Cavity	**4** Percutaneous Endoscopic	**G** Other Therapeutic Substance	**C** Other Substance
Y Pericardial Cavity	**7** Via Natural or Artificial Opening	**0** Antineoplastic	**4** Liquid Brachytherapy Radioisotope **5** Other Antineoplastic **M** Monoclonal Antibody
Y Pericardial Cavity	**7** Via Natural or Artificial Opening	**S** Gas	**F** Other Gas

3   **Administration**
E   **Physiological Systems and Anatomical Regions**
1   **Irrigation**   Definition: Putting in or on a cleansing substance

Body System/Region Character 4	Approach Character 5	Substance Character 6	Qualifier Character 7
0 Skin and Mucous Membranes **C** Eye	**3** Percutaneous **X** External	**8** Irrigating Substance	**X** Diagnostic **Z** No Qualifier
9 Nose **B** Ear **F** Respiratory Tract **G** Upper GI **H** Lower GI **J** Biliary and Pancreatic Tract **K** Genitourinary Tract **N** Male Reproductive ♂ **P** Female Reproductive ♀	**3** Percutaneous **7** Via Natural or Artificial Opening **8** Via Natural or Artificial Opening Endoscopic	**8** Irrigating Substance	**X** Diagnostic **Z** No Qualifier
L Pleural Cavity **Q** Cranial Cavity and Brain **R** Spinal Canal **S** Epidural Space **Y** Pericardial Cavity	**3** Percutaneous	**8** Irrigating Substance	**X** Diagnostic **Z** No Qualifier
M Peritoneal Cavity	**3** Percutaneous	**8** Irrigating Substance	**X** Diagnostic **Z** No Qualifier
M Peritoneal Cavity	**3** Percutaneous	**9** Dialysate	**Z** No Qualifier
M Peritoneal Cavity	**4** Percutaneous Endoscopic	**8** Irrigating Substance	**X** Diagnostic **Z** No Qualifier
U Joints	**3** Percutaneous **4** Percutaneous Endoscopic	**8** Irrigating Substance	**X** Diagnostic **Z** No Qualifier

♂   3E1N[3,7,8]8[X,Z]
♀   3E1P[3,7,8]8[X,Z]

NC Noncovered Procedure   **LC** Limited Coverage   **QA** Questionable OB Admit   **NT** New Tech Add-on   ⊞ Combination Member   ♂ Male   ♀ Female

ICD-10-PCS 2024   733

Measurement and Monitoring 4AØ–4BØ

AHA Coding Clinic for table 4AØ

2022, 1Q, 46	Internal cardioversion
2020, 4Q, 62	Measurement of intracranial arterial flow
2020, 4Q, 62	Percutaneous endoscopic measurement of portal venous pressure
2020, 4Q, 63	Intercompartmental pressure measurement
2019, 3Q, 32	Endomyocardial biopsy and right heart catheterization
2018, 1Q, 12	Percutaneous balloon valvuloplasty & cardiac catheterization with ventriculogram
2016, 3Q, 37	Fractional flow reserve
2015, 3Q, 29	Approach value for esophageal electrophysiology study

AHA Coding Clinic for table 4BØ

2021, 4Q, 55-56	Measurement of flow in a cerebral fluid shunt

AHA Coding Clinic for table 4A1

2019, 4Q, 38-39	Intraoperative fluorescence lymphatic mapping using Indocyanine green dye
2016, 4Q, 114	Fluorescence vascular angiography
2016, 2Q, 29	Decompressive craniectomy with cryopreservation and storage of bone flap
2016, 2Q, 33	Monitoring of arterial pressure & pulse
2015, 3Q, 35	Swan Ganz catheterization
2015, 2Q, 14	Intraoperative EMG monitoring via endotracheal tube
2015, 1Q, 26	Intraoperative monitoring using Sentio MMG®
2014, 4Q, 28	Removal and replacement of displaced growing rods

4   **Measurement and Monitoring**
A   **Physiological Systems**
Ø   **Measurement**   Definition: Determining the level of a physiological or physical function at a point in time

Body System Character 4	Approach Character 5	Function/Device Character 6	Qualifier Character 7
Ø Central Nervous	Ø Open	2 Conductivity 4 Electrical Activity B Pressure	Z No Qualifier
Ø Central Nervous	3 Percutaneous 7 Via Natural or Artificial Opening 8 Via Natural or Artificial Opening Endoscopic	4 Electrical Activity	Z No Qualifier
Ø Central Nervous	3 Percutaneous 7 Via Natural or Artificial Opening 8 Via Natural or Artificial Opening Endoscopic	B Pressure K Temperature R Saturation	D Intracranial
Ø Central Nervous	X External	2 Conductivity 4 Electrical Activity	Z No Qualifier
1 Peripheral Nervous	Ø Open 3 Percutaneous 7 Via Natural or Artificial Opening 8 Via Natural or Artificial Opening Endoscopic X External	2 Conductivity	9 Sensory B Motor
1 Peripheral Nervous	Ø Open 3 Percutaneous 7 Via Natural or Artificial Opening 8 Via Natural or Artificial Opening Endoscopic X External	4 Electrical Activity	Z No Qualifier
2 Cardiac	Ø Open 3 Percutaneous 7 Via Natural or Artificial Opening 8 Via Natural or Artificial Opening Endoscopic	4 Electrical Activity 9 Output C Rate F Rhythm H Sound P Action Currents	Z No Qualifier
2 Cardiac	Ø Open 3 Percutaneous 7 Via Natural or Artificial Opening 8 Via Natural or Artificial Opening Endoscopic	N Sampling and Pressure	6 Right Heart 7 Left Heart 8 Bilateral
2 Cardiac	X External	4 Electrical Activity	A Guidance Z No Qualifier
2 Cardiac	X External	9 Output C Rate F Rhythm H Sound P Action Currents	Z No Qualifier
2 Cardiac	X External	M Total Activity	4 Stress
3 Arterial	Ø Open 3 Percutaneous	5 Flow J Pulse	1 Peripheral 3 Pulmonary C Coronary
3 Arterial	Ø Open 3 Percutaneous	B Pressure	1 Peripheral 3 Pulmonary C Coronary F Other Thoracic

DRG Non-OR	4AØ2[3,7,8]FZ
DRG Non-OR	4AØ2[Ø,3,7,8]N[6,7,8]

4AØ Continued on next page

NC Noncovered Procedure   LC Limited Coverage   QA Questionable OB Admit   NT New Tech Add-on   ✚ Combination Member   ♂ Male   ♀ Female

Measurement and Monitoring

4A0 Continued

4   **Measurement and Monitoring**
A   **Physiological Systems**
Ø   **Measurement**   Definition: Determining the level of a physiological or physical function at a point in time

Body System Character 4	Approach Character 5	Function/Device Character 6	Qualifier Character 7
3 Arterial	Ø Open 3 Percutaneous	H Sound R Saturation	1 Peripheral
3 Arterial	X External	5 Flow	1 Peripheral D Intracranial
3 Arterial	X External	B Pressure H Sound J Pulse R Saturation	1 Peripheral
4 Venous	Ø Open 3 Percutaneous	5 Flow B Pressure J Pulse	Ø Central 1 Peripheral 2 Portal 3 Pulmonary
4 Venous	Ø Open 3 Percutaneous	R Saturation	1 Peripheral
4 Venous	4 Percutaneous Endoscopic	B Pressure	2 Portal
4 Venous	X External	5 Flow B Pressure J Pulse R Saturation	1 Peripheral
5 Circulatory	X External	L Volume	Z No Qualifier
6 Lymphatic	Ø Open 3 Percutaneous 7 Via Natural or Artificial Opening 8 Via Natural or Artificial Opening Endoscopic	5 Flow B Pressure	Z No Qualifier
7 Visual	X External	Ø Acuity 7 Mobility B Pressure	Z No Qualifier
8 Olfactory	X External	Ø Acuity	Z No Qualifier
9 Respiratory	7 Via Natural or Artificial Opening 8 Via Natural or Artificial Opening Endoscopic X External	1 Capacity 5 Flow C Rate D Resistance L Volume M Total Activity	Z No Qualifier
B Gastrointestinal	7 Via Natural or Artificial Opening 8 Via Natural or Artificial Opening Endoscopic	8 Motility B Pressure G Secretion	Z No Qualifier
C Biliary	3 Percutaneous 4 Percutaneous Endoscopic 7 Via Natural or Artificial Opening 8 Via Natural or Artificial Opening Endoscopic	5 Flow B Pressure	Z No Qualifier
D Urinary	7 Via Natural or Artificial Opening 8 Via Natural or Artificial Opening Endoscopic	3 Contractility 5 Flow B Pressure D Resistance L Volume	Z No Qualifier
F Musculoskeletal	3 Percutaneous	3 Contractility	Z No Qualifier
F Musculoskeletal	3 Percutaneous	B Pressure	E Compartment
F Musculoskeletal	X External	3 Contractility	Z No Qualifier
H Products of Conception, ♀ Cardiac	7 Via Natural or Artificial Opening 8 Via Natural or Artificial Opening Endoscopic X External	4 Electrical Activity C Rate F Rhythm H Sound	Z No Qualifier
J Products of Conception, ♀ Nervous	7 Via Natural or Artificial Opening 8 Via Natural or Artificial Opening Endoscopic X External	2 Conductivity 4 Electrical Activity B Pressure	Z No Qualifier
Z None	7 Via Natural or Artificial Opening	6 Metabolism K Temperature	Z No Qualifier
Z None	X External	6 Metabolism K Temperature Q Sleep	Z No Qualifier

Valid OR   4A06Ø[5,B]Z   ♀   4AØH[7,8,X][4,C,F,H]Z
Valid OR   4AØC4[5,B]Z   ♀   4AØJ[7,8,X][2,4,B]Z

Non-OR Procedure   DRG Non-OR Procedure   Valid OR Procedure   HAC Associated Procedure   Combination Only   New/Revised April   New/Revised October

736   ICD-10-PCS 2024

4   Measurement and Monitoring
A   Physiological Systems
1   Monitoring   Definition: Determining the level of a physiological or physical function repetitively over a period of time

Body System Character 4	Approach Character 5	Function/Device Character 6	Qualifier Character 7
Ø Central Nervous	Ø Open	2 Conductivity B Pressure	Z No Qualifier
Ø Central Nervous	Ø Open	4 Electrical Activity	G Intraoperative Z No Qualifier
Ø Central Nervous	3 Percutaneous 7 Via Natural or Artificial Opening 8 Via Natural or Artificial Opening Endoscopic	4 Electrical Activity	G Intraoperative Z No Qualifier
Ø Central Nervous	3 Percutaneous 7 Via Natural or Artificial Opening 8 Via Natural or Artificial Opening Endoscopic	B Pressure K Temperature R Saturation	D Intracranial
Ø Central Nervous	X External	2 Conductivity	Z No Qualifier
Ø Central Nervous	X External	4 Electrical Activity	G Intraoperative Z No Qualifier
1 Peripheral Nervous	Ø Open 3 Percutaneous 7 Via Natural or Artificial Opening 8 Via Natural or Artificial Opening Endoscopic X External	2 Conductivity	9 Sensory B Motor
1 Peripheral Nervous	Ø Open 3 Percutaneous 7 Via Natural or Artificial Opening 8 Via Natural or Artificial Opening Endoscopic X External	4 Electrical Activity	G Intraoperative Z No Qualifier
2 Cardiac	Ø Open 3 Percutaneous 7 Via Natural or Artificial Opening 8 Via Natural or Artificial Opening Endoscopic	4 Electrical Activity 9 Output C Rate F Rhythm H Sound	Z No Qualifier
2 Cardiac	X External	4 Electrical Activity	5 Ambulatory Z No Qualifier
2 Cardiac	X External	9 Output C Rate F Rhythm H Sound	Z No Qualifier
2 Cardiac	X External	M Total Activity	4 Stress
2 Cardiac	X External	S Vascular Perfusion	H Indocyanine Green Dye
3 Arterial	Ø Open 3 Percutaneous	5 Flow B Pressure J Pulse	1 Peripheral 3 Pulmonary C Coronary
3 Arterial	Ø Open 3 Percutaneous	H Sound R Saturation	1 Peripheral
3 Arterial	X External	5 Flow B Pressure H Sound J Pulse R Saturation	1 Peripheral
4 Venous	Ø Open 3 Percutaneous	5 Flow B Pressure J Pulse	Ø Central 1 Peripheral 2 Portal 3 Pulmonary
4 Venous	Ø Open 3 Percutaneous	R Saturation	Ø Central 2 Portal 3 Pulmonary
4 Venous	X External	5 Flow B Pressure J Pulse	1 Peripheral
6 Lymphatic	Ø Open 3 Percutaneous 7 Via Natural or Artificial Opening 8 Via Natural or Artificial Opening Endoscopic	5 Flow	H Indocyanine Green Dye Z No Qualifier

Valid OR   4A1605Z

4A1 Continued on next page

NC Noncovered Procedure   **LC** Limited Coverage   **QA** Questionable OB Admit   **NT** New Tech Add-on   ⊞ Combination Member   ♂ Male   ♀ Female

ICD-10-PCS 2024   737

4   Measurement and Monitoring
A   Physiological Systems
1   Monitoring   Definition: Determining the level of a physiological or physical function repetitively over a period of time

4A1 Continued

Body System Character 4	Approach Character 5	Function/Device Character 6	Qualifier Character 7
6 Lymphatic	Ø Open 3 Percutaneous 7 Via Natural or Artificial Opening 8 Via Natural or Artificial Opening Endoscopic	B Pressure	Z No Qualifier
9 Respiratory	7 Via Natural or Artificial Opening X External	1 Capacity 5 Flow C Rate D Resistance L Volume	Z No Qualifier
B Gastrointestinal	7 Via Natural or Artificial Opening 8 Via Natural or Artificial Opening Endoscopic	8 Motility B Pressure G Secretion	Z No Qualifier
B Gastrointestinal	X External	S Vascular Perfusion	H Indocyanine Green Dye
D Urinary	7 Via Natural or Artificial Opening 8 Via Natural or Artificial Opening Endoscopic	3 Contractility 5 Flow B Pressure D Resistance L Volume	Z No Qualifier
G Skin and Breast	X External	S Vascular Perfusion	H Indocyanine Green Dye
H Products of Conception, ♀ Cardiac	7 Via Natural or Artificial Opening 8 Via Natural or Artificial Opening Endoscopic X External	4 Electrical Activity C Rate F Rhythm H Sound	Z No Qualifier
J Products of Conception, ♀ Nervous	7 Via Natural or Artificial Opening 8 Via Natural or Artificial Opening Endoscopic X External	2 Conductivity 4 Electrical Activity B Pressure	Z No Qualifier
Z None	7 Via Natural or Artificial Opening	K Temperature	Z No Qualifier
Z None	X External	K Temperature Q Sleep	Z No Qualifier

Valid OR   4A16ØBZ
♀   4A1H[7,8,X][4,C,F,H]Z
♀   4A1J[7,8,X][2,4,B]Z

4   Measurement and Monitoring
B   Physiological Devices
Ø   Measurement   Definition: Determining the level of a physiological or physical function at a point in time

Body System Character 4	Approach Character 5	Function/Device Character 6	Qualifier Character 7
Ø Central Nervous	X External	V Stimulator	Z No Qualifier
Ø Central Nervous	X External	W Cerebrospinal Fluid Shunt	Ø Wireless Sensor
1 Peripheral Nervous F Musculoskeletal	X External	V Stimulator	Z No Qualifier
2 Cardiac	X External	S Pacemaker T Defibrillator	Z No Qualifier
9 Respiratory	X External	S Pacemaker	Z No Qualifier

Non-OR Procedure   DRG Non-OR Procedure   Valid OR Procedure   HAC Associated Procedure   Combination Only   New/Revised April   New/Revised October

738   ICD-10-PCS 2024

Extracorporeal or Systemic Assistance and Performance 5A0–5A2

AHA Coding Clinic for table 5A0

2022, 4Q, 61-62	Cardiac perfusion with intra-arterial supersaturated oxygen
2022, 3Q, 23	Placement of preCARDIA device
2021, 2Q, 12	Repositioning of displaced intra-aortic balloon pump
2020, 4Q, 64-65	Ventilatory assistance by high flow or high velocity nasal cannula devices
2020, 1Q, 10	Intermittent use of continuous positive airway pressure
2018, 2Q, 3-5	Intra-aortic balloon pump
2017, 4Q, 43-44	Insertion of external heart assist devices
2017, 3Q, 18	Intra-aortic balloon pump removal
2017, 1Q, 10-11	External heart assist device
2017, 1Q, 29	Newborn resuscitation using positive pressure ventilation
2017, 1Q, 29	Newborn noninvasive ventilation
2016, 4Q, 137-139	Heart assist device systems
2014, 4Q, 9	Mechanical ventilation
2014, 3Q, 19	Ablation of ventricular tachycardia with Impella® support
2013, 3Q, 18	Heart transplant surgery

AHA Coding Clinic for table 5A1

2022, 2Q, 25	Temporary-permanent pacemaker placement
2021, 4Q, 56	Automated chest compression
2019, 4Q, 39-41	Intraoperative extracorporeal membrane oxygenation
2019, 3Q, 19	Insertion of left ventricular catheter
2019, 3Q, 20	Removal and revision of ECMO component
2019, 3Q, 21	Exchange of extracorporeal membrane oxygenation component (oxygenator)

AHA Coding Clinic for table 5A1 (Continued)

2019, 2Q, 36	Veno-arterial extracorporeal membrane oxygenation via sternotomy
2019, 3Q, 22	Extracorporeal membrane oxygenation and Centrimag™ pump
2019, 3Q, 22	Extracorporeal membrane oxygenation transfers
2018, 4Q, 52-54	Percutaneous extracorporeal membrane oxygenation
2018, 1Q, 13	Mechanical ventilation using patient's equipment
2017, 4Q, 71-73	Hemodialysis and renal replacement therapy
2017, 3Q, 7	Senning procedure (arterial switch)
2017, 1Q, 19	Norwood Sano procedure
2016, 1Q, 27	Aortocoronary bypass graft utilizing Y-graft
2016, 1Q, 28	Extracorporeal liver assist device
2016, 1Q, 29	Duration of hemodialysis
2015, 4Q, 22-24	Congenital heart corrective procedures
2014, 4Q, 3-10	Mechanical ventilation
2014, 4Q, 11-15	Sequencing of mechanical ventilation with other procedures
2014, 3Q, 16	Repair of Tetralogy of Fallot
2014, 3Q, 20	MAZE procedure performed with coronary artery bypass graft
2014, 1Q, 10	Repair of thoracic aortic aneurysm & coronary artery bypass graft
2013, 3Q, 18	Heart transplant surgery

AHA Coding Clinic for table 5A2

2022, 1Q, 46	Internal cardioversion

5   Extracorporeal or Systemic Assistance and Performance
A   Physiological Systems
0   Assistance   Definition: Taking over a portion of a physiological function by extracorporeal means

Body System Character 4	Duration Character 5	Function Character 6	Qualifier Character 7
2 Cardiac	1 Intermittent	1 Output	0 Balloon Pump 5 Pulsatile Compression 6 Other Pump D Impeller Pump
2 Cardiac	2 Continuous	1 Output	0 Balloon Pump 5 Pulsatile Compression 6 Other Pump D Impeller Pump
2 Cardiac	2 Continuous	2 Oxygenation	C Supersaturated
5 Circulatory	1 Intermittent 2 Continuous	2 Oxygenation	1 Hyperbaric
9 Respiratory	2 Continuous	0 Filtration **NT**	Z No Qualifier
9 Respiratory	3 Less than 24 Consecutive Hours 4 24-96 Consecutive Hours 5 Greater than 96 Consecutive Hours	5 Ventilation	7 Continuous Positive Airway Pressure 8 Intermittent Positive Airway Pressure 9 Continuous Negative Airway Pressure A High Nasal Flow/Velocity B Intermittent Negative Airway Pressure Z No Qualifier
9 Respiratory	B Less than 8 Consecutive Hours C 8-24 Consecutive Hours D Greater than 24 Consecutive Hours	5 Ventilation	K Intubated Prone Positioning

Valid OR 5A0211[0,6,D]
Valid OR 5A0221[0,6,D]
NT 5A0920Z for Hemolung Respiratory Assist System (RAS)

Extracorporeal or Systemic Assistance and Performance (left margin, rotated)

5   Extracorporeal or Systemic Assistance and Performance
A   Physiological Systems
1   Performance   Definition: Completely taking over a physiological function by extracorporeal means

Body System Character 4	Duration Character 5	Function Character 6	Qualifier Character 7
2 Cardiac	Ø Single	1 Output	2 Manual
2 Cardiac	1 Intermittent	3 Pacing	Z No Qualifier
2 Cardiac	2 Continuous	1 Output	J Automated Z No Qualifier
2 Cardiac	2 Continuous	3 Pacing	Z No Qualifier
5 Circulatory	2 Continuous A Intraoperative	2 Oxygenation	F Membrane, Central G Membrane, Peripheral Veno-arterial H Membrane, Peripheral Veno-venous
9 Respiratory	Ø Single	5 Ventilation	4 Nonmechanical
9 Respiratory	3 Less than 24 Consecutive Hours 4 24-96 Consecutive Hours 5 Greater than 96 Consecutive Hours	5 Ventilation	Z No Qualifier
C Biliary	Ø Single 6 Multiple	Ø Filtration	Z No Qualifier
D Urinary	7 Intermittent, Less than 6 Hours per day 8 Prolonged Intermittent, 6-18 Hours per day 9 Continuous, Greater than 18 Hours per day	Ø Filtration	Z No Qualifier

Valid OR   5A1522F
DRG Non-OR   5A1522[G,H]
DRG Non-OR   5A19[3,4]5Z
DRG Non-OR   5A1955Z Length of stay must be > 4 consecutive days.
DRG Non-OR   5A1D[7,8,9]ØZ

5   Extracorporeal or Systemic Assistance and Performance
A   Physiological Systems
2   Restoration   Definition: Returning, or attempting to return, a physiological function to its original state by extracorporeal means.

Body System Character 4	Duration Character 5	Function Character 6	Qualifier Character 7
2 Cardiac	Ø Single	4 Rhythm	Z No Qualifier

Non-OR Procedure   DRG Non-OR Procedure   Valid OR Procedure   HAC Associated Procedure   Combination Only   New/Revised April   New/Revised October

740   ICD-10-PCS 2024

Extracorporeal or Systemic Therapies 6A0–6AB

AHA Coding Clinic for table 6A4
2019, 2Q, 17   Cryoamputation of lower leg

AHA Coding Clinic for table 6A5
2022, 1Q, 48   Umbilical cord blood sampling

AHA Coding Clinic for table 6A7
2014, 4Q, 19   Ultrasound accelerated thrombolysis

AHA Coding Clinic for table 6AB
2023, 2Q, 32   Preparation of donor organ before transplantation
2016, 4Q, 115   Donor organ perfusion

6   Extracorporeal or Systemic Therapies
A   Physiological Systems
0   Atmospheric Control   Definition: Extracorporeal control of atmospheric pressure and composition

Body System Character 4	Duration Character 5	Qualifier Character 6	Qualifier Character 7
Z None	0 Single 1 Multiple	Z No Qualifier	Z No Qualifier

6   Extracorporeal or Systemic Therapies
A   Physiological Systems
1   Decompression   Definition: Extracorporeal elimination of undissolved gas from body fluids

Body System Character 4	Duration Character 5	Qualifier Character 6	Qualifier Character 7
5 Circulatory	0 Single 1 Multiple	Z No Qualifier	Z No Qualifier

6   Extracorporeal or Systemic Therapies
A   Physiological Systems
2   Electromagnetic Therapy   Definition: Extracorporeal treatment by electromagnetic rays

Body System Character 4	Duration Character 5	Qualifier Character 6	Qualifier Character 7
1 Urinary 2 Central Nervous	0 Single 1 Multiple	Z No Qualifier	Z No Qualifier

6   Extracorporeal or Systemic Therapies
A   Physiological Systems
3   Hyperthermia   Definition: Extracorporeal raising of body temperature

Body System Character 4	Duration Character 5	Qualifier Character 6	Qualifier Character 7
Z None	0 Single 1 Multiple	Z No Qualifier	Z No Qualifier

6   Extracorporeal or Systemic Therapies
A   Physiological Systems
4   Hypothermia   Definition: Extracorporeal lowering of body temperature

Body System Character 4	Duration Character 5	Qualifier Character 6	Qualifier Character 7
Z None	0 Single 1 Multiple	Z No Qualifier	Z No Qualifier

6   Extracorporeal or Systemic Therapies
A   Physiological Systems
5   Pheresis   Definition: Extracorporeal separation of blood products

Body System Character 4	Duration Character 5	Qualifier Character 6	Qualifier Character 7
5 Circulatory	0 Single 1 Multiple	Z No Qualifier	0 Erythrocytes 1 Leukocytes 2 Platelets 3 Plasma T Stem Cells, Cord Blood V Stem Cells, Hematopoietic

NC Noncovered Procedure   LC Limited Coverage   QA Questionable OB Admit   NT New Tech Add-on   ⊞ Combination Member   ♂ Male   ♀ Female

ICD-10-PCS 2024   741

6   Extracorporeal or Systemic Therapies
A   Physiological Systems
6   Phototherapy   Definition: Extracorporeal treatment by light rays

Body System Character 4	Duration Character 5	Qualifier Character 6	Qualifier Character 7
Ø Skin 5 Circulatory	Ø Single 1 Multiple	Z No Qualifier	Z No Qualifier

6   Extracorporeal or Systemic Therapies
A   Physiological Systems
7   Ultrasound Therapy   Definition: Extracorporeal treatment by ultrasound

Body System Character 4	Duration Character 5	Qualifier Character 6	Qualifier Character 7
5 Circulatory	Ø Single 1 Multiple	Z No Qualifier	4 Head and Neck Vessels 5 Heart 6 Peripheral Vessels 7 Other Vessels Z No Qualifier

6   Extracorporeal or Systemic Therapies
A   Physiological Systems
8   Ultraviolet Light Therapy   Definition: Extracorporeal treatment by ultraviolet light

Body System Character 4	Duration Character 5	Qualifier Character 6	Qualifier Character 7
Ø Skin	Ø Single 1 Multiple	Z No Qualifier	Z No Qualifier

6   Extracorporeal or Systemic Therapies
A   Physiological Systems
9   Shock Wave Therapy   Definition: Extracorporeal treatment by shock waves

Body System Character 4	Duration Character 5	Qualifier Character 6	Qualifier Character 7
3 Musculoskeletal	Ø Single 1 Multiple	Z No Qualifier	Z No Qualifier

6   Extracorporeal or Systemic Therapies
A   Physiological Systems
B   Perfusion   Definition: Extracorporeal treatment by diffusion of therapeutic fluid

Body System Character 4	Duration Character 5	Qualifier Character 6	Qualifier Character 7
5 Circulatory B Respiratory System F Hepatobiliary System and Pancreas T Urinary System	Ø Single	B Donor Organ	Z No Qualifier

Non-OR Procedure   DRG Non-OR Procedure   Valid OR Procedure   HAC Associated Procedure   Combination Only   New/Revised April   New/Revised October

742   ICD-10-PCS 2024

Osteopathic 7W0

7   **Osteopathic**
W   **Anatomical Regions**
0   **Treatment**   Definition: Manual treatment to eliminate or alleviate somatic dysfunction and related disorders

Body Region Character 4	Approach Character 5	Method Character 6	Qualifier Character 7
0 Head	X External	0 Articulatory-Raising	Z None
1 Cervical		1 Fascial Release	
2 Thoracic		2 General Mobilization	
3 Lumbar		3 High Velocity-Low Amplitude	
4 Sacrum		4 Indirect	
5 Pelvis		5 Low Velocity-High Amplitude	
6 Lower Extremities		6 Lymphatic Pump	
7 Upper Extremities		7 Muscle Energy-Isometric	
8 Rib Cage		8 Muscle Energy-Isotonic	
9 Abdomen		9 Other Method	

NC Noncovered Procedure   **LC** Limited Coverage   **QA** Questionable OB Admit   **NT** New Tech Add-on   ⊞ Combination Member   ♂ Male   ♀ Female

ICD-10-PCS 2024   **743**

7W0–7W0

Other Procedures 8C0–8E0

AHA Coding Clinic for table 8E0

2021, 4Q, 49	Division of liver for staged hepatectomy
2021, 2Q, 19	Electromagnetic stealth guided ventriculoperitoneal shunt insertion with endoscopy
2020, 4Q, 53	Bypass pancreatic duct to stomach
2020, 4Q, 65-66	Near infrared spectroscopy for tissue viability assessment
2020, 4Q, 99	Robotic-assisted prostatectomy with extension of incision for specimen removal
2020, 4Q, 100	Robotic-assisted sigmoid colectomy with extension of incision for specimen removal
2019, 4Q, 41-42	Intraoperative fluorescence guidance
2019, 1Q, 30	Laparoscopic-assisted rectopexy with manual reduction of prolapse
2015, 1Q, 33	Robotic-assisted laparoscopic hysterectomy converted to open procedure
2014, 4Q, 33	Radical prostatectomy

8   Other Procedures
C   Indwelling Device
0   Other Procedures   Definition: Methodologies which attempt to remediate or cure a disorder or disease

Body Region Character 4	Approach Character 5	Method Character 6	Qualifier Character 7
1 Nervous System	X External	6 Collection	J Cerebrospinal Fluid L Other Fluid
2 Circulatory System	X External	6 Collection	K Blood L Other Fluid

NC Noncovered Procedure   LC Limited Coverage   QA Questionable OB Admit   NT New Tech Add-on   ⊞ Combination Member   ♂ Male   ♀ Female

ICD-10-PCS 2024   745

Other Procedures

8   Other Procedures
E   Physiological Systems and Anatomical Regions
0   Other Procedures   Definition: Methodologies which attempt to remediate or cure a disorder or disease

Body Region Character 4	Approach Character 5	Method Character 6	Qualifier Character 7
1 Nervous System	X External	Y Other Method	7 Examination
2 Circulatory System	3 Percutaneous X External	D Near Infrared Spectroscopy	Z No Qualifier
9 Head and Neck Region	0 Open	C Robotic Assisted Procedure	Z No Qualifier
9 Head and Neck Region	0 Open	E Fluorescence Guided Procedure	M Aminolevulinic Acid Z No Qualifier
9 Head and Neck Region	3 Percutaneous 4 Percutaneous Endoscopic 7 Via Natural or Artificial Opening 8 Via Natural or Artificial Opening Endoscopic	C Robotic Assisted Procedure E Fluorescence Guided Procedure	Z No Qualifier
9 Head and Neck Region	X External	B Computer Assisted Procedure	F With Fluoroscopy G With Computerized Tomography H With Magnetic Resonance Imaging Z No Qualifier
9 Head and Neck Region	X External	C Robotic Assisted Procedure	Z No Qualifier
9 Head and Neck Region	X External	Y Other Method	8 Suture Removal
H Integumentary System and Breast	3 Percutaneous	0 Acupuncture	0 Anesthesia Z No Qualifier
H Integumentary System and Breast ♀	X External	6 Collection	2 Breast Milk
H Integumentary System and Breast	X External	Y Other Method	9 Piercing
K Musculoskeletal System	X External	1 Therapeutic Massage	Z No Qualifier
K Musculoskeletal System	X External	Y Other Method	7 Examination
U Female Reproductive System ♀	0 Open 3 Percutaneous 4 Percutaneous Endoscopic 7 Via Natural or Artificial Opening 8 Via Natural or Artificial Opening Endoscopic	E Fluorescence Guided Procedure	N Pafolacianine
U Female Reproductive System ♀	X External	Y Other Method	7 Examination
V Male Reproductive System ♂	X External	1 Therapeutic Massage	C Prostate D Rectum
V Male Reproductive System ♂	X External	6 Collection	3 Sperm
W Trunk Region	0 Open 3 Percutaneous 4 Percutaneous Endoscopic 7 Via Natural or Artificial Opening 8 Via Natural or Artificial Opening Endoscopic	C Robotic Assisted Procedure	Z No Qualifier
W Trunk Region	0 Open 3 Percutaneous 4 Percutaneous Endoscopic 7 Via Natural or Artificial Opening 8 Via Natural or Artificial Opening Endoscopic	E Fluorescence Guided Procedure	N Pafolacianine Z No Qualifier
W Trunk Region	X External	B Computer Assisted Procedure	F With Fluoroscopy G With Computerized Tomography H With Magnetic Resonance Imaging Z No Qualifier
W Trunk Region	X External	C Robotic Assisted Procedure	Z No Qualifier
W Trunk Region	X External	Y Other Method	8 Suture Removal
X Upper Extremity Y Lower Extremity	0 Open 3 Percutaneous 4 Percutaneous Endoscopic	C Robotic Assisted Procedure E Fluorescence Guided Procedure	Z No Qualifier
X Upper Extremity Y Lower Extremity	X External	B Computer Assisted Procedure	F With Fluoroscopy G With Computerized Tomography H With Magnetic Resonance Imaging Z No Qualifier
X Upper Extremity Y Lower Extremity	X External	C Robotic Assisted Procedure	Z No Qualifier
X Upper Extremity Y Lower Extremity	X External	Y Other Method	8 Suture Removal
Z None	X External	Y Other Method	1 In Vitro Fertilization 4 Yoga Therapy 5 Meditation 6 Isolation

♂	8E0VX1C	♀	8E0UXY7
♂	8E0VX63	♀	8E0HX62

Non-OR Procedure   DRG Non-OR Procedure   Valid OR Procedure   HAC Associated Procedure   Combination Only   New/Revised April   New/Revised October

746   ICD-10-PCS 2024

Chiropractic 9WB

9   Chiropractic
W   Anatomical Regions
B   Manipulation   Definition: Manual procedure that involves a directed thrust to move a joint past the physiological range of motion, without exceeding the anatomical limit

Body Region Character 4	Approach Character 5	Method Character 6	Qualifier Character 7
Ø Head	X External	B Non-Manual	Z None
1 Cervical		C Indirect Visceral	
2 Thoracic		D Extra-Articular	
3 Lumbar		F Direct Visceral	
4 Sacrum		G Long Lever Specific Contact	
5 Pelvis		H Short Lever Specific Contact	
6 Lower Extremities		J Long and Short Lever Specific	
7 Upper Extremities		Contact	
8 Rib Cage		K Mechanically Assisted	
9 Abdomen		L Other Method	

NC Noncovered Procedure   LC Limited Coverage   QA Questionable OB Admit   NT New Tech Add-on   ⊞ Combination Member   ♂ Male   ♀ Female

ICD-10-PCS 2024   747

Imaging B00–BY4

AHA Coding Clinic for table B21
2018, 1Q, 12   Percutaneous balloon valvuloplasty & cardiac catheterization with ventriculogram
2016, 3Q, 36   Type of contrast medium for angiography (high osmolar, low osmolar, and other)

AHA Coding Clinic for table B41
2015, 3Q, 9   Aborted endovascular stenting of superficial femoral artery

AHA Coding Clinic for table B51
2015, 4Q, 30   Vascular access devices

AHA Coding Clinic for table BB3
2022, 4Q, 62   Hyperpolarized Xenon-129 gas for imaging of lung function

AHA Coding Clinic for table BF1
2021, 4Q, 57   Fluoroscopic guidance of hepatobiliary sites

AHA Coding Clinic for table BF4
2014, 3Q, 15   Drainage of pancreatic pseudocyst
2020, 4Q, 66   Other imaging type

AHA Coding Clinic for table BF5
2020, 4Q, 66   Other imaging type
2020, 4Q, 66-67   Fluorescence imaging of hepatobiliary system

AHA Coding Clinic for table BW5
2020, 4Q, 66   Other imaging type
2020, 4Q, 68   Bacterial autofluorescence detection

Contrast Agents

High Osmolar (Ø)	Low Osmolar (1)	Other Contrast (Y)
cholografin meglumine	hexabrix	iodixanol
conray	iohexol	iotrolan
cysto-conray II	iomeprol	isovist
cystografin	iomeron	visipaque
cystografin-dilute	iopamidol	
diatrizoate	iopromide	
gastrografin	ioversol	
hypaque	ioxaglate	
iothalamate	ioxilan	
isopaque	isovue	
md-76r	omnipaque	
metrizoate	optiray	
reno-dip	oxilan	
sinografin	ultravist	

B   **Imaging**
Ø   **Central Nervous System**
Ø   **Plain Radiography**   Definition: Planar display of an image developed from the capture of external ionizing radiation on photographic or photoconductive plate

Body Part Character 4	Contrast Character 5	Qualifier Character 6	Qualifier Character 7
B Spinal Cord	Ø High Osmolar 1 Low Osmolar Y Other Contrast Z None	Z None	Z None

B   **Imaging**
Ø   **Central Nervous System**
1   **Fluoroscopy**   Definition: Single plane or bi-plane real time display of an image developed from the capture of external ionizing radiation on a fluorescent screen. The image may also be stored by either digital or analog means.

Body Part Character 4	Contrast Character 5	Qualifier Character 6	Qualifier Character 7
B Spinal Cord	Ø High Osmolar 1 Low Osmolar Y Other Contrast Z None	Z None	Z None

NC Noncovered Procedure   **LC** Limited Coverage   **QA** Questionable OB Admit   **NT** New Tech Add-on   ✛ Combination Member   ♂ Male   ♀ Female

ICD-10-PCS 2024   749

B00–B01

B   Imaging
0   Central Nervous System
2   Computerized Tomography (CT Scan) Definition: Computer reformatted digital display of multiplanar images developed from the capture of multiple exposures of external ionizing radiation

Body Part Character 4	Contrast Character 5	Qualifier Character 6	Qualifier Character 7
0 Brain 7 Cisterna 8 Cerebral Ventricle(s) 9 Sella Turcica/Pituitary Gland B Spinal Cord	0 High Osmolar 1 Low Osmolar Y Other Contrast	0 Unenhanced and Enhanced Z None	Z None
0 Brain 7 Cisterna 8 Cerebral Ventricle(s) 9 Sella Turcica/Pituitary Gland B Spinal Cord	Z None	Z None	Z None

B   Imaging
0   Central Nervous System
3   Magnetic Resonance Imaging (MRI) Definition: Computer reformatted digital display of multiplanar images developed from the capture of radio-frequency signals emitted by nuclei in a body site excited within a magnetic field

Body Part Character 4	Contrast Character 5	Qualifier Character 6	Qualifier Character 7
0 Brain 9 Sella Turcica/Pituitary Gland B Spinal Cord C Acoustic Nerves	Y Other Contrast	0 Unenhanced and Enhanced Z None	Z None
0 Brain 9 Sella Turcica/Pituitary Gland B Spinal Cord C Acoustic Nerves	Z None	Z None	Z None

B   Imaging
0   Central Nervous System
4   Ultrasonography Definition: Real time display of images of anatomy or flow information developed from the capture of reflected and attenuated high frequency sound waves

Body Part Character 4	Contrast Character 5	Qualifier Character 6	Qualifier Character 7
0 Brain B Spinal Cord	Z None	Z None	Z None

B   Imaging
2   Heart
0   Plain Radiography Definition: Planar display of an image developed from the capture of external ionizing radiation on photographic or photoconductive plate

Body Part Character 4	Contrast Character 5	Qualifier Character 6	Qualifier Character 7
0 Coronary Artery, Single 1 Coronary Arteries, Multiple 2 Coronary Artery Bypass Graft, Single 3 Coronary Artery Bypass Grafts, Multiple 4 Heart, Right 5 Heart, Left 6 Heart, Right and Left 7 Internal Mammary Bypass Graft, Right 8 Internal Mammary Bypass Graft, Left F Bypass Graft, Other	0 High Osmolar 1 Low Osmolar Y Other Contrast	Z None	Z None

DRG Non-OR   All body part, contrast, and qualifier values

Non-OR Procedure   DRG Non-OR Procedure   Valid OR Procedure   HAC Associated Procedure   Combination Only   New/Revised April   New/Revised October

750   ICD-10-PCS 2024

B02–B20

B   Imaging
2   Heart
1   Fluoroscopy   Definition: Single plane or bi-plane real time display of an image developed from the capture of external ionizing radiation on a fluorescent screen. The image may also be stored by either digital or analog means.

Body Part Character 4	Contrast Character 5	Qualifier Character 6	Qualifier Character 7
Ø Coronary Artery, Single 1 Coronary Arteries, Multiple 2 Coronary Artery Bypass Graft, Single 3 Coronary Artery Bypass Grafts, Multiple	Ø High Osmolar 1 Low Osmolar Y Other Contrast	1 Laser	Ø Intraoperative
Ø Coronary Artery, Single 1 Coronary Arteries, Multiple 2 Coronary Artery Bypass Graft, Single 3 Coronary Artery Bypass Grafts, Multiple	Ø High Osmolar 1 Low Osmolar Y Other Contrast	Z None	Z None
4 Heart, Right 5 Heart, Left 6 Heart, Right and Left 7 Internal Mammary Bypass Graft, Right 8 Internal Mammary Bypass Graft, Left F Bypass Graft, Other	Ø High Osmolar 1 Low Osmolar Y Other Contrast	Z None	Z None

DRG Non-OR   B21[Ø,1,2,3][Ø,1,Y]ZZ
DRG Non-OR   B21[4,5,6,7,8,F][Ø,1,Y]ZZ

B   Imaging
2   Heart
2   Computerized Tomography (CT Scan)   Definition: Computer reformatted digital display of multiplanar images developed from the capture of multiple exposures of external ionizing radiation

Body Part Character 4	Contrast Character 5	Qualifier Character 6	Qualifier Character 7
1 Coronary Arteries, Multiple 3 Coronary Artery Bypass Grafts, Multiple 6 Heart, Right and Left	Ø High Osmolar 1 Low Osmolar Y Other Contrast	Ø Unenhanced and Enhanced Z None	Z None
1 Coronary Arteries, Multiple 3 Coronary Artery Bypass Grafts, Multiple 6 Heart, Right and Left	Z None	2 Intravascular Optical Coherence Z None	Z None

B   Imaging
2   Heart
3   Magnetic Resonance Imaging (MRI)   Definition: Computer reformatted digital display of multiplanar images developed from the capture of radio-frequency signals emitted by nuclei in a body site excited within a magnetic field

Body Part Character 4	Contrast Character 5	Qualifier Character 6	Qualifier Character 7
1 Coronary Arteries, Multiple 3 Coronary Artery Bypass Grafts, Multiple 6 Heart, Right and Left	Y Other Contrast	Ø Unenhanced and Enhanced Z None	Z None
1 Coronary Arteries, Multiple 3 Coronary Artery Bypass Grafts, Multiple 6 Heart, Right and Left	Z None	Z None	Z None

NC Noncovered Procedure   LC Limited Coverage   QA Questionable OB Admit   NT New Tech Add-on   ⊞ Combination Member   ♂ Male   ♀ Female
ICD-10-PCS 2024   751

B21–B23

B   **Imaging**
2   **Heart**
4   **Ultrasonography**   Definition: Real time display of images of anatomy or flow information developed from the capture of reflected and attenuated high frequency sound waves

Body Part Character 4	Contrast Character 5	Qualifier Character 6	Qualifier Character 7
Ø Coronary Artery, Single 1 Coronary Arteries, Multiple 4 Heart, Right 5 Heart, Left 6 Heart, Right and Left B Heart with Aorta C Pericardium D Pediatric Heart	Y Other Contrast	Z None	Z None
Ø Coronary Artery, Single 1 Coronary Arteries, Multiple 4 Heart, Right 5 Heart, Left 6 Heart, Right and Left B Heart with Aorta C Pericardium D Pediatric Heart	Z None	Z None	3 Intravascular 4 Transesophageal Z None

B   **Imaging**
3   **Upper Arteries**
Ø   **Plain Radiography**   Definition: Planar display of an image developed from the capture of external ionizing radiation on photographic or photoconductive plate

Body Part Character 4	Contrast Character 5	Qualifier Character 6	Qualifier Character 7
Ø Thoracic Aorta 1 Brachiocephalic-Subclavian Artery, Right 2 Subclavian Artery, Left 3 Common Carotid Artery, Right 4 Common Carotid Artery, Left 5 Common Carotid Arteries, Bilateral 6 Internal Carotid Artery, Right 7 Internal Carotid Artery, Left 8 Internal Carotid Arteries, Bilateral 9 External Carotid Artery, Right B External Carotid Artery, Left C External Carotid Arteries, Bilateral D Vertebral Artery, Right F Vertebral Artery, Left G Vertebral Arteries, Bilateral H Upper Extremity Arteries, Right J Upper Extremity Arteries, Left K Upper Extremity Arteries, Bilateral L Intercostal and Bronchial Arteries M Spinal Arteries N Upper Arteries, Other P Thoraco-Abdominal Aorta Q Cervico-Cerebral Arch R Intracranial Arteries S Pulmonary Artery, Right T Pulmonary Artery, Left	Ø High Osmolar 1 Low Osmolar Y Other Contrast Z None	Z None	Z None

Non-OR Procedure   DRG Non-OR Procedure   Valid OR Procedure   HAC Associated Procedure   Combination Only   New/Revised April   New/Revised October

752   ICD-10-PCS 2024

B24–B3Ø

B   Imaging
3   Upper Arteries
1   Fluoroscopy   Definition: Single plane or bi-plane real time display of an image developed from the capture of external ionizing radiation on a fluorescent screen. The image may also be stored by either digital or analog means.

Body Part Character 4	Contrast Character 5	Qualifier Character 6	Qualifier Character 7
Ø Thoracic Aorta 1 Brachiocephalic-Subclavian Artery, Right 2 Subclavian Artery, Left 3 Common Carotid Artery, Right 4 Common Carotid Artery, Left 5 Common Carotid Arteries, Bilateral 6 Internal Carotid Artery, Right 7 Internal Carotid Artery, Left 8 Internal Carotid Arteries, Bilateral 9 External Carotid Artery, Right B External Carotid Artery, Left C External Carotid Arteries, Bilateral D Vertebral Artery, Right F Vertebral Artery, Left G Vertebral Arteries, Bilateral H Upper Extremity Arteries, Right J Upper Extremity Arteries, Left K Upper Extremity Arteries, Bilateral L Intercostal and Bronchial Arteries M Spinal Arteries N Upper Arteries, Other P Thoraco-Abdominal Aorta Q Cervico-Cerebral Arch R Intracranial Arteries S Pulmonary Artery, Right T Pulmonary Artery, Left U Pulmonary Trunk	Ø High Osmolar 1 Low Osmolar Y Other Contrast	1 Laser	Ø Intraoperative
Ø Thoracic Aorta 1 Brachiocephalic-Subclavian Artery, Right 2 Subclavian Artery, Left 3 Common Carotid Artery, Right 4 Common Carotid Artery, Left 5 Common Carotid Arteries, Bilateral 6 Internal Carotid Artery, Right 7 Internal Carotid Artery, Left 8 Internal Carotid Arteries, Bilateral 9 External Carotid Artery, Right B External Carotid Artery, Left C External Carotid Arteries, Bilateral D Vertebral Artery, Right F Vertebral Artery, Left G Vertebral Arteries, Bilateral H Upper Extremity Arteries, Right J Upper Extremity Arteries, Left K Upper Extremity Arteries, Bilateral L Intercostal and Bronchial Arteries M Spinal Arteries N Upper Arteries, Other P Thoraco-Abdominal Aorta Q Cervico-Cerebral Arch R Intracranial Arteries S Pulmonary Artery, Right T Pulmonary Artery, Left U Pulmonary Trunk	Ø High Osmolar 1 Low Osmolar Y Other Contrast	Z None	Z None

B31 Continued on next page

NC Noncovered Procedure   LC Limited Coverage   QA Questionable OB Admit   NT New Tech Add-on   ⊞ Combination Member   ♂ Male   ♀ Female

ICD-10-PCS 2024

753

B31-B31

B   **Imaging**
3   **Upper Arteries**
1   **Fluoroscopy**   Definition: Single plane or bi-plane real time display of an image developed from the capture of external ionizing radiation on a fluorescent screen. The image may also be stored by either digital or analog means.

Body Part Character 4	Contrast Character 5	Qualifier Character 6	Qualifier Character 7
Ø Thoracic Aorta 1 Brachiocephalic-Subclavian Artery, Right 2 Subclavian Artery, Left 3 Common Carotid Artery, Right 4 Common Carotid Artery, Left 5 Common Carotid Arteries, Bilateral 6 Internal Carotid Artery, Right 7 Internal Carotid Artery, Left 8 Internal Carotid Arteries, Bilateral 9 External Carotid Artery, Right B External Carotid Artery, Left C External Carotid Arteries, Bilateral D Vertebral Artery, Right F Vertebral Artery, Left G Vertebral Arteries, Bilateral H Upper Extremity Arteries, Right J Upper Extremity Arteries, Left K Upper Extremity Arteries, Bilateral L Intercostal and Bronchial Arteries M Spinal Arteries N Upper Arteries, Other P Thoraco-Abdominal Aorta Q Cervico-Cerebral Arch R Intracranial Arteries S Pulmonary Artery, Right T Pulmonary Artery, Left U Pulmonary Trunk	Z None	Z None	Z None

B   **Imaging**
3   **Upper Arteries**
2   **Computerized Tomography (CT Scan)**   Definition: Computer reformatted digital display of multiplanar images developed from the capture of multiple exposures of external ionizing radiation

Body Part Character 4	Contrast Character 5	Qualifier Character 6	Qualifier Character 7
Ø Thoracic Aorta 5 Common Carotid Arteries, Bilateral 8 Internal Carotid Arteries, Bilateral G Vertebral Arteries, Bilateral R Intracranial Arteries S Pulmonary Artery, Right T Pulmonary Artery, Left	Ø High Osmolar 1 Low Osmolar Y Other Contrast	Z None	Z None
Ø Thoracic Aorta 5 Common Carotid Arteries, Bilateral 8 Internal Carotid Arteries, Bilateral G Vertebral Arteries, Bilateral R Intracranial Arteries S Pulmonary Artery, Right T Pulmonary Artery, Left	Z None	2 Intravascular Optical Coherence Z None	Z None

Non-OR Procedure   DRG Non-OR Procedure   Valid OR Procedure   HAC Associated Procedure   Combination Only   New/Revised April   New/Revised October

754   ICD-10-PCS 2024

B   **Imaging**
3   **Upper Arteries**
3   **Magnetic Resonance Imaging (MRI)**   Definition: Computer reformatted digital display of multiplanar images developed from the capture of radio-frequency signals emitted by nuclei in a body site excited within a magnetic field

Body Part Character 4	Contrast Character 5	Qualifier Character 6	Qualifier Character 7
Ø Thoracic Aorta 5 Common Carotid Arteries, Bilateral 8 Internal Carotid Arteries, Bilateral G Vertebral Arteries, Bilateral H Upper Extremity Arteries, Right J Upper Extremity Arteries, Left K Upper Extremity Arteries, Bilateral M Spinal Arteries Q Cervico-Cerebral Arch R Intracranial Arteries	Y Other Contrast	Ø Unenhanced and Enhanced Z None	Z None
Ø Thoracic Aorta 5 Common Carotid Arteries, Bilateral 8 Internal Carotid Arteries, Bilateral G Vertebral Arteries, Bilateral H Upper Extremity Arteries, Right J Upper Extremity Arteries, Left K Upper Extremity Arteries, Bilateral M Spinal Arteries Q Cervico-Cerebral Arch R Intracranial Arteries	Z None	Z None	Z None

B   **Imaging**
3   **Upper Arteries**
4   **Ultrasonography**   Definition: Real time display of images of anatomy or flow information developed from the capture of reflected and attenuated high frequency sound waves

Body Part Character 4	Contrast Character 5	Qualifier Character 6	Qualifier Character 7
Ø Thoracic Aorta 1 Brachiocephalic-Subclavian Artery, Right 2 Subclavian Artery, Left 3 Common Carotid Artery, Right 4 Common Carotid Artery, Left 5 Common Carotid Arteries, Bilateral 6 Internal Carotid Artery, Right 7 Internal Carotid Artery, Left 8 Internal Carotid Arteries, Bilateral H Upper Extremity Arteries, Right J Upper Extremity Arteries, Left K Upper Extremity Arteries, Bilateral R Intracranial Arteries S Pulmonary Artery, Right T Pulmonary Artery, Left V Ophthalmic Arteries	Z None	Z None	3 Intravascular Z None

B   **Imaging**
4   **Lower Arteries**
Ø   **Plain Radiography**   Definition: Planar display of an image developed from the capture of external ionizing radiation on photographic or photoconductive plate

Body Part Character 4	Contrast Character 5	Qualifier Character 6	Qualifier Character 7
Ø Abdominal Aorta 2 Hepatic Artery 3 Splenic Arteries 4 Superior Mesenteric Artery 5 Inferior Mesenteric Artery 6 Renal Artery, Right 7 Renal Artery, Left 8 Renal Arteries, Bilateral 9 Lumbar Arteries B Intra-Abdominal Arteries, Other C Pelvic Arteries D Aorta and Bilateral Lower Extremity Arteries F Lower Extremity Arteries, Right G Lower Extremity Arteries, Left J Lower Arteries, Other M Renal Artery Transplant	Ø High Osmolar 1 Low Osmolar Y Other Contrast	Z None	Z None

NC Noncovered Procedure   **LC** Limited Coverage   **QA** Questionable OB Admit   **NT** New Tech Add-on   ⊞ Combination Member   ♂ Male   ♀ Female

ICD-10-PCS 2024   755

B33–B4Ø

B Imaging
4 Lower Arteries
1 Fluoroscopy   Definition: Single plane or bi-plane real time display of an image developed from the capture of external ionizing radiation on a fluorescent screen. The image may also be stored by either digital or analog means.

Body Part Character 4	Contrast Character 5	Qualifier Character 6	Qualifier Character 7
Ø Abdominal Aorta 2 Hepatic Artery 3 Splenic Arteries 4 Superior Mesenteric Artery 5 Inferior Mesenteric Artery 6 Renal Artery, Right 7 Renal Artery, Left 8 Renal Arteries, Bilateral 9 Lumbar Arteries B Intra-Abdominal Arteries, Other C Pelvic Arteries D Aorta and Bilateral Lower Extremity Arteries F Lower Extremity Arteries, Right G Lower Extremity Arteries, Left J Lower Arteries, Other	Ø High Osmolar 1 Low Osmolar Y Other Contrast	1 Laser	Ø Intraoperative
Ø Abdominal Aorta 2 Hepatic Artery 3 Splenic Arteries 4 Superior Mesenteric Artery 5 Inferior Mesenteric Artery 6 Renal Artery, Right 7 Renal Artery, Left 8 Renal Arteries, Bilateral 9 Lumbar Arteries B Intra-Abdominal Arteries, Other C Pelvic Arteries D Aorta and Bilateral Lower Extremity Arteries F Lower Extremity Arteries, Right G Lower Extremity Arteries, Left J Lower Arteries, Other	Ø High Osmolar 1 Low Osmolar Y Other Contrast	Z None	Z None
Ø Abdominal Aorta 2 Hepatic Artery 3 Splenic Arteries 4 Superior Mesenteric Artery 5 Inferior Mesenteric Artery 6 Renal Artery, Right 7 Renal Artery, Left 8 Renal Arteries, Bilateral 9 Lumbar Arteries B Intra-Abdominal Arteries, Other C Pelvic Arteries D Aorta and Bilateral Lower Extremity Arteries F Lower Extremity Arteries, Right G Lower Extremity Arteries, Left J Lower Arteries, Other	Z None	Z None	Z None

Non-OR Procedure   DRG Non-OR Procedure   Valid OR Procedure   HAC Associated Procedure   Combination Only   New/Revised April   New/Revised October

756

ICD-10-PCS 2024

B   **Imaging**
4   **Lower Arteries**
2   **Computerized Tomography (CT Scan)** Definition: Computer reformatted digital display of multiplanar images developed from the capture of multiple exposures of external ionizing radiation

Body Part Character 4	Contrast Character 5	Qualifier Character 6	Qualifier Character 7
Ø Abdominal Aorta 1 Celiac Artery 4 Superior Mesenteric Artery 8 Renal Arteries, Bilateral C Pelvic Arteries F Lower Extremity Arteries, Right G Lower Extremity Arteries, Left H Lower Extremity Arteries, Bilateral M Renal Artery Transplant	Ø High Osmolar 1 Low Osmolar Y Other Contrast	Z None	Z None
Ø Abdominal Aorta 1 Celiac Artery 4 Superior Mesenteric Artery 8 Renal Arteries, Bilateral C Pelvic Arteries F Lower Extremity Arteries, Right G Lower Extremity Arteries, Left H Lower Extremity Arteries, Bilateral M Renal Artery Transplant	Z None	2 Intravascular Optical Coherence Z None	Z None

B   **Imaging**
4   **Lower Arteries**
3   **Magnetic Resonance Imaging (MRI)**   Definition: Computer reformatted digital display of multiplanar images developed from the capture of radio-frequency signals emitted by nuclei in a body site excited within a magnetic field

Body Part Character 4	Contrast Character 5	Qualifier Character 6	Qualifier Character 7
Ø Abdominal Aorta 1 Celiac Artery 4 Superior Mesenteric Artery 8 Renal Arteries, Bilateral C Pelvic Arteries F Lower Extremity Arteries, Right G Lower Extremity Arteries, Left H Lower Extremity Arteries, Bilateral	Y Other Contrast	Ø Unenhanced and Enhanced Z None	Z None
Ø Abdominal Aorta 1 Celiac Artery 4 Superior Mesenteric Artery 8 Renal Arteries, Bilateral C Pelvic Arteries F Lower Extremity Arteries, Right G Lower Extremity Arteries, Left H Lower Extremity Arteries, Bilateral	Z None	Z None	Z None

B   **Imaging**
4   **Lower Arteries**
4   **Ultrasonography**   Definition: Real time display of images of anatomy or flow information developed from the capture of reflected and attenuated high frequency sound waves

Body Part Character 4	Contrast Character 5	Qualifier Character 6	Qualifier Character 7
Ø Abdominal Aorta 4 Superior Mesenteric Artery 5 Inferior Mesenteric Artery 6 Renal Artery, Right 7 Renal Artery, Left 8 Renal Arteries, Bilateral B Intra-Abdominal Arteries, Other F Lower Extremity Arteries, Right G Lower Extremity Arteries, Left H Lower Extremity Arteries, Bilateral K Celiac and Mesenteric Arteries L Femoral Artery N Penile Arteries	Z None	Z None	3 Intravascular Z None

NC Noncovered Procedure   LC Limited Coverage   QA Questionable OB Admit   NT New Tech Add-on   ⊞ Combination Member   ♂ Male   ♀ Female
ICD-10-PCS 2024   757

B42–B44

B **Imaging**
5 **Veins**
Ø **Plain Radiography** Definition: Planar display of an image developed from the capture of external ionizing radiation on photographic or photoconductive plate

Body Part Character 4	Contrast Character 5	Qualifier Character 6	Qualifier Character 7
Ø Epidural Veins	Ø High Osmolar	Z None	Z None
1 Cerebral and Cerebellar Veins	1 Low Osmolar		
2 Intracranial Sinuses	Y Other Contrast		
3 Jugular Veins, Right			
4 Jugular Veins, Left			
5 Jugular Veins, Bilateral			
6 Subclavian Vein, Right			
7 Subclavian Vein, Left			
8 Superior Vena Cava			
9 Inferior Vena Cava			
B Lower Extremity Veins, Right			
C Lower Extremity Veins, Left			
D Lower Extremity Veins, Bilateral			
F Pelvic (Iliac) Veins, Right			
G Pelvic (Iliac) Veins, Left			
H Pelvic (Iliac) Veins, Bilateral			
J Renal Vein, Right			
K Renal Vein, Left			
L Renal Veins, Bilateral			
M Upper Extremity Veins, Right			
N Upper Extremity Veins, Left			
P Upper Extremity Veins, Bilateral			
Q Pulmonary Vein, Right			
R Pulmonary Vein, Left			
S Pulmonary Veins, Bilateral			
T Portal and Splanchnic Veins			
V Veins, Other			
W Dialysis Shunt/Fistula			

B **Imaging**
5 **Veins**
1 **Fluoroscopy** Definition: Single plane or bi-plane real time display of an image developed from the capture of external ionizing radiation on a fluorescent screen. The image may also be stored by either digital or analog means.

Body Part Character 4	Contrast Character 5	Qualifier Character 6	Qualifier Character 7
Ø Epidural Veins	Ø High Osmolar	Z None	A Guidance
1 Cerebral and Cerebellar Veins	1 Low Osmolar		Z None
2 Intracranial Sinuses	Y Other Contrast		
3 Jugular Veins, Right	Z None		
4 Jugular Veins, Left			
5 Jugular Veins, Bilateral			
6 Subclavian Vein, Right			
7 Subclavian Vein, Left			
8 Superior Vena Cava			
9 Inferior Vena Cava			
B Lower Extremity Veins, Right			
C Lower Extremity Veins, Left			
D Lower Extremity Veins, Bilateral			
F Pelvic (Iliac) Veins, Right			
G Pelvic (Iliac) Veins, Left			
H Pelvic (Iliac) Veins, Bilateral			
J Renal Vein, Right			
K Renal Vein, Left			
L Renal Veins, Bilateral			
M Upper Extremity Veins, Right			
N Upper Extremity Veins, Left			
P Upper Extremity Veins, Bilateral			
Q Pulmonary Vein, Right			
R Pulmonary Vein, Left			
S Pulmonary Veins, Bilateral			
T Portal and Splanchnic Veins			
V Veins, Other			
W Dialysis Shunt/Fistula			

Non-OR Procedure   DRG Non-OR Procedure   Valid OR Procedure   HAC Associated Procedure   Combination Only   New/Revised April   New/Revised October

758   ICD-10-PCS 2024

B5Ø–B51

B   **Imaging**
5   **Veins**
2   **Computerized Tomography (CT Scan)** Definition: Computer reformatted digital display of multiplanar images developed from the capture of multiple exposures of external ionizing radiation

Body Part Character 4	Contrast Character 5	Qualifier Character 6	Qualifier Character 7
2 Intracranial Sinuses **8** Superior Vena Cava **9** Inferior Vena Cava **F** Pelvic (Iliac) Veins, Right **G** Pelvic (Iliac) Veins, Left **H** Pelvic (Iliac) Veins, Bilateral **J** Renal Vein, Right **K** Renal Vein, Left **L** Renal Veins, Bilateral **Q** Pulmonary Vein, Right **R** Pulmonary Vein, Left **S** Pulmonary Veins, Bilateral **T** Portal and Splanchnic Veins	**Ø** High Osmolar **1** Low Osmolar **Y** Other Contrast	**Ø** Unenhanced and Enhanced **Z** None	**Z** None
2 Intracranial Sinuses **8** Superior Vena Cava **9** Inferior Vena Cava **F** Pelvic (Iliac) Veins, Right **G** Pelvic (Iliac) Veins, Left **H** Pelvic (Iliac) Veins, Bilateral **J** Renal Vein, Right **K** Renal Vein, Left **L** Renal Veins, Bilateral **Q** Pulmonary Vein, Right **R** Pulmonary Vein, Left **S** Pulmonary Veins, Bilateral **T** Portal and Splanchnic Veins	**Z** None	**2** Intravascular Optical Coherence **Z** None	**Z** None

B   **Imaging**
5   **Veins**
3   **Magnetic Resonance Imaging (MRI)**   Definition: Computer reformatted digital display of multiplanar images developed from the capture of radio-frequency signals emitted by nuclei in a body site excited within a magnetic field

Body Part Character 4	Contrast Character 5	Qualifier Character 6	Qualifier Character 7
1 Cerebral and Cerebellar Veins **2** Intracranial Sinuses **5** Jugular Veins, Bilateral **8** Superior Vena Cava **9** Inferior Vena Cava **B** Lower Extremity Veins, Right **C** Lower Extremity Veins, Left **D** Lower Extremity Veins, Bilateral **H** Pelvic (Iliac) Veins, Bilateral **L** Renal Veins, Bilateral **M** Upper Extremity Veins, Right **N** Upper Extremity Veins, Left **P** Upper Extremity Veins, Bilateral **S** Pulmonary Veins, Bilateral **T** Portal and Splanchnic Veins **V** Veins, Other	**Y** Other Contrast	**Ø** Unenhanced and Enhanced **Z** None	**Z** None
1 Cerebral and Cerebellar Veins **2** Intracranial Sinuses **5** Jugular Veins, Bilateral **8** Superior Vena Cava **9** Inferior Vena Cava **B** Lower Extremity Veins, Right **C** Lower Extremity Veins, Left **D** Lower Extremity Veins, Bilateral **H** Pelvic (Iliac) Veins, Bilateral **L** Renal Veins, Bilateral **M** Upper Extremity Veins, Right **N** Upper Extremity Veins, Left **P** Upper Extremity Veins, Bilateral **S** Pulmonary Veins, Bilateral **T** Portal and Splanchnic Veins **V** Veins, Other	**Z** None	**Z** None	**Z** None

NC Noncovered Procedure   **LC** Limited Coverage   **QA** Questionable OB Admit   **NT** New Tech Add-on   ⊞ Combination Member   ♂ Male   ♀ Female

ICD-10-PCS 2024   759

B52–B53

Imaging

B   Imaging
5   Veins
4   Ultrasonography   Definition: Real time display of images of anatomy or flow information developed from the capture of reflected and attenuated high frequency sound waves

Body Part Character 4	Contrast Character 5	Qualifier Character 6	Qualifier Character 7
3 Jugular Veins, Right 4 Jugular Veins, Left 6 Subclavian Vein, Right 7 Subclavian Vein, Left 8 Superior Vena Cava 9 Inferior Vena Cava B Lower Extremity Veins, Right C Lower Extremity Veins, Left D Lower Extremity Veins, Bilateral J Renal Vein, Right K Renal Vein, Left L Renal Veins, Bilateral M Upper Extremity Veins, Right N Upper Extremity Veins, Left P Upper Extremity Veins, Bilateral T Portal and Splanchnic Veins	Z None	Z None	3 Intravascular A Guidance Z None

B   Imaging
7   Lymphatic System
Ø   Plain Radiography   Definition: Planar display of an image developed from the capture of external ionizing radiation on photographic or photoconductive plate

Body Part Character 4	Contrast Character 5	Qualifier Character 6	Qualifier Character 7
Ø Abdominal/Retroperitoneal Lymphatics, Unilateral 1 Abdominal/Retroperitoneal Lymphatics, Bilateral 4 Lymphatics, Head and Neck 5 Upper Extremity Lymphatics, Right 6 Upper Extremity Lymphatics, Left 7 Upper Extremity Lymphatics, Bilateral 8 Lower Extremity Lymphatics, Right 9 Lower Extremity Lymphatics, Left B Lower Extremity Lymphatics, Bilateral C Lymphatics, Pelvic	Ø High Osmolar 1 Low Osmolar Y Other Contrast	Z None	Z None

B   Imaging
8   Eye
Ø   Plain Radiography   Definition: Planar display of an image developed from the capture of external ionizing radiation on photographic or photoconductive plate

Body Part Character 4	Contrast Character 5	Qualifier Character 6	Qualifier Character 7
Ø Lacrimal Duct, Right 1 Lacrimal Duct, Left 2 Lacrimal Ducts, Bilateral	Ø High Osmolar 1 Low Osmolar Y Other Contrast	Z None	Z None
3 Optic Foramina, Right 4 Optic Foramina, Left 5 Eye, Right 6 Eye, Left 7 Eyes, Bilateral	Z None	Z None	Z None

B   Imaging
8   Eye
2   Computerized Tomography (CT Scan)   Definition: Computer reformatted digital display of multiplanar images developed from the capture of multiple exposures of external ionizing radiation

Body Part Character 4	Contrast Character 5	Qualifier Character 6	Qualifier Character 7
5 Eye, Right 6 Eye, Left 7 Eyes, Bilateral	Ø High Osmolar 1 Low Osmolar Y Other Contrast	Ø Unenhanced and Enhanced Z None	Z None
5 Eye, Right 6 Eye, Left 7 Eyes, Bilateral	Z None	Z None	Z None

Non-OR Procedure   DRG Non-OR Procedure   Valid OR Procedure   HAC Associated Procedure   Combination Only   New/Revised April   New/Revised October

760   ICD-10-PCS 2024

B　Imaging
8　Eye
3　Magnetic Resonance Imaging (MRI)　Definition: Computer reformatted digital display of multiplanar images developed from the capture of radio-frequency signals emitted by nuclei in a body site excited within a magnetic field

Body Part Character 4	Contrast Character 5	Qualifier Character 6	Qualifier Character 7
5　Eye, Right 6　Eye, Left 7　Eyes, Bilateral	Y　Other Contrast	Ø　Unenhanced and Enhanced Z　None	Z　None
5　Eye, Right 6　Eye, Left 7　Eyes, Bilateral	Z　None	Z　None	Z　None

B　Imaging
8　Eye
4　Ultrasonography　Definition: Real time display of images of anatomy or flow information developed from the capture of reflected and attenuated high frequency sound waves

Body Part Character 4	Contrast Character 5	Qualifier Character 6	Qualifier Character 7
5　Eye, Right 6　Eye, Left 7　Eyes, Bilateral	Z　None	Z　None	Z　None

B　Imaging
9　Ear, Nose, Mouth and Throat
Ø　Plain Radiography　Definition: Planar display of an image developed from the capture of external ionizing radiation on photographic or photoconductive plate

Body Part Character 4	Contrast Character 5	Qualifier Character 6	Qualifier Character 7
2　Paranasal Sinuses F　Nasopharynx/Oropharynx H　Mastoids	Z　None	Z　None	Z　None
4　Parotid Gland, Right 5　Parotid Gland, Left 6　Parotid Glands, Bilateral 7　Submandibular Gland, Right 8　Submandibular Gland, Left 9　Submandibular Glands, Bilateral B　Salivary Gland, Right C　Salivary Gland, Left D　Salivary Glands, Bilateral	Ø　High Osmolar 1　Low Osmolar Y　Other Contrast	Z　None	Z　None

B　Imaging
9　Ear, Nose, Mouth and Throat
1　Fluoroscopy　Definition: Single plane or bi-plane real time display of an image developed from the capture of external ionizing radiation on a fluorescent screen. The image may also be stored by either digital or analog means.

Body Part Character 4	Contrast Character 5	Qualifier Character 6	Qualifier Character 7
G　Pharynx and Epiglottis J　Larynx	Y　Other Contrast Z　None	Z　None	Z　None

B　Imaging
9　Ear, Nose, Mouth and Throat
2　Computerized Tomography (CT Scan)　Definition: Computer reformatted digital display of multiplanar images developed from the capture of multiple exposures of external ionizing radiation

Body Part Character 4	Contrast Character 5	Qualifier Character 6	Qualifier Character 7
Ø　Ear 2　Paranasal Sinuses 6　Parotid Glands, Bilateral 9　Submandibular Glands, Bilateral D　Salivary Glands, Bilateral F　Nasopharynx/Oropharynx J　Larynx	Ø　High Osmolar 1　Low Osmolar Y　Other Contrast	Ø　Unenhanced and Enhanced Z　None	Z　None
Ø　Ear 2　Paranasal Sinuses 6　Parotid Glands, Bilateral 9　Submandibular Glands, Bilateral D　Salivary Glands, Bilateral F　Nasopharynx/Oropharynx J　Larynx	Z　None	Z　None	Z　None

NC Noncovered Procedure　　LC Limited Coverage　　QA Questionable OB Admit　　NT New Tech Add-on　　⊞ Combination Member　　♂ Male　　♀ Female

ICD-10-PCS 2024　　　　　　　　　　　　　　　　　　　　　　　　　　　761

B83–B92

B   **Imaging**
9   **Ear, Nose, Mouth and Throat**
3   **Magnetic Resonance Imaging (MRI)**   Definition: Computer reformatted digital display of multiplanar images developed from the capture of radio-frequency signals emitted by nuclei in a body site excited within a magnetic field

Body Part Character 4	Contrast Character 5	Qualifier Character 6	Qualifier Character 7
0 Ear 2 Paranasal Sinuses 6 Parotid Glands, Bilateral 9 Submandibular Glands, Bilateral D Salivary Glands, Bilateral F Nasopharynx/Oropharynx J Larynx	Y Other Contrast	0 Unenhanced and Enhanced Z None	Z None
0 Ear 2 Paranasal Sinuses 6 Parotid Glands, Bilateral 9 Submandibular Glands, Bilateral D Salivary Glands, Bilateral F Nasopharynx/Oropharynx J Larynx	Z None	Z None	Z None

B   **Imaging**
B   **Respiratory System**
0   **Plain Radiography**   Definition: Planar display of an image developed from the capture of external ionizing radiation on photographic or photoconductive plate

Body Part Character 4	Contrast Character 5	Qualifier Character 6	Qualifier Character 7
7 Tracheobronchial Tree, Right 8 Tracheobronchial Tree, Left 9 Tracheobronchial Trees, Bilateral	Y Other Contrast	Z None	Z None
D Upper Airways	Z None	Z None	Z None

B   **Imaging**
B   **Respiratory System**
1   **Fluoroscopy**   Definition: Single plane or bi-plane real time display of an image developed from the capture of external ionizing radiation on a fluorescent screen. The image may also be stored by either digital or analog means.

Body Part Character 4	Contrast Character 5	Qualifier Character 6	Qualifier Character 7
2 Lung, Right 3 Lung, Left 4 Lungs, Bilateral 6 Diaphragm C Mediastinum D Upper Airways	Z None	Z None	Z None
7 Tracheobronchial Tree, Right 8 Tracheobronchial Tree, Left 9 Tracheobronchial Trees, Bilateral	Y Other Contrast	Z None	Z None

B   **Imaging**
B   **Respiratory System**
2   **Computerized Tomography (CT Scan)**   Definition: Computer reformatted digital display of multiplanar images developed from the capture of multiple exposures of external ionizing radiation

Body Part Character 4	Contrast Character 5	Qualifier Character 6	Qualifier Character 7
4 Lungs, Bilateral 7 Tracheobronchial Tree, Right 8 Tracheobronchial Tree, Left 9 Tracheobronchial Trees, Bilateral F Trachea/Airways	0 High Osmolar 1 Low Osmolar Y Other Contrast	0 Unenhanced and Enhanced Z None	Z None
4 Lungs, Bilateral 7 Tracheobronchial Tree, Right 8 Tracheobronchial Tree, Left 9 Tracheobronchial Trees, Bilateral F Trachea/Airways	Z None	Z None	Z None

Non-OR Procedure   DRG Non-OR Procedure   Valid OR Procedure   HAC Associated Procedure   Combination Only   New/Revised April   New/Revised October

762   ICD-10-PCS 2024

B93–BB2

B　Imaging
B　Respiratory System
3　Magnetic Resonance Imaging (MRI)　Definition: Computer reformatted digital display of multiplanar images developed from the capture of radio-frequency signals emitted by nuclei in a body site excited within a magnetic field

Body Part Character 4	Contrast Character 5	Qualifier Character 6	Qualifier Character 7
4　Lungs, Bilateral	Z　None	3　Hyperpolarized Xenon 129 (Xe-129)	Z　None
G　Lung Apices	Y　Other Contrast	0　Unenhanced and Enhanced Z　None	Z　None
G　Lung Apices	Z　None	Z　None	Z　None

B　Imaging
B　Respiratory System
4　Ultrasonography　Definition: Real time display of images of anatomy or flow information developed from the capture of reflected and attenuated high frequency sound waves

Body Part Character 4	Contrast Character 5	Qualifier Character 6	Qualifier Character 7
B　Pleura C　Mediastinum	Z　None	Z　None	Z　None

B　Imaging
D　Gastrointestinal System
1　Fluoroscopy　Definition: Single plane or bi-plane real time display of an image developed from the capture of external ionizing radiation on a fluorescent screen. The image may also be stored by either digital or analog means.

Body Part Character 4	Contrast Character 5	Qualifier Character 6	Qualifier Character 7
1　Esophagus 2　Stomach 3　Small Bowel 4　Colon 5　Upper GI 6　Upper GI and Small Bowel 9　Duodenum B　Mouth/Oropharynx	Y　Other Contrast Z　None	Z　None	Z　None

B　Imaging
D　Gastrointestinal System
2　Computerized Tomography (CT Scan)　Definition: Computer reformatted digital display of multiplanar images developed from the capture of multiple exposures of external ionizing radiation

Body Part Character 4	Contrast Character 5	Qualifier Character 6	Qualifier Character 7
4　Colon	0　High Osmolar 1　Low Osmolar Y　Other Contrast	0　Unenhanced and Enhanced Z　None	Z　None
4　Colon	Z　None	Z　None	Z　None

B　Imaging
D　Gastrointestinal System
4　Ultrasonography　Definition: Real time display of images of anatomy or flow information developed from the capture of reflected and attenuated high frequency sound waves

Body Part Character 4	Contrast Character 5	Qualifier Character 6	Qualifier Character 7
1　Esophagus 2　Stomach 7　Gastrointestinal Tract 8　Appendix 9　Duodenum C　Rectum	Z　None	Z　None	Z　None

B　Imaging
F　Hepatobiliary System and Pancreas
0　Plain Radiography　Definition: Planar display of an image developed from the capture of external ionizing radiation on photographic or photoconductive plate

Body Part Character 4	Contrast Character 5	Qualifier Character 6	Qualifier Character 7
0　Bile Ducts 3　Gallbladder and Bile Ducts C　Hepatobiliary System, All	0　High Osmolar 1　Low Osmolar Y　Other Contrast	Z　None	Z　None

NC Noncovered Procedure　　**LC** Limited Coverage　　**QA** Questionable OB Admit　　**NT** New Tech Add-on　　⊞ Combination Member　　♂ Male　　♀ Female

ICD-10-PCS 2024　　　　　　　　　　　　　　　　　　　　　　　　　　　　763

BB3–BF0

B   Imaging
F   Hepatobiliary System and Pancreas
1   Fluoroscopy   Definition: Single plane or bi-plane real time display of an image developed from the capture of external ionizing radiation on a fluorescent screen. The image may also be stored by either digital or analog means.

Body Part Character 4	Contrast Character 5	Qualifier Character 6	Qualifier Character 7
Ø Bile Ducts 1 Biliary and Pancreatic Ducts 2 Gallbladder 3 Gallbladder and Bile Ducts 4 Gallbladder, Bile Ducts and Pancreatic Ducts 8 Pancreatic Ducts	Ø High Osmolar 1 Low Osmolar Y Other Contrast	Z None	Z None
5 Liver	Ø High Osmolar 1 Low Osmolar Y Other Contrast	Z None	Z None
5 Liver	Z None	Z None	A Guidance

B   Imaging
F   Hepatobiliary System and Pancreas
2   Computerized Tomography (CT Scan)   Definition: Computer reformatted digital display of multiplanar images developed from the capture of multiple exposures of external ionizing radiation

Body Part Character 4	Contrast Character 5	Qualifier Character 6	Qualifier Character 7
5 Liver 6 Liver and Spleen 7 Pancreas C Hepatobiliary System, All	Ø High Osmolar 1 Low Osmolar Y Other Contrast	Ø Unenhanced and Enhanced Z None	Z None
5 Liver 6 Liver and Spleen 7 Pancreas C Hepatobiliary System, All	Z None	Z None	Z None

B   Imaging
F   Hepatobiliary System and Pancreas
3   Magnetic Resonance Imaging (MRI)   Definition: Computer reformatted digital display of multiplanar images developed from the capture of radio-frequency signals emitted by nuclei in a body site excited within a magnetic field

Body Part Character 4	Contrast Character 5	Qualifier Character 6	Qualifier Character 7
5 Liver 6 Liver and Spleen 7 Pancreas	Y Other Contrast	Ø Unenhanced and Enhanced Z None	Z None
5 Liver 6 Liver and Spleen 7 Pancreas	Z None	Z None	Z None

B   Imaging
F   Hepatobiliary System and Pancreas
4   Ultrasonography   Definition: Real time display of images of anatomy or flow information developed from the capture of reflected and attenuated high frequency sound waves

Body Part Character 4	Contrast Character 5	Qualifier Character 6	Qualifier Character 7
Ø Bile Ducts 2 Gallbladder 3 Gallbladder and Bile Ducts 5 Liver 6 Liver and Spleen 7 Pancreas C Hepatobiliary System, All	Z None	Z None	Z None

B   Imaging
F   Hepatobiliary System and Pancreas
5   Other Imaging   Definition: Other specified modality for visualizing a body part

Body Part Character 4	Contrast Character 5	Qualifier Character 6	Qualifier Character 7
Ø Bile Ducts 2 Gallbladder 3 Gallbladder and Bile Ducts 5 Liver 6 Liver and Spleen 7 Pancreas C Hepatobiliary System, All	2 Fluorescing Agent	Ø Indocyanine Green Dye Z None	Ø Intraoperative Z None

Non-OR Procedure   DRG Non-OR Procedure   Valid OR Procedure   HAC Associated Procedure   Combination Only   New/Revised April   New/Revised October

764   ICD-10-PCS 2024

BF1–BF5

B　Imaging
G　Endocrine System
2　Computerized Tomography (CT Scan) Definition: Computer reformatted digital display of multiplanar images developed from the capture of multiple exposures of external ionizing radiation

Body Part Character 4	Contrast Character 5	Qualifier Character 6	Qualifier Character 7
2　Adrenal Glands, Bilateral 3　Parathyroid Glands 4　Thyroid Gland	Ø　High Osmolar 1　Low Osmolar Y　Other Contrast	Ø　Unenhanced and Enhanced Z　None	Z　None
2　Adrenal Glands, Bilateral 3　Parathyroid Glands 4　Thyroid Gland	Z　None	Z　None	Z　None

B　Imaging
G　Endocrine System
3　Magnetic Resonance Imaging (MRI) Definition: Computer reformatted digital display of multiplanar images developed from the capture of radio-frequency signals emitted by nuclei in a body site excited within a magnetic field

Body Part Character 4	Contrast Character 5	Qualifier Character 6	Qualifier Character 7
2　Adrenal Glands, Bilateral 3　Parathyroid Glands 4　Thyroid Gland	Y　Other Contrast	Ø　Unenhanced and Enhanced Z　None	Z　None
2　Adrenal Glands, Bilateral 3　Parathyroid Glands 4　Thyroid Gland	Z　None	Z　None	Z　None

B　Imaging
G　Endocrine System
4　Ultrasonography Definition: Real time display of images of anatomy or flow information developed from the capture of reflected and attenuated high frequency sound waves

Body Part Character 4	Contrast Character 5	Qualifier Character 6	Qualifier Character 7
Ø　Adrenal Gland, Right 1　Adrenal Gland, Left 2　Adrenal Glands, Bilateral 3　Parathyroid Glands 4　Thyroid Gland	Z　None	Z　None	Z　None

B　Imaging
H　Skin, Subcutaneous Tissue and Breast
Ø　Plain Radiography Definition: Planar display of an image developed from the capture of external ionizing radiation on photographic or photoconductive plate

Body Part Character 4	Contrast Character 5	Qualifier Character 6	Qualifier Character 7
Ø　Breast, Right 1　Breast, Left 2　Breasts, Bilateral	Z　None	Z　None	Z　None
3　Single Mammary Duct, Right 4　Single Mammary Duct, Left 5　Multiple Mammary Ducts, Right 6　Multiple Mammary Ducts, Left	Ø　High Osmolar 1　Low Osmolar Y　Other Contrast Z　None	Z　None	Z　None

B   **Imaging**
H   **Skin, Subcutaneous Tissue and Breast**
3   **Magnetic Resonance Imaging (MRI)**   Definition: Computer reformatted digital display of multiplanar images developed from the capture of radio-frequency signals emitted by nuclei in a body site excited within a magnetic field

Body Part Character 4	Contrast Character 5	Qualifier Character 6	Qualifier Character 7
0 Breast, Right **1** Breast, Left **2** Breasts, Bilateral **D** Subcutaneous Tissue, Head/Neck **F** Subcutaneous Tissue, Upper Extremity **G** Subcutaneous Tissue, Thorax **H** Subcutaneous Tissue, Abdomen and Pelvis **J** Subcutaneous Tissue, Lower Extremity	**Y** Other Contrast	**0** Unenhanced and Enhanced **Z** None	**Z** None
0 Breast, Right **1** Breast, Left **2** Breasts, Bilateral **D** Subcutaneous Tissue, Head/Neck **F** Subcutaneous Tissue, Upper Extremity **G** Subcutaneous Tissue, Thorax **H** Subcutaneous Tissue, Abdomen and Pelvis **J** Subcutaneous Tissue, Lower Extremity	**Z** None	**Z** None	**Z** None

B   **Imaging**
H   **Skin, Subcutaneous Tissue and Breast**
4   **Ultrasonography**   Definition: Real time display of images of anatomy or flow information developed from the capture of reflected and attenuated high frequency sound waves

Body Part Character 4	Contrast Character 5	Qualifier Character 6	Qualifier Character 7
0 Breast, Right **1** Breast, Left **2** Breasts, Bilateral **7** Extremity, Upper **8** Extremity, Lower **9** Abdominal Wall **B** Chest Wall **C** Head and Neck	**Z** None	**Z** None	**Z** None

B   **Imaging**
L   **Connective Tissue**
3   **Magnetic Resonance Imaging (MRI)**   Definition: Computer reformatted digital display of multiplanar images developed from the capture of radio-frequency signals emitted by nuclei in a body site excited within a magnetic field

Body Part Character 4	Contrast Character 5	Qualifier Character 6	Qualifier Character 7
0 Connective Tissue, Upper Extremity **1** Connective Tissue, Lower Extremity **2** Tendons, Upper Extremity **3** Tendons, Lower Extremity	**Y** Other Contrast	**0** Unenhanced and Enhanced **Z** None	**Z** None
0 Connective Tissue, Upper Extremity **1** Connective Tissue, Lower Extremity **2** Tendons, Upper Extremity **3** Tendons, Lower Extremity	**Z** None	**Z** None	**Z** None

B   **Imaging**
L   **Connective Tissue**
4   **Ultrasonography**   Definition: Real time display of images of anatomy or flow information developed from the capture of reflected and attenuated high frequency sound waves

Body Part Character 4	Contrast Character 5	Qualifier Character 6	Qualifier Character 7
0 Connective Tissue, Upper Extremity **1** Connective Tissue, Lower Extremity **2** Tendons, Upper Extremity **3** Tendons, Lower Extremity	**Z** None	**Z** None	**Z** None

B   **Imaging**
N   **Skull and Facial Bones**
Ø   **Plain Radiography**   Definition: Planar display of an image developed from the capture of external ionizing radiation on photographic or photoconductive plate

Body Part Character 4	Contrast Character 5	Qualifier Character 6	Qualifier Character 7
Ø Skull **1** Orbit, Right **2** Orbit, Left **3** Orbits, Bilateral **4** Nasal Bones **5** Facial Bones **6** Mandible **B** Zygomatic Arch, Right **C** Zygomatic Arch, Left **D** Zygomatic Arches, Bilateral **G** Tooth, Single **H** Teeth, Multiple **J** Teeth, All	**Z** None	**Z** None	**Z** None
7 Temporomandibular Joint, Right **8** Temporomandibular Joint, Left **9** Temporomandibular Joints, Bilateral	**Ø** High Osmolar **1** Low Osmolar **Y** Other Contrast **Z** None	**Z** None	**Z** None

B   **Imaging**
N   **Skull and Facial Bones**
1   **Fluoroscopy**   Definition: Single plane or bi-plane real time display of an image developed from the capture of external ionizing radiation on a fluorescent screen. The image may also be stored by either digital or analog means.

Body Part Character 4	Contrast Character 5	Qualifier Character 6	Qualifier Character 7
7 Temporomandibular Joint, Right **8** Temporomandibular Joint, Left **9** Temporomandibular Joints, Bilateral	**Ø** High Osmolar **1** Low Osmolar **Y** Other Contrast **Z** None	**Z** None	**Z** None

B   **Imaging**
N   **Skull and Facial Bones**
2   **Computerized Tomography (CT Scan)**   Definition: Computer reformatted digital display of multiplanar images developed from the capture of multiple exposures of external ionizing radiation

Body Part Character 4	Contrast Character 5	Qualifier Character 6	Qualifier Character 7
Ø Skull **3** Orbits, Bilateral **5** Facial Bones **6** Mandible **9** Temporomandibular Joints, Bilateral **F** Temporal Bones	**Ø** High Osmolar **1** Low Osmolar **Y** Other Contrast **Z** None	**Z** None	**Z** None

B   **Imaging**
N   **Skull and Facial Bones**
3   **Magnetic Resonance Imaging (MRI)**   Definition: Computer reformatted digital display of multiplanar images developed from the capture of radio-frequency signals emitted by nuclei in a body site excited within a magnetic field

Body Part Character 4	Contrast Character 5	Qualifier Character 6	Qualifier Character 7
9 Temporomandibular Joints, Bilateral	**Y** Other Contrast **Z** None	**Z** None	**Z** None

NC Noncovered Procedure   **LC** Limited Coverage   **QA** Questionable OB Admit   **NT** New Tech Add-on   ⊞ Combination Member   ♂ Male   ♀ Female

ICD-10-PCS 2024   767

B   **Imaging**
P   **Non-Axial Upper Bones**
0   **Plain Radiography**   Definition: Planar display of an image developed from the capture of external ionizing radiation on photographic or photoconductive plate

Body Part Character 4	Contrast Character 5	Qualifier Character 6	Qualifier Character 7
0 Sternoclavicular Joint, Right **1** Sternoclavicular Joint, Left **2** Sternoclavicular Joints, Bilateral **3** Acromioclavicular Joints, Bilateral **4** Clavicle, Right **5** Clavicle, Left **6** Scapula, Right **7** Scapula, Left **A** Humerus, Right **B** Humerus, Left **E** Upper Arm, Right **F** Upper Arm, Left **J** Forearm, Right **K** Forearm, Left **N** Hand, Right **P** Hand, Left **R** Finger(s), Right **S** Finger(s), Left **X** Ribs, Right **Y** Ribs, Left	**Z** None	**Z** None	**Z** None
8 Shoulder, Right **9** Shoulder, Left **C** Hand/Finger Joint, Right **D** Hand/Finger Joint, Left **G** Elbow, Right **H** Elbow, Left **L** Wrist, Right **M** Wrist, Left	**0** High Osmolar **1** Low Osmolar **Y** Other Contrast **Z** None	**Z** None	**Z** None

B   **Imaging**
P   **Non-Axial Upper Bones**
1   **Fluoroscopy**   Definition: Single plane or bi-plane real time display of an image developed from the capture of external ionizing radiation on a fluorescent screen. The image may also be stored by either digital or analog means.

Body Part Character 4	Contrast Character 5	Qualifier Character 6	Qualifier Character 7
0 Sternoclavicular Joint, Right **1** Sternoclavicular Joint, Left **2** Sternoclavicular Joints, Bilateral **3** Acromioclavicular Joints, Bilateral **4** Clavicle, Right **5** Clavicle, Left **6** Scapula, Right **7** Scapula, Left **A** Humerus, Right **B** Humerus, Left **E** Upper Arm, Right **F** Upper Arm, Left **J** Forearm, Right **K** Forearm, Left **N** Hand, Right **P** Hand, Left **R** Finger(s), Right **S** Finger(s), Left **X** Ribs, Right **Y** Ribs, Left	**Z** None	**Z** None	**Z** None
8 Shoulder, Right **9** Shoulder, Left **L** Wrist, Right **M** Wrist, Left	**0** High Osmolar **1** Low Osmolar **Y** Other Contrast **Z** None	**Z** None	**Z** None
C Hand/Finger Joint, Right **D** Hand/Finger Joint, Left **G** Elbow, Right **H** Elbow, Left	**0** High Osmolar **1** Low Osmolar **Y** Other Contrast	**Z** None	**Z** None

Non-OR Procedure   DRG Non-OR Procedure   Valid OR Procedure   HAC Associated Procedure   Combination Only   New/Revised April   New/Revised October

B   Imaging
P   Non-Axial Upper Bones
2   Computerized Tomography (CT Scan) Definition: Computer reformatted digital display of multiplanar images developed from the capture of multiple exposures of external ionizing radiation

Body Part Character 4	Contrast Character 5	Qualifier Character 6	Qualifier Character 7
Ø Sternoclavicular Joint, Right 1 Sternoclavicular Joint, Left W Thorax	Ø High Osmolar 1 Low Osmolar Y Other Contrast	Z None	Z None
2 Sternoclavicular Joints, Bilateral 3 Acromioclavicular Joints, Bilateral 4 Clavicle, Right 5 Clavicle, Left 6 Scapula, Right 7 Scapula, Left 8 Shoulder, Right 9 Shoulder, Left A Humerus, Right B Humerus, Left E Upper Arm, Right F Upper Arm, Left G Elbow, Right H Elbow, Left J Forearm, Right K Forearm, Left L Wrist, Right M Wrist, Left N Hand, Right P Hand, Left Q Hands and Wrists, Bilateral R Finger(s), Right S Finger(s), Left T Upper Extremity, Right U Upper Extremity, Left V Upper Extremities, Bilateral X Ribs, Right Y Ribs, Left	Ø High Osmolar 1 Low Osmolar Y Other Contrast Z None	Z None	Z None
C Hand/Finger Joint, Right D Hand/Finger Joint, Left	Z None	Z None	Z None

B   Imaging
P   Non-Axial Upper Bones
3   Magnetic Resonance Imaging (MRI) Definition: Computer reformatted digital display of multiplanar images developed from the capture of radio-frequency signals emitted by nuclei in a body site excited within a magnetic field

Body Part Character 4	Contrast Character 5	Qualifier Character 6	Qualifier Character 7
8 Shoulder, Right 9 Shoulder, Left C Hand/Finger Joint, Right D Hand/Finger Joint, Left E Upper Arm, Right F Upper Arm, Left G Elbow, Right H Elbow, Left J Forearm, Right K Forearm, Left L Wrist, Right M Wrist, Left	Y Other Contrast	Ø Unenhanced and Enhanced Z None	Z None
8 Shoulder, Right 9 Shoulder, Left C Hand/Finger Joint, Right D Hand/Finger Joint, Left E Upper Arm, Right F Upper Arm, Left G Elbow, Right H Elbow, Left J Forearm, Right K Forearm, Left L Wrist, Right M Wrist, Left	Z None	Z None	Z None

NC Noncovered Procedure   LC Limited Coverage   QA Questionable OB Admit   NT New Tech Add-on   ⊞ Combination Member   ♂Male   ♀Female

ICD-10-PCS 2024   769

Imaging

B Imaging
P Non-Axial Upper Bones
4 Ultrasonography Definition: Real time display of images of anatomy or flow information developed from the capture of reflected and attenuated high frequency sound waves

Body Part Character 4	Contrast Character 5	Qualifier Character 6	Qualifier Character 7
8 Shoulder, Right 9 Shoulder, Left G Elbow, Right H Elbow, Left L Wrist, Right M Wrist, Left N Hand, Right P Hand, Left	Z None	Z None	1 Densitometry Z None

B Imaging
Q Non-Axial Lower Bones
Ø Plain Radiography Definition: Planar display of an image developed from the capture of external ionizing radiation on photographic or photoconductive plate

Body Part Character 4	Contrast Character 5	Qualifier Character 6	Qualifier Character 7
Ø Hip, Right 1 Hip, Left	Ø High Osmolar 1 Low Osmolar Y Other Contrast	Z None	Z None
Ø Hip, Right 1 Hip, Left	Z None	Z None	1 Densitometry Z None
3 Femur, Right 4 Femur, Left	Z None	Z None	1 Densitometry Z None
7 Knee, Right 8 Knee, Left G Ankle, Right H Ankle, Left	Ø High Osmolar 1 Low Osmolar Y Other Contrast Z None	Z None	Z None
D Lower Leg, Right F Lower Leg, Left J Calcaneus, Right K Calcaneus, Left L Foot, Right M Foot, Left P Toe(s), Right Q Toe(s), Left V Patella, Right W Patella, Left	Z None	Z None	Z None
X Foot/Toe Joint, Right Y Foot/Toe Joint, Left	Ø High Osmolar 1 Low Osmolar Y Other Contrast	Z None	Z None

B Imaging
Q Non-Axial Lower Bones
1 Fluoroscopy Definition: Single plane or bi-plane real time display of an image developed from the capture of external ionizing radiation on a fluorescent screen. The image may also be stored by either digital or analog means.

Body Part Character 4	Contrast Character 5	Qualifier Character 6	Qualifier Character 7
Ø Hip, Right 1 Hip, Left 7 Knee, Right 8 Knee, Left G Ankle, Right H Ankle, Left X Foot/Toe Joint, Right Y Foot/Toe Joint, Left	Ø High Osmolar 1 Low Osmolar Y Other Contrast Z None	Z None	Z None
3 Femur, Right 4 Femur, Left D Lower Leg, Right F Lower Leg, Left J Calcaneus, Right K Calcaneus, Left L Foot, Right M Foot, Left P Toe(s), Right Q Toe(s), Left V Patella, Right W Patella, Left	Z None	Z None	Z None

Non-OR Procedure   DRG Non-OR Procedure   Valid OR Procedure   HAC Associated Procedure   Combination Only   New/Revised April   New/Revised October

B   Imaging
Q   Non-Axial Lower Bones
2   Computerized Tomography (CT Scan) Definition: Computer reformatted digital display of multiplanar images developed from the capture of multiple exposures of external ionizing radiation

Body Part Character 4	Contrast Character 5	Qualifier Character 6	Qualifier Character 7
Ø Hip, Right 1 Hip, Left 3 Femur, Right 4 Femur, Left 7 Knee, Right 8 Knee, Left D Lower Leg, Right F Lower Leg, Left G Ankle, Right H Ankle, Left J Calcaneus, Right K Calcaneus, Left L Foot, Right M Foot, Left P Toe(s), Right Q Toe(s), Left R Lower Extremity, Right S Lower Extremity, Left V Patella, Right W Patella, Left X Foot/Toe Joint, Right Y Foot/Toe Joint, Left	Ø High Osmolar 1 Low Osmolar Y Other Contrast Z None	Z None	Z None
B Tibia/Fibula, Right C Tibia/Fibula, Left	Ø High Osmolar 1 Low Osmolar Y Other Contrast	Z None	Z None

B   Imaging
Q   Non-Axial Lower Bones
3   Magnetic Resonance Imaging (MRI) Definition: Computer reformatted digital display of multiplanar images developed from the capture of radio-frequency signals emitted by nuclei in a body site excited within a magnetic field

Body Part Character 4	Contrast Character 5	Qualifier Character 6	Qualifier Character 7
Ø Hip, Right 1 Hip, Left 3 Femur, Right 4 Femur, Left 7 Knee, Right 8 Knee, Left D Lower Leg, Right F Lower Leg, Left G Ankle, Right H Ankle, Left J Calcaneus, Right K Calcaneus, Left L Foot, Right M Foot, Left P Toe(s), Right Q Toe(s), Left V Patella, Right W Patella, Left	Y Other Contrast	Ø Unenhanced and Enhanced Z None	Z None
Ø Hip, Right 1 Hip, Left 3 Femur, Right 4 Femur, Left 7 Knee, Right 8 Knee, Left D Lower Leg, Right F Lower Leg, Left G Ankle, Right H Ankle, Left J Calcaneus, Right K Calcaneus, Left L Foot, Right M Foot, Left P Toe(s), Right Q Toe(s), Left V Patella, Right W Patella, Left	Z None	Z None	Z None

NC Noncovered Procedure   LC Limited Coverage   QA Questionable OB Admit   NT New Tech Add-on   ⊞ Combination Member   ♂ Male   ♀ Female

ICD-10-PCS 2024   771

Imaging

B   **Imaging**
Q   **Non-Axial Lower Bones**
4   **Ultrasonography**   Definition: Real time display of images of anatomy or flow information developed from the capture of reflected and attenuated high frequency sound waves

Body Part Character 4	Contrast Character 5	Qualifier Character 6	Qualifier Character 7
0 Hip, Right 1 Hip, Left 2 Hips, Bilateral 7 Knee, Right 8 Knee, Left 9 Knees, Bilateral	Z None	Z None	Z None

B   **Imaging**
R   **Axial Skeleton, Except Skull and Facial Bones**
0   **Plain Radiography**   Definition: Planar display of an image developed from the capture of external ionizing radiation on photographic or photoconductive plate

Body Part Character 4	Contrast Character 5	Qualifier Character 6	Qualifier Character 7
0 Cervical Spine 7 Thoracic Spine 9 Lumbar Spine G Whole Spine	Z None	Z None	1 Densitometry Z None
1 Cervical Disc(s) 2 Thoracic Disc(s) 3 Lumbar Disc(s) 4 Cervical Facet Joint(s) 5 Thoracic Facet Joint(s) 6 Lumbar Facet Joint(s) D Sacroiliac Joints	0 High Osmolar 1 Low Osmolar Y Other Contrast Z None	Z None	Z None
8 Thoracolumbar Joint B Lumbosacral Joint C Pelvis F Sacrum and Coccyx H Sternum	Z None	Z None	Z None

B   **Imaging**
R   **Axial Skeleton, Except Skull and Facial Bones**
1   **Fluoroscopy**   Definition: Single plane or bi-plane real time display of an image developed from the capture of external ionizing radiation on a fluorescent screen. The image may also be stored by either digital or analog means.

Body Part Character 4	Contrast Character 5	Qualifier Character 6	Qualifier Character 7
0 Cervical Spine 1 Cervical Disc(s) 2 Thoracic Disc(s) 3 Lumbar Disc(s) 4 Cervical Facet Joint(s) 5 Thoracic Facet Joint(s) 6 Lumbar Facet Joint(s) 7 Thoracic Spine 8 Thoracolumbar Joint 9 Lumbar Spine B Lumbosacral Joint C Pelvis D Sacroiliac Joints F Sacrum and Coccyx G Whole Spine H Sternum	0 High Osmolar 1 Low Osmolar Y Other Contrast Z None	Z None	Z None

B   **Imaging**
R   **Axial Skeleton, Except Skull and Facial Bones**
2   **Computerized Tomography (CT Scan)**   Definition: Computer reformatted digital display of multiplanar images developed from the capture of multiple exposures of external ionizing radiation

Body Part Character 4	Contrast Character 5	Qualifier Character 6	Qualifier Character 7
0 Cervical Spine 7 Thoracic Spine 9 Lumbar Spine C Pelvis D Sacroiliac Joints F Sacrum and Coccyx	0 High Osmolar 1 Low Osmolar Y Other Contrast Z None	Z None	Z None

Non-OR Procedure   DRG Non-OR Procedure   Valid OR Procedure   HAC Associated Procedure   Combination Only   New/Revised April   New/Revised October

772   ICD-10-PCS 2024

BQ4–BR2

B　Imaging
R　Axial Skeleton, Except Skull and Facial Bones
3　Magnetic Resonance Imaging (MRI)　Definition: Computer reformatted digital display of multiplanar images developed from the capture of radio-frequency signals emitted by nuclei in a body site excited within a magnetic field

Body Part Character 4	Contrast Character 5	Qualifier Character 6	Qualifier Character 7
Ø　Cervical Spine 1　Cervical Disc(s) 2　Thoracic Disc(s) 3　Lumbar Disc(s) 7　Thoracic Spine 9　Lumbar Spine C　Pelvis F　Sacrum and Coccyx	Y　Other Contrast	Ø　Unenhanced and Enhanced Z　None	Z　None
Ø　Cervical Spine 1　Cervical Disc(s) 2　Thoracic Disc(s) 3　Lumbar Disc(s) 7　Thoracic Spine 9　Lumbar Spine C　Pelvis F　Sacrum and Coccyx	Z　None	Z　None	Z　None

B　Imaging
R　Axial Skeleton, Except Skull and Facial Bones
4　Ultrasonography　Definition: Real time display of images of anatomy or flow information developed from the capture of reflected and attenuated high frequency sound waves

Body Part Character 4	Contrast Character 5	Qualifier Character 6	Qualifier Character 7
Ø　Cervical Spine 7　Thoracic Spine 9　Lumbar Spine F　Sacrum and Coccyx	Z　None	Z　None	Z　None

B　Imaging
T　Urinary System
Ø　Plain Radiography　Definition: Planar display of an image developed from the capture of external ionizing radiation on photographic or photoconductive plate

Body Part Character 4	Contrast Character 5	Qualifier Character 6	Qualifier Character 7
Ø　Bladder 1　Kidney, Right 2　Kidney, Left 3　Kidneys, Bilateral 4　Kidneys, Ureters and Bladder 5　Urethra 6　Ureter, Right 7　Ureter, Left 8　Ureters, Bilateral B　Bladder and Urethra C　Ileal Diversion Loop	Ø　High Osmolar 1　Low Osmolar Y　Other Contrast Z　None	Z　None	Z　None

B　Imaging
T　Urinary System
1　Fluoroscopy　Definition: Single plane or bi-plane real time display of an image developed from the capture of external ionizing radiation on a fluorescent screen. The image may also be stored by either digital or analog means.

Body Part Character 4	Contrast Character 5	Qualifier Character 6	Qualifier Character 7
Ø　Bladder 1　Kidney, Right 2　Kidney, Left 3　Kidneys, Bilateral 4　Kidneys, Ureters and Bladder 5　Urethra 6　Ureter, Right 7　Ureter, Left B　Bladder and Urethra C　Ileal Diversion Loop D　Kidney, Ureter and Bladder, Right F　Kidney, Ureter and Bladder, Left G　Ileal Loop, Ureters and Kidneys	Ø　High Osmolar 1　Low Osmolar Y　Other Contrast Z　None	Z　None	Z　None

🅽🅲 Noncovered Procedure　　🅻🅲 Limited Coverage　　🆀🅰 Questionable OB Admit　　🅽🆃 New Tech Add-on　　⊞ Combination Member　　♂ Male　　♀ Female
ICD-10-PCS 2024　　　　　　　　　　　　　　　　　　　　　　　　　　　　　　　　　　　　　　　773

BR3–BT1

B　**Imaging**
T　**Urinary System**
2　**Computerized Tomography (CT Scan)**　Definition: Computer reformatted digital display of multiplanar images developed from the capture of multiple exposures of external ionizing radiation

Body Part Character 4	Contrast Character 5	Qualifier Character 6	Qualifier Character 7
Ø Bladder 1 Kidney, Right 2 Kidney, Left 3 Kidneys, Bilateral 9 Kidney Transplant	Ø High Osmolar 1 Low Osmolar Y Other Contrast	Ø Unenhanced and Enhanced Z None	Z None
Ø Bladder 1 Kidney, Right 2 Kidney, Left 3 Kidneys, Bilateral 9 Kidney Transplant	Z None	Z None	Z None

B　**Imaging**
T　**Urinary System**
3　**Magnetic Resonance Imaging (MRI)**　Definition: Computer reformatted digital display of multiplanar images developed from the capture of radio-frequency signals emitted by nuclei in a body site excited within a magnetic field

Body Part Character 4	Contrast Character 5	Qualifier Character 6	Qualifier Character 7
Ø Bladder 1 Kidney, Right 2 Kidney, Left 3 Kidneys, Bilateral 9 Kidney Transplant	Y Other Contrast	Ø Unenhanced and Enhanced Z None	Z None
Ø Bladder 1 Kidney, Right 2 Kidney, Left 3 Kidneys, Bilateral 9 Kidney Transplant	Z None	Z None	Z None

B　**Imaging**
T　**Urinary System**
4　**Ultrasonography**　Definition: Real time display of images of anatomy or flow information developed from the capture of reflected and attenuated high frequency sound waves

Body Part Character 4	Contrast Character 5	Qualifier Character 6	Qualifier Character 7
Ø Bladder 1 Kidney, Right 2 Kidney, Left 3 Kidneys, Bilateral 5 Urethra 6 Ureter, Right 7 Ureter, Left 8 Ureters, Bilateral 9 Kidney Transplant J Kidneys and Bladder	Z None	Z None	Z None

B　**Imaging**
U　**Female Reproductive System**
Ø　**Plain Radiography**　Definition: Planar display of an image developed from the capture of external ionizing radiation on photographic or photoconductive plate

Body Part Character 4	Contrast Character 5	Qualifier Character 6	Qualifier Character 7
Ø Fallopian Tube, Right ♀ 1 Fallopian Tube, Left ♀ 2 Fallopian Tubes, Bilateral ♀ 6 Uterus ♀ 8 Uterus and Fallopian Tubes ♀ 9 Vagina ♀	Ø High Osmolar 1 Low Osmolar Y Other Contrast	Z None	Z None

♀　All body part, contrast, and qualifier values

Non-OR Procedure　　DRG Non-OR Procedure　　Valid OR Procedure　　HAC Associated Procedure　　Combination Only　　New/Revised April　　New/Revised October

774　　　　　　　　　　　　　　　　　　　　　　　　　　　　　　　　　　　　　ICD-10-PCS 2024

B   **Imaging**
U   **Female Reproductive System**
1   **Fluoroscopy**   Definition: Single plane or bi-plane real time display of an image developed from the capture of external ionizing radiation on a fluorescent screen. The image may also be stored by either digital or analog means.

Body Part Character 4		Contrast Character 5		Qualifier Character 6	Qualifier Character 7
Ø Fallopian Tube, Right	♀	Ø High Osmolar		Z None	Z None
1 Fallopian Tube, Left	♀	1 Low Osmolar			
2 Fallopian Tubes, Bilateral	♀	Y Other Contrast			
6 Uterus	♀	Z None			
8 Uterus and Fallopian Tubes	♀				
9 Vagina	♀				

   ♀   All body part, contrast, and qualifier values

B   **Imaging**
U   **Female Reproductive System**
3   **Magnetic Resonance Imaging (MRI)**   Definition: Computer reformatted digital display of multiplanar images developed from the capture of radio-frequency signals emitted by nuclei in a body site excited within a magnetic field

Body Part Character 4		Contrast Character 5	Qualifier Character 6	Qualifier Character 7
3 Ovary, Right	♀	Y Other Contrast	Ø Unenhanced and Enhanced	Z None
4 Ovary, Left	♀		Z None	
5 Ovaries, Bilateral	♀			
6 Uterus	♀			
9 Vagina	♀			
B Pregnant Uterus	♀			
C Uterus and Ovaries	♀			
3 Ovary, Right	♀	Z None	Z None	Z None
4 Ovary, Left	♀			
5 Ovaries, Bilateral	♀			
6 Uterus	♀			
9 Vagina	♀			
B Pregnant Uterus	♀			
C Uterus and Ovaries	♀			

   ♀   All body part, contrast, and qualifier values

B   **Imaging**
U   **Female Reproductive System**
4   **Ultrasonography**   Definition: Real time display of images of anatomy or flow information developed from the capture of reflected and attenuated high frequency sound waves

Body Part Character 4		Contrast Character 5	Qualifier Character 6	Qualifier Character 7
Ø Fallopian Tube, Right	♀	Y Other Contrast	Z None	Z None
1 Fallopian Tube, Left	♀	Z None		
2 Fallopian Tubes, Bilateral	♀			
3 Ovary, Right	♀			
4 Ovary, Left	♀			
5 Ovaries, Bilateral	♀			
6 Uterus	♀			
C Uterus and Ovaries	♀			

   ♀   All body part, contrast, and qualifier values

B   **Imaging**
V   **Male Reproductive System**
Ø   **Plain Radiography**   Definition: Planar display of an image developed from the capture of external ionizing radiation on photographic or photoconductive plate

Body Part Character 4		Contrast Character 5	Qualifier Character 6	Qualifier Character 7
Ø Corpora Cavernosa	♂	Ø High Osmolar	Z None	Z None
1 Epididymis, Right	♂	1 Low Osmolar		
2 Epididymis, Left	♂	Y Other Contrast		
3 Prostate	♂			
5 Testicle, Right	♂			
6 Testicle, Left	♂			
8 Vasa Vasorum	♂			

   ♂   All body part, contrast, and qualifier values

NC Noncovered Procedure   **LC** Limited Coverage   **QA** Questionable OB Admit   **NT** New Tech Add-on   ⊞ Combination Member   ♂ Male   ♀ Female

ICD-10-PCS 2024   775

Imaging

B   **Imaging**
V   **Male Reproductive System**
1   **Fluoroscopy**   Definition: Single plane or bi-plane real time display of an image developed from the capture of external ionizing radiation on a fluorescent screen. The image may also be stored by either digital or analog means.

Body Part Character 4	Contrast Character 5	Qualifier Character 6	Qualifier Character 7
Ø Corpora Cavernosa ♂ 8 Vasa Vasorum ♂	Ø High Osmolar 1 Low Osmolar Y Other Contrast Z None	Z None	Z None

♂   All body part, contrast, and qualifier values

B   **Imaging**
V   **Male Reproductive System**
2   **Computerized Tomography (CT Scan)**   Definition: Computer reformatted digital display of multiplanar images developed from the capture of multiple exposures of external ionizing radiation

Body Part Character 4	Contrast Character 5	Qualifier Character 6	Qualifier Character 7
3 Prostate ♂	Ø High Osmolar 1 Low Osmolar Y Other Contrast	Ø Unenhanced and Enhanced Z None	Z None
3 Prostate ♂	Z None	Z None	Z None

♂   BV23[Ø,Y][Ø,Z]Z
♂   BV231ØZ
♂   BV23ZZZ

B   **Imaging**
V   **Male Reproductive System**
3   **Magnetic Resonance Imaging (MRI)**   Definition: Computer reformatted digital display of multiplanar images developed from the capture of radio-frequency signals emitted by nuclei in a body site excited within a magnetic field

Body Part Character 4	Contrast Character 5	Qualifier Character 6	Qualifier Character 7
Ø Corpora Cavernosa ♂ 3 Prostate ♂ 4 Scrotum ♂ 5 Testicle, Right ♂ 6 Testicle, Left ♂ 7 Testicles, Bilateral ♂	Y Other Contrast	Ø Unenhanced and Enhanced Z None	Z None
Ø Corpora Cavernosa ♂ 3 Prostate ♂ 4 Scrotum ♂ 5 Testicle, Right ♂ 6 Testicle, Left ♂ 7 Testicles, Bilateral ♂	Z None	Z None	Z None

♂   All body part, contrast, and qualifier values

B   **Imaging**
V   **Male Reproductive System**
4   **Ultrasonography**   Definition: Real time display of images of anatomy or flow information developed from the capture of reflected and attenuated high frequency sound waves

Body Part Character 4	Contrast Character 5	Qualifier Character 6	Qualifier Character 7
4 Scrotum ♂ 9 Prostate and Seminal Vesicles ♂ B Penis ♂	Z None	Z None	Z None

♂   All body part, contrast, and qualifier values

B   **Imaging**
W   **Anatomical Regions**
Ø   **Plain Radiography**   Definition: Planar display of an image developed from the capture of external ionizing radiation on photographic or photoconductive plate

Body Part Character 4	Contrast Character 5	Qualifier Character 6	Qualifier Character 7
Ø Abdomen 1 Abdomen and Pelvis 3 Chest B Long Bones, All C Lower Extremity J Upper Extremity K Whole Body L Whole Skeleton M Whole Body, Infant	Z None	Z None	Z None

Non-OR Procedure   DRG Non-OR Procedure   Valid OR Procedure   HAC Associated Procedure   Combination Only   New/Revised April   New/Revised October

B　Imaging
W　Anatomical Regions
1　Fluoroscopy　Definition: Single plane or bi-plane real time display of an image developed from the capture of external ionizing radiation on a fluorescent screen. The image may also be stored by either digital or analog means.

Body Part Character 4	Contrast Character 5	Qualifier Character 6	Qualifier Character 7
1　Abdomen and Pelvis 9　Head and Neck C　Lower Extremity J　Upper Extremity	Ø　High Osmolar 1　Low Osmolar Y　Other Contrast Z　None	Z　None	Z　None

B　Imaging
W　Anatomical Regions
2　Computerized Tomography (CT Scan)　Definition: Computer reformatted digital display of multiplanar images developed from the capture of multiple exposures of external ionizing radiation

Body Part Character 4	Contrast Character 5	Qualifier Character 6	Qualifier Character 7
Ø　Abdomen 1　Abdomen and Pelvis 4　Chest and Abdomen 5　Chest, Abdomen and Pelvis 8　Head 9　Head and Neck F　Neck G　Pelvic Region	Ø　High Osmolar 1　Low Osmolar Y　Other Contrast	Ø　Unenhanced and Enhanced Z　None	Z　None
Ø　Abdomen 1　Abdomen and Pelvis 4　Chest and Abdomen 5　Chest, Abdomen and Pelvis 8　Head 9　Head and Neck F　Neck G　Pelvic Region	Z　None	Z　None	Z　None

B　Imaging
W　Anatomical Regions
3　Magnetic Resonance Imaging (MRI)　Definition: Computer reformatted digital display of multiplanar images developed from the capture of radio-frequency signals emitted by nuclei in a body site excited within a magnetic field

Body Part Character 4	Contrast Character 5	Qualifier Character 6	Qualifier Character 7
Ø　Abdomen 8　Head F　Neck G　Pelvic Region H　Retroperitoneum P　Brachial Plexus	Y　Other Contrast	Ø　Unenhanced and Enhanced Z　None	Z　None
Ø　Abdomen 8　Head F　Neck G　Pelvic Region H　Retroperitoneum P　Brachial Plexus	Z　None	Z　None	Z　None
3　Chest	Y　Other Contrast	Ø　Unenhanced and Enhanced Z　None	Z　None

B　Imaging
W　Anatomical Regions
4　Ultrasonography　Definition: Real time display of images of anatomy or flow information developed from the capture of reflected and attenuated high frequency sound waves

Body Part Character 4	Contrast Character 5	Qualifier Character 6	Qualifier Character 7
Ø　Abdomen 1　Abdomen and Pelvis F　Neck G　Pelvic Region	Z　None	Z　None	Z　None

NC Noncovered Procedure　　LC Limited Coverage　　QA Questionable OB Admit　　NT New Tech Add-on　　✚ Combination Member　　♂ Male　　♀ Female

ICD-10-PCS 2024

777

BW1–BW4

B Imaging
W Anatomical Regions
5 Other Imaging Definition: Other specified modality for visualizing a body part

Body Part Character 4	Contrast Character 5	Qualifier Character 6	Qualifier Character 7
2 Trunk 9 Head and Neck C Lower Extremity J Upper Extremity	Z None	1 Bacterial Autofluorescence	Z None

B Imaging
Y Fetus and Obstetrical
3 Magnetic Resonance Imaging (MRI) Definition: Computer reformatted digital display of multiplanar images developed from the capture of radio-frequency signals emitted by nuclei in a body site excited within a magnetic field

Body Part Character 4	Contrast Character 5	Qualifier Character 6	Qualifier Character 7
0 Fetal Head ♀ 1 Fetal Heart ♀ 2 Fetal Thorax ♀ 3 Fetal Abdomen ♀ 4 Fetal Spine ♀ 5 Fetal Extremities ♀ 6 Whole Fetus ♀	Y Other Contrast	0 Unenhanced and Enhanced Z None	Z None
0 Fetal Head ♀ 1 Fetal Heart ♀ 2 Fetal Thorax ♀ 3 Fetal Abdomen ♀ 4 Fetal Spine ♀ 5 Fetal Extremities ♀ 6 Whole Fetus ♀	Z None	Z None	Z None

♀ BY3[0,1,2,3,5,6]Y[0,Z]Z
♀ BY34YZZ
♀ BY3[0,1,2,3,4,5,6]ZZZ

B Imaging
Y Fetus and Obstetrical
4 Ultrasonography Definition: Real time display of images of anatomy or flow information developed from the capture of reflected and attenuated high frequency sound waves

Body Part Character 4	Contrast Character 5	Qualifier Character 6	Qualifier Character 7
7 Fetal Umbilical Cord ♀ 8 Placenta ♀ 9 First Trimester, Single Fetus ♀ B First Trimester, Multiple Gestation ♀ C Second Trimester, Single Fetus ♀ D Second Trimester, Multiple Gestation ♀ F Third Trimester, Single Fetus ♀ G Third Trimester, Multiple Gestation ♀	Z None	Z None	Z None

♀ All body part, contrast, and qualifier values

Nuclear Medicine CØ1–CW7

C   **Nuclear Medicine**
Ø   **Central Nervous System**
1   **Planar Nuclear Medicine Imaging**   Definition: Introduction of radioactive materials into the body for single plane display of images developed from the capture of radioactive emissions

Body Part Character 4	Radionuclide Character 5	Qualifier Character 6	Qualifier Character 7
Ø Brain	1 Technetium 99m (Tc-99m) Y Other Radionuclide	Z None	Z None
5 Cerebrospinal Fluid	D Indium 111 (In-111) Y Other Radionuclide	Z None	Z None
Y Central Nervous System	Y Other Radionuclide	Z None	Z None

C   **Nuclear Medicine**
Ø   **Central Nervous System**
2   **Tomographic (Tomo) Nuclear Medicine Imaging**   Definition: Introduction of radioactive materials into the body for three dimensional display of images developed from the capture of radioactive emissions

Body Part Character 4	Radionuclide Character 5	Qualifier Character 6	Qualifier Character 7
Ø Brain	1 Technetium 99m (Tc-99m) F Iodine 123 (I-123) S Thallium 201 (Tl-201) Y Other Radionuclide	Z None	Z None
5 Cerebrospinal Fluid	D Indium 111 (In-111) Y Other Radionuclide	Z None	Z None
Y Central Nervous System	Y Other Radionuclide	Z None	Z None

C   **Nuclear Medicine**
Ø   **Central Nervous System**
3   **Positron Emission Tomographic (PET) Imaging**   Definition: Introduction of radioactive materials into the body for three dimensional display of images developed from the simultaneous capture, 180 degrees apart, of radioactive emissions

Body Part Character 4	Radionuclide Character 5	Qualifier Character 6	Qualifier Character 7
Ø Brain	B Carbon 11 (C-11) K Fluorine 18 (F-18) M Oxygen 15 (O-15) Y Other Radionuclide	Z None	Z None
Y Central Nervous System	Y Other Radionuclide	Z None	Z None

C   **Nuclear Medicine**
Ø   **Central Nervous System**
5   **Nonimaging Nuclear Medicine Probe**   Definition: Introduction of radioactive materials into the body for the study of distribution and fate of certain substances by the detection of radioactive emissions; or, alternatively, measurement of absorption of radioactive emissions from an external source

Body Part Character 4	Radionuclide Character 5	Qualifier Character 6	Qualifier Character 7
Ø Brain	V Xenon 133 (Xe-133) Y Other Radionuclide	Z None	Z None
Y Central Nervous System	Y Other Radionuclide	Z None	Z None

C   **Nuclear Medicine**
2   **Heart**
1   **Planar Nuclear Medicine Imaging**   Definition: Introduction of radioactive materials into the body for single plane display of images developed from the capture of radioactive emissions

Body Part Character 4	Radionuclide Character 5	Qualifier Character 6	Qualifier Character 7
6 Heart, Right and Left	1 Technetium 99m (Tc-99m) Y Other Radionuclide	Z None	Z None
G Myocardium	1 Technetium 99m (Tc-99m) D Indium 111 (In-111) S Thallium 201 (Tl-201) Y Other Radionuclide Z None	Z None	Z None
Y Heart	Y Other Radionuclide	Z None	Z None

Nuclear Medicine (side margin)

C   **Nuclear Medicine**
2   **Heart**
2   **Tomographic (Tomo) Nuclear Medicine Imaging**   Definition: Introduction of radioactive materials into the body for three dimensional display of images developed from the capture of radioactive emissions

Body Part Character 4	Radionuclide Character 5	Qualifier Character 6	Qualifier Character 7
6 Heart, Right and Left	1 Technetium 99m (Tc-99m) Y Other Radionuclide	Z None	Z None
G Myocardium	1 Technetium 99m (Tc-99m) D Indium 111 (In-111) K Fluorine 18 (F-18) S Thallium 201 (Tl-201) Y Other Radionuclide Z None	Z None	Z None
Y Heart	Y Other Radionuclide	Z None	Z None

C   **Nuclear Medicine**
2   **Heart**
3   **Positron Emission Tomographic (PET) Imaging**   Definition: Introduction of radioactive materials into the body for three dimensional display of images developed from the simultaneous capture, 180 degrees apart, of radioactive emissions

Body Part Character 4	Radionuclide Character 5	Qualifier Character 6	Qualifier Character 7
G Myocardium	K Fluorine 18 (F-18) M Oxygen 15 (O-15) Q Rubidium 82 (Rb-82) R Nitrogen 13 (N-13) Y Other Radionuclide	Z None	Z None
Y Heart	Y Other Radionuclide	Z None	Z None

C   **Nuclear Medicine**
2   **Heart**
5   **Nonimaging Nuclear Medicine Probe**   Definition: Introduction of radioactive materials into the body for the study of distribution and fate of certain substances by the detection of radioactive emissions; or, alternatively, measurement of absorption of radioactive emissions from an external source

Body Part Character 4	Radionuclide Character 5	Qualifier Character 6	Qualifier Character 7
6 Heart, Right and Left	1 Technetium 99m (Tc-99m) Y Other Radionuclide	Z None	Z None
Y Heart	Y Other Radionuclide	Z None	Z None

C   **Nuclear Medicine**
5   **Veins**
1   **Planar Nuclear Medicine Imaging**   Definition: Introduction of radioactive materials into the body for single plane display of images developed from the capture of radioactive emissions

Body Part Character 4	Radionuclide Character 5	Qualifier Character 6	Qualifier Character 7
B Lower Extremity Veins, Right C Lower Extremity Veins, Left D Lower Extremity Veins, Bilateral N Upper Extremity Veins, Right P Upper Extremity Veins, Left Q Upper Extremity Veins, Bilateral R Central Veins	1 Technetium 99m (Tc-99m) Y Other Radionuclide	Z None	Z None
Y Veins	Y Other Radionuclide	Z None	Z None

C   **Nuclear Medicine**
7   **Lymphatic and Hematologic System**
1   **Planar Nuclear Medicine Imaging**   Definition: Introduction of radioactive materials into the body for single plane display of images developed from the capture of radioactive emissions

Body Part Character 4	Radionuclide Character 5	Qualifier Character 6	Qualifier Character 7
Ø Bone Marrow	1 Technetium 99m (Tc-99m) D Indium 111 (In-111) Y Other Radionuclide	Z None	Z None
2 Spleen 5 Lymphatics, Head and Neck D Lymphatics, Pelvic J Lymphatics, Head K Lymphatics, Neck L Lymphatics, Upper Chest M Lymphatics, Trunk N Lymphatics, Upper Extremity P Lymphatics, Lower Extremity	1 Technetium 99m (Tc-99m) Y Other Radionuclide	Z None	Z None
3 Blood	D Indium 111 (In-111) Y Other Radionuclide	Z None	Z None
Y Lymphatic and Hematologic System	Y Other Radionuclide	Z None	Z None

C   **Nuclear Medicine**
7   **Lymphatic and Hematologic System**
2   **Tomographic (Tomo) Nuclear Medicine Imaging**   Definition: Introduction of radioactive materials into the body for three dimensional display of images developed from the capture of radioactive emissions

Body Part Character 4	Radionuclide Character 5	Qualifier Character 6	Qualifier Character 7
2 Spleen	1 Technetium 99m (Tc-99m) Y Other Radionuclide	Z None	Z None
Y Lymphatic and Hematologic System	Y Other Radionuclide	Z None	Z None

C   **Nuclear Medicine**
7   **Lymphatic and Hematologic System**
5   **Nonimaging Nuclear Medicine Probe**   Definition: Introduction of radioactive materials into the body for the study of distribution and fate of certain substances by the detection of radioactive emissions; or, alternatively, measurement of absorption of radioactive emissions from an external source

Body Part Character 4	Radionuclide Character 5	Qualifier Character 6	Qualifier Character 7
5 Lymphatics, Head and Neck D Lymphatics, Pelvic J Lymphatics, Head K Lymphatics, Neck L Lymphatics, Upper Chest M Lymphatics, Trunk N Lymphatics, Upper Extremity P Lymphatics, Lower Extremity	1 Technetium 99m (Tc-99m) Y Other Radionuclide	Z None	Z None
Y Lymphatic and Hematologic System	Y Other Radionuclide	Z None	Z None

C   **Nuclear Medicine**
7   **Lymphatic and Hematologic System**
6   **Nonimaging Nuclear Medicine Assay**   Definition: Introduction of radioactive materials into the body for the study of body fluids and blood elements, by the detection of radioactive emissions

Body Part Character 4	Radionuclide Character 5	Qualifier Character 6	Qualifier Character 7
3 Blood	1 Technetium 99m (Tc-99m) 7 Cobalt 58 (Co-58) C Cobalt 57 (Co-57) D Indium 111 (In-111) H Iodine 125 (I-125) W Chromium (Cr-51) Y Other Radionuclide	Z None	Z None
Y Lymphatic and Hematologic System	Y Other Radionuclide	Z None	Z None

C   Nuclear Medicine
8   Eye
1   Planar Nuclear Medicine Imaging   Definition: Introduction of radioactive materials into the body for single plane display of images developed from the capture of radioactive emissions

Body Part Character 4	Radionuclide Character 5	Qualifier Character 6	Qualifier Character 7
9 Lacrimal Ducts, Bilateral	1 Technetium 99m (Tc-99m) Y Other Radionuclide	Z None	Z None
Y Eye	Y Other Radionuclide	Z None	Z None

C   Nuclear Medicine
9   Ear, Nose, Mouth and Throat
1   Planar Nuclear Medicine Imaging   Definition: Introduction of radioactive materials into the body for single plane display of images developed from the capture of radioactive emissions

Body Part Character 4	Radionuclide Character 5	Qualifier Character 6	Qualifier Character 7
B Salivary Glands, Bilateral	1 Technetium 99m (Tc-99m) Y Other Radionuclide	Z None	Z None
Y Ear, Nose, Mouth and Throat	Y Other Radionuclide	Z None	Z None

C   Nuclear Medicine
B   Respiratory System
1   Planar Nuclear Medicine Imaging   Definition: Introduction of radioactive materials into the body for single plane display of images developed from the capture of radioactive emissions

Body Part Character 4	Radionuclide Character 5	Qualifier Character 6	Qualifier Character 7
2 Lungs and Bronchi	1 Technetium 99m (Tc-99m) 9 Krypton (Kr-81m) T Xenon 127 (Xe-127) V Xenon 133 (Xe-133) Y Other Radionuclide	Z None	Z None
Y Respiratory System	Y Other Radionuclide	Z None	Z None

C   Nuclear Medicine
B   Respiratory System
2   Tomographic (Tomo) Nuclear Medicine Imaging   Definition: Introduction of radioactive materials into the body for three dimensional display of images developed from the capture of radioactive emissions

Body Part Character 4	Radionuclide Character 5	Qualifier Character 6	Qualifier Character 7
2 Lungs and Bronchi	1 Technetium 99m (Tc-99m) 9 Krypton (Kr-81m) Y Other Radionuclide	Z None	Z None
Y Respiratory System	Y Other Radionuclide	Z None	Z None

C   Nuclear Medicine
B   Respiratory System
3   Positron Emission Tomographic (PET) Imaging   Definition: Introduction of radioactive materials into the body for three dimensional display of images developed from the simultaneous capture, 180 degrees apart, of radioactive emissions

Body Part Character 4	Radionuclide Character 5	Qualifier Character 6	Qualifier Character 7
2 Lungs and Bronchi	K Fluorine 18 (F-18) Y Other Radionuclide	Z None	Z None
Y Respiratory System	Y Other Radionuclide	Z None	Z None

C   Nuclear Medicine
D   Gastrointestinal System
1   Planar Nuclear Medicine Imaging   Definition: Introduction of radioactive materials into the body for single plane display of images developed from the capture of radioactive emissions

Body Part Character 4	Radionuclide Character 5	Qualifier Character 6	Qualifier Character 7
5 Upper Gastrointestinal Tract 7 Gastrointestinal Tract	1 Technetium 99m (Tc-99m) D Indium 111 (In-111) Y Other Radionuclide	Z None	Z None
Y Digestive System	Y Other Radionuclide	Z None	Z None

Non-OR Procedure   DRG Non-OR Procedure   Valid OR Procedure   HAC Associated Procedure   Combination Only   New/Revised April   New/Revised October

782   ICD-10-PCS 2024

C81–CD1

C   **Nuclear Medicine**
D   **Gastrointestinal System**
2   **Tomographic (Tomo) Nuclear Medicine Imaging**   Definition: Introduction of radioactive materials into the body for three dimensional display of images developed from the capture of radioactive emissions

Body Part Character 4	Radionuclide Character 5	Qualifier Character 6	Qualifier Character 7
7 Gastrointestinal Tract	1 Technetium 99m (Tc-99m) D Indium 111 (In-111) Y Other Radionuclide	Z None	Z None
Y Digestive System	Y Other Radionuclide	Z None	Z None

C   **Nuclear Medicine**
F   **Hepatobiliary System and Pancreas**
1   **Planar Nuclear Medicine Imaging**   Definition: Introduction of radioactive materials into the body for single plane display of images developed from the capture of radioactive emissions

Body Part Character 4	Radionuclide Character 5	Qualifier Character 6	Qualifier Character 7
4 Gallbladder 5 Liver 6 Liver and Spleen C Hepatobiliary System, All	1 Technetium 99m (Tc-99m) Y Other Radionuclide	Z None	Z None
Y Hepatobiliary System and Pancreas	Y Other Radionuclide	Z None	Z None

C   **Nuclear Medicine**
F   **Hepatobiliary System and Pancreas**
2   **Tomographic (Tomo) Nuclear Medicine Imaging**   Definition: Introduction of radioactive materials into the body for three dimensional display of images developed from the capture of radioactive emissions

Body Part Character 4	Radionuclide Character 5	Qualifier Character 6	Qualifier Character 7
4 Gallbladder 5 Liver 6 Liver and Spleen	1 Technetium 99m (Tc-99m) Y Other Radionuclide	Z None	Z None
Y Hepatobiliary System and Pancreas	Y Other Radionuclide	Z None	Z None

C   **Nuclear Medicine**
G   **Endocrine System**
1   **Planar Nuclear Medicine Imaging**   Definition: Introduction of radioactive materials into the body for single plane display of images developed from the capture of radioactive emissions

Body Part Character 4	Radionuclide Character 5	Qualifier Character 6	Qualifier Character 7
1 Parathyroid Glands	1 Technetium 99m (Tc-99m) S Thallium 201 (Tl-201) Y Other Radionuclide	Z None	Z None
2 Thyroid Gland	1 Technetium 99m (Tc-99m) F Iodine 123 (I-123) G Iodine 131 (I-131) Y Other Radionuclide	Z None	Z None
4 Adrenal Glands, Bilateral	G Iodine 131 (I-131) Y Other Radionuclide	Z None	Z None
Y Endocrine System	Y Other Radionuclide	Z None	Z None

C   **Nuclear Medicine**
G   **Endocrine System**
2   **Tomographic (Tomo) Nuclear Medicine Imaging**   Definition: Introduction of radioactive materials into the body for three dimensional display of images developed from the capture of radioactive emissions

Body Part Character 4	Radionuclide Character 5	Qualifier Character 6	Qualifier Character 7
1 Parathyroid Glands	1 Technetium 99m (Tc-99m) S Thallium 201 (Tl-201) Y Other Radionuclide	Z None	Z None
Y Endocrine System	Y Other Radionuclide	Z None	Z None

NC Noncovered Procedure   LC Limited Coverage   QA Questionable OB Admit   NT New Tech Add-on   ✛ Combination Member   ♂ Male   ♀ Female

ICD-10-PCS 2024   783

Nuclear Medicine *(side tab)*

C   **Nuclear Medicine**
G   **Endocrine System**
4   **Nonimaging Nuclear Medicine Uptake**   Definition: Introduction of radioactive materials into the body for measurements of organ function, from the detection of radioactive emissions

Body Part Character 4	Radionuclide Character 5	Qualifier Character 6	Qualifier Character 7
2 Thyroid Gland	1 Technetium 99m (Tc-99m) F Iodine 123 (I-123) G Iodine 131 (I-131) Y Other Radionuclide	Z None	Z None
Y Endocrine System	Y Other Radionuclide	Z None	Z None

C   **Nuclear Medicine**
H   **Skin, Subcutaneous Tissue and Breast**
1   **Planar Nuclear Medicine Imaging**   Definition: Introduction of radioactive materials into the body for single plane display of images developed from the capture of radioactive emissions

Body Part Character 4	Radionuclide Character 5	Qualifier Character 6	Qualifier Character 7
Ø Breast, Right 1 Breast, Left 2 Breasts, Bilateral	1 Technetium 99m (Tc-99m) S Thallium 201 (Tl-201) Y Other Radionuclide	Z None	Z None
Y Skin, Subcutaneous Tissue and Breast	Y Other Radionuclide	Z None	Z None

C   **Nuclear Medicine**
H   **Skin, Subcutaneous Tissue and Breast**
2   **Tomographic (Tomo) Nuclear Medicine Imaging**   Definition: Introduction of radioactive materials into the body for three dimensional display of images developed from the capture of radioactive emissions

Body Part Character 4	Radionuclide Character 5	Qualifier Character 6	Qualifier Character 7
Ø Breast, Right 1 Breast, Left 2 Breasts, Bilateral	1 Technetium 99m (Tc-99m) S Thallium 201 (Tl-201) Y Other Radionuclide	Z None	Z None
Y Skin, Subcutaneous Tissue and Breast	Y Other Radionuclide	Z None	Z None

C   **Nuclear Medicine**
P   **Musculoskeletal System**
1   **Planar Nuclear Medicine Imaging**   Definition: Introduction of radioactive materials into the body for single plane display of images developed from the capture of radioactive emissions

Body Part Character 4	Radionuclide Character 5	Qualifier Character 6	Qualifier Character 7
1 Skull 4 Thorax 5 Spine 6 Pelvis 7 Spine and Pelvis 8 Upper Extremity, Right 9 Upper Extremity, Left B Upper Extremities, Bilateral C Lower Extremity, Right D Lower Extremity, Left F Lower Extremities, Bilateral Z Musculoskeletal System, All	1 Technetium 99m (Tc-99m) Y Other Radionuclide	Z None	Z None
Y Musculoskeletal System, Other	Y Other Radionuclide	Z None	Z None

C   Nuclear Medicine
P   Musculoskeletal System
2   Tomographic (Tomo) Nuclear Medicine Imaging   Definition: Introduction of radioactive materials into the body for three dimensional display of images developed from the capture of radioactive emissions

Body Part Character 4	Radionuclide Character 5	Qualifier Character 6	Qualifier Character 7
1 Skull 2 Cervical Spine 3 Skull and Cervical Spine 4 Thorax 6 Pelvis 7 Spine and Pelvis 8 Upper Extremity, Right 9 Upper Extremity, Left B Upper Extremities, Bilateral C Lower Extremity, Right D Lower Extremity, Left F Lower Extremities, Bilateral G Thoracic Spine H Lumbar Spine J Thoracolumbar Spine	1 Technetium 99m (Tc-99m) Y Other Radionuclide	Z None	Z None
Y Musculoskeletal System, Other	Y Other Radionuclide	Z None	Z None

C   Nuclear Medicine
P   Musculoskeletal System
5   Nonimaging Nuclear Medicine Probe   Definition: Introduction of radioactive materials into the body for the study of distribution and fate of certain substances by the detection of radioactive emissions; or, alternatively, measurement of absorption of radioactive emissions from an external source

Body Part Character 4	Radionuclide Character 5	Qualifier Character 6	Qualifier Character 7
5 Spine N Upper Extremities P Lower Extremities	Z None	Z None	Z None
Y Musculoskeletal System, Other	Y Other Radionuclide	Z None	Z None

C   Nuclear Medicine
T   Urinary System
1   Planar Nuclear Medicine Imaging   Definition: Introduction of radioactive materials into the body for single plane display of images developed from the capture of radioactive emissions

Body Part Character 4	Radionuclide Character 5	Qualifier Character 6	Qualifier Character 7
3 Kidneys, Ureters and Bladder	1 Technetium 99m (Tc-99m) F Iodine 123 (I-123) G Iodine 131 (I-131) Y Other Radionuclide	Z None	Z None
H Bladder and Ureters	1 Technetium 99m (Tc-99m) Y Other Radionuclide	Z None	Z None
Y Urinary System	Y Other Radionuclide	Z None	Z None

C   Nuclear Medicine
T   Urinary System
2   Tomographic (Tomo) Nuclear Medicine Imaging   Definition: Introduction of radioactive materials into the body for three dimensional display of images developed from the capture of radioactive emissions

Body Part Character 4	Radionuclide Character 5	Qualifier Character 6	Qualifier Character 7
3 Kidneys, Ureters and Bladder	1 Technetium 99m (Tc-99m) Y Other Radionuclide	Z None	Z None
Y Urinary System	Y Other Radionuclide	Z None	Z None

C   Nuclear Medicine
T   Urinary System
6   Nonimaging Nuclear Medicine Assay   Definition: Introduction of radioactive materials into the body for the study of body fluids and blood elements, by the detection of radioactive emissions

Body Part Character 4	Radionuclide Character 5	Qualifier Character 6	Qualifier Character 7
3 Kidneys, Ureters and Bladder	1 Technetium 99m (Tc-99m) F Iodine 123 (I-123) G Iodine 131 (I-131) H Iodine 125 (I-125) Y Other Radionuclide	Z None	Z None
Y Urinary System	Y Other Radionuclide	Z None	Z None

NC Noncovered Procedure   **LC** Limited Coverage   **QA** Questionable OB Admit   **NT** New Tech Add-on   ⊞ Combination Member   ♂ Male   ♀ Female

ICD-10-PCS 2024   785

CP2–CT6

Nuclear Medicine

C   **Nuclear Medicine**
V   **Male Reproductive System**
1   **Planar Nuclear Medicine Imaging**   Definition: Introduction of radioactive materials into the body for single plane display of images developed from the capture of radioactive emissions

Body Part Character 4	Radionuclide Character 5	Qualifier Character 6	Qualifier Character 7
9 Testicles, Bilateral ♂	1 Technetium 99m (Tc-99m) Y Other Radionuclide	Z None	Z None
Y Male Reproductive System ♂	Y Other Radionuclide	Z None	Z None

♂   All body part, radionuclide, and qualifier values

C   **Nuclear Medicine**
W   **Anatomical Regions**
1   **Planar Nuclear Medicine Imaging**   Definition: Introduction of radioactive materials into the body for single plane display of images developed from the capture of radioactive emissions

Body Part Character 4	Radionuclide Character 5	Qualifier Character 6	Qualifier Character 7
Ø Abdomen 1 Abdomen and Pelvis 4 Chest and Abdomen 6 Chest and Neck B Head and Neck D Lower Extremity J Pelvic Region M Upper Extremity N Whole Body	1 Technetium 99m (Tc-99m) D Indium 111 (In-111) F Iodine 123 (I-123) G Iodine 131 (I-131) L Gallium 67 (Ga-67) S Thallium 201 (Tl-201) Y Other Radionuclide	Z None	Z None
3 Chest	1 Technetium 99m (Tc-99m) D Indium 111 (In-111) F Iodine 123 (I-123) G Iodine 131 (I-131) K Fluorine 18 (F-18) L Gallium 67 (Ga-67) S Thallium 201 (Tl-201) Y Other Radionuclide	Z None	Z None
Y Anatomical Regions, Multiple	Y Other Radionuclide	Z None	Z None
Z Anatomical Region, Other	Z None	Z None	Z None

C   **Nuclear Medicine**
W   **Anatomical Regions**
2   **Tomographic (Tomo) Nuclear Medicine Imaging**   Definition: Introduction of radioactive materials into the body for three dimensional display of images developed from the capture of radioactive emissions

Body Part Character 4	Radionuclide Character 5	Qualifier Character 6	Qualifier Character 7
Ø Abdomen 1 Abdomen and Pelvis 3 Chest 4 Chest and Abdomen 6 Chest and Neck B Head and Neck D Lower Extremity J Pelvic Region M Upper Extremity	1 Technetium 99m (Tc-99m) D Indium 111 (In-111) F Iodine 123 (I-123) G Iodine 131 (I-131) K Fluorine 18 (F-18) L Gallium 67 (Ga-67) S Thallium 201 (Tl-201) Y Other Radionuclide	Z None	Z None
Y Anatomical Regions, Multiple	Y Other Radionuclide	Z None	Z None

C   **Nuclear Medicine**
W   **Anatomical Regions**
3   **Positron Emission Tomographic (PET) Imaging**   Definition: Introduction of radioactive materials into the body for three dimensional display of images developed from the simultaneous capture, 180 degrees apart, of radioactive emissions

Body Part Character 4	Radionuclide Character 5	Qualifier Character 6	Qualifier Character 7
N Whole Body	Y Other Radionuclide	Z None	Z None

C Nuclear Medicine
W Anatomical Regions
5 Nonimaging Nuclear Medicine Probe Definition: Introduction of radioactive materials into the body for the study of distribution and fate of certain substances by the detection of radioactive emissions; or, alternatively, measurement of absorption of radioactive emissions from an external source

Body Part Character 4	Radionuclide Character 5	Qualifier Character 6	Qualifier Character 7
Ø Abdomen 1 Abdomen and Pelvis 3 Chest 4 Chest and Abdomen 6 Chest and Neck B Head and Neck D Lower Extremity J Pelvic Region M Upper Extremity	1 Technetium 99m (Tc-99m) D Indium 111 (In-111) Y Other Radionuclide	Z None	Z None

C Nuclear Medicine
W Anatomical Regions
7 Systemic Nuclear Medicine Therapy Definition: Introduction of unsealed radioactive materials into the body for treatment

Body Part Character 4	Radionuclide Character 5	Qualifier Character 6	Qualifier Character 7
Ø Abdomen 3 Chest	N Phosphorus 32 (P-32) Y Other Radionuclide	Z None	Z None
G Thyroid	G Iodine 131 (I-131) Y Other Radionuclide	Z None	Z None
N Whole Body	8 Samarium 153 (Sm-153) G Iodine 131 (I-131) N Phosphorus 32 (P-32) P Strontium 89 (Sr-89) Y Other Radionuclide	Z None	Z None
Y Anatomical Regions, Multiple	Y Other Radionuclide	Z None	Z None

Radiation Therapy D00–DWY

AHA Coding Clinic for table D01
2020, 4Q, 43-44   Insertion of radioactive element
2020, 4Q, 69-70   Cesium 131 brachytherapy
2019, 4Q, 42-44   Unidirectional source brachytherapy

AHA Coding Clinic for table D0Y
2022, 4Q, 62   Deletion of qualifier value for laser interstitial thermal therapy
2020, 4Q, 70   Intraoperative radiation therapy

AHA Coding Clinic for table D71
2020, 4Q, 43-44   Insertion of radioactive element
2020, 4Q, 69-70   Cesium 131 brachytherapy
2019, 4Q, 42-44   Unidirectional source brachytherapy

AHA Coding Clinic for table D81
2020, 4Q, 43-44   Insertion of radioactive element
2020, 4Q, 69-70   Cesium 131 brachytherapy
2019, 4Q, 42-44   Unidirectional source brachytherapy

AHA Coding Clinic for table D91
2020, 4Q, 43-44   Insertion of radioactive element
2020, 4Q, 69-70   Cesium 131 brachytherapy
2019, 4Q, 42-44   Unidirectional source brachytherapy

AHA Coding Clinic for table DB1
2020, 4Q, 43-44   Insertion of radioactive element
2020, 4Q, 69-70   Cesium 131 brachytherapy
2019, 4Q, 42-44   Unidirectional source brachytherapy

AHA Coding Clinic for table DBY
2022, 4Q, 62   Deletion of qualifier value for laser interstitial thermal therapy

AHA Coding Clinic for table DD1
2020, 4Q, 43-44   Insertion of radioactive element
2020, 4Q, 69-70   Cesium 131 brachytherapy
2019, 4Q, 42-44   Unidirectional source brachytherapy

AHA Coding Clinic for table DDY
2022, 4Q, 62   Deletion of qualifier value for laser interstitial thermal therapy

AHA Coding Clinic for table DF1
2022, 2Q, 26   Radioembolization of right hepatic lobe
2020, 4Q, 43-44   Insertion of radioactive element
2020, 4Q, 69-70   Cesium 131 brachytherapy
2019, 4Q, 42-44   Unidirectional source brachytherapy

AHA Coding Clinic for table DFY
2022, 4Q, 62   Deletion of qualifier value for laser interstitial thermal therapy

AHA Coding Clinic for table DG1
2020, 4Q, 43-44   Insertion of radioactive element
2020, 4Q, 69-70   Cesium 131 brachytherapy
2019, 4Q, 42-44   Unidirectional source brachytherapy

AHA Coding Clinic for table DGY
2022, 4Q, 62   Deletion of qualifier value for laser interstitial thermal therapy

AHA Coding Clinic for table DM1
2020, 4Q, 43-44   Insertion of radioactive element
2020, 4Q, 69-70   Cesium 131 brachytherapy
2019, 4Q, 42-44   Unidirectional source brachytherapy

AHA Coding Clinic for table DMY
2022, 4Q, 62   Deletion of qualifier value for laser interstitial thermal therapy

AHA Coding Clinic for table DT1
2020, 4Q, 43-44   Insertion of radioactive element
2020, 4Q, 69-70   Cesium 131 brachytherapy
2019, 4Q, 42-44   Unidirectional source brachytherapy

AHA Coding Clinic for table DU1
2020, 4Q, 43-44   Insertion of radioactive element
2020, 4Q, 69-70   Cesium 131 brachytherapy
2019, 4Q, 42-44   Unidirectional source brachytherapy
2017, 4Q, 104   Intrauterine brachytherapy & placement of tandems & ovoids

AHA Coding Clinic for table DV1
2020, 4Q, 43-44   Insertion of radioactive element
2020, 4Q, 69-70   Cesium 131 brachytherapy
2019, 4Q, 42-44   Unidirectional source brachytherapy

AHA Coding Clinic for table DVY
2022, 4Q, 62   Deletion of qualifier value for laser interstitial thermal therapy

AHA Coding Clinic for table DW1
2020, 4Q, 43-44   Insertion of radioactive element
2020, 4Q, 69-70   Cesium 131 brachytherapy
2019, 4Q, 42-44   Unidirectional source brachytherapy

AHA Coding Clinic for table DWY
2019, 4Q, 37   Hyperthermic antineoplastic chemotherapy

D   **Radiation Therapy**
0   **Central and Peripheral Nervous System**
0   **Beam Radiation**

Treatment Site Character 4	Modality Qualifier Character 5	Isotope Character 6	Qualifier Character 7
0 Brain 1 Brain Stem 6 Spinal Cord 7 Peripheral Nerve	0 Photons <1 MeV 1 Photons 1- 10 MeV 2 Photons >10 MeV 4 Heavy Particles (Protons, Ions) 5 Neutrons 6 Neutron Capture	Z None	Z None
0 Brain 1 Brain Stem 6 Spinal Cord 7 Peripheral Nerve	3 Electrons	Z None	0 Intraoperative Z None

NC Noncovered Procedure   **LC** Limited Coverage   **QA** Questionable OB Admit   **NT** New Tech Add-on   ✚ Combination Member   ♂ Male   ♀ Female

ICD-10-PCS 2024   **789**

D00–D00

D   Radiation Therapy
Ø   Central and Peripheral Nervous System
1   Brachytherapy

Treatment Site Character 4	Modality Qualifier Character 5	Isotope Character 6	Qualifier Character 7
Ø Brain 1 Brain Stem 6 Spinal Cord 7 Peripheral Nerve	9 High Dose Rate (HDR)	7 Cesium 137 (Cs-137) 8 Iridium 192 (Ir-192) 9 Iodine 125 (I-125) B Palladium 103 (Pd-103) C Californium 252 (Cf-252) Y Other Isotope	Z None
Ø Brain 1 Brain Stem 6 Spinal Cord 7 Peripheral Nerve	B Low Dose Rate (LDR)	6 Cesium 131 (Cs-131) 7 Cesium 137 (Cs-137) 8 Iridium 192 (Ir-192) 9 Iodine 125 (I-125) C Californium 252 (Cf-252) Y Other Isotope	Z None
Ø Brain 1 Brain Stem 6 Spinal Cord 7 Peripheral Nerve	B Low Dose Rate (LDR)	B Palladium 103 (Pd-103)	1 Unidirectional Source Z None

D   Radiation Therapy
Ø   Central and Peripheral Nervous System
2   Stereotactic Radiosurgery

Treatment Site Character 4	Modality Qualifier Character 5	Isotope Character 6	Qualifier Character 7
Ø Brain 1 Brain Stem 6 Spinal Cord 7 Peripheral Nerve	D Stereotactic Other Photon Radiosurgery H Stereotactic Particulate Radiosurgery J Stereotactic Gamma Beam Radiosurgery	Z None	Z None

DRG Non-OR   All treatment site, modality, isotope, and qualifier values

D   Radiation Therapy
Ø   Central and Peripheral Nervous System
Y   Other Radiation

Treatment Site Character 4	Modality Qualifier Character 5	Isotope Character 6	Qualifier Character 7
Ø Brain 1 Brain Stem 6 Spinal Cord 7 Peripheral Nerve	7 Contact Radiation 8 Hyperthermia C Intraoperative Radiation Therapy (IORT) F Plaque Radiation	Z None	Z None

D   Radiation Therapy
7   Lymphatic and Hematologic System
Ø   Beam Radiation

Treatment Site Character 4	Modality Qualifier Character 5	Isotope Character 6	Qualifier Character 7
Ø Bone Marrow 1 Thymus 2 Spleen 3 Lymphatics, Neck 4 Lymphatics, Axillary 5 Lymphatics, Thorax 6 Lymphatics, Abdomen 7 Lymphatics, Pelvis 8 Lymphatics, Inguinal	Ø Photons <1 MeV 1 Photons 1- 10 MeV 2 Photons >10 MeV 4 Heavy Particles (Protons, Ions) 5 Neutrons 6 Neutron Capture	Z None	Z None
Ø Bone Marrow 1 Thymus 2 Spleen 3 Lymphatics, Neck 4 Lymphatics, Axillary 5 Lymphatics, Thorax 6 Lymphatics, Abdomen 7 Lymphatics, Pelvis 8 Lymphatics, Inguinal	3 Electrons	Z None	Ø Intraoperative Z None

Non-OR Procedure   DRG Non-OR Procedure   Valid OR Procedure   HAC Associated Procedure   Combination Only   New/Revised April   New/Revised October

790   ICD-10-PCS 2024

D01–D70

D Radiation Therapy
7 Lymphatic and Hematologic System
1 Brachytherapy

Treatment Site Character 4	Modality Qualifier Character 5	Isotope Character 6	Qualifier Character 7
Ø Bone Marrow 1 Thymus 2 Spleen 3 Lymphatics, Neck 4 Lymphatics, Axillary 5 Lymphatics, Thorax 6 Lymphatics, Abdomen 7 Lymphatics, Pelvis 8 Lymphatics, Inguinal	9 High Dose Rate (HDR)	7 Cesium 137 (Cs-137) 8 Iridium 192 (Ir-192) 9 Iodine 125 (I-125) B Palladium 103 (Pd-103) C Californium 252 (Cf-252) Y Other Isotope	Z None
Ø Bone Marrow 1 Thymus 2 Spleen 3 Lymphatics, Neck 4 Lymphatics, Axillary 5 Lymphatics, Thorax 6 Lymphatics, Abdomen 7 Lymphatics, Pelvis 8 Lymphatics, Inguinal	B Low Dose Rate (LDR)	6 Cesium 131 (Cs-131) 7 Cesium 137 (Cs-137) 8 Iridium 192 (Ir-192) 9 Iodine 125 (I-125) C Californium 252 (Cf-252) Y Other Isotope	Z None
Ø Bone Marrow 1 Thymus 2 Spleen 3 Lymphatics, Neck 4 Lymphatics, Axillary 5 Lymphatics, Thorax 6 Lymphatics, Abdomen 7 Lymphatics, Pelvis 8 Lymphatics, Inguinal	B Low Dose Rate (LDR)	B Palladium 103 (Pd-103)	1 Unidirectional Source Z None

D Radiation Therapy
7 Lymphatic and Hematologic System
2 Stereotactic Radiosurgery

Treatment Site Character 4	Modality Qualifier Character 5	Isotope Character 6	Qualifier Character 7
Ø Bone Marrow 1 Thymus 2 Spleen 3 Lymphatics, Neck 4 Lymphatics, Axillary 5 Lymphatics, Thorax 6 Lymphatics, Abdomen 7 Lymphatics, Pelvis 8 Lymphatics, Inguinal	D Stereotactic Other Photon Radiosurgery H Stereotactic Particulate Radiosurgery J Stereotactic Gamma Beam Radiosurgery	Z None	Z None

DRG Non-OR All treatment site, modality, isotope, and qualifier values

D Radiation Therapy
7 Lymphatic and Hematologic System
Y Other Radiation

Treatment Site Character 4	Modality Qualifier Character 5	Isotope Character 6	Qualifier Character 7
Ø Bone Marrow 1 Thymus 2 Spleen 3 Lymphatics, Neck 4 Lymphatics, Axillary 5 Lymphatics, Thorax 6 Lymphatics, Abdomen 7 Lymphatics, Pelvis 8 Lymphatics, Inguinal	8 Hyperthermia F Plaque Radiation	Z None	Z None

NC Noncovered Procedure   LC Limited Coverage   QA Questionable OB Admit   NT New Tech Add-on   ⊞ Combination Member   ♂ Male   ♀ Female

ICD-10-PCS 2024   791

D71–D7Y

Radiation Therapy

D Radiation Therapy
8 Eye
Ø Beam Radiation

Treatment Site Character 4	Modality Qualifier Character 5	Isotope Character 6	Qualifier Character 7
Ø Eye	Ø Photons <1 MeV 1 Photons 1- 10 MeV 2 Photons >10 MeV 4 Heavy Particles (Protons, Ions) 5 Neutrons 6 Neutron Capture	Z None	Z None
Ø Eye	3 Electrons	Z None	Ø Intraoperative Z None

D Radiation Therapy
8 Eye
1 Brachytherapy

Treatment Site Character 4	Modality Qualifier Character 5	Isotope Character 6	Qualifier Character 7
Ø Eye	9 High Dose Rate (HDR)	7 Cesium 137 (Cs-137) 8 Iridium 192 (Ir-192) 9 Iodine 125 (I-125) B Palladium 103 (Pd-103) C Californium 252 (Cf-252) Y Other Isotope	Z None
Ø Eye	B Low Dose Rate (LDR)	6 Cesium 131 (Cs-131) 7 Cesium 137 (Cs-137) 8 Iridium 192 (Ir-192) 9 Iodine 125 (I-125) C Californium 252 (Cf-252) Y Other Isotope	Z None
Ø Eye	B Low Dose Rate (LDR)	B Palladium 103 (Pd-103)	1 Unidirectional Source Z None

D Radiation Therapy
8 Eye
2 Stereotactic Radiosurgery

Treatment Site Character 4	Modality Qualifier Character 5	Isotope Character 6	Qualifier Character 7
Ø Eye	D Stereotactic Other Photon Radiosurgery H Stereotactic Particulate Radiosurgery J Stereotactic Gamma Beam Radiosurgery	Z None	Z None

DRG Non-OR All treatment site, modality, isotope, and qualifier values

D Radiation Therapy
8 Eye
Y Other Radiation

Treatment Site Character 4	Modality Qualifier Character 5	Isotope Character 6	Qualifier Character 7
Ø Eye	7 Contact Radiation 8 Hyperthermia F Plaque Radiation	Z None	Z None

D Radiation Therapy
9 Ear, Nose, Mouth and Throat
Ø Beam Radiation

Treatment Site Character 4	Modality Qualifier Character 5	Isotope Character 6	Qualifier Character 7
Ø Ear 1 Nose 3 Hypopharynx 4 Mouth 5 Tongue 6 Salivary Glands 7 Sinuses 8 Hard Palate 9 Soft Palate B Larynx D Nasopharynx F Oropharynx	Ø Photons <1 MeV 1 Photons 1- 10 MeV 2 Photons >10 MeV 4 Heavy Particles (Protons, Ions) 5 Neutrons 6 Neutron Capture	Z None	Z None
Ø Ear 1 Nose 3 Hypopharynx 4 Mouth 5 Tongue 6 Salivary Glands 7 Sinuses 8 Hard Palate 9 Soft Palate B Larynx D Nasopharynx F Oropharynx	3 Electrons	Z None	Ø Intraoperative Z None

D Radiation Therapy
9 Ear, Nose, Mouth and Throat
1 Brachytherapy

Treatment Site Character 4	Modality Qualifier Character 5	Isotope Character 6	Qualifier Character 7
Ø Ear 1 Nose 3 Hypopharynx 4 Mouth 5 Tongue 6 Salivary Glands 7 Sinuses 8 Hard Palate 9 Soft Palate B Larynx D Nasopharynx F Oropharynx	9 High Dose Rate (HDR)	7 Cesium 137 (Cs-137) 8 Iridium 192 (Ir-192) 9 Iodine 125 (I-125) B Palladium 103 (Pd-103) C Californium 252 (Cf-252) Y Other Isotope	Z None
Ø Ear 1 Nose 3 Hypopharynx 4 Mouth 5 Tongue 6 Salivary Glands 7 Sinuses 8 Hard Palate 9 Soft Palate B Larynx D Nasopharynx F Oropharynx	B Low Dose Rate (LDR)	6 Cesium 131 (Cs-131) 7 Cesium 137 (Cs-137) 8 Iridium 192 (Ir-192) 9 Iodine 125 (I-125) C Californium 252 (Cf-252) Y Other Isotope	Z None
Ø Ear 1 Nose 3 Hypopharynx 4 Mouth 5 Tongue 6 Salivary Glands 7 Sinuses 8 Hard Palate 9 Soft Palate B Larynx D Nasopharynx F Oropharynx	B Low Dose Rate (LDR)	B Palladium 103 (Pd-103)	1 Unidirectional Source Z None

---

NC Noncovered Procedure   LC Limited Coverage   QA Questionable OB Admit   NT New Tech Add-on   ⊞ Combination Member   ♂ Male   ♀ Female

Radiation Therapy

D Radiation Therapy
9 Ear, Nose, Mouth and Throat
2 Stereotactic Radiosurgery

Treatment Site Character 4	Modality Qualifier Character 5	Isotope Character 6	Qualifier Character 7
Ø Ear 1 Nose 4 Mouth 5 Tongue 6 Salivary Glands 7 Sinuses 8 Hard Palate 9 Soft Palate B Larynx C Pharynx D Nasopharynx	D Stereotactic Other Photon Radiosurgery H Stereotactic Particulate Radiosurgery J Stereotactic Gamma Beam Radiosurgery	Z None	Z None

DRG Non-OR All treatment site, modality, isotope, and qualifier values

D Radiation Therapy
9 Ear, Nose, Mouth and Throat
Y Other Radiation

Treatment Site Character 4	Modality Qualifier Character 5	Isotope Character 6	Qualifier Character 7
Ø Ear 1 Nose 5 Tongue 6 Salivary Glands 7 Sinuses 8 Hard Palate 9 Soft Palate	7 Contact Radiation 8 Hyperthermia F Plaque Radiation	Z None	Z None
3 Hypopharynx F Oropharynx	7 Contact Radiation 8 Hyperthermia	Z None	Z None
4 Mouth B Larynx D Nasopharynx	7 Contact Radiation 8 Hyperthermia C Intraoperative Radiation Therapy (IORT) F Plaque Radiation	Z None	Z None
C Pharynx	C Intraoperative Radiation Therapy (IORT) F Plaque Radiation	Z None	Z None

D Radiation Therapy
B Respiratory System
Ø Beam Radiation

Treatment Site Character 4	Modality Qualifier Character 5	Isotope Character 6	Qualifier Character 7
Ø Trachea 1 Bronchus 2 Lung 5 Pleura 6 Mediastinum 7 Chest Wall 8 Diaphragm	Ø Photons <1 MeV 1 Photons 1- 10 MeV 2 Photons >10 MeV 4 Heavy Particles (Protons, Ions) 5 Neutrons 6 Neutron Capture	Z None	Z None
Ø Trachea 1 Bronchus 2 Lung 5 Pleura 6 Mediastinum 7 Chest Wall 8 Diaphragm	3 Electrons	Z None	Ø Intraoperative Z None

Non-OR Procedure   DRG Non-OR Procedure   Valid OR Procedure   HAC Associated Procedure   Combination Only   New/Revised April   New/Revised October

794

ICD-10-PCS 2024

D92–DBØ

D   Radiation Therapy
B   Respiratory System
1   Brachytherapy

Treatment Site Character 4	Modality Qualifier Character 5	Isotope Character 6	Qualifier Character 7
Ø Trachea 1 Bronchus 2 Lung 5 Pleura 6 Mediastinum 7 Chest Wall 8 Diaphragm	9 High Dose Rate (HDR)	7 Cesium 137 (Cs-137) 8 Iridium 192 (Ir-192) 9 Iodine 125 (I-125) B Palladium 103 (Pd-103) C Californium 252 (Cf-252) Y Other Isotope	Z None
Ø Trachea 1 Bronchus 2 Lung 5 Pleura 6 Mediastinum 7 Chest Wall 8 Diaphragm	B Low Dose Rate (LDR)	6 Cesium 131 (Cs-131) 7 Cesium 137 (Cs-137) 8 Iridium 192 (Ir-192) 9 Iodine 125 (I-125) C Californium 252 (Cf-252) Y Other Isotope	Z None
Ø Trachea 1 Bronchus 2 Lung 5 Pleura 6 Mediastinum 7 Chest Wall 8 Diaphragm	B Low Dose Rate (LDR)	B Palladium 103 (Pd-103)	1 Unidirectional Source Z None

D   Radiation Therapy
B   Respiratory System
2   Stereotactic Radiosurgery

Treatment Site Character 4	Modality Qualifier Character 5	Isotope Character 6	Qualifier Character 7
Ø Trachea 1 Bronchus 2 Lung 5 Pleura 6 Mediastinum 7 Chest Wall 8 Diaphragm	D Stereotactic Other Photon Radiosurgery H Stereotactic Particulate Radiosurgery J Stereotactic Gamma Beam Radiosurgery	Z None	Z None

DRG Non-OR   All treatment site, modality, isotope, and qualifier values

D   Radiation Therapy
B   Respiratory System
Y   Other Radiation

Treatment Site Character 4	Modality Qualifier Character 5	Isotope Character 6	Qualifier Character 7
Ø Trachea 1 Bronchus 2 Lung 5 Pleura 6 Mediastinum 7 Chest Wall 8 Diaphragm	7 Contact Radiation 8 Hyperthermia F Plaque Radiation	Z None	Z None

NC Noncovered Procedure   LC Limited Coverage   QA Questionable OB Admit   NT New Tech Add-on   ⊞ Combination Member   ♂ Male   ♀ Female

ICD-10-PCS 2024   795

Radiation Therapy

DB1–DBY

Radiation Therapy

D   **Radiation Therapy**
D   **Gastrointestinal System**
Ø   **Beam Radiation**

Treatment Site Character 4	Modality Qualifier Character 5	Isotope Character 6	Qualifier Character 7
Ø Esophagus 1 Stomach 2 Duodenum 3 Jejunum 4 Ileum 5 Colon 7 Rectum	Ø Photons <1 MeV 1 Photons 1- 10 MeV 2 Photons >10 MeV 4 Heavy Particles (Protons, Ions) 5 Neutrons 6 Neutron Capture	Z None	Z None
Ø Esophagus 1 Stomach 2 Duodenum 3 Jejunum 4 Ileum 5 Colon 7 Rectum	3 Electrons	Z None	Ø Intraoperative Z None

D   **Radiation Therapy**
D   **Gastrointestinal System**
1   **Brachytherapy**

Treatment Site Character 4	Modality Qualifier Character 5	Isotope Character 6	Qualifier Character 7
Ø Esophagus 1 Stomach 2 Duodenum 3 Jejunum 4 Ileum 5 Colon 7 Rectum	9 High Dose Rate (HDR)	7 Cesium 137 (Cs-137) 8 Iridium 192 (Ir-192) 9 Iodine 125 (I-125) B Palladium 103 (Pd-103) C Californium 252 (Cf-252) Y Other Isotope	Z None
Ø Esophagus 1 Stomach 2 Duodenum 3 Jejunum 4 Ileum 5 Colon 7 Rectum	B Low Dose Rate (LDR)	6 Cesium 131 (Cs-131) 7 Cesium 137 (Cs-137) 8 Iridium 192 (Ir-192) 9 Iodine 125 (I-125) C Californium 252 (Cf-252) Y Other Isotope	Z None
Ø Esophagus 1 Stomach 2 Duodenum 3 Jejunum 4 Ileum 5 Colon 7 Rectum	B Low Dose Rate (LDR)	B Palladium 103 (Pd-103)	1 Unidirectional Source Z None

D   **Radiation Therapy**
D   **Gastrointestinal System**
2   **Stereotactic Radiosurgery**

Treatment Site Character 4	Modality Qualifier Character 5	Isotope Character 6	Qualifier Character 7
Ø Esophagus 1 Stomach 2 Duodenum 3 Jejunum 4 Ileum 5 Colon 7 Rectum	D Stereotactic Other Photon Radiosurgery H Stereotactic Particulate Radiosurgery J Stereotactic Gamma Beam Radiosurgery	Z None	Z None

DRG Non-OR   All treatment site, modality, isotope, and qualifier values

Non-OR Procedure   DRG Non-OR Procedure   Valid OR Procedure   HAC Associated Procedure   Combination Only   New/Revised April   New/Revised October

796   ICD-10-PCS 2024

D Radiation therapy
D Gastrointestinal System
Y Other Radiation

Treatment Site Character 4	Modality Qualifier Character 5	Isotope Character 6	Qualifier Character 7
Ø Esophagus	7 Contact Radiation 8 Hyperthermia F Plaque Radiation	Z None	Z None
1 Stomach 2 Duodenum 3 Jejunum 4 Ileum 5 Colon 7 Rectum	7 Contact Radiation 8 Hyperthermia C Intraoperative Radiation Therapy (IORT) F Plaque Radiation	Z None	Z None
8 Anus	C Intraoperative Radiation Therapy (IORT) F Plaque Radiation	Z None	Z None

D Radiation Therapy
F Hepatobiliary System and Pancreas
Ø Beam Radiation

Treatment Site Character 4	Modality Qualifier Character 5	Isotope Character 6	Qualifier Character 7
Ø Liver 1 Gallbladder 2 Bile Ducts 3 Pancreas	Ø Photons <1 MeV 1 Photons 1- 10 MeV 2 Photons >10 MeV 4 Heavy Particles (Protons, Ions) 5 Neutrons 6 Neutron Capture	Z None	Z None
Ø Liver 1 Gallbladder 2 Bile Ducts 3 Pancreas	3 Electrons	Z None	Ø Intraoperative Z None

D Radiation Therapy
F Hepatobiliary System and Pancreas
1 Brachytherapy

Treatment Site Character 4	Modality Qualifier Character 5	Isotope Character 6	Qualifier Character 7
Ø Liver 1 Gallbladder 2 Bile Ducts 3 Pancreas	9 High Dose Rate (HDR)	7 Cesium 137 (Cs-137) 8 Iridium 192 (Ir-192) 9 Iodine 125 (I-125) B Palladium 103 (Pd-103) C Californium 252 (Cf-252) Y Other Isotope	Z None
Ø Liver 1 Gallbladder 2 Bile Ducts 3 Pancreas	B Low Dose Rate (LDR)	6 Cesium 131 (Cs-131) 7 Cesium 137 (Cs-137) 8 Iridium 192 (Ir-192) 9 Iodine 125 (I-125) C Californium 252 (Cf-252) Y Other Isotope	Z None
Ø Liver 1 Gallbladder 2 Bile Ducts 3 Pancreas	B Low Dose Rate (LDR)	B Palladium 103 (Pd-103)	1 Unidirectional Source Z None

D Radiation Therapy
F Hepatobiliary System and Pancreas
2 Stereotactic Radiosurgery

Treatment Site Character 4	Modality Qualifier Character 5	Isotope Character 6	Qualifier Character 7
Ø Liver 1 Gallbladder 2 Bile Ducts 3 Pancreas	D Stereotactic Other Photon Radiosurgery H Stereotactic Particulate Radiosurgery J Stereotactic Gamma Beam Radiosurgery	Z None	Z None

DRG Non-OR All treatment site, modality, isotope, and qualifier values

NC Noncovered Procedure   **LC** Limited Coverage   **QA** Questionable OB Admit   **NT** New Tech Add-on   ⊞ Combination Member   ♂ Male   ♀ Female

ICD-10-PCS 2024   797

DDY–DF2

Radiation Therapy

D Radiation Therapy
F Hepatobiliary System and Pancreas
Y Other Radiation

Treatment Site Character 4	Modality Qualifier Character 5	Isotope Character 6	Qualifier Character 7
Ø Liver 1 Gallbladder 2 Bile Ducts 3 Pancreas	7 Contact Radiation 8 Hyperthermia C Intraoperative Radiation Therapy (IORT) F Plaque Radiation	Z None	Z None

D Radiation Therapy
G Endocrine System
Ø Beam Radiation

Treatment Site Character 4	Modality Qualifier Character 5	Isotope Character 6	Qualifier Character 7
Ø Pituitary Gland 1 Pineal Body 2 Adrenal Glands 4 Parathyroid Glands 5 Thyroid	Ø Photons <1 MeV 1 Photons 1- 10 MeV 2 Photons >10 MeV 5 Neutrons 6 Neutron Capture	Z None	Z None
Ø Pituitary Gland 1 Pineal Body 2 Adrenal Glands 4 Parathyroid Glands 5 Thyroid	3 Electrons	Z None	Ø Intraoperative Z None

D Radiation Therapy
G Endocrine System
1 Brachytherapy

Treatment Site Character 4	Modality Qualifier Character 5	Isotope Character 6	Qualifier Character 7
Ø Pituitary Gland 1 Pineal Body 2 Adrenal Glands 4 Parathyroid Glands 5 Thyroid	9 High Dose Rate (HDR)	7 Cesium 137 (Cs-137) 8 Iridium 192 (Ir-192) 9 Iodine 125 (I-125) B Palladium 103 (Pd-103) C Californium 252 (Cf-252) Y Other Isotope	Z None
Ø Pituitary Gland 1 Pineal Body 2 Adrenal Glands 4 Parathyroid Glands 5 Thyroid	B Low Dose Rate (LDR)	6 Cesium 131 (Cs-131) 7 Cesium 137 (Cs-137) 8 Iridium 192 (Ir-192) 9 Iodine 125 (I-125) C Californium 252 (Cf-252) Y Other Isotope	Z None
Ø Pituitary Gland 1 Pineal Body 2 Adrenal Glands 4 Parathyroid Glands 5 Thyroid	B Low Dose Rate (LDR)	B Palladium 103 (Pd-103)	1 Unidirectional Source Z None

D Radiation Therapy
G Endocrine System
2 Stereotactic Radiosurgery

Treatment Site Character 4	Modality Qualifier Character 5	Isotope Character 6	Qualifier Character 7
Ø Pituitary Gland 1 Pineal Body 2 Adrenal Glands 4 Parathyroid Glands 5 Thyroid	D Stereotactic Other Photon Radiosurgery H Stereotactic Particulate Radiosurgery J Stereotactic Gamma Beam Radiosurgery	Z None	Z None

DRG Non-OR All treatment site, modality, isotope, and qualifier values

Non-OR Procedure   DRG Non-OR Procedure   Valid OR Procedure   HAC Associated Procedure   Combination Only   New/Revised April   New/Revised October

798   ICD-10-PCS 2024

D   Radiation therapy
G   Endocrine System
Y   Other Radiation

Treatment Site Character 4	Modality Qualifier Character 5	Isotope Character 6	Qualifier Character 7
Ø Pituitary Gland 1 Pineal Body 2 Adrenal Glands 4 Parathyroid Glands 5 Thyroid	7 Contact Radiation 8 Hyperthermia F Plaque Radiation	Z None	Z None

D   Radiation Therapy
H   Skin
Ø   Beam Radiation

Treatment Site Character 4	Modality Qualifier Character 5	Isotope Character 6	Qualifier Character 7
2 Skin, Face 3 Skin, Neck 4 Skin, Arm 6 Skin, Chest 7 Skin, Back 8 Skin, Abdomen 9 Skin, Buttock B Skin, Leg	Ø Photons <1 MeV 1 Photons 1- 10 MeV 2 Photons >10 MeV 4 Heavy Particles (Protons, Ions) 5 Neutrons 6 Neutron Capture	Z None	Z None
2 Skin, Face 3 Skin, Neck 4 Skin, Arm 6 Skin, Chest 7 Skin, Back 8 Skin, Abdomen 9 Skin, Buttock B Skin, Leg	3 Electrons	Z None	Ø Intraoperative Z None

D   Radiation Therapy
H   Skin
Y   Other Radiation

Treatment Site Character 4	Modality Qualifier Character 5	Isotope Character 6	Qualifier Character 7
2 Skin, Face 3 Skin, Neck 4 Skin, Arm 6 Skin, Chest 7 Skin, Back 8 Skin, Abdomen 9 Skin, Buttock B Skin, Leg	7 Contact Radiation 8 Hyperthermia F Plaque Radiation	Z None	Z None
5 Skin, Hand C Skin, Foot	F Plaque Radiation	Z None	Z None

D   Radiation Therapy
M   Breast
Ø   Beam Radiation

Treatment Site Character 4	Modality Qualifier Character 5	Isotope Character 6	Qualifier Character 7
Ø Breast, Left 1 Breast, Right	Ø Photons <1 MeV 1 Photons 1- 10 MeV 2 Photons >10 MeV 4 Heavy Particles (Protons, Ions) 5 Neutrons 6 Neutron Capture	Z None	Z None
Ø Breast, Left 1 Breast, Right	3 Electrons	Z None	Ø Intraoperative Z None

NC Noncovered Procedure   LC Limited Coverage   QA Questionable OB Admit   NT New Tech Add-on   ⊞ Combination Member   ♂ Male   ♀ Female

ICD-10-PCS 2024   799

Radiation Therapy

DGY–DMØ

Radiation Therapy *(left margin)*

D　Radiation Therapy
M　Breast
1　Brachytherapy

Treatment Site Character 4	Modality Qualifier Character 5	Isotope Character 6	Qualifier Character 7
Ø　Breast, Left 1　Breast, Right	9　High Dose Rate (HDR)	7　Cesium 137 (Cs-137) 8　Iridium 192 (Ir-192) 9　Iodine 125 (I-125) B　Palladium 103 (Pd-103) C　Californium 252 (Cf-252) Y　Other Isotope	Z　None
Ø　Breast, Left 1　Breast, Right	B　Low Dose Rate (LDR)	6　Cesium 131 (Cs-131) 7　Cesium 137 (Cs-137) 8　Iridium 192 (Ir-192) 9　Iodine 125 (I-125) C　Californium 252 (Cf-252) Y　Other Isotope	Z　None
Ø　Breast, Left 1　Breast, Right	B　Low Dose Rate (LDR)	B　Palladium 103 (Pd-103)	1　Unidirectional Source Z　None

D　Radiation Therapy
M　Breast
2　Stereotactic Radiosurgery

Treatment Site Character 4	Modality Qualifier Character 5	Isotope Character 6	Qualifier Character 7
Ø　Breast, Left 1　Breast, Right	D　Stereotactic Other Photon 　　Radiosurgery H　Stereotactic Particulate 　　Radiosurgery J　Stereotactic Gamma Beam 　　Radiosurgery	Z　None	Z　None

DRG Non-OR　All treatment site, modality, isotope, and qualifier values

D　Radiation Therapy
M　Breast
Y　Other Radiation

Treatment Site Character 4	Modality Qualifier Character 5	Isotope Character 6	Qualifier Character 7
Ø　Breast, Left 1　Breast, Right	7　Contact Radiation 8　Hyperthermia F　Plaque Radiation	Z　None	Z　None

D　Radiation Therapy
P　Musculoskeletal System
Ø　Beam Radiation

Treatment Site Character 4	Modality Qualifier Character 5	Isotope Character 6	Qualifier Character 7
Ø　Skull 2　Maxilla 3　Mandible 4　Sternum 5　Rib(s) 6　Humerus 7　Radius/Ulna 8　Pelvic Bones 9　Femur B　Tibia/Fibula C　Other Bone	Ø　Photons <1 MeV 1　Photons 1- 10 MeV 2　Photons >10 MeV 4　Heavy Particles (Protons, Ions) 5　Neutrons 6　Neutron Capture	Z　None	Z　None
Ø　Skull 2　Maxilla 3　Mandible 4　Sternum 5　Rib(s) 6　Humerus 7　Radius/Ulna 8　Pelvic Bones 9　Femur B　Tibia/Fibula C　Other Bone	3　Electrons	Z　None	Ø　Intraoperative Z　None

*(left margin)* DM1–DPØ

D   Radiation Therapy
P   Musculoskeletal System
Y   Other Radiation

Treatment Site Character 4	Modality Qualifier Character 5	Isotope Character 6	Qualifier Character 7
Ø Skull 2 Maxilla 3 Mandible 4 Sternum 5 Rib(s) 6 Humerus 7 Radius/Ulna 8 Pelvic Bones 9 Femur B Tibia/Fibula C Other Bone	7 Contact Radiation 8 Hyperthermia F Plaque Radiation	Z None	Z None

D   Radiation Therapy
T   Urinary System
Ø   Beam Radiation

Treatment Site Character 4	Modality Qualifier Character 5	Isotope Character 6	Qualifier Character 7
Ø Kidney 1 Ureter 2 Bladder 3 Urethra	Ø Photons <1 MeV 1 Photons 1- 10 MeV 2 Photons >10 MeV 4 Heavy Particles (Protons, Ions) 5 Neutrons 6 Neutron Capture	Z None	Z None
Ø Kidney 1 Ureter 2 Bladder 3 Urethra	3 Electrons	Z None	Ø Intraoperative Z None

D   Radiation Therapy
T   Urinary System
1   Brachytherapy

Treatment Site Character 4	Modality Qualifier Character 5	Isotope Character 6	Qualifier Character 7
Ø Kidney 1 Ureter 2 Bladder 3 Urethra	9 High Dose Rate (HDR)	7 Cesium 137 (Cs-137) 8 Iridium 192 (Ir-192) 9 Iodine 125 (I-125) B Palladium 103 (Pd-103) C Californium 252 (Cf-252) Y Other Isotope	Z None
Ø Kidney 1 Ureter 2 Bladder 3 Urethra	B Low Dose Rate (LDR)	6 Cesium 131 (Cs-131) 7 Cesium 137 (Cs-137) 8 Iridium 192 (Ir-192) 9 Iodine 125 (I-125) C Californium 252 (Cf-252) Y Other Isotope	Z None
Ø Kidney 1 Ureter 2 Bladder 3 Urethra	B Low Dose Rate (LDR)	B Palladium 103 (Pd-103)	1 Unidirectional Source Z None

D   Radiation Therapy
T   Urinary System
2   Stereotactic Radiosurgery

Treatment Site Character 4	Modality Qualifier Character 5	Isotope Character 6	Qualifier Character 7
Ø Kidney 1 Ureter 2 Bladder 3 Urethra	D Stereotactic Other Photon Radiosurgery H Stereotactic Particulate Radiosurgery J Stereotactic Gamma Beam Radiosurgery	Z None	Z None

DRG Non-OR   All treatment site, modality, isotope, and qualifier values

NC Noncovered Procedure   LC Limited Coverage   QA Questionable OB Admit   NT New Tech Add-on   ✚ Combination Member   ♂ Male   ♀ Female

ICD-10-PCS 2024   801

Radiation Therapy

D Radiation Therapy
T Urinary System
Y Other Radiation

Treatment Site Character 4	Modality Qualifier Character 5	Isotope Character 6	Qualifier Character 7
Ø Kidney 1 Ureter 2 Bladder 3 Urethra	7 Contact Radiation 8 Hyperthermia C Intraoperative Radiation Therapy (IORT) F Plaque Radiation	Z None	Z None

D Radiation Therapy
U Female Reproductive System
Ø Beam Radiation

Treatment Site Character 4	Modality Qualifier Character 5	Isotope Character 6	Qualifier Character 7
Ø Ovary ♀ 1 Cervix ♀ 2 Uterus ♀	Ø Photons <1 MeV 1 Photons 1- 10 MeV 2 Photons >10 MeV 4 Heavy Particles (Protons, Ions) 5 Neutrons 6 Neutron Capture	Z None	Z None
Ø Ovary ♀ 1 Cervix ♀ 2 Uterus ♀	3 Electrons	Z None	Ø Intraoperative Z None

♀   All treatment site, modality, isotope, and qualifier values

D Radiation Therapy
U Female Reproductive System
1 Brachytherapy

Treatment Site Character 4	Modality Qualifier Character 5	Isotope Character 6	Qualifier Character 7
Ø Ovary ♀ 1 Cervix ♀ 2 Uterus ♀	9 High Dose Rate (HDR)	7 Cesium 137 (Cs-137) 8 Iridium 192 (Ir-192) 9 Iodine 125 (I-125) B Palladium 103 (Pd-103) C Californium 252 (Cf-252) Y Other Isotope	Z None
Ø Ovary ♀ 1 Cervix ♀ 2 Uterus ♀	B Low Dose Rate (LDR)	6 Cesium 131 (Cs-131) 7 Cesium 137 (Cs-137) 8 Iridium 192 (Ir-192) 9 Iodine 125 (I-125) C Californium 252 (Cf-252) Y Other Isotope	Z None
Ø Ovary ♀ 1 Cervix ♀ 2 Uterus ♀	B Low Dose Rate (LDR)	B Palladium 103 (Pd-103)	1 Unidirectional Source Z None

♀   All treatment site, modality, isotope, and qualifier values

D Radiation Therapy
U Female Reproductive System
2 Stereotactic Radiosurgery

Treatment Site Character 4	Modality Qualifier Character 5	Isotope Character 6	Qualifier Character 7
Ø Ovary ♀ 1 Cervix ♀ 2 Uterus ♀	D Stereotactic Other Photon Radiosurgery H Stereotactic Particulate Radiosurgery J Stereotactic Gamma Beam Radiosurgery	Z None	Z None

DRG Non-OR   All treatment site, modality, isotope, and qualifier values
♀   All treatment site, modality, isotope, and qualifier values

Non-OR Procedure   DRG Non-OR Procedure   Valid OR Procedure   HAC Associated Procedure   Combination Only   New/Revised April   New/Revised October

802   ICD-10-PCS 2024

DTY–DU2

D   Radiation Therapy
U   Female Reproductive System
Y   Other Radiation

Treatment Site Character 4		Modality Qualifier Character 5	Isotope Character 6	Qualifier Character 7
Ø Ovary	♀	7 Contact Radiation	Z None	Z None
1 Cervix	♀	8 Hyperthermia		
2 Uterus	♀	C Intraoperative Radiation Therapy (IORT)		
		F Plaque Radiation		

♀   All treatment site, modality, isotope, and qualifier values

D   Radiation Therapy
V   Male Reproductive System
Ø   Beam Radiation

Treatment Site Character 4		Modality Qualifier Character 5	Isotope Character 6	Qualifier Character 7
Ø Prostate	♂	Ø Photons <1 MeV	Z None	Z None
1 Testis	♂	1 Photons 1- 10 MeV		
		2 Photons >10 MeV		
		4 Heavy Particles (Protons, Ions)		
		5 Neutrons		
		6 Neutron Capture		
Ø Prostate	♂	3 Electrons	Z None	Ø Intraoperative
1 Testis	♂			Z None

♂   All treatment site, modality, isotope, and qualifier values

D   Radiation Therapy
V   Male Reproductive System
1   Brachytherapy

Treatment Site Character 4		Modality Qualifier Character 5	Isotope Character 6	Qualifier Character 7
Ø Prostate	♂	9 High Dose Rate (HDR)	7 Cesium 137 (Cs-137)	Z None
1 Testis	♂		8 Iridium 192 (Ir-192)	
			9 Iodine 125 (I-125)	
			B Palladium 103 (Pd-103)	
			C Californium 252 (Cf-252)	
			Y Other Isotope	
Ø Prostate	♂	B Low Dose Rate (LDR)	6 Cesium 131 (Cs-131)	Z None
1 Testis	♂		7 Cesium 137 (Cs-137)	
			8 Iridium 192 (Ir-192)	
			9 Iodine 125 (I-125)	
			C Californium 252 (Cf-252)	
			Y Other Isotope	
Ø Prostate	♂	B Low Dose Rate (LDR)	B Palladium 103 (Pd-103)	1 Unidirectional Source
1 Testis	♂			Z None

♂   All treatment site, modality, isotope, and qualifier values

D   Radiation Therapy
V   Male Reproductive System
2   Stereotactic Radiosurgery

Treatment Site Character 4		Modality Qualifier Character 5	Isotope Character 6	Qualifier Character 7
Ø Prostate	♂	D Stereotactic Other Photon Radiosurgery	Z None	Z None
1 Testis	♂	H Stereotactic Particulate Radiosurgery		
		J Stereotactic Gamma Beam Radiosurgery		

DRG Non-OR   All treatment site, modality, isotope, and qualifier values
♂   All treatment site, modality, isotope, and qualifier values

NC Noncovered Procedure   LC Limited Coverage   QA Questionable OB Admit   NT New Tech Add-on   ⊞ Combination Member   ♂ Male   ♀ Female

ICD-10-PCS 2024   803

DUY–DV2

Radiation Therapy

D   **Radiation Therapy**
V   **Male Reproductive System**
Y   **Other Radiation**

Treatment Site Character 4	Modality Qualifier Character 5	Isotope Character 6	Qualifier Character 7
Ø Prostate ♂	7 Contact Radiation 8 Hyperthermia C Intraoperative Radiation Therapy (IORT) F Plaque Radiation	Z None	Z None
1 Testis ♂	7 Contact Radiation 8 Hyperthermia F Plaque Radiation	Z None	Z None
♂ All treatment site, modality, isotope, and qualifier values			

D   **Radiation Therapy**
W   **Anatomical Regions**
Ø   **Beam Radiation**

Treatment Site Character 4	Modality Qualifier Character 5	Isotope Character 6	Qualifier Character 7
1 Head and Neck 2 Chest 3 Abdomen 4 Hemibody 5 Whole Body 6 Pelvic Region	Ø Photons <1 MeV 1 Photons 1- 10 MeV 2 Photons >10 MeV 4 Heavy Particles (Protons, Ions) 5 Neutrons 6 Neutron Capture	Z None	Z None
1 Head and Neck 2 Chest 3 Abdomen 4 Hemibody 5 Whole Body 6 Pelvic Region	3 Electrons	Z None	Ø Intraoperative Z None

D   **Radiation Therapy**
W   **Anatomical Regions**
1   **Brachytherapy**

Treatment Site Character 4	Modality Qualifier Character 5	Isotope Character 6	Qualifier Character 7
Ø Cranial Cavity K Upper Back L Lower Back P Gastrointestinal Tract Q Respiratory Tract R Genitourinary Tract X Upper Extremity Y Lower Extremity	B Low Dose Rate (LDR)	B Palladium 103 (Pd-103)	1 Unidirectional Source Z None
1 Head and Neck 2 Chest 3 Abdomen 6 Pelvic Region	9 High Dose Rate (HDR)	7 Cesium 137 (Cs-137) 8 Iridium 192 (Ir-192) 9 Iodine 125 (I-125) B Palladium 103 (Pd-103) C Californium 252 (Cf-252) Y Other Isotope	Z None
1 Head and Neck 2 Chest 3 Abdomen 6 Pelvic Region	B Low Dose Rate (LDR)	6 Cesium 131 (Cs-131) 7 Cesium 137 (Cs-137) 8 Iridium 192 (Ir-192) 9 Iodine 125 (I-125) C Californium 252 (Cf-252) Y Other Isotope	Z None
1 Head and Neck 2 Chest 3 Abdomen 6 Pelvic Region	B Low Dose Rate (LDR)	B Palladium 103 (Pd-103)	1 Unidirectional Source Z None

Non-OR Procedure   DRG Non-OR Procedure   Valid OR Procedure   HAC Associated Procedure   Combination Only   New/Revised April   New/Revised October

D Radiation Therapy
W Anatomical Regions
2 Stereotactic Radiosurgery

Treatment Site Character 4	Modality Qualifier Character 5	Isotope Character 6	Qualifier Character 7
1 Head and Neck 2 Chest 3 Abdomen 6 Pelvic Region	D Stereotactic Other Photon 　Radiosurgery H Stereotactic Particulate 　Radiosurgery J Stereotactic Gamma Beam 　Radiosurgery	Z None	Z None

DRG Non-OR All treatment site, modality, isotope, and qualifier values

D Radiation Therapy
W Anatomical Regions
Y Other Radiation

Treatment Site Character 4	Modality Qualifier Character 5	Isotope Character 6	Qualifier Character 7
1 Head and Neck 2 Chest 3 Abdomen 4 Hemibody 6 Pelvic Region	7 Contact Radiation 8 Hyperthermia F Plaque Radiation	Z None	Z None
5 Whole Body	7 Contact Radiation 8 Hyperthermia F Plaque Radiation	Z None	Z None
5 Whole Body	G Isotope Administration	D Iodine 131 (I-131) F Phosphorus 32 (P-32) G Strontium 89 (Sr-89) H Strontium 90 (Sr-90) Y Other Isotope	Z None

Physical Rehabilitation and Diagnostic Audiology F00–F15

F   **Physical Rehabilitation and Diagnostic Audiology**
Ø   **Rehabilitation**
Ø   **Speech Assessment**   Definition: Measurement of speech and related functions

Body System/Region Character 4	Type Qualifier Character 5	Equipment Character 6	Qualifier Character 7
3 Neurological System - Whole Body	**G** Communicative/Cognitive Integration Skills	**K** Audiovisual **M** Augmentative / Alternative Communication **P** Computer **Y** Other Equipment **Z** None	**Z** None
Z None	**Ø** Filtered Speech **3** Staggered Spondaic Word **Q** Performance Intensity Phonetically Balanced Speech Discrimination **R** Brief Tone Stimuli **S** Distorted Speech **T** Dichotic Stimuli **V** Temporal Ordering of Stimuli **W** Masking Patterns	**1** Audiometer **2** Sound Field / Booth **K** Audiovisual **Z** None	**Z** None
Z None	**1** Speech Threshold **2** Speech/Word Recognition	**1** Audiometer **2** Sound Field / Booth **9** Cochlear Implant **K** Audiovisual **Z** None	**Z** None
Z None	**4** Sensorineural Acuity Level	**1** Audiometer **2** Sound Field / Booth **Z** None	**Z** None
Z None	**5** Synthetic Sentence Identification	**1** Audiometer **2** Sound Field / Booth **9** Cochlear Implant **K** Audiovisual	**Z** None
Z None	**6** Speech and/or Language Screening **7** Nonspoken Language **8** Receptive/Expressive Language **C** Aphasia **G** Communicative/Cognitive Integration Skills **L** Augmentative/Alternative Communication System	**K** Audiovisual **M** Augmentative / Alternative Communication **P** Computer **Y** Other Equipment **Z** None	**Z** None
Z None	**9** Articulation/Phonology	**K** Audiovisual **P** Computer **Q** Speech Analysis **Y** Other Equipment **Z** None	**Z** None
Z None	**B** Motor Speech	**K** Audiovisual **N** Biosensory Feedback **P** Computer **Q** Speech Analysis **T** Aerodynamic Function **Y** Other Equipment **Z** None	**Z** None
Z None	**D** Fluency	**K** Audiovisual **N** Biosensory Feedback **P** Computer **Q** Speech Analysis **S** Voice Analysis **T** Aerodynamic Function **Y** Other Equipment **Z** None	**Z** None
Z None	**F** Voice	**K** Audiovisual **N** Biosensory Feedback **P** Computer **S** Voice Analysis **T** Aerodynamic Function **Y** Other Equipment **Z** None	**Z** None

DRG Non-OR   All body system/region, type qualifier, equipment, and qualifier values

F00 Continued on next page

Physical Rehabilitation and Diagnostic Audiology (sidebar)

F   **Physical Rehabilitation and Diagnostic Audiology**   *F00 Continued*
Ø   **Rehabilitation**
Ø   **Speech Assessment**   Definition: Measurement of speech and related functions

Body System/Region Character 4	Type Qualifier Character 5	Equipment Character 6	Qualifier Character 7
Z None	H Bedside Swallowing and Oral Function P Oral Peripheral Mechanism	Y Other Equipment Z None	Z None
Z None	J Instrumental Swallowing and Oral Function	T Aerodynamic Function W Swallowing Y Other Equipment	Z None
Z None	K Orofacial Myofunctional	K Audiovisual P Computer Y Other Equipment Z None	Z None
Z None	M Voice Prosthetic	K Audiovisual P Computer S Voice Analysis V Speech Prosthesis Y Other Equipment Z None	Z None
Z None	N Non-invasive Instrumental Status	N Biosensory Feedback P Computer Q Speech Analysis S Voice Analysis T Aerodynamic Function Y Other Equipment	Z None
Z None	X Other Specified Central Auditory Processing	Z None	Z None

DRG Non-OR   All body system/region, type qualifier, equipment, and qualifier values

F   **Physical Rehabilitation and Diagnostic Audiology**
Ø   **Rehabilitation**
1   **Motor and/or Nerve Function Assessment**   Definition: Measurement of motor, nerve, and related functions

Body System/Region Character 4	Type Qualifier Character 5	Equipment Character 6	Qualifier Character 7
Ø Neurological System - Head and Neck 1 Neurological System - Upper Back/ Upper Extremity 2 Neurological System - Lower Back/ Lower Extremity 3 Neurological System - Whole Body	Ø Muscle Performance	E Orthosis F Assistive, Adaptive, Supportive or Protective U Prosthesis Y Other Equipment Z None	Z None
Ø Neurological System - Head and Neck 1 Neurological System - Upper Back/ Upper Extremity 2 Neurological System - Lower Back/ Lower Extremity 3 Neurological System - Whole Body	1 Integumentary Integrity 3 Coordination/Dexterity 4 Motor Function G Reflex Integrity	Z None	Z None
Ø Neurological System - Head and Neck 1 Neurological System - Upper Back/ Upper Extremity 2 Neurological System - Lower Back/ Lower Extremity 3 Neurological System - Whole Body	5 Range of Motion and Joint Integrity 6 Sensory Awareness/Processing/ Integrity	Y Other Equipment Z None	Z None
D Integumentary System - Head and Neck F Integumentary System - Upper Back/ Upper Extremity G Integumentary System - Lower Back/ Lower Extremity H Integumentary System - Whole Body J Musculoskeletal System - Head and Neck K Musculoskeletal System - Upper Back/ Upper Extremity L Musculoskeletal System - Lower Back/ Lower Extremity M Musculoskeletal System - Whole Body	Ø Muscle Performance	E Orthosis F Assistive, Adaptive, Supportive or Protective U Prosthesis Y Other Equipment Z None	Z None

DRG Non-OR   All body system/region, type qualifier, equipment, and qualifier values

F01 Continued on next page

Non-OR Procedure   DRG Non-OR Procedure   Valid OR Procedure   HAC Associated Procedure   Combination Only   New/Revised April   New/Revised October
808   ICD-10-PCS 2024

F00–F01 (sidebar)

F   Physical Rehabilitation and Diagnostic Audiology
Ø   Rehabilitation
1   Motor and/or Nerve Function Assessment   Definition: Measurement of motor, nerve, and related functions

F01 Continued

Body System/Region Character 4	Type Qualifier Character 5	Equipment Character 6	Qualifier Character 7
D Integumentary System - Head and Neck F Integumentary System - Upper Back/ Upper Extremity G Integumentary System - Lower Back/ Lower Extremity H Integumentary System - Whole Body J Musculoskeletal System - Head and Neck K Musculoskeletal System - Upper Back/ Upper Extremity L Musculoskeletal System - Lower Back/ Lower Extremity M Musculoskeletal System - Whole Body	1 Integumentary Integrity	Z None	Z None
D Integumentary System - Head and Neck F Integumentary System - Upper Back/ Upper Extremity G Integumentary System - Lower Back/ Lower Extremity H Integumentary System - Whole Body J Musculoskeletal System - Head and Neck K Musculoskeletal System - Upper Back/ Upper Extremity L Musculoskeletal System - Lower Back/ Lower Extremity M Musculoskeletal System - Whole Body	5 Range of Motion and Joint Integrity 6 Sensory Awareness/Processing/ Integrity	Y Other Equipment Z None	Z None
N Genitourinary System	Ø Muscle Performance	E Orthosis F Assistive, Adaptive, Supportive or Protective U Prosthesis Y Other Equipment Z None	Z None
Z None	2 Visual Motor Integration	K Audiovisual M Augmentative / Alternative Communication N Biosensory Feedback P Computer Q Speech Analysis S Voice Analysis Y Other Equipment Z None	Z None
Z None	7 Facial Nerve Function	7 Electrophysiologic	Z None
Z None	9 Somatosensory Evoked Potentials	J Somatosensory	Z None
Z None	B Bed Mobility C Transfer F Wheelchair Mobility	E Orthosis F Assistive, Adaptive, Supportive or Protective U Prosthesis Z None	Z None
Z None	D Gait and/or Balance	E Orthosis F Assistive, Adaptive, Supportive or Protective U Prosthesis Y Other Equipment Z None	Z None

DRG Non-OR   All body system/region, type qualifier, equipment, and qualifier values

NC Noncovered Procedure   LC Limited Coverage   QA Questionable OB Admit   NT New Tech Add-on   ⊞ Combination Member   ♂ Male   ♀ Female

F   Physical Rehabilitation and Diagnostic Audiology
Ø   Rehabilitation
2   Activities of Daily Living Assessment   Definition: Measurement of functional level for activities of daily living

Body System/Region Character 4	Type Qualifier Character 5	Equipment Character 6	Qualifier Character 7
Ø Neurological System - Head and Neck	9 Cranial Nerve Integrity D Neuromotor Development	Y Other Equipment Z None	Z None
1 Neurological System - Upper Back/Upper Extremity 2 Neurological System - Lower Back/Lower Extremity 3 Neurological System - Whole Body	D Neuromotor Development	Y Other Equipment Z None	Z None
4 Circulatory System - Head and Neck 5 Circulatory System - Upper Back/Upper Extremity 6 Circulatory System - Lower Back/Lower Extremity 8 Respiratory System - Head and Neck 9 Respiratory System - Upper Back/Upper Extremity B Respiratory System - Lower Back/Lower Extremity	G Ventilation, Respiration and Circulation	C Mechanical G Aerobic Endurance and Conditioning Y Other Equipment Z None	Z None
7 Circulatory System - Whole Body C Respiratory System - Whole Body	7 Aerobic Capacity and Endurance	E Orthosis G Aerobic Endurance and Conditioning U Prosthesis Y Other Equipment Z None	Z None
7 Circulatory System - Whole Body C Respiratory System - Whole Body	G Ventilation, Respiration and Circulation	C Mechanical G Aerobic Endurance and Conditioning Y Other Equipment Z None	Z None
Z None	Ø Bathing/Showering 1 Dressing 3 Grooming/Personal Hygiene 4 Home Management	E Orthosis F Assistive, Adaptive, Supportive or Protective U Prosthesis Z None	Z None
Z None	2 Feeding/Eating 8 Anthropometric Characteristics F Pain	Y Other Equipment Z None	Z None
Z None	5 Perceptual Processing	K Audiovisual M Augmentative / Alternative Communication N Biosensory Feedback P Computer Q Speech Analysis S Voice Analysis Y Other Equipment Z None	Z None
Z None	6 Psychosocial Skills	Z None	Z None
Z None	B Environmental, Home and Work Barriers C Ergonomics and Body Mechanics	E Orthosis F Assistive, Adaptive, Supportive or Protective U Prosthesis Y Other Equipment Z None	Z None
Z None	H Vocational Activities and Functional Community or Work Reintegration Skills	E Orthosis F Assistive, Adaptive, Supportive or Protective G Aerobic Endurance and Conditioning U Prosthesis Y Other Equipment Z None	Z None

DRG Non-OR   All body system/region, type qualifier, equipment, and qualifier values

Non-OR Procedure   DRG Non-OR Procedure   Valid OR Procedure   HAC Associated Procedure   Combination Only   New/Revised April   New/Revised October

F   Physical Rehabilitation and Diagnostic Audiology
Ø   Rehabilitation
6   Speech Treatment   Definition: Application of techniques to improve, augment, or compensate for speech and related functional impairment

Body System/Region Character 4	Type Qualifier Character 5	Equipment Character 6	Qualifier Character 7
3 Neurological System - Whole Body	6 Communicative/Cognitive Integration Skills	K Audiovisual M Augmentative / Alternative Communication P Computer Y Other Equipment Z None	Z None
Z None	Ø Nonspoken Language 3 Aphasia 6 Communicative/Cognitive Integration Skills	K Audiovisual M Augmentative / Alternative Communication P Computer Y Other Equipment Z None	Z None
Z None	1 Speech-Language Pathology and Related Disorders Counseling 2 Speech-Language Pathology and Related Disorders Prevention	K Audiovisual Z None	Z None
Z None	4 Articulation/Phonology	K Audiovisual P Computer Q Speech Analysis T Aerodynamic Function Y Other Equipment Z None	Z None
Z None	5 Aural Rehabilitation	K Audiovisual L Assistive Listening M Augmentative / Alternative Communication N Biosensory Feedback P Computer Q Speech Analysis S Voice Analysis Y Other Equipment Z None	Z None
Z None	7 Fluency	4 Electroacoustic Immitance / Acoustic Reflex K Audiovisual N Biosensory Feedback Q Speech Analysis S Voice Analysis T Aerodynamic Function Y Other Equipment Z None	Z None
Z None	8 Motor Speech	K Audiovisual N Biosensory Feedback P Computer Q Speech Analysis S Voice Analysis T Aerodynamic Function Y Other Equipment Z None	Z None
Z None	9 Orofacial Myofunctional	K Audiovisual P Computer Y Other Equipment Z None	Z None
Z None	B Receptive/Expressive Language	K Audiovisual L Assistive Listening M Augmentative / Alternative Communication P Computer Y Other Equipment Z None	Z None

DRG Non-OR   All body system/region, type qualifier, equipment, and qualifier values

F06 Continued on next page

NC Noncovered Procedure   **LC** Limited Coverage   **QA** Questionable OB Admit   **NT** New Tech Add-on   ⊞ Combination Member   ♂ Male   ♀ Female

F   **Physical Rehabilitation and Diagnostic Audiology**   *F06 Continued*
Ø   **Rehabilitation**
6   **Speech Treatment**   Definition: Application of techniques to improve, augment, or compensate for speech and related functional impairment

Body System/Region Character 4	Type Qualifier Character 5	Equipment Character 6	Qualifier Character 7
Z None	C Voice	K Audiovisual N Biosensory Feedback P Computer S Voice Analysis T Aerodynamic Function V Speech Prosthesis Y Other Equipment Z None	Z None
Z None	D Swallowing Dysfunction	M Augmentative / Alternative Communication T Aerodynamic Function V Speech Prosthesis Y Other Equipment Z None	Z None

DRG Non-OR   All body system/region, type qualifier, equipment, and qualifier values

F   **Physical Rehabilitation and Diagnostic Audiology**
Ø   **Rehabilitation**
7   **Motor Treatment**   Definition: Exercise or activities to increase or facilitate motor function

Body System/Region Character 4	Type Qualifier Character 5	Equipment Character 6	Qualifier Character 7
Ø Neurological System - Head and Neck 1 Neurological System - Upper Back/Upper Extremity 2 Neurological System - Lower Back/Lower Extremity 3 Neurological System - Whole Body D Integumentary System - Head and Neck F Integumentary System - Upper Back/ Upper Extremity G Integumentary System - Lower Back/ Lower Extremity H Integumentary System - Whole Body J Musculoskeletal System - Head and Neck K Musculoskeletal System - Upper Back/ Upper Extremity L Musculoskeletal System - Lower Back/ Lower Extremity M Musculoskeletal System - Whole Body	Ø Range of Motion and Joint Mobility 1 Muscle Performance 2 Coordination/Dexterity 3 Motor Function	E Orthosis F Assistive, Adaptive, Supportive or Protective U Prosthesis Y Other Equipment Z None	Z None
Ø Neurological System - Head and Neck 1 Neurological System - Upper Back/Upper Extremity 2 Neurological System - Lower Back/Lower Extremity 3 Neurological System - Whole Body D Integumentary System - Head and Neck F Integumentary System - Upper Back/ Upper Extremity G Integumentary System - Lower Back/ Lower Extremity H Integumentary System - Whole Body J Musculoskeletal System - Head and Neck K Musculoskeletal System - Upper Back/ Upper Extremity L Musculoskeletal System - Lower Back/ Lower Extremity M Musculoskeletal System - Whole Body	6 Therapeutic Exercise	B Physical Agents C Mechanical D Electrotherapeutic E Orthosis F Assistive, Adaptive, Supportive or Protective G Aerobic Endurance and Conditioning H Mechanical or Electromechanical U Prosthesis Y Other Equipment Z None	Z None

DRG Non-OR   All body system/region, type qualifier, equipment, and qualifier values

F07 Continued on next page

F   **Physical Rehabilitation and Diagnostic Audiology**   *F07 Continued*
Ø   **Rehabilitation**
7   **Motor Treatment**   Definition: Exercise or activities to increase or facilitate motor function

Body System/Region Character 4	Type Qualifier Character 5	Equipment Character 6	Qualifier Character 7
Ø Neurological System - Head and Neck 1 Neurological System - Upper Back/Upper Extremity 2 Neurological System - Lower Back/Lower Extremity 3 Neurological System - Whole Body D Integumentary System - Head and Neck F Integumentary System - Upper Back/ Upper Extremity G Integumentary System - Lower Back/ Lower Extremity H Integumentary System - Whole Body J Musculoskeletal System - Head and Neck K Musculoskeletal System - Upper Back/ Upper Extremity L Musculoskeletal System - Lower Back/ Lower Treatment M Musculoskeletal System - Whole Body	7 Manual Therapy Techniques	Z None	Z None
4 Circulatory System - Head and Neck 5 Circulatory System - Upper Back / Upper Extremity 6 Circulatory System - Lower Back / Lower Extremity 7 Circulatory System - Whole Body 8 Respiratory System - Head and Neck 9 Respiratory System - Upper Back / Upper Extremity B Respiratory System - Lower Back / Lower Extremity C Respiratory System - Whole Body	6 Therapeutic Exercise	B Physical Agents C Mechanical D Electrotherapeutic E Orthosis F Assistive, Adaptive, Supportive or Protective G Aerobic Endurance and Conditioning H Mechanical or Electromechanical U Prosthesis Y Other Equipment Z None	Z None
N Genitourinary System	1 Muscle Performance	E Orthosis F Assistive, Adaptive, Supportive or Protective U Prosthesis Y Other Equipment Z None	Z None
N Genitourinary System	6 Therapeutic Exercise	B Physical Agents C Mechanical D Electrotherapeutic E Orthosis F Assistive, Adaptive, Supportive or Protective G Aerobic Endurance and Conditioning H Mechanical or Electromechanical U Prosthesis Y Other Equipment Z None	Z None
Z None	4 Wheelchair Mobility	D Electrotherapeutic E Orthosis F Assistive, Adaptive, Supportive or Protective U Prosthesis Y Other Equipment Z None	Z None
Z None	5 Bed Mobility	C Mechanical E Orthosis F Assistive, Adaptive, Supportive or Protective U Prosthesis Y Other Equipment Z None	Z None
Z None	8 Transfer Training	C Mechanical D Electrotherapeutic E Orthosis F Assistive, Adaptive, Supportive or Protective U Prosthesis Y Other Equipment Z None	Z None

DRG Non-OR   All body system/region, type qualifier, equipment, and qualifier values

F07 Continued on next page

NC Noncovered Procedure   LC Limited Coverage   QA Questionable OB Admit   NT New Tech Add-on   ⊞ Combination Member   ♂ Male   ♀ Female

Physical Rehabilitation and Diagnostic Audiology

F07 Continued

F   Physical Rehabilitation and Diagnostic Audiology
0   Rehabilitation
7   Motor Treatment   Definition: Exercise or activities to increase or facilitate motor function

Body System/Region Character 4	Type Qualifier Character 5	Equipment Character 6	Qualifier Character 7
Z None	9 Gait Training/Functional Ambulation	C Mechanical D Electrotherapeutic E Orthosis F Assistive, Adaptive, Supportive or Protective G Aerobic Endurance and Conditioning U Prosthesis Y Other Equipment Z None	Z None

DRG Non-OR All body system/region, type qualifier, equipment, and qualifier values

F   Physical Rehabilitation and Diagnostic Audiology
0   Rehabilitation
8   Activities of Daily Living Treatment   Definition: Exercise or activities to facilitate functional competence for activities of daily living

Body System/Region Character 4	Type Qualifier Character 5	Equipment Character 6	Qualifier Character 7
D Integumentary System - Head and Neck F Integumentary System - Upper Back/Upper Extremity G Integumentary System - Lower Back/Lower Extremity H Integumentary System - Whole Body J Musculoskeletal System - Head and Neck K Musculoskeletal System - Upper Back/Upper Extremity L Musculoskeletal System - Lower Back/Lower Extremity M Musculoskeletal System - Whole Body	5 Wound Management	B Physical Agents C Mechanical D Electrotherapeutic E Orthosis F Assistive, Adaptive, Supportive or Protective U Prosthesis Y Other Equipment Z None	Z None
Z None	0 Bathing/Showering Techniques 1 Dressing Techniques 2 Grooming/Personal Hygiene	E Orthosis F Assistive, Adaptive, Supportive or Protective U Prosthesis Y Other Equipment Z None	Z None
Z None	3 Feeding/Eating	C Mechanical D Electrotherapeutic E Orthosis F Assistive, Adaptive, Supportive or Protective U Prosthesis Y Other Equipment Z None	Z None
Z None	4 Home Management	D Electrotherapeutic E Orthosis F Assistive, Adaptive, Supportive or Protective U Prosthesis Y Other Equipment Z None	Z None
Z None	6 Psychosocial Skills	Z None	Z None
Z None	7 Vocational Activities and Functional Community or Work Reintegration Skills	B Physical Agents C Mechanical D Electrotherapeutic E Orthosis F Assistive, Adaptive, Supportive or Protective G Aerobic Endurance and Conditioning U Prosthesis Y Other Equipment Z None	Z None

DRG Non-OR All body system/region, type qualifier, equipment, and qualifier values

Non-OR Procedure   DRG Non-OR Procedure   Valid OR Procedure   HAC Associated Procedure   Combination Only   New/Revised April   New/Revised October

F   Physical Rehabilitation and Diagnostic Audiology
0   Rehabilitation
9   Hearing Treatment   Definition: Application of techniques to improve, augment, or compensate for hearing and related functional impairment

Body System/Region Character 4	Type Qualifier Character 5	Equipment Character 6	Qualifier Character 7
Z None	0 Hearing and Related Disorders Counseling 1 Hearing and Related Disorders Prevention	K Audiovisual Z None	Z None
Z None	2 Auditory Processing	K Audiovisual L Assistive Listening P Computer Y Other Equipment Z None	Z None
Z None	3 Cerumen Management	X Cerumen Management Z None	Z None

DRG Non-OR All body system/region, type qualifier, equipment, and qualifier values

F   Physical Rehabilitation and Diagnostic Audiology
0   Rehabilitation
B   Cochlear Implant Treatment   Definition: Application of techniques to improve the communication abilities of individuals with cochlear implant

Body System/Region Character 4	Type Qualifier Character 5	Equipment Character 6	Qualifier Character 7
Z None	0 Cochlear Implant Rehabilitation	1 Audiometer 2 Sound Field / Booth 9 Cochlear Implant K Audiovisual P Computer Y Other Equipment	Z None

DRG Non-OR All body system/region, type qualifier, equipment, and qualifier values

F   Physical Rehabilitation and Diagnostic Audiology
0   Rehabilitation
C   Vestibular Treatment   Definition: Application of techniques to improve, augment, or compensate for vestibular and related functional impairment

Body System/Region Character 4	Type Qualifier Character 5	Equipment Character 6	Qualifier Character 7
3 Neurological System - Whole Body H Integumentary System - Whole Body M Musculoskeletal System - Whole Body	3 Postural Control	E Orthosis F Assistive, Adaptive, Supportive or Protective U Prosthesis Y Other Equipment Z None	Z None
Z None	0 Vestibular	8 Vestibular / Balance Z None	Z None
Z None	1 Perceptual Processing 2 Visual Motor Integration	K Audiovisual L Assistive Listening N Biosensory Feedback P Computer Q Speech Analysis S Voice Analysis T Aerodynamic Function Y Other Equipment Z None	Z None

DRG Non-OR All body system/region, type qualifier, equipment, and qualifier values

F   Physical Rehabilitation and Diagnostic Audiology
Ø   Rehabilitation
D   Device Fitting   Definition: Fitting of a device designed to facilitate or support achievement of a higher level of function

Body System/Region Character 4	Type Qualifier Character 5	Equipment Character 6	Qualifier Character 7
Z None	Ø Tinnitus Masker	5 Hearing Aid Selection / Fitting / Test Z None	Z None
Z None	1 Monaural Hearing Aid 2 Binaural Hearing Aid 5 Assistive Listening Device	1 Audiometer 2 Sound Field / Booth 5 Hearing Aid Selection / Fitting / Test K Audiovisual L Assistive Listening Z None	Z None
Z None	3 Augmentative/Alternative Communication System	M Augmentative / Alternative Communication	Z None
Z None	4 Voice Prosthetic	S Voice Analysis V Speech Prosthesis	Z None
Z None	6 Dynamic Orthosis 7 Static Orthosis 8 Prosthesis 9 Assistive, Adaptive, Supportive or Protective Devices	E Orthosis F Assistive, Adaptive, Supportive or Protective U Prosthesis Z None	Z None

DRG Non-OR   FØDZØ[5,Z]Z
DRG Non-OR   FØDZ[1, 2,5][1,2,5, K,L,Z]Z
DRG Non-OR   FØDZ3MZ
DRG Non-OR   FØDZ4[S,V]Z
DRG Non-OR   FØDZ[6,7][E,F,U,Z]Z
DRG Non-OR   FØDZ8[E,F,U]Z

F   Physical Rehabilitation and Diagnostic Audiology
Ø   Rehabilitation
F   Caregiver Training   Definition: Training in activities to support patient's optimal level of function

Body System/Region Character 4	Type Qualifier Character 5	Equipment Character 6	Qualifier Character 7
Z None	Ø Bathing/Showering Technique 1 Dressing 2 Feeding and Eating 3 Grooming/Personal Hygiene 4 Bed Mobility 5 Transfer 6 Wheelchair Mobility 7 Therapeutic Exercise 8 Airway Clearance Techniques 9 Wound Management B Vocational Activities and Functional Community or Work Reintegration Skills C Gait Training/Functional Ambulation D Application, Proper Use and Care of Devices F Application, Proper Use and Care of Orthoses G Application, Proper Use and Care of Prosthesis H Home Management	E Orthosis F Assistive, Adaptive, Supportive or Protective U Prosthesis Z None	Z None
Z None	J Communication Skills	K Audiovisual L Assistive Listening M Augmentative / Alternative Communication P Computer Z None	Z None

DRG Non-OR   All body system/region, type qualifier, equipment, and qualifier values

Non-OR Procedure   DRG Non-OR Procedure   Valid OR Procedure   HAC Associated Procedure   Combination Only   New/Revised April   New/Revised October

816   ICD-10-PCS 2024

F   Physical Rehabilitation and Diagnostic Audiology
1   Diagnostic Audiology
3   Hearing Assessment   Definition: Measurement of hearing and related functions

Body System/Region Character 4	Type Qualifier Character 5	Equipment Character 6	Qualifier Character 7
Z None	Ø Hearing Screening	Ø Occupational Hearing 1 Audiometer 2 Sound Field / Booth 3 Tympanometer 8 Vestibular / Balance 9 Cochlear Implant Z None	Z None
Z None	1 Pure Tone Audiometry, Air 2 Pure Tone Audiometry, Air and Bone	Ø Occupational Hearing 1 Audiometer 2 Sound Field / Booth Z None	Z None
Z None	3 Bekesy Audiometry 6 Visual Reinforcement Audiometry 9 Short Increment Sensitivity Index B Stenger C Pure Tone Stenger	1 Audiometer 2 Sound Field / Booth Z None	Z None
Z None	4 Conditioned Play Audiometry 5 Select Picture Audiometry	1 Audiometer 2 Sound Field / Booth K Audiovisual Z None	Z None
Z None	7 Alternate Binaural or Monaural Loudness Balance	1 Audiometer K Audiovisual Z None	Z None
Z None	8 Tone Decay D Tympanometry F Eustachian Tube Function G Acoustic Reflex Patterns H Acoustic Reflex Threshold J Acoustic Reflex Decay	3 Tympanometer 4 Electroacoustic Immitance / Acoustic Reflex Z None	Z None
Z None	K Electrocochleography L Auditory Evoked Potentials	7 Electrophysiologic Z None	Z None

Z None	M Evoked Otoacoustic Emissions,
	    Screening
	N Evoked Otoacoustic Emissions,
	    Diagnostic
		6 Otoacoustic Emission (OAE)
		Z None
			Z None

Z None	P Aural Rehabilitation Status	1 Audiometer 2 Sound Field / Booth 4 Electroacoustic Immitance / Acoustic Reflex 9 Cochlear Implant K Audiovisual L Assistive Listening P Computer Z None	Z None
Z None	Q Auditory Processing	K Audiovisual P Computer Y Other Equipment Z None	Z None

NC Noncovered Procedure   **LC** Limited Coverage   **QA** Questionable OB Admit   **NT** New Tech Add-on   ⊞ Combination Member   ♂ Male   ♀ Female

ICD-10-PCS 2024   817

F   Physical Rehabilitation and Diagnostic Audiology
1   Diagnostic Audiology
4   Hearing Aid Assessment   Definition: Measurement of the appropriateness and/or effectiveness of a hearing device

Body System/Region Character 4	Type Qualifier Character 5	Equipment Character 6	Qualifier Character 7
Z None	0 Cochlear Implant	1 Audiometer 2 Sound Field / Booth 3 Tympanometer 4 Electroacoustic Immitance / Acoustic Reflex 5 Hearing Aid Selection / Fitting / Test 7 Electrophysiologic 9 Cochlear Implant K Audiovisual L Assistive Listening P Computer Y Other Equipment Z None	Z None
Z None	1 Ear Canal Probe Microphone 6 Binaural Electroacoustic Hearing Aid Check 8 Monaural Electroacoustic Hearing Aid Check	5 Hearing Aid Selection / Fitting / Test Z None	Z None
Z None	2 Monaural Hearing Aid 3 Binaural Hearing Aid	1 Audiometer 2 Sound Field / Booth 3 Tympanometer 4 Electroacoustic Immitance / Acoustic Reflex 5 Hearing Aid Selection / Fitting / Test K Audiovisual L Assistive Listening P Computer Z None	Z None
Z None	4 Assistive Listening System/Device Selection	1 Audiometer 2 Sound Field / Booth 3 Tympanometer 4 Electroacoustic Immitance / Acoustic Reflex K Audiovisual L Assistive Listening Z None	Z None
Z None	5 Sensory Aids	1 Audiometer 2 Sound Field / Booth 3 Tympanometer 4 Electroacoustic Immitance / Acoustic Reflex 5 Hearing Aid Selection / Fitting / Test K Audiovisual L Assistive Listening Z None	Z None
Z None	7 Ear Protector Attentuation	0 Occupational Hearing Z None	Z None

F   Physical Rehabilitation and Diagnostic Audiology
1   Diagnostic Audiology
5   Vestibular Assessment   Definition: Measurement of the vestibular system and related functions

Body System/Region Character 4	Type Qualifier Character 5	Equipment Character 6	Qualifier Character 7
Z None	0 Bithermal, Binaural Caloric Irrigation 1 Bithermal, Monaural Caloric Irrigation 2 Unithermal Binaural Screen 3 Oscillating Tracking 4 Sinusoidal Vertical Axis Rotational 5 Dix-Hallpike Dynamic 6 Computerized Dynamic Posturography	8 Vestibular / Balance Z None	Z None
Z None	7 Tinnitus Masker	5 Hearing Aid Selection / Fitting / Test Z None	Z None

Non-OR Procedure   DRG Non-OR Procedure   Valid OR Procedure   HAC Associated Procedure   Combination Only   New/Revised April   New/Revised October

818   ICD-10-PCS 2024

Mental Health GZ1–GZJ

G   Mental Health
Z   None
1   Psychological Tests   Definition: The administration and interpretation of standardized psychological tests and measurement instruments for the assessment of psychological function

Qualifier Character 4	Qualifier Character 5	Qualifier Character 6	Qualifier Character 7
0 Developmental 1 Personality and Behavioral 2 Intellectual and Psychoeducational 3 Neuropsychological 4 Neurobehavioral and Cognitive Status	Z None	Z None	Z None

G   Mental Health
Z   None
2   Crisis Intervention   Definition: Treatment of a traumatized, acutely disturbed or distressed individual for the purpose of short-term stabilization

Qualifier Character 4	Qualifier Character 5	Qualifier Character 6	Qualifier Character 7
Z None	Z None	Z None	Z None

G   Mental Health
Z   None
3   Medication Management   Definition: Monitoring and adjusting the use of medications for the treatment of a mental health disorder

Qualifier Character 4	Qualifier Character 5	Qualifier Character 6	Qualifier Character 7
Z None	Z None	Z None	Z None

G   Mental Health
Z   None
5   Individual Psychotherapy   Definition: Treatment of an individual with a mental health disorder by behavioral, cognitive, psychoanalytic, psychodynamic or psychophysiological means to improve functioning or well-being

Qualifier Character 4	Qualifier Character 5	Qualifier Character 6	Qualifier Character 7
0 Interactive 1 Behavioral 2 Cognitive 3 Interpersonal 4 Psychoanalysis 5 Psychodynamic 6 Supportive 8 Cognitive-Behavioral 9 Psychophysiological	Z None	Z None	Z None

G   Mental Health
Z   None
6   Counseling   Definition: The application of psychological methods to treat an individual with normal developmental issues and psychological problems in order to increase function, improve well-being, alleviate distress, maladjustment or resolve crises

Qualifier Character 4	Qualifier Character 5	Qualifier Character 6	Qualifier Character 7
0 Educational 1 Vocational 3 Other Counseling	Z None	Z None	Z None

G   Mental Health
Z   None
7   Family Psychotherapy   Definition: Treatment that includes one or more family members of an individual with a mental health disorder by behavioral, cognitive, psychoanalytic, psychodynamic or psychophysiological means to improve functioning or well-being

Explanation: Remediation of emotional or behavioral problems presented by one or more family members in cases where psychotherapy with more than one family member is indicated

Qualifier Character 4	Qualifier Character 5	Qualifier Character 6	Qualifier Character 7
2 Other Family Psychotherapy	Z None	Z None	Z None

NC Noncovered Procedure   LC Limited Coverage   QA Questionable OB Admit   NT New Tech Add-on   ⊞ Combination Member   ♂ Male   ♀ Female

ICD-10-PCS 2024   819

GZ1–GZ7

Mental Health

G   **Mental Health**
Z   **None**
B   **Electroconvulsive Therapy**   Definition: The application of controlled electrical voltages to treat a mental health disorder

Qualifier Character 4	Qualifier Character 5	Qualifier Character 6	Qualifier Character 7
Ø Unilateral-Single Seizure 1 Unilateral-Multiple Seizure 2 Bilateral-Single Seizure 3 Bilateral-Multiple Seizure 4 Other Electroconvulsive Therapy	Z None	Z None	Z None

G   **Mental Health**
Z   **None**
C   **Biofeedback**   Definition: Provision of information from the monitoring and regulating of physiological processes in conjunction with cognitive-behavioral techniques to improve patient functioning or well-being

Qualifier Character 4	Qualifier Character 5	Qualifier Character 6	Qualifier Character 7
9 Other Biofeedback	Z None	Z None	Z None

G   **Mental Health**
Z   **None**
F   **Hypnosis**   Definition: Induction of a state of heightened suggestibility by auditory, visual and tactile techniques to elicit an emotional or behavioral response

Qualifier Character 4	Qualifier Character 5	Qualifier Character 6	Qualifier Character 7
Z None	Z None	Z None	Z None

G   **Mental Health**
Z   **None**
G   **Narcosynthesis**   Definition: Administration of intravenous barbiturates in order to release suppressed or repressed thoughts

Qualifier Character 4	Qualifier Character 5	Qualifier Character 6	Qualifier Character 7
Z None	Z None	Z None	Z None

G   **Mental Health**
Z   **None**
H   **Group Psychotherapy**   Definition: Treatment of two or more individuals with a mental health disorder by behavioral, cognitive, psychoanalytic, psychodynamic or psychophysiological means to improve functioning or well-being

Qualifier Character 4	Qualifier Character 5	Qualifier Character 6	Qualifier Character 7
Z None	Z None	Z None	Z None

G   **Mental Health**
Z   **None**
J   **Light Therapy**   Definition: Application of specialized light treatments to improve functioning or well-being

Qualifier Character 4	Qualifier Character 5	Qualifier Character 6	Qualifier Character 7
Z None	Z None	Z None	Z None

Substance Abuse Treatment HZ2–HZ9

AHA Coding Clinic for table HZ2

2020, 1Q, 21   Inpatient detoxification services

AHA Coding Clinic for table HZ9

2020, 1Q, 21   Inpatient detoxification services

H   **Substance Abuse Treatment**
Z   **None**
2   **Detoxification Services**   Definition: Detoxification from alcohol and/or drugs

                         Explanation: Not a treatment modality, but helps the patient stabilize physically and psychologically until the body becomes free of drugs and the effects of alcohol

Qualifier Character 4	Qualifier Character 5	Qualifier Character 6	Qualifier Character 7
Z None	**Z** None	**Z** None	**Z** None

H   **Substance Abuse Treatment**
Z   **None**
3   **Individual Counseling**   Definition: The application of psychological methods to treat an individual with addictive behavior

                         Explanation: Comprised of several different techniques, which apply various strategies to address drug addiction

Qualifier Character 4	Qualifier Character 5	Qualifier Character 6	Qualifier Character 7
Ø Cognitive 1 Behavioral 2 Cognitive-Behavioral 3 12-Step 4 Interpersonal 5 Vocational 6 Psychoeducation 7 Motivational Enhancement 8 Confrontational 9 Continuing Care B Spiritual C Pre/Post-Test Infectious Disease	**Z** None	**Z** None	**Z** None

DRG Non-OR   HZ3[Ø,1,2,3,4,5,6,7,8,9,B]ZZZ

H   **Substance Abuse Treatment**
Z   **None**
4   **Group Counseling**   Definition: The application of psychological methods to treat two or more individuals with addictive behavior

                         Explanation: Provides structured group counseling sessions and healing power through the connection with others

Qualifier Character 4	Qualifier Character 5	Qualifier Character 6	Qualifier Character 7
Ø Cognitive 1 Behavioral 2 Cognitive-Behavioral 3 12-Step 4 Interpersonal 5 Vocational 6 Psychoeducation 7 Motivational Enhancement 8 Confrontational 9 Continuing Care B Spiritual C Pre/Post-Test Infectious Disease	**Z** None	**Z** None	**Z** None

DRG Non-OR   HZ4[Ø,1,2,3,4,5,6,7,8,9,B]ZZZ

NC Noncovered Procedure   **LC** Limited Coverage   **QA** Questionable OB Admit   **NT** New Tech Add-on   ⊞ Combination Member   ♂ Male   ♀ Female

ICD-10-PCS 2024   821

Substance Abuse Treatment (side margin)

H Substance Abuse Treatment
Z None
5 Individual Psychotherapy   Definition: Treatment of an individual with addictive behavior by behavioral, cognitive, psychoanalytic, psychodynamic or psychophysiological means

Qualifier Character 4	Qualifier Character 5	Qualifier Character 6	Qualifier Character 7
Ø Cognitive	Z None	Z None	Z None
1 Behavioral			
2 Cognitive-Behavioral			
3 12-Step			
4 Interpersonal			
5 Interactive			
6 Psychoeducation			
7 Motivational Enhancement			
8 Confrontational			
9 Supportive			
B Psychoanalysis			
C Psychodynamic			
D Psychophysiological			

DRG Non-OR For all qualifier values

H Substance Abuse Treatment
Z None
6 Family Counseling   Definition: The application of psychological methods that includes one or more family members to treat an individual with addictive behavior

Explanation: Provides support and education for family members of addicted individuals. Family member participation is seen as a critical area of substance abuse treatment

Qualifier Character 4	Qualifier Character 5	Qualifier Character 6	Qualifier Character 7
3 Other Family Counseling	Z None	Z None	Z None

H Substance Abuse Treatment
Z None
8 Medication Management   Definition: Monitoring or adjusting the use of replacement medications for the treatment of addiction

Qualifier Character 4	Qualifier Character 5	Qualifier Character 6	Qualifier Character 7
Ø Nicotine Replacement	Z None	Z None	Z None
1 Methadone Maintenance			
2 Levo-alpha-acetyl-methadol (LAAM)			
3 Antabuse			
4 Naltrexone			
5 Naloxone			
6 Clonidine			
7 Bupropion			
8 Psychiatric Medication			
9 Other Replacement Medication			

H Substance Abuse Treatment
Z None
9 Pharmacotherapy   Definition: The use of replacement medications for the treatment of addiction

Qualifier Character 4	Qualifier Character 5	Qualifier Character 6	Qualifier Character 7
Ø Nicotine Replacement	Z None	Z None	Z None
1 Methadone Maintenance			
2 Levo-alpha-acetyl-methadol (LAAM)			
3 Antabuse			
4 Naltrexone			
5 Naloxone			
6 Clonidine			
7 Bupropion			
8 Psychiatric Medication			
9 Other Replacement Medication			

New Technology XØ5–XYØ

AHA Coding Clinic for all tables in the New Technology Section
2015, 4Q, 8-11   New Section X codes - New Technology procedures

AHA Coding Clinic for table XØH
2022, 4Q, 63-64   Implantation of sphenopalatine ganglion stimulator for ischemic stroke
2022, 4Q, 64-65   Implantation of paired vagus nerve stimulator using an external controller

AHA Coding Clinic for table XØZ
2022, 4Q, 65-66   Computer-assisted transcranial magnetic stimulation of the prefrontal cortex

AHA Coding Clinic for table X27
2019, 4Q, 45-46   Sustained released drug-eluting stent

AHA Coding Clinic for table X2A
2022, 4Q, 66   Pressure-controlled intermittent coronary sinus occlusion
2021, 1Q, 16   Placement of Sentinel™ embolic protection device with deployment of single filter
2020, 4Q, 70-71   Cerebral embolic filtration extracorporeal flow reversal circuit
2019, 4Q, 46   Cerebral embolic filtration
2016, 4Q, 115-116 Cerebral embolic filtration

AHA Coding Clinic for table X2C
2021, 4Q, 58-59   Computer-aided mechanical aspiration thrombectomy
2016, 4Q, 82-83   Coronary artery, number of arteries
2015, 4Q, 8-14   New Section X codes—New Technology procedures

AHA Coding Clinic for table X2J
2021, 4Q, 59   Transthoracic echocardiography with computer-aided image acquisition

AHA Coding Clinic for table X2K
2021, 4Q, 60   Percutaneous creation of arteriovenous fistula using thermal resistance energy

AHA Coding Clinic for table X2R
2022, 4Q, 54-55   Rapid deployment technique for replacement of aortic valve using zooplastic tissue
2021, 4Q, 61-62   Replacement combined with restriction of descending thoracic aorta
2016, 4Q, 116   Aortic valve rapid deployment
2015, 4Q, 8-12   New Section X codes—New Technology procedures

AHA Coding Clinic for table X2V
2021, 4Q, 61-62   Replacement combined with restriction of descending thoracic aorta
2021, 4Q, 63   Restriction of coronary sinus

AHA Coding Clinic for table XD2
2021, 4Q, 63-64   Monitoring of tissue oxygen saturation in gastrointestinal tract

AHA Coding Clinic for table XDP
2021, 4Q, 64-65   Colonic irrigation for colonoscopy

AHA Coding Clinic for table XF5
2022, 4Q, 67   Extracorporeal histotripsy of targeted liver tissue using ultrasound-guided cavitation

AHA Coding Clinic for table XFJ
2021, 4Q, 65-66   Single-use duodenoscope during endoscopic retrograde cholangiopancreatography

AHA Coding Clinic for table XHR
2021, 4Q, 66   Application of bioengineered allogeneic construct
2016, 4Q, 116   Application of wound matrix

AHA Coding Clinic for table XKØ
2017, 4Q, 74   Intramuscular autologous bone marrow cell therapy

AHA Coding Clinic for table XKU
2022, 4Q, 67-68   Posterior vertebral body tethering

AHA Coding Clinic for table XNH
2022, 4Q, 69   Internal fixation device with Tulip connector

AHA Coding Clinic for table XNS
2021, 4Q, 67   Posterior dynamic distraction
2017, 4Q, 74-75   Magnetic growth rods
2016, 4Q, 117   Placement of magnetic growth rods

AHA Coding Clinic for table XNU
2020, 4Q, 72   Implantation of vertebral mechanically expandable device

AHA Coding Clinic for table XRG
2022, 4Q, 69   Internal fixation device with Tulip connector
2021, 4Q, 68   Customizable interbody fusion
2017, 4Q, 76   Radiolucent porous interbody fusion device

AHA Coding Clinic for table XRH
2022, 4Q, 70   Insertion of posterior spinal motion preservation device

AHA Coding Clinic for table XRR
2022, 4Q, 70-71   Replacement of synthetic substitute meniscus of knee

AHA Coding Clinic for table XT2
2019, 4Q, 46-47   Renal function monitoring

AHA Coding Clinic for table XV5
2018, 4Q, 55   Robotic waterjet ablation

AHA Coding Clinic for table XWØ
2023, 2Q, 26   Control of bleeding with Hemospray®
2023, 1Q, 12   REGN-COV2 monoclonal antibody
2023, 1Q, 12   Sabizabulin
2022, 4Q, 60-61   Introduction of other therapeutic monoclonal antibody
2022, 4Q, 71-72   Spesolimab monoclonal antibody
2022, 4Q, 72   Daratumumab and hyaluronidase-fihj
2022, 4Q, 72   Maribavir anti-infective
2022, 4Q, 72   Teclistamab antineoplastic
2022, 4Q, 72-73   Mosunetuzumab antineoplatic
2022, 4Q, 73   Afamitresgene autoleucel immunotherapy
2022, 4Q, 73   Tabelecleucel immunotherapy
2022, 4Q, 74   Treosulfan
2022, 4Q, 74   Inebilizumab-cdon
2022, 4Q, 74   Engineered allogeneic thymus tissue
2022, 4Q, 74   Broad consortium microbiota-based live biotherapeutic suspension
2022, 3Q, 26   Tumor-infiltrating lymphocyte therapy
2022, 1Q, 5-6   COVID-19 vaccine administration
2022, 1Q, 7   Fostamatinib
2022, 1Q, 7-8   Tixagevimab and cilgavimab
2022, 1Q, 8   Other monoclonal antibody
2021, 4Q, 69-71   Introduction of new therapeutic substances
2021, 4Q, 71-74   Chimeric antigen receptor T-cell immunotherapy
2021, 4Q, 74-75   Antibiotic-eluting bone void filler
2021, 4Q, 110   New/revised frequently asked questions regarding ICD-10-CM/PCS coding for COVID-19
2021, 1Q, 49   Frequently asked questions regarding ICD-10-CM and ICD-10-PCS coding for COVID-19
2020, 4Q, 72-76   Introduction of new therapeutic substances
2020, 4Q, 95   Frequently asked questions regarding ICD-10-PCS coding for COVID-19
2020, 3Q, 17-21   New procedure codes for introduction or infusion of therapeutics
2019, 4Q, 47-50   New therapeutic substances
2018, 4Q, 56   New therapeutic substances
2015, 4Q, 8-15   New Section X codes—New Technology procedures

AHA Coding Clinic for table XW1
2023, 1Q, 13   Exagamglogene autotemcel
2022, 4Q, 75   Betibeglogene autotemcel
2022, 4Q, 75   Omidubicel
2022, 4Q, 76   OTL-103
2022, 4Q, 76   OTL-200
2021, 4Q, 76   Transfusion of hyperimmune globulin and high-dose immune globulin
2020, 3Q, 17-21   New procedure codes for introduction or infusion of therapeutics

AHA Coding Clinic for table XWH
2021, 4Q, 76-77   Pharyngeal electrical stimulation

AHA Coding Clinic for table XXE
2022, 4Q, 76   Computer-aided analysis for the detection and classification of epileptic events
2022, 4Q, 77   Quantitative flow rate for noninvasive analysis of coronary angiography
2022, 4Q, 77   Simulation for assessment of coronary obstruction risk
2022, 4Q, 78   Gene expression assay
2021, 4Q, 77   Computer-aided assessment of intracranial vascular activity
2021, 4Q, 77-78   Computer-aided triage and notification of pulmonary artery flow
2021, 4Q, 78-79   Mechanical initial specimen diversion of whole blood using active negative pressure
2021, 4Q, 79-80   Concurrent measurement of mRNA, PCR test and detection of antibodies
2020, 4Q, 78-79   Measurement of infection
2020, 4Q, 78-79   Positive blood culture fluorescence hybridization
2020, 4Q, 79   Nucleic acid-base microbial detection
2019, 4Q, 50-51   Whole blood nucleic acid-base microbial detection

AHA Coding Clinic for table XYØ
2022, 4Q, 78   Extracorporeal antimicrobial administration during renal replacement therapy
2021, 4Q, 80   Regional anticoagulation for renal replacement therapy
2017, 4Q, 78   Intraoperative treatment of vascular grafts

NC Noncovered Procedure   **LC** Limited Coverage   **QA** Questionable OB Admit   **NT** New Tech Add-on   ⊞ Combination Member   ♂ Male   ♀ Female

X **New Technology**
Ø **Nervous System**
5 **Destruction** Definition: Physical eradication of all or a portion of a body part by the direct use of energy, force, or a destructive agent
Explanation: None

Body Part Character 4	Approach Character 5	Device/Substance/Technology Character 6	Qualifier Character 7
1 Renal Sympathetic Nerve(s)	3 Percutaneous	2 Ultrasound Ablation	9 New Technology Group 9

X **New Technology**
Ø **Nervous System**
H **Insertion** Definition: Putting in a nonbiological appliance that monitors, assists, performs, or prevents a physiological function but does not physically take the place of a body part
Explanation: None

Body Part Character 4	Approach Character 5	Device/Substance/Technology Character 6	Qualifier Character 7
K Sphenopalatine Ganglion	3 Percutaneous	Q Neurostimulator Lead	8 New Technology Group 8
Q Vagus Nerve ⊞	3 Percutaneous	R Neurostimulator Lead with ⁿᵗ Paired Stimulation System	8 New Technology Group 8

Valid OR All body part, approach, device/substance/technology, and qualifier values   **See Appendix L for Procedure Combinations**
NT XØHQ3R8 for ViviStim® Paired VNS System   ⊞   XØHQ3R8

X **New Technology**
Ø **Nervous System**
Z **Other Procedures** Definition: Methodologies which attempt to remediate or cure a disorder or disease
Explanation: None

Body Part Character 4	Approach Character 5	Device/Substance/Technology Character 6	Qualifier Character 7
Ø Prefrontal Cortex	X External	1 Computer-assisted Transcranial Magnetic Stimulation	8 New Technology Group 8

X **New Technology**
2 **Cardiovascular System**
7 **Dilation** Definition: Expanding an orifice or the lumen of a tubular body part
Explanation: The orifice can be a natural orifice or an artificially created orifice. Accomplished by stretching a tubular body part using intraluminal pressure or by cutting part of the orifice or wall of the tubular body part.

Body Part Character 4	Approach Character 5	Device/Substance/Technology Character 6	Qualifier Character 7
H Femoral Artery, Right J Femoral Artery, Left K Popliteal Artery, Proximal Right L Popliteal Artery, Proximal Left M Popliteal Artery, Distal Right N Popliteal Artery, Distal Left P Anterior Tibial Artery, Right Q Anterior Tibial Artery, Left R Posterior Tibial Artery, Right S Posterior Tibial Artery, Left T Peroneal Artery, Right U Peroneal Artery, Left	3 Percutaneous	8 Intraluminal Device, Sustained Release Drug-eluting 9 Intraluminal Device, Sustained Release Drug-eluting, Two B Intraluminal Device, Sustained Release Drug-eluting, Three C Intraluminal Device, Sustained Release Drug-eluting, Four or More	5 New Technology Group 5

Valid OR All body part, approach, device/substance/technology, and qualifier values

X **New Technology**
2 **Cardiovascular System**
A **Assistance** Definition: Taking over a portion of a physiological function by extracorporeal means
Explanation: None

Body Part Character 4	Approach Character 5	Device/Substance/Technology Character 6	Qualifier Character 7
5 Innominate Artery and Left Common Carotid Artery	3 Percutaneous	1 Cerebral Embolic Filtration, Dual Filter	2 New Technology Group 2
6 Aortic Arch	3 Percutaneous	2 Cerebral Embolic Filtration, Single Deflection Filter	5 New Technology Group 5
7 Coronary Sinus	3 Percutaneous	5 Intermittent Coronary Sinus Occlusion	8 New Technology Group 8
H Common Carotid Artery, Right J Common Carotid Artery, Left	3 Percutaneous	3 Cerebral Embolic Filtration, Extracorporeal Flow Reversal Circuit	6 New Technology Group 6

DRG Non-OR X2A7358

Non-OR Procedure   DRG Non-OR Procedure   Valid OR Procedure   HAC Associated Procedure   Combination Only   New/Revised April   New/Revised October

X   New Technology
2   Cardiovascular System
C   Extirpation   Definition: Taking or cutting out solid matter from a body part

Explanation: The solid matter may be an abnormal byproduct of a biological function or a foreign body; it may be imbedded in a body part or in the lumen of a tubular body part. The solid matter may or may not have been previously broken into pieces.

Body Part Character 4	Approach Character 5	Device/Substance/Technology Character 6	Qualifier Character 7
P Abdominal Aorta Q Upper Extremity Vein, Right R Upper Extremity Vein, Left S Lower Extremity Artery, Right T Lower Extremity Artery, Left U Lower Extremity Vein, Right V Lower Extremity Vein, Left Y Great Vessel	3 Percutaneous	T Computer-aided Mechanical Aspiration	7 New Technology Group 7

Valid OR   All body part, approach, device/substance/technology, and qualifier values

X   New Technology
2   Cardiovascular System
H   Insertion   Definition: Putting in a nonbiological appliance that monitors, assists, performs, or prevents a physiological function but does not physically take the place of a body part

Explanation: None

Body Part Character 4	Approach Character 5	Device/Substance/Technology Character 6	Qualifier Character 7
0 Inferior Vena Cava 1 Superior Vena Cava	3 Percutaneous	R Intraluminal Device, Bioprosthetic Valve	9 New Technology Group 9
2 Femoral Vein, Right 3 Femoral Vein, Left	0 Open	R Intraluminal Device, Bioprosthetic Valve	9 New Technology Group 9
6 Atrium, Right K Ventricle, Right	3 Percutaneous	V Intracardiac Pacemaker, Dual-Chamber	9 New Technology Group 9
L Axillary Artery, Right M Axillary Artery, Left X Thoracic Aorta, Ascending	0 Open	F Conduit to Short-term External Heart Assist System	9 New Technology Group 9

Valid OR   X2H13R9

X   New Technology
2   Cardiovascular System
J   Inspection   Definition: Visually and/or manually exploring a body part

Explanation: None

Body Part Character 4	Approach Character 5	Device/Substance/Technology Character 6	Qualifier Character 7
A Heart	X External	4 Transthoracic Echocardiography, Computer-aided Guidance **NT**	7 New Technology Group 7

NT   X2JAX47 for Caption Guidance™

X   New Technology
2   Cardiovascular System
K   Bypass   Definition: Altering the route of passage of the contents of a tubular body part

Explanation: None

Body Part Character 4	Approach Character 5	Device/Substance/Technology Character 6	Qualifier Character 7
B Radial Artery, Right C Radial Artery, Left	3 Percutaneous	1 Thermal Resistance Energy	7 New Technology Group 7
H Femoral Artery, Right J Femoral Artery, Left	3 Percutaneous	D Conduit through Femoral Vein to Superficial Femoral Artery E Conduit through Femoral Vein to Popliteal Artery	9 New Technology Group 9

Valid OR   All body part, approach, device/substance/technology, and qualifier values

X   New Technology
2   Cardiovascular System
R   Replacement   Definition: Putting in or on biological or synthetic material that physically takes the place and/or function of all or a portion of a body part

Explanation: None

Body Part Character 4	Approach Character 5	Device/Substance/Technology Character 6	Qualifier Character 7
X Thoracic Aorta, Arch	0 Open	N Branched Synthetic Substitute **NT** with Intraluminal Device	7 New Technology Group 7

Valid OR   All body part, approach, device/substance/technology, and qualifier values
NT   X2RX0N7 with X2VW0N7 for Thoraflex™ Hybrid System

NC Noncovered Procedure   **LC** Limited Coverage   **QA** Questionable OB Admit   **NT** New Tech Add-on   ⊞ Combination Member   ♂ Male   ♀ Female

X   **New Technology**
2   **Cardiovascular System**
U   **Supplememt**   Definition: Putting in or on biological or synthetic material that physically reinforces and/or augments the function of a portion of a body part
       Explanation: None

Body Part Character 4	Approach Character 5	Device/Substance/Technology Character 6	Qualifier Character 7
4 Coronary Artery/Arteries	Ø Open	7 Vein Graft Extraluminal Support Device(s)	9 New Technology Group 9
Q Upper Extremity Vein, Right R Upper Extremity Vein, Left	Ø Open	P Synthetic Substitute, Extraluminal Support Device	9 New Technology Group 9

Valid OR   X2U[Q,R]ØP9

X   **New Technology**
2   **Cardiovascular System**
V   **Restriction**   Definition: Partially closing an orifice or the lumen of a tubular body part
       Explanation: None

Body Part Character 4	Approach Character 5	Device/Substance/Technology Character 6	Qualifier Character 7
7 Coronary Sinus	3 Percutaneous	Q Reduction Device	7 New Technology Group 7
W Thoracic Aorta, Descending	Ø Open	N Branched Synthetic Substitute **NT** with Intraluminal Device	7 New Technology Group 7

Valid OR   All body part, approach, device/substance/technology, and qualifier values
NT   X2VWØN7 with X2RXØN7 for Thoraflex™ Hybrid System

X   **New Technology**
D   **Gastrointestinal System**
2   **Monitoring**   Definition: Determining the level of a physiological or physical function repetitively over a period of time
       Explanation: None

Body Part Character 4	Approach Character 5	Device/Substance/Technology Character 6	Qualifier Character 7
G Upper GI H Lower GI	4 Percutaneous Endoscopic 8 Via Natural or Artificial Opening Endoscopic	V Oxygen Saturation	7 New Technology Group 7

X   **New Technology**
D   **Gastrointestinal System**
P   **Irrigation**   Definition: Putting in or on a cleansing substance
       Explanation: None

Body Part Character 4	Approach Character 5	Device/Substance/Technology Character 6	Qualifier Character 7
H Lower GI	8 Via Natural or Artificial Opening Endoscopic	K Intraoperative Single-use Oversleeve	7 New Technology Group 7

X   **New Technology**
F   **Hepatobiliary System and Pancreas**
5   **Destruction**   Definition: Physical eradication of all or a portion of a body part by the direct use of energy, force, or a destructive agent
       Explanation: None of the body part is physically taken out

Body Part Character 4	Approach Character 5	Device/Substance/Technology Character 6	Qualifier Character 7
Ø Liver 1 Liver, Right Lobe 2 Liver, Left Lobe	X External	Ø Ultrasound-guided Cavitation	8 New Technology Group 8

DRG Non-OR   All body part, approach, device/substance/technology, and qualifier values

---

X   **New Technology**
F   **Hepatobiliary System and Pancreas**
J   **Inspection**   Definition: Visually and/or manually exploring a body part
       Explanation: None

Body Part Character 4	Approach Character 5	Device/Substance/Technology Character 6	Qualifier Character 7
B Hepatobiliary Duct D Pancreatic Duct	8 Via Natural or Artificial Opening Endoscopic	A Single-use Duodenoscope **NT**	7 New Technology Group 7

NT   XFJ[B,D]8A7 for aScope® Duodeno

X   **New Technology**
H   **Skin, Subcutaneous Tissue, Fascia and Breast**
R   **Replacement**   Definition: Putting in or on biological or synthetic material that physically takes the place and/or function of all or a portion of a body part
       Explanation: None

Body Part Character 4	Approach Character 5	Device/Substance/Technology Character 6	Qualifier Character 7
P Skin	X External	F Bioengineered Allogeneic **NT** Construct	7 New Technology Group 7

Valid OR   XHRPXF7
NT   XHRPXF7 for StrataGraft®

Non-OR Procedure   DRG Non-OR Procedure   Valid OR Procedure   HAC Associated Procedure   Combination Only   New/Revised April   New/Revised October

X   **New Technology**
K   **Muscles, Tendons, Bursae and Ligaments**
U   **Supplement**   Definition: Putting in or on biological or synthetic material that physically reinforces and/or augments the function of a portion of a body part
                             Explanation: None

Body Part Character 4	Approach Character 5	Device/Substance/Technology Character 6	Qualifier Character 7
C Upper Spine Bursa and Ligament D Lower Spine Bursa and Ligament	Ø Open	6 Posterior Vertebral Tether	8 New Technology Group 8

Valid OR   All body part, approach, device/substance/technology, and qualifier values

---

X   **New Technology**
N   **Bones**
H   **Insertion**   Definition: Putting in a nonbiological appliance that monitors, assists, performs, or prevents a physiological function but does not physically take the place of a body part
                           Explanation: None

Body Part Character 4	Approach Character 5	Device/Substance/Technology Character 6	Qualifier Character 7
6 Pelvic Bone, Right 7 Pelvic Bone, Left	Ø Open 3 Percutaneous	5 Internal Fixation Device with **NT** Tulip Connector	8 New Technology Group 8
G Tibia, Right H Tibia, Left	Ø Open	F Tibial Extension with Motion Sensors	9 New Technology Group 9

Valid OR   All body part, approach, device/substance/technology, and qualifier values
NT   XNH[6,7][Ø,3]58 for iFuse Bedrock Granite Implant System

---

X   **New Technology**
N   **Bones**
R   **Replacement**   Definition: Putting in or on biological or synthetic material that physically takes the place and/or function of all or a portion of a body part
                           Explanation: None

Body Part Character 4	Approach Character 5	Device/Substance/Technology Character 6	Qualifier Character 7
8 Skull	Ø Open	D Synthetic Substitute, Ultrasound Penetrable	9 New Technology Group 9
L Tarsal, Right M Tarsal, Left	Ø Open	9 Synthetic Substitute, Talar Prosthesis	9 New Technology Group 9

Valid OR   XNR8ØD9

X   **New Technology**
N   **Bones**
S   **Reposition**   Definition: Moving to its normal location, or other suitable location, all or a portion of a body part
                           Explanation: The body part is moved to a new location from an abnormal location, or from a normal location where it is not functioning correctly. The body part may or may not be cut out or off to be moved to the new location.

Body Part Character 4	Approach Character 5	Device/Substance/Technology Character 6	Qualifier Character 7
Ø Lumbar Vertebra	Ø Open	3 Magnetically Controlled Growth Rod(s)	2 New Technology Group 2
Ø Lumbar Vertebra	Ø Open	C Posterior (Dynamic) Distraction Device	7 New Technology Group 7
Ø Lumbar Vertebra	3 Percutaneous	3 Magnetically Controlled Growth Rod(s)	2 New Technology Group 2
Ø Lumbar Vertebra	3 Percutaneous	C Posterior (Dynamic) Distraction Device	7 New Technology Group 7
3 Cervical Vertebra	Ø Open 3 Percutaneous	3 Magnetically Controlled Growth Rod(s)	2 New Technology Group 2
4 Thoracic Vertebra	Ø Open	3 Magnetically Controlled Growth Rod(s)	2 New Technology Group 2
4 Thoracic Vertebra	Ø Open	C Posterior (Dynamic) Distraction Device	7 New Technology Group 7
4 Thoracic Vertebra	3 Percutaneous	3 Magnetically Controlled Growth Rod(s)	2 New Technology Group 2
4 Thoracic Vertebra	3 Percutaneous	C Posterior (Dynamic) Distraction Device	7 New Technology Group 7

Valid OR   All body part, approach, device/substance/technology, and qualifier values

---

X   **New Technology**
N   **Bones**
U   **Supplement**   Definition: Putting in or on biological or synthetic material that physically reinforces and/or augments the function of a portion of a body part
                           Explanation: None

Body Part Character 4	Approach Character 5	Device/Substance/Technology Character 6	Qualifier Character 7
Ø Lumbar Vertebra 4 Thoracic Vertebra	3 Percutaneous	5 Synthetic Substitute, Mechanically Expandable (Paired)	6 New Technology Group 6

Valid OR   XNU[Ø,4]356

NC Noncovered Procedure   **LC** Limited Coverage   **QA** Questionable OB Admit   **NT** New Tech Add-on   ⊞ Combination Member   ♂ Male   ♀ Female

ICD-10-PCS 2024   827

XKU–XNU

X   **New Technology**
R   **Joints**
G   **Fusion**   Definition: Joining together portions of an articular body part rendering the articular body part immobile
           Explanation: None

Body Part Character 4	Approach Character 5	Device/Substance/Technology Character 6	Qualifier Character 7

A Thoracolumbar Vertebral Joint
B Lumbar Vertebral Joint
C Lumbar Vertebral Joints, ⊞
   2 or more
D Lumbosacral Joint
	Ø Open
	3 Percutaneous
	4 Percutaneous Endoscopic
		R Interbody Fusion Device, **NT**
		   Custom-Made Anatomically
		   Designed
			7 New Technology Group 7

E Sacroiliac Joint, Right F Sacroiliac Joint, Left	Ø Open 3 Percutaneous	5 Internal Fixation Device with **NT** Tulip Connector	8 New Technology Group 8
J Ankle Joint, Right K Ankle Joint, Left L Tarsal Joint, Right M Tarsal Joint, Left	Ø Open	B Internal Fixation Device, Open-truss Design	9 New Technology Group 9

Valid OR   All body part, approach, device/substance/technology, and qualifier values

HAC   XRG[A,B,C,D][Ø,3,4]R7 when reported with SDx K68.11 or T81.4Ø-T81.49, T84.6Ø-T84.619, T84.63-T84.7 with 7th character A

HAC   XRG[E,F][Ø,3]58 when reported with SDx K68.11 or T81.4Ø-T81.49, T84.6Ø-T84.619, T84.63-T84.7 with 7th character A

NT   XRG[A,B,C,D][Ø,3,4]R7 for aprevo® Intervertebral Body Fusion Device

NT   XRG[E,F][Ø,3]58 for iFuse Bedrock Granit Implant System

See Appendix L for Procedure Combinations
   ⊞   XRGC[Ø,3,4]R7

X   **New Technology**
R   **Joints**
H   **Insertion**   Definition: Putting in a nonbiological appliance that monitors, assists, performs, or prevents a physiological function but does not physically take the place of a body part
           Explanation: None

Body Part Character 4	Approach Character 5	Device/Substance/Technology Character 6	Qualifier Character 7
B Lumbar Vertebral Joint D Lumbosacral Joint	Ø Open	1 Posterior Spinal Motion Preservation Device	8 New Technology Group 8

Valid OR   All body part, approach, device/substance/technology, and qualifier values

---

X   **New Technology**
R   **Joints**
R   **Replacement**   Definition: Putting in or on biological or synthetic material that physically takes the place and/or function of all or a portion of a body part
           Explanation: None

Body Part Character 4	Approach Character 5	Device/Substance/Technology Character 6	Qualifier Character 7

G Knee Joint, Right ⊞
H Knee Joint, Left ⊞
	Ø Open	L Synthetic Substitute, Lateral
		   Meniscus
		M Synthetic Substitute, Medial
		   Meniscus
			8 New Technology Group 8

Valid OR   All body part, approach, device/substance/technology, and qualifier values

HAC   XRR[G,H]Ø[L,M]8 when reported with SDx of I26.Ø2-I26.Ø9, I26.92-I26.99, or I82.4Ø1-I82.4Z9

See Appendix L for Procedure Combinations
   ⊞   XRR[G,H]Ø[L,M]8

X   **New Technology**
T   **Urinary System**
2   **Monitoring**   Definition: Determining the level of a physiological or physical function repetitively over a period of time
           Explanation: None

Body Part Character 4	Approach Character 5	Device/Substance/Technology Character 6	Qualifier Character 7
5 Kidney	X External	E Fluorescent Pyrazine	5 New Technology Group 5

X New Technology
W Anatomical Regions
Ø Introduction   Definition: Putting in or on a therapeutic, diagnostic, nutritional, physiological, or prophylactic substance except blood or blood products
Explanation: None

Body Part Character 4	Approach Character 5	Device/Substance/Technology Character 6	Qualifier Character 7
Ø Skin	X External	2 Anacaulase-bcdb	7 New Technology Group 7
1 Subcutaneous Tissue	3 Percutaneous	1 Daratumumab and Hyaluronidase-fihj **NT** 4 Teclistamab Antineoplastic	8 New Technology Group 8
1 Subcutaneous Tissue	3 Percutaneous	9 Satralizumab-mwge	7 New Technology Group 7
1 Subcutaneous Tissue	3 Percutaneous	F Other New Technology Therapeutic Substance	5 New Technology Group 5
1 Subcutaneous Tissue	3 Percutaneous	G REGN-COV2 Monoclonal Antibody H Other New Technology Monoclonal Antibody K Leronlimab Monoclonal Antibody	6 New Technology Group 6
1 Subcutaneous Tissue	3 Percutaneous	L Elranatamab Antineoplastic	9 New Technology Group 9
1 Subcutaneous Tissue	3 Percutaneous	S COVID-19 Vaccine Dose 1	6 New Technology Group 6
1 Subcutaneous Tissue	3 Percutaneous	S Epcoritamab Monoclonal Antibody	9 New Technology Group 9
1 Subcutaneous Tissue	3 Percutaneous	T COVID-19 Vaccine Dose 2 U COVID-19 Vaccine	6 New Technology Group 6
1 Subcutaneous Tissue	3 Percutaneous	V COVID-19 Vaccine Dose 3	7 New Technology Group 7
1 Subcutaneous Tissue	3 Percutaneous	W Caplacizumab	5 New Technology Group 5
1 Subcutaneous Tissue	3 Percutaneous	W COVID-19 Vaccine Booster	7 New Technology Group 7
1 Subcutaneous Tissue	X External	2 Anacaulase-bcdb	7 New Technology Group 7
2 Muscle	Ø Open	D Engineered Allogeneic Thymus Tissue	8 New Technology Group 8
2 Muscle	3 Percutaneous	S COVID-19 Vaccine Dose 1 T COVID-19 Vaccine Dose 2 U COVID-19 Vaccine	6 New Technology Group 6
2 Muscle	3 Percutaneous	V COVID-19 Vaccine Dose 3 W COVID-19 Vaccine Booster X Tixagevimab and Cilgavimab Monoclonal Antibody Y Other New Technology Monoclonal Antibody	7 New Technology Group 7
3 Peripheral Vein	3 Percutaneous	Ø Brexanolone	6 New Technology Group 6
3 Peripheral Vein	3 Percutaneous	Ø Spesolimab Monoclonal Antibody	8 New Technology Group 8
3 Peripheral Vein	3 Percutaneous	2 Nerinitide 3 Durvalumab Antineoplastic	6 New Technology Group 6
3 Peripheral Vein	3 Percutaneous	5 Narsoplimab Monoclonal Antibody	7 New Technology Group 7
3 Peripheral Vein	3 Percutaneous	5 Mosunetuzumab Antineoplastic	8 New Technology Group 8
3 Peripheral Vein	3 Percutaneous	6 Lefamulin Anti-infective	6 New Technology Group 6
3 Peripheral Vein	3 Percutaneous	6 Terlipressin	7 New Technology Group 7
3 Peripheral Vein	3 Percutaneous	6 Afamitresgene Autoleucel Immunotherapy	8 New Technology Group 8
3 Peripheral Vein	3 Percutaneous	7 Coagulation Factor Xa, Inactivated	2 New Technology Group 2
3 Peripheral Vein	3 Percutaneous	7 Trilaciclib **NT**	7 New Technology Group 7
3 Peripheral Vein	3 Percutaneous	7 Tabelecleucel Immunotherapy	8 New Technology Group 8
3 Peripheral Vein	3 Percutaneous	8 Lurbinectedin **NT**	7 New Technology Group 7
3 Peripheral Vein	3 Percutaneous	8 Treosulfan	8 New Technology Group 8
3 Peripheral Vein	3 Percutaneous	9 Ceftolozane/Tazobactam Anti-infective	6 New Technology Group 6
3 Peripheral Vein	3 Percutaneous	9 Inebilizumab-cdon	8 New Technology Group 8
3 Peripheral Vein	3 Percutaneous	A Cefiderocol Anti-infective **NT**	6 New Technology Group 6
3 Peripheral Vein	3 Percutaneous	A Ciltacabtagene Autoleucel **NT**	7 New Technology Group 7
3 Peripheral Vein	3 Percutaneous	B Cytarabine and Daunorubicin Liposome Antineoplastic	3 New Technology Group 3
3 Peripheral Vein	3 Percutaneous	B Omadacycline Anti-infective	6 New Technology Group 6
3 Peripheral Vein	3 Percutaneous	B Amivantamab Monoclonal Antibody **NT**	7 New Technology Group 7
3 Peripheral Vein	3 Percutaneous	C Eculizumab	6 New Technology Group 6
3 Peripheral Vein	3 Percutaneous	C Engineered Chimeric Antigen Receptor T-cell Immunotherapy, Autologous	7 New Technology Group 7
3 Peripheral Vein	3 Percutaneous	D Atezolizumab Antineoplastic	6 New Technology Group 6
3 Peripheral Vein	3 Percutaneous	E Remdesivir Anti-infective	5 New Technology Group 5
3 Peripheral Vein	3 Percutaneous	E Etesevimab Monoclonal Antibody	6 New Technology Group 6
3 Peripheral Vein	3 Percutaneous	F Other New Technology Therapeutic Substance	3 New Technology Group 3

Valid OR   XWØ2ØD8
DRG Non-OR   XWØ3368
DRG Non-OR   XWØ3378
DRG Non-OR   XWØ33A7
DRG Non-OR   XWØ33C7

NT XWØ1318 in combination with code E85.81
NT XWØ3377
NT XWØ3387
NT XWØ33A6 in combination with code Y95 and one of the following: J14, J15.Ø, J15.1, J15.5, J15.6, J15.8, OR code J95.851 and one of the following: B96.1, B96.2Ø, B96.21, B96.22, B96.23, B96.29, B96.3, B96.5, or B96.89
NT XWØ33A7
NT XWØ33B7
* For all codes with NT icon *see* Appendix I for registered or trade name of substance

XWØ Continued on next page

NC Noncovered Procedure   **LC** Limited Coverage   **QA** Questionable OB Admit   **NT** New Tech Add-on   ⊞ Combination Member   ♂ Male   ♀ Female

New Technology

XWØ Continued

X	**New Technology**
W	**Anatomical Regions**
Ø	**Introduction**

Definition: Putting in or on a therapeutic, diagnostic, nutritional, physiological, or prophylactic substance except blood or blood products

Explanation: None

Body Part Character 4		Approach Character 5		Device/Substance/Technology Character 6		Qualifier Character 7	
3	Peripheral Vein	3	Percutaneous	F	Other New Technology Therapeutic Substance	5	New Technology Group 5
3	Peripheral Vein	3	Percutaneous	F	Bamlanivimab Monoclonal Antibody	6	New Technology Group 6
3	Peripheral Vein	3	Percutaneous	G	Sarilumab	5	New Technology Group 5
3	Peripheral Vein	3	Percutaneous	G	REGN-COV2 Monoclonal Antibody	6	New Technology Group 6
3	Peripheral Vein	3	Percutaneous	G	Engineered Chimeric Antigen Receptor T-cell Immunotherapy, Allogeneic	7	New Technology Group 7
3	Peripheral Vein	3	Percutaneous	H	Tocilizumab	5	New Technology Group 5
3	Peripheral Vein	3	Percutaneous	H	Other New Technology Monoclonal Antibody	6	New Technology Group 6
3	Peripheral Vein	3	Percutaneous	H	Axicabtagene Ciloleucel Immunotherapy	7	New Technology Group 7
				J	Tisagenlecleucel Immunotherapy		
3	Peripheral Vein	3	Percutaneous	K	Fosfomycin Anti-infective	5	New Technology Group 5
3	Peripheral Vein	3	Percutaneous	K	Idecabtagene Vicleucel Immunotherapy [NT]	7	New Technology Group 7
3	Peripheral Vein	3	Percutaneous	K	Sulbactam-Durlobactam	9	New Technology Group 9
3	Peripheral Vein	3	Percutaneous	L	CD24Fc Immunomodulator	6	New Technology Group 6
3	Peripheral Vein	3	Percutaneous	L	Lifileucel Immunotherapy	7	New Technology Group 7
				M	Brexucabtagene Autoleucel Immunotherapy [NT]		
3	Peripheral Vein	3	Percutaneous	N	Meropenem-vaborbactam Anti-infective	5	New Technology Group 5
3	Peripheral Vein	3	Percutaneous	N	Lisocabtagene Maraleucel Immunotherapy	7	New Technology Group 7
3	Peripheral Vein	3	Percutaneous	P	Glofitamab Antineoplastic	9	New Technology Group 9
3	Peripheral Vein	3	Percutaneous	Q	Tagraxofusp-erzs Antineoplastic	5	New Technology Group 5
3	Peripheral Vein	3	Percutaneous	Q	Posoleucel	9	New Technology Group 9
				R	Rezafungin		
3	Peripheral Vein	3	Percutaneous	S	Iobenguane I-131 Antineoplastic	5	New Technology Group 5
				U	Imipenem-cilastatin-relebactam Anti-infective [NT]		
				W	Caplacizumab		
4	Central Vein	3	Percutaneous	Ø	Brexanolone	6	New Technology Group 6
4	Central Vein	3	Percutaneous	Ø	Spesolimab Monoclonal Antibody	8	New Technology Group 8
4	Central Vein	3	Percutaneous	2	Nerinitide	6	New Technology Group 6
				3	Durvalumab Antineoplastic		
4	Central Vein	3	Percutaneous	5	Narsoplimab Monoclonal Antibody	7	New Technology Group 7
4	Central Vein	3	Percutaneous	5	Mosunetuzumab Antineoplastic	8	New Technology Group 8
4	Central Vein	3	Percutaneous	6	Lefamulin Anti-infective	6	New Technology Group 6
4	Central Vein	3	Percutaneous	6	Terlipressin	7	New Technology Group 7
4	Central Vein	3	Percutaneous	6	Afamitresgene Autoleucel Immunotherapy	8	New Technology Group 8
4	Central Vein	3	Percutaneous	7	Coagulation Factor Xa, Inactivated	2	New Technology Group 2
4	Central Vein	3	Percutaneous	7	Trilaciclib [NT]	7	New Technology Group 7
4	Central Vein	3	Percutaneous	7	Tabelecleucel Immunotherapy	8	New Technology Group 8
4	Central Vein	3	Percutaneous	8	Lurbinectedin [NT]	7	New Technology Group 7
4	Central Vein	3	Percutaneous	8	Treosulfan	8	New Technology Group 8
4	Central Vein	3	Percutaneous	9	Ceftolozane/Tazobactam Anti-infective	6	New Technology Group 6
4	Central Vein	3	Percutaneous	9	Inebilizumab-cdon	8	New Technology Group 8
4	Central Vein	3	Percutaneous	A	Cefiderocol Anti-infective [NT]	6	New Technology Group 6
4	Central Vein	3	Percutaneous	A	Ciltacabtagene Autoleucel [NT]	7	New Technology Group 7
4	Central Vein	3	Percutaneous	B	Cytarabine and Daunorubicin Liposome Antineoplastic	3	New Technology Group 3
4	Central Vein	3	Percutaneous	B	Omadacycline Anti-infective	6	New Technology Group 6
4	Central Vein	3	Percutaneous	B	Amivantamab Monoclonal Antibody [NT]	7	New Technology Group 7
4	Central Vein	3	Percutaneous	C	Eculizumab	6	New Technology Group 6
4	Central Vein	3	Percutaneous	C	Engineered Chimeric Antigen Receptor T-cell Immunotherapy, Autologous	7	New Technology Group 7
4	Central Vein	3	Percutaneous	D	Atezolizumab Antineoplastic	6	New Technology Group 6

DRG Non-OR	XWØ33G7	[NT]	XWØ33K7
DRG Non-OR	XWØ33[H,J]7	[NT]	XWØ33M7
DRG Non-OR	XWØ33K7	[NT]	XWØ33U5 in combination with code Y95 and one of the following: J14, J15.Ø, J15.1, J15.5, J15.6, J15.8, OR code
DRG Non-OR	XWØ33[L,M]7		J95.851 and one of the following: B96.1, B96.2Ø, B96.21, B96.22, B96.23, B96.29, B96.3, B96.5, or B96.89
DRG Non-OR	XWØ33N7	[NT]	XWØ4377
DRG Non-OR	XWØ4368	[NT]	XWØ4387
DRG Non-OR	XWØ4378	[NT]	XWØ43A6 in combination with code Y95 and one of the following: J14, J15.Ø, J15.1, J15.5, J15.6, J15.8 OR code
DRG Non-OR	XWØ43A7		J95.851 and one of the following: B96.1, B96.2Ø, B96.21, B96.22, B96.23, B96.29, B96.3, B96.5, or B96.89
DRG Non-OR	XWØ43C7	[NT]	XWØ43A7
		[NT]	XWØ43B7

* For all codes with NT icon *see* Appendix I for registered or trade name of substance

XWØ Continued on next page

Non-OR Procedure   DRG Non-OR Procedure   Valid OR Procedure   HAC Associated Procedure   Combination Only   New/Revised April   New/Revised October

830   ICD-10-PCS 2024

XWØ–XWØ

X   **New Technology**
W   **Anatomical Regions**
Ø   **Introduction**   Definition: Putting in or on a therapeutic, diagnostic, nutritional, physiological, or prophylactic substance except blood or blood products
                    Explanation: None

XWØ Continued

Body Part Character 4		Approach Character 5		Device/Substance/Technology Character 6		Qualifier Character 7	
4	Central Vein	3	Percutaneous	E	Remdesivir Anti-infective	5	New Technology Group 5
4	Central Vein	3	Percutaneous	E	Etesevimab Monoclonal Antibody	6	New Technology Group 6
4	Central Vein	3	Percutaneous	F	Other New Technology Therapeutic Substance	3	New Technology Group 3
4	Central Vein	3	Percutaneous	F	Other New Technology Therapeutic Substance	5	New Technology Group 5
4	Central Vein	3	Percutaneous	F	Bamlanivimab Monoclonal Antibody	6	New Technology Group 6
4	Central Vein	3	Percutaneous	G	Sarilumab	5	New Technology Group 5
4	Central Vein	3	Percutaneous	G	REGN-COV2 Monoclonal Antibody	6	New Technology Group 6
4	Central Vein	3	Percutaneous	G	Engineered Chimeric Antigen Receptor T-cell Immunotherapy, Allogeneic	7	New Technology Group 7
4	Central Vein	3	Percutaneous	H	Tocilizumab	5	New Technology Group 5
4	Central Vein	3	Percutaneous	H	Other New Technology Monoclonal Antibody	6	New Technology Group 6
4	Central Vein	3	Percutaneous	H	Axicabtagene Ciloleucel Immunotherapy J Tisagenlecleucel Immunotherapy	7	New Technology Group 7
4	Central Vein	3	Percutaneous	K	Fosfomycin Anti-infective	5	New Technology Group 5
4	Central Vein	3	Percutaneous	K	Idecabtagene Vicleucel Immunotherapy **NT**	7	New Technology Group 7
4	Central Vein	3	Percutaneous	K	Sulbactam-Durlobactam	9	New Technology Group 9
4	Central Vein	3	Percutaneous	L	CD24Fc Immunomodulator	6	New Technology Group 6
4	Central Vein	3	Percutaneous	L	Lifileucel Immunotherapy M Brexucabtagene Autoleucel Immunotherapy **NT**	7	New Technology Group 7
4	Central Vein	3	Percutaneous	N	Meropenem-vaborbactam Anti-infective	5	New Technology Group 5
4	Central Vein	3	Percutaneous	N	Lisocabtagene Maraleucel Immunotherapy	7	New Technology Group 7
4	Central Vein	3	Percutaneous	P	Glofitamab Antineoplastic	9	New Technology Group 9
4	Central Vein	3	Percutaneous	Q	Tagraxofusp-erzs Antineoplastic	5	New Technology Group 5
4	Central Vein	3	Percutaneous	Q	Posoleucel R Rezafungin	9	New Technology Group 9
4	Central Vein	3	Percutaneous	S	Iobenguane I-131 Antineoplastic U Imipenem-cilastatin-relebactam Anti-infective **NT** W Caplacizumab	5	New Technology Group 5
5	Peripheral Artery	3	Percutaneous	T	Melphalan Hydrochloride Antineoplastic	9	New Technology Group 9
9	Nose	7	Via Natural or Artificial Opening	M	Esketamine Hydrochloride	5	New Technology Group 5
D	Mouth and Pharynx	X	External	3	Maribavir Anti-infective **NT**	8	New Technology Group 8
D	Mouth and Pharynx	X	External	6	Lefamulin Anti-infective	6	New Technology Group 6
D	Mouth and Pharynx	X	External	8	Uridine Triacetate	2	New Technology Group 2
D	Mouth and Pharynx	X	External	F	Other New Technology Therapeutic Substance J Apalutamide Antineoplastic	5	New Technology Group 5
D	Mouth and Pharynx	X	External	J	Quizartinib Antineoplastic	9	New Technology Group 9
D	Mouth and Pharynx	X	External	K	Sabizabulin	8	New Technology Group 8
D	Mouth and Pharynx	X	External	L	Erdafitinib Antineoplastic	5	New Technology Group 5
D	Mouth and Pharynx	X	External	M	Baricitinib	6	New Technology Group 6
D	Mouth and Pharynx	X	External	N	SER-109	9	New Technology Group 9
D	Mouth and Pharynx	X	External	R	Venetoclax Antineoplastic	5	New Technology Group 5
D	Mouth and Pharynx	X	External	R	Fostamatinib	7	New Technology Group 7
D	Mouth and Pharynx	X	External	T	Ruxolitinib V Gilteritinib Antineoplastic	5	New Technology Group 5
G	Upper GI	7	Via Natural or Artificial Opening	3	Maribavir Anti-infective **NT** K Sabizabulin	8	New Technology Group 8
G	Upper GI	7	Via Natural or Artificial Opening	M	Baricitinib	6	New Technology Group 6
G	Upper GI	7	Via Natural or Artificial Opening	R	Fostamatinib	7	New Technology Group 7
G	Upper GI	8	Via Natural or Artificial Opening Endoscopic	8	Mineral-based Topical Hemostatic Agent	6	New Technology Group 6

DRG Non-OR   XWØ43G7
DRG Non-OR   XWØ43[H,J]7
DRG Non-OR   XWØ43K7
DRG Non-OR   XWØ43[L,M]7
DRG Non-OR   XWØ43N7

NT   XWØ43K7
NT   XWØ43M7
NT   XWØ43U5 in combination with code Y95 and one of the following: J14, J15.Ø, J15.1, J15.5, J15.6, J15.8, OR code J95.851 and one of the following: B96.1, B96.2Ø, B96.21, B96.22, B96.23, B96.29, B96.3, B96.5, or B96.89
NT   XWØDX38
NT   XWØG738
    * For all codes with NT icon *see* Appendix I for registered or trade name of substance

XWØ Continued on next page

XWØ Continued

X New Technology
W Anatomical Regions
Ø Introduction Definition: Putting in or on a therapeutic, diagnostic, nutritional, physiological, or prophylactic substance except blood or blood products
Explanation: None

Body Part Character 4		Approach Character 5		Device/Substance/Technology Character 6		Qualifier Character 7
H Lower GI	7	Via Natural or Artificial Opening	3	Maribavir Anti-infective NT	8	New Technology Group 8
			K	Sabizabulin		
H Lower GI	7	Via Natural or Artificial Opening	M	Baricitinib	6	New Technology Group 6
H Lower GI	7	Via Natural or Artificial Opening	R	Fostamatinib	7	New Technology Group 7
H Lower GI	7	Via Natural or Artificial Opening	X	Broad Consortium Microbiota-based Live Biotherapeutic Suspension	8	New Technology Group 8
H Lower GI	8	Via Natural or Artificial Opening Endoscopic	8	Mineral-based Topical HemostaticAgent	6	New Technology Group 6
Q Cranial Cavity and Brain	3	Percutaneous	1	Eladocagene exuparvovec	6	New Technology Group 6
V Bones	Ø	Open	P	Antibiotic-eluting Bone Void Filler NT	7	New Technology Group 7

Valid OR	XWØQ316
NT	XWØH738
NT	XWØVØP7 for Cerament® G

X New Technology
W Anatomical Regions
1 Transfusion Definition: Putting in blood or blood products
Explanation: None

Body Part Character 4		Approach Character 5		Device/Substance/Technology Character 6		Qualifier Character 7
3 Peripheral Vein	3	Percutaneous	2	Plasma, Convalescent (Nonautologous)	5	New Technology Group 5
3 Peripheral Vein	3	Percutaneous	B	Betibeglogene Autotemcel	8	New Technology Group 8
			C	Omidubicel		
3 Peripheral Vein	3	Percutaneous	D	High-Dose Intravenous Immune Globulin	7	New Technology Group 7
			E	Hyperimmune Globulin		
3 Peripheral Vein	3	Percutaneous	F	OTL-103	8	New Technology Group 8
			G	OTL-200		
3 Peripheral Vein	3	Percutaneous	H	Lovotibeglogene Autotemcel	9	New Technology Group 9
3 Peripheral Vein	3	Percutaneous	J	Exagamglogene Autotemcel	8	New Technology Group 8
4 Central Vein	3	Percutaneous	2	Plasma, Convalescent (Nonautologous)	5	New Technology Group 5
4 Central Vein	3	Percutaneous	B	Betibeglogene Autotemcel	8	New Technology Group 8
			C	Omidubicel		
4 Central Vein	3	Percutaneous	D	High-Dose Intravenous Immune Globulin	7	New Technology Group 7
			E	Hyperimmune Globulin		
4 Central Vein	3	Percutaneous	F	OTL-103	8	New Technology Group 8
			G	OTL-200		
4 Central Vein	3	Percutaneous	H	Lovotibeglogene Autotemcel	9	New Technology Group 9
4 Central Vein	3	Percutaneous	J	Exagamglogene Autotemcel	8	New Technology Group 8

DRG Non-OR	XW133[B,C]8
DRG Non-OR	XW133[F,G]8
DRG Non-OR	XW133H9
DRG Non-OR	XW133J8
DRG Non-OR	XW143[B,C]8
DRG Non-OR	XW143[F,G]8
DRG Non-OR	XW143H9
DRG Non-OR	XW143J8

X New Technology
W Anatomical Regions
H Insertion Definition: Putting in a nonbiological appliance that monitors, assists, performs, or prevents a physiological function but does not physically take the place of a body part
Explanation: None

Body Part Character 4		Approach Character 5		Device/Substance/Technology Character 6		Qualifier Character 7
D Mouth and Pharynx	7	Via Natural or Artificial Opening	Q	Neurostimulator Lead	7	New Technology Group 7

Non-OR Procedure   DRG Non-OR Procedure   Valid OR Procedure   HAC Associated Procedure   Combination Only   New/Revised April   New/Revised October

X New Technology
X Physiological Systems
2 Monitoring   Definition: Determining the level of a physiological or physical function repetitively over a period of time
         Explanation: None

Body Part Character 4	Approach Character 5	Device/Substance/Technology Character 6	Qualifier Character 7
Ø Central Nervous	X External	8 Brain Electrical Activity, Computer-aided Detection and Notification	9 New Technology Group 9
F Musculoskeletal	3 Percutaneous	W Muscle Compartment Pressure, Micro-Electro-Mechanical System	9 New Technology Group 9

X New Technology
X Physiological Systems
E Measurement   Definition: Determining the level of a physiological or physical function at a point in time
         Explanation: None

Body Part Character 4	Approach Character 5	Device/Substance/Technology Character 6	Qualifier Character 7
Ø Central Nervous	X External	Ø Intracranial Vascular Activity, Computer-aided Assessment	7 New Technology Group 7
Ø Central Nervous	X External	4 Brain Electrical Activity, Computer-aided Semiologic Analysis	8 New Technology Group 8
2 Cardiac	X External	1 Output, Computer-aided Assessment	9 New Technology Group 9
3 Arterial	X External	2 Pulmonary Artery Flow, Computer-aided Triage and Notification	7 New Technology Group 7
3 Arterial	X External	5 Coronary Artery Flow, Quantitative Flow Ratio Analysis 6 Coronary Artery Flow, Computer-aided Valve Modeling and Notification	8 New Technology Group 8
5 Circulatory	X External	3 Infection, Whole Blood Reverse Transcription and Quantitative Real-time Polymerase Chain Reaction	8 New Technology Group 8
5 Circulatory	X External	M Infection, Whole Blood Nucleic Acid-base Microbial Detection	5 New Technology Group 5
5 Circulatory	X External	N Infection, Positive Blood Culture Fluorescence Hybridization for Organism Identification, Concentration and Susceptibility	6 New Technology Group 6
5 Circulatory	X External	R Infection, Mechanical Initial Specimen Diversion Technique Using Active Negative Pressure T Intracranial Arterial Flow, Whole Blood mRNA V Infection, Serum/Plasma Nanoparticle Fluorescence SARS-CoV-2 Antibody Detection	7 New Technology Group 7
5 Circulatory	X External	Y Infection, Other Positive Blood/Isolated Colonies Bimodal Phenotypic Susceptibility Technology	9 New Technology Group 9
9 Nose	7 Via Natural or Artificial Opening	U Infection, Nasopharyngeal Fluid SARS-CoV-2 Polymerase Chain Reaction	7 New Technology Group 7
B Respiratory	X External	Q Infection, Lower Respiratory Fluid Nucleic Acid-base Microbial Detection	6 New Technology Group 6

X New Technology
Y Extracorporeal
Ø Introduction   Definition: Putting in or on a therapeutic, diagnostic, nutritional, physiological, or prophylactic substance except blood or blood products
         Explanation: None

Body Part Character 4	Approach Character 5	Device/Substance/Technology Character 6	Qualifier Character 7
V Vein Graft	X External	8 Endothelial Damage Inhibitor	3 New Technology Group 3
Y Extracorporeal	X External	2 Taurolidine Anti-infective and Heparin Anticoagulant [NT]	8 New Technology Group 8
Y Extracorporeal	X External	3 Nafamostat Anticoagulant	7 New Technology Group 7

[NT]   XYØYX28 for DefenCath™

Appendixes

Appendix A: Components of the Medical and Surgical Approach Definitions

ICD-10-PCS Value	Definition	Access Location	Method	Type of Instrumentation	Example
Open (Ø)	Cutting through the skin or mucous membrane and any other body layers necessary to expose the site of the procedure	Skin or mucous membrane, any other body layers	Cutting	None	Abdominal hysterectomy
Percutaneous (3)	Entry, by puncture or minor incision, of instrumentation through the skin or mucous membrane and any other body layers necessary to reach the site of the procedure	Skin or mucous membrane, any other body layers	Puncture or minor incision	Without visualization	Needle biopsy of liver, Liposuction
Percutaneous endoscopic (4)	Entry, by puncture or minor incision, of instrumentation through the skin or mucous membrane and any other body layers necessary to reach and visualize the site of the procedure	Skin or mucous membrane, any other body layers	Puncture or minor incision	With visualization	Arthroscopy, Laparoscopic cholecystectomy
Via natural or artificial opening (7)	Entry of instrumentation through a natural or artificial external opening to reach the site of the procedure	Natural or artificial external opening	Direct entry	Without visualization	Endotracheal tube insertion, Foley catheter placement
Via natural or artificial opening endoscopic (8)	Entry of instrumentation through a natural or artificial external opening to reach and visualize the site of the procedure	Natural or artificial external opening	Direct entry	With visualization	Sigmoidoscopy, EGD, ERCP
Via natural or artificial opening with percutaneous endoscopic assistance (F)	Entry of instrumentation through a natural or artificial external opening and entry, by puncture or minor incision, of instrumentation through the skin or mucous membrane and any other body layers necessary to aid in the performance of the procedure	Skin or mucous membrane, any other body layers	Direct entry with puncture or minor incision for instrumentation only	With visualization	Laparoscopic-assisted vaginal hysterectomy
External (X)	Procedures performed directly on the skin or mucous membrane and procedures performed indirectly by the application of external force through the skin or mucous membrane	Skin or mucous membrane	Direct or indirect application	None	Closed fracture reduction, Resection of tonsils

The approach comprises three components: the access location, method, and type of instrumentation.

Access location: For procedures performed on an internal body part, the access location specifies the external site through which the site of the procedure is reached. There are two general types of access locations: skin or mucous membranes, and external orifices. Every approach value except external includes one of these two access locations. The skin or mucous membrane can be cut or punctured to reach the procedure site. All open and percutaneous approach values use this access location. The site of a procedure can also be reached through an external opening. External openings can be natural (e.g., mouth) or artificial (e.g., colostomy stoma).

Method: For procedures performed on an internal body part, the method specifies how the external access location is entered. An open method specifies cutting through the skin or mucous membrane and any other intervening body layers necessary to expose the site of the procedure. An instrumentation method specifies the entry of instrumentation through the access location to the internal procedure site. Instrumentation can be introduced by puncture or minor incision, or through an external opening. The puncture or minor incision does not constitute an open approach because it does not expose the site of the procedure. An approach can define multiple methods. For example, Via Natural or Artificial Opening with Percutaneous Endoscopic Assistance includes both the initial entry of instrumentation to reach the site of the procedure, and the placement of additional percutaneous instrumentation into the body part to visualize and assist in the performance of the procedure.

Type of instrumentation: For procedures performed on an internal body part, instrumentation means that specialized equipment is used to perform the procedure. Instrumentation is used in all internal approaches other than the basic open approach. Instrumentation may or may not include the capacity to visualize the procedure site. For example, the instrumentation used to perform a sigmoidoscopy permits the internal site of the procedure to be visualized, while the instrumentation used to perform a needle biopsy of the liver does not. The term "endoscopic" as used in approach values refers to instrumentation that permits a site to be visualized.

Procedures performed directly on the skin or mucous membrane are identified by the external approach (e.g., skin excision). Procedures performed indirectly by the application of external force are also identified by the external approach (e.g., closed reduction of fracture).

Appendix A: Components of the Medical and Surgical Approach Definitions

Open (Ø)

Percutaneous (3)

Percutaneous Endoscopic (4)

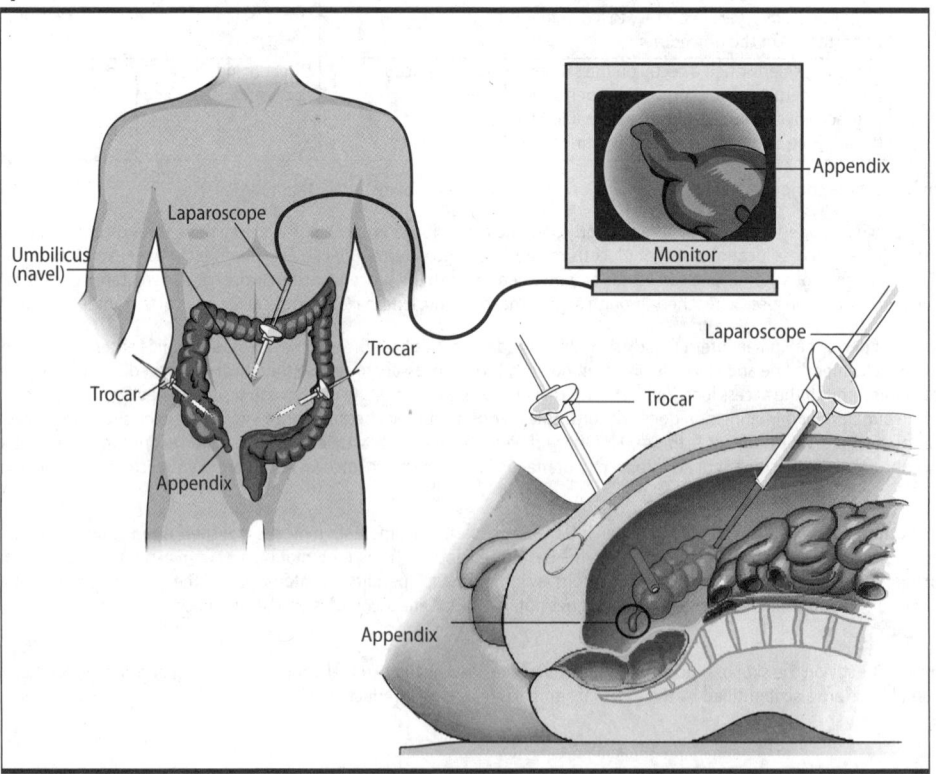

Via Natural or Artificial Opening (7)

Via Natural or Artificial Opening, Endoscopic (8)

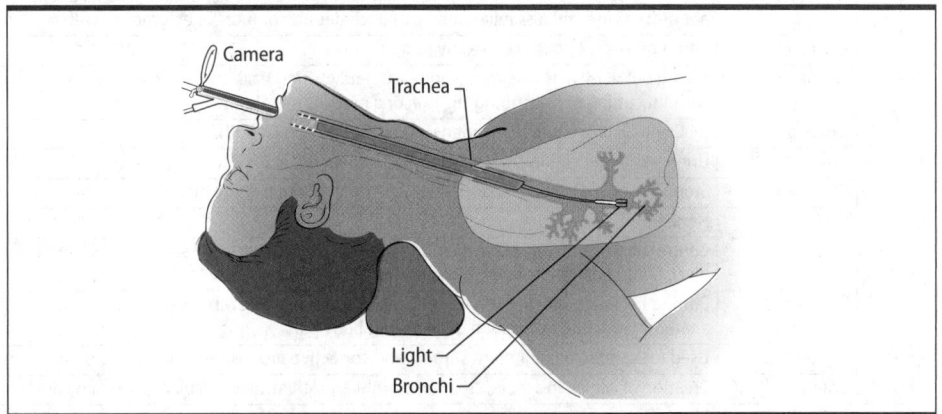

Via Natural or Artificial Opening with Percutaneous Endoscopic Assistance (F)

External (X)

Appendix B: Root Operation Definitions

The character 3 value in the Medical and Surgical section (0) and the Medical and Surgical-related sections (1-9) represents the root operation. This resource provides each root operation (character 3) value, found in sections 0-9, as well as their associated definition, explanation, and examples, where applicable. The Ancillary sections (B-H) do not include root operations; instead, the character 3 value represents the type of procedure performed with additional detail provided by the character 4 or 5 value, when applicable. For the character 3, character 4, and character 5 values used in the Ancillary sections of B-H, along with their definitions, see appendix J.

Ø	Medical and Surgical		
ICD-10-PCS Value			**Definition**
Ø	Alteration	Definition:	Modifying the anatomic structure of a body part without affecting the function of the body part
		Explanation:	Principal purpose is to improve appearance
		Examples:	Face lift, breast augmentation
1	Bypass	Definition:	Altering the route of passage of the contents of a tubular body part
		Explanation:	Rerouting contents of a body part to a downstream area of the normal route, to a similar route and body part, or to an abnormal route and dissimilar body part. Includes one or more anastomoses, with or without the use of a device.
		Examples:	Coronary artery bypass, colostomy formation
2	Change	Definition:	Taking out or off a device from a body part and putting back an identical or similar device in or on the same body part without cutting or puncturing the skin or a mucous membrane
		Explanation:	All CHANGE procedures are coded using the approach EXTERNAL
		Examples:	Urinary catheter change, gastrostomy tube change
3	Control	Definition:	Stopping, or attempting to stop, postprocedural or other acute bleeding
		Explanation:	None
		Examples:	Control of post-prostatectomy hemorrhage, control of intracranial subdural hemorrhage, control of bleeding duodenal ulcer, control of retroperitoneal hemorrhage
4	Creation	Definition:	Putting in or on biological or synthetic material to form a new body part that to the extent possible replicates the anatomic structure or function of an absent body part
		Explanation:	Used for gender reassignment surgery and corrective procedures in individuals with congenital anomalies
		Examples:	Creation of vagina in a male, creation of right and left atrioventricular valve from common atrioventricular valve
5	Destruction	Definition:	Physical eradication of all or a portion of a body part by the direct use of energy, force, or a destructive agent
		Explanation:	None of the body part is physically taken out
		Examples:	Fulguration of rectal polyp, cautery of skin lesion
6	Detachment	Definition:	Cutting off all or a portion of the upper or lower extremities
		Explanation:	The body part value is the site of the detachment, with a qualifier if applicable to further specify the level where the extremity was detached
		Examples:	Below knee amputation, disarticulation of shoulder
7	Dilation	Definition:	Expanding an orifice or the lumen of a tubular body part
		Explanation:	The orifice can be a natural orifice or an artificially created orifice. Accomplished by stretching a tubular body part using intraluminal pressure or by cutting part of the orifice or wall of the tubular body part.
		Examples:	Percutaneous transluminal angioplasty, internal urethrotomy
8	Division	Definition:	Cutting into a body part, without draining fluids and/or gases from the body part, in order to separate or transect a body part
		Explanation:	All or a portion of the body part is separated into two or more portions
		Examples:	Spinal cordotomy, osteotomy
9	Drainage	Definition:	Taking or letting out fluids and/or gases from a body part
		Explanation:	The qualifier DIAGNOSTIC is used to identify drainage procedures that are biopsies
		Examples:	Thoracentesis, incision and drainage
B	Excision	Definition:	Cutting out or off, without replacement, a portion of a body part
		Explanation:	The qualifier DIAGNOSTIC is used to identify excision procedures that are biopsies
		Examples:	Partial nephrectomy, liver biopsy
C	Extirpation	Definition:	Taking or cutting out solid matter from a body part
		Explanation:	The solid matter may be an abnormal byproduct of a biological function or a foreign body; it may be imbedded in a body part or in the lumen of a tubular body part. The solid matter may or may not have been previously broken into pieces.
		Examples:	Thrombectomy, choledocholithotomy
D	Extraction	Definition:	Pulling or stripping out or off all or a portion of a body part by the use of force
		Explanation:	The qualifier DIAGNOSTIC is used to identify extractions that are biopsies
		Examples:	Dilation and curettage, vein stripping

Continued on next page

Ø	**Medical and Surgical**		*Continued from previous page*
ICD-10-PCS Value			**Definition**
F	Fragmentation	Definition:	Breaking solid matter in a body part into pieces
		Explanation:	Physical force (e.g., manual, ultrasonic) applied directly or indirectly is used to break the solid matter into pieces. The solid matter may be an abnormal byproduct of a biological function or a foreign body. The pieces of solid matter are not taken out.
		Examples:	Extracorporeal shockwave lithotripsy, transurethral lithotripsy
G	Fusion	Definition:	Joining together portions of an articular body part rendering the articular body part immobile
		Explanation:	The body part is joined together by fixation device, bone graft, or other means
		Examples:	Spinal fusion, ankle arthrodesis
H	Insertion	Definition:	Putting in a nonbiological appliance that monitors, assists, performs, or prevents a physiological function but does not physically take the place of a body part
		Explanation:	None
		Examples:	Insertion of radioactive implant, insertion of central venous catheter
J	Inspection	Definition:	Visually and/or manually exploring a body part
		Explanation:	Visual exploration may be performed with or without optical instrumentation. Manual exploration may be performed directly or through intervening body layers.
		Examples:	Diagnostic arthroscopy, exploratory laparotomy
K	Map	Definition:	Locating the route of passage of electrical impulses and/or locating functional areas in a body part
		Explanation:	Applicable only to the cardiac conduction mechanism and the central nervous system
		Examples:	Cardiac mapping, cortical mapping
L	Occlusion	Definition:	Completely closing an orifice or lumen of a tubular body part
		Explanation:	The orifice can be a natural orifice or an artificially created orifice
		Examples:	Fallopian tube ligation, ligation of inferior vena cava
M	Reattachment	Definition:	Putting back in or on all or a portion of a separated body part to its normal location or other suitable location
		Explanation:	Vascular circulation and nervous pathways may or may not be reestablished
		Examples:	Reattachment of hand, reattachment of avulsed kidney
N	Release	Definition:	Freeing a body part from an abnormal physical constraint by cutting or by use of force
		Explanation:	Some of the restraining tissue may be taken out but none of the body part is taken out
		Examples:	Adhesiolysis, carpal tunnel release
P	Removal	Definition:	Taking out or off a device from a body part
		Explanation:	If a device is taken out and a similar device put in without cutting or puncturing the skin or mucous membrane, the procedure is coded to the root operation CHANGE. Otherwise, the procedure for taking out a device is coded to the root operation REMOVAL.
		Examples:	Drainage tube removal, cardiac pacemaker removal
Q	Repair	Definition:	Restoring, to the extent possible, a body part to its normal anatomic structure and function
		Explanation:	Used only when the method to accomplish the repair is not one of the other root operations
		Examples:	Colostomy takedown, suture of laceration
R	Replacement	Definition:	Putting in or on biological or synthetic material that physically takes the place and/or function of all or a portion of a body part
		Explanation:	The body part may have been taken out or replaced, or may be taken out, physically eradicated, or rendered nonfunctional during the REPLACEMENT procedure. A REMOVAL procedure is coded for taking out the device used in a previous replacement procedure.
		Examples:	Total hip replacement, bone graft, free skin graft
S	Reposition	Definition:	Moving to its normal location, or other suitable location, all or a portion of a body part
		Explanation:	The body part is moved to a new location from an abnormal location, or from a normal location where it is not functioning correctly. The body part may or may not be cut out or off to be moved to the new location.
		Examples:	Reposition of undescended testicle, fracture reduction
T	Resection	Definition:	Cutting out or off, without replacement, all of a body part
		Explanation:	None
		Examples:	Total nephrectomy, total lobectomy of lung
V	Restriction	Definition:	Partially closing an orifice or the lumen of a tubular body part
		Explanation:	The orifice can be a natural orifice or an artificially created orifice
		Examples:	Esophagogastric fundoplication, cervical cerclage
W	Revision	Definition:	Correcting, to the extent possible, a portion of a malfunctioning device or the position of a displaced device
		Explanation:	Revision can include correcting a malfunctioning or displaced device by taking out or putting in components of the device such as a screw or pin
		Examples:	Adjustment of position of pacemaker lead, recementing of hip prosthesis

Continued on next page

Ø	**Medical and Surgical**			*Continued from previous page*
ICD-10-PCS Value			**Definition**	
U	Supplement	Definition:	Putting in or on biological or synthetic material that physically reinforces and/or augments the function of a portion of a body part	
		Explanation:	The biological material is non-living, or is living and from the same individual. The body part may have been previously replaced, and the SUPPLEMENT procedure is performed to physically reinforce and/or augment the function of the replaced body part.	
		Examples:	Herniorrhaphy using mesh, mitral valve ring annuloplasty, put a new acetabular liner in a previous hip replacement	
X	Transfer	Definition:	Moving, without taking out, all or a portion of a body part to another location to take over the function of all or a portion of a body part	
		Explanation:	The body part transferred remains connected to its vascular and nervous supply	
		Examples:	Tendon transfer, skin pedicle flap transfer	
Y	Transplantation	Definition:	Putting in or on all or a portion of a living body part taken from another individual or animal to physically take the place and/or function of all or a portion of a similar body part	
		Explanation:	The native body part may or may not be taken out, and the transplanted body part may take over all or a portion of its function	
		Examples:	Kidney transplant, heart transplant	

Root Operation Definitions for Other Sections

1	**Obstetrics**		
ICD-10-PCS Value			**Definition**
2	Change	Definition:	Taking out or off a device from a body part and putting back an identical or similar device in or on the same body part without cutting or puncturing the skin or a mucous membrane
		Explanation:	None
		Example:	Replacement of fetal scalp electrode
9	Drainage	Definition:	Taking or letting out fluids and/or gases from a body part
		Explanation:	None
		Example:	Biopsy of amniotic fluid
A	Abortion	Definition:	Artificially terminating a pregnancy
		Explanation:	None
		Example:	Transvaginal abortion using vacuum aspiration technique
D	Extraction	Definition:	Pulling or stripping out or off all or a portion of a body part by the use of force
		Explanation:	None
		Example:	Low-transverse C-section
E	Delivery	Definition:	Assisting the passage of the products of conception from the genital canal
		Explanation:	None
		Example:	Manually-assisted delivery
H	Insertion	Definition:	Putting in a nonbiological appliance that monitors, assists, performs, or prevents a physiological function but does not physically take the place of a body part
		Explanation:	None
		Example:	Placement of fetal scalp electrode
J	Inspection	Definition:	Visually and/or manually exploring a body part
		Explanation:	Visual exploration may be performed with or without optical instrumentation. Manual exploration may be performed directly or through intervening body layers.
		Example:	Bimanual pregnancy exam
P	Removal	Definition:	Taking out or off a device from a body part, region or orifice
		Explanation:	If a device is taken out and a similar device put in without cutting or puncturing the skin or mucous membrane, the procedure is coded to the root operation CHANGE. Otherwise, the procedure for taking out a device is coded to the root operation REMOVAL.
		Example:	Removal of fetal monitoring electrode
Q	Repair	Definition:	Restoring, to the extent possible, a body part to its normal anatomic structure and function
		Explanation:	Used only when the method to accomplish the repair is not one of the other root operations
		Example:	In utero repair of congenital diaphragmatic hernia
S	Reposition	Definition:	Moving to its normal location, or other suitable location, all or a portion of a body part
		Explanation:	The body part is moved to a new location from an abnormal location, or from a normal location where it is not functioning correctly. The body part may or may not be cut out or off to be moved to the new location.
		Example:	External version of fetus
T	Resection	Definition:	Cutting out or off, without replacement, all of a body part
		Explanation:	None
		Example:	Total excision of tubal pregnancy

Continued on next page

1	Obstetrics		*Continued from previous page*
ICD-10-PCS Value			**Definition**
Y	Transplantation	Definition:	Putting in or on all or a portion of a living body part taken from another individual or animal to physically take the place and/or function of all or a portion of a similar body part
		Explanation:	The native body part may or may not be taken out, and the transplanted body part may take over all or a portion of its function
		Example:	In utero fetal kidney transplant

2	Placement		
ICD-10-PCS Value			**Definition**
Ø	Change	Definition:	Taking out or off a device from a body part and putting back an identical or similar device in or on the same body part without cutting or puncturing the skin or a mucous membrane
		Example:	Change of vaginal packing
1	Compression	Definition:	Putting pressure on a body region
		Example:	Placement of pressure dressing on abdominal wall
2	Dressing	Definition:	Putting material on a body region for protection
		Example:	Application of sterile dressing to head wound
3	Immobilization	Definition:	Limiting or preventing motion of a body region
		Example:	Placement of splint on left finger
4	Packing	Definition:	Putting material in a body region or orifice
		Example:	Placement of nasal packing
5	Removal	Definition:	Taking out or off a device from a body part
		Example:	Removal of stereotactic head frame
6	Traction	Definition:	Exerting a pulling force on a body region in a distal direction
		Example:	Lumbar traction using motorized split-traction table

3	Administration		
ICD-10-PCS Value			**Definition**
Ø	Introduction	Definition:	Putting in or on a therapeutic, diagnostic, nutritional, physiological, or prophylactic substance except blood or blood products
		Example:	Nerve block injection to median nerve
1	Irrigation	Definition:	Putting in or on a cleansing substance
		Example:	Flushing of eye
2	Transfusion	Definition:	Putting in blood or blood products
		Example:	Transfusion of cell saver red cells into central venous line

4	Measurement and Monitoring		
ICD-10-PCS Value			**Definition**
Ø	Measurement	Definition:	Determining the level of a physiological or physical function at a point in time
		Example:	External electrocardiogram(EKG), single reading
1	Monitoring	Definition:	Determining the level of a physiological or physical function repetitively over a period of time
		Example:	Urinary pressure monitoring

5	Extracorporeal or Systemic Assistance and Performance		
ICD-10-PCS Value			**Definition**
Ø	Assistance	Definition:	Taking over a portion of a physiological function by extracorporeal means
		Example:	Hyperbaric oxygenation of wound
1	Performance	Definition:	Completely taking over a physiological function by extracorporeal means
		Example:	Cardiopulmonary bypass in conjunction with CABG
2	Restoration	Definition:	Returning, or attempting to return, a physiological function to its original state by extracorporeal means
		Example:	Attempted cardiac defibrillation, unsuccessful

6   Extracorporeal or Systemic Therapies

ICD-10-PCS Value		Definition	
Ø	Atmospheric Control	Definition:	Extracorporeal control of atmospheric pressure and composition
		Example:	Antigen-free air conditioning, series treatment
1	Decompression	Definition:	Extracorporeal elimination of undissolved gas from body fluids
		Example:	Hyperbaric decompression treatment, single
2	Electromagnetic Therapy	Definition:	Extracorporeal treatment by electromagnetic rays
		Example:	TMS (transcranial magnetic stimulation), series treatment
3	Hyperthermia	Definition:	Extracorporeal raising of body temperature
		Example:	None
4	Hypothermia	Definition:	Extracorporeal lowering of body temperature
		Example:	Whole body hypothermia treatment for temperature imbalances, series
5	Pheresis	Definition:	Extracorporeal separation of blood products
		Example:	Therapeutic leukopheresis, single treatment
6	Phototherapy	Definition:	Extracorporeal treatment by light rays
		Example:	Phototherapy of circulatory system, series treatment
7	Ultrasound Therapy	Definition:	Extracorporeal treatment by ultrasound
		Example:	Therapeutic ultrasound of peripheral vessels, single treatment
8	Ultraviolet Light Therapy	Definition:	Extracorporeal treatment by ultraviolet light
		Example:	Ultraviolet light phototherapy, series treatment
9	Shock Wave Therapy	Definition:	Extracorporeal treatment by shock waves
		Example:	Shockwave therapy of plantar fascia, single treatment
B	Perfusion	Definition:	Extracorporeal treatment by diffusion of therapeutic fluid
		Example:	Perfusion of donor liver while preparing transplant patient

7   Osteopathic

ICD-10-PCS Value		Definition	
Ø	Treatment	Definition:	Manual treatment to eliminate or alleviate somatic dysfunction and related disorders
		Examples:	Fascial release of abdomen, osteopathic treatment

8   Other Procedures

ICD-10-PCS Value		Definition	
Ø	Other Procedures	Definition:	Methodologies which attempt to remediate or cure a disorder or disease
		Examples:	Acupuncture, yoga therapy

9   Chiropractic

ICD-10-PCS Value		Definition	
B	Manipulation	Definition:	Manual procedure that involves a directed thrust to move a joint past the physiological range of motion, without exceeding the anatomical limit
		Example:	Chiropractic treatment of cervical spine, short lever specific contact

Appendix C: Comparison of Medical and Surgical Root Operations

Note: The character associated with each operation appears in parentheses after its title.

Procedures That Take Out Some or All of a Body Part

Root Operation	Objective of Procedure	Site of Procedure	Example
Destruction (5)	Eradicating without taking out or replacement	Some/all of a body part	Fulguration of endometrium
Detachment (6)	Cutting out/off without replacement	Extremity only, any level	Amputation above elbow
Excision (B)	Cutting out/off without replacement	Some of a body part	Breast lumpectomy
Extraction (D)	Pulling out/off without replacement	Some/all of a body part	Suction D&C
Resection (T)	Cutting out/off without replacement	All of a body part	Total mastectomy

Procedures That Put In/Put Back or Move Some/All of a Body Part

Root Operation	Objective of Procedure	Site of Procedure	Example
Reattachment (M)	Putting back a detached body part	Some/all of a body part	Reattach finger
Reposition (S)	Moving a body part to normal or other suitable location	Some/all of a body part	Move undescended testicle
Transfer (X)	Moving a body part to function for a similar body part	Some/all of a body part	Skin pedicle transfer flap
Transplantation (Y)	Putting in a living body part from a person/animal	Some/all of a body part	Kidney transplant

Procedures That Take Out or Eliminate Solid Matter, Fluids, or Gases From a Body Part

Root Operation	Objective of Procedure	Site of Procedure	Example
Drainage (9)	Taking or letting out	Fluids and/or gases from a body part	Incision and drainage
Extirpation (C)	Taking or cutting out	Solid matter in a body part	Thrombectomy
Fragmentation (F)	Breaking into pieces	Solid matter within a body part	Lithotripsy

Procedures That Involve Only Examination of Body Parts and Regions

Root Operation	Objective of Procedure	Site of Procedure	Example
Inspection (J)	Visual/manual exploration	Some/all of a body part	Diagnostic cystoscopy Exploratory laparoscopy
Map (K)	Locating electrical impulse route/functional areas	Brain/cardiac conduction mechanism	Cardiac mapping

Procedures That Alter the Diameter/Route of a Tubular Body Part

Root Operation	Objective of Procedure	Site of Procedure	Example
Bypass (1)	Altering route of passage of contents	Tubular body part	Coronary artery bypass graft (CABG)
Dilation (7)	Expanding natural or artificially created orifice/lumen	Tubular body part	Percutaneous transluminal coronary angioplasty (PTCA)
Occlusion (L)	Completely closing natural or artificially created orifice/lumen	Tubular body part	Fallopian tube ligation
Restriction (V)	Partially closing natural or artificially created orifice/lumen	Tubular body part	Gastroesophageal fundoplication

Procedures That Always Involve Devices

Root Operation		Objective of Procedure	Site of Procedure	Example
Change (2)	DVC	Exchanging device w/out cutting/puncturing	In/on a body part	Gastrostomy tube change
Insertion (H)	DVC	Putting in nonbiological device	In/on a body part	Central line insertion
Removal (P)	DVC	Taking out device	In/on a body part	Central line removal
Replacement (R)	DVC	Putting in device that replaces a body part	Some/all of a body part	Total hip replacement
Revision (W)	DVC	Correcting a malfunctioning/displaced device	In/on a body part	Revision of pacemaker
Supplement (U)	DVC	Putting in device that reinforces or augments a body part	In/on a body part	Abdominal wall herniorrhaphy using mesh

DVC = Device involved in root operation

Procedures Involving Cutting or Separation Only

Root Operation	Objective of Procedure	Site of Procedure	Example
Division (8)	Cutting into/separating	A body part	Neurotomy
Release (N)	Freeing a body part from constraint	Around a body part	Adhesiolysis

Procedures That Define Other Repairs

Root Operation	Objective of Procedure	Site of Procedure	Example
Control (3)	Stopping/attempting to stop postprocedural or other acute bleeding	Anatomical region or nasal mucosa/soft tissue	Post-prostatectomy bleeding control, control subdural hemorrhage, bleeding ulcer, retroperitoneal hemorrhage
Repair (Q)	Restoring body part to its normal structure/function	Some/all of a body part	Suture laceration

Procedures That Define Other Objectives

Root Operation	Objective of Procedure	Site of Procedure	Example
Alteration (Ø)	Modifying body part for cosmetic purposes without affecting function	Some/all of a body part	Face lift
Creation (4)	Using biological or synthetic material to form a new body part that replicates the anatomic structure or function of a missing body part	Perineum, valve	Sex change/artificial vagina/penis, atrioventricular valve creation
Fusion (G)	Unification or immobilization	Joint or articular body part	Spinal fusion

Appendix D: Body Part Key

Term	ICD-10-PCS Value
Abdominal aortic plexus	Abdominal Sympathetic Nerve
Abdominal cavity	Peritoneal Cavity
Abdominal esophagus	Esophagus, Lower
Abductor hallucis muscle	Foot Muscle, Right
	Foot Muscle, Left
Accessory cephalic vein	Cephalic Vein, Right
	Cephalic Vein, Left
Accessory obturator nerve	Lumbar Plexus
Accessory phrenic nerve	Phrenic nerve
Accessory spleen	Spleen
Acetabulofemoral joint	Hip Joint, Right
	Hip Joint, Left
Achilles tendon	Lower Leg Tendon, Right
	Lower Leg Tendon, Left
Acromioclavicular ligament	Shoulder Bursa and Ligament, Right
	Shoulder Bursa and Ligament, Left
Acromion (process)	Scapula, Right
	Scapula, Left
Adductor brevis muscle	Upper Leg Muscle, Right
	Upper Leg Muscle, Left
Adductor hallucis muscle	Foot Muscle, Right
	Foot Muscle, Left
Adductor longus muscle	Upper Leg Muscle, Right
	Upper Leg Muscle, Left
Adductor magnus muscle	Upper Leg Muscle, Right
	Upper Leg Muscle, Left
Adenohypophysis	Pituitary Gland
Alar ligament of axis	Head and Neck Bursa and Ligament
Alveolar process of mandible	Mandible, Right
	Mandible, Left
Alveolar process of maxilla	Maxilla
Anal orifice	Anus
Anatomical snuffbox	Lower Arm and Wrist Muscle, Right
	Lower Arm and Wrist Muscle, Left
Angular artery	Face Artery
Angular vein	Face Vein, Right
	Face Vein, Left
Annular ligament	Elbow Bursa and Ligament, Right
	Elbow Bursa and Ligament, Left
Anorectal junction	Rectum
Ansa cervicalis	Cervical Plexus
Antebrachial fascia	Subcutaneous Tissue and Fascia, Right Lower Arm
	Subcutaneous Tissue and Fascia, Left Lower Arm
Anterior (pectoral) lymph node	Lymphatic, Right Axillary
	Lymphatic, Left Axillary
Anterior cerebral artery	Intracranial Artery
Anterior cerebral vein	Intracranial Vein
Anterior choroidal artery	Intracranial Artery
Anterior circumflex humeral artery	Axillary Artery, Right
	Axillary Artery, Left
Anterior communicating artery	Intracranial Artery
Anterior cruciate ligament (ACL)	Knee Bursa and Ligament, Right
	Knee Bursa and Ligament, Left
Anterior crural nerve	Femoral Nerve

Term	ICD-10-PCS Value
Anterior facial vein	Face Vein, Right
	Face Vein, Left
Anterior intercostal artery	Internal Mammary Artery, Right
	Internal Mammary Artery, Left
Anterior interosseous nerve	Median Nerve
Anterior lateral malleolar artery	Anterior Tibial Artery, Right
	Anterior Tibial Artery, Left
Anterior lingual gland	Minor Salivary Gland
Anterior medial malleolar artery	Anterior Tibial Artery, Right
	Anterior Tibial Artery, Left
Anterior spinal artery	Vertebral Artery, Right
	Vertebral Artery, Left
Anterior tibial recurrent artery	Anterior Tibial Artery, Right
	Anterior Tibial Artery, Left
Anterior ulnar recurrent artery	Ulnar Artery, Right
	Ulnar Artery, Left
Anterior vagal trunk	Vagus Nerve
Anterior vertebral muscle	Neck Muscle, Right
	Neck Muscle, Left
Antihelix	External Ear, Right
	External Ear, Left
	External Ear, Bilateral
Antitragus	External Ear, Right
	External Ear, Left
	External Ear, Bilateral
Antrum of Highmore	Maxillary Sinus, Right
	Maxillary Sinus, Left
Aortic annulus	Aortic Valve
Aortic arch	Thoracic Aorta, Ascending/Arch
Aortic intercostal artery	Upper Artery
Apical (subclavicular) lymph node	Lymphatic, Right Axillary
	Lymphatic, Left Axillary
Apneustic center	Pons
Appendiceal orifice	Appendix
Aqueduct of Sylvius	Cerebral Ventricle
Aqueous humour	Anterior Chamber, Right
	Anterior Chamber, Left
Arachnoid mater, intracranial	Cerebral Meninges
Arachnoid mater, spinal	Spinal Meninges
Arcuate artery	Foot Artery, Right
	Foot Artery, Left
Areola	Nipple, Right
	Nipple, Left
Arterial canal (duct)	Pulmonary Artery, Left
Aryepiglottic fold	Larynx
Arytenoid cartilage	Larynx
Arytenoid muscle	Neck Muscle, Right
	Neck Muscle, Left
Ascending aorta	Thoracic Aorta, Ascending/Arch
Ascending palatine artery	Face Artery
Ascending pharyngeal artery	External Carotid Artery, Right
	External Carotid Artery, Left
Atlantoaxial joint	Cervical Vertebral Joint
Atrioventricular node	Conduction Mechanism
Atrium dextrum cordis	Atrium, Right
Atrium pulmonale	Atrium, Left

Term	ICD-10-PCS Value
Auditory tube	Eustachian Tube, Right
	Eustachian Tube, Left
Auerbach's (myenteric) plexus	Abdominal Sympathetic Nerve
Auricle	External Ear, Right
	External Ear, Left
	External Ear, Bilateral
Auricularis muscle	Head Muscle
Axillary fascia	Subcutaneous Tissue and Fascia, Right Upper Arm
	Subcutaneous Tissue and Fascia, Left Upper Arm
Axillary nerve	Brachial Plexus
Bartholin's (greater vestibular) gland	Vestibular Gland
Basal (internal) cerebral vein	Intracranial Vein
Basal nuclei	Basal Ganglia
Base of tongue	Pharynx
Basilar artery	Intracranial Artery
Basis pontis	Pons
Biceps brachii muscle	Upper Arm Muscle, Right
	Upper Arm Muscle, Left
Biceps femoris muscle	Upper Leg Muscle, Right
	Upper Leg Muscle, Left
Bicipital aponeurosis	Subcutaneous Tissue and Fascia, Right Lower Arm
	Subcutaneous Tissue and Fascia, Left Lower Arm
Bicuspid valve	Mitral Valve
Body of femur	Femoral Shaft, Right
	Femoral Shaft, Left
Body of fibula	Fibula, Right
	Fibula, Left
Bony labyrinth	Inner Ear, Right
	Inner Ear, Left
Bony orbit	Orbit, Right
	Orbit, Left
Bony vestibule	Inner Ear, Right
	Inner Ear, Left
Botallo's duct	Pulmonary Artery, Left
Brachial (lateral) lymph node	Lymphatic, Right Axillary
	Lymphatic, Left Axillary
Brachialis muscle	Upper Arm Muscle, Right
	Upper Arm Muscle, Left
Brachiocephalic artery	Innominate Artery
Brachiocephalic trunk	Innominate Artery
Brachiocephalic vein	Innominate Vein, Right
	Innominate Vein, Left
Brachioradialis muscle	Lower Arm and Wrist Muscle, Right
	Lower Arm and Wrist Muscle, Left
Breast procedures, skin only	Skin, Chest
Broad ligament	Uterine Supporting Structure
Bronchial artery	Upper Artery
Bronchus intermedius	Main Bronchus, Right
Buccal gland	Buccal Mucosa
Buccinator lymph node	Lymphatic, Head
Buccinator muscle	Facial Muscle
Bulbospongiosus muscle	Perineum Muscle
Bulbourethral (Cowper's) gland	Urethra
Bundle of His	Conduction Mechanism

Term	ICD-10-PCS Value
Bundle of Kent	Conduction Mechanism
Calcaneocuboid joint	Tarsal Joint, Right
	Tarsal Joint, Left
Calcaneocuboid ligament	Foot Bursa and Ligament, Right
	Foot Bursa and Ligament, Left
Calcaneofibular ligament	Ankle Bursa and Ligament, Right
	Ankle Bursa and Ligament, Left
Calcaneus	Tarsal, Right
	Tarsal, Left
Capitate bone	Carpal, Right
	Carpal, Left
Cardia	Esophagogastric Junction
Cardiac plexus	Thoracic Sympathetic Nerve
Cardioesophageal junction	Esophagogastric Junction
Caroticotympanic artery	Internal Carotid Artery, Right
	Internal Carotid Artery, Left
Carotid glomus	Carotid Body, Right
	Carotid Body, Left
	Carotid Bodies, Bilateral
Carotid sinus	Internal Carotid Artery, Right
	Internal Carotid Artery, Left
Carotid sinus nerve	Glossopharyngeal Nerve
Carpometacarpal ligament	Hand Bursa and Ligament, Right
	Hand Bursa and Ligament, Left
Cauda equina	Lumbar Spinal Cord
Cavernous plexus	Head and Neck Sympathetic Nerve
Cavoatrial junction	Superior Vena Cava
Celiac ganglion	Abdominal Sympathetic Nerve
Celiac (solar) plexus	Abdominal Sympathetic Nerve
Celiac lymph node	Lymphatic, Aortic
Celiac trunk	Celiac Artery
Central axillary lymph node	Lymphatic, Right Axillary
	Lymphatic, Left Axillary
Cerebral aqueduct (Sylvius)	Cerebral Ventricle
Cerebrum	Brain
Cervical esophagus	Esophagus, Upper
Cervical facet joint	Cervical Vertebral Joint
	Cervical Vertebral Joints, 2 or more
Cervical ganglion	Head and Neck Sympathetic Nerve
Cervical interspinous ligament	Head and Neck Bursa and Ligament
Cervical intertransverse ligament	Head and Neck Bursa and Ligament
Cervical ligamentum flavum	Head and Neck Bursa and Ligament
Cervical lymph node	Lymphatic, Right Neck
	Lymphatic, Left Neck
Cervicothoracic facet joint	Cervicothoracic Vertebral Joint
Chin	Subcutaneous Tissue and Fascia, Face
Choana	Nasopharynx
Chondroglossus muscle	Tongue, Palate, Pharynx Muscle
Chorda tympani	Facial Nerve
Choroid plexus	Cerebral Ventricle
Ciliary body	Eye, Right
	Eye, Left
Ciliary ganglion	Head and Neck Sympathetic Nerve
Circle of Willis	Intracranial Artery
Circumflex iliac artery	Femoral Artery, Right
	Femoral Artery, Left
Claustrum	Basal Ganglia
Coccygeal body	Coccygeal Glomus

Term	ICD-10-PCS Value
Coccygeus muscle	Trunk Muscle, Right
	Trunk Muscle, Left
Cochlea	Inner Ear, Right
	Inner Ear, Left
Cochlear nerve	Acoustic Nerve
Columella	Nasal Mucosa and Soft Tissue
Common digital vein	Foot Vein, Right
	Foot Vein, Left
Common facial vein	Face Vein, Right
	Face Vein, Left
Common fibular nerve	Peroneal Nerve
Common hepatic artery	Hepatic Artery
Common iliac (subaortic) lymph node	Lymphatic, Pelvis
Common interosseous artery	Ulnar Artery, Right
	Ulnar Artery, Left
Common peroneal nerve	Peroneal Nerve
Condyloid process	Mandible, Right
	Mandible, Left
Conus arteriosus	Ventricle, Right
Conus medullaris	Lumbar Spinal Cord
Coracoacromial ligament	Shoulder Bursa and Ligament, Right
	Shoulder Bursa and Ligament, Left
Coracobrachialis muscle	Upper Arm Muscle, Right
	Upper Arm Muscle, Left
Coracoclavicular ligament	Shoulder Bursa and Ligament, Right
	Shoulder Bursa and Ligament, Left
Coracohumeral ligament	Shoulder Bursa and Ligament, Right
	Shoulder Bursa and Ligament, Left
Coracoid process	Scapula, Right
	Scapula, Left
Corniculate cartilage	Larynx
Corpus callosum	Brain
Corpus cavernosum	Penis
Corpus spongiosum	Penis
Corpus striatum	Basal Ganglia
Corrugator supercilii muscle	Facial Muscle
Costocervical trunk	Subclavian Artery, Right
	Subclavian Artery, Left
Costoclavicular ligament	Shoulder Bursa and Ligament, Right
	Shoulder Bursa and Ligament, Left
Costotransverse joint	Thoracic Vertebral Joint
Costotransverse ligament	Rib(s) Bursa and Ligament
Costovertebral joint	Thoracic Vertebral Joint
Costoxiphoid ligament	Sternum Bursa and Ligament
Cowper's (bulbourethral) gland	Urethra
Cremaster muscle	Perineum Muscle
Cribriform plate	Ethmoid Bone, Right
	Ethmoid Bone, Left
Cricoid cartilage	Trachea
Cricothyroid artery	Thyroid Artery, Right
	Thyroid Artery, Left
Cricothyroid muscle	Neck Muscle, Right
	Neck Muscle, Left
Crural fascia	Subcutaneous Tissue and Fascia, Right Upper Leg
	Subcutaneous Tissue and Fascia, Left Upper Leg
Cubital lymph node	Lymphatic, Right Upper Extremity
	Lymphatic, Left Upper Extremity

Term	ICD-10-PCS Value
Cubital nerve	Ulnar Nerve
Cuboid bone	Tarsal, Right
	Tarsal, Left
Cuboideonavicular joint	Tarsal Joint, Right
	Tarsal Joint, Left
Culmen	Cerebellum
Cuneiform cartilage	Larynx
Cuneonavicular joint	Tarsal Joint, Right
	Tarsal Joint, Left
Cuneonavicular ligament	Foot Bursa and Ligament, Right
	Foot Bursa and Ligament, Left
Cutaneous (transverse) cervical nerve	Cervical Plexus
Deep cervical fascia	Subcutaneous Tissue and Fascia, Right Neck
	Subcutaneous Tissue and Fascia, Left Neck
Deep cervical vein	Vertebral Vein, Right
	Vertebral Vein, Left
Deep circumflex iliac artery	External Iliac Artery, Right
	External Iliac Artery, Left
Deep facial vein	Face Vein, Right
	Face Vein, Left
Deep femoral artery	Femoral Artery, Right
	Femoral Artery, Left
Deep femoral (profunda femoris) vein	Femoral Vein, Right
	Femoral Vein, Left
Deep palmar arch	Hand Artery, Right
	Hand Artery, Left
Deep transverse perineal muscle	Perineum Muscle
Deferential artery	Internal Iliac Artery, Right
	Internal Iliac Artery, Left
Deltoid fascia	Subcutaneous Tissue and Fascia, Right Upper Arm
	Subcutaneous Tissue and Fascia, Left Upper Arm
Deltoid ligament	Ankle Bursa and Ligament, Right
	Ankle Bursa and Ligament, Left
Deltoid muscle	Shoulder Muscle, Right
	Shoulder Muscle, Left
Deltopectoral (infraclavicular) lymph node	Lymphatic, Right Upper Extremity
	Lymphatic, Left Upper Extremity
Dens	Cervical Vertebra
Denticulate (dentate) ligament	Spinal Meninges
Depressor anguli oris muscle	Facial Muscle
Depressor labii inferioris muscle	Facial Muscle
Depressor septi nasi muscle	Facial Muscle
Depressor supercilii muscle	Facial Muscle
Dermis	Skin
Descending genicular artery	Femoral Artery, Right
	Femoral Artery, Left
Diaphragma sellae	Dura Mater
Distal humerus	Humeral Shaft, Right
	Humeral Shaft, Left
Distal humerus, involving joint	Elbow Joint, Right
	Elbow Joint, Left
Distal radioulnar joint	Wrist Joint, Right
	Wrist Joint, Left
Dorsal digital nerve	Radial Nerve

Appendix D: Body Part Key

Term	ICD-10-PCS Value
Dorsal metacarpal vein	Hand Vein, Right
	Hand Vein, Left
Dorsal metatarsal artery	Foot Artery, Right
	Foot Artery, Left
Dorsal metatarsal vein	Foot Vein, Right
	Foot Vein, Left
Dorsal root ganglion	Cervical Spinal Cord
	Lumbar Spinal Cord
	Spinal Cord
	Thoracic Spinal Cord
Dorsal scapular artery	Subclavian Artery, Right
	Subclavian Artery, Left
Dorsal scapular nerve	Brachial Plexus
Dorsal venous arch	Foot Vein, Right
	Foot Vein, Left
Dorsalis pedis artery	Anterior Tibial Artery, Right
	Anterior Tibial Artery, Left
Duct of Santorini	Pancreatic Duct, Accessory
Duct of Wirsung	Pancreatic Duct
Ductus deferens	Vas Deferens, Right
	Vas Deferens, Left
	Vas Deferens, Bilateral
	Vas Deferens
Duodenal ampulla	Ampulla of Vater
Duodenojejunal flexure	Jejunum
Dura mater, intracranial	Dura Mater
Dura mater, spinal	Spinal Meninges
Dural venous sinus	Intracranial Vein
Earlobe	External Ear, Right
	External Ear, Left
	External Ear, Bilateral
Eighth cranial nerve	Acoustic Nerve
Ejaculatory duct	Vas Deferens, Right
	Vas Deferens, Left
	Vas Deferens, Bilateral
	Vas Deferens
Eleventh cranial nerve	Accessory Nerve
Encephalon	Brain
Ependyma	Cerebral Ventricle
Epidermis	Skin
Epidural space, spinal	Spinal Canal
Epiploic foramen	Peritoneum
Epithalamus	Thalamus
Epitrochlear lymph node	Lymphatic, Right Upper Extremity
	Lymphatic, Left Upper Extremity
Erector spinae muscle	Trunk Muscle, Right
	Trunk Muscle, Left
Esophageal artery	Upper Artery
Esophageal plexus	Thoracic Sympathetic Nerve
Ethmoidal air cell	Ethmoid Sinus, Right
	Ethmoid Sinus, Left
Extensor carpi radialis muscle	Lower Arm and Wrist Muscle, Right
	Lower Arm and Wrist Muscle, Left
Extensor carpi ulnaris muscle	Lower Arm and Wrist Muscle, Right
	Lower Arm and Wrist Muscle, Left
Extensor digitorum brevis muscle	Foot Muscle, Right
	Foot Muscle, Left
Extensor digitorum longus muscle	Lower Leg Muscle, Right
	Lower Leg Muscle, Left

Term	ICD-10-PCS Value
Extensor hallucis brevis muscle	Foot Muscle, Right
	Foot Muscle, Left
Extensor hallucis longus muscle	Lower Leg Muscle, Right
	Lower Leg Muscle, Left
External anal sphincter	Anal Sphincter
External auditory meatus	External Auditory Canal, Right
	External Auditory Canal, Left
External maxillary artery	Face Artery
External naris	Nasal Mucosa and Soft Tissue
External oblique aponeurosis	Subcutaneous Tissue and Fascia, Trunk
External oblique muscle	Abdomen Muscle, Right
	Abdomen Muscle, Left
External popliteal nerve	Peroneal Nerve
External pudendal artery	Femoral Artery, Right
	Femoral Artery, Left
External pudendal vein	Saphenous Vein, Right
	Saphenous Vein, Left
External urethral sphincter	Urethra
Extradural space, intracranial	Epidural Space, Intracranial
Extradural space, spinal	Spinal Canal
Facial artery	Face Artery
False vocal cord	Larynx
Falx cerebri	Dura Mater
Fascia lata	Subcutaneous Tissue and Fascia, Right Upper Leg
	Subcutaneous Tissue and Fascia, Left Upper Leg
Femoral head	Upper Femur, Right
	Upper Femur, Left
Femoral lymph node	Lymphatic, Right Lower Extremity
	Lymphatic, Left Lower Extremity
Femoropatellar joint	Knee Joint, Right
	Knee Joint, Left
	Knee Joint, Femoral Surface, Right
	Knee Joint, Femoral Surface, Left
Femorotibial joint	Knee Joint, Right
	Knee Joint, Left
	Knee Joint, Tibial Surface, Right
	Knee Joint, Tibial Surface, Left
Fibular artery	Peroneal Artery, Right
	Peroneal Artery, Left
Fibular sesamoid	Metatarsal, Right
	Metatarsal, Left
Fibularis brevis muscle	Lower Leg Muscle, Right
	Lower Leg Muscle, Left
Fibularis longus muscle	Lower Leg Muscle, Right
	Lower Leg Muscle, Left
Fifth cranial nerve	Trigeminal Nerve
Filum terminale	Spinal Meninges
First cranial nerve	Olfactory Nerve
First intercostal nerve	Brachial Plexus
Flexor carpi radialis muscle	Lower Arm and Wrist Muscle, Right
	Lower Arm and Wrist Muscle, Left
Flexor carpi ulnaris muscle	Lower Arm and Wrist Muscle, Right
	Lower Arm and Wrist Muscle, Left
Flexor digitorum brevis muscle	Foot Muscle, Right
	Foot Muscle, Left
Flexor digitorum longus muscle	Lower Leg Muscle, Right
	Lower Leg Muscle, Left
Flexor hallucis brevis muscle	Foot Muscle, Right
	Foot Muscle, Left

Term	ICD-10-PCS Value
Flexor hallucis longus muscle	Lower Leg Muscle, Right
	Lower Leg Muscle, Left
Flexor pollicis longus muscle	Lower Arm and Wrist Muscle, Right
	Lower Arm and Wrist Muscle, Left
Foramen magnum	Occipital Bone
Foramen of Monro (intraventricular)	Cerebral Ventricle
Foreskin	Prepuce
Fossa of Rosenmuller	Nasopharynx
Fourth cranial nerve	Trochlear Nerve
Fourth ventricle	Cerebral Ventricle
Fovea	Retina, Right
	Retina, Left
Frenulum labii inferioris	Lower Lip
Frenulum labii superioris	Upper Lip
Frenulum linguae	Tongue
Frontal lobe	Cerebral Hemisphere
Frontal vein	Face Vein, Right
	Face Vein, Left
Fundus uteri	Uterus
Galea aponeurotica	Subcutaneous Tissue and Fascia, Scalp
Ganglion impar (ganglion of Walther)	Sacral Sympathetic Nerve
Gasserian ganglion	Trigeminal Nerve
Gastric lymph node	Lymphatic, Aortic
Gastric plexus	Abdominal Sympathetic Nerve
Gastrocnemius muscle	Lower Leg Muscle, Right
	Lower Leg Muscle, Left
Gastrocolic ligament	Omentum
Gastrocolic omentum	Omentum
Gastroduodenal artery	Hepatic Artery
Gastroesophageal (GE) junction	Esophagogastric Junction
Gastrohepatic omentum	Omentum
Gastrophrenic ligament	Omentum
Gastrosplenic ligament	Omentum
Gemellus muscle	Hip Muscle, Right
	Hip Muscle, Left
Geniculate ganglion	Facial Nerve
Geniculate nucleus	Thalamus
Genioglossus muscle	Tongue, Palate, Pharynx Muscle
Genitofemoral nerve	Lumbar Plexus
Glans penis	Prepuce
Glenohumeral joint	Shoulder Joint, Right
	Shoulder Joint, Left
Glenohumeral ligament	Shoulder Bursa and Ligament, Right
	Shoulder Bursa and Ligament, Left
Glenoid fossa (of scapula)	Glenoid Cavity, Right
	Glenoid Cavity, Left
Glenoid ligament (labrum)	Shoulder Joint, Right
	Shoulder Joint, Left
Globus pallidus	Basal Ganglia
Glossoepiglottic fold	Epiglottis
Glottis	Larynx
Gluteal lymph node	Lymphatic, Pelvis
Gluteal vein	Hypogastric Vein, Right
	Hypogastric Vein, Left
Gluteus maximus muscle	Hip Muscle, Right
	Hip Muscle, Left
Gluteus medius muscle	Hip Muscle, Right
	Hip Muscle, Left

Term	ICD-10-PCS Value
Gluteus minimus muscle	Hip Muscle, Right
	Hip Muscle, Left
Gracilis muscle	Upper Leg Muscle, Right
	Upper Leg Muscle, Left
Great auricular nerve	Cervical Plexus
Great cerebral vein	Intracranial Vein
Great(er) saphenous vein	Saphenous Vein, Right
	Saphenous Vein, Left
Greater alar cartilage	Nasal Mucosa and Soft Tissue
Greater occipital nerve	Cervical Nerve
Greater omentum	Omentum
Greater splanchnic nerve	Thoracic Sympathetic Nerve
Greater superficial petrosal nerve	Facial Nerve
Greater trochanter	Upper Femur, Right
	Upper Femur, Left
Greater tuberosity	Humeral Head, Right
	Humeral Head, Left
Greater vestibular (Bartholin's) gland	Vestibular Gland
Greater wing	Sphenoid Bone
Hallux	1st Toe, Right
	1st Toe, Left
Hamate bone	Carpal, Right
	Carpal, Left
Head of fibula	Fibula, Right
	Fibula, Left
Helix	External Ear, Right
	External Ear, Left
	External Ear, Bilateral
Hepatic artery proper	Hepatic Artery
Hepatic flexure	Transverse Colon
Hepatic lymph node	Lymphatic, Aortic
Hepatic plexus	Abdominal Sympathetic Nerve
Hepatic portal vein	Portal Vein
Hepatogastric ligament	Omentum
Hepatopancreatic ampulla	Ampulla of Vater
Humeroradial joint	Elbow Joint, Right
	Elbow Joint, Left
Humeroulnar joint	Elbow Joint, Right
	Elbow Joint, Left
Humerus, distal	Humeral Shaft, Right
	Humeral Shaft, Left
Hyoglossus muscle	Tongue, Palate, Pharynx Muscle
Hyoid artery	Thyroid Artery, Right
	Thyroid Artery, Left
Hypogastric artery	Internal Iliac Artery, Right
	Internal Iliac Artery, Left
Hypopharynx	Pharynx
Hypophysis	Pituitary Gland
Hypothenar muscle	Hand Muscle, Right
	Hand Muscle, Left
Ileal artery	Superior Mesenteric Artery
Ileocolic artery	Superior Mesenteric Artery
Ileocolic vein	Colic Vein
Iliac crest	Pelvic Bone, Right
	Pelvic Bone, Left
Iliac fascia	Subcutaneous Tissue and Fascia, Right Upper Leg
	Subcutaneous Tissue and Fascia, Left Upper Leg

Term	ICD-10-PCS Value
Iliac lymph node	Lymphatic, Pelvis
Iliacus muscle	Hip Muscle, Right
	Hip Muscle, Left
Iliofemoral ligament	Hip Bursa and Ligament, Right
	Hip Bursa and Ligament, Left
Iliohypogastric nerve	Lumbar Plexus
Ilioinguinal nerve	Lumbar Plexus
Iliolumbar artery	Internal Iliac Artery, Right
	Internal Iliac Artery, Left
Iliolumbar ligament	Lower Spine Bursa and Ligament
Iliotibial tract (band)	Subcutaneous Tissue and Fascia, Right Upper Leg
	Subcutaneous Tissue and Fascia, Left Upper Leg
Ilium	Pelvic Bone, Right
	Pelvic Bone, Left
Incus	Auditory Ossicle, Right
	Auditory Ossicle, Left
Inferior cardiac nerve	Thoracic Sympathetic Nerve
Inferior cerebellar vein	Intracranial Vein
Inferior cerebral vein	Intracranial Vein
Inferior epigastric artery	External Iliac Artery, Right
	External Iliac Artery, Left
Inferior epigastric lymph node	Lymphatic, Pelvis
Inferior genicular artery	Popliteal Artery, Right
	Popliteal Artery, Left
Inferior gluteal artery	Internal Iliac Artery, Right
	Internal Iliac Artery, Left
Inferior gluteal nerve	Sacral Plexus
Inferior hypogastric plexus	Abdominal Sympathetic Nerve
Inferior labial artery	Face Artery
Inferior longitudinal muscle	Tongue, Palate, Pharynx Muscle
Inferior mesenteric ganglion	Abdominal Sympathetic Nerve
Inferior mesenteric lymph node	Lymphatic, Mesenteric
Inferior mesenteric plexus	Abdominal Sympathetic Nerve
Inferior oblique muscle	Extraocular Muscle, Right
	Extraocular Muscle, Left
Inferior pancreaticoduodenal artery	Superior Mesenteric Artery
Inferior phrenic artery	Abdominal Aorta
Inferior rectus muscle	Extraocular Muscle, Right
	Extraocular Muscle, Left
Inferior suprarenal artery	Renal Artery, Right
	Renal Artery, Left
Inferior tarsal plate	Lower Eyelid, Right
	Lower Eyelid, Left
Inferior thyroid vein	Innominate Vein, Right
	Innominate Vein, Left
Inferior tibiofibular joint	Ankle Joint, Right
	Ankle Joint, Left
Inferior turbinate	Nasal Turbinate
Inferior ulnar collateral artery	Brachial Artery, Right
	Brachial Artery, Left
Inferior vesical artery	Internal Iliac Artery, Right
	Internal Iliac Artery, Left
Infraauricular lymph node	Lymphatic, Head
Infraclavicular (deltopectoral) lymph node	Lymphatic, Right Upper Extremity
	Lymphatic, Left Upper Extremity

Term	ICD-10-PCS Value
Infrahyoid muscle	Neck Muscle, Right
	Neck Muscle, Left
Infraparotid lymph node	Lymphatic, Head
Infraspinatus fascia	Subcutaneous Tissue and Fascia, Right Upper Arm
	Subcutaneous Tissue and Fascia, Left Upper Arm
Infraspinatus muscle	Shoulder Muscle, Right
	Shoulder Muscle, Left
Infundibulopelvic ligament	Uterine Supporting Structure
Inguinal canal	Inguinal Region, Right
	Inguinal Region, Left
	Inguinal Region, Bilateral
Inguinal triangle	Inguinal Region, Right
	Inguinal Region, Left
	Inguinal Region, Bilateral
Interatrial septum	Atrial Septum
Intercarpal joint	Carpal Joint, Right
	Carpal Joint, Left
Intercarpal ligament	Hand Bursa and Ligament, Right
	Hand Bursa and Ligament, Left
Interclavicular ligament	Shoulder Bursa and Ligament, Right
	Shoulder Bursa and Ligament, Left
Intercostal lymph node	Lymphatic, Thorax
Intercostal muscle	Thorax Muscle, Right
	Thorax Muscle, Left
Intercostal nerve	Thoracic Nerve
Intercostobrachial nerve	Thoracic Nerve
Intercuneiform joint	Tarsal Joint, Right
	Tarsal Joint, Left
Intercuneiform ligament	Foot Bursa and Ligament, Right
	Foot Bursa and Ligament, Left
Intermediate bronchus	Main Bronchus, Right
Intermediate cuneiform bone	Tarsal, Right
	Tarsal, Left
Internal anal sphincter	Anal Sphincter
Internal (basal) cerebral vein	Intracranial Vein
Internal carotid artery, intracranial portion	Intracranial Artery
Internal carotid plexus	Head and Neck Sympathetic Nerve
Internal iliac vein	Hypogastric Vein, Right
	Hypogastric Vein, Left
Internal maxillary artery	External Carotid Artery, Right
	External Carotid Artery, Left
Internal naris	Nasal Mucosa and Soft Tissue
Internal oblique muscle	Abdomen Muscle, Right
	Abdomen Muscle, Left
Internal pudendal artery	Internal Iliac Artery, Right
	Internal Iliac Artery, Left
Internal pudendal vein	Hypogastric Vein, Right
	Hypogastric Vein, Left
Internal thoracic artery	Internal Mammary Artery, Right
	Internal Mammary Artery, Left
	Subclavian Artery, Right
	Subclavian Artery, Left
Internal urethral sphincter	Urethra
Interphalangeal (IP) joint	Finger Phalangeal Joint, Right
	Finger Phalangeal Joint, Left
	Toe Phalangeal Joint, Right
	Toe Phalangeal Joint, Left

Term	ICD-10-PCS Value	Term	ICD-10-PCS Value
Interphalangeal ligament	Foot Bursa and Ligament, Right	Lateral femoral cutaneous nerve	Lumbar Plexus
	Foot Bursa and Ligament, Left	Lateral malleolus	Fibula, Right
	Hand Bursa and Ligament, Right		Fibula, Left
	Hand Bursa and Ligament, Left	Lateral meniscus	Knee Joint, Right
Interspinalis muscle	Trunk Muscle, Right		Knee Joint, Left
	Trunk Muscle, Left	Lateral nasal cartilage	Nasal Mucosa and Soft Tissue
Interspinous ligament, cervical	Head and Neck Bursa and Ligament	Lateral plantar artery	Foot Artery, Right
			Foot Artery, Left
Interspinous ligament, lumbar	Lower Spine Bursa and Ligament	Lateral plantar nerve	Tibial Nerve
		Lateral rectus muscle	Extraocular Muscle, Right
Interspinous ligament, thoracic	Upper Spine Bursa and Ligament		Extraocular Muscle, Left
Intertransversarius muscle	Trunk Muscle, Right	Lateral sacral artery	Internal Iliac Artery, Right
	Trunk Muscle, Left		Internal Iliac Artery, Left
Intertransverse ligament, cervical	Head and Neck Bursa and Ligament	Lateral sacral vein	Hypogastric Vein, Right
			Hypogastric Vein, Left
Intertransverse ligament, lumbar	Lower Spine Bursa and Ligament	Lateral sural cutaneous nerve	Peroneal Nerve
Intertransverse ligament, thoracic	Upper Spine Bursa and Ligament	Lateral tarsal artery	Foot Artery, Right
			Foot Artery, Left
Interventricular foramen (Monro)	Cerebral Ventricle	Lateral temporo- mandibular ligament	Head and Neck Bursa and Ligament
Interventricular septum	Ventricular Septum		
Intestinal lymphatic trunk	Cisterna Chyli	Lateral thoracic artery	Axillary Artery, Right
Ischiatic nerve	Sciatic Nerve		Axillary Artery, Left
Ischiocavernosus muscle	Perineum Muscle	Latissimus dorsi muscle	Trunk Muscle, Right
Ischiofemoral ligament	Hip Bursa and Ligament, Right		Trunk Muscle, Left
	Hip Bursa and Ligament, Left	Least splanchnic nerve	Thoracic Sympathetic Nerve
Ischium	Pelvic Bone, Right	Left ascending lumbar vein	Hemiazygos Vein
	Pelvic Bone, Left	Left atrioventricular valve	Mitral Valve
Jejunal artery	Superior Mesenteric Artery	Left auricular appendix	Atrium, Left
Jugular body	Glomus Jugulare	Left colic vein	Colic Vein
Jugular lymph node	Lymphatic, Right Neck	Left coronary sulcus	Heart, Left
	Lymphatic, Left Neck	Left gastric artery	Gastric Artery
Labia majora	Vulva	Left gastroepiploic artery	Splenic Artery
Labia minora	Vulva	Left gastroepiploic vein	Splenic Vein
Labial gland	Upper Lip	Left inferior phrenic vein	Renal Vein, Left
	Lower Lip	Left inferior pulmonary vein	Pulmonary Vein, Left
Lacrimal canaliculus	Lacrimal Duct, Right	Left jugular trunk	Thoracic Duct
	Lacrimal Duct, Left	Left lateral ventricle	Cerebral Ventricle
Lacrimal punctum	Lacrimal Duct, Right	Left ovarian vein	Renal Vein, Left
	Lacrimal Duct, Left	Left second lumbar vein	Renal Vein, Left
Lacrimal sac	Lacrimal Duct, Right	Left subclavian trunk	Thoracic Duct
	Lacrimal Duct, Left	Left subcostal vein	Hemiazygos Vein
Laryngopharynx	Pharynx	Left superior pulmonary vein	Pulmonary Vein, Left
Lateral (brachial) lymph node	Lymphatic, Right Axillary	Left suprarenal vein	Renal Vein, Left
	Lymphatic, Left Axillary	Left testicular vein	Renal Vein, Left
Lateral canthus	Upper Eyelid, Right	Leptomeninges, intracranial	Cerebral Meninges
	Upper Eyelid, Left	Leptomeninges, spinal	Spinal Meninges
Lateral collateral ligament (LCL)	Knee Bursa and Ligament, Right	Lesser alar cartilage	Nasal Mucosa and Soft Tissue
	Knee Bursa and Ligament, Left	Lesser occipital nerve	Cervical Plexus
Lateral condyle of femur	Lower Femur, Right	Lesser omentum	Omentum
	Lower Femur, Left	Lesser saphenous vein	Saphenous Vein, Right
Lateral condyle of tibia	Tibia, Right		Saphenous Vein, Left
	Tibia, Left	Lesser splanchnic nerve	Thoracic Sympathetic Nerve
Lateral cuneiform bone	Tarsal, Right	Lesser trochanter	Upper Femur, Right
	Tarsal, Left		Upper Femur, Left
Lateral epicondyle of femur	Lower Femur, Right	Lesser tuberosity	Humeral Head, Right
	Lower Femur, Left		Humeral Head, Left
Lateral epicondyle of humerus	Humeral Shaft, Right	Lesser wing	Sphenoid Bone
	Humeral Shaft, Left	Levator anguli oris muscle	Facial Muscle
		Levator ani muscle	Perineum Muscle

Term	ICD-10-PCS Value	Term	ICD-10-PCS Value
Levator labii superioris alaeque nasi muscle	Facial Muscle	Medial canthus	Lower Eyelid, Right
			Lower Eyelid, Left
Levator labii superioris muscle	Facial Muscle	Medial collateral ligament (MCL)	Knee Bursa and Ligament, Right
			Knee Bursa and Ligament, Left
Levator palpebrae superioris muscle	Upper Eyelid, Right	Medial condyle of femur	Lower Femur, Right
	Upper Eyelid, Left		Lower Femur, Left
Levator scapulae muscle	Neck Muscle, Right	Medial condyle of tibia	Tibia, Right
	Neck Muscle, Left		Tibia, Left
Levator veli palatini muscle	Tongue, Palate, Pharynx Muscle	Medial cuneiform bone	Tarsal, Right
Levatores costarum muscle	Thorax Muscle, Right		Tarsal, Left
	Thorax Muscle, Left	Medial epicondyle of femur	Lower Femur, Right
Ligament of head of fibula	Knee Bursa and Ligament, Right		Lower Femur, Left
	Knee Bursa and Ligament, Left	Medial epicondyle of humerus	Humeral Shaft, Right
Ligament of the lateral malleolus	Ankle Bursa and Ligament, Right		Humeral Shaft, Left
	Ankle Bursa and Ligament, Left	Medial malleolus	Tibia, Right
Ligamentum flavum, cervical	Head and Neck Bursa and Ligament		Tibia, Left
Ligamentum flavum, lumbar	Lower Spine Bursa and Ligament	Medial meniscus	Knee Joint, Right
Ligamentum flavum, thoracic	Upper Spine Bursa and Ligament		Knee Joint, Left
Lingual artery	External Carotid Artery, Right	Medial plantar artery	Foot Artery, Right
	External Carotid Artery, Left		Foot Artery, Left
Lingual tonsil	Pharynx	Medial plantar nerve	Tibial Nerve
Locus ceruleus	Pons	Medial popliteal nerve	Tibial Nerve
Long thoracic nerve	Brachial Plexus	Medial rectus muscle	Extraocular Muscle, Right
Lumbar artery	Abdominal Aorta		Extraocular Muscle, Left
Lumbar facet joint	Lumbar Vertebral Joint	Medial sural cutaneous nerve	Tibial Nerve
Lumbar ganglion	Lumbar Sympathetic Nerve	Median antebrachial vein	Basilic Vein, Right
Lumbar lymph node	Lymphatic, Aortic		Basilic Vein, Left
Lumbar lymphatic trunk	Cisterna Chyli	Median cubital vein	Basilic Vein, Right
Lumbar splanchnic nerve	Lumbar Sympathetic Nerve		Basilic Vein, Left
Lumbosacral facet joint	Lumbosacral Joint	Median sacral artery	Abdominal Aorta
Lumbosacral trunk	Lumbar Nerve	Mediastinal cavity	Mediastinum
Lunate bone	Carpal, Right	Mediastinal lymph node	Lymphatic, Thorax
	Carpal, Left	Mediastinal space	Mediastinum
Lunotriquetral ligament	Hand Bursa and Ligament, Right	Meissner's (submucous) plexus	Abdominal Sympathetic Nerve
	Hand Bursa and Ligament, Left	Membranous urethra	Urethra
Macula	Retina, Right	Mental foramen	Mandible, Right
	Retina, Left		Mandible, Left
Malleus	Auditory Ossicle, Right	Mentalis muscle	Facial Muscle
	Auditory Ossicle, Left	Mesoappendix	Mesentery
Mammary duct	Breast, Right	Mesocolon	Mesentery
	Breast, Left	Metacarpal ligament	Hand Bursa and Ligament, Right
	Breast, Bilateral		Hand Bursa and Ligament, Left
Mammary gland	Breast, Right	Metacarpophalangeal ligament	Hand Bursa and Ligament, Right
	Breast, Left		Hand Bursa and Ligament, Left
	Breast, Bilateral	Metatarsal ligament	Foot Bursa and Ligament, Right
Mammillary body	Hypothalamus		Foot Bursa and Ligament, Left
Mandibular nerve	Trigeminal Nerve	Metatarsophalangeal ligament	Foot Bursa and Ligament, Right
Mandibular notch	Mandible, Right		Foot Bursa and Ligament, Left
	Mandible, Left	Metatarsophalangeal (MTP) joint	Metatarsal-Phalangeal Joint, Right
Manubrium	Sternum		Metatarsal-Phalangeal Joint, Left
Masseter muscle	Head Muscle	Metathalamus	Thalamus
Masseteric fascia	Subcutaneous Tissue and Fascia, Face	Midcarpal joint	Carpal Joint, Right
Mastoid (postauricular) lymph node	Lymphatic, Right Neck		Carpal Joint, Left
	Lymphatic, Left Neck	Middle cardiac nerve	Thoracic Sympathetic Nerve
Mastoid air cells	Mastoid Sinus, Right	Middle cerebral artery	Intracranial Artery
	Mastoid Sinus, Left	Middle cerebral vein	Intracranial Vein
Mastoid process	Temporal Bone, Right	Middle colic vein	Colic Vein
	Temporal Bone, Left	Middle genicular artery	Popliteal Artery, Right
Maxillary artery	External Carotid Artery, Right		Popliteal Artery, Left
	External Carotid Artery, Left		
Maxillary nerve	Trigeminal Nerve		

Term	ICD-10-PCS Value
Middle hemorrhoidal vein	Hypogastric Vein, Right
	Hypogastric Vein, Left
Middle meningeal artery, intracranial portion	Intracranial Artery
Middle rectal artery	Internal Iliac Artery, Right
	Internal Iliac Artery, Left
Middle suprarenal artery	Abdominal Aorta
Middle temporal artery	Temporal Artery, Right
	Temporal Artery, Left
Middle turbinate	Nasal Turbinate
Mitral annulus	Mitral Valve
Molar gland	Buccal Mucosa
Musculocutaneous nerve	Brachial Plexus
Musculophrenic artery	Internal Mammary Artery, Right
	Internal Mammary Artery, Left
Musculospiral nerve	Radial Nerve
Myelencephalon	Medulla Oblongata
Myenteric (Auerbach's) plexus	Abdominal Sympathetic Nerve
Myometrium	Uterus
Nail bed	Finger Nail
	Toe Nail
Nail plate	Finger Nail
	Toe Nail
Nasal cavity	Nasal Mucosa and Soft Tissue
Nasal concha	Nasal Turbinate
Nasalis muscle	Facial Muscle
Nasolacrimal duct	Lacrimal Duct, Right
	Lacrimal Duct, Left
Navicular bone	Tarsal, Right
	Tarsal, Left
Neck of femur	Upper Femur, Right
	Upper Femur, Left
Neck of humerus (anatomical) (surgical)	Humeral Head, Right
	Humeral Head, Left
Nerve to the stapedius	Facial Nerve
Neurohypophysis	Pituitary Gland
Ninth cranial nerve	Glossopharyngeal Nerve
Nostril	Nasal Mucosa and Soft Tissue
Obturator artery	Internal Iliac Artery, Right
	Internal Iliac Artery, Left
Obturator lymph node	Lymphatic, Pelvis
Obturator muscle	Hip Muscle, Right
	Hip Muscle, Left
Obturator nerve	Lumbar Plexus
Obturator vein	Hypogastric Vein, Right
	Hypogastric Vein, Left
Obtuse margin	Heart, Left
Occipital artery	External Carotid Artery, Right
	External Carotid Artery, Left
Occipital lobe	Cerebral Hemisphere
Occipital lymph node	Lymphatic, Right Neck
	Lymphatic, Left Neck
Occipitofrontalis muscle	Facial Muscle
Odontoid process	Cervical Vertebra
Olecranon bursa	Elbow Bursa and Ligament, Right
	Elbow Bursa and Ligament, Left
Olecranon process	Ulna, Right
	Ulna, Left
Olfactory bulb	Olfactory Nerve

Term	ICD-10-PCS Value
Ophthalmic artery	Intracranial Artery
Ophthalmic nerve	Trigeminal Nerve
Ophthalmic vein	Intracranial Vein
Optic chiasma	Optic Nerve
Optic disc	Retina, Right
	Retina, Left
Optic foramen	Sphenoid Bone
Orbicularis oculi muscle	Upper Eyelid, Right
	Upper Eyelid, Left
Orbicularis oris muscle	Facial Muscle
Orbital fascia	Subcutaneous Tissue and Fascia, Face
Orbital portion of ethmoid bone	Orbit, Right
	Orbit, Left
Orbital portion of frontal bone	Orbit, Right
	Orbit, Left
Orbital portion of lacrimal bone	Orbit, Right
	Orbit, Left
Orbital portion of maxilla	Orbit, Right
	Orbit, Left
Orbital portion of palatine bone	Orbit, Right
	Orbit, Left
Orbital portion of sphenoid bone	Orbit, Right
	Orbit, Left
Orbital portion of zygomatic bone	Orbit, Right
	Orbit, Left
Oropharynx	Pharynx
Otic ganglion	Head and Neck Sympathetic Nerve
Oval window	Middle Ear, Right
	Middle Ear, Left
Ovarian artery	Abdominal Aorta
Ovarian ligament	Uterine Supporting Structure
Oviduct	Fallopian Tube, Right
	Fallopian Tube, Left
Palatine gland	Buccal Mucosa
Palatine tonsil	Tonsils
Palatine uvula	Uvula
Palatoglossal muscle	Tongue, Palate, Pharynx Muscle
Palatopharyngeal muscle	Tongue, Palate, Pharynx Muscle
Palmar (volar) digital vein	Hand Vein, Right
	Hand Vein, Left
Palmar (volar) metacarpal vein	Hand Vein, Right
	Hand Vein, Left
Palmar cutaneous nerve	Median Nerve
	Radial Nerve
Palmar fascia (aponeurosis)	Subcutaneous Tissue and Fascia, Right Hand
	Subcutaneous Tissue and Fascia, Left Hand
Palmar interosseous muscle	Hand Muscle, Right
	Hand Muscle, Left
Palmar ulnocarpal ligament	Wrist Bursa and Ligament, Right
	Wrist Bursa and Ligament, Left
Palmaris longus muscle	Lower Arm and Wrist Muscle, Right
	Lower Arm and Wrist Muscle, Left
Pancreatic artery	Splenic Artery
Pancreatic plexus	Abdominal Sympathetic Nerve
Pancreatic vein	Splenic Vein
Pancreaticosplenic lymph node	Lymphatic, Aortic
Paraaortic lymph node	Lymphatic, Aortic
Parapharyngeal space	Neck
Pararectal lymph node	Lymphatic, Mesenteric

Term	ICD-10-PCS Value
Parasternal lymph node	Lymphatic, Thorax
Paratracheal lymph node	Lymphatic, Thorax
Paraurethral (Skene's) gland	Vestibular Gland
Parietal lobe	Cerebral Hemisphere
Parotid lymph node	Lymphatic, Head
Parotid plexus	Facial Nerve
Pars flaccida	Tympanic Membrane, Right
	Tympanic Membrane, Left
Patellar ligament	Knee Bursa and Ligament, Right
	Knee Bursa and Ligament, Left
Patellar tendon	Knee Tendon, Right
	Knee Tendon, Left
Patellofemoral joint	Knee Joint, Right
	Knee Joint, Left
	Knee Joint, Femoral Surface, Right
	Knee Joint, Femoral Surface, Left
Pectineus muscle	Upper Leg Muscle, Right
	Upper Leg Muscle, Left
Pectoral (anterior) lymph node	Lymphatic, Right Axillary
	Lymphatic, Left Axillary
Pectoral fascia	Subcutaneous Tissue and Fascia, Chest
Pectoralis major muscle	Thorax Muscle, Right
	Thorax Muscle, Left
Pectoralis minor muscle	Thorax Muscle, Right
	Thorax Muscle, Left
Pelvic splanchnic nerve	Abdominal Sympathetic Nerve
	Sacral Sympathetic Nerve
Penile urethra	Urethra
Perianal skin	Skin, Perineum
Pericardiophrenic artery	Internal Mammary Artery, Right
	Internal Mammary Artery, Left
Perimetrium	Uterus
Peroneus brevis muscle	Lower Leg Muscle, Right
	Lower Leg Muscle, Left
Peroneus longus muscle	Lower Leg Muscle, Right
	Lower Leg Muscle, Left
Petrous part of temporal bone	Temporal Bone, Right
	Temporal Bone, Left
Pharyngeal constrictor muscle	Tongue, Palate, Pharynx Muscle
Pharyngeal plexus	Vagus Nerve
Pharyngeal recess	Nasopharynx
Pharyngeal tonsil	Adenoids
Pharyngotympanic tube	Eustachian Tube, Right
	Eustachian Tube, Left
Pia mater, intracranial	Cerebral Meninges
Pia mater, spinal	Spinal Meninges
Pinna	External Ear, Right
	External Ear, Left
	External Ear, Bilateral
Piriform recess (sinus)	Pharynx
Piriformis muscle	Hip Muscle, Right
	Hip Muscle, Left
Pisiform bone	Carpal, Right
	Carpal, Left
Pisohamate ligament	Hand Bursa and Ligament, Right
	Hand Bursa and Ligament, Left
Pisometacarpal ligament	Hand Bursa and Ligament, Right
	Hand Bursa and Ligament, Left

Term	ICD-10-PCS Value
Plantar digital vein	Foot Vein, Right
	Foot Vein, Left
Plantar fascia (aponeurosis)	Subcutaneous Tissue and Fascia, Right Foot
	Subcutaneous Tissue and Fascia, Left Foot
Plantar metatarsal vein	Foot Vein, Right
	Foot Vein, Left
Plantar venous arch	Foot Vein, Right
	Foot Vein, Left
Platysma muscle	Neck Muscle, Right
	Neck Muscle, Left
Plica semilunaris	Conjunctiva, Right
	Conjunctiva, Left
Pneumogastric nerve	Vagus Nerve
Pneumotaxic center	Pons
Pontine tegmentum	Pons
Popliteal ligament	Knee Bursa and Ligament, Right
	Knee Bursa and Ligament, Left
Popliteal lymph node	Lymphatic, Left Lower Extremity
	Lymphatic, Right Lower Extremity
Popliteal vein	Femoral Vein, Right
	Femoral Vein, Left
Popliteus muscle	Lower Leg Muscle, Right
	Lower Leg Muscle, Left
Postauricular (mastoid) lymph node	Lymphatic, Right Neck
	Lymphatic, Left Neck
Postcava	Inferior Vena Cava
Posterior (subscapular) lymph node	Lymphatic, Right Axillary
	Lymphatic, Left Axillary
Posterior auricular artery	External Carotid Artery, Right
	External Carotid Artery, Left
Posterior auricular nerve	Facial Nerve
Posterior auricular vein	External Jugular Vein, Right
	External Jugular Vein, Left
Posterior cerebral artery	Intracranial Artery
Posterior chamber	Eye, Right
	Eye, Left
Posterior circumflex humeral artery	Axillary Artery, Right
	Axillary Artery, Left
Posterior communicating artery	Intracranial Artery
Posterior cruciate ligament (PCL)	Knee Bursa and Ligament, Right
	Knee Bursa and Ligament, Left
Posterior facial (retromandibular) vein	Face Vein, Right
	Face Vein, Left
Posterior femoral cutaneous nerve	Sacral Plexus
Posterior inferior cerebellar artery (PICA)	Intracranial Artery
Posterior interosseous nerve	Radial Nerve
Posterior labial nerve	Pudendal Nerve
Posterior scrotal nerve	Pudendal Nerve
Posterior spinal artery	Vertebral Artery, Right
	Vertebral Artery, Left
Posterior tibial recurrent artery	Anterior Tibial Artery, Right
	Anterior Tibial Artery, Left
Posterior ulnar recurrent artery	Ulnar Artery, Right
	Ulnar Artery, Left
Posterior vagal trunk	Vagus Nerve
Preauricular lymph node	Lymphatic, Head
Precava	Superior Vena Cava

Appendix D: Body Part Key

Term	ICD-10-PCS Value
Prepatellar bursa	Knee Bursa and Ligament, Right
	Knee Bursa and Ligament, Left
Pretracheal fascia	Subcutaneous Tissue and Fascia, Right Neck
	Subcutaneous Tissue and Fascia, Left Neck
Prevertebral fascia	Subcutaneous Tissue and Fascia, Right Neck
	Subcutaneous Tissue and Fascia, Left Neck
Princeps pollicis artery	Hand Artery, Right
	Hand Artery, Left
Procerus muscle	Facial Muscle
Profunda brachii	Brachial Artery, Right
	Brachial Artery, Left
Profunda femoris (deep femoral) vein	Femoral Vein, Right
	Femoral Vein, Left
Pronator quadratus muscle	Lower Arm and Wrist Muscle, Right
	Lower Arm and Wrist Muscle, Left
Pronator teres muscle	Lower Arm and Wrist Muscle, Right
	Lower Arm and Wrist Muscle, Left
Prostatic artery	Internal Iliac Artery, Right
	Internal Iliac Artery, Left
Prostatic urethra	Urethra
Proximal radioulnar joint	Elbow Joint, Right
	Elbow Joint, Left
Psoas muscle	Hip Muscle, Right
	Hip Muscle, Left
Pterygoid muscle	Head Muscle
Pterygoid process	Sphenoid Bone
Pterygopalatine (sphenopalatine) ganglion	Head and Neck Sympathetic Nerve
Pubis	Pelvic Bone, Right
	Pelvic Bone, Left
Pubofemoral ligament	Hip Bursa and Ligament, Right
	Hip Bursa and Ligament, Left
Pudendal nerve	Sacral Plexus
Pulmoaortic canal	Pulmonary Artery, Left
Pulmonary annulus	Pulmonary Valve
Pulmonary plexus	Thoracic Sympathetic Nerve
	Vagus Nerve
Pulmonic valve	Pulmonary Valve
Pulvinar	Thalamus
Pyloric antrum	Stomach, Pylorus
Pyloric canal	Stomach, Pylorus
Pyloric sphincter	Stomach, Pylorus
Pyramidalis muscle	Abdomen Muscle, Right
	Abdomen Muscle, Left
Quadrangular cartilage	Nasal Septum
Quadrate lobe	Liver
Quadratus femoris muscle	Hip Muscle, Right
	Hip Muscle, Left
Quadratus lumborum muscle	Trunk Muscle, Right
	Trunk Muscle, Left
Quadratus plantae muscle	Foot Muscle, Right
	Foot Muscle, Left
Quadriceps (femoris)	Upper Leg Muscle, Right
	Upper Leg Muscle, Left
Radial collateral carpal ligament	Wrist Bursa and Ligament, Right
	Wrist Bursa and Ligament, Left
Radial collateral ligament	Elbow Bursa and Ligament, Right
	Elbow Bursa and Ligament, Left
Radial notch	Ulna, Right
	Ulna, Left

Term	ICD-10-PCS Value
Radial recurrent artery	Radial Artery, Right
	Radial Artery, Left
Radial vein	Brachial Vein, Right
	Brachial Vein, Left
Radialis indicis	Hand Artery, Right
	Hand Artery, Left
Radiocarpal joint	Wrist Joint, Right
	Wrist Joint, Left
Radiocarpal ligament	Wrist Bursa and Ligament, Right
	Wrist Bursa and Ligament, Left
Radioulnar ligament	Wrist Bursa and Ligament, Right
	Wrist Bursa and Ligament, Left
Rectosigmoid junction	Sigmoid Colon
Rectus abdominis muscle	Abdomen Muscle, Right
	Abdomen Muscle, Left
Rectus femoris muscle	Upper Leg Muscle, Right
	Upper Leg Muscle, Left
Recurrent laryngeal nerve	Vagus Nerve
Renal calyx	Kidney, Right
	Kidney, Left
	Kidneys, Bilateral
	Kidney
Renal capsule	Kidney, Right
	Kidney, Left
	Kidneys, Bilateral
	Kidney
Renal cortex	Kidney, Right
	Kidney, Left
	Kidneys, Bilateral
	Kidney
Renal nerve	Abdominal sympathetic Nerve
Renal plexus	Abdominal Sympathetic Nerve
Renal segment	Kidney, Right
	Kidney, Left
	Kidneys, Bilateral
	Kidney
Renal segmental artery	Renal Artery, Right
	Renal Artery, Left
Retroperitoneal cavity	Retroperitoneum
Retroperitoneal lymph node	Lymphatic, Aortic
Retroperitoneal space	Retroperitoneum
Retropharyngeal lymph node	Lymphatic, Right Neck
	Lymphatic, Left Neck
Retropharyngeal space	Neck
Retropubic space	Pelvic Cavity
Rhinopharynx	Nasopharynx
Rhomboid major muscle	Trunk Muscle, Right
	Trunk Muscle, Left
Rhomboid minor muscle	Trunk Muscle, Right
	Trunk Muscle, Left
Right ascending lumbar vein	Azygos Vein
Right atrioventricular valve	Tricuspid Valve
Right auricular appendix	Atrium, Right
Right colic vein	Colic Vein
Right coronary sulcus	Heart, Right
Right gastric artery	Gastric Artery
Right gastroepiploic vein	Superior Mesenteric Vein
Right inferior phrenic vein	Inferior Vena Cava
Right inferior pulmonary vein	Pulmonary Vein, Right
Right jugular trunk	Lymphatic, Right Neck

Appendix D: Body Part Key

Term	ICD-10-PCS Value
Right lateral ventricle	Cerebral Ventricle
Right lymphatic duct	Lymphatic, Right Neck
Right ovarian vein	Inferior Vena Cava
Right second lumbar vein	Inferior Vena Cava
Right subclavian trunk	Lymphatic, Right Neck
Right subcostal vein	Azygos Vein
Right superior pulmonary vein	Pulmonary Vein, Right
Right suprarenal vein	Inferior Vena Cava
Right testicular vein	Inferior Vena Cava
Rima glottidis	Larynx
Risorius muscle	Facial Muscle
Round ligament of uterus	Uterine Supporting Structure
Round window	Inner Ear, Right
	Inner Ear, Left
Sacral ganglion	Sacral Sympathetic Nerve
Sacral lymph node	Lymphatic, Pelvis
Sacral splanchnic nerve	Sacral Sympathetic Nerve
Sacrococcygeal ligament	Lower Spine Bursa and Ligament
Sacrococcygeal symphysis	Sacrococcygeal Joint
Sacroiliac ligament	Lower Spine Bursa and Ligament
Sacrospinous ligament	Lower Spine Bursa and Ligament
Sacrotuberous ligament	Lower Spine Bursa and Ligament
Salpingopharyngeus muscle	Tongue, Palate, Pharynx Muscle
Salpinx	Fallopian Tube, Right
	Fallopian Tube, Left
Saphenous nerve	Femoral Nerve
Sartorius muscle	Upper Leg Muscle, Right
	Upper Leg Muscle, Left
Scalene muscle	Neck Muscle, Right
	Neck Muscle, Left
Scaphoid bone	Carpal, Right
	Carpal, Left
Scapholunate ligament	Wrist Bursa and Ligament, Right
	Wrist Bursa and Ligament, Left
Scaphotrapezium ligament	Hand Bursa and Ligament, Right
	Hand Bursa and Ligament, Left
Scarpa's (vestibular) ganglion	Acoustic Nerve
Sebaceous gland	Skin
Second cranial nerve	Optic Nerve
Sella turcica	Sphenoid Bone
Semicircular canal	Inner Ear, Right
	Inner Ear, Left
Semimembranosus muscle	Upper Leg Muscle, Right
	Upper Leg Muscle, Left
Semitendinosus muscle	Upper Leg Muscle, Right
	Upper Leg Muscle, Left
Septal cartilage	Nasal Septum
Serratus anterior muscle	Thorax Muscle, Right
	Thorax Muscle, Left
Serratus posterior muscle	Trunk Muscle, Right
	Trunk Muscle, Left
Seventh cranial nerve	Facial Nerve
Short gastric artery	Splenic Artery
Sigmoid artery	Inferior Mesenteric Artery
Sigmoid flexure	Sigmoid Colon
Sigmoid vein	Inferior Mesenteric Vein
Sinoatrial node	Conduction Mechanism
Sinus venosus	Atrium, Right
Sixth cranial nerve	Abducens Nerve

Term	ICD-10-PCS Value
Skene's (paraurethral) gland	Vestibular Gland
Small saphenous vein	Saphenous Vein, Right
	Saphenous Vein, Left
Solar (celiac) plexus	Abdominal Sympathetic Nerve
Soleus muscle	Lower Leg Muscle, Right
	Lower Leg Muscle, Left
Space of Retzius	Pelvic Cavity
Sphenomandibular ligament	Head and Neck Bursa and Ligament
Sphenopalatine (pterygopalatine) ganglion	Head and Neck Sympathetic Nerve
Spinal nerve, cervical	Cervical Nerve
Spinal nerve, lumbar	Lumbar Nerve
Spinal nerve, sacral	Sacral Nerve
Spinal nerve, thoracic	Thoracic Nerve
Spinous process	Cervical Vertebra
	Lumbar Vertebra
	Thoracic Vertebra
Spiral ganglion	Acoustic Nerve
Splenic flexure	Transverse Colon
Splenic plexus	Abdominal Sympathetic Nerve
Splenius capitis muscle	Head Muscle
Splenius cervicis muscle	Neck Muscle, Right
	Neck Muscle, Left
Stapes	Auditory Ossicle, Right
	Auditory Ossicle, Left
Stellate ganglion	Head and Neck Sympathetic Nerve
Stensen's duct	Parotid Duct, Right
	Parotid Duct, Left
Sternoclavicular ligament	Shoulder Bursa and Ligament, Right
	Shoulder Bursa and Ligament, Left
Sternocleidomastoid artery	Thyroid Artery, Right
	Thyroid Artery, Left
Sternocleidomastoid muscle	Neck Muscle, Right
	Neck Muscle, Left
Sternocostal ligament	Sternum Bursa and Ligament
Styloglossus muscle	Tongue, Palate, Pharynx Muscle
Stylomandibular ligament	Head and Neck Bursa and Ligament
Stylopharyngeus muscle	Tongue, Palate, Pharynx Muscle
Subacromial bursa	Shoulder Bursa and Ligament, Right
	Shoulder Bursa and Ligament, Left
Subaortic (common iliac) lymph node	Lymphatic, Pelvis
Subarachnoid space, spinal	Spinal Canal
Subclavicular (apical) lymph node	Lymphatic, Right Axillary
	Lymphatic, Left Axillary
Subclavius muscle	Thorax Muscle, Right
	Thorax Muscle, Left
Subclavius nerve	Brachial Plexus
Subcostal artery	Upper Artery
Subcostal muscle	Thorax Muscle, Right
	Thorax Muscle, Left
Subcostal nerve	Thoracic Nerve
Subdural space, spinal	Spinal Canal
Submandibular ganglion	Facial Nerve
	Head and Neck Sympathetic Nerve
Submandibular gland	Submaxillary Gland, Right
	Submaxillary Gland, Left
Submandibular lymph node	Lymphatic, Head
Submandibular space	Subcutaneous Tissue and Fascia, Face
Submaxillary ganglion	Head and Neck Sympathetic Nerve
Submaxillary lymph node	Lymphatic, Head

Term	ICD-10-PCS Value
Submental artery	Face Artery
Submental lymph node	Lymphatic, Head
Submucous (Meissner's) plexus	Abdominal Sympathetic Nerve
Suboccipital nerve	Cervical Nerve
Suboccipital venous plexus	Vertebral Vein, Right
	Vertebral Vein, Left
Subparotid lymph node	Lymphatic, Head
Subscapular aponeurosis	Subcutaneous Tissue and Fascia, Right Upper Arm
	Subcutaneous Tissue and Fascia, Left Upper Arm
Subscapular artery	Axillary Artery, Right
	Axillary Artery, Left
Subscapular (posterior) lymph node	Lymphatic, Right Axillary
	Lymphatic, Left Axillary
Subscapularis muscle	Shoulder Muscle, Right
	Shoulder Muscle, Left
Substantia nigra	Basal Ganglia
Subtalar (talocalcaneal) joint	Tarsal Joint, Right
	Tarsal Joint, Left
Subtalar ligament	Foot Bursa and Ligament, Right
	Foot Bursa and Ligament, Left
Subthalamic nucleus	Basal Ganglia
Superficial circumflex iliac vein	Saphenous Vein, Right
	Saphenous Vein, Left
Superficial epigastric artery	Femoral Artery, Right
	Femoral Artery, Left
Superficial epigastric vein	Saphenous Vein, Right
	Saphenous Vein, Left
Superficial palmar arch	Hand Artery, Right
	Hand Artery, Left
Superficial palmar venous arch	Hand Vein, Right
	Hand Vein, Left
Superficial temporal artery	Temporal Artery, Right
	Temporal Artery, Left
Superficial transverse perineal muscle	Perineum Muscle
Superior cardiac nerve	Thoracic Sympathetic Nerve
Superior cerebellar vein	Intracranial Vein
Superior cerebral vein	Intracranial Vein
Superior clunic (cluneal) nerve	Lumbar Nerve
Superior epigastric artery	Internal Mammary Artery, Right
	Internal Mammary Artery, Left
Superior genicular artery	Popliteal Artery, Right
	Popliteal Artery, Left
Superior gluteal artery	Internal Iliac Artery, Right
	Internal Iliac Artery, Left
Superior gluteal nerve	Lumbar Plexus
Superior hypogastric plexus	Abdominal Sympathetic Nerve
Superior labial artery	Face Artery
Superior laryngeal artery	Thyroid Artery, Right
	Thyroid Artery, Left
Superior laryngeal nerve	Vagus Nerve
Superior longitudinal muscle	Tongue, Palate, Pharynx Muscle
Superior mesenteric ganglion	Abdominal Sympathetic Nerve
Superior mesenteric lymph node	Lymphatic, Mesenteric
Superior mesenteric plexus	Abdominal Sympathetic Nerve

Term	ICD-10-PCS Value
Superior oblique muscle	Extraocular Muscle, Right
	Extraocular Muscle, Left
Superior olivary nucleus	Pons
Superior rectal artery	Inferior Mesenteric Artery
Superior rectal vein	Inferior Mesenteric Vein
Superior rectus muscle	Extraocular Muscle, Right
	Extraocular Muscle, Left
Superior tarsal plate	Upper Eyelid, Right
	Upper Eyelid, Left
Superior thoracic artery	Axillary Artery, Right
	Axillary Artery, Left
Superior thyroid artery	External Carotid Artery, Right
	External Carotid Artery, Left
	Thyroid Artery, Right
	Thyroid Artery, Left
Superior turbinate	Nasal Turbinate
Superior ulnar collateral artery	Brachial Artery, Right
	Brachial Artery, Left
Superior vesical artery	Internal Iliac Artery, Right
	Internal Iliac Artery, Left
Supraclavicular nerve	Cervical Plexus
Supraclavicular (Virchow's) lymph node	Lymphatic, Right Neck
	Lymphatic, Left Neck
Suprahyoid lymph node	Lymphatic, Head
Suprahyoid muscle	Neck Muscle, Right
	Neck Muscle, Left
Suprainguinal lymph node	Lymphatic, Pelvis
Supraorbital vein	Face Vein, Right
	Face Vein, Left
Suprarenal gland	Adrenal Gland, Right
	Adrenal Gland, Left
	Adrenal Glands, Bilateral
	Adrenal Gland
Suprarenal plexus	Abdominal Sympathetic Nerve
Suprascapular nerve	Brachial Plexus
Supraspinatus fascia	Subcutaneous Tissue and Fascia, Right Upper Arm
	Subcutaneous Tissue and Fascia, Left Upper Arm
Supraspinatus muscle	Shoulder Muscle, Right
	Shoulder Muscle, Left
Supraspinous ligament	Upper Spine Bursa and Ligament
	Lower Spine Bursa and Ligament
Suprasternal notch	Sternum
Supratrochlear lymph node	Lymphatic, Right Upper Extremity
	Lymphatic, Left Upper Extremity
Sural artery	Popliteal Artery, Right
	Popliteal Artery, Left
Sweat gland	Skin
Talocalcaneal ligament	Foot Bursa and Ligament, Right
	Foot Bursa and Ligament, Left
Talocalcaneal (subtalar) joint	Tarsal Joint, Right
	Tarsal Joint, Left
Talocalcaneonavicular joint	Tarsal Joint, Right
	Tarsal Joint, Left
Talocalcaneonavicular ligament	Foot Bursa and Ligament, Right
	Foot Bursa and Ligament, Left
Talocrural joint	Ankle Joint, Right
	Ankle Joint, Left
Talofibular ligament	Ankle Bursa and Ligament, Right
	Ankle Bursa and Ligament, Left

Term	ICD-10-PCS Value
Talus bone	Tarsal, Right
	Tarsal, Left
Tarsometatarsal ligament	Foot Bursa and Ligament, Right
	Foot Bursa and Ligament, Left
Temporal lobe	Cerebral Hemisphere
Temporalis muscle	Head Muscle
Temporoparietalis muscle	Head Muscle
Tensor fasciae latae muscle	Hip Muscle, Right
	Hip Muscle, Left
Tensor veli palatini muscle	Tongue, Palate, Pharynx Muscle
Tenth cranial nerve	Vagus Nerve
Tentorium cerebelli	Dura Mater
Teres major muscle	Shoulder Muscle, Right
	Shoulder Muscle, Left
Teres minor muscle	Shoulder Muscle, Right
	Shoulder Muscle, Left
Testicular artery	Abdominal Aorta
Thenar muscle	Hand Muscle, Right
	Hand Muscle, Left
Third cranial nerve	Oculomotor Nerve
Third occipital nerve	Cervical Nerve
Third ventricle	Cerebral Ventricle
Thoracic aortic plexus	Thoracic Sympathetic Nerve
Thoracic esophagus	Esophagus, Middle
Thoracic facet joint	Thoracic Vertebral Joint
Thoracic ganglion	Thoracic Sympathetic Nerve
Thoracoacromial artery	Axillary Artery, Right
	Axillary Artery, Left
Thoracolumbar facet joint	Thoracolumbar Vertebral Joint
Thymus gland	Thymus
Thyroarytenoid muscle	Neck Muscle, Right
	Neck Muscle, Left
Thyrocervical trunk	Thyroid Artery, Right
	Thyroid Artery, Left
Thyroid cartilage	Larynx
Tibial sesamoid	Metatarsal, Right
	Metatarsal, Left
Tibialis anterior muscle	Lower Leg Muscle, Right
	Lower Leg Muscle, Left
Tibialis posterior muscle	Lower Leg Muscle, Right
	Lower Leg Muscle, Left
Tibiofemoral joint	Knee Joint, Right
	Knee Joint, Left
	Knee Joint, Tibial Surface, Right
	Knee Joint, Tibial Surface, Left
Tibioperoneal trunk	Popliteal Artery, Right
	Popliteal Artery, Left
Tongue, base of	Pharynx
Tracheobronchial lymph node	Lymphatic, Thorax
Tragus	External Ear, Right
	External Ear, Left
	External Ear, Bilateral
Transversalis fascia	Subcutaneous Tissue and Fascia, Trunk
Transverse acetabular ligament	Hip Bursa and Ligament, Right
	Hip Bursa and Ligament, Left
Transverse (cutaneous) cervical nerve	Cervical Plexus
Transverse facial artery	Temporal Artery, Right
	Temporal Artery, Left
Transverse foramen	Cervical Vertebra

Term	ICD-10-PCS Value
Transverse humeral ligament	Shoulder Bursa and Ligament, Right
	Shoulder Bursa and Ligament, Left
Transverse ligament of atlas	Head and Neck Bursa and Ligament
Transverse process	Cervical Vertebra
	Thoracic Vertebra
	Lumbar Vertebra
Transverse scapular ligament	Shoulder Bursa and Ligament, Right
	Shoulder Bursa and Ligament, Left
Transverse thoracis muscle	Thorax Muscle, Right
	Thorax Muscle, Left
Transversospinalis muscle	Trunk Muscle, Right
	Trunk Muscle, Left
Transversus abdominis muscle	Abdomen Muscle, Right
	Abdomen Muscle, Left
Trapezium bone	Carpal, Right
	Carpal, Left
Trapezius muscle	Trunk Muscle, Right
	Trunk Muscle, Left
Trapezoid bone	Carpal, Right
	Carpal, Left
Triceps brachii muscle	Upper Arm Muscle, Right
	Upper Arm Muscle, Left
Tricuspid annulus	Tricuspid Valve
Trifacial nerve	Trigeminal Nerve
Trigone of bladder	Bladder
Triquetral bone	Carpal, Right
	Carpal, Left
Trochanteric bursa	Hip Bursa and Ligament, Right
	Hip Bursa and Ligament, Left
Twelfth cranial nerve	Hypoglossal Nerve
Tympanic cavity	Middle Ear, Right
	Middle Ear, Left
Tympanic nerve	Glossopharyngeal Nerve
Tympanic part of temoporal bone	Temporal Bone, Right
	Temporal Bone, Left
Ulnar collateral carpal ligament	Wrist Bursa and Ligament, Right
	Wrist Bursa and Ligament, Left
Ulnar collateral ligament	Elbow Bursa and Ligament, Right
	Elbow Bursa and Ligament, Left
Ulnar notch	Radius, Right
	Radius, Left
Ulnar vein	Brachial Vein, Right
	Brachial Vein, Left
Umbilical artery	Internal Iliac Artery, Right
	Internal Iliac Artery, Left
	Lower Artery
Ureteral orifice	Ureter, Right
	Ureter, Left
	Ureters, Bilateral
	Ureter
Ureteropelvic junction (UPJ)	Kidney Pelvis, Right
	Kidney Pelvis, Left
Ureterovesical orifice	Ureter, Right
	Ureter, Left
	Ureters, Bilateral
	Ureter
Uterine artery	Internal Iliac Artery, Right
	Internal Iliac Artery, Left
Uterine cornu	Uterus

Term	ICD-10-PCS Value
Uterine tube	Fallopian Tube, Right
	Fallopian Tube, Left
Uterine vein	Hypogastric Vein, Right
	Hypogastric Vein, Left
Vaginal artery	Internal Iliac Artery, Right
	Internal Iliac Artery, Left
Vaginal vein	Hypogastric Vein, Right
	Hypogastric Vein, Left
Vastus intermedius muscle	Upper Leg Muscle, Right
	Upper Leg Muscle, Left
Vastus lateralis muscle	Upper Leg Muscle, Right
	Upper Leg Muscle, Left
Vastus medialis muscle	Upper Leg Muscle, Right
	Upper Leg Muscle, Left
Ventricular fold	Larynx
Vermiform appendix	Appendix
Vermilion border	Upper Lip
	Lower Lip
Vertebral arch	Cervical Vertebra
	Lumbar Vertebra
	Thoracic Vertebra
Vertebral artery, intracranial portion	Intracranial Artery
Vertebral body	Cervical Vertebra
	Lumbar Vertebra
	Thoracic Vertebra
Vertebral canal	Spinal Canal
Vertebral foramen	Cervical Vertebra
	Lumbar Vertebra
	Thoracic Vertebra
Vertebral lamina	Cervical Vertebra
	Lumbar Vertebra
	Thoracic Vertebra
Vertebral pedicle	Cervical Vertebra
	Lumbar Vertebra
	Thoracic Vertebra

Term	ICD-10-PCS Value
Vesical vein	Hypogastric Vein, Right
	Hypogastric Vein, Left
Vestibular (Scarpa's) ganglion	Acoustic Nerve
Vestibular nerve	Acoustic Nerve
Vestibulocochlear nerve	Acoustic Nerve
Virchow's (supraclavicular) lymph node	Lymphatic, Right Neck
	Lymphatic, Left Neck
Vitreous body	Vitreous, Right
	Vitreous, Left
Vocal fold	Vocal Cord, Right
	Vocal Cord, Left
Volar (palmar) digital vein	Hand Vein, Right
	Hand Vein, Left
Volar (palmar) metacarpal vein	Hand Vein, Right
	Hand Vein, Left
Vomer bone	Nasal Septum
Vomer of nasal septum	Nasal Bone
Xiphoid process	Sternum
Zonule of Zinn	Lens, Right
	Lens, Left
Zygomatic process of frontal bone	Frontal Bone
Zygomatic process of temporal bone	Temporal Bone, Right
	Temporal Bone, Left
Zygomaticus muscle	Facial Muscle

Appendix E: Body Part Definitions

ICD-10-PCS Value	Definition
1st Toe, Left 1st Toe, Right	Hallux
Abdomen Muscle, Left Abdomen Muscle, Right	External oblique muscle Internal oblique muscle Pyramidalis muscle Rectus abdominis muscle Transversus abdominis muscle
Abdominal Aorta	Inferior phrenic artery Lumbar artery Median sacral artery Middle suprarenal artery Ovarian artery Testicular artery
Abdominal Sympathetic Nerve	Abdominal aortic plexus Auerbach's (myenteric) plexus Celiac (solar) plexus Celiac ganglion Gastric plexus Hepatic plexus Inferior hypogastric plexus Inferior mesenteric ganglion Inferior mesenteric plexus Meissner's (submucous) plexus Myenteric (Auerbach's) plexus Pancreatic plexus Pelvic splanchnic nerve Renal nerve Renal plexus Solar (celiac) plexus Splenic plexus Submucous (Meissner's) plexus Superior hypogastric plexus Superior mesenteric ganglion Superior mesenteric plexus Suprarenal plexus
Abducens Nerve	Sixth cranial nerve
Accessory Nerve	Eleventh cranial nerve
Acoustic Nerve	Cochlear nerve Eighth cranial nerve Scarpa's (vestibular) ganglion Spiral ganglion Vestibular (Scarpa's) ganglion Vestibular nerve Vestibulocochlear nerve
Adenoids	Pharyngeal tonsil
Adrenal Gland Adrenal Gland, Left Adrenal Gland, Right Adrenal Glands, Bilateral	Suprarenal gland
Ampulla of Vater	Duodenal ampulla Hepatopancreatic ampulla
Anal Sphincter	External anal sphincter Internal anal sphincter
Ankle Bursa and Ligament, Left Ankle Bursa and Ligament, Right	Calcaneofibular ligament Deltoid ligament Ligament of the lateral malleolus Talofibular ligament
Ankle Joint, Left Ankle Joint, Right	Inferior tibiofibular joint Talocrural joint
Anterior Chamber, Left Anterior Chamber, Right	Aqueous humour
Anterior Tibial Artery, Left Anterior Tibial Artery, Right	Anterior lateral malleolar artery Anterior medial malleolar artery Anterior tibial recurrent artery Dorsalis pedis artery Posterior tibial recurrent artery

ICD-10-PCS Value	Definition
Anus	Anal orifice
Aortic Valve	Aortic annulus
Appendix	Appendiceal orifice Vermiform appendix
Atrial Septum	Interatrial septum
Atrium, Left	Atrium pulmonale Left auricular appendix
Atrium, Right	Atrium dextrum cordis Right auricular appendix Sinus venosus
Auditory Ossicle, Left Auditory Ossicle, Right	Incus Malleus Stapes
Axillary Artery, Left Axillary Artery, Right	Anterior circumflex humeral artery Lateral thoracic artery Posterior circumflex humeral artery Subscapular artery Superior thoracic artery Thoracoacromial artery
Azygos Vein	Right ascending lumbar vein Right subcostal vein
Basal Ganglia	Basal nuclei Claustrum Corpus striatum Globus pallidus Substantia nigra Subthalamic nucleus
Basilic Vein, Left Basilic Vein, Right	Median antebrachial vein Median cubital vein
Bladder	Trigone of bladder
Brachial Artery, Left Brachial Artery, Right	Inferior ulnar collateral artery Profunda brachii Superior ulnar collateral artery
Brachial Plexus	Axillary nerve Dorsal scapular nerve First intercostal nerve Long thoracic nerve Musculocutaneous nerve Subclavius nerve Suprascapular nerve
Brachial Vein, Left Brachial Vein, Right	Radial vein Ulnar vein
Brain	Cerebrum Corpus callosum Encephalon
Breast, Bilateral Breast, Left Breast, Right	Mammary duct Mammary gland
Buccal Mucosa	Buccal gland Molar gland Palatine gland
Carotid Bodies, Bilateral Carotid Body, Left Carotid Body, Right	Carotid glomus
Carpal Joint, Left Carpal Joint, Right	Intercarpal joint Midcarpal joint
Carpal, Left Carpal, Right	Capitate bone Hamate bone Lunate bone Pisiform bone Scaphoid bone Trapezium bone Trapezoid bone Triquetral bone
Celiac Artery	Celiac trunk

ICD-10-PCS Value	Definition
Cephalic Vein, Left Cephalic Vein, Right	Accessory cephalic vein
Cerebellum	Culmen
Cerebral Hemisphere	Frontal lobe Occipital lobe Parietal lobe Temporal lobe
Cerebral Meninges	Arachnoid mater, intracranial Leptomeninges, intracranial Pia mater, intracranial
Cerebral Ventricle	Aqueduct of Sylvius Cerebral aqueduct (Sylvius) Choroid plexus Ependyma Foramen of Monro (intraventricular) Fourth ventricle Interventricular foramen (Monro) Left lateral ventricle Right lateral ventricle Third ventricle
Cervical Nerve	Greater occipital nerve Spinal nerve, cervical Suboccipital nerve Third occipital nerve
Cervical Plexus	Ansa cervicalis Cutaneous (transverse) cervical nerve Great auricular nerve Lesser occipital nerve Supraclavicular nerve Transverse (cutaneous) cervical nerve
Cervical Spinal Cord	Dorsal root ganglion
Cervical Vertebra	Dens Odontoid process Spinous process Transverse foramen Transverse process Vertebral arch Vertebral body Vertebral foramen Vertebral lamina Vertebral pedicle
Cervical Vertebral Joint	Atlantoaxial joint Cervical facet joint
Cervical Vertebral Joints, 2 or more	Cervical facet joint
Cervicothoracic Vertebral Joint	Cervicothoracic facet joint
Cisterna Chyli	Intestinal lymphatic trunk Lumbar lymphatic trunk
Coccygeal Glomus	Coccygeal body
Colic Vein	Ileocolic vein Left colic vein Middle colic vein Right colic vein
Conduction Mechanism	Atrioventricular node Bundle of His Bundle of Kent Sinoatrial node
Conjunctiva, Left Conjunctiva, Right	Plica semilunaris
Dura Mater	Diaphragma sellae Dura mater, intracranial Falx cerebri Tentorium cerebelli
Elbow Bursa and Ligament, Left Elbow Bursa and Ligament, Right	Annular ligament Olecranon bursa Radial collateral ligament Ulnar collateral ligament

ICD-10-PCS Value	Definition
Elbow Joint, Left Elbow Joint, Right	Distal humerus, involving joint Humeroradial joint Humeroulnar joint Proximal radioulnar joint
Epidural Space, Intracranial	Extradural space, intracranial
Epiglottis	Glossoepiglottic fold
Esophagogastric Junction	Cardia Cardioesophageal junction Gastroesophageal (GE) junction
Esophagus, Lower	Abdominal esophagus
Esophagus, Middle	Thoracic esophagus
Esophagus, Upper	Cervical esophagus
Ethmoid Bone, Left Ethmoid Bone, Right	Cribriform plate
Ethmoid Sinus, Left Ethmoid Sinus, Right	Ethmoidal air cell
Eustachian Tube, Left Eustachian Tube, Right	Auditory tube Pharyngotympanic tube
External Auditory Canal, Left External Auditory Canal, Right	External auditory meatus
External Carotid Artery, Left External Carotid Artery, Right	Ascending pharyngeal artery Internal maxillary artery Lingual artery Maxillary artery Occipital artery Posterior auricular artery Superior thyroid artery
External Ear, Bilateral External Ear, Left External Ear, Right	Antihelix Antitragus Auricle Earlobe Helix Pinna Tragus
External Iliac Artery, Left External Iliac Artery, Right	Deep circumflex iliac artery Inferior epigastric artery
External Jugular Vein, Left External Jugular Vein, Right	Posterior auricular vein
Extraocular Muscle, Left Extraocular Muscle, Right	Inferior oblique muscle Inferior rectus muscle Lateral rectus muscle Medial rectus muscle Superior oblique muscle Superior rectus muscle
Eye, Left Eye, Right	Ciliary body Posterior chamber
Face Artery	Angular artery Ascending palatine artery External maxillary artery Facial artery Inferior labial artery Submental artery Superior labial artery
Face Vein, Left Face Vein, Right	Angular vein Anterior facial vein Common facial vein Deep facial vein Frontal vein Posterior facial (retromandibular) vein Supraorbital vein

ICD-10-PCS Value	Definition
Facial Muscle	Buccinator muscle Corrugator supercilii muscle Depressor anguli oris muscle Depressor labii inferioris muscle Depressor septi nasi muscle Depressor supercilii muscle Levator anguli oris muscle Levator labii superioris alaeque nasi muscle Levator labii superioris muscle Mentalis muscle Nasalis muscle Occipitofrontalis muscle Orbicularis oris muscle Procerus muscle Risorius muscle Zygomaticus muscle
Facial Nerve	Chorda tympani Geniculate ganglion Greater superficial petrosal nerve Nerve to the stapedius Parotid plexus Posterior auricular nerve Seventh cranial nerve Submandibular ganglion
Fallopian Tube, Left Fallopian Tube, Right	Oviduct Salpinx Uterine tube
Femoral Artery, Left Femoral Artery, Right	Circumflex iliac artery Deep femoral artery Descending genicular artery External pudendal artery Superficial epigastric artery
Femoral Nerve	Anterior crural nerve Saphenous nerve
Femoral Shaft, Left Femoral Shaft, Right	Body of femur
Femoral Vein, Left Femoral Vein, Right	Deep femoral (profunda femoris) vein Popliteal vein Profunda femoris (deep femoral) vein
Fibula, Left Fibula, Right	Body of fibula Head of fibula Lateral malleolus
Finger Nail	Nail bed Nail plate
Finger Phalangeal Joint, Left Finger Phalangeal Joint, Right	Interphalangeal (IP) joint
Foot Artery, Left Foot Artery, Right	Arcuate artery Dorsal metatarsal artery Lateral plantar artery Lateral tarsal artery Medial plantar artery
Foot Bursa and Ligament, Left Foot Bursa and Ligament, Right	Calcaneocuboid ligament Cuneonavicular ligament Intercuneiform ligament Interphalangeal ligament Metatarsal ligament Metatarsophalangeal ligament Subtalar ligament Talocalcaneal ligament Talocalcaneonavicular ligament Tarsometatarsal ligament
Foot Muscle, Left Foot Muscle, Right	Abductor hallucis muscle Adductor hallucis muscle Extensor digitorum brevis muscle Extensor hallucis brevis muscle Flexor digitorum brevis muscle Flexor hallucis brevis muscle Quadratus plantae muscle

ICD-10-PCS Value	Definition
Foot Vein, Left Foot Vein, Right	Common digital vein Dorsal metatarsal vein Dorsal venous arch Plantar digital vein Plantar metatarsal vein Plantar venous arch
Frontal Bone	Zygomatic process of frontal bone
Gastric Artery	Left gastric artery Right gastric artery
Glenoid Cavity, Left Glenoid Cavity, Right	Glenoid fossa (of scapula)
Glomus Jugulare	Jugular body
Glossopharyngeal Nerve	Carotid sinus nerve Ninth cranial nerve Tympanic nerve
Hand Artery, Left Hand Artery, Right	Deep palmar arch Princeps pollicis artery Radialis indicis Superficial palmar arch
Hand Bursa and Ligament, Left Hand Bursa and Ligament, Right	Carpometacarpal ligament Intercarpal ligament Interphalangeal ligament Lunotriquetral ligament Metacarpal ligament Metacarpophalangeal ligament Pisohamate ligament Pisometacarpal ligament Scaphotrapezium ligament
Hand Muscle, Left Hand Muscle, Right	Hypothenar muscle Palmar interosseous muscle Thenar muscle
Hand Vein, Left Hand Vein, Right	Dorsal metacarpal vein Palmar (volar) digital vein Palmar (volar) metacarpal vein Superficial palmar venous arch Volar (palmar) digital vein Volar (palmar) metacarpal vein
Head and Neck Bursa and Ligament	Alar ligament of axis Cervical interspinous ligament Cervical intertransverse ligament Cervical ligamentum flavum Interspinous ligament, cervical Intertransverse ligament, cervical Lateral temporomandibular ligament Ligamentum flavum, cervical Sphenomandibular ligament Stylomandibular ligament Transverse ligament of atlas
Head and Neck Sympathetic Nerve	Cavernous plexus Cervical ganglion Ciliary ganglion Internal carotid plexus Otic ganglion Pterygopalatine (sphenopalatine) ganglion Sphenopalatine (pterygopalatine) ganglion Stellate ganglion Submandibular ganglion Submaxillary ganglion
Head Muscle	Auricularis muscle Masseter muscle Pterygoid muscle Splenius capitis muscle Temporalis muscle Temporoparietalis muscle
Heart, Left	Left coronary sulcus Obtuse margin
Heart, Right	Right coronary sulcus
Hemiazygos Vein	Left ascending lumbar vein Left subcostal vein

ICD-10-PCS Value	Definition
Hepatic Artery	Common hepatic artery Gastroduodenal artery Hepatic artery proper
Hip Bursa and Ligament, Left **Hip Bursa and Ligament, Right**	Iliofemoral ligament Ischiofemoral ligament Pubofemoral ligament Transverse acetabular ligament Trochanteric bursa
Hip Joint, Left **Hip Joint, Right**	Acetabulofemoral joint
Hip Muscle, Left **Hip Muscle, Right**	Gemellus muscle Gluteus maximus muscle Gluteus medius muscle Gluteus minimus muscle Iliacus muscle Obturator muscle Piriformis muscle Psoas muscle Quadratus femoris muscle Tensor fasciae latae muscle
Humeral Head, Left **Humeral Head, Right**	Greater tuberosity Lesser tuberosity Neck of humerus (anatomical)(surgical)
Humeral Shaft, Left **Humeral Shaft, Right**	Distal humerus Humerus, distal Lateral epicondyle of humerus Medial epicondyle of humerus
Hypogastric Vein, Left **Hypogastric Vein, Right**	Gluteal vein Internal iliac vein Internal pudendal vein Lateral sacral vein Middle hemorrhoidal vein Obturator vein Uterine vein Vaginal vein Vesical vein
Hypoglossal Nerve	Twelfth cranial nerve
Hypothalamus	Mammillary body
Inferior Mesenteric Artery	Sigmoid artery Superior rectal artery
Inferior Mesenteric Vein	Sigmoid vein Superior rectal vein
Inferior Vena Cava	Postcava Right inferior phrenic vein Right ovarian vein Right second lumbar vein Right suprarenal vein Right testicular vein
Inguinal Region, Bilateral **Inguinal Region, Left** **Inguinal Region, Right**	Inguinal canal Inguinal triangle
Inner Ear, Left **Inner Ear, Right**	Bony labyrinth Bony vestibule Cochlea Round window Semicircular canal
Innominate Artery	Brachiocephalic artery Brachiocephalic trunk
Innominate Vein, Left **Innominate Vein, Right**	Brachiocephalic vein Inferior thyroid vein
Internal Carotid Artery, Left **Internal Carotid Artery, Right**	Caroticotympanic artery Carotid sinus

ICD-10-PCS Value	Definition
Internal Iliac Artery, Left **Internal Iliac Artery, Right**	Deferential artery Hypogastric artery Iliolumbar artery Inferior gluteal artery Inferior vesical artery Internal pudendal artery Lateral sacral artery Middle rectal artery Obturator artery Prostatic artery Superior gluteal artery Superior vesical artery Umbilical artery Uterine artery Vaginal artery
Internal Mammary Artery, Left **Internal Mammary Artery, Right**	Anterior intercostal artery Internal thoracic artery Musculophrenic artery Pericardiophrenic artery Superior epigastric artery
Intracranial Artery	Anterior cerebral artery Anterior choroidal artery Anterior communicating artery Basilar artery Circle of Willis Internal carotid artery, intracranial portion Middle cerebral artery Middle meningeal artery, intracranial portion Ophthalmic artery Posterior cerebral artery Posterior communicating artery Posterior inferior cerebellar artery (PICA) Vertebral artery, intracranial portion
Intracranial Vein	Anterior cerebral vein Basal (internal) cerebral vein Dural venous sinus Great cerebral vein Inferior cerebellar vein Inferior cerebral vein Internal (basal) cerebral vein Middle cerebral vein Ophthalmic vein Superior cerebellar vein Superior cerebral vein
Jejunum	Duodenojejunal flexure
Kidney	Renal calyx Renal capsule Renal cortex Renal segment
Kidney Pelvis, Left **Kidney Pelvis, Right**	Ureteropelvic junction (UPJ)
Kidney, Left **Kidney, Right** **Kidneys, Bilateral**	Renal calyx Renal capsule Renal cortex Renal segment
Knee Bursa and Ligament, Left **Knee Bursa and Ligament, Right**	Anterior cruciate ligament (ACL) Lateral collateral ligament (LCL) Ligament of head of fibula Medial collateral ligament (MCL) Patellar ligament Popliteal ligament Posterior cruciate ligament (PCL) Prepatellar bursa
Knee Joint, Femoral Surface, Left **Knee Joint, Femoral Surface, Right**	Femoropatellar joint Patellofemoral joint

ICD-10-PCS Value	Definition
Knee Joint, Left Knee Joint, Right	Femoropatellar joint Femorotibial joint Lateral meniscus Medial meniscus Patellofemoral joint Tibiofemoral joint
Knee Joint, Tibial Surface, Left Knee Joint, Tibial Surface, Right	Femorotibial joint Tibiofemoral joint
Knee Tendon, Left Knee Tendon, Right	Patellar tendon
Lacrimal Duct, Left Lacrimal Duct, Right	Lacrimal canaliculus Lacrimal punctum Lacrimal sac Nasolacrimal duct
Larynx	Aryepiglottic fold Arytenoid cartilage Corniculate cartilage Cuneiform cartilage False vocal cord Glottis Rima glottidis Thyroid cartilage Ventricular fold
Lens, Left Lens, Right	Zonule of Zinn
Liver	Quadrate lobe
Lower Arm and Wrist Muscle, Left Lower Arm and Wrist Muscle, Right	Anatomical snuffbox Brachioradialis muscle Extensor carpi radialis muscle Extensor carpi ulnaris muscle Flexor carpi radialis muscle Flexor carpi ulnaris muscle Flexor pollicis longus muscle Palmaris longus muscle Pronator quadratus muscle Pronator teres muscle
Lower Artery	Umbilical artery
Lower Eyelid, Left Lower Eyelid, Right	Inferior tarsal plate Medial canthus
Lower Femur, Left Lower Femur, Right	Lateral condyle of femur Lateral epicondyle of femur Medial condyle of femur Medial epicondyle of femur
Lower Leg Muscle, Left Lower Leg Muscle, Right	Extensor digitorum longus muscle Extensor hallucis longus muscle Fibularis brevis muscle Fibularis longus muscle Flexor digitorum longus muscle Flexor hallucis longus muscle Gastrocnemius muscle Peroneus brevis muscle Peroneus longus muscle Popliteus muscle Soleus muscle Tibialis anterior muscle Tibialis posterior muscle
Lower Leg Tendon, Left Lower Leg Tendon, Right	Achilles tendon
Lower Lip	Frenulum labii inferioris Labial gland Vermilion border
Lower Spine Bursa and Ligament	Iliolumbar ligament Interspinous ligament, lumbar Intertransverse ligament, lumbar Ligamentum flavum, lumbar Sacrococcygeal ligament Sacroiliac ligament Sacrospinous ligament Sacrotuberous ligament Supraspinous ligament

ICD-10-PCS Value	Definition
Lumbar Nerve	Lumbosacral trunk Spinal nerve, lumbar Superior clunic (cluneal) nerve
Lumbar Plexus	Accessory obturator nerve Genitofemoral nerve Iliohypogastric nerve Ilioinguinal nerve Lateral femoral cutaneous nerve Obturator nerve Superior gluteal nerve
Lumbar Spinal Cord	Cauda equina Conus medullaris Dorsal root ganglion
Lumbar Sympathetic Nerve	Lumbar ganglion Lumbar splanchnic nerve
Lumbar Vertebra	Spinous process Transverse process Vertebral arch Vertebral body Vertebral foramen Vertebral lamina Vertebral pedicle
Lumbar Vertebral Joint	Lumbar facet joint
Lumbosacral Joint	Lumbosacral facet joint
Lymphatic, Aortic	Celiac lymph node Gastric lymph node Hepatic lymph node Lumbar lymph node Pancreaticosplenic lymph node Paraaortic lymph node Retroperitoneal lymph node
Lymphatic, Head	Buccinator lymph node Infraauricular lymph node Infraparotid lymph node Parotid lymph node Preauricular lymph node Submandibular lymph node Submaxillary lymph node Submental lymph node Subparotid lymph node Suprahyoid lymph node
Lymphatic, Left Axillary	Anterior (pectoral) lymph node Apical (subclavicular) lymph node Brachial (lateral) lymph node Central axillary lymph node Lateral (brachial) lymph node Pectoral (anterior) lymph node Posterior (subscapular) lymph node Subclavicular (apical) lymph node Subscapular (posterior) lymph node
Lymphatic, Left Lower Extremity	Femoral lymph node Popliteal lymph node
Lymphatic, Left Neck	Cervical lymph node Jugular lymph node Mastoid (postauricular) lymph node Occipital lymph node Postauricular (mastoid) lymph node Retropharyngeal lymph node Supraclavicular (Virchow's) lymph node Virchow's (supraclavicular) lymph node
Lymphatic, Left Upper Extremity	Cubital lymph node Deltopectoral (infraclavicular) lymph node Epitrochlear lymph node Infraclavicular (deltopectoral) lymph node Supratrochlear lymph node
Lymphatic, Mesenteric	Inferior mesenteric lymph node Pararectal lymph node Superior mesenteric lymph node

ICD-10-PCS Value	Definition	ICD-10-PCS Value	Definition
Lymphatic, Pelvis	Common iliac (subaortic) lymph node Gluteal lymph node Iliac lymph node Inferior epigastric lymph node Obturator lymph node Sacral lymph node Subaortic (common iliac) lymph node Suprainguinal lymph node	Mitral Valve	Bicuspid valve Left atrioventricular valve Mitral annulus
		Nasal Bone	Vomer of nasal septum
Lymphatic, Right Axillary	Anterior (pectoral) lymph node Apical (subclavicular) lymph node Brachial (lateral) lymph node Central axillary lymph node Lateral (brachial) lymph node Pectoral (anterior) lymph node Posterior (subscapular) lymph node Subclavicular (apical) lymph node Subscapular (posterior) lymph node	Nasal Mucosa and Soft Tissue	Columella External naris Greater alar cartilage Internal naris Lateral nasal cartilage Lesser alar cartilage Nasal cavity Nostril
		Nasal Septum	Quadrangular cartilage Septal cartilage Vomer bone
Lymphatic, Right Lower Extremity	Femoral lymph node Popliteal lymph node	Nasal Turbinate	Inferior turbinate Middle turbinate Nasal concha Superior turbinate
Lymphatic, Right Neck	Cervical lymph node Jugular lymph node Mastoid (postauricular) lymph node Occipital lymph node Postauricular (mastoid) lymph node Retropharyngeal lymph node Right jugular trunk Right lymphatic duct Right subclavian trunk Supraclavicular (Virchow's) lymph node Virchow's (supraclavicular) lymph node	Nasopharynx	Choana Fossa of Rosenmuller Pharyngeal recess Rhinopharynx
		Neck	Parapharyngeal space Retropharyngeal space
Lymphatic, Right Upper Extremity	Cubital lymph node Deltopectoral (infraclavicular) lymph node Epitrochlear lymph node Infraclavicular (deltopectoral) lymph node Supratrochlear lymph node	Neck Muscle, Left Neck Muscle, Right	Anterior vertebral muscle Arytenoid muscle Cricothyroid muscle Infrahyoid muscle Levator scapulae muscle Platysma muscle Scalene muscle Splenius cervicis muscle Sternocleidomastoid muscle Suprahyoid muscle Thyroarytenoid muscle
Lymphatic, Thorax	Intercostal lymph node Mediastinal lymph node Parasternal lymph node Paratracheal lymph node Tracheobronchial lymph node		
		Nipple, Left Nipple, Right	Areola
Main Bronchus, Right	Bronchus intermedius Intermediate bronchus	Occipital Bone	Foramen magnum
		Oculomotor Nerve	Third cranial nerve
Mandible, Left Mandible, Right	Alveolar process of mandible Condyloid process Mandibular notch Mental foramen	Olfactory Nerve	First cranial nerve Olfactory bulb
Mastoid Sinus, Left Mastoid Sinus, Right	Mastoid air cells	Omentum	Gastrocolic ligament Gastrocolic omentum Gastrohepatic omentum Gastrophrenic ligament Gastrosplenic ligament Greater Omentum Hepatogastric ligament Lesser Omentum
Metatarsal, Left Metatarsal, Right	Fibular sesamoid Tibial sesamoid		
Maxilla	Alveolar process of maxilla		
Maxillary Sinus, Left Maxillary Sinus, Right	Antrum of Highmore	Optic Nerve	Optic chiasma Second cranial nerve
Median Nerve	Anterior interosseous nerve Palmar cutaneous nerve	Orbit, Left Orbit, Right	Bony orbit Orbital portion of ethmoid bone Orbital portion of frontal bone Orbital portion of lacrimal bone Orbital portion of maxilla Orbital portion of palatine bone Orbital portion of sphenoid bone Orbital portion of zygomatic bone
Mediastinum	Mediastinal cavity Mediastinal space		
Medulla Oblongata	Myelencephalon		
Mesentery	Mesoappendix Mesocolon	Pancreatic Duct	Duct of Wirsung
Metatarsal, Right Metatarsal, Left	Fibular sesamoid Tibial sesamoid	Pancreatic Duct, Accessory	Duct of Santorini
Metatarsal-Phalangeal Joint, Left Metatarsal-Phalangeal Joint, Right	Metatarsophalangeal (MTP) joint	Parotid Duct, Left Parotid Duct, Right	Stensen's duct
		Pelvic Bone, Left Pelvic Bone, Right	Iliac crest Ilium Ischium Pubis
Middle Ear, Left Middle Ear, Right	Oval window Tympanic cavity		
Minor Salivary Gland	Anterior lingual gland	Pelvic Cavity	Retropubic space Space of Retzius

Appendix E: Body Part Definitions

ICD-10-PCS Value	Definition
Penis	Corpus cavernosum Corpus spongiosum
Perineum Muscle	Bulbospongiosus muscle Cremaster muscle Deep transverse perineal muscle Ischiocavernosus muscle Levator ani muscle Superficial transverse perineal muscle
Peritoneal Cavity	Abdominal cavity
Peritoneum	Epiploic foramen
Peroneal Artery, Left Peroneal Artery, Right	Fibular artery
Peroneal Nerve	Common fibular nerve Common peroneal nerve External popliteal nerve Lateral sural cutaneous nerve
Pharynx	Base of Tongue Hypopharynx Laryngopharynx Lingual tonsil Oropharynx Piriform recess (sinus) Tongue, base of
Phrenic Nerve	Accessory phrenic nerve
Pituitary Gland	Adenohypophysis Hypophysis Neurohypophysis
Pons	Apneustic center Basis pontis Locus ceruleus Pneumotaxic center Pontine tegmentum Superior olivary nucleus
Popliteal Artery, Left Popliteal Artery, Right	Inferior genicular artery Middle genicular artery Superior genicular artery Sural artery Tibioperoneal trunk
Portal Vein	Hepatic portal vein
Prepuce	Foreskin Glans penis
Pudendal Nerve	Posterior labial nerve Posterior scrotal nerve
Pulmonary Artery, Left	Arterial canal (duct) Botallo's duct Pulmoaortic canal
Pulmonary Valve	Pulmonary annulus Pulmonic valve
Pulmonary Vein, Left	Left inferior pulmonary vein Left superior pulmonary vein
Pulmonary Vein, Right	Right inferior pulmonary vein Right superior pulmonary vein
Radial Artery, Left Radial Artery, Right	Radial recurrent artery
Radial Nerve	Dorsal digital nerve Musculospiral nerve Palmar cutaneous nerve Posterior interosseous nerve
Radius, Left Radius, Right	Ulnar notch
Rectum	Anorectal junction
Renal Artery, Left Renal Artery, Right	Inferior suprarenal artery Renal segmental artery
Renal Vein, Left	Left inferior phrenic vein Left ovarian vein Left second lumbar vein Left suprarenal vein Left testicular vein

ICD-10-PCS Value	Definition
Retina, Left Retina, Right	Fovea Macula Optic disc
Retroperitoneum	Retroperitoneal cavity Retroperitoneal space
Rib(s) Bursa and Ligament	Costotransverse ligament
Sacral Nerve	Spinal nerve, sacral
Sacral Plexus	Inferior gluteal nerve Posterior femoral cutaneous nerve Pudendal nerve
Sacral Sympathetic Nerve	Ganglion impar (ganglion of Walther) Pelvic splanchnic nerve Sacral ganglion Sacral splanchnic nerve
Sacrococcygeal Joint	Sacrococcygeal symphysis
Saphenous Vein, Left Saphenous Vein, Right	External pudendal vein Great(er) saphenous vein Lesser saphenous vein Small saphenous vein Superficial circumflex iliac vein Superficial epigastric vein
Scapula, Left Scapula, Right	Acromion (process) Coracoid process
Sciatic Nerve	Ischiatic nerve
Shoulder Bursa and Ligament, Left Shoulder Bursa and Ligament, Right	Acromioclavicular ligament Coracoacromial ligament Coracoclavicular ligament Coracohumeral ligament Costoclavicular ligament Glenohumeral ligament Interclavicular ligament Sternoclavicular ligament Subacromial bursa Transverse humeral ligament Transverse scapular ligament
Shoulder Joint, Left Shoulder Joint, Right	Glenohumeral joint Glenoid ligament (labrum)
Shoulder Muscle, Left Shoulder Muscle, Right	Deltoid muscle Infraspinatus muscle Subscapularis muscle Supraspinatus muscle Teres major muscle Teres minor muscle
Sigmoid Colon	Rectosigmoid junction Sigmoid flexure
Skin	Dermis Epidermis Sebaceous gland Sweat gland
Skin, Chest	Breast procedures, skin only
Skin, Perineum	Perianal skin
Sphenoid Bone	Greater wing Lesser wing Optic foramen Pterygoid process Sella turcica
Spinal Canal	Epidural space, spinal Extradural space, spinal Subarachnoid space, spinal Subdural space, spinal Vertebral canal
Spinal Cord	Dorsal root ganglion
Spinal Meninges	Arachnoid mater, spinal Denticulate (dentate) ligament Dura mater, spinal Filum terminale Leptomeninges, spinal Pia mater, spinal

ICD-10-PCS Value	Definition
Spleen	Accessory spleen
Splenic Artery	Left gastroepiploic artery Pancreatic artery Short gastric artery
Splenic Vein	Left gastroepiploic vein Pancreatic vein
Sternum	Manubrium Suprasternal notch Xiphoid process
Sternum Bursa and Ligament	Costoxiphoid ligament Sternocostal ligament
Stomach, Pylorus	Pyloric antrum Pyloric canal Pyloric sphincter
Subclavian Artery, Left Subclavian Artery, Right	Costocervical trunk Dorsal scapular artery Internal thoracic artery
Subcutaneous Tissue and Fascia, Chest	Pectoral fascia
Subcutaneous Tissue and Fascia, Face	Chin Masseteric fascia Orbital fascia Submandibular space
Subcutaneous Tissue and Fascia, Left Foot	Plantar fascia (aponeurosis)
Subcutaneous Tissue and Fascia, Left Hand	Palmar fascia (aponeurosis)
Subcutaneous Tissue and Fascia, Left Lower Arm	Antebrachial fascia Bicipital aponeurosis
Subcutaneous Tissue and Fascia, Left Neck	Deep cervical fascia Pretracheal fascia Prevertebral fascia
Subcutaneous Tissue and Fascia, Left Upper Arm	Axillary fascia Deltoid fascia Infraspinatus fascia Subscapular aponeurosis Supraspinatus fascia
Subcutaneous Tissue and Fascia, Left Upper Leg	Crural fascia Fascia lata Iliac fascia Iliotibial tract (band)
Subcutaneous Tissue and Fascia, Right Foot	Plantar fascia (aponeurosis)
Subcutaneous Tissue and Fascia, Right Hand	Palmar fascia (aponeurosis)
Subcutaneous Tissue and Fascia, Right Lower Arm	Antebrachial fascia Bicipital aponeurosis
Subcutaneous Tissue and Fascia, Right Neck	Deep cervical fascia Pretracheal fascia Prevertebral fascia
Subcutaneous Tissue and Fascia, Right Upper Arm	Axillary fascia Deltoid fascia Infraspinatus fascia Subscapular aponeurosis Supraspinatus fascia
Subcutaneous Tissue and Fascia, Right Upper Leg	Crural fascia Fascia lata Iliac fascia Iliotibial tract (band)
Subcutaneous Tissue and Fascia, Scalp	Galea aponeurotica
Subcutaneous Tissue and Fascia, Trunk	External oblique aponeurosis Transversalis fascia
Submaxillary Gland, Left Submaxillary Gland, Right	Submandibular gland

ICD-10-PCS Value	Definition
Superior Mesenteric Artery	Ileal artery Ileocolic artery Inferior pancreaticoduodenal artery Jejunal artery
Superior Mesenteric Vein	Right gastroepiploic vein
Superior Vena Cava	Cavoatrial junction Precava
Tarsal Joint, Left Tarsal Joint, Right	Calcaneocuboid joint Cuboideonavicular joint Cuneonavicular joint Intercuneiform joint Subtalar (talocalcaneal) joint Talocalcaneal (subtalar) joint Talocalcaneonavicular joint
Tarsal, Left Tarsal, Right	Calcaneus Cuboid bone Intermediate cuneiform bone Lateral cuneiform bone Medial cuneiform bone Navicular bone Talus bone
Temporal Artery, Left Temporal Artery, Right	Middle temporal artery Superficial temporal artery Transverse facial artery
Temporal Bone, Left Temporal Bone, Right	Mastoid process Petrous part of temporal bone Tympanic part of temporal bone Zygomatic process of temporal bone
Thalamus	Epithalamus Geniculate nucleus Metathalamus Pulvinar
Thoracic Aorta, Ascending/Arch	Aortic arch Ascending aorta
Thoracic Duct	Left jugular trunk Left subclavian trunk
Thoracic Nerve	Intercostal nerve Intercostobrachial nerve Spinal nerve, thoracic Subcostal nerve
Thoracic Spinal Cord	Dorsal root ganglion
Thoracic Sympathetic Nerve	Cardiac plexus Esophageal plexus Greater splanchnic nerve Inferior cardiac nerve Least splanchnic nerve Lesser splanchnic nerve Middle cardiac nerve Pulmonary plexus Superior cardiac nerve Thoracic aortic plexus Thoracic ganglion
Thoracic Vertebra	Spinous process Transverse process Vertebral arch Vertebral body Vertebral foramen Vertebral lamina Vertebral pedicle
Thoracic Vertebral Joint	Costotransverse joint Costovertebral joint Thoracic facet joint
Thoracolumbar Vertebral Joint	Thoracolumbar facet joint

ICD-10-PCS Value	Definition
Thorax Muscle, Left **Thorax Muscle, Right**	Intercostal muscle Levatores costarum muscle Pectoralis major muscle Pectoralis minor muscle Serratus anterior muscle Subclavius muscle Subcostal muscle Transverse thoracis muscle
Thymus	Thymus gland
Thyroid Artery, Left **Thyroid Artery, Right**	Cricothyroid artery Hyoid artery Sternocleidomastoid artery Superior laryngeal artery Superior thyroid artery Thyrocervical trunk
Tibia, Left **Tibia, Right**	Lateral condyle of tibia Medial condyle of tibia Medial malleolus
Tibial Nerve	Lateral plantar nerve Medial plantar nerve Medial popliteal nerve Medial sural cutaneous nerve
Toe Nail	Nail bed Nail plate
Toe Phalangeal Joint, Left **Toe Phalangeal Joint, Right**	Interphalangeal (IP) joint
Tongue	Frenulum linguae
Tongue, Palate, Pharynx Muscle	Chondroglossus muscle Genioglossus muscle Hyoglossus muscle Inferior longitudinal muscle Levator veli palatini muscle Palatoglossal muscle Palatopharyngeal muscle Pharyngeal constrictor muscle Salpingopharyngeus muscle Styloglossus muscle Stylopharyngeus muscle Superior longitudinal muscle Tensor veli palatini muscle
Tonsils	Palatine tonsil
Trachea	Cricoid cartilage
Transverse Colon	Hepatic flexure Splenic flexure
Tricuspid Valve	Right atrioventricular valve Tricuspid annulus
Trigeminal Nerve	Fifth cranial nerve Gasserian ganglion Mandibular nerve Maxillary nerve Ophthalmic nerve Trifacial nerve
Trochlear Nerve	Fourth cranial nerve
Trunk Muscle, Left **Trunk Muscle, Right**	Coccygeus muscle Erector spinae muscle Interspinalis muscle Intertransversarius muscle Latissimus dorsi muscle Quadratus lumborum muscle Rhomboid major muscle Rhomboid minor muscle Serratus posterior muscle Transversospinalis muscle Trapezius muscle
Tympanic Membrane, Left **Tympanic Membrane, Right**	Pars flaccida
Ulna, Left **Ulna, Right**	Olecranon process Radial notch

ICD-10-PCS Value	Definition
Ulnar Artery, Left **Ulnar Artery, Right**	Anterior ulnar recurrent artery Common interosseous artery Posterior ulnar recurrent artery
Ulnar Nerve	Cubital nerve
Upper Arm Muscle, Left **Upper Arm Muscle, Right**	Biceps brachii muscle Brachialis muscle Coracobrachialis muscle Triceps brachii muscle
Upper Artery	Aortic intercostal artery Bronchial artery Esophageal artery Subcostal artery
Upper Eyelid, Left **Upper Eyelid, Right**	Lateral canthus Levator palpebrae superioris muscle Orbicularis oculi muscle Superior tarsal plate
Upper Femur, Left **Upper Femur, Right**	Femoral head Greater trochanter Lesser trochanter Neck of femur
Upper Leg Muscle, Left **Upper Leg Muscle, Right**	Adductor brevis muscle Adductor longus muscle Adductor magnus muscle Biceps femoris muscle Gracilis muscle Pectineus muscle Quadriceps (femoris) Rectus femoris muscle Sartorius muscle Semimembranosus muscle Semitendinosus muscle Vastus intermedius muscle Vastus lateralis muscle Vastus medialis muscle
Upper Lip	Frenulum labii superioris Labial gland Vermilion border
Upper Spine Bursa and Ligament	Interspinous ligament, thoracic Intertransverse ligament, thoracic Ligamentum flavum, thoracic Supraspinous ligament
Ureter **Ureter, Left** **Ureter, Right** **Ureters, Bilateral**	Ureteral orifice Ureterovesical orifice
Urethra	Bulbourethral (Cowper's) gland Cowper's (bulbourethral) gland External urethral sphincter Internal urethral sphincter Membranous urethra Penile urethra Prostatic urethra
Uterine Supporting Structure	Broad ligament Infundibulopelvic ligament Ovarian ligament Round ligament of uterus
Uterus	Fundus uteri Myometrium Perimetrium Uterine cornu
Uvula	Palatine uvula
Vagus Nerve	Anterior vagal trunk Pharyngeal plexus Pneumogastric nerve Posterior vagal trunk Pulmonary plexus Recurrent laryngeal nerve Superior laryngeal nerve Tenth cranial nerve

ICD-10-PCS Value	Definition
Vas Deferens **Vas Deferens, Bilateral** **Vas Deferens, Left** **Vas Deferens, Right**	Ductus deferens Ejaculatory duct
Ventricle, Right	Conus arteriosus
Ventricular Septum	Interventricular septum
Vertebral Artery, Left **Vertebral Artery, Right**	Anterior spinal artery Posterior spinal artery
Vertebral Vein, Left **Vertebral Vein, Right**	Deep cervical vein Suboccipital venous plexus
Vestibular Gland	Bartholin's (greater vestibular) gland Greater vestibular (Bartholin's) gland Paraurethral (Skene's) gland Skene's (paraurethral) gland
Vitreous, Left **Vitreous, Right**	Vitreous body

ICD-10-PCS Value	Definition
Vocal Cord, Left **Vocal Cord, Right**	Vocal fold
Vulva	Labia majora Labia minora
Wrist Bursa and Ligament, Left **Wrist Bursa and Ligament, Right**	Palmar ulnocarpal ligament Radial collateral carpal ligament Radiocarpal ligament Radioulnar ligament Scapholunate ligament Ulnar collateral carpal ligament
Wrist Joint, Left **Wrist Joint, Right**	Distal radioulnar joint Radiocarpal joint

Appendix F: Device Classification

In most PCS codes, the sixth character of the code classifies the device. The sixth character device value "defines the material or appliance used to accomplish the objective of the procedure that remains in or on the procedure site at the end of the procedure." If the device is the means by which the procedural objective is accomplished, then a specific device value is coded in the sixth character. If no device is used to accomplish the objective of the procedure, the device value *No Device* is coded in the sixth character. In limited root operations, the classification provides the qualifier values *Temporary* and *Intraoperative*, for specific procedures involving clinically significant devices whose purpose is brief use during the procedure or current inpatient stay.

Material that is classified as a PCS device is distinguished from material classified as a PCS substance by its having a specific location. A device is intended to maintain a fixed location at the procedure site where it was put, whereas a substance is intended to disperse or be absorbed in the body. There are circumstances in which a device does not stay where it was put and may need to be "revised" in a subsequent procedure to move the device back to its intended location.

Material classified as a PCS device is also distinguishable by the fact that it is removable. Although it may not be practical to remove some types of devices, once they become established at the site, it is physically possible to remove a device for some time after the procedure. A skin graft, for example, once it "takes," may be nearly indistinguishable from the surrounding skin and so is no longer clearly identifiable as a device. Nevertheless, procedures that involve material coded as a device can for the most part be "reversed" by removing the device from the procedure site.

General Device Types

Device Type	Definition	Examples
Grafts	Biological or synthetic material that **takes the place of all or a portion of a body part.**	Full- or partial-thickness skin grafts: • Autologous • Nonautologous • Synthetic • Zooplastic Other tissue grafts: • Bone • Tendon • Vascular
Prosthesis	Biological or synthetic material that **takes the place of all or a portion of a body part.**	Joint prosthesis: • Autologous • Nonautologous • Synthetic
Implants	**Therapeutic** material that is not absorbed by, eliminated by, or incorporated into a body part.	External fixation device Internal fixation device: • Orthopaedic pins • Intramedullary rods Radioactive element implant Mesh
Simple or mechanical appliances	Biological or synthetic material that **assists or prevents a physiological function.**	Drainage device Extraluminal device Endobrachial device Fusion device Intraluminal device (can be temporary) Tracheostomy device IUD
Electronic appliances	Electronic appliances used to **assist, monitor, take the pace of, or prevent a physiological function.**	Cardiac leads Diaphragmatic pacemaker External heart assist system Short-term external heart assist system (Intraoperative) Fetal monitoring Hearing device Monitoring device Neurostimulator
External appliances	Performed without making an incision or a puncture, external appliances are used for the purpose of **protection, immobilization, stretching, compression, or packing.**	Bandage Cast Packing material Pressure dressing Traction apparatus

Transplant/Grafting Tissue Type Terminology

Tissue Type	Terminology
Tissue or organ transferred into a new position in **the body of the same individual**	Autograft Autologous Autoplastic
Having to do with individuals or tissues that have **identical genes**, such as identical twins	Isograft Isologous Syngeneic Syngraft
Tissue or organ taken from **different individuals** of the same species	Allogeneic Allograft Homologous Homograft
Tissue or organ from a **cadaver**	Nonautologous
Tissue or organ from individuals of **different species**	Heterogeneic Heterologous Xenogeneic Xenograft Zooplastic

Appendix G: Device Key and Aggregation Table

This **NT** symbol next to a device in the Term column identifies that the device has been approved for NTAP (new technology add-on payment). CMS provides incremental payment, in addition to the DRG payment, for technologies that have received an NTAP designation.

Device Key

Terms	ICD-10-PCS Value
3f (Aortic) Bioprosthesis valve	Zooplastic Tissue in Heart and Great Vessels
AbioCor® Total Replacement Heart	Synthetic Substitute
Absolute Pro Vascular (OTW) Self-Expanding Stent System	Intraluminal Device
Acculink (RX) Carotid Stent System	Intraluminal Device
Acellular Hydrated Dermis	Nonautologous Tissue Substitute
Acetabular cup	Liner in Lower Joints
Activa PC neurostimulator	Stimulator Generator, Multiple Array for Insertion in Subcutaneous Tissue and Fascia
Activa RC neurostimulator	Stimulator Generator, Multiple Array Rechargeable for Insertion in Subcutaneous Tissue and Fascia
Activa SC neurostimulator	Stimulator Generator, Single Array for Insertion in Subcutaneous Tissue and Fascia
ACUITY™ Steerable Lead	Cardiac Lead, Pacemaker for Insertion in Heart and Great Vessels Cardiac Lead, Defibrillator for Insertion in Heart and Great Vessels
Advisa (MRI)	Pacemaker, Dual Chamber for Insertion in Subcutaneous Tissue and Fascia
AFX® Endovascular AAA System	Intraluminal Device
Alfapump® system	Other Device
AMPLATZER® Muscular VSD Occluder	Synthetic Substitute
AMS 800® Urinary Control System	Artificial Sphincter in Urinary System
AneuRx® AAA Advantage®	Intraluminal Device
Ankle Truss System™ (ATS)	Internal Fixation Device, Open-truss Design in New Technology
Annuloplasty ring	Synthetic Substitute
Aortix™ System	Short-term External Heart Assist System in Heart and Great Vessels
ApiFix® Minimally Invasive Deformity Correction (MID-C) System (C)	Posterior (Dynamic) Distraction Device in New Technology
aprevo™	Interbody Fusion Device, Custom-made Anatomically Designed in New Technology
Articulating Spacer (Antibiotic)	Articulating Spacer in Lower Joints
Artificial anal sphincter (AAS)	Artificial Sphincter in Gastrointestinal System
Artificial bowel sphincter (neosphincter)	Artificial Sphincter in Gastrointestinal System
Artificial urinary sphincter (AUS)	Artificial Sphincter in Urinary System
Ascenda Intrathecal Catheter	Infusion Device
Assurant (Cobalt) stent	Intraluminal Device
AtriClip LAA Exclusion System	Extraluminal Device
Attain Ability® Lead	Cardiac Lead, Pacemaker for Insertion in Heart and Great Vessels Cardiac Lead, Defibrillator for Insertion in Heart and Great Vessels

Terms	ICD-10-PCS Value
Attain StarFix® (OTW) Lead	Cardiac Lead, Pacemaker for Insertion in Heart and Great Vessels Cardiac Lead, Defibrillator for Insertion in Heart and Great Vessels
Autograft	Autologous Tissue Substitute
Autologous artery graft	Autologous Arterial Tissue in Heart and Great Vessels Autologous Arterial Tissue in Upper Arteries Autologous Arterial Tissue in Lower Arteries Autologous Arterial Tissue in Upper Veins Autologous Arterial Tissue in Lower Veins
Autologous vein graft	Autologous Venous Tissue in Heart and Great Vessels Autologous Venous Tissue in Upper Arteries Autologous Venous Tissue in Lower Arteries Autologous Venous Tissue in Upper Veins Autologous Venous Tissue in Lower Veins
Aveir™ AR, as dual chamber	Intracardiac Pacemaker, Dual-Chamber in New Technology
Aveir™ DR, dual chamber	Intracardiac Pacemaker, Dual-Chamber in New Technology
Aveir™ VR, as single chamber	Intracardiac Pacemaker in the Heart and Great Vessels
Axial Lumbar Interbody Fusion System	Interbody Fusion Device in Lower Joints
AxiaLIF® System	Interbody Fusion Device in Lower Joints
BAK/C® Interbody Cervical Fusion System	Interbody Fusion Device in Upper Joints
Bard® Composix® (E/X)(LP) mesh	Synthetic Substitute
Bard® Composix® Kugel® patch	Synthetic Substitute
Bard® Dulex™ mesh	Synthetic Substitute
Bard® Ventralex™ hernia patch	Synthetic Substitute
Baroreflex Activation Therapy® (BAT®)	Stimulator Lead in Upper Arteries Stimulator Generator in Subcutaneous Tissue and Fascia
Barricaid® Annular Closure Device (ACD)	Synthetic Substitute
Berlin Heart Ventricular Assist Device	Implantable Heart Assist System in Heart and Great Vessels
Bioactive embolization coil(s)	Intraluminal Device, Bioactive in Upper Arteries
Biventricular external heart assist system	Short-term External Heart Assist System in Heart and Great Vessels
Blood glucose monitoring system	Monitoring Device
Bone anchored hearing device	Hearing Device, Bone Conduction for Insertion in Ear, Nose, Sinus Hearing Device, in Head and Facial Bones
Bone bank bone graft	Nonautologous Tissue Substitute
Bone screw (interlocking)(lag)(pedicle) (recessed)	Internal Fixation Device in Head and Facial Bones Internal Fixation Device in Upper Bones Internal Fixation Device in Lower Bones
Bovine pericardial valve	Zooplastic Tissue in Heart and Great Vessels
Bovine pericardium graft	Zooplastic Tissue in Heart and Great Vessels
Brachytherapy seeds	Radioactive Element
BRYAN® Cervical Disc System	Synthetic Substitute
BVS 5000 Ventricular Assist Device	Short-term External Heart Assist System in Heart and Great Vessels

Terms	ICD-10-PCS Value
Canturio™ te (Tibial Extension)	Tibial Extension with Motion Sensors in New Technology
Cardiac contractility modulation lead	Cardiac Lead in Heart and Great Vessels
Cardiac event recorder	Monitoring Device
Cardiac resynchronization therapy (CRT) lead	Cardiac Lead, Pacemaker for Insertion in Heart and Great Vessels Cardiac Lead, Defibrillator for Insertion in Heart and Great Vessels
CardioMEMS® pressure sensor	Monitoring Device, Pressure Sensor for Insertion in Heart and Great Vessels
Carmat total artificial heart (TAH)	Biologic with Synthetic Substitute, Autoregulated Electrohydraulic for Replacement in Heart and Great Vessels
Carotid (artery) sinus (baroreceptor) lead	Stimulator Lead in Upper Arteries
Carotid WALLSTENT® Monorail® Endoprosthesis	Intraluminal Device
Centrimag® Blood Pump	Short-term External Heart Assist System in Heart and Great Vessels
Ceramic on ceramic bearing surface	Synthetic Substitute, Ceramic for Replacement in Lower Joints
Cesium-131 Collagen Implant	Radioactive Element, Cesium-131 Collagen Implant for Insertion in Central Nervous System and Cranial Nerves
CivaSheet®	Radioactive Element
Clamp and rod internal fixation system (CRIF)	Internal Fixation Device in Upper Bones Internal Fixation Device in Lower Bones
COALESCE® radiolucent interbody fusion device	Interbody Fusion Device in Upper Joints Interbody Fusion Device in Lower Joints
CoAxia NeuroFlo catheter	Intraluminal Device
Cobalt/chromium head and polyethylene socket	Synthetic Substitute, Metal on Polyethylene for Replacement in Lower Joints
Cobalt/chromium head and socket	Synthetic Substitute, Metal for Replacement in Lower Joints
Cochlear implant (CI), multiple channel (electrode)	Hearing Device, Multiple Channel Cochlear Prosthesis for Insertion in Ear, Nose, Sinus
Cochlear implant (CI), single channel (electrode)	Hearing Device, Single Channel Cochlear Prosthesis for Insertion in Ear, Nose, Sinus
COGNIS® CRT-D	Cardiac Resynchronization Defibrillator Pulse Generator for Insertion in Subcutaneous Tissue and Fascia
COHERE® radiolucent interbody fusion device	Interbody Fusion Device in Upper Joints Interbody Fusion Device in Lower Joints
Colonic Z-Stent®	Intraluminal Device
Complete (SE) stent	Intraluminal Device
Concerto II CRT-D	Cardiac Resynchronization Defibrillator Pulse Generator for Insertion in Subcutaneous Tissue and Fascia
CONSERVE® PLUS Total Resurfacing Hip System	Resurfacing Device in Lower Joints
Consulta CRT-D	Cardiac Resynchronization Defibrillator Pulse Generator for Insertion in Subcutaneous Tissue and Fascia
Consulta CRT-P	Cardiac Resynchronization Pacemaker Pulse Generator for Insertion in Subcutaneous Tissue and Fascia
CONTAK RENEWAL® 3 RF (HE) CRT-D	Cardiac Resynchronization Defibrillator Pulse Generator for Insertion in Subcutaneous Tissue and Fascia
Contegra Pulmonary Valved Conduit	Zooplastic Tissue in Heart and Great Vessels
Continuous Glucose Monitoring (CGM) device	Monitoring Device
Cook Biodesign® Fistula Plug(s)	Nonautologous Tissue Substitute
Cook Biodesign® Hernia Graft(s)	Nonautologous Tissue Substitute

Terms	ICD-10-PCS Value
Cook Biodesign® Layered Graft(s)	Nonautologous Tissue Substitute
Cook Zenapro™ Layered Graft(s)	Nonautologous Tissue Substitute
Cook Zenith AAA Endovascular Graft	Intraluminal Device
Cook Zenith® Fenestrated AAA Endovascular Graft	Intraluminal Device, Branched or Fenestrated, One or Two Arteries for Restriction in Lower Arteries Intraluminal Device, Branched or Fenestrated, Three or More Arteries for Restriction in Lower Arteries
CoreValve transcatheter aortic valve	Zooplastic Tissue in Heart and Great Vessels
Cormet Hip Resurfacing System	Resurfacing Device in Lower Joints
CoRoent® XL	Interbody Fusion Device in Lower Joints
Corox (OTW) Bipolar Lead	Cardiac Lead, Pacemaker for Insertion in Heart and Great Vessels Cardiac Lead, Defibrillator for Insertion in Heart and Great Vessels
Cortical strip neurostimulator lead	Neurostimulator Lead in Central Nervous System and Cranial Nerves
Corvia IASD®	Synthetic Substitute
Cultured epidermal cell autograft	Autologous Tissue Substitute
CYPHER® Stent	Intraluminal Device, Drug-eluting in Heart and Great Vessels
Cystostomy tube	Drainage Device
DBS lead	Neurostimulator Lead in Central Nervous System and Cranial Nerves
DeBakey Left Ventricular Assist Device	Implantable Heart Assist System in Heart and Great Vessels
Deep brain neurostimulator lead	Neurostimulator Lead in Central Nervous System and Cranial Nerves
Delta frame external fixator	External Fixation Device, Hybrid for Insertion in Upper Bones External Fixation Device, Hybrid for Reposition in Upper Bones External Fixation Device, Hybrid for Insertion in Lower Bones External Fixation Device, Hybrid for Reposition in Lower Bones
Delta III Reverse shoulder prosthesis	Synthetic Substitute, Reverse Ball and Socket for Replacement in Upper Joints
DETOUR® System	Conduit through Femoral Vein to Popliteal Artery in New Technology Conduit through Femoral Vein to Superficial Femoral Artery in New Technology
Diaphragmatic pacemaker generator	Stimulator Generator in Subcutaneous Tissue and Fascia
Direct Lateral Interbody Fusion (DLIF) device	Interbody Fusion Device in Lower Joints
Driver stent (RX) (OTW)	Intraluminal Device
DuraHeart Left Ventricular Assist System	Implantable Heart Assist System in Heart and Great Vessels
Durata® Defibrillation Lead	Cardiac Lead, Defibrillator for Insertion in Heart and Great Vessels
DynaClip® (Forte)	Internal Fixation Device, Sustained Compression for Fusion in Upper Joints Internal Fixation Device, Sustained Compression for Fusion in Lower Joints
DynaNail® (Helix) (Hybrid) (Mini)	Internal Fixation Device, Sustained Compression for Fusion in Upper Joints Internal Fixation Device, Sustained Compression for Fusion in Lower Joints

Appendix G: Device Key and Aggregation Table

Terms	ICD-10-PCS Value
Dynesys® Dynamic Stabilization System	Spinal Stabilization Device, Pedicle-Based for Insertion in Upper Joints Spinal Stabilization Device, Pedicle-Based for Insertion in Lower Joints
E-Luminexx™ (Biliary) (Vascular) Stent	Intraluminal Device
Electrical bone growth stimulator (EBGS)	Bone Growth Stimulator in Head and Facial Bones Bone Growth Stimulator in Upper Bones Bone Growth Stimulator in Lower Bones
Electrical muscle stimulation (EMS) lead	Stimulator Lead in Muscles
Electronic muscle stimulator lead	Stimulator Lead in Muscles
Eluvia™ Drug-eluting Vascular Stent System	Intraluminal Device, Sustained Release Drug-eluting in New Technology Intraluminal Device, Sustained Release Drug-eluting, Two in New Technology Intraluminal Device, Sustained Release Drug-eluting, Three in New Technology Intraluminal Device, Sustained Release Drug-eluting, Four or More in New Technology
Embolization coil(s)	Intraluminal Device
Endeavor® (III) (IV) (Sprint) Zotarolimus-eluting Coronary Stent System	Intraluminal Device, Drug-eluting in Heart and Great Vessels
Endologix AFX® Endovascular AAA System	Intraluminal Device
EndoSure® sensor	Monitoring Device, Pressure Sensor for Insertion in Heart and Great Vessels
ENDOTAK RELIANCE® (G) Defibrillation Lead	Cardiac Lead, Defibrillator for Insertion in Heart and Great Vessels
Endotracheal tube (cuffed) (double-lumen)	Intraluminal Device, Endotracheal Airway in Respiratory System
Endurant® Endovascular Stent Graft	Intraluminal Device
Endurant® II AAA stent graft system	Intraluminal Device
EnRhythm	Pacemaker, Dual Chamber for Insertion in Subcutaneous Tissue and Fascia
Enterra gastric neurostimulator	Stimulator Generator, Multiple Array for Insertion in Subcutaneous Tissue and Fascia
Epic™ Stented Tissue Valve (aortic)	Zooplastic Tissue in Heart and Great Vessels
Epicel® cultured epidermal autograft	Autologous Tissue Substitute
Esophageal obturator airway (EOA)	Intraluminal Device, Airway in Gastrointestinal System
Esteem® implantable hearing system	Hearing Device in Ear, Nose, Sinus
EV ICD System (Extravascular implantable defibrillator lead)	Defibrillator Lead in Anatomical Regions, General
Evera (XT)(S)(DR/VR)	Defibrillator Generator for Insertion in Subcutaneous Tissue and Fascia
Everolimus-eluting coronary stent	Intraluminal Device, Drug-eluting in Heart and Great Vessels
Ex-PRESS™ mini glaucoma shunt	Synthetic Substitute
EXCLUDER® AAA Endoprosthesis	Intraluminal Device Intraluminal Device, Branched or Fenestrated, One or Two Arteries for Restriction in Lower Arteries Intraluminal Device, Branched or Fenestrated, Three or More Arteries for Restriction in Lower Arteries

Terms	ICD-10-PCS Value
EXCLUDER® IBE Endoprosthesis	Intraluminal Device, Branched or Fenestrated, One or Two Arteries for Restriction in Lower Arteries
Express® (LD) Premounted Stent System	Intraluminal Device
Express® Biliary SD Monorail® Premounted Stent System	Intraluminal Device
Express® SD Renal Monorail® Premounted Stent System	Intraluminal Device
External fixator	External Fixation Device in Head and Facial Bones External Fixation Device in Upper Bones External Fixation Device in Lower Bones External Fixation Device in Upper Joints External Fixation Device in Lower Joints
EXtreme Lateral Interbody Fusion (XLIF) device	Interbody Fusion Device in Lower Joints
Facet replacement spinal stabilization device	Spinal Stabilization Device, Facet Replacement for Insertion in Upper Joints Spinal Stabilization Device, Facet Replacement for Insertion in Lower Joints
FLAIR® Endovascular Stent Graft	Intraluminal Device
Flexible Composite Mesh	Synthetic Substitute
Flourish® Pediatric Esophageal Atresia Device	Magnetic Lengthening Device in Gastrointestinal System
Flow Diverter embolization device	Intraluminal Device, Flow Diverter for Restriction in Upper Arteries
Foley catheter	Drainage Device
Formula™ Balloon-Expandable Renal Stent System	Intraluminal Device
Freestyle (Stentless) Aortic Root Bioprosthesis	Zooplastic Tissue in Heart and Great Vessels
Fusion screw (compression)(lag)(locking)	Internal Fixation Device in Upper Joints Internal Fixation Device in Lower Joints
GammaTile™	Radioactive Element, Cesium-131 Collagen Implant for Insertion in Central Nervous System and Cranial Nerves
Gastric electrical stimulation (GES) lead	Stimulator Lead in Gastrointestinal System
Gastric pacemaker lead	Stimulator Lead in Gastrointestinal System
GORE EXCLUDER® AAA Endoprosthesis	Intraluminal Device Intraluminal Device, Branched or Fenestrated, One or Two Arteries for Restriction in Lower Arteries Intraluminal Device, Branched or Fenestrated, Three or More Arteries for Restriction in Lower Arteries
GORE EXCLUDER® IBE Endoprosthesis	Intraluminal Device, Branched or Fenestrated, One or Two Arteries for Restriction in Lower Arteries
GORE TAG® Thoracic Endoprosthesis [NT]	Intraluminal Device
GORE® DUALMESH®	Synthetic Substitute
Guedel airway	Intraluminal Device, Airway in Mouth and Throat
Hancock Bioprosthesis (aortic)(mitral) valve	Zooplastic Tissue in Heart and Great Vessels
Hancock Bioprosthetic Valved Conduit	Zooplastic Tissue in Heart and Great Vessels
HeartMate 3™ LVAS	Implantable Heart Assist System in Heart and Great Vessels
HeartMate II® Left Ventricular Assist Device (LVAD)	Implantable Heart Assist System in Heart and Great Vessels
HeartMate XVE® Left Ventricular Assist Device (LVAD)	Implantable Heart Assist System in Heart and Great Vessels

Terms	ICD-10-PCS Value
Herculink (RX) Elite Renal Stent System	Intraluminal Device
Hip (joint) liner	Liner in Lower Joints
Holter valve ventricular shunt	Synthetic Substitute
IASD® (InterAtrial Shunt Device), Corvia	Synthetic Substitute
iFuse Bedrock™ Granite Implant System **NT**	Internal Fixation Device with Tulip Connector in New Technology
Ilizarov external fixator	External Fixation Device, Ring for Insertion in Upper Bones External Fixation Device, Ring for Reposition in Upper Bones External Fixation Device, Ring for Insertion in Lower Bones External Fixation Device, Ring for Reposition in Lower Bones
Ilizarov-Vecklich device	External Fixation Device, Limb Lengthening for Insertion in Upper Bones External Fixation Device, Limb Lengthening for Insertion in Lower Bones
Impella® 5.5 with SmartAssist® System	Conduit To Short-term External Heart Assist System in New Technology
Impella® heart pump	Short-term External Heart Assist System in Heart and Great Vessels
Implantable cardioverter-defibrillator (ICD)	Defibrillator Generator for Insertion in Subcutaneous Tissue and Fascia
Implantable drug infusion pump (anti-spasmodic) (chemotherapy)(pain)	Infusion Device, Pump in Subcutaneous Tissue and Fascia
Implantable glucose monitoring device	Monitoring Device
Implantable hemodynamic monitor (IHM)	Monitoring Device, Hemodynamic for Insertion in Subcutaneous Tissue and Fascia
Implantable hemodynamic monitoring system (IHMS)	Monitoring Device, Hemodynamic for Insertion in Subcutaneous Tissue and Fascia
Implantable Miniature Telescope™ (IMT)	Synthetic Substitute, Intraocular Telescope for Replacement in Eye
Implanted (venous)(access) port	Vascular Access Device, Totally Implantable in Subcutaneous Tissue and Fascia
InDura, intrathecal catheter (1P) (spinal)	Infusion Device
Injection reservoir, port	Vascular Access Device, Totally Implantable in Subcutaneous Tissue and Fascia
Injection reservoir, pump	Infusion Device, Pump in Subcutaneous Tissue and Fascia
Intellis™ neurostimulator	Stimulator Generator, Multiple Array Rechargeable for Insertion in Subcutaneous Tissue and Fascia
InterAtrial Shunt Device IASD®, Corvia	Synthetic Substitute
Interbody fusion (spine) cage	Interbody Fusion Device in Upper Joints Interbody Fusion Device in Lower Joints
Interspinous process spinal stabilization device	Spinal Stabilization Device, Interspinous Process for Insertion in Upper Joints Spinal Stabilization Device, Interspinous Process for Insertion in Lower Joints
InterStim™ Micro Therapy neurostimulator	Stimulator Generator, Single Array Rechargeable for Insertion in Subcutaneous Tissue and Fascia
InterStim® Therapy lead	Neurostimulator Lead in Peripheral Nervous System
InterStim™ II Therapy neurostimulator	Stimulator Generator, Single Array for Insertion in Subcutaneous Tissue and Fascia

Terms	ICD-10-PCS Value
Intramedullary (IM) rod (nail)	Internal Fixation Device, Intramedullary in Upper Bones Internal Fixation Device, Intramedullary in Lower Bones
Intramedullary skeletal kinetic distractor (ISKD)	Internal Fixation Device, Intramedullary in Upper Bones Internal Fixation Device, Intramedullary in Lower Bones
Intrauterine Device (IUD)	Contraceptive Device in Female Reproductive System
Ischemic Stroke System (ISS500)	Neurostimulator Lead in New Technology
ISS500 (Ischemic Stroke System)	Neurostimulator Lead in New Technology
Itrel (3)(4) neurostimulator	Stimulator Generator, Single Array for Insertion in Subcutaneous Tissue and Fascia
Joint fixation plate	Internal Fixation Device in Upper Joints Internal Fixation Device in Lower Joints
Joint liner (insert)	Liner in Lower Joints
Joint spacer (antibiotic)	Spacer in Upper Joints Spacer in Lower Joints
Kappa	Pacemaker, Dual Chamber for Insertion in Subcutaneous Tissue and Fascia
Kirschner wire (K-wire)	Internal Fixation Device in Head and Facial Bones Internal Fixation Device in Upper Bones Internal Fixation Device in Lower Bones Internal Fixation Device in Upper Joints Internal Fixation Device in Lower Joints
Knee (implant) insert	Liner in Lower Joints
Kuntscher nail	Internal Fixation Device, Intramedullary in Upper Bones Internal Fixation Device, Intramedullary in Lower Bones
LAP-BAND® adjustable gastric banding system	Extraluminal Device
LifeStent® (Flexstar)(XL) Vascular Stent System	Intraluminal Device
LigaPASS 2.0™ PJK Prevention System	Posterior Vertebral Tether in New Technology
LIVIAN™ CRT-D	Cardiac Resynchronization Defibrillator Pulse Generator for Insertion in Subcutaneous Tissue and Fascia
Longeviti ClearFit® Cranial Implant	Synthetic Substitute, Ultrasound Penetrable in New Technology
Longeviti ClearFit® OTS Cranial Implant	Synthetic Substitute, Ultrasound Penetrable in New Technology
Loop recorder, implantable	Monitoring Device
MAGEC® Spinal Bracing and Distraction System	Magnetically Controlled Growth Rod(s) in New Technology
Mark IV Breathing Pacemaker System	Stimulator Generator in Subcutaneous Tissue and Fascia
Maximo II DR (VR)	Defibrillator Generator for Insertion in Subcutaneous Tissue and Fascia
Maximo II DR CRT-D	Cardiac Resynchronization Defibrillator Pulse Generator for Insertion in Subcutaneous Tissue and Fascia
Medtronic Endurant® II AAA stent graft system	Intraluminal Device
Melody® transcatheter pulmonary valve	Zooplastic Tissue in Heart and Great Vessels
Metal on metal bearing surface	Synthetic Substitute, Metal for Replacement in Lower Joints
Micro-Driver stent (RX) (OTW)	Intraluminal Device
MicroMed HeartAssist	Implantable Heart Assist System in Heart and Great Vessels

Appendix G: Device Key and Aggregation Table

Terms	ICD-10-PCS Value
Micrus CERECYTE microcoil	Intraluminal Device, Bioactive in Upper Arteries
MIRODERM™ Biologic Wound Matrix	Nonautologous Tissue Substitute
MitraClip valve repair system	Synthetic Substitute
Mitroflow® Aortic Pericardial Heart Valve	Zooplastic Tissue in Heart and Great Vessels
Mosaic Bioprosthesis (aortic) (mitral) valve	Zooplastic Tissue in Heart and Great Vessels
MULTI-LINK (VISION)(MINI-VISION)(ULTRA) Coronary Stent System	Intraluminal Device
nanoLOCK™ interbody fusion device	Interbody Fusion Device in Upper Joints Interbody Fusion Device in Lower Joints
Nasopharyngeal airway (NPA)	Intraluminal Device, Airway in Ear, Nose, Sinus
Neovasc Reducer™	Reduction Device in New Technology
Neuromuscular electrical stimulation (NEMS) lead	Stimulator Lead in Muscles
Neurostimulator generator, multiple channel	Stimulator Generator, Multiple Array for Insertion in Subcutaneous Tissue and Fascia
Neurostimulator generator, multiple channel rechargeable	Stimulator Generator, Multiple Array Rechargeable for Insertion in Subcutaneous Tissue and Fascia
Neurostimulator generator, single channel	Stimulator Generator, Single Array for Insertion in Subcutaneous Tissue and Fascia
Neurostimulator generator, single channel rechargeable	Stimulator Generator, Single Array Rechargeable for Insertion in Subcutaneous Tissue and Fascia
Neutralization plate	Internal Fixation Device in Head and Facial Bones Internal Fixation Device in Upper Bones Internal Fixation Device in Lower Bones
Nitinol framed polymer mesh	Synthetic Substitute
Non-tunneled central venous catheter	Infusion Device
Novacor Left Ventricular Assist Device	Implantable Heart Assist System in Heart and Great Vessels
Novation® Ceramic AHS® (Articulation Hip System)	Synthetic Substitute, Ceramic for Replacement in Lower Joints
NUsurface® Meniscus Implant	Synthetic Substitute, Lateral Meniscus in New Technology Synthetic Substitute, Medial Meniscus in New Technology
Omnilink Elite Vascular Balloon Expandable Stent System	Intraluminal Device
Open Pivot Aortic Valve Graft (AVG)	Synthetic Substitute
Open Pivot (mechanical) Valve	Synthetic Substitute
Optimizer™ III implantable pulse generator	Contractility Modulation Device for Insertion in Subcutaneous Tissue and Fascia
Oropharyngeal airway (OPA)	Intraluminal Device, Airway in Mouth and Throat
Ovatio™ CRT-D	Cardiac Resynchronization Defibrillator Pulse Generator for Insertion in Subcutaneous Tissue and Fascia
OXINIUM	Synthetic Substitute, Oxidized Zirconium on Polyethylene for Replacement in Lower Joints
Paclitaxel-eluting coronary stent	Intraluminal Device, Drug-eluting in Heart and Great Vessels
Paclitaxel-eluting peripheral stent	Intraluminal Device, Drug-eluting in Upper Arteries Intraluminal Device, Drug-eluting in Lower Arteries
Partially absorbable mesh	Synthetic Substitute

Terms	ICD-10-PCS Value
Pedicle-based dynamic stabilization device	Spinal Stabilization Device, Pedicle-Based for Insertion in Upper Joints Spinal Stabilization Device, Pedicle-Based for Insertion in Lower Joints
PERCEPT™ PC neurostimulator	Stimulator Generator, Multiple Array for Insertion in Subcutaneous Tissue and Fascia
Percutaneous endoscopic gastrojejunostomy (PEG/J) tube	Feeding Device in Gastrointestinal System
Percutaneous endoscopic gastrostomy (PEG) tube	Feeding Device in Gastrointestinal System
Percutaneous nephrostomy catheter	Drainage Device
Peripherally inserted central catheter (PICC)	Infusion Device
Pessary ring	Intraluminal Device, Pessary in Female Reproductive System
Phrenic nerve stimulator generator	Stimulator Generator in Subcutaneous Tissue and Fascia
Phrenic nerve stimulator lead	Diaphragmatic Pacemaker Lead in Respiratory System
PHYSIOMESH™ Flexible Composite Mesh	Synthetic Substitute
Pipeline™ (Flex) embolization device	Intraluminal Device, Flow Diverter for Restriction in Upper Arteries
Polyethylene socket	Synthetic Substitute, Polyethylene for Replacement in Lower Joints
Polymethylmethacrylate (PMMA)	Synthetic Substitute
Polypropylene mesh	Synthetic Substitute
Porcine (bioprosthetic) valve	Zooplastic Tissue in Heart and Great Vessels
PRECICE intramedullary limb lengthening system	Internal Fixation Device, Intramedullary Limb Lengthening for Insertion in Upper Bones Internal Fixation Device, Intramedullary Limb Lengthening for Insertion in Lower Bones
PRESTIGE® Cervical Disc	Synthetic Substitute
PrimeAdvanced neurostimulator (SureScan)(MRI Safe)	Stimulator Generator, Multiple Array for Insertion in Subcutaneous Tissue and Fascia
PROCEED™ Ventral Patch	Synthetic Substitute
Prodisc-C	Synthetic Substitute
Prodisc-L	Synthetic Substitute
PROLENE Polypropylene Hernia System (PHS)	Synthetic Substitute
Protecta XT CRT-D	Cardiac Resynchronization Defibrillator Pulse Generator for Insertion in Subcutaneous Tissue and Fascia
Protecta XT DR (XT VR)	Defibrillator Generator for Insertion in Subcutaneous Tissue and Fascia
Protégé® RX Carotid Stent System	Intraluminal Device
Pump reservoir	Infusion Device, Pump in Subcutaneous Tissue and Fascia
REALIZE® Adjustable Gastric Band	Extraluminal Device
Rebound HRD® (Hernia Repair Device)	Synthetic Substitute
Reducer™ System	Reduction Device in New Technology
RestoreAdvanced neurostimulator (SureScan)(MRI Safe)	Stimulator Generator, Multiple Array Rechargeable for Insertion in Subcutaneous Tissue and Fascia
RestoreSensor neurostimulator (SureScan)(MRI Safe)	Stimulator Generator, Multiple Array Rechargeable for Insertion in Subcutaneous Tissue and Fascia

Terms	ICD-10-PCS Value
RestoreUltra neurostimulator (SureScan)(MRI Safe)	Stimulator Generator, Multiple Array Rechargeable for Insertion in Subcutaneous Tissue and Fascia
Reveal (LINQ)(DX)(XT)	Monitoring Device
Reverse® Shoulder Prosthesis	Synthetic Substitute, Reverse Ball and Socket for Replacement in Upper Joints
Revo MRI™ SureScan® pacemaker	Pacemaker, Dual Chamber for Insertion in Subcutaneous Tissue and Fascia
Rheos® System device	Stimulator Generator in Subcutaneous Tissue and Fascia
Rheos® System lead	Stimulator Lead in Upper Arteries
RNS System lead	Neurostimulator Lead in Central Nervous System and Cranial Nerves
RNS system neurostimulator generator	Neurostimulator Generator in Head and Facial Bones
S-ICD™ lead	Subcutaneous Defibrillator Lead in Subcutaneous Tissue and Fascia
Sacral nerve modulation (SNM) lead	Stimulator Lead in Urinary System
Sacral neuromodulation lead	Stimulator Lead in Urinary System
SAPIEN transcatheter aortic valve	Zooplastic Tissue in Heart and Great Vessels
SAVAL below-the-knee (BTK) drug-eluting stent system	Intraluminal Device, Sustained Release Drug-eluting in New Technology Intraluminal Device, Sustained Release Drug-eluting, Two in New Technology Intraluminal Device, Sustained Release Drug-eluting, Three in New Technology Intraluminal Device, Sustained Release Drug-eluting, Four or More in New Technology
Secura (DR) (VR)	Defibrillator Generator for Insertion in Subcutaneous Tissue and Fascia
Sheffield hybrid external fixator	External Fixation Device, Hybrid for Insertion in Upper Bones External Fixation Device, Hybrid for Reposition in Upper Bones External Fixation Device, Hybrid for Insertion in Lower Bones External Fixation Device, Hybrid for Reposition in Lower Bones
Sheffield ring external fixator	External Fixation Device, Ring for Insertion in Upper Bones External Fixation Device, Ring for Reposition in Upper Bones External Fixation Device, Ring for Insertion in Lower Bones External Fixation Device, Ring for Reposition in Lower Bones
Single lead pacemaker (atrium)(ventricle)	Pacemaker, Single Chamber for Insertion in Subcutaneous Tissue and Fascia
Single lead rate responsive pacemaker (atrium)(ventricle)	Pacemaker, Single Chamber Rate Responsive for Insertion in Subcutaneous Tissue and Fascia
Sirolimus-eluting coronary stent	Intraluminal Device, Drug-eluting in Heart and Great Vessels
SJM Biocor® Stented Valve System	Zooplastic Tissue in Heart and Great Vessels
Spacer, Articulating (Antibiotic)	Articulating Spacer in Lower Joints
Spacer, Static (Antibiotic)	Spacer in Lower Joints
Spinal cord neurostimulator lead	Neurostimulator Lead in Central Nervous System and Cranial Nerves
Spinal growth rods, magnetically controlled	Magnetically Controlled Growth Rod(s) in New Technology
SpineJack® system	Synthetic Substitute, Mechanically Expandable (Paired) in New Technology

Terms	ICD-10-PCS Value
Spiration IBV™ Valve System	Intraluminal Device, Endobronchial Valve in Respiratory System
Static Spacer (Antibiotic)	Spacer in Lower Joints
Stent, intraluminal (cardiovascular) (gastrointestinal) (hepatobiliary)(urinary)	Intraluminal Device
Stented tissue valve	Zooplastic Tissue in Heart and Great Vessels
Stratos LV	Cardiac Resynchronization Pacemaker Pulse Generator for Insertion in Subcutaneous Tissue and Fascia
Subcutaneous injection reservoir, port	Vascular Access Device, Totally Implantable in Subcutaneous Tissue and Fascia
Subcutaneous injection reservoir, pump	Infusion Device, Pump in Subcutaneous Tissue and Fascia
Subdermal progesterone implant	Contraceptive Device in Subcutaneous Tissue and Fascia
Surpass Streamline™ Flow Diverter	Intraluminal Device, Flow Diverter for Restriction in Upper Arteries
SynCardia (temporary) Total Artificial Heart (TAH)	Synthetic Substitute, Pneumatic for Replacement in Heart and Great Vessels
SynCardia Total Artificial Heart	Synthetic Substitute
Synchra CRT-P	Cardiac Resynchronization Pacemaker Pulse Generator for Insertion in Subcutaneous Tissue and Fascia
SynchroMed Pump	Infusion Device, Pump in Subcutaneous Tissue and Fascia
Talent® Converter	Intraluminal Device
Talent® Occluder	Intraluminal Device
Talent® Stent Graft (abdominal)(thoracic)	Intraluminal Device
TandemHeart® System	Short-term External Heart Assist System in Heart and Great Vessels
TAXUS® Liberté® Paclitaxel-eluting Coronary Stent System	Intraluminal Device, Drug-eluting in Heart and Great Vessels
Therapeutic occlusion coil(s)	Intraluminal Device
Thoracostomy tube	Drainage Device
Thoraflex™ Hybrid device **NT**	Branched Synthetic Substitute with Intraluminal Device in New Technology
Thoratec IVAD (Implantable Ventricular Assist Device)	Implantable Heart Assist System in Heart and Great Vessels
Thoratec Paracorporeal Ventricular Assist Device	Short-term External Heart Assist System in Heart and Great Vessels
Tibial insert	Liner in Lower Joints
Tissue bank graft	Nonautologous Tissue Substitute
Tissue expander (inflatable)(injectable)	Tissue Expander in Skin and Breast Tissue Expander in Subcutaneous Tissue and Fascia
Titan Endoskeleton™	Interbody Fusion Device in Upper Joints Interbody Fusion Device in Lower Joints
Titanium Sternal Fixation System (TSFS)	Internal Fixation Device, Rigid Plate for Insertion in Upper Bones Internal Fixation Device, Rigid Plate for Reposition in Upper Bones
TOPS™ System	Posterior Spinal Motion Preservation Device in New Technology
Total Ankle Talar Replacement™ (TATR)	Synthetic Substitute, Talar Prosthesis in New Technology
Total artificial (replacement) heart	Synthetic Substitute
Tracheostomy tube	Tracheostomy Device in Respiratory System
TricValve® Transcatheter Bicaval Valve System	Intraluminal Device, Bioprosthetic Valve in New Technology
Trifecta™ Valve (aortic)	Zooplastic Tissue in Heart and Great Vessels

Appendix G: Device Key and Aggregation Table

Terms	ICD-10-PCS Value
Tunneled central venous catheter	Vascular Access Device, Tunneled in Subcutaneous Tissue and Fascia
Tunneled spinal (intrathecal) catheter	Infusion Device
Two lead pacemaker	Pacemaker, Dual Chamber for Insertion in Subcutaneous Tissue and Fascia
Ultraflex™ Precision Colonic Stent System	Intraluminal Device
ULTRAPRO Hernia System (UHS)	Synthetic Substitute
ULTRAPRO Partially Absorbable Lightweight Mesh	Synthetic Substitute
ULTRAPRO Plug	Synthetic Substitute
Ultrasonic osteogenic stimulator	Bone Growth Stimulator in Head and Facial Bones Bone Growth Stimulator in Upper Bones Bone Growth Stimulator in Lower Bones
Ultrasound bone healing system	Bone Growth Stimulator in Head and Facial Bones Bone Growth Stimulator in Upper Bones Bone Growth Stimulator in Lower Bones
Uniplanar external fixator	External Fixation Device, Monoplanar for Insertion in Upper Bones External Fixation Device, Monoplanar for Reposition in Upper Bones External Fixation Device, Monoplanar for Insertion in Lower Bones External Fixation Device, Monoplanar for Reposition in Lower Bones
Urinary incontinence stimulator lead	Stimulator Lead in Urinary System
V-Wave Interatrial Shunt System	Synthetic Substitute
Vaginal pessary	Intraluminal Device, Pessary in Female Reproductive System
Valiant Thoracic Stent Graft	Intraluminal Device
Vanta™ PC neurostimulator	Stimulator Generator, Multiple Array for Insertion in Subcutaneous Tissue and Fascia
VasQ™ External Support device	Synthetic Substitute, Extraluminal Support Device in New Technology
Vectra® Vascular Access Graft	Vascular Access Device, Tunneled in Subcutaneous Tissue and Fascia
VenoValve®	Intraluminal Device, Bioprosthetic Valve in New Technology
Ventrio™ Hernia Patch	Synthetic Substitute

Terms	ICD-10-PCS Value
Versa	Pacemaker, Dual Chamber for Insertion in Subcutaneous Tissue and Fascia
VEST™ Venous External Support device	Vein Graft Extraluminal Support Device(s) in New Technology
Virtuoso (II) (DR) (VR)	Defibrillator Generator for Insertion in Subcutaneous Tissue and Fascia
Viva(XT)(S)	Cardiac Resynchronization Defibrillator Pulse Generator for Insertion in Subcutaneous Tissue and Fascia
Vivistim® Paired VNS System Lead **NT**	Neurostimulator Lead with Paired Stimulation System in New Technology
WALLSTENT® Endoprosthesis	Intraluminal Device
X-Spine Axle Cage	Spinal Stabilization Device, Interspinous Process for Insertion in Upper Joints Spinal Stabilization Device, Interspinous Process for Insertion in Lower Joints
X-STOP® Spacer	Spinal Stabilization Device, Interspinous Process for Insertion in Upper Joints Spinal Stabilization Device, Interspinous Process for Insertion in Lower Joints
Xact Carotid Stent System	Intraluminal Device
Xenograft	Zooplastic Tissue in Heart and Great Vessels
XIENCE Everolimus Eluting Coronary Stent System	Intraluminal Device, Drug-eluting in Heart and Great Vessels
XLIF® System	Interbody Fusion Device in Lower Joints
Zenith AAA Endovascular Graft	Intraluminal Device
Zenith® Fenestrated AAA Endovascular Graft	Intraluminal Device, Branched or Fenestrated, One or Two Arteries for Restriction in Lower Arteries Intraluminal Device, Branched or Fenestrated, Three or More Arteries for Restriction in Lower Arteries
Zenith Flex® AAA Endovascular Graft	Intraluminal Device
Zenith® Renu™ AAA Ancillary Graft	Intraluminal Device
Zenith TX2® TAA Endovascular Graft	Intraluminal Device
Zilver® PTX® (paclitaxel) Drug-Eluting Peripheral Stent	Intraluminal Device, Drug-eluting in Upper Arteries Intraluminal Device, Drug-eluting in Lower Arteries
Zimmer® NexGen® LPS Mobile Bearing Knee	Synthetic Substitute
Zimmer® NexGen® LPS-Flex Mobile Knee	Synthetic Substitute
Zotarolimus-eluting coronary stent	Intraluminal Device, Drug-eluting in Heart and Great Vessels

Device Aggregation Table

This table crosswalks specific device character value definitions for specific root operations in a specific body system to the more general device character value to be used when the root operation covers a wide range of body parts and the device character represents an entire family of devices.

Specific Device	for Operation	in Body System	General Device	
Autologous Arterial Tissue (A)	All applicable	Heart and Great Vessels Lower Arteries Lower Veins Upper Arteries Upper Veins	7	Autologous Tissue Substitute
Autologous Venous Tissue (9)	All applicable	Heart and Great Vessels Lower Arteries Lower Veins Upper Arteries Upper Veins	7	Autologous Tissue Substitute
Cardiac Lead, Defibrillator (K)	Insertion	Heart and Great Vessels	M	Cardiac Lead
Cardiac Lead, Pacemaker (J)	Insertion	Heart and Great Vessels	M	Cardiac Lead
Cardiac Resynchronization Defibrillator Pulse Generator (9)	Insertion	Subcutaneous Tissue and Fascia	P	Cardiac Rhythm Related Device
Cardiac Resynchronization Pacemaker Pulse Generator (7)	Insertion	Subcutaneous Tissue and Fascia	P	Cardiac Rhythm Related Device
Contractility Modulation Device (A)	Insertion	Subcutaneous Tissue and Fascia	P	Cardiac Rhythm Related Device
Defibrillator Generator (8)	Insertion	Subcutaneous Tissue and Fascia	P	Cardiac Rhythm Related Device
Epiretinal Visual Prosthesis (5)	All applicable	Eye	J	Synthetic Substitute
External Fixation Device, Hybrid (D)	Insertion	Lower Bones Upper Bones	5	External Fixation Device
External Fixation Device, Hybrid (D)	Reposition	Lower Bones Upper Bones	5	External Fixation Device
External Fixation Device, Limb Lengthening (8)	Insertion	Lower Bones Upper Bones	5	External Fixation Device
External Fixation Device, Monoplanar (B)	Insertion	Lower Bones Upper Bones	5	External Fixation Device
External Fixation Device, Monoplanar (B)	Reposition	Lower Bones Upper Bones	5	External Fixation Device
External Fixation Device, Ring (C)	Insertion	Lower Bones Upper Bones	5	External Fixation Device
External Fixation Device, Ring (C)	Reposition	Lower Bones Upper Bones	5	External Fixation Device
Hearing Device, Bone Conduction (4)	Insertion	Ear, Nose, Sinus	S	Hearing Device
Hearing Device, Multiple Channel Cochlear Prosthesis (6)	Insertion	Ear, Nose, Sinus	S	Hearing Device
Hearing Device, Single Channel Cochlear Prosthesis (5)	Insertion	Ear, Nose, Sinus	S	Hearing Device
Internal Fixation Device, Intramedullary (6)	All applicable	Lower Bones Upper Bones	4	Internal Fixation Device
Internal Fixation Device, Intramedullary Limb Lengthening (7)	Insertion	Lower Bones Upper Bones	6	Internal Fixation Device, Intramedullary
Internal Fixation Device, Rigid Plate (Ø)	Insertion	Upper Bones	4	Internal Fixation Device
Internal Fixation Device, Rigid Plate (Ø)	Reposition	Upper Bones	4	Internal Fixation Device
Intraluminal Device, Airway (B)	All applicable	Ear, Nose, Sinus Gastrointestinal System Mouth and Throat	D	Intraluminal Device
Intraluminal Device, Bioactive (B)	All applicable	Upper Arteries	D	Intraluminal Device
Intraluminal Device, Branched or Fenestrated, One or Two Arteries (E)	Restriction	Heart and Great Vessels Lower Arteries	D	Intraluminal Device
Intraluminal Device, Branched or Fenestrated, Three or More Arteries (F)	Restriction	Heart and Great Vessels Lower Arteries	D	Intraluminal Device
Intraluminal Device, Drug-eluting (4)	All applicable	Heart and Great Vessels Lower Arteries Upper Arteries	D	Intraluminal Device
Intraluminal Device, Drug-eluting, Four or More (7)	All applicable	Heart and Great Vessels Lower Arteries Upper Arteries	D	Intraluminal Device
Intraluminal Device, Drug-eluting, Three (6)	All applicable	Heart and Great Vessels Lower Arteries Upper Arteries	D	Intraluminal Device
Intraluminal Device, Drug-eluting, Two (5)	All applicable	Heart and Great Vessels Lower Arteries Upper Arteries	D	Intraluminal Device
Intraluminal Device, Endobronchial Valve (G)	All applicable	Respiratory System	D	Intraluminal Device
Intraluminal Device, Endotracheal Airway (E)	All applicable	Respiratory System	D	Intraluminal Device

Specific Device	for Operation	in Body System	General Device	
Intraluminal Device, Flow Diverter (H)	Restriction	Upper Arteries	D	Intraluminal Device
Intraluminal Device, Four or More (G)	All applicable	Heart and Great Vessels Lower Arteries Upper Arteries	D	Intraluminal Device
Intraluminal Device, Pessary (G)	All applicable	Female Reproductive System	D	Intraluminal Device
Intraluminal Device, Radioactive (T)	All applicable	Heart and Great Vessels	D	Intraluminal Device
Intraluminal Device, Three (F)	All applicable	Heart and Great Vessels Lower Arteries Upper Arteries	D	Intraluminal Device
Intraluminal Device, Two (E)	All applicable	Heart and Great Vessels Lower Arteries Upper Arteries	D	Intraluminal Device
Monitoring Device, Hemodynamic (Ø)	Insertion	Subcutaneous Tissue and Fascia	2	Monitoring Device
Monitoring Device, Pressure Sensor (Ø)	Insertion	Heart and Great Vessels	2	Monitoring Device
Pacemaker, Dual Chamber (6)	Insertion	Subcutaneous Tissue and Fascia	P	Cardiac Rhythm Related Device
Pacemaker, Single Chamber (4)	Insertion	Subcutaneous Tissue and Fascia	P	Cardiac Rhythm Related Device
Pacemaker, Single Chamber Rate Responsive (5)	Insertion	Subcutaneous Tissue and Fascia	P	Cardiac Rhythm Related Device
Spinal Stabilization Device, Facet Replacement (D)	Insertion	Lower Joints Upper Joints	4	Internal Fixation Device
Spinal Stabilization Device, Interspinous Process (B)	Insertion	Lower Joints Upper Joints	4	Internal Fixation Device
Spinal Stabilization Device, Pedicle-Based (C)	Insertion	Lower Joints Upper Joints	4	Internal Fixation Device
Spinal Stabilization Device, Vertebral Body Tether (3)	Reposition	Lower Bones Upper Bones	4	Internal Fixation Device
Stimulator Generator, Multiple Array (D)	Insertion	Subcutaneous Tissue and Fascia	M	Stimulator Generator
Stimulator Generator, Multiple Array Rechargeable (E)	Insertion	Subcutaneous Tissue and Fascia	M	Stimulator Generator
Stimulator Generator, Single Array (B)	Insertion	Subcutaneous Tissue and Fascia	M	Stimulator Generator
Stimulator Generator, Single Array Rechargeable (C)	Insertion	Subcutaneous Tissue and Fascia	M	Stimulator Generator
Synthetic Substitute, Ceramic (3)	Replacement	Lower Joints	J	Synthetic Substitute
Synthetic Substitute, Ceramic on Polyethylene (4)	Replacement	Lower Joints	J	Synthetic Substitute
Synthetic Substitute, Intraocular Telescope (Ø)	Replacement	Eye	J	Synthetic Substitute
Synthetic Substitute, Metal (1)	Replacement	Lower Joints	J	Synthetic Substitute
Synthetic Substitute, Metal on Polyethylene (2)	Replacement	Lower Joints	J	Synthetic Substitute
Synthetic Substitute, Oxidized Zirconium on Polyethylene (6)	Replacement	Lower Joints	J	Synthetic Substitute
Synthetic Substitute, Polyethylene (Ø)	Replacement	Lower Joints	J	Synthetic Substitute
Synthetic Substitute, Reverse Ball and Socket (Ø)	Replacement	Upper Joints	J	Synthetic Substitute

Appendix H: Device Definitions

This **NT** symbol next to a device in the Definition column identifies that the device has been approved for NTAP (new technology add-on payment). CMS provides incremental payment, in addition to the DRG payment, for technologies that have received an NTAP designation.

ICD-10-PCS Value	Definition
Articulating Spacer in Lower Joints	Articulating Spacer (Antibiotic) Spacer, Articulating (Antibiotic)
Artificial Sphincter in Gastrointestinal System	Artificial anal sphincter (AAS) Artificial bowel sphincter (neosphincter)
Artificial Sphincter in Urinary System	AMS 800® Urinary Control System Artificial urinary sphincter (AUS)
Autologous Arterial Tissue in Heart and Great Vessels	Autologous artery graft
Autologous Arterial Tissue in Lower Arteries	Autologous artery graft
Autologous Arterial Tissue in Lower Veins	Autologous artery graft
Autologous Arterial Tissue in Upper Arteries	Autologous artery graft
Autologous Arterial Tissue in Upper Veins	Autologous artery graft
Autologous Tissue Substitute	Autograft Cultured epidermal cell autograft Epicel® cultured epidermal autograft
Autologous Venous Tissue in Heart and Great Vessels	Autologous vein graft
Autologous Venous Tissue in Lower Arteries	Autologous vein graft
Autologous Venous Tissue in Lower Veins	Autologous vein graft
Autologous Venous Tissue in Upper Arteries	Autologous vein graft
Autologous Venous Tissue in Upper Veins	Autologous vein graft
Biologic with Synthetic Substitute, Autoregulated Electrohydraulic Replacement in Heart and Great Vessels	Carmat total artificial heart (TAH)
Bone Growth Stimulator in Head and Facial Bones	Electrical bone growth stimulator (EBGS) Ultrasonic osteogenic stimulator Ultrasound bone healing system
Bone Growth Stimulator in Lower Bones	Electrical bone growth stimulator (EBGS) Ultrasonic osteogenic stimulator Ultrasound bone healing system
Bone Growth Stimulator in Upper Bones	Electrical bone growth stimulator (EBGS) Ultrasonic osteogenic stimulator Ultrasound bone healing system
Branched Synthetic Substitute with Intraluminal Device in New Technology	Thoraflex™ Hybrid device **NT**
Cardiac Lead in Heart and Great Vessels	Cardiac contractility modulation lead
Cardiac Lead, Defibrillator for Insertion in Heart and Great Vessels	ACUITY™ Steerable Lead Attain Ability® lead Attain StarFix® (OTW) lead Cardiac resynchronization therapy (CRT) lead Corox (OTW) Bipolar Lead Durata® Defibrillation Lead ENDOTAK RELIANCE® (G) Defibrillation Lead
Cardiac Lead, Pacemaker for Insertion in Heart and Great Vessels	ACUITY™ Steerable Lead Attain Ability® lead Attain StarFix® (OTW) lead Cardiac resynchronization therapy (CRT) lead Corox (OTW) Bipolar Lead

ICD-10-PCS Value	Definition
Cardiac Resynchronization Defibrillator Pulse Generator for Insertion in Subcutaneous Tissue and Fascia	COGNIS® CRT-D Concerto II CRT-D Consulta CRT-D CONTAK RENEWA® 3 RF (HE) CRT-D LIVIAN™ CRT-D Maximo II DR CRT-D Ovatio™ CRT-D Protecta XT CRT-D Viva (XT)(S)
Cardiac Resynchronization Pacemaker Pulse Generator for Insertion in Subcutaneous Tissue and Fascia	Consulta CRT-P Stratos LV Synchra CRT-P
Conduit through Femoral Vein to Popliteal Artery in New Technology	DETOUR® System
Conduit through Femoral Vein to Superficial Femoral Artery in New Technology	DETOUR® System
Conduit to Short-term External Heart Assist System in New Technology	Impella® 5.5 with SmartAssist® System
Contraceptive Device in Female Reproductive System	Intrauterine device (IUD)
Contraceptive Device in Subcutaneous Tissue and Fascia	Subdermal progesterone implant
Contractility Modulation Device for Insertion in Subcutaneous Tissue and Fascia	Optimizer™ III implantable pulse generator
Defibrillator Generator for Insertion in Subcutaneous Tissue and Fascia	Evera (XT)(S)(DR/VR) Implantable cardioverter-defibrillator (ICD) Maximo II DR (VR) Protecta XT DR (XT VR) Secura (DR) (VR) Virtuoso (II) (DR) (VR)
Defibrillator Lead in Anatomical Regions, General	EV ICD System (Extravascular implantable defibrillator lead)
Diaphragmatic Pacemaker Lead in Respiratory System	Phrenic nerve stimulator lead
Drainage Device	Cystostomy tube Foley catheter Percutaneous nephrostomy catheter Thoracostomy tube
External Fixation Device in Head and Facial Bones	External fixator
External Fixation Device in Lower Bones	External fixator
External Fixation Device in Lower Joints	External fixator
External Fixation Device in Upper Bones	External fixator
External Fixation Device in Upper Joints	External fixator
External Fixation Device, Hybrid for Insertion in Lower Bones	Delta frame external fixator Sheffield hybrid external fixator
External Fixation Device, Hybrid for Insertion in Upper Bones	Delta frame external fixator Sheffield hybrid external fixator

ICD-10-PCS Value	Definition
External Fixation Device, Hybrid for Reposition in Lower Bones	Delta frame external fixator Sheffield hybrid external fixator
External Fixation Device, Hybrid for Reposition in Upper Bones	Delta frame external fixator Sheffield hybrid external fixator
External Fixation Device, Limb Lengthening for Insertion in Lower Bones	Ilizarov-Vecklich device
External Fixation Device, Limb Lengthening for Insertion in Upper Bones	Ilizarov-Vecklich device
External Fixation Device, Monoplanar for Insertion in Lower Bones	Uniplanar external fixator
External Fixation Device, Monoplanar for Insertion in Upper Bones	Uniplanar external fixator
External Fixation Device, Monoplanar for Reposition in Lower Bones	Uniplanar external fixator
External Fixation Device, Monoplanar for Reposition in Upper Bones	Uniplanar external fixator
External Fixation Device, Ring for Insertion in Lower Bones	Ilizarov external fixator Sheffield ring external fixator
External Fixation Device, Ring for Insertion in Upper Bones	Ilizarov external fixator Sheffield ring external fixator
External Fixation Device, Ring for Reposition in Lower Bones	Ilizarov external fixator Sheffield ring external fixator
External Fixation Device, Ring for Reposition in Upper Bones	Ilizarov external fixator Sheffield ring external fixator
Extraluminal Device	AtriClip LAA Exclusion System LAP-BAND® adjustable gastric banding system REALIZE® Adjustable Gastric Band
Feeding Device in Gastrointestinal System	Percutaneous endoscopic gastrojejunostomy (PEG/J) tube Percutaneous endoscopic gastrostomy (PEG) tube
Hearing Device in Ear, Nose, Sinus	Esteem® implantable hearing system
Hearing Device in Head and Facial Bones	Bone anchored hearing device
Hearing Device, Bone Conduction for Insertion in Ear, Nose, Sinus	Bone anchored hearing device
Hearing Device, Multiple Channel Cochlear Prosthesis for Insertion in Ear, Nose, Sinus	Cochlear implant (CI), multiple channel (electrode)
Hearing Device, Single Channel Cochlear Prosthesis for Insertion in Ear, Nose, Sinus	Cochlear implant (CI), single channel (electrode)

ICD-10-PCS Value	Definition
Implantable Heart Assist System in Heart and Great Vessels	Berlin Heart Ventricular Assist Device DeBakey Left Ventricular Assist Device DuraHeart Left Ventricular Assist System HeartMate 3™ LVAS HeartMate II® Left Ventricular Assist Device (LVAD) HeartMate XVE® Left Ventricular Assist Device (LVAD) MicroMed HeartAssist Novacor Left Ventricular Assist Device Thoratec IVAD (Implantable Ventricular Assist Device)
Infusion Device	Ascenda Intrathecal Catheter InDura, intrathecal catheter (1P) (spinal) Non-tunneled central venous catheter Peripherally inserted central catheter (PICC) Tunneled spinal (intrathecal) catheter
Infusion Device, Pump in Subcutaneous Tissue and Fascia	Implantable drug infusion pump (anti-spasmodic)(chemotherapy)(pain) Injection reservoir, pump Pump reservoir Subcutaneous injection reservoir, pump SynchroMed pump
Interbody Fusion Device, Custom-made Anatomically Designedin New Technology	aprevo™
Interbody Fusion Device in Lower Joints	Axial Lumbar Interbody Fusion System AxiaLIF® System COALESCE® radiolucent interbody fusion device COHERE® radiolucent interbody fusion device CoRoent® XL Direct Lateral Interbody Fusion (DLIF) device EXtreme Lateral Interbody Fusion (XLIF) device Interbody fusion (spine) cage nanoLOCK™ interbody fusion device Titan Endoskeleton™ XLIF® System
Interbody Fusion Device in Upper Joints	BAK/C® Interbody Cervical Fusion System COALESCE® radiolucent interbody fusion device COHERE® radiolucent interbody fusion device Interbody fusion (spine) cage nanoLOCK™ interbody fusion device Titan Endoskeleton™
Internal Fixation Device in Head and Facial Bones	Bone screw (interlocking)(lag)(pedicle) (recessed) Kirschner wire (K-wire) Neutralization plate
Internal Fixation Device in Lower Bones	Bone screw (interlocking)(lag)(pedicle) (recessed) Clamp and rod internal fixation system (CRIF) Kirschner wire (K-wire) Neutralization plate
Internal Fixation Device in Lower Joints	Fusion screw (compression)(lag)(locking) Joint fixation plate Kirschner wire (K-wire)
Internal Fixation Device in Upper Bones	Bone screw (interlocking)(lag)(pedicle) (recessed) Clamp and rod internal fixation system (CRIF) Kirschner wire (K-wire) Neutralization plate
Internal Fixation Device in Upper Joints	Fusion screw (compression)(lag)(locking) Joint fixation plate Kirschner wire (K-wire)
Internal Fixation Device, Intramedullary in Lower Bones	Intramedullary (IM) rod (nail) Intramedullary skeletal kinetic distractor (ISKD) Kuntscher nail

ICD-10-PCS Value	Definition
Internal Fixation Device, Intramedullary in Upper Bones	Intramedullary (IM) rod (nail) Intramedullary skeletal kinetic distractor (ISKD) Kuntscher nail
Internal Fixation Device Intramedullary Limb Lengthening for Insertion in Lower Bones	PRECICE intramedullary limb lengthening system
Internal Fixation Device Intramedullary Limb Lengthening for Insertion in Upper Bones	PRECICE intramedullary limb lengthening system
Internal Fixation Device, Open-truss Design in New Technology	Ankle Truss System™ (ATS)
Internal Fixation Device, Rigid Plate for Insertion in Upper Bones	Titanium Sternal Fixation System (TSFS)
Internal Fixation Device, Rigid Plate for Reposition in Upper Bones	Titanium Sternal Fixation System (TSFS)
Internal Fixation Device, Sustained Compression for Fusion in Lower Joints	DynaClip® (Forte) DynaNail® (Helix) (Hybrid) (Mini)
Internal Fixation Device, Sustained Compression for Fusion in Upper Joints	DynaClip® (Forte) DynaNail® (Helix) (Hybrid) (Mini)
Internal Fixation Device with Tulip Connector in New Technology	iFuse Bedrock™ Granite Implant System ᴺᵀ
Intracardiac Pacemaker, Dual-Chamber in New Technology	Aveir™ AR, as dual chamber Aveir™ DR, dual chamber
Intracardiac Pacemaker in Heart and Great Vessels	Aveir™ VR, as single chamber

ICD-10-PCS Value	Definition
Intraluminal Device	Absolute Pro Vascular (OTW) Self-Expanding Stent System Acculink (RX) Carotid Stent System AFX® Endovascular AAA System AneuRx® AAA Advantage® Assurant (Cobalt) stent Carotid WALLSTENT® Monorail® Endoprosthesis CoAxia NeuroFlo catheter Colonic Z-Stent® Complete (SE) stent Cook Zenith AAA Endovascular Graft Driver stent (RX) (OTW) E-Luminexx™ (Biliary)(Vascular) Stent Embolization coil(s) Endologix AFX® Endovascular AAA System Endurant® Endovascular Stent Graft Endurant® II AAA stent graft system EXCLUDER® AAA Endoprosthesis Express® (LD) Premounted Stent System Express® Biliary SD Monorail® Premounted Stent System Express® SD Renal Monorail® Premounted Stent System FLAIR® Endovascular Stent Graft Formula™ Balloon-Expandable Renal Stent System GORE EXCLUDER® AAA Endoprosthesis GORE TAG® Thoracic Endoprosthesis ᴺᵀ Herculink (RX) Elite Renal Stent System LifeStent® (Flexstar)(XL) Vascular Stent System Medtronic Endurant® II AAA stent graft system Micro-Driver stent (RX) (OTW) MULTI-LINK (VISION)(MINI-VISION)(ULTRA) Coronary Stent System Omnilink Elite Vascular Balloon Expandable Stent System Protege® RX Carotid Stent System Stent, intraluminal (cardiovascular) (gastrointestinal)(hepatobiliary) (urinary) Talent® Converter Talent® Occluder Talent® Stent Graft (abdominal)(thoracic) Therapeutic occlusion coil(s) Ultraflex™ Precision Colonic Stent System Valiant Thoracic Stent Graft WALLSTENT® Endoprosthesis Xact Carotid Stent System Zenith AAA Endovascular Graft Zenith Flex® AAA Endovascular Graft Zenith TX2® TAA Endovascular Graft Zenith® Renu™ AAA Ancillary Graft
Intraluminal Device, Airway in Ear, Nose, Sinus	Nasopharyngeal airway (NPA)
Intraluminal Device, Airway in Gastrointestinal System	Esophageal obturator airway (EOA)
Intraluminal Device, Airway in Mouth and Throat	Guedel airway Oropharyngeal airway (OPA)
Intraluminal Device, Bioactive in Upper Arteries	Bioactive embolization coil(s) Micrus CERECYTE microcoil
Intraluminal Device, Bioprosthetic Valve in New Technology	TricValve® Transcatheter Bicaval Valve System VenoValve®
Intraluminal Device, Branched or Fenestrated, One or Two Arteries for Restriction in Lower Arteries	Cook Zenith® Fenestrated AAA Endovascular Graft EXCLUDER® AAA Endoprosthesis EXCLUDER® IBE Endoprosthesis GORE EXCLUDER® AAA Endoprosthesis GORE EXCLUDER®IBE Endoprosthesis Zenith® Fenestrated AAA Endovascular Graft

Appendix H: Device Definitions

ICD-10-PCS Value	Definition
Intraluminal Device, Branched or Fenestrated, Three or More Arteries for Restriction in Lower Arteries	Cook Zenith® Fenestrated AAA Endovascular Graft EXCLUDER® AAA Endoprosthesis GORE EXCLUDER® AAA Endoprosthesis Zenith® Fenestrated AAA Endovascular Graft
Intraluminal Device, Drug-eluting in Heart and Great Vessels	CYPHER® Stent Endeavor® (III)(IV) (Sprint) Zotarolimus-eluting Coronary Stent System Everolimus-eluting coronary stent Paclitaxel-eluting coronary stent Sirolimus-eluting coronary stent TAXUS® Liberte® Paclitaxel-eluting Coronary Stent System XIENCE Everolimus Eluting Coronary Stent System Zotarolimus-eluting coronary stent
Intraluminal Device, Drug-eluting in Lower Arteries	Paclitaxel-eluting peripheral stent Zilver® PTX® (paclitaxel) Drug-Eluting Peripheral Stent
Intraluminal Device, Drug-eluting in Upper Arteries	Paclitaxel-eluting peripheral stent Zilver® PTX® (paclitaxel) Drug-Eluting Peripheral Stent
Intraluminal Device, Endobronchial Valve in Respiratory System	Spiration IBV™ Valve System
Intraluminal Device, Endotracheal Airway in Respiratory System	Endotracheal tube (cuffed)(double-lumen)
Intraluminal Device, Flow Diverter for Restriction in Upper Arteries	Flow Diverter embolization device Pipeline™ (Flex) embolization device Surpass Streamline™ Flow Diverter
Intraluminal Device, Pessary in Female Reproductive System	Pessary ring Vaginal pessary
Intraluminal Device, Sustained Release Drug-eluting in New Technology	Eluvia™ Drug-eluting Vascular Stent System SAVAL below-the-knee (BTK) drug-eluting stent system
Intraluminal Device, Sustained Release Drug-eluting, Four or More in New Technology	Eluvia™ Drug-eluting Vascular Stent System SAVAL below-the-knee (BTK) drug-eluting stent system
Intraluminal Device, Sustained Release Drug-eluting, Three in New Technology	Eluvia™ Drug-eluting Vascular Stent System SAVAL below-the-knee (BTK) drug-eluting stent system
Intraluminal Device, Sustained Release Drug-eluting, Two in New Technology	Eluvia™ Drug-eluting Vascular Stent System SAVAL below-the-knee (BTK) drug-eluting stent system
Liner in Lower Joints	Acetabular cup Hip (joint) liner Joint liner (insert) Knee (implant) insert Tibial insert
Magnetically Controlled Growth Rod(s) in New Technology	MAGEC® Spinal Bracing and Distraction System Spinal growth rods, magnetically controlled
Magnetic Lengthening Device in Gastrointestinal System	Flourish® Pediatric Esophageal Atresia Device
Monitoring Device	Blood glucose monitoring system Cardiac event recorder Continuous Glucose Monitoring (CGM) device Implantable glucose monitoring device Loop recorder, implantable Reveal (LINQ)(DX)(XT)

ICD-10-PCS Value	Definition
Monitoring Device, Hemodynamic for Insertion in Subcutaneous Tissue and Fascia	Implantable hemodynamic monitor (IHM) Implantable hemodynamic monitoring system (IHMS)
Monitoring Device, Pressure Sensor for Insertion in Heart and Great Vessels	CardioMEMS® pressure sensor EndoSure® sensor
Neurostimulator Generator in Head and Facial Bones	RNS system neurostimulator generator
Neurostimulator Lead in Central Nervous System and Cranial Nerves	Cortical strip neurostimulator lead DBS lead Deep brain neurostimulator lead RNS System lead Spinal cord neurostimulator lead
Neurostimulator Lead in Peripheral Nervous System	InterStim® Therapy lead
Neurostimulator Lead in New Technology	Ischemic Stroke System (ISS500) ISS500 (Ischemic Stroke System)
Neurostimulator Lead with Paired Stimulation System in New Technology	Vivistim® Paired VNS System Lead **NT**
Nonautologous Tissue Substitute	Acellular Hydrated Dermis Bone bank bone graft Cook Biodesign® Fistula Plug(s) Cook Biodesign® Hernia Graft(s) Cook Biodesign® Layered Graft(s) Cook Zenapro™ Layered Graft(s) MIRODERM™ Biologic Wound Matrix Tissue bank graft
Other Device	Alfapump® system
Pacemaker, Dual Chamber for Insertion in Subcutaneous Tissue and Fascia	Advisa (MRI) EnRhythm Kappa Revo MRI™ SureScan® pacemaker Two lead pacemaker Versa
Pacemaker, Single Chamber for Insertion in Subcutaneous Tissue and Fascia	Single lead pacemaker (atrium)(ventricle)
Pacemaker, Single Chamber Rate Responsive for Insertion in Subcutaneous Tissue and Fascia	Single lead rate responsive pacemaker (atrium)(ventricle)
Posterior (Dynamic) Distraction Device in New Technology	ApiFix® Minimally Invasive Deformity Correction (MID-C) System
Posterior Spinal Motion Preservation Device in New Technology	TOPS™ System
Posterior Vertebral Tether in New Technology	LigaPASS 2.0™ PJK Prevention System
Radioactive Element	Brachytherapy seeds CivaSheet®
Radioactive Element, Cesium-131 Collagen Implant for Insertion in Central Nervous System and Cranial Nerves	Cesium-131 Collagen Implant GammaTile™
Reduction Device in New Technology	Neovasc Reducer™ Reducer™ System
Resurfacing Device in Lower Joints	CONSERVE® PLUS Total Resurfacing Hip System Cormet Hip Resurfacing System

ICD-10-PCS Value	Definition
Short-term External Heart Assist System in Heart and Great Vessels	Aortix™ System Biventricular external heart assist system BVS 5000 Ventricular Assist Device Centrimag® Blood Pump Impella® heart pump TandemHeart® System Thoratec Paracorporeal Ventricular Assist Device
Spacer in Lower Joints	Joint spacer (antibiotic) Spacer, Static (Antibiotic) Static Spacer (Antibiotic)
Spacer in Upper Joints	Joint spacer (antibiotic)
Spinal Stabilization Device, Facet Replacement for Insertion in Lower Joints	Facet replacement spinal stabilization device
Spinal Stabilization Device, Facet Replacement for Insertion in Upper Joints	Facet replacement spinal stabilization device
Spinal Stabilization Device, Interspinous Process for Insertion in Lower Joints	Interspinous process spinal stabilization device X-Spine Axle Cage X-STOP® Spacer
Spinal Stabilization Device, Interspinous Process for Insertion in Upper Joints	Interspinous process spinal stabilization device X-Spine Axle Cage X-STOP® Spacer
Spinal Stabilization Device, Pedicle- Based for Insertion in Lower Joints	Dynesys® Dynamic Stabilization System Pedicle-based dynamic stabilization device
Spinal Stabilization Device, Pedicle-Based for Insertion in Upper Joints	Dynesys® Dynamic Stabilization System Pedicle-based dynamic stabilization device
Stimulator Generator in Subcutaneous Tissue and Fascia	Baroreflex Activation Therapy® (BAT®) Diaphragmatic pacemaker generator Mark IV Breathing Pacemaker System Phrenic nerve stimulator generator Rheos® System device
Stimulator Generator, Multiple Array for Insertion in Subcutaneous Tissue and Fascia	Activa PC neurostimulator Enterra gastric neurostimulator Neurostimulator generator, multiple channel PERCEPT™ PC neurostimulator PrimeAdvanced neurostimulator (SureScan)(MRI Safe) Vanta™ PC neurostimulator
Stimulator Generator, Multiple Array Rechargeable for Insertion in Subcutaneous Tissue and Fascia	Activa RC neurostimulator Intellis™ neurostimulator Neurostimulator generator, multiple channel rechargeable RestoreAdvanced neurostimulator (SureScan)(MRI Safe) RestoreSensor neurostimulator (SureScan)(MRI Safe) RestoreUltra neurostimulator (SureScan)(MRI Safe)
Stimulator Generator, Single Array for Insertion in Subcutaneous Tissue and Fascia	Activa SC neurostimulator InterStim™ II Therapy neurostimulator Itrel (3)(4) neurostimulator Neurostimulator generator, single channel
Stimulator Generator, Single Array Rechargeable for Insertion in Subcutaneous Tissue and Fascia	InterStim™ Micro Therapy neurostimulator Neurostimulator generator, single channel rechargeable
Stimulator Lead in Gastrointestinal System	Gastric electrical stimulation (GES) lead Gastric pacemaker lead
Stimulator Lead in Muscles	Electrical muscle stimulation (EMS) lead Electronic muscle stimulator lead Neuromuscular electrical stimulation (NEMS) lead

ICD-10-PCS Value	Definition
Stimulator Lead in Upper Arteries	Baroreflex Activation Therapy® (BAT®) Carotid (artery) sinus (baroreceptor) lead Rheos® System lead
Stimulator Lead in Urinary System	Sacral nerve modulation (SNM) lead Sacral neuromodulation lead Urinary incontinence stimulator lead
Subcutaneous Defibrillator Lead in Subcutaneous Tissue and Fascia	S-ICD™ lead
Synthetic Substitute	AbioCor® Total Replacement Heart AMPLATZER® Muscular VSD Occluder Annuloplasty ring Bard® Composix® (E/X) (LP) mesh Bard® Composix® Kugel® patch Bard® Dulex® mesh Bard® Ventralex™ hernia patch Barricaid® Annular Closure Device (ACD) BRYAN® Cervical Disc System Corvia IASD® Ex-PRESS™ mini glaucoma shunt Flexible Composite Mesh GORE® DUALMESH® Holter valve ventricular shunt IASD® (InterAtrial Shunt Device), Corvia InterAtrial Shunt Device IASD®, Corvia MitraClip valve repair system Nitinol framed polymer mesh Open Pivot (mechanical) valve Open Pivot Aortic Valve Graft (AVG) Partially absorbable mesh PHYSIOMESH™ Flexible Composite Mesh Polymethylmethacrylate (PMMA) Polypropylene mesh PRESTIGE® Cervical Disc PROCEED™ Ventral Patch Prodisc-C Prodisc-L PROLENE Polypropylene Hernia System (PHS) Rebound HRD® (Hernia Repair Device) SynCardia Total Artificial Heart Total artificial (replacement) heart ULTRAPRO Hernia System (UHS) ULTRAPRO Partially Absorbable Lightweight Mesh ULTRAPRO Plug V-Wave Interatrial Shunt System Ventrio™ Hernia Patch Zimmer® NexGen® LPS Mobile Bearing Knee Zimmer® NexGen® LPS-Flex Mobile Knee
Synthetic Substitute, Ceramic for Replacement in Lower Joints	Ceramic on ceramic bearing surface Novation® Ceramic AHS® (Articulation Hip System)
Synthetic Substitute, Extraluminal Support Device in New Technology	VasQ™ External Support device
Synthetic Substitute, Intraocular Telescope for Replacement in Eye	Implantable Miniature Telescope™ (IMT)
Synthetic Substitute, Lateral Meniscus in New Technology	NUsurface® Meniscus Implant
Synthetic Substitute, Mechanically Expandable (Paired) in New Technology	SpineJack® system
Synthetic Substitute, Medial Meniscus in New Technology	NUsurface® Meniscus Implant
Synthetic Substitute, Metal for Replacement in Lower Joints	Cobalt/chromium head and socket Metal on metal bearing surface
Synthetic Substitute, Metal on Polyethylene for Replacement in Lower Joints	Cobalt/chromium head and polyethylene socket

ICD-10-PCS Value	Definition
Synthetic Substitute, Oxidized Zirconium on Polyethylene for Replacement in Lower Joints	OXINIUM
Synthetic Substitute, Pneumatic for Replacement in Heart and Great Vessels	SynCardia (temporary) total artificial heart (TAH)
Synthetic Substitute, Polyethylene for Replacement in Lower Joints	Polyethylene socket
Synthetic Substitute, Reverse Ball and Socket for Replacement in Upper Joints	Delta III Reverse shoulder prosthesis Reverse® Shoulder Prosthesis
Synthetic Substitute, Talar Prosthesis in New Technology	Total Ankle Talar Replacement™ (TATR)
Synthetic Substitute, Ultrasound Penetrable in New Technology	Longeviti ClearFit® Cranial Implant Longeviti ClearFit® OTS Cranial Implant
Tibial Extension with Motion Sensors in New Technology	Canturio™ te (Tibial Extension)
Tissue Expander in Skin and Breast	Tissue expander (inflatable) (injectable)
Tissue Expander in Subcutaneous Tissue and Fascia	Tissue expander (inflatable) (injectable)
Tracheostomy Device in Respiratory System	Tracheostomy tube

ICD-10-PCS Value	Definition
Vascular Access Device, Totally Implantable in Subcutaneous Tissue and Fascia	Implanted (venous)(access) port Injection reservoir, port Subcutaneous injection reservoir, port
Vascular Access Device, Tunneled in Subcutaneous Tissue and Fascia	Tunneled central venous catheter Vectra® Vascular Access Graft
Vein Graft Extraluminal Support Device(s) in New Technology	VEST™ Venous External Support device
Zooplastic Tissue in Heart and Great Vessels	3f (Aortic) Bioprosthesis valve Bovine pericardial valve Bovine pericardium graft Contegra Pulmonary Valved Conduit CoreValve transcatheter aortic valve Epic™ Stented Tissue Valve (aortic) Freestyle (Stentless) Aortic Root Bioprosthesis Hancock Bioprosthesis (aortic) (mitral) valve Hancock Bioprosthetic Valved Conduit Melody® transcatheter pulmonary valve Mitroflow® Aortic Pericardial Heart Valve Mosaic Bioprosthesis (aortic) (mitral) valve Porcine (bioprosthetic) valve SAPIEN transcatheter aortic valve SJM Biocor® Stented Valve System Stented tissue valve Trifecta™ Valve (aortic) Xenograft

Appendix I: Substance Key/Substance Definitions

Substance Key

This table crosswalks a specific substance, listed by trade name or synonym, to the PCS value that would be used to represent that substance in either the Administration or New Technology section. The ICD-10-PCS value may be located in either the 6th-character Substance column or the 7th-character Qualifier column depending on the section/table to which it is classified. The most specific character is listed in the table.

This **NT** symbol next to a substance/technology in the Trade Name or Synonym column identifies that the substance/technology has been approved for NTAP (new technology add-on payment). CMS provides incremental payment, in addition to the DRG payment, for technologies that have received an NTAP designation.

Substances denoted by an asterisk (*) in the Trade Name or Synonym column, although not included in the official ICD-10-PCS classification, were added based on information provided in the FY 2024 IPPS proposed rule.

Trade Name or Synonym	ICD-10-PCS Value	PCS Section
ABECMA® **NT**	Idecabtagene Vicleucel Immunotherapy (K)	New Technology (X)
ACTEMRA®	Tocilizumab (H)	New Technology (X)
afami-cel	Afamitresgene Autoleucel Immunotherapy (6)	New Technology (X)
AIGISRx Antibacterial Envelope	Anti-Infective Envelope (A)	Administration (3)
Andexanet Alfa, Factor Xa Inhibitor Reversal Agent	Coagulation Factor Xa, Inactivated (7)	New Technology (X)
Andexxa	Coagulation Factor Xa, Inactivated (7)	New Technology (X)
Angiotensin II	Vasopressor (X)	Administration (3)
Antibacterial Envelope (TYRX) (AIGISRx)	Anti-Infective Envelope (A)	Administration (3)
Antimicrobial envelope	Anti-Infective Envelope (A)	Administration (3)
Anti-SARS-CoV-2 hyperimmune globulin	Hyperimmune Globulin (E)	New Technology (X)
AVYCAZ® (ceftazidime-avibactam)	Other Anti-infective (9)	Administration (3)
Axicabtagene Ciloleucel	Axicabtagene Ciloleucel Immunotherapy (H)	New Technology (X)
AZEDRA®	Iobenguane I-131 Antineoplastic (S)	New Technology (X)
*Balversa™	Erdafitinib Antineoplastic (L)	New Technology (X)
beti-cel	Betibeglogene Autotemcel (B)	New Technology (X)
Blinatumomab	Other Antineoplastic (5)	Administration (3)
BLINCYTO® (blinatumomab)	Other Antineoplastic (5)	Administration (3)
Bone morphogenetic protein 2 (BMP 2)	Recombinant Bone Morphogenetic Protein (B)	Administration (3)
Brexucabtagene Autoleucel	Brexucabtagene Autoleucel Immunotherapy (4)	New Technology (X)
Breyanzi®	Lisocabtagene Maraleucel Immunotherapy (N)	New Technology (X)
Bromelain-enriched Proteolytic Enzyme	Anacaulase-bcdb (2)	New Technology (X)
*CABLIVI®	Caplacizumab (W)	New Technology (X)
CARVYKTI™ **NT**	Ciltacabtagene Autoleucel (A)	New Technology (X)
Casirivimab (REGN10933) and Imdevimab (REGN10987)	REGN-COV2 Monoclonal Antibody (G)	New Technology (X)
CBMA (Concentrated Bone Marrow Aspirate)	Other Substance (C)	Administration (3)
Ceftazidime-avibactam	Other Anti-infective (9)	Administration (3)
CERAMENT® G **NT**	Antibiotic-eluting Bone Void Filler (P)	New Technology (X)
cilta-cel	Ciltacabtagene Autoleucel (A)	New Technology (X)
Clolar	Clofarabine (P)	Administration (3)
Coagulation Factor Xa, (Recombinant) Inactivated	Coagulation Factor Xa, Inactivated (7)	New Technology (X)
COMIRNATY®	COVID-19 Vaccine (U) COVID-19 Booster (W) COVID-19 Vaccine Dose 1 (S) COVID-19 Vaccine Dose 2 (T) COVID-19 Vaccine Dose 3 (V)	New Technology (X)
CONTEPO™	Fosfomycin Anti-infective (K)	New Technology (X)
COSELA™ **NT**	Trilaciclib (7)	New Technology (X)
CRESEMBA® (isavuconazonium sulfate)	Other Anti-infective (9)	Administration (3)
CTX001™	Exagamglogene Autotemcel (J)	New Technology (X)
Darzalex Faspro® **NT**	Daratumumab and Hyaluronidase-fihj (1)	New Technology (X)
DefenCath™ **NT**	Taurolidine Anti-infective and Heparin Anticoagulant (2)	New Technology (X)
Defitelio	Other Substance (C)	Administration (3)
DuraGraft® Endothelial Damage Inhibitor	Endothelial Damage Inhibitor (8)	New Technology (X)
ELZONRIS™	Tagraxofusp-erzs Antineoplastic (Q)	New Technology (X)
ENSPRYNG™	Satralizumab-mwge (9)	New Technology (X)
ERLEADA™	Apalutamide Antineoplastic (J)	New Technology (X)
EVUSHELD™	Tixagevimab and Cilgavimab Monoclonal Antibody (X)	New Technology (X)
Factor Xa Inhibitor Reversal Agent, Andexanet Alfa	Coagulation Factor Xa, Inactivated (7)	New Technology (X)
FETROJA® **NT**	Cefiderocol Anti-infective (A)	New Technology (X)

Trade Name or Synonym	ICD-10-PCS Value	PCS Section
Fosfomycin injection	Fosfomycin Anti-infective (K)	New Technology (X)
Gammaglobulin	Globulin (S)	Administration (3)
GAMUNEX-C, for COVID-19 treatment	High-Dose Intravenous Immune Globulin (D)	New Technology (X)
GIAPREZA™	Vasopressor (X)	Administration (3)
GS-5734	Remdesivir Anti-infective (E)	New Technology (X)
hdIVIG (high-dose intravenous immunoglobulin), for COVID-19 treatment	High-Dose Intravenous Immune Globulin (D)	New Technology (X)
Hemospray® Endoscopic Hemostat	Mineral-based Topical Hemostatic Agent (8)	New Technology (X)
HEPZATO™ KIT (melphalan hydrochloride Hepatic Delivery System)	Melphalan Hydrochloride Antineoplastic (T)	New Technology (X)
HIG (hyperimmune globulin), for COVID-19 treatment	Hyperimmune Globulin (E)	New Technology (X)
High-dose intravenous immunoglobulin (hdIVIG), for COVID-19 treatment	High-Dose Intravenous Immune Globulin (D)	New Technology (X)
hIVIG (hyperimmune intravenous immunoglobulin), for COVID-19 treatment	Hyperimmune Globulin (E)	New Technology (X)
Human angiotensin II, synthetic	Vasopressor (X)	Administration (3)
Hyperimmune globulin	Globulin (S)	Administration (3)
Hyperimmune intravenous immunoglobulin (hIVIG), for COVID-19 treatment	Hyperimmune Globulin (E)	New Technology (X)
Idarucizumab, Pradaxa® (dabigatran) reversal agent	Other Therapeutic Substance (G)	Administration (3)
Idecabtagene Vicleucel	Idecabtagene Vicleucel Immunotherapy (K)	New Technology (X)
Ide-cel	Idecabtagene Vicleucel Immunotherapy (K)	New Technology (X)
IGIV-C, for COVID-19 treatment	Hyperimmune Globulin (E)	New Technology (X)
Imdevimab (REGN10987) and Casirivimab (REGN10933)	REGN-COV2 Monoclonal Antibody (G)	New Technology (X)
IMFINZI®	Durvalumab Antineoplastic (3)	New Technology (X)
IMI/REL	Imipenem-cilastatin-relebactam Anti-infective (U)	New Technology (X)
Immunoglobulin	Globulin (S)	Administration (3)
INTERCEPT Blood System for Plasma Pathogen Reduced Cryoprecipitated Fibrinogen Complex	Pathogen Reduced Cryoprecipitated Fibrinogen Complex (D)	Administration (3)
INTERCEPT Fibrinogen Complex	Pathogen Reduced Cryoprecipitated Fibrinogen Complex (D)	Administration (3)
Iobenguane I-131, High Specific Activity (HSA)	Iobenguane I-131 Antineoplastic (S)	New Technology (X)
Isavuconazole (isavuconazonium sulfate)	Other Anti-infective (9)	Administration (3)
Jakafi®	Ruxolitinib (T)	New Technology (X)
Kcentra	4-Factor Prothrombin Complex Concentrate (B)	Administration (3)
KEVZARA®	Sarilumab (G)	New Technology (X)
KYMRIAH®	Tisagenlecleucel Immunotherapy (J)	New Technology (X)
Lifileucel	Lifileucel Immunotherapy (L)	New Technology (X)
Lisocabtagene Maraleucel	Lisocabtagene Maraleucel Immunotherapy (7)	New Technology (X)
LIVTENCITY™ [NT]	Maribavir Anti-infective (3)	New Technology (X)
LTX Regional Anticoagulant	Nafamostat Anticoagulant (3)	New Technology (X)
LUNSUMIO™	Mosunetuzumab Antineoplastic (5)	New Technology (X)
MarrowStim™ PAD Kit for CBMA (Concentrated Bone Marrow Aspirate)	Other Substance (C)	Administration (3)
NA-1 (Nerinitide)	Nerinitide (2)	New Technology (X)
Nesiritide	Human B-type Natriuretic Peptide (H)	Administration (3)
NexoBrid™	Anacaulase-bcdb (2)	New Technology (X)
Niyad™	Nafamostat Anticoagulant (3)	New Technology (X)
NUZYRA™	Omadacycline Anti-infective (B)	New Technology (X)
Octagam 10%, for COVID-19 treatment	High-Dose Intravenous Immune Globulin (D)	New Technology (X)
Olumiant®	Baricitinib (M)	New Technology (X)
OTL-101	Hematopoietic Stem/Progenitor Cells, Genetically Modified (C)	Administration (3)
Plazomicin	Other Anti-infective (9)	Administration (3)
Polyclonal hyperimmune globulin	Globulin (S)	Administration (3)
Praxbind® (idarucizumab), Pradaxa® (dabigatran) reversal agent	Other Therapeutic Substance (G)	Administration (3)
REBYOTA®	Broad Consortium Microbiota-based Live Biotherapeutic Suspension (X)	New Technology (X)
*RECARBRIO™ [NT]	Imipenem-cilastatin-relebactam Anti-infective (U)	New Technology (X)
RETHYMIC®	Engineered Allogeneic Thymus Tissue (D)	New Technology (X)
rhBMP-2	Recombinant Bone Morphogenetic Protein (B)	Administration (3)
RYBREVANT™ [NT]	Amivantamab Monoclonal Antibody (B)	New Technology (X)

Trade Name or Synonym	ICD-10-PCS Value	PCS Section
Seprafilm	Adhesion Barrier (5)	Administration (3)
Soliris®	Eculizumab (C)	New Technology (X)
SPIKEVAX™	COVID-19 Vaccine (U) COVID-19 Booster (W) COVID-19 Vaccine Dose 1 (S) COVID-19 Vaccine Dose 2 (T) COVID-19 Vaccine Dose 3 (V)	New Technology (X)
SPRAVATO™	Esketamine Hydrochloride (M)	New Technology (X)
STELARA®	Other New Technology Therapeutic Substance (F)	New Technology (X)
StrataGraft® NT	Bioengineered Allogeneic Construct (F)	New Technology (X)
SUL-DUR	Sulbactam-Durlobactam (K)	New Technology (X)
tab-cel®	Tabelecleucel Immunotherapy (7)	New Technology (X)
TECARTUS™ NT	Brexucabtagene Autoleucel Immunotherapy (M)	New Technology (X)
TECENTRIQ®	Atezolizumab Antineoplastic (D)	New Technology (X)
TERLIVAZ®	Terlipressin (6)	New Technology (X)
Tisagenlecleucel	Tisagenlecleucel Immunotherapy (J)	New Technology (X)
Tissue Plasminogen Activator (tPA)(r-tPA)	Other Thrombolytic (7)	Administration (3)
TYRX Antibacterial Envelope	Anti-Infective Envelope (A)	Administration (3)
UPLIZNA®	Inebilizumab-cdon (9)	New Technology (X)
Ustekinumab	Other New Technology Therapeutic Substance (F)	New Technology (X)
Vabomere™	Meropenem-vaborbactam Anti-infective (N)	New Technology (X)
Veklury	Remdesivir Anti-infective (E)	New Technology (X)
Venclexta®	Venetoclax Antineoplastic (R)	New Technology (X)
Vistogard®	Uridine Triacetate (8)	New Technology (X)
Voraxaze	Glucarpidase (Q)	Administration (3)
VYXEOS™	Cytarabine and Daunorubicin Liposome Antineoplastic (B)	New Technology (X)
XENLETA™	Lefamulin Anti-infective (6)	New Technology (X)
XOSPATA®	Gilteritinib Antineoplastic (V)	New Technology (X)
Yescarta®	Axicabtagene Ciloleucel Immunotherapy (H)	New Technology (X)
*ZEMDRI®	Plazomicin Anti-infective (6)	New Technology (X)
ZEPZELCA™ NT	Lurbinectedin (8)	New Technology (X)
ZERBAXA®	Ceftolozane/Tazobactam Anti-infective (9)	New Technology (X)
ZULRESSO™	Brexanolone (Ø)	New Technology (X)
ZYNTEGLO®	Betibeglogene Autotemcel (B)	New Technology (X)
Zyvox	Oxazolidinones (8)	Administration (3)

Substance Definitions

This table crosswalks a PCS value, used in the Administration or New Technology section, to a specific substance. The specific substances are listed by trade name or synonym. The ICD-10-PCS value may be located in either the 6th-character Substance column or the 7th-character Qualifier column depending on the section/table to which it is classified.

This **NT** symbol next to a substance/technology in the Trade Name or Synonym column identifies that the substance/technology has been approved for NTAP (new technology add-on payment). CMS provides incremental payment, in addition to the DRG payment, for technologies that have received an NTAP designation.

Substances denoted by an asterisk (*) in the Trade Name or Synonym column, although not included in the official ICD-10-PCS classification, were added based on information provided in the FY 2024 IPPS proposed rule.

ICD-10-PCS Value	Trade Name or Synonym	PCS Section
4-Factor Prothrombin Complex Concentrate (B)	Kcentra	Administration (3)
Afamitresgene Autoleucel Immunotherapy (6)	afami-cel	New Technology (X)
Adhesion Barrier (5)	Seprafilm	Administration (3)
Amivantamab Monoclonal Antibody (B)	RYBREVANT™ NT	New Technology (X)
Anacaulase-bcdb (2)	Bromelain-enriched Proteolytic Enzyme NexoBrid™	New Technology (X)
Antibiotic-eluting Bone Void Filler (P)	CERAMENT® G NT	New Technology (X)
Anti-Infective Envelope (A)	AIGISRx Antibacterial Envelope Antibacterial Envelope (TYRX) (AIGISRx) Antimicrobial envelope TYRX Antibacterial Envelope	Administration (3)
Apalutamide Antineoplastic (J)	ERLEADA™	New Technology (X)
Atezolizumab Antineoplastic (D)	TECENTRIQ®	New Technology (X)
Axicabtagene Ciloleucel Immunotherapy (H)	Axicabtagene Ciloleucel Yescarta®	New Technology (X)
Baricitinib (M)	Olumiant®	New Technology (X)

ICD-10-PCS Value	Trade Name or Synonym	PCS Section
Betibeglogene Autotemcel (B)	beti-cel ZYNTEGLO®	New Technology (X)
Bioengineered Allogeneic Construct (F)	StrataGraft® **NT**	New Technology (X)
Brexanolone (0)	ZULRESSO™	New Technology (X)
Brexucabtagene Autoleucel Immunotherapy (M)	TECARTUS™ **NT**	New Technology (X)
Broad Consortium Microbiota-based Live Biotherapeutic Suspension (X)	REBYOTA®	New Technology (X)
Caplacizumab (W)	*CABLIVI®	New Technology (X)
Cefiderocol Anti-infective (A)	FETROJA® **NT**	New Technology (X)
Ceftolozane/Tazobactam Anti- infective (9)	ZERBAXA®	New Technology (X)
Ciltacabtagene Autoleucel (A)	CARVYKTI™ **NT** cilta-cel	New Technology (X)
Clofarabine (P)	Clolar	Administration (3)
Coagulation Factor Xa, Inactivated (7)	Andexanet Alfa, Factor Xa Inhibitor Reversal Agent Andexxa Coagulation Factor Xa, (Recombinant) Inactivated Factor Xa Inhibitor Reversal Agent, Andexanet Alfa	New Technology (X)
COVID-19 Vaccine (U)	COMIRNATY® SPIKEVAX™	New Technology (X)
COVID-19 Booster (W)	COMIRNATY® SPIKEVAX™	New Technology (X)
COVID-19 Vaccine Dose 1 (S)	COMIRNATY® SPIKEVAX™	New Technology (X)
COVID-19 Vaccine Dose 2 (T)	COMIRNATY® SPIKEVAX™	New Technology (X)
COVID-19 Vaccine Dose 3 (V)	COMIRNATY® SPIKEVAX™	New Technology (X)
Cytarabine and Daunorubicin Liposome Antineoplastic (B)	VYXEOS™	New Technology (X)
Daratumumab and Hyaluronidase-fihj (1)	Darzalex Faspro® **NT**	New Technology (X)
Durvalumab Antineoplastic (3)	IMFINZI®	New Technology (X)
Eculizumab (C)	Soliris®	New Technology (X)
Endothelial Damage Inhibitor (8)	DuraGraft® Endothelial Damage Inhibitor	New Technology (X)
Erdafitinib Antineoplastic (L)	*Balversa™	New Technology (X)
Engineered Allogeneic Thymus Tissue (D)	RETHYMIC®	New Technology (X)
Esketamine Hydrochloride (M)	SPRAVATO™	New Technology (X)
Exagamglogene Autotemcel (J)	CTX001™	New Technology (X)
Fosfomycin Anti-infective (K)	CONTEPO™ Fosfomycin injection	New Technology (X)
Gilteritinib Antineoplastic (V)	XOSPATA®	New Technology (X)
Globulin (S)	Gammaglobulin Hyperimmune globulin Immunoglobulin Polyclonal hyperimmune globulin	Administration (3)
Glucarpidase (Q)	Voraxaze	Administration (3)
Hematopoietic Stem/Progenitor Cells, Genetically Modified (C)	OTL-101	Administration (3)
High-Dose Intravenous Immune Globulin (D)	GAMUNEX-C, for COVID-19 treatment hdIVIG (high-dose intravenous immunoglobulin), for COVID-19 treatment High-dose intravenous immunoglobulin (hdIVIG), for COVID-19 treatment Octagam 10%, for COVID-19 treatment	New Technology (X)
Human B-type Natriuretic Peptide (H)	Nesiritide	Administration (3)
Hyperimmune Globulin (E)	Anti-SARS-CoV-2 hyperimmune globulin HIG (hyperimmune globulin), for COVID-19 treatment hIVIG (hyperimmune intravenous immunoglobulin), for COVID-19 treatment Hyperimmune intravenous immunoglobulin (hIVIG), for COVID-19 treatment IGIV-C, for COVID-19 treatment	New Technology (X)
Idecabtagene Vicleucel Immunotherapy (K)	ABECMA® **NT** Idecabtagene Vicleucel Ide-cel	New Technology (X)
Imipenem-cilastatin-relebactam Anti-infective (U)	IMI/REL *RECARBRIO™ **NT**	New Technology (X)
Inebilizumab-cdon (9)	UPLIZNA®	New Technology (X)

ICD-10-PCS Value	Trade Name or Synonym	PCS Section
Iobenguane I-131 Antineoplastic (S)	AZEDRA® Iobenguane I-131, High Specific Activity (HSA)	New Technology (X)
Lefamulin Anti-infective (6)	XENLETA™	New Technology (X)
Lifileucel Immunotherapy (L)	Lifileucel	New Technology (X)
Lisocabtagene Maraleucel Immunotherapy (7)	Breyanzi® Lisocabtagene Maraleucel	New Technology (X)
Lurbinectedin (8)	ZEPZELCA™　　　　　　　　　　　　　NT	New Technology (X)
Maribavir Anti-infective (3)	LIVTENCITY™　　　　　　　　　　　　NT	New Technology (X)
Melphalan Hydrochloride Antineoplastic (T)	HEPZATO™ KIT (melphalan hydrochloride Hepatic Delivery System)	New Technology (X)
Meropenem-vaborbactam Anti-infective (N)	Vabomere™	New Technology (X)
Mineral-based Topical Hemostatic Agent (8)	Hemospray® Endoscopic Hemostat	New Technology (X)
Mosunetuzumab Antineoplastic (5)	LUNSUMIO™	New Technology (X)
Nafamostat Anticoagulant (3)	LTX Regional Anticoagulant Niyad™	New Technology (X)
Nerinitide (2)	NA-1 (Nerinitide)	New Technology (X)
Omadacycline Anti-infective (B)	NUZYRA™	New Technology (X)
Other Anti-infective (9)	AVYCAZ® (ceftazidime-avibactam) Ceftazidime-avibactam CRESEMBA® (isavuconazonium sulfate) Isavuconazole (isavuconazonium sulfate) Plazomicin *ZEMDRI	Administration (3)
Other Antineoplastic (5)	Blinatumomab BLINCYTO® (blinatumomab)	Administration (3)
Other New Technology Therapeutic Substance (F)	STELARA® Ustekinumab	New Technology (X)
Other Substance (C)	CBMA (Concentrated Bone Marrow Aspirate) Defitelio MarrowStim™ PAD Kit for CBMA (Concentrated Bone Marrow Aspirate)	Administration (3)
Other Therapeutic Substance (G)	Idarucizumab, Pradaxa® (dabigatran) reversal agent Praxbind® (idarucizumab), Pradaxa® (dabigatran) reversal agent	Administration (3)
Other Thrombolytic (7)	Tissue Plasminogen Activator (tPA)(r-tPA)	Administration (3)
Oxazolidinones (8)	Zyvox	Administration (3)
Pathogen Reduced Cryoprecipitated Fibrinogen Complex (D)	INTERCEPT Blood System for Plasma Pathogen Reduced Cryoprecipitated Fibrinogen Complex INTERCEPT Fibrinogen Complex	Administration (3)
Recombinant Bone Morphogenetic Protein (B)	Bone morphogenetic protein 2 (BMP 2) rhBMP-2	Administration (3)
REGN-COV2 Monoclonal Antibody (G)	Casirivimab (REGN10933) and Imdevimab (REGN10987) Imdevimab (REGN10987) and Casirivimab (REGN10933)	New Technology (X)
Remdesivir Anti-infective (E)	GS-5734 Veklury　　　　　　　　　　　　　　NT	New Technology (X)
Ruxolitinib (T)	Jakafi®	New Technology (X)
Sarilumab (G)	KEVZARA®	New Technology (X)
Satralizumab-mwge (9)	ENSPRYNG™	New Technology (X)
Sulbactam-Durlobactam (K)	SUL-DUR	New Technology (X)
Tabelecleucel Immunotherapy (7)	tab-cel®	New Technology (X)
Tagraxofusp-erzs Antineoplastic (Q)	ELZONRIS™	New Technology (X)
Taurolidine Anti-infective and Heparin Anticoagulant (2)	DefenCath™　　　　　　　　　　　　NT	New Technology (X)
Terlipressin (6)	TERLIVAZ®	New Technology (X)
Tisagenlecleucel Immunotherapy (J)	KYMRIAH® Tisagenlecleucel	New Technology (X)
Tixagevimab and Cilgavimab Monoclonal Antibody (X)	EVUSHELD™	New Technology (X)
Tocilizumab (H)	ACTEMRA®	New Technology (X)
Trilaciclib (7)	COSELA™　　　　　　　　　　　　　NT	New Technology (X)
Uridine Triacetate (8)	Vistogard®	New Technology (X)
Vasopressor (X)	Angiotensin II GIAPREZA™ Human angiotensin II, synthetic	Administration (3)
Venetoclax Antineoplastic (R)	Venclexta®	New Technology (X)

Appendix J: Sections B–H Character Definitions

Sections B-H (Imaging through Substance Abuse Treatment) do not include root operations. Instead, the character 3 value represents the type of procedure performed with additional details about that procedure provided by the character 4 or 5 value, when appropriate. This resource provides the specific ICD-10-PCS value and its associated definition for the character 3, character 4, and character 5 values in the ancillary sections of B-H.

Section B–Imaging

ICD-10-PCS Value (Character 3)	Definition
Computerized Tomography (CT Scan) (2)	Computer reformatted digital display of multiplanar images developed from the capture of multiple exposures of external ionizing radiation
Fluoroscopy (1)	Single plane or bi-plane real time display of an image developed from the capture of external ionizing radiation on a fluorescent screen. The image may also be stored by either digital or analog means.
Magnetic Resonance Imaging (MRI) (3)	Computer reformatted digital display of multiplanar images developed from the capture of radiofrequency signals emitted by nuclei in a body site excited within a magnetic field
Other Imaging (5)	Other specified modality for visualizing a body part
Plain Radiography (Ø)	Planar display of an image developed from the capture of external ionizing radiation on photographic or photoconductive plate
Ultrasonography (4)	Real time display of images of anatomy or flow information developed from the capture of reflected and attenuated high frequency sound waves

Section C–Nuclear Medicine

ICD-10-PCS Value (Character 3)	Definition
Nonimaging Nuclear Medicine Assay (6)	Introduction of radioactive materials into the body for the study of body fluids and blood elements, by the detection of radioactive emissions
Nonimaging Nuclear Medicine Probe (5)	Introduction of radioactive materials into the body for the study of distribution and fate of certain substances by the detection of radioactive emissions; or, alternatively, measurement of absorption of radioactive emissions from an external source
Nonimaging Nuclear Medicine Uptake (4)	Introduction of radioactive materials into the body for measurements of organ function, from the detection of radioactive emissions
Planar Nuclear Medicine Imaging (1)	Introduction of radioactive materials into the body for single plane display of images developed from the capture of radioactive emissions
Positron Emission Tomographic (PET) Imaging (3)	Introduction of radioactive materials into the body for three dimensional display of images developed from the simultaneous capture, 18Ø degrees apart, of radioactive emissions
Systemic Nuclear Medicine Therapy (7)	Introduction of unsealed radioactive materials into the body for treatment
Tomographic (Tomo) Nuclear Medicine Imaging (2)	Introduction of radioactive materials into the body for three dimensional display of images developed from the capture of radioactive emissions

Section F–Physical Rehabilitation and Diagnostic Audiology

ICD-10-PCS Value (Character 3)	Definition
Activities of Daily Living Assessment (2)	Measurement of functional level for activities of daily living
Activities of Daily Living Treatment (8)	Exercise or activities to facilitate functional competence for activities of daily living
Caregiver Training (F)	Training in activities to support patient's optimal level of function
Cochlear Implant Treatment (B)	Application of techniques to improve the communication abilities of individuals with cochlear implant
Device Fitting (D)	Fitting of a device designed to facilitate or support achievement of a higher level of function
Hearing Aid Assessment (4)	Measurement of the appropriateness and/or effectiveness of a hearing device
Hearing Assessment (3)	Measurement of hearing and related functions
Hearing Treatment (9)	Application of techniques to improve, augment, or compensate for hearing and related functional impairment
Motor and/or Nerve Function Assessment (1)	Measurement of motor, nerve, and related functions
Motor Treatment (7)	Exercise or activities to increase or facilitate motor function
Speech Assessment (Ø)	Measurement of speech and related functions

Continued on next page

Section F–Physical Rehabilitation and Diagnostic Audiology

Continued from previous page

ICD-10-PCS Value (Character 3)	Definition
Speech Treatment (6)	Application of techniques to improve, augment, or compensate for speech and related functional impairment
Vestibular Assessment (5)	Measurement of the vestibular system and related functions
Vestibular Treatment (C)	Application of techniques to improve, augment, or compensate for vestibular and related functional impairment

Section F–Physical Rehabilitation and Diagnostic Audiology

ICD-10-PCS Value Qualifier (Character 5)	Definition
Acoustic Reflex Decay (J)	Measures reduction in size/strength of acoustic reflex over time Includes/Examples: Includes site of lesion test
Acoustic Reflex Patterns (G)	Defines site of lesion based upon presence/absence of acoustic reflexes with ipsilateral vs. contralateral stimulation
Acoustic Reflex Threshold (H)	Determines minimal intensity that acoustic reflex occurs with ipsilateral and/or contralateral stimulation
Aerobic Capacity and Endurance (7)	Measures autonomic responses to positional changes; perceived exertion, dyspnea or angina during activity; performance during exercise protocols; standard vital signs; and blood gas analysis or oxygen consumption
Alternate Binaural or Monaural Loudness Balance (7)	Determines auditory stimulus parameter that yields the same objective sensation Includes/Examples: Sound intensities that yield same loudness perception
Anthropometric Characteristics (B)	Measures edema, body fat composition, height, weight, length and girth
Aphasia (Assessment) (C)	Measures expressive and receptive speech and language function including reading and writing
Aphasia (Treatment) (3)	Applying techniques to improve, augment, or compensate for receptive/ expressive language impairments
Articulation/Phonology (Assessment) (9)	Measures speech production
Articulation/Phonology (Treatment) (4)	Applying techniques to correct, improve, or compensate for speech productive impairment
Assistive Listening Device (5)	Assists in use of effective and appropriate assistive listening device/system
Assistive Listening System/Device Selection (4)	Measures the effectiveness and appropriateness of assistive listening systems/devices
Assistive, Adaptive, Supportive or Protective Devices (9)	Explanation: Devices to facilitate or support achievement of a higher level of function in wheelchair mobility; bed mobility; transfer or ambulation ability; bath and showering ability; dressing; grooming; personal hygiene; play or leisure
Auditory Evoked Potentials (L)	Measures electric responses produced by the VIIIth cranial nerve and brainstem following auditory stimulation
Auditory Processing (Assessment) (Q)	Evaluates ability to receive and process auditory information and comprehension of spoken language
Auditory Processing (Treatment) (2)	Applying techniques to improve the receiving and processing of auditory information and comprehension of spoken language
Augmentative/Alternative Communication System (Assessment) (L)	Determines the appropriateness of aids, techniques, symbols, and/or strategies to augment or replace speech and enhance communication Includes/Examples: Includes the use of telephones, writing equipment, emergency equipment, and TDD
Augmentative/Alternative Communication System (Treatment) (3)	Includes/Examples: Includes augmentative communication devices and aids
Aural Rehabilitation (5)	Applying techniques to improve the communication abilities associated with hearing loss
Aural Rehabilitation Status (P)	Measures impact of a hearing loss including evaluation of receptive and expressive communication skills
Bathing/Showering (Ø)	Includes/Examples: Includes obtaining and using supplies; soaping, rinsing, and drying body parts; maintaining bathing position; and transferring to and from bathing positions
Bathing/Showering Techniques (Ø)	Activities to facilitate obtaining and using supplies, soaping, rinsing and drying body parts, maintaining bathing position, and transferring to and from bathing positions
Bed Mobility (Assessment) (B)	Transitional movement within bed
Bed Mobility (Treatment) (5)	Exercise or activities to facilitate transitional movements within bed
Bedside Swallowing and Oral Function (H)	Includes/Examples: Bedside swallowing includes assessment of sucking, masticating, coughing, and swallowing. Oral function includes assessment of musculature for controlled movements, structures, and functions to determine coordination and phonation.

Continued on next page

Section F–Physical Rehabilitation and Diagnostic Audiology   *Continued from previous page*

ICD-10-PCS Value Qualifier (Character 5)	Definition
Bekesy Audiometry (3)	Uses an instrument that provides a choice of discrete or continuously varying pure tones; choice of pulsed or continuous signal
Binaural Electroacoustic Hearing Aid Check (6)	Determines mechanical and electroacoustic function of bilateral hearing aids using hearing aid test box
Binaural Hearing Aid (Assessment) (3)	Measures the candidacy, effectiveness, and appropriateness of a hearing aid Explanation: Measures bilateral fit
Binaural Hearing Aid (Treatment) (2).	Explanation: Assists in achieving maximum understanding and performance
Bithermal, Binaural Caloric Irrigation (Ø)	Measures the rhythmic eye movements stimulated by changing the temperature of the vestibular system
Bithermal, Monaural Caloric Irrigation (1)	Measures the rhythmic eye movements stimulated by changing the temperature of the vestibular system in one ear
Brief Tone Stimuli (R)	Measures specific central auditory process
Cerumen Management (3)	Includes examination of external auditory canal and tympanic membrane and removal of cerumen from external ear canal
Cochlear Implant (Ø)	Measures candidacy for cochlear implant
Cochlear Implant Rehabilitation (Ø)	Applying techniques to improve the communication abilities of individuals with cochlear implant; includes programming the device, providing patients/families with information
Communicative/Cognitive Integration Skills (Assessment) (G)	Measures ability to use higher cortical functions Includes/Examples: Includes orientation, recognition, attention span, initiation and termination of activity, memory, sequencing, categorizing, concept formation, spatial operations, judgment, problem solving, generalization and pragmatic communication
Communicative/Cognitive Integration Skills (Treatment) (6)	Activities to facilitate the use of higher cortical functions Includes/Examples: Includes level of arousal, orientation, recognition, attention span, initiation and termination of activity, memory sequencing, judgment and problem solving, learning and generalization, and pragmatic communication
Computerized Dynamic Posturography (6)	Measures the status of the peripheral and central vestibular system and the sensory/motor component of balance; evaluates the efficacy of vestibular rehabilitation
Conditioned Play Audiometry (4)	Behavioral measures using nonspeech and speech stimuli to obtain frequency-specific and ear-specific information on auditory status from the patient Explanation: Obtains speech reception threshold by having patient point to pictures of spondaic words
Coordination/Dexterity (Assessment) (3)	Measures large and small muscle groups for controlled goal-directed movements Explanation: Dexterity includes object manipulation
Coordination/Dexterity (Treatment) (2)	Exercise or activities to facilitate gross coordination and fine coordination
Cranial Nerve Integrity (9)	Measures cranial nerve sensory and motor functions, including tastes, smell and facial expression
Dichotic Stimuli (T)	Measures specific central auditory process
Distorted Speech (S)	Measures specific central auditory process
Dix-Hallpike Dynamic (5)	Measures nystagmus following Dix-Hallpike maneuver
Dressing (1)	Includes/Examples: Includes selecting clothing and accessories, obtaining clothing from storage, dressing, fastening and adjusting clothing and shoes, and applying and removing personal devices, prosthesis or orthosis
Dressing Techniques (1)	Activities to facilitate selecting clothing and accessories, dressing and undressing, adjusting clothing and shoes, applying and removing devices, prostheses or orthoses
Dynamic Orthosis (6)	Includes/Examples: Includes customized and prefabricated splints, inhibitory casts, spinal and other braces, and protective devices; allows motion through transfer of movement from other body parts or by use of outside forces
Ear Canal Probe Microphone (1)	Real ear measures
Ear Protector Attentuation (7)	Measures ear protector fit and effectiveness
Electrocochleography (K)	Measures the VIIIth cranial nerve action potential
Environmental, Home, Work Barriers (B)	Measures current and potential barriers to optimal function, including safety hazards, access problems and home or office design
Ergonomics and Body Mechanics (C)	Ergonomic measurement of job tasks, work hardening or work conditioning needs; functional capacity; and body mechanics
Eustachian Tube Function (F)	Measures eustachian tube function and patency of eustachian tube

Continued on next page

Section F–Physical Rehabilitation and Diagnostic Audiology

Continued from previous page

ICD-10-PCS Value Qualifier (Character 5)	Definition
Evoked Otoacoustic Emissions, Diagnostic (N)	Measures auditory evoked potentials in a diagnostic format
Evoked Otoacoustic Emissions, Screening (M)	Measures auditory evoked potentials in a screening format
Facial Nerve Function (7)	Measures electrical activity of the VIIth cranial nerve (facial nerve)
Feeding/Eating (Assessment) (2)	Includes/Examples: Includes setting up food, selecting and using utensils and tableware, bringing food or drink to mouth, cleaning face, hands, and clothing, and management of alternative methods of nourishment
Feeding/Eating (Treatment) (3)	Exercise or activities to facilitate setting up food, selecting and using utensils and tableware, bringing food or drink to mouth, cleaning face, hands, and clothing, and management of alternative methods of nourishment
Filtered Speech (Ø)	Uses high or low pass filtered speech stimuli to assess central auditory processing disorders, site of lesion testing
Fluency (Assessment) (D)	Measures speech fluency or stuttering
Fluency (Treatment) (7)	Applying techniques to improve and augment fluent speech
Gait and/or Balance (D)	Measures biomechanical, arthrokinematic and other spatial and temporal characteristics of gait and balance
Gait Training/Functional Ambulation (9)	Exercise or activities to facilitate ambulation on a variety of surfaces and in a variety of environments
Grooming/Personal Hygiene (Assessment) (3)	Includes/Examples: Includes ability to obtain and use supplies in a sequential fashion, general grooming, oral hygiene, toilet hygiene, personal care devices, including care for artificial airways
Grooming/Personal Hygiene (Treatment) (2)	Activities to facilitate obtaining and using supplies in a sequential fashion: general grooming, oral hygiene, toilet hygiene, cleaning body, and personal care devices, including artificial airways
Hearing and Related Disorders Counseling (Ø)	Provides patients/families/caregivers with information, support, referrals to facilitate recovery from a communication disorder Includes/Examples: Includes strategies for psychosocial adjustment to hearing loss for clients and families/caregivers
Hearing and Related Disorders Prevention (1)	Provides patients/families/caregivers with information and support to prevent communication disorders
Hearing Screening (Ø)	Pass/refer measures designed to identify need for further audiologic assessment
Home Management (Assessment) (4)	Obtaining and maintaining personal and household possessions and environment Includes/Examples: Includes clothing care, cleaning, meal preparation and cleanup, shopping, money management, household maintenance, safety procedures, and childcare/parenting
Home Management (Treatment) (4)	Activities to facilitate obtaining and maintaining personal household possessions and environment Includes/Examples: Includes clothing care, cleaning, meal preparation and clean-up, shopping, money management, household maintenance, safety procedures, childcare/parenting
Instrumental Swallowing and Oral Function (J)	Measures swallowing function using instrumental diagnostic procedures Explanation: Methods include videofluoroscopy, ultrasound, manometry, endoscopy
Integumentary Integrity (1)	Includes/Examples: Includes burns, skin conditions, ecchymosis, bleeding, blisters, scar tissue, wounds and other traumas, tissue mobility, turgor and texture
Manual Therapy Techniques (7)	Techniques in which the therapist uses his/her hands to administer skilled movements Includes/Examples: Includes connective tissue massage, joint mobilization and manipulation, manual lymph drainage, manual traction, soft tissue mobilization and manipulation
Masking Patterns (W)	Measures central auditory processing status
Monaural Electroacoustic Hearing Aid Check (8)	Determines mechanical and electroacoustic function of one hearing aid using hearing aid test box
Monaural Hearing Aid (Assessment) (2)	Measures the candidacy, effectiveness, and appropriateness of a hearing aid Explanation: Measures unilateral fit
Monaural Hearing Aid (Treatment) (1)	Explanation: Assists in achieving maximum understanding and performance
Motor Function (Assessment) (4)	Measures the body's functional and versatile movement patterns Includes/Examples: Includes motor assessment scales, analysis of head, trunk and limb movement, and assessment of motor learning
Motor Function (Treatment) (3)	Exercise or activities to facilitate crossing midline, laterality, bilateral integration, praxis, neuromuscular relaxation, inhibition, facilitation, motor function and motor learning
Motor Speech (Assessment) (B)	Measures neurological motor aspects of speech production
Motor Speech (Treatment) (8)	Applying techniques to improve and augment the impaired neurological motor aspects of speech production

Continued on next page

Section F–Physical Rehabilitation and Diagnostic Audiology

Continued from previous page

ICD-10-PCS Value Qualifier (Character 5)	Definition
Muscle Performance (Assessment) (Ø)	Measures muscle strength, power and endurance using manual testing, dynamometry or computer-assisted electromechanical muscle test; functional muscle strength, power and endurance; muscle pain, tone, or soreness; or pelvic-floor musculature Explanation: Muscle endurance refers to the ability to contract a muscle repeatedly over time
Muscle Performance (Treatment) (1)	Exercise or activities to increase the capacity of a muscle to do work in terms of strength, power, and/or endurance Explanation: Muscle strength is the force exerted to overcome resistance in one maximal effort. Muscle power is work produced per unit of time, or the product of strength and speed. Muscle endurance is the ability to contract a muscle repeatedly over time.
Neuromotor Development (D)	Measures motor development, righting and equilibrium reactions, and reflex and equilibrium reactions
Non-invasive Instrumental Status (N)	Instrumental measures of oral, nasal, vocal, and velopharyngeal functions as they pertain to speech production
Nonspoken Language (Assessment) (7)	Measures nonspoken language (print, sign, symbols) for communication
Nonspoken Language (Treatment) (Ø)	Applying techniques that improve, augment, or compensate spoken communication
Oral Peripheral Mechanism (P)	Structural measures of face, jaw, lips, tongue, teeth, hard and soft palate, pharynx as related to speech production
Orofacial Myofunctional (Assessment) (K)	Measures orofacial myofunctional patterns for speech and related functions
Orofacial Myofunctional (Treatment) (9)	Applying techniques to improve, alter, or augment impaired orofacial myofunctional patterns and related speech production errors
Oscillating Tracking (3)	Measures ability to visually track
Pain (F)	Measures muscle soreness, pain and soreness with joint movement, and pain perception Includes/Examples: Includes questionnaires, graphs, symptom magnification scales or visual analog scales
Perceptual Processing (Assessment) (5)	Measures stereognosis, kinesthesia, body schema, right-left discrimination, form constancy, position in space, visual closure, figure-ground, depth perception, spatial relations and topographical orientation
Perceptual Processing (Treatment) (1)	Exercise and activities to facilitate perceptual processing Explanation: Includes stereognosis, kinesthesia, body schema, right-left discrimination, form constancy, position in space, visual closure, figure-ground, depth perception, spatial relations, and topographical orientation Includes/Examples: Includes stereognosis, kinesthesia, body schema, right-left discrimination, form constancy, position in space, visual closure, figure-ground, depth perception, spatial relations, and topographical orientation
Performance Intensity Phonetically Balanced Speech Discrimination (Q)	Measures word recognition over varying intensity levels
Postural Control (3)	Exercise or activities to increase postural alignment and control
Prosthesis (8)	Explanation: Artificial substitutes for missing body parts that augment performance or function Includes/Examples: Limb prosthesis, ocular prosthesis
Psychosocial Skills (Assessment) (6)	The ability to interact in society and to process emotions Includes/Examples: Includes psychological (values, interests, self-concept); social (role performance, social conduct, interpersonal skills, self expression); self-management (coping skills, time management, self-control)
Psychosocial Skills (Treatment) (6)	The ability to interact in society and to process emotions Includes/Examples: Includes psychological (values, interests, self-concept); social (role performance, social conduct, interpersonal skills, self expression); self-management (coping skills, time management, self-control)
Pure Tone Audiometry, Air (1)	Air-conduction pure tone threshold measures with appropriate masking
Pure Tone Audiometry, Air and Bone (2)	Air-conduction and bone-conduction pure tone threshold measures with appropriate masking
Pure Tone Stenger (C)	Measures unilateral nonorganic hearing loss based on simultaneous presentation of pure tones of differing volume
Range of Motion and Joint Integrity (5)	Measures quantity, quality, grade, and classification of joint movement and/or mobility Explanation: Range of Motion is the space, distance or angle through which movement occurs at a joint or series of joints. Joint integrity is the conformance of joints to expected anatomic, biomechanical and kinematic norms.
Range of Motion and Joint Mobility (Ø)	Exercise or activities to increase muscle length and joint mobility
Receptive/Expressive Language (Assessment) (8)	Measures receptive and expressive language
Receptive/Expressive Language (Treatment) (B)	Applying techniques to improve and augment receptive/expressive language
Reflex Integrity (G)	Measures the presence, absence, or exaggeration of developmentally appropriate, pathologic or normal reflexes

Continued on next page

Section F–Physical Rehabilitation and Diagnostic Audiology

Continued from previous page

ICD-10-PCS Value Qualifier (Character 5)	Definition
Select Picture Audiometry (5)	Establishes hearing threshold levels for speech using pictures
Sensorineural Acuity Level (4)	Measures sensorineural acuity masking presented via bone conduction
Sensory Aids (5)	Determines the appropriateness of a sensory prosthetic device, other than a hearing aid or assistive listening system/device
Sensory Awareness/ Processing/ Integrity (6)	Includes/Examples: Includes light touch, pressure, temperature, pain, sharp/dull, proprioception, vestibular, visual, auditory, gustatory, and olfactory
Short Increment Sensitivity Index (9)	Measures the ear's ability to detect small intensity changes; site of lesion test requiring a behavioral response
Sinusoidal Vertical Axis Rotational (4)	Measures nystagmus following rotation
Somatosensory Evoked Potentials (9)	Measures neural activity from sites throughout the body
Speech/Language Screening (6)	Identifies need for further speech and/or language evaluation
Speech Threshold (1)	Measures minimal intensity needed to repeat spondaic words
Speech-Language Pathology and Related Disorders Counseling (1)	Provides patients/families with information, support, referrals to facilitate recovery from a communication disorder
Speech-Language Pathology and Related Disorders Prevention (2)	Applying techniques to avoid or minimize onset and/or development of a communication disorder
Speech/Word Recognition (2)	Measures ability to repeat/identify single syllable words; scores given as a percentage; includes word recognition/speech discrimination
Staggered Spondaic Word (3)	Measures central auditory processing site of lesion based upon dichotic presentation of spondaic words
Static Orthosis (7)	Includes/Examples: Includes customized and prefabricated splints, inhibitory casts, spinal and other braces, and protective devices; has no moving parts, maintains joint(s) in desired position
Stenger (B)	Measures unilateral nonorganic hearing loss based on simultaneous presentation of signals of differing volume
Swallowing Dysfunction (D)	Activities to improve swallowing function in coordination with respiratory function Includes/Examples: Includes function and coordination of sucking, mastication, coughing, swallowing
Synthetic Sentence Identification (5)	Measures central auditory dysfunction using identification of third order approximations of sentences and competing messages
Temporal Ordering of Stimuli (V)	Measures specific central auditory process
Therapeutic Exercise (6)	Exercise or activities to facilitate sensory awareness, sensory processing, sensory integration, balance training, conditioning, reconditioning Includes/Examples: Includes developmental activities, breathing exercises, aerobic endurance activities, aquatic exercises, stretching and ventilatory muscle training
Tinnitus Masker (Assessment) (7)	Determines candidacy for tinnitus masker
Tinnitus Masker (Treatment) (Ø)	Explanation: Used to verify physical fit, acoustic appropriateness, and benefit; assists in achieving maximum benefit
Tone Decay (8)	Measures decrease in hearing sensitivity to a tone; site of lesion test requiring a behavioral response
Transfer (C)	Transitional movement from one surface to another
Transfer Training (8)	Exercise or activities to facilitate movement from one surface to another
Tympanometry (D)	Measures the integrity of the middle ear; measures ease at which sound flows through the tympanic membrane while air pressure against the membrane is varied
Unithermal Binaural Screen (2)	Measures the rhythmic eye movements stimulated by changing the temperature of the vestibular system in both ears using warm water, screening format
Ventilation/Respiration/Circulation (G)	Measures ventilatory muscle strength, power and endurance, pulmonary function and ventilatory mechanics Includes/Examples: Includes ability to clear airway, activities that aggravate or relieve edema, pain, dyspnea or other symptoms, chest wall mobility, cardiopulmonary response to performance of ADL and IAD, cough and sputum, standard vital signs
Vestibular (Ø)	Applying techniques to compensate for balance disorders; includes habituation, exercise therapy, and balance retraining
Visual Motor Integration (Assessment) (2)	Coordinating the interaction of information from the eyes with body movement during activity

Continued on next page

Section F–Physical Rehabilitation and Diagnostic Audiology

Continued from previous page

ICD-10-PCS Value Qualifier (Character 5)	Definition
Visual Motor Integration (Treatment) (2)	Exercise or activities to facilitate coordinating the interaction of information from eyes with body movement during activity
Visual Reinforcement Audiometry (6)	Behavioral measures using nonspeech and speech stimuli to obtain frequency/ear-specific information on auditory status Includes/Examples: Includes a conditioned response of looking toward a visual reinforcer (e.g., lights, animated toy) every time auditory stimuli are heard
Vocational Activities and Functional Community or Work Reintegration Skills (Assessment) (H)	Measures environmental, home, work (job/school/play) barriers that keep patients from functioning optimally in their environment Includes/Examples: Includes assessment of vocational skills and interests, environment of work (job/school/play), injury potential and injury prevention or reduction, ergonomic stressors, transportation skills, and ability to access and use community resources
Vocational Activities and Functional Community or Work Reintegration Skills (Treatment) (7)	Activities to facilitate vocational exploration, body mechanics training, job acquisition, and environmental or work (job/school/play) task adaptation Includes/Examples: Includes injury prevention and reduction, ergonomic stressor reduction, job coaching and simulation, work hardening and conditioning, driving training, transportation skills, and use of community resources
Voice (Assessment) (F)	Measures vocal structure, function and production
Voice (Treatment) (C)	Applying techniques to improve voice and vocal function
Voice Prosthetic (Assessment) (M)	Determines the appropriateness of voice prosthetic/adaptive device to enhance or facilitate communication
Voice Prosthetic (Treatment) (4)	Includes/Examples: Includes electrolarynx, and other assistive, adaptive, supportive devices
Wheelchair Mobility (Assessment) (F)	Measures fit and functional abilities within wheelchair in a variety of environments
Wheelchair Mobility (Treatment) (4)	Management, maintenance and controlled operation of a wheelchair, scooter or other device, in and on a variety of surfaces and environments
Wound Management (5)	Includes/Examples: Includes non-selective and selective debridement (enzymes, autolysis, sharp debridement), dressings (wound coverings, hydrogel, vacuum-assisted closure), topical agents, etc.

Section G–Mental Health

ICD-10-PCS Value (Character 3)	Definition
Biofeedback (C)	Provision of information from the monitoring and regulating of physiological processes in conjunction with cognitive-behavioral techniques to improve patient functioning or well-being Includes/Examples: Includes EEG, blood pressure, skin temperature or peripheral blood flow, ECG, electrooculogram, EMG, respirometry or capnometry, GSR/EDR, perineometry to monitor/regulate bowel/bladder activity, electrogastrogram to monitor/regulate gastric motility
Counseling (6)	The application of psychological methods to treat an individual with normal developmental issues and psychological problems in order to increase function, improve well-being, alleviate distress, maladjustment or resolve crises
Crisis Intervention (2)	Treatment of a traumatized, acutely disturbed or distressed individual for the purpose of short-term stabilization Includes/Examples: Includes defusing, debriefing, counseling, psychotherapy and/or coordination of care with other providers or agencies
Electroconvulsive Therapy (B)	The application of controlled electrical voltages to treat a mental health disorder Includes/Examples: Includes appropriate sedation and other preparation of the individual
Family Psychotherapy (7)	Treatment that includes one or more family members of an individual with a mental health disorder by behavioral, cognitive, psychoanalytic, psychodynamic or psychophysiological means to improve functioning or well-being Explanation: Remediation of emotional or behavioral problems presented by one or more family members in cases where psychotherapy with more than one family member is indicated
Group Psychotherapy (H)	Treatment of two or more individuals with a mental health disorder by behavioral, cognitive, psychoanalytic, psychodynamic or psychophysiological means to improve functioning or well-being
Hypnosis (F)	Induction of a state of heightened suggestibility by auditory, visual and tactile techniques to elicit an emotional or behavioral response
Individual Psychotherapy (5)	Treatment of an individual with a mental health disorder by behavioral, cognitive, psychoanalytic, psychodynamic or psychophysiological means to improve functioning or well-being
Light Therapy (J)	Application of specialized light treatments to improve functioning or well-being
Medication Management (3)	Monitoring and adjusting the use of medications for the treatment of a mental health disorder
Narcosynthesis (G)	Administration of intravenous barbiturates in order to release suppressed or repressed thoughts
Psychological Tests (1)	The administration and interpretation of standardized psychological tests and measurement instruments for the assessment of psychological function

Continued on next page

Section G–Mental Health

Continued from previous page

ICD-10-PCS Value (Character 3)	Definition
Behavioral (1)	Primarily to modify behavior Includes/Examples: Includes modeling and role playing, positive reinforcement of target behaviors, response cost, and training of self-management skills
Cognitive (2)	Primarily to correct cognitive distortions and errors
Cognitive-Behavioral (8)	Combining cognitive and behavioral treatment strategies to improve functioning Explanation: Maladaptive responses are examined to determine how cognitions relate to behavior patterns in response to an event. Uses learning principles and information-processing models.
Developmental (Ø)	Age-normed developmental status of cognitive, social and adaptive behavior skills
Intellectual and Psychoeducational (2)	Intellectual abilities, academic achievement and learning capabilities (including behaviors and emotional factors affecting learning)
Interactive (Ø)	Uses primarily physical aids and other forms of non-oral interaction with a patient who is physically, psychologically or developmentally unable to use ordinary language for communication Includes/Examples: Includes the use of toys in symbolic play
Interpersonal (3)	Helps an individual make changes in interpersonal behaviors to reduce psychological dysfunction Includes/Examples: Includes exploratory techniques, encouragement of affective expression, clarification of patient statements, analysis of communication patterns, use of therapy relationship and behavior change techniques
Neurobehavioral and Cognitive Status (4)	Includes neurobehavioral status exam, interview(s), and observation for the clinical assessment of thinking, reasoning and judgment, acquired knowledge, attention, memory, visual spatial abilities, language functions, and planning
Neuropsychological (3)	Thinking, reasoning and judgment, acquired knowledge, attention, memory, visual spatial abilities, language functions, planning
Personality and Behavioral (1)	Mood, emotion, behavior, social functioning, psychopathological conditions, personality traits and characteristics
Psychoanalysis (4)	Methods of obtaining a detailed account of past and present mental and emotional experiences to determine the source and eliminate or diminish the undesirable effects of unconscious conflicts Explanation: Accomplished by making the individual aware of their existence, origin, and inappropriate expression in emotions and behavior
Psychodynamic (5)	Exploration of past and present emotional experiences to understand motives and drives using insight-oriented techniques to reduce the undesirable effects of internal conflicts on emotions and behavior Explanation: Techniques include empathetic listening, clarifying self-defeating behavior patterns, and exploring adaptive alternatives
Psychophysiological (9)	Monitoring and alteration of physiological processes to help the individual associate physiological reactions combined with cognitive and behavioral strategies to gain improved control of these processes to help the individual cope more effectively
Supportive (6)	Formation of therapeutic relationship primarily for providing emotional support to prevent further deterioration in functioning during periods of particular stress Explanation: Often used in conjunction with other therapeutic approaches
Vocational (1)	Exploration of vocational interests, aptitudes and required adaptive behavior skills to develop and carry out a plan for achieving a successful vocational placement Includes/Examples: Includes enhancing work related adjustment and/or pursuing viable options in training education or preparation

Section H–Substance Abuse Treatment

ICD-10-PCS Value (Character 3)	Definition
Detoxification Services (2)	Detoxification from alcohol and/or drugs Explanation: Not a treatment modality, but helps the patient stabilize physically and psychologically until the body becomes free of drugs and the effects of alcohol
Family Counseling (6)	The application of psychological methods that includes one or more family members to treat an individual with addictive behavior Explanation: Provides support and education for family members of addicted individuals. Family member participation is seen as a critical area of substance abuse treatment.
Group Counseling (4)	The application of psychological methods to treat two or more individuals with addictive behavior Explanation: Provides structured group counseling sessions and healing power through the connection with others
Individual Counseling (3)	The application of psychological methods to treat an individual with addictive behavior Explanation: Comprised of several different techniques, which apply various strategies to address drug addiction
Individual Psychotherapy (5)	Treatment of an individual with addictive behavior by behavioral, cognitive, psychoanalytic, psychodynamic or psychophysiological means
Medication Management (8)	Monitoring and adjusting the use of replacement medications for the treatment of addiction
Pharmacotherapy (9)	The use of replacement medications for the treatment of addiction

Appendix K: Hospital Acquired Conditions

Hospital acquired conditions (HACs) are conditions considered reasonably preventable through the application of evidence-based guidelines. Although it is the ICD-10-CM diagnosis code that drives a HAC designation, in some cases a specific ICD-10-PCS procedure code must also be present before that diagnosis code can be considered a HAC. This resource provides only those HAC categories that require both an ICD-10-PCS code and an ICD-10-CM diagnosis code. The official descriptions for each code are also provided. To see all 14 HAC categories and their corresponding codes, refer to Optum's *ICD-10-CM Expert for Hospitals*.

Note: The resource used to compile this list is the proposed, version 40, MS-DRG Grouper software and Definitions Manual files published with the fiscal 2024 IPPS proposed rule. For the most current files, refer to the following:
https://www.cms.gov/Medicare/Medicare-Fee-for-Service-Payment/AcuteInpatientPPS/MS-DRG-Classifications-and-Software.

HAC 08: Surgical Site Infection of Mediastinitis After Coronary Bypass Graft (CABG) Procedures

Secondary diagnosis not POA:

J98.51   Mediastinitis

J98.59   Other diseases of mediastinum, not elsewhere classified

AND

Any of the following procedures:

0210083   Bypass Coronary Artery, One Artery from Coronary Artery with Zooplastic Tissue, Open Approach

0210088   Bypass Coronary Artery, One Artery from Right Internal Mammary with Zooplastic Tissue, Open Approach

0210089   Bypass Coronary Artery, One Artery from Left Internal Mammary with Zooplastic Tissue, Open Approach

021008C   Bypass Coronary Artery, One Artery from Thoracic Artery with Zooplastic Tissue, Open Approach

021008F   Bypass Coronary Artery, One Artery from Abdominal Artery with Zooplastic Tissue, Open Approach

021008W   Bypass Coronary Artery, One Artery from Aorta with Zooplastic Tissue, Open Approach

0210093   Bypass Coronary Artery, One Artery from Coronary Artery with Autologous Venous Tissue, Open Approach

0210098   Bypass Coronary Artery, One Artery from Right Internal Mammary with Autologous Venous Tissue, Open Approach

0210099   Bypass Coronary Artery, One Artery from Left Internal Mammary with Autologous Venous Tissue, Open Approach

021009C   Bypass Coronary Artery, One Artery from Thoracic Artery with Autologous Venous Tissue, Open Approach

021009F   Bypass Coronary Artery, One Artery from Abdominal Artery with Autologous Venous Tissue, Open Approach

021009W   Bypass Coronary Artery, One Artery from Aorta with Autologous Venous Tissue, Open Approach

02100A3   Bypass Coronary Artery, One Artery from Coronary Artery with Autologous Arterial Tissue, Open Approach

02100A8   Bypass Coronary Artery, One Artery from Right Internal Mammary with Autologous Arterial Tissue, Open Approach

02100A9   Bypass Coronary Artery, One Artery from Left Internal Mammary with Autologous Arterial Tissue, Open Approach

02100AC   Bypass Coronary Artery, One Artery from Thoracic Artery with Autologous Arterial Tissue, Open Approach

02100AF   Bypass Coronary Artery, One Artery from Abdominal Artery with Autologous Arterial Tissue, Open Approach

02100AW   Bypass Coronary Artery, One Artery from Aorta with Autologous Arterial Tissue, Open Approach

02100J3   Bypass Coronary Artery, One Artery from Coronary Artery with Synthetic Substitute, Open Approach

02100J8   Bypass Coronary Artery, One Artery from Right Internal Mammary with Synthetic Substitute, Open Approach

02100J9   Bypass Coronary Artery, One Artery from Left Internal Mammary with Synthetic Substitute, Open Approach

02100JC   Bypass Coronary Artery, One Artery from Thoracic Artery with Synthetic Substitute, Open Approach

02100JF   Bypass Coronary Artery, One Artery from Abdominal Artery with Synthetic Substitute, Open Approach

02100JW   Bypass Coronary Artery, One Artery from Aorta with Synthetic Substitute, Open Approach

02100K3   Bypass Coronary Artery, One Artery from Coronary Artery with Nonautologous Tissue Substitute, Open Approach

02100K8   Bypass Coronary Artery, One Artery from Right Internal Mammary with Nonautologous Tissue Substitute, Open Approach

02100K9   Bypass Coronary Artery, One Artery from Left Internal Mammary with Nonautologous Tissue Substitute, Open Approach

02100KC   Bypass Coronary Artery, One Artery from Thoracic Artery with Nonautologous Tissue Substitute, Open Approach

02100KF   Bypass Coronary Artery, One Artery from Abdominal Artery with Nonautologous Tissue Substitute, Open Approach

02100KW   Bypass Coronary Artery, One Artery from Aorta with Nonautologous Tissue Substitute, Open Approach

02100Z3   Bypass Coronary Artery, One Artery from Coronary Artery, Open Approach

02100Z8   Bypass Coronary Artery, One Artery from Right Internal Mammary, Open Approach

02100Z9   Bypass Coronary Artery, One Artery from Left Internal Mammary, Open Approach

02100ZC   Bypass Coronary Artery, One Artery from Thoracic Artery, Open Approach

02100ZF   Bypass Coronary Artery, One Artery from Abdominal Artery, Open Approach

0210483   Bypass Coronary Artery, One Artery from Coronary Artery with Zooplastic Tissue, Percutaneous Endoscopic Approach

0210488   Bypass Coronary Artery, One Artery from Right Internal Mammary with Zooplastic Tissue, Percutaneous Endoscopic Approach

0210489   Bypass Coronary Artery, One Artery from Left Internal Mammary with Zooplastic Tissue, Percutaneous Endoscopic Approach

021048C   Bypass Coronary Artery, One Artery from Thoracic Artery with Zooplastic Tissue, Percutaneous Endoscopic Approach

021048F   Bypass Coronary Artery, One Artery from Abdominal Artery with Zooplastic Tissue, Percutaneous Endoscopic Approach

021048W   Bypass Coronary Artery, One Artery from Aorta with Zooplastic Tissue, Percutaneous Endoscopic Approach

0210493   Bypass Coronary Artery, One Artery from Coronary Artery with Autologous Venous Tissue, Percutaneous Endoscopic Approach

0210498   Bypass Coronary Artery, One Artery from Right Internal Mammary with Autologous Venous Tissue, Percutaneous Endoscopic Approach

0210499   Bypass Coronary Artery, One Artery from Left Internal Mammary with Autologous Venous Tissue, Percutaneous Endoscopic Approach

021049C   Bypass Coronary Artery, One Artery from Thoracic Artery with Autologous Venous Tissue, Percutaneous Endoscopic Approach

021049F   Bypass Coronary Artery, One Artery from Abdominal Artery with Autologous Venous Tissue, Percutaneous Endoscopic Approach

021049W   Bypass Coronary Artery, One Artery from Aorta with Autologous Venous Tissue, Percutaneous Endoscopic Approach

02104A3   Bypass Coronary Artery, One Artery from Coronary Artery with Autologous Arterial Tissue, Percutaneous Endoscopic Approach

02104A8   Bypass Coronary Artery, One Artery from Right Internal Mammary with Autologous Arterial Tissue, Percutaneous Endoscopic Approach

02104A9   Bypass Coronary Artery, One Artery from Left Internal Mammary with Autologous Arterial Tissue, Percutaneous Endoscopic Approach

02104AC   Bypass Coronary Artery, One Artery from Thoracic Artery with Autologous Arterial Tissue, Percutaneous Endoscopic Approach

02104AF   Bypass Coronary Artery, One Artery from Abdominal Artery with Autologous Arterial Tissue, Percutaneous Endoscopic Approach

02104AW   Bypass Coronary Artery, One Artery from Aorta with Autologous Arterial Tissue, Percutaneous Endoscopic Approach

02104J3   Bypass Coronary Artery, One Artery from Coronary Artery with Synthetic Substitute, Percutaneous Endoscopic Approach

02104J8   Bypass Coronary Artery, One Artery from Right Internal Mammary with Synthetic Substitute, Percutaneous Endoscopic Approach

02104J9   Bypass Coronary Artery, One Artery from Left Internal Mammary with Synthetic Substitute, Percutaneous Endoscopic Approach

HAC 08: Surgical Site Infection of Mediastinitis After Coronary Bypass Graft (CABG) Procedures (continued)

02104JC　Bypass Coronary Artery, One Artery from Thoracic Artery with Synthetic Substitute, Percutaneous Endoscopic Approach

02104JF　Bypass Coronary Artery, One Artery from Abdominal Artery with Synthetic Substitute, Percutaneous Endoscopic Approach

02104JW　Bypass Coronary Artery, One Artery from Aorta with Synthetic Substitute, Percutaneous Endoscopic Approach

02104K3　Bypass Coronary Artery, One Artery from Coronary Artery with Nonautologous Tissue Substitute, Percutaneous Endoscopic Approach

02104K8　Bypass Coronary Artery, One Artery from Right Internal Mammary with Nonautologous Tissue Substitute, Percutaneous Endoscopic Approach

02104K9　Bypass Coronary Artery, One Artery from Left Internal Mammary with Nonautologous Tissue Substitute, Percutaneous Endoscopic Approach

02104KC　Bypass Coronary Artery, One Artery from Thoracic Artery with Nonautologous Tissue Substitute, Percutaneous Endoscopic Approach

02104KF　Bypass Coronary Artery, One Artery from Abdominal Artery with Nonautologous Tissue Substitute, Percutaneous Endoscopic Approach

02104KW　Bypass Coronary Artery, One Artery from Aorta with Nonautologous Tissue Substitute, Percutaneous Endoscopic Approach

02104Z3　Bypass Coronary Artery, One Artery from Coronary Artery, Percutaneous Endoscopic Approach

02104Z8　Bypass Coronary Artery, One Artery from Right Internal Mammary, Percutaneous Endoscopic Approach

02104Z9　Bypass Coronary Artery, One Artery from Left Internal Mammary, Percutaneous Endoscopic Approach

02104ZC　Bypass Coronary Artery, One Artery from Thoracic Artery, Percutaneous Endoscopic Approach

02104ZF　Bypass Coronary Artery, One Artery from Abdominal Artery, Percutaneous Endoscopic Approach

0211083　Bypass Coronary Artery, Two Arteries from Coronary Artery with Zooplastic Tissue, Open Approach

0211088　Bypass Coronary Artery, Two Arteries from Right Internal Mammary with Zooplastic Tissue, Open Approach

0211089　Bypass Coronary Artery, Two Arteries from Left Internal Mammary with Zooplastic Tissue, Open Approach

021108C　Bypass Coronary Artery, Two Arteries from Thoracic Artery with Zooplastic Tissue, Open Approach

021108F　Bypass Coronary Artery, Two Arteries from Abdominal Artery with Zooplastic Tissue, Open Approach

021108W　Bypass Coronary Artery, Two Arteries from Aorta with Zooplastic Tissue, Open Approach

0211093　Bypass Coronary Artery, Two Arteries from Coronary Artery with Autologous Venous Tissue, Open Approach

0211098　Bypass Coronary Artery, Two Arteries from Right Internal Mammary with Autologous Venous Tissue, Open Approach

0211099　Bypass Coronary Artery, Two Arteries from Left Internal Mammary with Autologous Venous Tissue, Open Approach

021109C　Bypass Coronary Artery, Two Arteries from Thoracic Artery with Autologous Venous Tissue, Open Approach

021109F　Bypass Coronary Artery, Two Arteries from Abdominal Artery with Autologous Venous Tissue, Open Approach

021109W　Bypass Coronary Artery, Two Arteries from Aorta with Autologous Venous Tissue, Open Approach

02110A3　Bypass Coronary Artery, Two Arteries from Coronary Artery with Autologous Arterial Tissue, Open Approach

02110A8　Bypass Coronary Artery, Two Arteries from Right Internal Mammary with Autologous Arterial Tissue, Open Approach

02110A9　Bypass Coronary Artery, Two Arteries from Left Internal Mammary with Autologous Arterial Tissue, Open Approach

02110AC　Bypass Coronary Artery, Two Arteries from Thoracic Artery with Autologous Arterial Tissue, Open Approach

02110AF　Bypass Coronary Artery, Two Arteries from Abdominal Artery with Autologous Arterial Tissue, Open Approach

02110AW　Bypass Coronary Artery, Two Arteries from Aorta with Autologous Arterial Tissue, Open Approach

02110J3　Bypass Coronary Artery, Two Arteries from Coronary Artery with Synthetic Substitute, Open Approach

02110J8　Bypass Coronary Artery, Two Arteries from Right Internal Mammary with Synthetic Substitute, Open Approach

02110J9　Bypass Coronary Artery, Two Arteries from Left Internal Mammary with Synthetic Substitute, Open Approach

02110JC　Bypass Coronary Artery, Two Arteries from Thoracic Artery with Synthetic Substitute, Open Approach

02110JF　Bypass Coronary Artery, Two Arteries from Abdominal Artery with Synthetic Substitute, Open Approach

02110JW　Bypass Coronary Artery, Two Arteries from Aorta with Synthetic Substitute, Open Approach

02110K3　Bypass Coronary Artery, Two Arteries from Coronary Artery with Nonautologous Tissue Substitute, Open Approach

02110K8　Bypass Coronary Artery, Two Arteries from Right Internal Mammary with Nonautologous Tissue Substitute, Open Approach

02110K9　Bypass Coronary Artery, Two Arteries from Left Internal Mammary with Nonautologous Tissue Substitute, Open Approach

02110KC　Bypass Coronary Artery, Two Arteries from Thoracic Artery with Nonautologous Tissue Substitute, Open Approach

02110KF　Bypass Coronary Artery, Two Arteries from Abdominal Artery with Nonautologous Tissue Substitute, Open Approach

02110KW　Bypass Coronary Artery, Two Arteries from Aorta with Nonautologous Tissue Substitute, Open Approach

02110Z3　Bypass Coronary Artery, Two Arteries from Coronary Artery, Open Approach

02110Z8　Bypass Coronary Artery, Two Arteries from Right Internal Mammary, Open Approach

02110Z9　Bypass Coronary Artery, Two Arteries from Left Internal Mammary, Open Approach

02110ZC　Bypass Coronary Artery, Two Arteries from Thoracic Artery, Open Approach

02110ZF　Bypass Coronary Artery, Two Arteries from Abdominal Artery, Open Approach

0211483　Bypass Coronary Artery, Two Arteries from Coronary Artery with Zooplastic Tissue, Percutaneous Endoscopic Approach

0211488　Bypass Coronary Artery, Two Arteries from Right Internal Mammary with Zooplastic Tissue, Percutaneous Endoscopic Approach

0211489　Bypass Coronary Artery, Two Arteries from Left Internal Mammary with Zooplastic Tissue, Percutaneous Endoscopic Approach

021148C　Bypass Coronary Artery, Two Arteries from Thoracic Artery with Zooplastic Tissue, Percutaneous Endoscopic Approach

021148F　Bypass Coronary Artery, Two Arteries from Abdominal Artery with Zooplastic Tissue, Percutaneous Endoscopic Approach

021148W　Bypass Coronary Artery, Two Arteries from Aorta with Zooplastic Tissue, Percutaneous Endoscopic Approach

0211493　Bypass Coronary Artery, Two Arteries from Coronary Artery with Autologous Venous Tissue, Percutaneous Endoscopic Approach

0211498　Bypass Coronary Artery, Two Arteries from Right Internal Mammary with Autologous Venous Tissue, Percutaneous Endoscopic Approach

0211499　Bypass Coronary Artery, Two Arteries from Left Internal Mammary with Autologous Venous Tissue, Percutaneous Endoscopic Approach

021149C　Bypass Coronary Artery, Two Arteries from Thoracic Artery with Autologous Venous Tissue, Percutaneous Endoscopic Approach

021149F　Bypass Coronary Artery, Two Arteries from Abdominal Artery with Autologous Venous Tissue, Percutaneous Endoscopic Approach

021149W　Bypass Coronary Artery, Two Arteries from Aorta with Autologous Venous Tissue, Percutaneous Endoscopic Approach

02114A3　Bypass Coronary Artery, Two Arteries from Coronary Artery with Autologous Arterial Tissue, Percutaneous Endoscopic Approach

02114A8　Bypass Coronary Artery, Two Arteries from Right Internal Mammary with Autologous Arterial Tissue, Percutaneous Endoscopic Approach

02114A9　Bypass Coronary Artery, Two Arteries from Left Internal Mammary with Autologous Arterial Tissue, Percutaneous Endoscopic Approach

02114AC　Bypass Coronary Artery, Two Arteries from Thoracic Artery with Autologous Arterial Tissue, Percutaneous Endoscopic Approach

02114AF　Bypass Coronary Artery, Two Arteries from Abdominal Artery with Autologous Arterial Tissue, Percutaneous Endoscopic Approach

02114AW　Bypass Coronary Artery, Two Arteries from Aorta with Autologous Arterial Tissue, Percutaneous Endoscopic Approach

02114J3　Bypass Coronary Artery, Two Arteries from Coronary Artery with Synthetic Substitute, Percutaneous Endoscopic Approach

02114J8　Bypass Coronary Artery, Two Arteries from Right Internal Mammary with Synthetic Substitute, Percutaneous Endoscopic Approach

Appendix K: Hospital Acquired Conditions

HAC 08: Surgical Site Infection of Mediastinitis After Coronary Bypass Graft (CABG) Procedures (continued)

Ø2114J9   Bypass Coronary Artery, Two Arteries from Left Internal Mammary with Synthetic Substitute, Percutaneous Endoscopic Approach

Ø2114JC   Bypass Coronary Artery, Two Arteries from Thoracic Artery with Synthetic Substitute, Percutaneous Endoscopic Approach

Ø2114JF   Bypass Coronary Artery, Two Arteries from Abdominal Artery with Synthetic Substitute, Percutaneous Endoscopic Approach

Ø2114JW   Bypass Coronary Artery, Two Arteries from Aorta with Synthetic Substitute, Percutaneous Endoscopic Approach

Ø2114K3   Bypass Coronary Artery, Two Arteries from Coronary Artery with Nonautologous Tissue Substitute, Percutaneous Endoscopic Approach

Ø2114K8   Bypass Coronary Artery, Two Arteries from Right Internal Mammary with Nonautologous Tissue Substitute, Percutaneous Endoscopic Approach

Ø2114K9   Bypass Coronary Artery, Two Arteries from Left Internal Mammary with Nonautologous Tissue Substitute, Percutaneous Endoscopic Approach

Ø2114KC   Bypass Coronary Artery, Two Arteries from Thoracic Artery with Nonautologous Tissue Substitute, Percutaneous Endoscopic Approach

Ø2114KF   Bypass Coronary Artery, Two Arteries from Abdominal Artery with Nonautologous Tissue Substitute, Percutaneous Endoscopic Approach

Ø2114KW   Bypass Coronary Artery, Two Arteries from Aorta with Nonautologous Tissue Substitute, Percutaneous Endoscopic Approach

Ø2114Z3   Bypass Coronary Artery, Two Arteries from Coronary Artery, Percutaneous Endoscopic Approach

Ø2114Z8   Bypass Coronary Artery, Two Arteries from Right Internal Mammary, Percutaneous Endoscopic Approach

Ø2114Z9   Bypass Coronary Artery, Two Arteries from Left Internal Mammary, Percutaneous Endoscopic Approach

Ø2114ZC   Bypass Coronary Artery, Two Arteries from Thoracic Artery, Percutaneous Endoscopic Approach

Ø2114ZF   Bypass Coronary Artery, Two Arteries from Abdominal Artery, Percutaneous Endoscopic Approach

Ø212Ø83   Bypass Coronary Artery, Three Arteries from Coronary Artery with Zooplastic Tissue, Open Approach

Ø212Ø88   Bypass Coronary Artery, Three Arteries from Right Internal Mammary with Zooplastic Tissue, Open Approach

Ø212Ø89   Bypass Coronary Artery, Three Arteries from Left Internal Mammary with Zooplastic Tissue, Open Approach

Ø212Ø8C   Bypass Coronary Artery, Three Arteries from Thoracic Artery with Zooplastic Tissue, Open Approach

Ø212Ø8F   Bypass Coronary Artery, Three Arteries from Abdominal Artery with Zooplastic Tissue, Open Approach

Ø212Ø8W   Bypass Coronary Artery, Three Arteries from Aorta with Zooplastic Tissue, Open Approach

Ø212Ø93   Bypass Coronary Artery, Three Arteries from Coronary Artery with Autologous Venous Tissue, Open Approach

Ø212Ø98   Bypass Coronary Artery, Three Arteries from Right Internal Mammary with Autologous Venous Tissue, Open Approach

Ø212Ø99   Bypass Coronary Artery, Three Arteries from Left Internal Mammary with Autologous Venous Tissue, Open Approach

Ø212Ø9C   Bypass Coronary Artery, Three Arteries from Thoracic Artery with Autologous Venous Tissue, Open Approach

Ø212Ø9F   Bypass Coronary Artery, Three Arteries from Abdominal Artery with Autologous Venous Tissue, Open Approach

Ø212Ø9W   Bypass Coronary Artery, Three Arteries from Aorta with Autologous Venous Tissue, Open Approach

Ø212ØA3   Bypass Coronary Artery, Three Arteries from Coronary Artery with Autologous Arterial Tissue, Open Approach

Ø212ØA8   Bypass Coronary Artery, Three Arteries from Right Internal Mammary with Autologous Arterial Tissue, Open Approach

Ø212ØA9   Bypass Coronary Artery, Three Arteries from Left Internal Mammary with Autologous Arterial Tissue, Open Approach

Ø212ØAC   Bypass Coronary Artery, Three Arteries from Thoracic Artery with Autologous Arterial Tissue, Open Approach

Ø212ØAF   Bypass Coronary Artery, Three Arteries from Abdominal Artery with Autologous Arterial Tissue, Open Approach

Ø212ØAW   Bypass Coronary Artery, Three Arteries from Aorta with Autologous Arterial Tissue, Open Approach

Ø212ØJ3   Bypass Coronary Artery, Three Arteries from Coronary Artery with Synthetic Substitute, Open Approach

Ø212ØJ8   Bypass Coronary Artery, Three Arteries from Right Internal Mammary with Synthetic Substitute, Open Approach

Ø212ØJ9   Bypass Coronary Artery, Three Arteries from Left Internal Mammary with Synthetic Substitute, Open Approach

Ø212ØJC   Bypass Coronary Artery, Three Arteries from Thoracic Artery with Synthetic Substitute, Open Approach

Ø212ØJF   Bypass Coronary Artery, Three Arteries from Abdominal Artery with Synthetic Substitute, Open Approach

Ø212ØJW   Bypass Coronary Artery, Three Arteries from Aorta with Synthetic Substitute, Open Approach

Ø212ØK3   Bypass Coronary Artery, Three Arteries from Coronary Artery with Nonautologous Tissue Substitute, Open Approach

Ø212ØK8   Bypass Coronary Artery, Three Arteries from Right Internal Mammary with Nonautologous Tissue Substitute, Open Approach

Ø212ØK9   Bypass Coronary Artery, Three Arteries from Left Internal Mammary with Nonautologous Tissue Substitute, Open Approach

Ø212ØKC   Bypass Coronary Artery, Three Arteries from Thoracic Artery with Nonautologous Tissue Substitute, Open Approach

Ø212ØKF   Bypass Coronary Artery, Three Arteries from Abdominal Artery with Nonautologous Tissue Substitute, Open Approach

Ø212ØKW   Bypass Coronary Artery, Three Arteries from Aorta with Nonautologous Tissue Substitute, Open Approach

Ø212ØZ3   Bypass Coronary Artery, Three Arteries from Coronary Artery, Open Approach

Ø212ØZ8   Bypass Coronary Artery, Three Arteries from Right Internal Mammary, Open Approach

Ø212ØZ9   Bypass Coronary Artery, Three Arteries from Left Internal Mammary, Open Approach

Ø212ØZC   Bypass Coronary Artery, Three Arteries from Thoracic Artery, Open Approach

Ø212ØZF   Bypass Coronary Artery, Three Arteries from Abdominal Artery, Open Approach

Ø212483   Bypass Coronary Artery, Three Arteries from Coronary Artery with Zooplastic Tissue, Percutaneous Endoscopic Approach

Ø212488   Bypass Coronary Artery, Three Arteries from Right Internal Mammary with Zooplastic Tissue, Percutaneous Endoscopic Approach

Ø212489   Bypass Coronary Artery, Three Arteries from Left Internal Mammary with Zooplastic Tissue, Percutaneous Endoscopic Approach

Ø21248C   Bypass Coronary Artery, Three Arteries from Thoracic Artery with Zooplastic Tissue, Percutaneous Endoscopic Approach

Ø21248F   Bypass Coronary Artery, Three Arteries from Abdominal Artery with Zooplastic Tissue, Percutaneous Endoscopic Approach

Ø21248W   Bypass Coronary Artery, Three Arteries from Aorta with Zooplastic Tissue, Percutaneous Endoscopic Approach

Ø212493   Bypass Coronary Artery, Three Arteries from Coronary Artery with Autologous Venous Tissue, Percutaneous Endoscopic Approach

Ø212498   Bypass Coronary Artery, Three Arteries from Right Internal Mammary with Autologous Venous Tissue, Percutaneous Endoscopic Approach

Ø212499   Bypass Coronary Artery, Three Arteries from Left Internal Mammary with Autologous Venous Tissue, Percutaneous Endoscopic Approach

Ø21249C   Bypass Coronary Artery, Three Arteries from Thoracic Artery with Autologous Venous Tissue, Percutaneous Endoscopic Approach

Ø21249F   Bypass Coronary Artery, Three Arteries from Abdominal Artery with Autologous Venous Tissue, Percutaneous Endoscopic Approach

Ø21249W   Bypass Coronary Artery, Three Arteries from Aorta with Autologous Venous Tissue, Percutaneous Endoscopic Approach

Ø2124A3   Bypass Coronary Artery, Three Arteries from Coronary Artery with Autologous Arterial Tissue, Percutaneous Endoscopic Approach

Ø2124A8   Bypass Coronary Artery, Three Arteries from Right Internal Mammary with Autologous Arterial Tissue, Percutaneous Endoscopic Approach

Ø2124A9   Bypass Coronary Artery, Three Arteries from Left Internal Mammary with Autologous Arterial Tissue, Percutaneous Endoscopic Approach

HAC 08: Surgical Site Infection of Mediastinitis After Coronary Bypass Graft (CABG) Procedures (continued)

02124AC Bypass Coronary Artery, Three Arteries from Thoracic Artery with Autologous Arterial Tissue, Percutaneous Endoscopic Approach

02124AF Bypass Coronary Artery, Three Arteries from Abdominal Artery with Autologous Arterial Tissue, Percutaneous Endoscopic Approach

02124AW Bypass Coronary Artery, Three Arteries from Aorta with Autologous Arterial Tissue, Percutaneous Endoscopic Approach

02124J3 Bypass Coronary Artery, Three Arteries from Coronary Artery with Synthetic Substitute, Percutaneous Endoscopic Approach

02124J8 Bypass Coronary Artery, Three Arteries from Right Internal Mammary with Synthetic Substitute, Percutaneous Endoscopic Approach

02124J9 Bypass Coronary Artery, Three Arteries from Left Internal Mammary with Synthetic Substitute, Percutaneous Endoscopic Approach

02124JC Bypass Coronary Artery, Three Arteries from Thoracic Artery with Synthetic Substitute, Percutaneous Endoscopic Approach

02124JF Bypass Coronary Artery, Three Arteries from Abdominal Artery with Synthetic Substitute, Percutaneous Endoscopic Approach

02124JW Bypass Coronary Artery, Three Arteries from Aorta with Synthetic Substitute, Percutaneous Endoscopic Approach

02124K3 Bypass Coronary Artery, Three Arteries from Coronary Artery with Nonautologous Tissue Substitute, Percutaneous Endoscopic Approach

02124K8 Bypass Coronary Artery, Three Arteries from Right Internal Mammary with Nonautologous Tissue Substitute, Percutaneous Endoscopic Approach

02124K9 Bypass Coronary Artery, Three Arteries from Left Internal Mammary with Nonautologous Tissue Substitute, Percutaneous Endoscopic Approach

02124KC Bypass Coronary Artery, Three Arteries from Thoracic Artery with Nonautologous Tissue Substitute, Percutaneous Endoscopic Approach

02124KF Bypass Coronary Artery, Three Arteries from Abdominal Artery with Nonautologous Tissue Substitute, Percutaneous Endoscopic Approach

02124KW Bypass Coronary Artery, Three Arteries from Aorta with Nonautologous Tissue Substitute, Percutaneous Endoscopic Approach

02124Z3 Bypass Coronary Artery, Three Arteries from Coronary Artery, Percutaneous Endoscopic Approach

02124Z8 Bypass Coronary Artery, Three Arteries from Right Internal Mammary, Percutaneous Endoscopic Approach

02124Z9 Bypass Coronary Artery, Three Arteries from Left Internal Mammary, Percutaneous Endoscopic Approach

02124ZC Bypass Coronary Artery, Three Arteries from Thoracic Artery, Percutaneous Endoscopic Approach

02124ZF Bypass Coronary Artery, Three Arteries from Abdominal Artery, Percutaneous Endoscopic Approach

0213083 Bypass Coronary Artery, Four or More Arteries from Coronary Artery with Zooplastic Tissue, Open Approach

0213088 Bypass Coronary Artery, Four or More Arteries from Right Internal Mammary with Zooplastic Tissue, Open Approach

0213089 Bypass Coronary Artery, Four or More Arteries from Left Internal Mammary with Zooplastic Tissue, Open Approach

021308C Bypass Coronary Artery, Four or More Arteries from Thoracic Artery with Zooplastic Tissue, Open Approach

021308F Bypass Coronary Artery, Four or More Arteries from Abdominal Artery with Zooplastic Tissue, Open Approach

021308W Bypass Coronary Artery, Four or More Arteries from Aorta with Zooplastic Tissue, Open Approach

0213093 Bypass Coronary Artery, Four or More Arteries from Coronary Artery with Autologous Venous Tissue, Open Approach

0213098 Bypass Coronary Artery, Four or More Arteries from Right Internal Mammary with Autologous Venous Tissue, Open Approach

0213099 Bypass Coronary Artery, Four or More Arteries from Left Internal Mammary with Autologous Venous Tissue, Open Approach

021309C Bypass Coronary Artery, Four or More Arteries from Thoracic Artery with Autologous Venous Tissue, Open Approach

021309F Bypass Coronary Artery, Four or More Arteries from Abdominal Artery with Autologous Venous Tissue, Open Approach

021309W Bypass Coronary Artery, Four or More Arteries from Aorta with Autologous Venous Tissue, Open Approach

02130A3 Bypass Coronary Artery, Four or More Arteries from Coronary Artery with Autologous Arterial Tissue, Open Approach

02130A8 Bypass Coronary Artery, Four or More Arteries from Right Internal Mammary with Autologous Arterial Tissue, Open Approach

02130A9 Bypass Coronary Artery, Four or More Arteries from Left Internal Mammary with Autologous Arterial Tissue, Open Approach

02130AC Bypass Coronary Artery, Four or More Arteries from Thoracic Artery with Autologous Arterial Tissue, Open Approach

02130AF Bypass Coronary Artery, Four or More Arteries from Abdominal Artery with Autologous Arterial Tissue, Open Approach

02130AW Bypass Coronary Artery, Four or More Arteries from Aorta with Autologous Arterial Tissue, Open Approach

02130J3 Bypass Coronary Artery, Four or More Arteries from Coronary Artery with Synthetic Substitute, Open Approach

02130J8 Bypass Coronary Artery, Four or More Arteries from Right Internal Mammary with Synthetic Substitute, Open Approach

02130J9 Bypass Coronary Artery, Four or More Arteries from Left Internal Mammary with Synthetic Substitute, Open Approach

02130JC Bypass Coronary Artery, Four or More Arteries from Thoracic Artery with Synthetic Substitute, Open Approach

02130JF Bypass Coronary Artery, Four or More Arteries from Abdominal Artery with Synthetic Substitute, Open Approach

02130JW Bypass Coronary Artery, Four or More Arteries from Aorta with Synthetic Substitute, Open Approach

02130K3 Bypass Coronary Artery, Four or More Arteries from Coronary Artery with Nonautologous Tissue Substitute, Open Approach

02130K8 Bypass Coronary Artery, Four or More Arteries from Right Internal Mammary with Nonautologous Tissue Substitute, Open Approach

02130K9 Bypass Coronary Artery, Four or More Arteries from Left Internal Mammary with Nonautologous Tissue Substitute, Open Approach

02130KC Bypass Coronary Artery, Four or More Arteries from Thoracic Artery with Nonautologous Tissue Substitute, Open Approach

02130KF Bypass Coronary Artery, Four or More Arteries from Abdominal Artery with Nonautologous Tissue Substitute, Open Approach

02130KW Bypass Coronary Artery, Four or More Arteries from Aorta with Nonautologous Tissue Substitute, Open Approach

02130Z3 Bypass Coronary Artery, Four or More Arteries from Coronary Artery, Open Approach

02130Z8 Bypass Coronary Artery, Four or More Arteries from Right Internal Mammary, Open Approach

02130Z9 Bypass Coronary Artery, Four or More Arteries from Left Internal Mammary, Open Approach

02130ZC Bypass Coronary Artery, Four or More Arteries from Thoracic Artery, Open Approach

02130ZF Bypass Coronary Artery, Four or More Arteries from Abdominal Artery, Open Approach

0213483 Bypass Coronary Artery, Four or More Arteries from Coronary Artery with Zooplastic Tissue, Percutaneous Endoscopic Approach

0213488 Bypass Coronary Artery, Four or More Arteries from Right Internal Mammary with Zooplastic Tissue, Percutaneous Endoscopic Approach

0213489 Bypass Coronary Artery, Four or More Arteries from Left Internal Mammary with Zooplastic Tissue, Percutaneous Endoscopic Approach

021348C Bypass Coronary Artery, Four or More Arteries from Thoracic Artery with Zooplastic Tissue, Percutaneous Endoscopic Approach

021348F Bypass Coronary Artery, Four or More Arteries from Abdominal Artery with Zooplastic Tissue, Percutaneous Endoscopic Approach

021348W Bypass Coronary Artery, Four or More Arteries from Aorta with Zooplastic Tissue, Percutaneous Endoscopic Approach

0213493 Bypass Coronary Artery, Four or More Arteries from Coronary Artery with Autologous Venous Tissue, Percutaneous Endoscopic Approach

HAC 08: Surgical Site Infection of Mediastinitis After Coronary Bypass Graft (CABG) Procedures (continued)

0213498 Bypass Coronary Artery, Four or More Arteries from Right Internal Mammary with Autologous Venous Tissue, Percutaneous Endoscopic Approach

0213499 Bypass Coronary Artery, Four or More Arteries from Left Internal Mammary with Autologous Venous Tissue, Percutaneous Endoscopic Approach

021349C Bypass Coronary Artery, Four or More Arteries from Thoracic Artery with Autologous Venous Tissue, Percutaneous Endoscopic Approach

021349F Bypass Coronary Artery, Four or More Arteries from Abdominal Artery with Autologous Venous Tissue, Percutaneous Endoscopic Approach

021349W Bypass Coronary Artery, Four or More Arteries from Aorta with Autologous Venous Tissue, Percutaneous Endoscopic Approach

02134A3 Bypass Coronary Artery, Four or More Arteries from Coronary Artery with Autologous Arterial Tissue, Percutaneous Endoscopic Approach

02134A8 Bypass Coronary Artery, Four or More Arteries from Right Internal Mammary with Autologous Arterial Tissue, Percutaneous Endoscopic Approach

02134A9 Bypass Coronary Artery, Four or More Arteries from Left Internal Mammary with Autologous Arterial Tissue, Percutaneous Endoscopic Approach

02134AC Bypass Coronary Artery, Four or More Arteries from Thoracic Artery with Autologous Arterial Tissue, Percutaneous Endoscopic Approach

02134AF Bypass Coronary Artery, Four or More Arteries from Abdominal Artery with Autologous Arterial Tissue, Percutaneous Endoscopic Approach

02134AW Bypass Coronary Artery, Four or More Arteries from Aorta with Autologous Arterial Tissue, Percutaneous Endoscopic Approach

02134J3 Bypass Coronary Artery, Four or More Arteries from Coronary Artery with Synthetic Substitute, Percutaneous Endoscopic Approach

02134J8 Bypass Coronary Artery, Four or More Arteries from Right Internal Mammary with Synthetic Substitute, Percutaneous Endoscopic Approach

02134J9 Bypass Coronary Artery, Four or More Arteries from Left Internal Mammary with Synthetic Substitute, Percutaneous Endoscopic Approach

02134JC Bypass Coronary Artery, Four or More Arteries from Thoracic Artery with Synthetic Substitute, Percutaneous Endoscopic Approach

02134JF Bypass Coronary Artery, Four or More Arteries from Abdominal Artery with Synthetic Substitute, Percutaneous Endoscopic Approach

02134JW Bypass Coronary Artery, Four or More Arteries from Aorta with Synthetic Substitute, Percutaneous Endoscopic Approach

02134K3 Bypass Coronary Artery, Four or More Arteries from Coronary Artery with Nonautologous Tissue Substitute, Percutaneous Endoscopic Approach

02134K8 Bypass Coronary Artery, Four or More Arteries from Right Internal Mammary with Nonautologous Tissue Substitute, Percutaneous Endoscopic Approach

02134K9 Bypass Coronary Artery, Four or More Arteries from Left Internal Mammary with Nonautologous Tissue Substitute, Percutaneous Endoscopic Approach

02134KC Bypass Coronary Artery, Four or More Arteries from Thoracic Artery with Nonautologous Tissue Substitute, Percutaneous Endoscopic Approach

02134KF Bypass Coronary Artery, Four or More Arteries from Abdominal Artery with Nonautologous Tissue Substitute, Percutaneous Endoscopic Approach

02134KW Bypass Coronary Artery, Four or More Arteries from Aorta with Nonautologous Tissue Substitute, Percutaneous Endoscopic Approach

02134Z3 Bypass Coronary Artery, Four or More Arteries from Coronary Artery, Percutaneous Endoscopic Approach

02134Z8 Bypass Coronary Artery, Four or More Arteries from Right Internal Mammary, Percutaneous Endoscopic Approach

02134Z9 Bypass Coronary Artery, Four or More Arteries from Left Internal Mammary, Percutaneous Endoscopic Approach

02134ZC Bypass Coronary Artery, Four or More Arteries from Thoracic Artery, Percutaneous Endoscopic Approach

02134ZF Bypass Coronary Artery, Four or More Arteries from Abdominal Artery, Percutaneous Endoscopic Approach

HAC 10: Deep Vein Thrombosis (DVT) or Pulmonary Embolism (PE) with Total Knee or Hip Replacement

Secondary diagnosis not POA:

I26.02 Saddle embolus of pulmonary artery with acute cor pulmonale

I26.09 Other pulmonary embolism with acute cor pulmonale

I26.92 Saddle embolus of pulmonary artery without acute cor pulmonale

I26.93 Single subsegmental pulmonary embolism without acute cor pulmonale

I26.94 Multiple subsegmental pulmonary emboli without acute cor pulmonale

I26.99 Other pulmonary embolism without acute cor pulmonale

I82.401 Acute embolism and thrombosis of unspecified deep veins of right lower extremity

I82.402 Acute embolism and thrombosis of unspecified deep veins of left lower extremity

I82.403 Acute embolism and thrombosis of unspecified deep veins of lower extremity, bilateral

I82.409 Acute embolism and thrombosis of unspecified deep veins of unspecified lower extremity

I82.411 Acute embolism and thrombosis of right femoral vein

I82.412 Acute embolism and thrombosis of left femoral vein

I82.413 Acute embolism and thrombosis of femoral vein, bilateral

I82.419 Acute embolism and thrombosis of unspecified femoral vein

I82.421 Acute embolism and thrombosis of right iliac vein

I82.422 Acute embolism and thrombosis of left iliac vein

I82.423 Acute embolism and thrombosis of iliac vein, bilateral

I82.429 Acute embolism and thrombosis of unspecified iliac vein

I82.431 Acute embolism and thrombosis of right popliteal vein

I82.432 Acute embolism and thrombosis of left popliteal vein

I82.433 Acute embolism and thrombosis of popliteal vein, bilateral

I82.439 Acute embolism and thrombosis of unspecified popliteal vein

I82.441 Acute embolism and thrombosis of right tibial vein

I82.442 Acute embolism and thrombosis of left tibial vein

I82.443 Acute embolism and thrombosis of tibial vein, bilateral

I82.449 Acute embolism and thrombosis of unspecified tibial vein

I82.451 Acute embolism and thrombosis of right peroneal vein

I82.452 Acute embolism and thrombosis of left peroneal vein

I82.453 Acute embolism and thrombosis of peroneal vein, bilateral

I82.459 Acute embolism and thrombosis of unspecified peroneal vein

I82.491 Acute embolism and thrombosis of other specified deep vein of right lower extremity

I82.492 Acute embolism and thrombosis of other specified deep vein of left lower extremity

I82.493 Acute embolism and thrombosis of other specified deep vein of lower extremity, bilateral

I82.499 Acute embolism and thrombosis of other specified deep vein of unspecified lower extremity

I82.4Y1 Acute embolism and thrombosis of unspecified deep veins of right proximal lower extremity

I82.4Y2 Acute embolism and thrombosis of unspecified deep veins of left proximal lower extremity

I82.4Y3 Acute embolism and thrombosis of unspecified deep veins of proximal lower extremity, bilateral

I82.4Y9 Acute embolism and thrombosis of unspecified deep veins of unspecified proximal lower extremity

I82.4Z1 Acute embolism and thrombosis of unspecified deep veins of right distal lower extremity

I82.4Z2 Acute embolism and thrombosis of unspecified deep veins of left distal lower extremity

I82.4Z3 Acute embolism and thrombosis of unspecified deep veins of distal lower extremity, bilateral

I82.4Z9 Acute embolism and thrombosis of unspecified deep veins of unspecified distal lower extremity

AND

Any of the following procedures:

0SR9019 Replacement of Right Hip Joint with Metal Synthetic Substitute, Cemented, Open Approach

0SR901A Replacement of Right Hip Joint with Metal Synthetic Substitute, Uncemented, Open Approach

0SR901Z Replacement of Right Hip Joint with Metal Synthetic Substitute, Open Approach

0SR9029 Replacement of Right Hip Joint with Metal on Polyethylene Synthetic Substitute, Cemented, Open Approach

HAC 10: Deep Vein Thrombosis (DVT) or Pulmonary Embolism (PE) with Total Knee or Hip Replacement (continued)

ØSR9Ø2A Replacement of Right Hip Joint with Metal on Polyethylene Synthetic Substitute, Uncemented, Open Approach

ØSR9Ø2Z Replacement of Right Hip Joint with Metal on Polyethylene Synthetic Substitute, Open Approach

ØSR9Ø39 Replacement of Right Hip Joint with Ceramic Synthetic Substitute, Cemented, Open Approach

ØSR9Ø3A Replacement of Right Hip Joint with Ceramic Synthetic Substitute, Uncemented, Open Approach

ØSR9Ø3Z Replacement of Right Hip Joint with Ceramic Synthetic Substitute, Open Approach

ØSR9Ø49 Replacement of Right Hip Joint with Ceramic on Polyethylene Synthetic Substitute, Cemented, Open Approach

ØSR9Ø4A Replacement of Right Hip Joint with Ceramic on Polyethylene Synthetic Substitute, Uncemented, Open Approach

ØSR9Ø4Z Replacement of Right Hip Joint with Ceramic on Polyethylene Synthetic Substitute, Open Approach

ØSR9Ø69 Replacement of Right Hip Joint with Oxidized Zirconium on Polyethylene Synthetic Substitute, Cemented, Open Approach

ØSR9Ø6A Replacement of Right Hip Joint with Oxidized Zirconium on Polyethylene Synthetic Substitute, Uncemented, Open Approach

ØSR9Ø6Z Replacement of Right Hip Joint with Oxidized Zirconium on Polyethylene Synthetic Substitute, Open Approach

ØSR9Ø7Z Replacement of Right Hip Joint with Autologous Tissue Substitute, Open Approach

ØSR9ØEZ Replacement of Right Hip Joint with Articulating Spacer, Open Approach

ØSR9ØJ9 Replacement of Right Hip Joint with Synthetic Substitute, Cemented, Open Approach

ØSR9ØJA Replacement of Right Hip Joint with Synthetic Substitute, Uncemented, Open Approach

ØSR9ØJZ Replacement of Right Hip Joint with Synthetic Substitute, Open Approach

ØSR9ØKZ Replacement of Right Hip Joint with Nonautologous Tissue Substitute, Open Approach

ØSRAØØ9 Replacement of Right Hip Joint, Acetabular Surface with Polyethylene Synthetic Substitute, Cemented, Open Approach

ØSRAØØA Replacement of Right Hip Joint, Acetabular Surface with Polyethylene Synthetic Substitute, Uncemented, Open Approach

ØSRAØØZ Replacement of Right Hip Joint, Acetabular Surface with Polyethylene Synthetic Substitute, Open Approach

ØSRAØ19 Replacement of Right Hip Joint, Acetabular Surface with Metal Synthetic Substitute, Cemented, Open Approach

ØSRAØ1A Replacement of Right Hip Joint, Acetabular Surface with Metal Synthetic Substitute, Uncemented, Open Approach

ØSRAØ1Z Replacement of Right Hip Joint, Acetabular Surface with Metal Synthetic Substitute, Open Approach

ØSRAØ39 Replacement of Right Hip Joint, Acetabular Surface with Ceramic Synthetic Substitute, Cemented, Open Approach

ØSRAØ3A Replacement of Right Hip Joint, Acetabular Surface with Ceramic Synthetic Substitute, Uncemented, Open Approach

ØSRAØ3Z Replacement of Right Hip Joint, Acetabular Surface with Ceramic Synthetic Substitute, Open Approach

ØSRAØ7Z Replacement of Right Hip Joint, Acetabular Surface with Autologous Tissue Substitute, Open Approach

ØSRAØJ9 Replacement of Right Hip Joint, Acetabular Surface with Synthetic Substitute, Cemented, Open Approach

ØSRAØJA Replacement of Right Hip Joint, Acetabular Surface with Synthetic Substitute, Uncemented, Open Approach

ØSRAØJZ Replacement of Right Hip Joint, Acetabular Surface with Synthetic Substitute, Open Approach

ØSRAØKZ Replacement of Right Hip Joint, Acetabular Surface with Nonautologous Tissue Substitute, Open Approach

ØSRBØ19 Replacement of Left Hip Joint with Metal Synthetic Substitute, Cemented, Open Approach

ØSRBØ1A Replacement of Left Hip Joint with Metal Synthetic Substitute, Uncemented, Open Approach

ØSRBØ1Z Replacement of Left Hip Joint with Metal Synthetic Substitute, Open Approach

ØSRBØ29 Replacement of Left Hip Joint with Metal on Polyethylene Synthetic Substitute, Cemented, Open Approach

ØSRBØ2A Replacement of Left Hip Joint with Metal on Polyethylene Synthetic Substitute, Uncemented, Open Approach

ØSRBØ2Z Replacement of Left Hip Joint with Metal on Polyethylene Synthetic Substitute, Open Approach

ØSRBØ39 Replacement of Left Hip Joint with Ceramic Synthetic Substitute, Cemented, Open Approach

ØSRBØ3A Replacement of Left Hip Joint with Ceramic Synthetic Substitute, Uncemented, Open Approach

ØSRBØ3Z Replacement of Left Hip Joint with Ceramic Synthetic Substitute, Open Approach

ØSRBØ49 Replacement of Left Hip Joint with Ceramic on Polyethylene Synthetic Substitute, Cemented, Open Approach

ØSRBØ4A Replacement of Left Hip Joint with Ceramic on Polyethylene Synthetic Substitute, Uncemented, Open Approach

ØSRBØ4Z Replacement of Left Hip Joint with Ceramic on Polyethylene Synthetic Substitute, Open Approach

ØSRBØ69 Replacement of Left Hip Joint with Oxidized Zirconium on Polyethylene Synthetic Substitute, Cemented, Open Approach

ØSRBØ6A Replacement of Left Hip Joint with Oxidized Zirconium on Polyethylene Synthetic Substitute, Uncemented, Open Approach

ØSRBØ6Z Replacement of Left Hip Joint with Oxidized Zirconium on Polyethylene Synthetic Substitute, Open Approach

ØSRBØ7Z Replacement of Left Hip Joint with Autologous Tissue Substitute, Open Approach

ØSRBØEZ Replacement of Left Hip Joint with Articulating Spacer, Open Approach

ØSRBØJ9 Replacement of Left Hip Joint with Synthetic Substitute, Cemented, Open Approach

ØSRBØJA Replacement of Left Hip Joint with Synthetic Substitute, Uncemented, Open Approach

ØSRBØJZ Replacement of Left Hip Joint with Synthetic Substitute, Open Approach

ØSRBØKZ Replacement of Left Hip Joint with Nonautologous Tissue Substitute, Open Approach

ØSRCØ69 Replacement of Right Knee Joint with Oxidized Zirconium on Polyethylene Synthetic Substitute, Cemented, Open Approach

ØSRCØ6A Replacement of Right Knee Joint with Oxidized Zirconium on Polyethylene Synthetic Substitute, Uncemented, Open Approach

ØSRCØ6Z Replacement of Right Knee Joint with Oxidized Zirconium on Polyethylene Synthetic Substitute, Open Approach

ØSRCØ7Z Replacement of Right Knee Joint with Autologous Tissue Substitute, Open Approach

ØSRCØEZ Replacement of Right Knee Joint with Articulating Spacer, Open Approach

ØSRCØJ9 Replacement of Right Knee Joint with Synthetic Substitute, Cemented, Open Approach

ØSRCØJA Replacement of Right Knee Joint with Synthetic Substitute, Uncemented, Open Approach

ØSRCØJZ Replacement of Right Knee Joint with Synthetic Substitute, Open Approach

ØSRCØKZ Replacement of Right Knee Joint with Nonautologous Tissue Substitute, Open Approach

ØSRCØL9 Replacement of Right Knee Joint with Medial Unicondylar Synthetic Substitute, Cemented, Open Approach

ØSRCØLA Replacement of Right Knee Joint with Medial Unicondylar Synthetic Substitute, Uncemented, Open Approach

ØSRCØLZ Replacement of Right Knee Joint with Medial Unicondylar Synthetic Substitute, Open Approach

ØSRCØM9 Replacement of Right Knee Joint with Lateral Unicondylar Synthetic Substitute, Cemented, Open Approach

ØSRCØMA Replacement of Right Knee Joint with Lateral Unicondylar Synthetic Substitute, Uncemented, Open Approach

ØSRCØMZ Replacement of Right Knee Joint with Lateral Unicondylar Synthetic Substitute, Open Approach

ØSRCØN9 Replacement of Right Knee Joint with Patellofemoral Synthetic Substitute, Cemented, Open Approach

ØSRCØNA Replacement of Right Knee Joint with Patellofemoral Synthetic Substitute, Uncemented, Open Approach

ØSRCØNZ Replacement of Right Knee Joint with Patellofemoral Synthetic Substitute, Open Approach

ØSRDØ69 Replacement of Left Knee Joint with Oxidized Zirconium on Polyethylene Synthetic Substitute, Cemented, Open Approach

ØSRDØ6A Replacement of Left Knee Joint with Oxidized Zirconium on Polyethylene Synthetic Substitute, Uncemented, Open Approach

ØSRDØ6Z Replacement of Left Knee Joint with Oxidized Zirconium on Polyethylene Synthetic Substitute, Open Approach

ØSRDØ7Z Replacement of Left Knee Joint with Autologous Tissue Substitute, Open Approach

HAC 10: Deep Vein Thrombosis (DVT) or Pulmonary Embolism (PE) with Total Knee or Hip Replacement (continued)

ØSRDØEZ	Replacement of Left Knee Joint with Articulating Spacer, Open Approach

ØSRDØJ9	Replacement of Left Knee Joint with Synthetic Substitute, Cemented, Open Approach

ØSRDØJA	Replacement of Left Knee Joint with Synthetic Substitute, Uncemented, Open Approach

ØSRDØJZ	Replacement of Left Knee Joint with Synthetic Substitute, Open Approach

ØSRDØKZ	Replacement of Left Knee Joint with Nonautologous Tissue Substitute, Open Approach

ØSRDØL9	Replacement of Left Knee Joint with Medial Unicondylar Synthetic Substitute, Cemented, Open Approach

ØSRDØLA	Replacement of Left Knee Joint with Medial Unicondylar Synthetic Substitute, Uncemented, Open Approach

ØSRDØLZ	Replacement of Left Knee Joint with Medial Unicondylar Synthetic Substitute, Open Approach

ØSRDØM9	Replacement of Left Knee Joint with Lateral Unicondylar Synthetic Substitute, Cemented, Open Approach

ØSRDØMA	Replacement of Left Knee Joint with Lateral Unicondylar Synthetic Substitute, Uncemented, Open Approach

ØSRDØMZ	Replacement of Left Knee Joint with Lateral Unicondylar Synthetic Substitute, Open Approach

ØSRDØN9	Replacement of Left Knee Joint with Patellofemoral Synthetic Substitute, Cemented, Open Approach

ØSRDØNA	Replacement of Left Knee Joint with Patellofemoral Synthetic Substitute, Uncemented, Open Approach

ØSRDØNZ	Replacement of Left Knee Joint with Patellofemoral Synthetic Substitute, Open Approach

ØSRE009	Replacement of Left Hip Joint, Acetabular Surface with Polyethylene Synthetic Substitute, Cemented, Open Approach

ØSRE00A	Replacement of Left Hip Joint, Acetabular Surface with Polyethylene Synthetic Substitute, Uncemented, Open Approach

ØSRE00Z	Replacement of Left Hip Joint, Acetabular Surface with Polyethylene Synthetic Substitute, Open Approach

ØSRE019	Replacement of Left Hip Joint, Acetabular Surface with Metal Synthetic Substitute, Cemented, Open Approach

ØSRE01A	Replacement of Left Hip Joint, Acetabular Surface with Metal Synthetic Substitute, Uncemented, Open Approach

ØSRE01Z	Replacement of Left Hip Joint, Acetabular Surface with Metal Synthetic Substitute, Open Approach

ØSRE039	Replacement of Left Hip Joint, Acetabular Surface with Ceramic Synthetic Substitute, Cemented, Open Approach

ØSRE03A	Replacement of Left Hip Joint, Acetabular Surface with Ceramic Synthetic Substitute, Uncemented, Open Approach

ØSRE03Z	Replacement of Left Hip Joint, Acetabular Surface with Ceramic Synthetic Substitute, Open Approach

ØSRE07Z	Replacement of Left Hip Joint, Acetabular Surface with Autologous Tissue Substitute, Open Approach

ØSRE0J9	Replacement of Left Hip Joint, Acetabular Surface with Synthetic Substitute, Cemented, Open Approach

ØSREØJA	Replacement of Left Hip Joint, Acetabular Surface with Synthetic Substitute, Uncemented, Open Approach

ØSREØJZ	Replacement of Left Hip Joint, Acetabular Surface with Synthetic Substitute, Open Approach

ØSREØKZ	Replacement of Left Hip Joint, Acetabular Surface with Nonautologous Tissue Substitute, Open Approach

ØSRR019	Replacement of Right Hip Joint, Femoral Surface with Metal Synthetic Substitute, Cemented, Open Approach

ØSRR01A	Replacement of Right Hip Joint, Femoral Surface with Metal Synthetic Substitute, Uncemented, Open Approach

ØSRR01Z	Replacement of Right Hip Joint, Femoral Surface with Metal Synthetic Substitute, Open Approach

ØSRR039	Replacement of Right Hip Joint, Femoral Surface with Ceramic Synthetic Substitute, Cemented, Open Approach

ØSRR03A	Replacement of Right Hip Joint, Femoral Surface with Ceramic Synthetic Substitute, Uncemented, Open Approach

ØSRR03Z	Replacement of Right Hip Joint, Femoral Surface with Ceramic Synthetic Substitute, Open Approach

ØSRR07Z	Replacement of Right Hip Joint, Femoral Surface with Autologous Tissue Substitute, Open Approach

ØSRRØJ9	Replacement of Right Hip Joint, Femoral Surface with Synthetic Substitute, Cemented, Open Approach

ØSRRØJA	Replacement of Right Hip Joint, Femoral Surface with Synthetic Substitute, Uncemented, Open Approach

ØSRRØJZ	Replacement of Right Hip Joint, Femoral Surface with Synthetic Substitute, Open Approach

ØSRRØKZ	Replacement of Right Hip Joint, Femoral Surface with Nonautologous Tissue Substitute, Open Approach

ØSRS019	Replacement of Left Hip Joint, Femoral Surface with Metal Synthetic Substitute, Cemented, Open Approach

ØSRS01A	Replacement of Left Hip Joint, Femoral Surface with Metal Synthetic Substitute, Uncemented, Open Approach

ØSRS01Z	Replacement of Left Hip Joint, Femoral Surface with Metal Synthetic Substitute, Open Approach

ØSRS039	Replacement of Left Hip Joint, Femoral Surface with Ceramic Synthetic Substitute, Cemented, Open Approach

ØSRS03A	Replacement of Left Hip Joint, Femoral Surface with Ceramic Synthetic Substitute, Uncemented, Open Approach

ØSRS03Z	Replacement of Left Hip Joint, Femoral Surface with Ceramic Synthetic Substitute, Open Approach

ØSRS07Z	Replacement of Left Hip Joint, Femoral Surface with Autologous Tissue Substitute, Open Approach

ØSRS0J9	Replacement of Left Hip Joint, Femoral Surface with Synthetic Substitute, Cemented, Open Approach

ØSRSØJA	Replacement of Left Hip Joint, Femoral Surface with Synthetic Substitute, Uncemented, Open Approach

ØSRSØJZ	Replacement of Left Hip Joint, Femoral Surface with Synthetic Substitute, Open Approach

ØSRSØKZ	Replacement of Left Hip Joint, Femoral Surface with Nonautologous Tissue Substitute, Open Approach

ØSRT07Z	Replacement of Right Knee Joint, Femoral Surface with Autologous Tissue Substitute, Open Approach

ØSRT0J9	Replacement of Right Knee Joint, Femoral Surface with Synthetic Substitute, Cemented, Open Approach

ØSRTØJA	Replacement of Right Knee Joint, Femoral Surface with Synthetic Substitute, Uncemented, Open Approach

ØSRTØJZ	Replacement of Right Knee Joint, Femoral Surface with Synthetic Substitute, Open Approach

ØSRTØKZ	Replacement of Right Knee Joint, Femoral Surface with Nonautologous Tissue Substitute, Open Approach

ØSRU07Z	Replacement of Left Knee Joint, Femoral Surface with Autologous Tissue Substitute, Open Approach

ØSRUØJ9	Replacement of Left Knee Joint, Femoral Surface with Synthetic Substitute, Cemented, Open Approach

ØSRUØJA	Replacement of Left Knee Joint, Femoral Surface with Synthetic Substitute, Uncemented, Open Approach

ØSRUØJZ	Replacement of Left Knee Joint, Femoral Surface with Synthetic Substitute, Open Approach

ØSRUØKZ	Replacement of Left Knee Joint, Femoral Surface with Nonautologous Tissue Substitute, Open Approach

ØSRV07Z	Replacement of Right Knee Joint, Tibial Surface with Autologous Tissue Substitute, Open Approach

ØSRVØJ9	Replacement of Right Knee Joint, Tibial Surface with Synthetic Substitute, Cemented, Open Approach

ØSRVØJA	Replacement of Right Knee Joint, Tibial Surface with Synthetic Substitute, Uncemented, Open Approach

ØSRVØJZ	Replacement of Right Knee Joint, Tibial Surface with Synthetic Substitute, Open Approach

ØSRVØKZ	Replacement of Right Knee Joint, Tibial Surface with Nonautologous Tissue Substitute, Open Approach

ØSRW07Z	Replacement of Left Knee Joint, Tibial Surface with Autologous Tissue Substitute, Open Approach

ØSRWØJ9	Replacement of Left Knee Joint, Tibial Surface with Synthetic Substitute, Cemented, Open Approach

ØSRWØJA	Replacement of Left Knee Joint, Tibial Surface with Synthetic Substitute, Uncemented, Open Approach

ØSRWØJZ	Replacement of Left Knee Joint, Tibial Surface with Synthetic Substitute, Open Approach

ØSRWØKZ	Replacement of Left Knee Joint, Tibial Surface with Nonautologous Tissue Substitute, Open Approach

ØSU90BZ	Supplement Right Hip Joint with Resurfacing Device, Open Approach

ØSUAØBZ	Supplement Right Hip Joint, Acetabular Surface with Resurfacing Device, Open Approach

ØSUBØBZ	Supplement Left Hip Joint with Resurfacing Device, Open Approach

ØSUEØBZ	Supplement Left Hip Joint, Acetabular Surface with Resurfacing Device, Open Approach

ØSURØBZ	Supplement Right Hip Joint, Femoral Surface with Resurfacing Device, Open Approach

ØSUSØBZ	Supplement Left Hip Joint, Femoral Surface with Resurfacing Device, Open Approach

HAC 10: Deep Vein Thrombosis (DVT) or Pulmonary Embolism (PE) with Total Knee or Hip Replacement (continued)

XRRGØL8 Replacement of Right Knee Joint with Synthetic Substitute, Lateral Meniscus, Open Approach, New Technology Group 8

XRRGØM8 Replacement of Right Knee Joint with Synthetic Substitute, Medial Meniscus, Open Approach, New Technology Group 8

XRRHØL8 Replacement of Left Knee Joint with Synthetic Substitute, Lateral Meniscus, Open Approach, New Technology Group 8

XRRHØM8 Replacement of Left Knee Joint with Synthetic Substitute, Medial Meniscus, Open Approach, New Technology Group 8

HAC 11: Surgical Site Infection-Bariatric Surgery

Principal diagnosis of:

E66.Ø1 Morbid (severe) obesity due to excess calories

AND

Secondary diagnosis not POA:

K68.11 Postprocedural retroperitoneal abscess
K95.Ø1 Infection due to gastric band procedure
K95.81 Infection due to other bariatric procedure
T81.4ØXA Infection following a procedure, unspecified, initial encounter
T81.41XA Infection following a procedure, superficial incisional surgical site, initial encounter
T81.42XA Infection following a procedure, deep incisional surgical site, initial encounter
T81.43XA Infection following a procedure, organ and space surgical site, initial encounter
T81.44XA Sepsis following a procedure, initial encounter
T81.49XA Infection following a procedure, other surgical site, initial encounter

AND

Any of the following procedures:

ØD16Ø79 Bypass Stomach to Duodenum with Autologous Tissue Substitute, Open Approach
ØD16Ø7A Bypass Stomach to Jejunum with Autologous Tissue Substitute, Open Approach
ØD16Ø7B Bypass Stomach to Ileum with Autologous Tissue Substitute, Open Approach
ØD16Ø7L Bypass Stomach to Transverse Colon with Autologous Tissue Substitute, Open Approach
ØD16ØJ9 Bypass Stomach to Duodenum with Synthetic Substitute, Open Approach
ØD16ØJA Bypass Stomach to Jejunum with Synthetic Substitute, Open Approach
ØD16ØJB Bypass Stomach to Ileum with Synthetic Substitute, Open Approach
ØD16ØJL Bypass Stomach to Transverse Colon with Synthetic Substitute, Open Approach
ØD16ØK9 Bypass Stomach to Duodenum with Nonautologous Tissue Substitute, Open Approach
ØD16ØKA Bypass Stomach to Jejunum with Nonautologous Tissue Substitute, Open Approach
ØD16ØKB Bypass Stomach to Ileum with Nonautologous Tissue Substitute, Open Approach
ØD16ØKL Bypass Stomach to Transverse Colon with Nonautologous Tissue Substitute, Open Approach
ØD16ØZ9 Bypass Stomach to Duodenum, Open Approach
ØD16ØZA Bypass Stomach to Jejunum, Open Approach
ØD16ØZB Bypass Stomach to Ileum, Open Approach

ØD16ØZL Bypass Stomach to Transverse Colon, Open Approach
ØD16479 Bypass Stomach to Duodenum with Autologous Tissue Substitute, Percutaneous Endoscopic Approach
ØD1647A Bypass Stomach to Jejunum with Autologous Tissue Substitute, Percutaneous Endoscopic Approach
ØD1647B Bypass Stomach to Ileum with Autologous Tissue Substitute, Percutaneous Endoscopic Approach
ØD1647L Bypass Stomach to Transverse Colon with Autologous Tissue Substitute, Percutaneous Endoscopic Approach
ØD164J9 Bypass Stomach to Duodenum with Synthetic Substitute, Percutaneous Endoscopic Approach
ØD164JA Bypass Stomach to Jejunum with Synthetic Substitute, Percutaneous Endoscopic Approach
ØD164JB Bypass Stomach to Ileum with Synthetic Substitute, Percutaneous Endoscopic Approach
ØD164JL Bypass Stomach to Transverse Colon with Synthetic Substitute, Percutaneous Endoscopic Approach
ØD164K9 Bypass Stomach to Duodenum with Nonautologous Tissue Substitute, Percutaneous Endoscopic Approach
ØD164KA Bypass Stomach to Jejunum with Nonautologous Tissue Substitute, Percutaneous Endoscopic Approach
ØD164KB Bypass Stomach to Ileum with Nonautologous Tissue Substitute, Percutaneous Endoscopic Approach
ØD164KL Bypass Stomach to Transverse Colon with Nonautologous Tissue Substitute, Percutaneous Endoscopic Approach
ØD164Z9 Bypass Stomach to Duodenum, Percutaneous Endoscopic Approach
ØD164ZA Bypass Stomach to Jejunum, Percutaneous Endoscopic Approach
ØD164ZB Bypass Stomach to Ileum, Percutaneous Endoscopic Approach
ØD164ZL Bypass Stomach to Transverse Colon, Percutaneous Endoscopic Approach
ØD16879 Bypass Stomach to Duodenum with Autologous Tissue Substitute, Via Natural or Artificial Opening Endoscopic
ØD1687A Bypass Stomach to Jejunum with Autologous Tissue Substitute, Via Natural or Artificial Opening Endoscopic
ØD1687B Bypass Stomach to Ileum with Autologous Tissue Substitute, Via Natural or Artificial Opening Endoscopic
ØD1687L Bypass Stomach to Transverse Colon with Autologous Tissue Substitute, Via Natural or Artificial Opening Endoscopic
ØD168J9 Bypass Stomach to Duodenum with Synthetic Substitute, Via Natural or Artificial Opening Endoscopic
ØD168JA Bypass Stomach to Jejunum with Synthetic Substitute, Via Natural or Artificial Opening Endoscopic
ØD168JB Bypass Stomach to Ileum with Synthetic Substitute, Via Natural or Artificial Opening Endoscopic
ØD168JL Bypass Stomach to Transverse Colon with Synthetic Substitute, Via Natural or Artificial Opening Endoscopic
ØD168K9 Bypass Stomach to Duodenum with Nonautologous Tissue Substitute, Via Natural or Artificial Opening Endoscopic
ØD168KA Bypass Stomach to Jejunum with Nonautologous Tissue Substitute, Via Natural or Artificial Opening Endoscopic

ØD168KB Bypass Stomach to Ileum with Nonautologous Tissue Substitute, Via Natural or Artificial Opening Endoscopic
ØD168KL Bypass Stomach to Transverse Colon with Nonautologous Tissue Substitute, Via Natural or Artificial Opening Endoscopic
ØD168Z9 Bypass Stomach to Duodenum, Via Natural or Artificial Opening Endoscopic
ØD168ZA Bypass Stomach to Jejunum, Via Natural or Artificial Opening Endoscopic
ØD168ZB Bypass Stomach to Ileum, Via Natural or Artificial Opening Endoscopic
ØD168ZL Bypass Stomach to Transverse Colon, Via Natural or Artificial Opening Endoscopic
ØDV64CZ Restriction of Stomach with Extraluminal Device, Percutaneous Endoscopic Approach

HAC 12: Surgical Site Infection-Certain Orthopedic Procedures of the Spine, Shoulder, and Elbow

Secondary diagnosis not POA:

K68.11 Postprocedural retroperitoneal abscess
T81.4ØXA Infection following a procedure, unspecified, initial encounter
T81.41XA Infection following a procedure, superficial incisional surgical site, initial encounter
T81.42XA Infection following a procedure, deep incisional surgical site, initial encounter
T81.43XA Infection following a procedure, organ and space surgical site, initial encounter
T81.44XA Sepsis following a procedure, initial encounter
T81.49XA Infection following a procedure, other surgical site, initial encounter
T84.6ØXA Infection and inflammatory reaction due to internal fixation device of unspecified site, initial encounter
T84.61ØA Infection and inflammatory reaction due to internal fixation device of right humerus, initial encounter
T84.611A Infection and inflammatory reaction due to internal fixation device of left humerus, initial encounter
T84.612A Infection and inflammatory reaction due to internal fixation device of right radius, initial encounter
T84.613A Infection and inflammatory reaction due to internal fixation device of left radius, initial encounter
T84.614A Infection and inflammatory reaction due to internal fixation device of right ulna, initial encounter
T84.615A Infection and inflammatory reaction due to internal fixation device of left ulna, initial encounter
T84.619A Infection and inflammatory reaction due to internal fixation device of unspecified bone of arm, initial encounter
T84.63XA Infection and inflammatory reaction due to internal fixation device of spine, initial encounter
T84.69XA Infection and inflammatory reaction due to internal fixation device of other site, initial encounter
T84.7XXA Infection and inflammatory reaction due to other internal orthopedic prosthetic devices, implants and grafts, initial encounter

AND

Any of the following procedures:

ØRGØØ7Ø Fusion of Occipital-cervical Joint with Autologous Tissue Substitute, Anterior Approach, Anterior Column, Open Approach

HAC 12: Surgical Site Infection-Certain Orthopedic Procedures of the Spine, Shoulder, and Elbow (continued)

ØRG0071 Fusion of Occipital-cervical Joint with Autologous Tissue Substitute, Posterior Approach, Posterior Column, Open Approach

ØRG007J Fusion of Occipital-cervical Joint with Autologous Tissue Substitute, Posterior Approach, Anterior Column, Open Approach

ØRG00A0 Fusion of Occipital-cervical Joint with Interbody Fusion Device, Anterior Approach, Anterior Column, Open Approach

ØRG00AJ Fusion of Occipital-cervical Joint with Interbody Fusion Device, Posterior Approach, Anterior Column, Open Approach

ØRG00J0 Fusion of Occipital-cervical Joint with Synthetic Substitute, Anterior Approach, Anterior Column, Open Approach

ØRG00J1 Fusion of Occipital-cervical Joint with Synthetic Substitute, Posterior Approach, Posterior Column, Open Approach

ØRG00JJ Fusion of Occipital-cervical Joint with Synthetic Substitute, Posterior Approach, Anterior Column, Open Approach

ØRG00K0 Fusion of Occipital-cervical Joint with Nonautologous Tissue Substitute, Anterior Approach, Anterior Column, Open Approach

ØRG00K1 Fusion of Occipital-cervical Joint with Nonautologous Tissue Substitute, Posterior Approach, Posterior Column, Open Approach

ØRG00KJ Fusion of Occipital-cervical Joint with Nonautologous Tissue Substitute, Posterior Approach, Anterior Column, Open Approach

ØRG0370 Fusion of Occipital-cervical Joint with Autologous Tissue Substitute, Anterior Approach, Anterior Column, Percutaneous Approach

ØRG0371 Fusion of Occipital-cervical Joint with Autologous Tissue Substitute, Posterior Approach, Posterior Column, Percutaneous Approach

ØRG037J Fusion of Occipital-cervical Joint with Autologous Tissue Substitute, Posterior Approach, Anterior Column, Percutaneous Approach

ØRG03A0 Fusion of Occipital-cervical Joint with Interbody Fusion Device, Anterior Approach, Anterior Column, Percutaneous Approach

ØRG03AJ Fusion of Occipital-cervical Joint with Interbody Fusion Device, Posterior Approach, Anterior Column, Percutaneous Approach

ØRG03J0 Fusion of Occipital-cervical Joint with Synthetic Substitute, Anterior Approach, Anterior Column, Percutaneous Approach

ØRG03J1 Fusion of Occipital-cervical Joint with Synthetic Substitute, Posterior Approach, Posterior Column, Percutaneous Approach

ØRG03JJ Fusion of Occipital-cervical Joint with Synthetic Substitute, Posterior Approach, Anterior Column, Percutaneous Approach

ØRG03K0 Fusion of Occipital-cervical Joint with Nonautologous Tissue Substitute, Anterior Approach, Anterior Column, Percutaneous Approach

ØRG03K1 Fusion of Occipital-cervical Joint with Nonautologous Tissue Substitute, Posterior Approach, Posterior Column, Percutaneous Approach

ØRG03KJ Fusion of Occipital-cervical Joint with Nonautologous Tissue Substitute, Posterior Approach, Anterior Column, Percutaneous Approach

ØRG0470 Fusion of Occipital-cervical Joint with Autologous Tissue Substitute, Anterior Approach, Anterior Column, Percutaneous Endoscopic Approach

ØRG0471 Fusion of Occipital-cervical Joint with Autologous Tissue Substitute, Posterior Approach, Posterior Column, Percutaneous Endoscopic Approach

ØRG047J Fusion of Occipital-cervical Joint with Autologous Tissue Substitute, Posterior Approach, Anterior Column, Percutaneous Endoscopic Approach

ØRG04A0 Fusion of Occipital-cervical Joint with Interbody Fusion Device, Anterior Approach, Anterior Column, Percutaneous Endoscopic Approach

ØRG04AJ Fusion of Occipital-cervical Joint with Interbody Fusion Device, Posterior Approach, Anterior Column, Percutaneous Endoscopic Approach

ØRG04J0 Fusion of Occipital-cervical Joint with Synthetic Substitute, Anterior Approach, Anterior Column, Percutaneous Endoscopic Approach

ØRG04J1 Fusion of Occipital-cervical Joint with Synthetic Substitute, Posterior Approach, Posterior Column, Percutaneous Endoscopic Approach

ØRG04JJ Fusion of Occipital-cervical Joint with Synthetic Substitute, Posterior Approach, Anterior Column, Percutaneous Endoscopic Approach

ØRG04K0 Fusion of Occipital-cervical Joint with Nonautologous Tissue Substitute, Anterior Approach, Anterior Column, Percutaneous Endoscopic Approach

ØRG04K1 Fusion of Occipital-cervical Joint with Nonautologous Tissue Substitute, Posterior Approach, Posterior Column, Percutaneous Endoscopic Approach

ØRG04KJ Fusion of Occipital-cervical Joint with Nonautologous Tissue Substitute, Posterior Approach, Anterior Column, Percutaneous Endoscopic Approach

ØRG1070 Fusion of Cervical Vertebral Joint with Autologous Tissue Substitute, Anterior Approach, Anterior Column, Open Approach

ØRG1071 Fusion of Cervical Vertebral Joint with Autologous Tissue Substitute, Posterior Approach, Posterior Column, Open Approach

ØRG107J Fusion of Cervical Vertebral Joint with Autologous Tissue Substitute, Posterior Approach, Anterior Column, Open Approach

ØRG10A0 Fusion of Cervical Vertebral Joint with Interbody Fusion Device, Anterior Approach, Anterior Column, Open Approach

ØRG10AJ Fusion of Cervical Vertebral Joint with Interbody Fusion Device, Posterior Approach, Anterior Column, Open Approach

ØRG10J0 Fusion of Cervical Vertebral Joint with Synthetic Substitute, Anterior Approach, Anterior Column, Open Approach

ØRG10J1 Fusion of Cervical Vertebral Joint with Synthetic Substitute, Posterior Approach, Posterior Column, Open Approach

ØRG10JJ Fusion of Cervical Vertebral Joint with Synthetic Substitute, Posterior Approach, Anterior Column, Open Approach

ØRG10K0 Fusion of Cervical Vertebral Joint with Nonautologous Tissue Substitute, Anterior Approach, Anterior Column, Open Approach

ØRG10K1 Fusion of Cervical Vertebral Joint with Nonautologous Tissue Substitute, Posterior Approach, Posterior Column, Open Approach

ØRG10KJ Fusion of Cervical Vertebral Joint with Nonautologous Tissue Substitute, Posterior Approach, Anterior Column, Open Approach

ØRG1370 Fusion of Cervical Vertebral Joint with Autologous Tissue Substitute, Anterior Approach, Anterior Column, Percutaneous Approach

ØRG1371 Fusion of Cervical Vertebral Joint with Autologous Tissue Substitute, Posterior Approach, Posterior Column, Percutaneous Approach

ØRG137J Fusion of Cervical Vertebral Joint with Autologous Tissue Substitute, Posterior Approach, Anterior Column, Percutaneous Approach

ØRG13A0 Fusion of Cervical Vertebral Joint with Interbody Fusion Device, Anterior Approach, Anterior Column, Percutaneous Approach

ØRG13AJ Fusion of Cervical Vertebral Joint with Interbody Fusion Device, Posterior Approach, Anterior Column, Percutaneous Approach

ØRG13J0 Fusion of Cervical Vertebral Joint with Synthetic Substitute, Anterior Approach, Anterior Column, Percutaneous Approach

ØRG13J1 Fusion of Cervical Vertebral Joint with Synthetic Substitute, Posterior Approach, Posterior Column, Percutaneous Approach

ØRG13JJ Fusion of Cervical Vertebral Joint with Synthetic Substitute, Posterior Approach, Anterior Column, Percutaneous Approach

ØRG13K0 Fusion of Cervical Vertebral Joint with Nonautologous Tissue Substitute, Anterior Approach, Anterior Column, Percutaneous Approach

ØRG13K1 Fusion of Cervical Vertebral Joint with Nonautologous Tissue Substitute, Posterior Approach, Posterior Column, Percutaneous Approach

ØRG13KJ Fusion of Cervical Vertebral Joint with Nonautologous Tissue Substitute, Posterior Approach, Anterior Column, Percutaneous Approach

ØRG1470 Fusion of Cervical Vertebral Joint with Autologous Tissue Substitute, Anterior Approach, Anterior Column, Percutaneous Endoscopic Approach

ØRG1471 Fusion of Cervical Vertebral Joint with Autologous Tissue Substitute, Posterior Approach, Posterior Column, Percutaneous Endoscopic Approach

ØRG147J Fusion of Cervical Vertebral Joint with Autologous Tissue Substitute, Posterior Approach, Anterior Column, Percutaneous Endoscopic Approach

ØRG14A0 Fusion of Cervical Vertebral Joint with Interbody Fusion Device, Anterior Approach, Anterior Column, Percutaneous Endoscopic Approach

HAC 12: Surgical Site Infection-Certain Orthopedic Procedures of the Spine, Shoulder, and Elbow (continued)

ØRG14AJ Fusion of Cervical Vertebral Joint with Interbody Fusion Device, Posterior Approach, Anterior Column, Percutaneous Endoscopic Approach

ØRG14JØ Fusion of Cervical Vertebral Joint with Synthetic Substitute, Anterior Approach, Anterior Column, Percutaneous Endoscopic Approach

ØRG14J1 Fusion of Cervical Vertebral Joint with Synthetic Substitute, Posterior Approach, Posterior Column, Percutaneous Endoscopic Approach

ØRG14JJ Fusion of Cervical Vertebral Joint with Synthetic Substitute, Posterior Approach, Anterior Column, Percutaneous Endoscopic Approach

ØRG14KØ Fusion of Cervical Vertebral Joint with Nonautologous Tissue Substitute, Anterior Approach, Anterior Column, Percutaneous Endoscopic Approach

ØRG14K1 Fusion of Cervical Vertebral Joint with Nonautologous Tissue Substitute, Posterior Approach, Posterior Column, Percutaneous Endoscopic Approach

ØRG14KJ Fusion of Cervical Vertebral Joint with Nonautologous Tissue Substitute, Posterior Approach, Anterior Column, Percutaneous Endoscopic Approach

ØRG2Ø7Ø Fusion of 2 or more Cervical Vertebral Joints with Autologous Tissue Substitute, Anterior Approach, Anterior Column, Open Approach

ØRG2Ø71 Fusion of 2 or more Cervical Vertebral Joints with Autologous Tissue Substitute, Posterior Approach, Posterior Column, Open Approach

ØRG2Ø7J Fusion of 2 or more Cervical Vertebral Joints with Autologous Tissue Substitute, Posterior Approach, Anterior Column, Open Approach

ØRG2ØAØ Fusion of 2 or more Cervical Vertebral Joints with Interbody Fusion Device, Anterior Approach, Anterior Column, Open Approach

ØRG2ØAJ Fusion of 2 or more Cervical Vertebral Joints with Interbody Fusion Device, Posterior Approach, Anterior Column, Open Approach

ØRG2ØJØ Fusion of 2 or more Cervical Vertebral Joints with Synthetic Substitute, Anterior Approach, Anterior Column, Open Approach

ØRG2ØJ1 Fusion of 2 or more Cervical Vertebral Joints with Synthetic Substitute, Posterior Approach, Posterior Column, Open Approach

ØRG2ØJJ Fusion of 2 or more Cervical Vertebral Joints with Synthetic Substitute, Posterior Approach, Anterior Column, Open Approach

ØRG2ØKØ Fusion of 2 or more Cervical Vertebral Joints with Nonautologous Tissue Substitute, Anterior Approach, Anterior Column, Open Approach

ØRG2ØK1 Fusion of 2 or more Cervical Vertebral Joints with Nonautologous Tissue Substitute, Posterior Approach, Posterior Column, Open Approach

ØRG2ØKJ Fusion of 2 or more Cervical Vertebral Joints with Nonautologous Tissue Substitute, Posterior Approach, Anterior Column, Open Approach

ØRG237Ø Fusion of 2 or more Cervical Vertebral Joints with Autologous Tissue Substitute, Anterior Approach, Anterior Column, Percutaneous Approach

ØRG2371 Fusion of 2 or more Cervical Vertebral Joints with Autologous Tissue Substitute, Posterior Approach, Posterior Column, Percutaneous Approach

ØRG237J Fusion of 2 or more Cervical Vertebral Joints with Autologous Tissue Substitute, Posterior Approach, Anterior Column, Percutaneous Approach

ØRG23AØ Fusion of 2 or more Cervical Vertebral Joints with Interbody Fusion Device, Anterior Approach, Anterior Column, Percutaneous Approach

ØRG23AJ Fusion of 2 or more Cervical Vertebral Joints with Interbody Fusion Device, Posterior Approach, Anterior Column, Percutaneous Approach

ØRG23JØ Fusion of 2 or more Cervical Vertebral Joints with Synthetic Substitute, Anterior Approach, Anterior Column, Percutaneous Approach

ØRG23J1 Fusion of 2 or more Cervical Vertebral Joints with Synthetic Substitute, Posterior Approach, Posterior Column, Percutaneous Approach

ØRG23JJ Fusion of 2 or more Cervical Vertebral Joints with Synthetic Substitute, Posterior Approach, Anterior Column, Percutaneous Approach

ØRG23KØ Fusion of 2 or more Cervical Vertebral Joints with Nonautologous Tissue Substitute, Anterior Approach, Anterior Column, Percutaneous Approach

ØRG23K1 Fusion of 2 or more Cervical Vertebral Joints with Nonautologous Tissue Substitute, Posterior Approach, Posterior Column, Percutaneous Approach

ØRG23KJ Fusion of 2 or more Cervical Vertebral Joints with Nonautologous Tissue Substitute, Posterior Approach, Anterior Column, Percutaneous Approach

ØRG247Ø Fusion of 2 or more Cervical Vertebral Joints with Autologous Tissue Substitute, Anterior Approach, Anterior Column, Percutaneous Endoscopic Approach

ØRG2471 Fusion of 2 or more Cervical Vertebral Joints with Autologous Tissue Substitute, Posterior Approach, Posterior Column, Percutaneous Endoscopic Approach

ØRG247J Fusion of 2 or more Cervical Vertebral Joints with Autologous Tissue Substitute, Posterior Approach, Anterior Column, Percutaneous Endoscopic Approach

ØRG24AØ Fusion of 2 or more Cervical Vertebral Joints with Interbody Fusion Device, Anterior Approach, Anterior Column, Percutaneous Endoscopic Approach

ØRG24AJ Fusion of 2 or more Cervical Vertebral Joints with Interbody Fusion Device, Posterior Approach, Anterior Column, Percutaneous Endoscopic Approach

ØRG24JØ Fusion of 2 or more Cervical Vertebral Joints with Synthetic Substitute, Anterior Approach, Anterior Column, Percutaneous Endoscopic Approach

ØRG24J1 Fusion of 2 or more Cervical Vertebral Joints with Synthetic Substitute, Posterior Approach, Posterior Column, Percutaneous Endoscopic Approach

ØRG24JJ Fusion of 2 or more Cervical Vertebral Joints with Synthetic Substitute, Posterior Approach, Anterior Column, Percutaneous Endoscopic Approach

ØRG24KØ Fusion of 2 or more Cervical Vertebral Joints with Nonautologous Tissue Substitute, Anterior Approach, Anterior Column, Percutaneous Endoscopic Approach

ØRG24K1 Fusion of 2 or more Cervical Vertebral Joints with Nonautologous Tissue Substitute, Posterior Approach, Posterior Column, Percutaneous Endoscopic Approach

ØRG24KJ Fusion of 2 or more Cervical Vertebral Joints with Nonautologous Tissue Substitute, Posterior Approach, Anterior Column, Percutaneous Endoscopic Approach

ØRG4Ø7Ø Fusion of Cervicothoracic Vertebral Joint with Autologous Tissue Substitute, Anterior Approach, Anterior Column, Open Approach

ØRG4Ø71 Fusion of Cervicothoracic Vertebral Joint with Autologous Tissue Substitute, Posterior Approach, Posterior Column, Open Approach

ØRG4Ø7J Fusion of Cervicothoracic Vertebral Joint with Autologous Tissue Substitute, Posterior Approach, Anterior Column, Open Approach

ØRG4ØAØ Fusion of Cervicothoracic Vertebral Joint with Interbody Fusion Device, Anterior Approach, Anterior Column, Open Approach

ØRG4ØAJ Fusion of Cervicothoracic Vertebral Joint with Interbody Fusion Device, Posterior Approach, Anterior Column, Open Approach

ØRG4ØJØ Fusion of Cervicothoracic Vertebral Joint with Synthetic Substitute, Anterior Approach, Anterior Column, Open Approach

ØRG4ØJ1 Fusion of Cervicothoracic Vertebral Joint with Synthetic Substitute, Posterior Approach, Posterior Column, Open Approach

ØRG4ØJJ Fusion of Cervicothoracic Vertebral Joint with Synthetic Substitute, Posterior Approach, Anterior Column, Open Approach

ØRG4ØKØ Fusion of Cervicothoracic Vertebral Joint with Nonautologous Tissue Substitute, Anterior Approach, Anterior Column, Open Approach

ØRG4ØK1 Fusion of Cervicothoracic Vertebral Joint with Nonautologous Tissue Substitute, Posterior Approach, Posterior Column, Open Approach

ØRG4ØKJ Fusion of Cervicothoracic Vertebral Joint with Nonautologous Tissue Substitute, Posterior Approach, Anterior Column, Open Approach

ØRG437Ø Fusion of Cervicothoracic Vertebral Joint with Autologous Tissue Substitute, Anterior Approach, Anterior Column, Percutaneous Approach

ØRG4371 Fusion of Cervicothoracic Vertebral Joint with Autologous Tissue Substitute, Posterior Approach, Posterior Column, Percutaneous Approach

ØRG437J Fusion of Cervicothoracic Vertebral Joint with Autologous Tissue Substitute, Posterior Approach, Anterior Column, Percutaneous Approach

ØRG43AØ Fusion of Cervicothoracic Vertebral Joint with Interbody Fusion Device, Anterior Approach, Anterior Column, Percutaneous Approach

HAC 12: Surgical Site Infection-Certain Orthopedic Procedures of the Spine, Shoulder, and Elbow (continued)

ØRG43AJ Fusion of Cervicothoracic Vertebral Joint with Interbody Fusion Device, Posterior Approach, Anterior Column, Percutaneous Approach

ØRG43J0 Fusion of Cervicothoracic Vertebral Joint with Synthetic Substitute, Anterior Approach, Anterior Column, Percutaneous Approach

ØRG43J1 Fusion of Cervicothoracic Vertebral Joint with Synthetic Substitute, Posterior Approach, Posterior Column, Percutaneous Approach

ØRG43JJ Fusion of Cervicothoracic Vertebral Joint with Synthetic Substitute, Posterior Approach, Anterior Column, Percutaneous Approach

ØRG43K0 Fusion of Cervicothoracic Vertebral Joint with Nonautologous Tissue Substitute, Anterior Approach, Anterior Column, Percutaneous Approach

ØRG43K1 Fusion of Cervicothoracic Vertebral Joint with Nonautologous Tissue Substitute, Posterior Approach, Posterior Column, Percutaneous Approach

ØRG43KJ Fusion of Cervicothoracic Vertebral Joint with Nonautologous Tissue Substitute, Posterior Approach, Anterior Column, Percutaneous Approach

ØRG4470 Fusion of Cervicothoracic Vertebral Joint with Autologous Tissue Substitute, Anterior Approach, Anterior Column, Percutaneous Endoscopic Approach

ØRG4471 Fusion of Cervicothoracic Vertebral Joint with Autologous Tissue Substitute, Posterior Approach, Posterior Column, Percutaneous Endoscopic Approach

ØRG447J Fusion of Cervicothoracic Vertebral Joint with Autologous Tissue Substitute, Posterior Approach, Anterior Column, Percutaneous Endoscopic Approach

ØRG44A0 Fusion of Cervicothoracic Vertebral Joint with Interbody Fusion Device, Anterior Approach, Anterior Column, Percutaneous Endoscopic Approach

ØRG44AJ Fusion of Cervicothoracic Vertebral Joint with Interbody Fusion Device, Posterior Approach, Anterior Column, Percutaneous Endoscopic Approach

ØRG44J0 Fusion of Cervicothoracic Vertebral Joint with Synthetic Substitute, Anterior Approach, Anterior Column, Percutaneous Endoscopic Approach

ØRG44J1 Fusion of Cervicothoracic Vertebral Joint with Synthetic Substitute, Posterior Approach, Posterior Column, Percutaneous Endoscopic Approach

ØRG44JJ Fusion of Cervicothoracic Vertebral Joint with Synthetic Substitute, Posterior Approach, Anterior Column, Percutaneous Endoscopic Approach

ØRG44K0 Fusion of Cervicothoracic Vertebral Joint with Nonautologous Tissue Substitute, Anterior Approach, Anterior Column, Percutaneous Endoscopic Approach

ØRG44K1 Fusion of Cervicothoracic Vertebral Joint with Nonautologous Tissue Substitute, Posterior Approach, Posterior Column, Percutaneous Endoscopic Approach

ØRG44KJ Fusion of Cervicothoracic Vertebral Joint with Nonautologous Tissue Substitute, Posterior Approach, Anterior Column, Percutaneous Endoscopic Approach

ØRG6070 Fusion of Thoracic Vertebral Joint with Autologous Tissue Substitute, Anterior Approach, Anterior Column, Open Approach

ØRG6071 Fusion of Thoracic Vertebral Joint with Autologous Tissue Substitute, Posterior Approach, Posterior Column, Open Approach

ØRG607J Fusion of Thoracic Vertebral Joint with Autologous Tissue Substitute, Posterior Approach, Anterior Column, Open Approach

ØRG60A0 Fusion of Thoracic Vertebral Joint with Interbody Fusion Device, Anterior Approach, Anterior Column, Open Approach

ØRG60AJ Fusion of Thoracic Vertebral Joint with Interbody Fusion Device, Posterior Approach, Anterior Column, Open Approach

ØRG60J0 Fusion of Thoracic Vertebral Joint with Synthetic Substitute, Anterior Approach, Anterior Column, Open Approach

ØRG60J1 Fusion of Thoracic Vertebral Joint with Synthetic Substitute, Posterior Approach, Posterior Column, Open Approach

ØRG60JJ Fusion of Thoracic Vertebral Joint with Synthetic Substitute, Posterior Approach, Anterior Column, Open Approach

ØRG60K0 Fusion of Thoracic Vertebral Joint with Nonautologous Tissue Substitute, Anterior Approach, Anterior Column, Open Approach

ØRG60K1 Fusion of Thoracic Vertebral Joint with Nonautologous Tissue Substitute, Posterior Approach, Posterior Column, Open Approach

ØRG60KJ Fusion of Thoracic Vertebral Joint with Nonautologous Tissue Substitute, Posterior Approach, Anterior Column, Open Approach

ØRG6370 Fusion of Thoracic Vertebral Joint with Autologous Tissue Substitute, Anterior Approach, Anterior Column, Percutaneous Approach

ØRG6371 Fusion of Thoracic Vertebral Joint with Autologous Tissue Substitute, Posterior Approach, Posterior Column, Percutaneous Approach

ØRG637J Fusion of Thoracic Vertebral Joint with Autologous Tissue Substitute, Posterior Approach, Anterior Column, Percutaneous Approach

ØRG63A0 Fusion of Thoracic Vertebral Joint with Interbody Fusion Device, Anterior Approach, Anterior Column, Percutaneous Approach

ØRG63AJ Fusion of Thoracic Vertebral Joint with Interbody Fusion Device, Posterior Approach, Anterior Column, Percutaneous Approach

ØRG63J0 Fusion of Thoracic Vertebral Joint with Synthetic Substitute, Anterior Approach, Anterior Column, Percutaneous Approach

ØRG63J1 Fusion of Thoracic Vertebral Joint with Synthetic Substitute, Posterior Approach, Posterior Column, Percutaneous Approach

ØRG63JJ Fusion of Thoracic Vertebral Joint with Synthetic Substitute, Posterior Approach, Anterior Column, Percutaneous Approach

ØRG63K0 Fusion of Thoracic Vertebral Joint with Nonautologous Tissue Substitute, Anterior Approach, Anterior Column, Percutaneous Approach

ØRG63K1 Fusion of Thoracic Vertebral Joint with Nonautologous Tissue Substitute, Posterior Approach, Posterior Column, Percutaneous Approach

ØRG63KJ Fusion of Thoracic Vertebral Joint with Nonautologous Tissue Substitute, Posterior Approach, Anterior Column, Percutaneous Approach

ØRG6470 Fusion of Thoracic Vertebral Joint with Autologous Tissue Substitute, Anterior Approach, Anterior Column, Percutaneous Endoscopic Approach

ØRG6471 Fusion of Thoracic Vertebral Joint with Autologous Tissue Substitute, Posterior Approach, Posterior Column, Percutaneous Endoscopic Approach

ØRG647J Fusion of Thoracic Vertebral Joint with Autologous Tissue Substitute, Posterior Approach, Anterior Column, Percutaneous Endoscopic Approach

ØRG64A0 Fusion of Thoracic Vertebral Joint with Interbody Fusion Device, Anterior Approach, Anterior Column, Percutaneous Endoscopic Approach

ØRG64AJ Fusion of Thoracic Vertebral Joint with Interbody Fusion Device, Posterior Approach, Anterior Column, Percutaneous Endoscopic Approach

ØRG64J0 Fusion of Thoracic Vertebral Joint with Synthetic Substitute, Anterior Approach, Anterior Column, Percutaneous Endoscopic Approach

ØRG64J1 Fusion of Thoracic Vertebral Joint with Synthetic Substitute, Posterior Approach, Posterior Column, Percutaneous Endoscopic Approach

ØRG64JJ Fusion of Thoracic Vertebral Joint with Synthetic Substitute, Posterior Approach, Anterior Column, Percutaneous Endoscopic Approach

ØRG64K0 Fusion of Thoracic Vertebral Joint with Nonautologous Tissue Substitute, Anterior Approach, Anterior Column, Percutaneous Endoscopic Approach

ØRG64K1 Fusion of Thoracic Vertebral Joint with Nonautologous Tissue Substitute, Posterior Approach, Posterior Column, Percutaneous Endoscopic Approach

ØRG64KJ Fusion of Thoracic Vertebral Joint with Nonautologous Tissue Substitute, Posterior Approach, Anterior Column, Percutaneous Endoscopic Approach

ØRG7070 Fusion of 2 to 7 Thoracic Vertebral Joints with Autologous Tissue Substitute, Anterior Approach, Anterior Column, Open Approach

ØRG7071 Fusion of 2 to 7 Thoracic Vertebral Joints with Autologous Tissue Substitute, Posterior Approach, Posterior Column, Open Approach

ØRG707J Fusion of 2 to 7 Thoracic Vertebral Joints with Autologous Tissue Substitute, Posterior Approach, Anterior Column, Open Approach

ØRG70A0 Fusion of 2 to 7 Thoracic Vertebral Joints with Interbody Fusion Device, Anterior Approach, Anterior Column, Open Approach

ØRG70AJ Fusion of 2 to 7 Thoracic Vertebral Joints with Interbody Fusion Device, Posterior Approach, Anterior Column, Open Approach

ØRG70J0 Fusion of 2 to 7 Thoracic Vertebral Joints with Synthetic Substitute, Anterior Approach, Anterior Column, Open Approach

HAC 12: Surgical Site Infection-Certain Orthopedic Procedures of the Spine, Shoulder, and Elbow (continued)

ØRG7ØJ1 Fusion of 2 to 7 Thoracic Vertebral Joints with Synthetic Substitute, Posterior Approach, Posterior Column, Open Approach

ØRG7ØJJ Fusion of 2 to 7 Thoracic Vertebral Joints with Synthetic Substitute, Posterior Approach, Anterior Column, Open Approach

ØRG7ØKØ Fusion of 2 to 7 Thoracic Vertebral Joints with Nonautologous Tissue Substitute, Anterior Approach, Anterior Column, Open Approach

ØRG7ØK1 Fusion of 2 to 7 Thoracic Vertebral Joints with Nonautologous Tissue Substitute, Posterior Approach, Posterior Column, Open Approach

ØRG7ØKJ Fusion of 2 to 7 Thoracic Vertebral Joints with Nonautologous Tissue Substitute, Posterior Approach, Anterior Column, Open Approach

ØRG737Ø Fusion of 2 to 7 Thoracic Vertebral Joints with Autologous Tissue Substitute, Anterior Approach, Anterior Column, Percutaneous Approach

ØRG7371 Fusion of 2 to 7 Thoracic Vertebral Joints with Autologous Tissue Substitute, Posterior Approach, Posterior Column, Percutaneous Approach

ØRG737J Fusion of 2 to 7 Thoracic Vertebral Joints with Autologous Tissue Substitute, Posterior Approach, Anterior Column, Percutaneous Approach

ØRG73AØ Fusion of 2 to 7 Thoracic Vertebral Joints with Interbody Fusion Device, Anterior Approach, Anterior Column, Percutaneous Approach

ØRG73AJ Fusion of 2 to 7 Thoracic Vertebral Joints with Interbody Fusion Device, Posterior Approach, Anterior Column, Percutaneous Approach

ØRG73JØ Fusion of 2 to 7 Thoracic Vertebral Joints with Synthetic Substitute, Anterior Approach, Anterior Column, Percutaneous Approach

ØRG73J1 Fusion of 2 to 7 Thoracic Vertebral Joints with Synthetic Substitute, Posterior Approach, Posterior Column, Percutaneous Approach

ØRG73JJ Fusion of 2 to 7 Thoracic Vertebral Joints with Synthetic Substitute, Posterior Approach, Anterior Column, Percutaneous Approach

ØRG73KØ Fusion of 2 to 7 Thoracic Vertebral Joints with Nonautologous Tissue Substitute, Anterior Approach, Anterior Column, Percutaneous Approach

ØRG73K1 Fusion of 2 to 7 Thoracic Vertebral Joints with Nonautologous Tissue Substitute, Posterior Approach, Posterior Column, Percutaneous Approach

ØRG73KJ Fusion of 2 to 7 Thoracic Vertebral Joints with Nonautologous Tissue Substitute, Posterior Approach, Anterior Column, Percutaneous Approach

ØRG747Ø Fusion of 2 to 7 Thoracic Vertebral Joints with Autologous Tissue Substitute, Anterior Approach, Anterior Column, Percutaneous Endoscopic Approach

ØRG7471 Fusion of 2 to 7 Thoracic Vertebral Joints with Autologous Tissue Substitute, Posterior Approach, Posterior Column, Percutaneous Endoscopic Approach

ØRG747J Fusion of 2 to 7 Thoracic Vertebral Joints with Autologous Tissue Substitute, Posterior Approach, Anterior Column, Percutaneous Endoscopic Approach

ØRG74AØ Fusion of 2 to 7 Thoracic Vertebral Joints with Interbody Fusion Device, Anterior Approach, Anterior Column, Percutaneous Endoscopic Approach

ØRG74AJ Fusion of 2 to 7 Thoracic Vertebral Joints with Interbody Fusion Device, Posterior Approach, Anterior Column, Percutaneous Endoscopic Approach

ØRG74JØ Fusion of 2 to 7 Thoracic Vertebral Joints with Synthetic Substitute, Anterior Approach, Anterior Column, Percutaneous Endoscopic Approach

ØRG74J1 Fusion of 2 to 7 Thoracic Vertebral Joints with Synthetic Substitute, Posterior Approach, Posterior Column, Percutaneous Endoscopic Approach

ØRG74JJ Fusion of 2 to 7 Thoracic Vertebral Joints with Synthetic Substitute, Posterior Approach, Anterior Column, Percutaneous Endoscopic Approach

ØRG74KØ Fusion of 2 to 7 Thoracic Vertebral Joints with Nonautologous Tissue Substitute, Anterior Approach, Anterior Column, Percutaneous Endoscopic Approach

ØRG74K1 Fusion of 2 to 7 Thoracic Vertebral Joints with Nonautologous Tissue Substitute, Posterior Approach, Posterior Column, Percutaneous Endoscopic Approach

ØRG74KJ Fusion of 2 to 7 Thoracic Vertebral Joints with Nonautologous Tissue Substitute, Posterior Approach, Anterior Column, Percutaneous Endoscopic Approach

ØRG8Ø7Ø Fusion of 8 or More Thoracic Vertebral Joints with Autologous Tissue Substitute, Anterior Approach, Anterior Column, Open Approach

ØRG8Ø71 Fusion of 8 or More Thoracic Vertebral Joints with Autologous Tissue Substitute, Posterior Approach, Posterior Column, Open Approach

ØRG8Ø7J Fusion of 8 or More Thoracic Vertebral Joints with Autologous Tissue Substitute, Posterior Approach, Anterior Column, Open Approach

ØRG8ØAØ Fusion of 8 or More Thoracic Vertebral Joints with Interbody Fusion Device, Anterior Approach, Anterior Column, Open Approach

ØRG8ØAJ Fusion of 8 or More Thoracic Vertebral Joints with Interbody Fusion Device, Posterior Approach, Anterior Column, Open Approach

ØRG8ØJØ Fusion of 8 or More Thoracic Vertebral Joints with Synthetic Substitute, Anterior Approach, Anterior Column, Open Approach

ØRG8ØJ1 Fusion of 8 or More Thoracic Vertebral Joints with Synthetic Substitute, Posterior Approach, Posterior Column, Open Approach

ØRG8ØJJ Fusion of 8 or More Thoracic Vertebral Joints with Synthetic Substitute, Posterior Approach, Anterior Column, Open Approach

ØRG8ØKØ Fusion of 8 or More Thoracic Vertebral Joints with Nonautologous Tissue Substitute, Anterior Approach, Anterior Column, Open Approach

ØRG8ØK1 Fusion of 8 or More Thoracic Vertebral Joints with Nonautologous Tissue Substitute, Posterior Approach, Posterior Column, Open Approach

ØRG8ØKJ Fusion of 8 or More Thoracic Vertebral Joints with Nonautologous Tissue Substitute, Posterior Approach, Anterior Column, Open Approach

ØRG837Ø Fusion of 8 or More Thoracic Vertebral Joints with Autologous Tissue Substitute, Anterior Approach, Anterior Column, Percutaneous Approach

ØRG8371 Fusion of 8 or More Thoracic Vertebral Joints with Autologous Tissue Substitute, Posterior Approach, Posterior Column, Percutaneous Approach

ØRG837J Fusion of 8 or More Thoracic Vertebral Joints with Autologous Tissue Substitute, Posterior Approach, Anterior Column, Percutaneous Approach

ØRG83AØ Fusion of 8 or More Thoracic Vertebral Joints with Interbody Fusion Device, Anterior Approach, Anterior Column, Percutaneous Approach

ØRG83AJ Fusion of 8 or More Thoracic Vertebral Joints with Interbody Fusion Device, Posterior Approach, Anterior Column, Percutaneous Approach

ØRG83JØ Fusion of 8 or More Thoracic Vertebral Joints with Synthetic Substitute, Anterior Approach, Anterior Column, Percutaneous Approach

ØRG83J1 Fusion of 8 or More Thoracic Vertebral Joints with Synthetic Substitute, Posterior Approach, Posterior Column, Percutaneous Approach

ØRG83JJ Fusion of 8 or More Thoracic Vertebral Joints with Synthetic Substitute, Posterior Approach, Anterior Column, Percutaneous Approach

ØRG83KØ Fusion of 8 or More Thoracic Vertebral Joints with Nonautologous Tissue Substitute, Anterior Approach, Anterior Column, Percutaneous Approach

ØRG83K1 Fusion of 8 or More Thoracic Vertebral Joints with Nonautologous Tissue Substitute, Posterior Approach, Posterior Column, Percutaneous Approach

ØRG83KJ Fusion of 8 or More Thoracic Vertebral Joints with Nonautologous Tissue Substitute, Posterior Approach, Anterior Column, Percutaneous Approach

ØRG847Ø Fusion of 8 or More Thoracic Vertebral Joints with Autologous Tissue Substitute, Anterior Approach, Anterior Column, Percutaneous Endoscopic Approach

ØRG8471 Fusion of 8 or More Thoracic Vertebral Joints with Autologous Tissue Substitute, Posterior Approach, Posterior Column, Percutaneous Endoscopic Approach

ØRG847J Fusion of 8 or More Thoracic Vertebral Joints with Autologous Tissue Substitute, Posterior Approach, Anterior Column, Percutaneous Endoscopic Approach

ØRG84AØ Fusion of 8 or More Thoracic Vertebral Joints with Interbody Fusion Device, Anterior Approach, Anterior Column, Percutaneous Endoscopic Approach

ØRG84AJ Fusion of 8 or More Thoracic Vertebral Joints with Interbody Fusion Device, Posterior Approach, Anterior Column, Percutaneous Endoscopic Approach

ØRG84JØ Fusion of 8 or More Thoracic Vertebral Joints with Synthetic Substitute, Anterior Approach, Anterior Column, Percutaneous Endoscopic Approach

ØRG84J1 Fusion of 8 or More Thoracic Vertebral Joints with Synthetic Substitute, Posterior Approach, Posterior Column, Percutaneous Endoscopic Approach

HAC 12: Surgical Site Infection-Certain Orthopedic Procedures of the Spine, Shoulder, and Elbow (continued)

ØRG84JJ   Fusion of 8 or More Thoracic Vertebral Joints with Synthetic Substitute, Posterior Approach, Anterior Column, Percutaneous Endoscopic Approach

ØRG84KØ   Fusion of 8 or More Thoracic Vertebral Joints with Nonautologous Tissue Substitute, Anterior Approach, Anterior Column, Percutaneous Endoscopic Approach

ØRG84K1   Fusion of 8 or More Thoracic Vertebral Joints with Nonautologous Tissue Substitute, Posterior Approach, Posterior Column, Percutaneous Endoscopic Approach

ØRG84KJ   Fusion of 8 or More Thoracic Vertebral Joints with Nonautologous Tissue Substitute, Posterior Approach, Anterior Column, Percutaneous Endoscopic Approach

ØRGAØ7Ø   Fusion of Thoracolumbar Vertebral Joint with Autologous Tissue Substitute, Anterior Approach, Anterior Column, Open Approach

ØRGAØ71   Fusion of Thoracolumbar Vertebral Joint with Autologous Tissue Substitute, Posterior Approach, Posterior Column, Open Approach

ØRGAØ7J   Fusion of Thoracolumbar Vertebral Joint with Autologous Tissue Substitute, Posterior Approach, Anterior Column, Open Approach

ØRGAØAØ   Fusion of Thoracolumbar Vertebral Joint with Interbody Fusion Device, Anterior Approach, Anterior Column, Open Approach

ØRGAØAJ   Fusion of Thoracolumbar Vertebral Joint with Interbody Fusion Device, Posterior Approach, Anterior Column, Open Approach

ØRGAØJØ   Fusion of Thoracolumbar Vertebral Joint with Synthetic Substitute, Anterior Approach, Anterior Column, Open Approach

ØRGAØJ1   Fusion of Thoracolumbar Vertebral Joint with Synthetic Substitute, Posterior Approach, Posterior Column, Open Approach

ØRGAØJJ   Fusion of Thoracolumbar Vertebral Joint with Synthetic Substitute, Posterior Approach, Anterior Column, Open Approach

ØRGAØKØ   Fusion of Thoracolumbar Vertebral Joint with Nonautologous Tissue Substitute, Anterior Approach, Anterior Column, Open Approach

ØRGAØK1   Fusion of Thoracolumbar Vertebral Joint with Nonautologous Tissue Substitute, Posterior Approach, Posterior Column, Open Approach

ØRGAØKJ   Fusion of Thoracolumbar Vertebral Joint with Nonautologous Tissue Substitute, Posterior Approach, Anterior Column, Open Approach

ØRGA37Ø   Fusion of Thoracolumbar Vertebral Joint with Autologous Tissue Substitute, Anterior Approach, Anterior Column, Percutaneous Approach

ØRGA371   Fusion of Thoracolumbar Vertebral Joint with Autologous Tissue Substitute, Posterior Approach, Posterior Column, Percutaneous Approach

ØRGA37J   Fusion of Thoracolumbar Vertebral Joint with Autologous Tissue Substitute, Posterior Approach, Anterior Column, Percutaneous Approach

ØRGA3AØ   Fusion of Thoracolumbar Vertebral Joint with Interbody Fusion Device, Anterior Approach, Anterior Column, Percutaneous Approach

ØRGA3AJ   Fusion of Thoracolumbar Vertebral Joint with Interbody Fusion Device, Posterior Approach, Anterior Column, Percutaneous Approach

ØRGA3JØ   Fusion of Thoracolumbar Vertebral Joint with Synthetic Substitute, Anterior Approach, Anterior Column, Percutaneous Approach

ØRGA3J1   Fusion of Thoracolumbar Vertebral Joint with Synthetic Substitute, Posterior Approach, Posterior Column, Percutaneous Approach

ØRGA3JJ   Fusion of Thoracolumbar Vertebral Joint with Synthetic Substitute, Posterior Approach, Anterior Column, Percutaneous Approach

ØRGA3KØ   Fusion of Thoracolumbar Vertebral Joint with Nonautologous Tissue Substitute, Anterior Approach, Anterior Column, Percutaneous Approach

ØRGA3K1   Fusion of Thoracolumbar Vertebral Joint with Nonautologous Tissue Substitute, Posterior Approach, Posterior Column, Percutaneous Approach

ØRGA3KJ   Fusion of Thoracolumbar Vertebral Joint with Nonautologous Tissue Substitute, Posterior Approach, Anterior Column, Percutaneous Approach

ØRGA47Ø   Fusion of Thoracolumbar Vertebral Joint with Autologous Tissue Substitute, Anterior Approach, Anterior Column, Percutaneous Endoscopic Approach

ØRGA471   Fusion of Thoracolumbar Vertebral Joint with Autologous Tissue Substitute, Posterior Approach, Posterior Column, Percutaneous Endoscopic Approach

ØRGA47J   Fusion of Thoracolumbar Vertebral Joint with Autologous Tissue Substitute, Posterior Approach, Anterior Column, Percutaneous Endoscopic Approach

ØRGA4AØ   Fusion of Thoracolumbar Vertebral Joint with Interbody Fusion Device, Anterior Approach, Anterior Column, Percutaneous Endoscopic Approach

ØRGA4AJ   Fusion of Thoracolumbar Vertebral Joint with Interbody Fusion Device, Posterior Approach, Anterior Column, Percutaneous Endoscopic Approach

ØRGA4JØ   Fusion of Thoracolumbar Vertebral Joint with Synthetic Substitute, Anterior Approach, Anterior Column, Percutaneous Endoscopic Approach

ØRGA4J1   Fusion of Thoracolumbar Vertebral Joint with Synthetic Substitute, Posterior Approach, Posterior Column, Percutaneous Endoscopic Approach

ØRGA4JJ   Fusion of Thoracolumbar Vertebral Joint with Synthetic Substitute, Posterior Approach, Anterior Column, Percutaneous Endoscopic Approach

ØRGA4KØ   Fusion of Thoracolumbar Vertebral Joint with Nonautologous Tissue Substitute, Anterior Approach, Anterior Column, Percutaneous Endoscopic Approach

ØRGA4K1   Fusion of Thoracolumbar Vertebral Joint with Nonautologous Tissue Substitute, Posterior Approach, Posterior Column, Percutaneous Endoscopic Approach

ØRGA4KJ   Fusion of Thoracolumbar Vertebral Joint with Nonautologous Tissue Substitute, Posterior Approach, Anterior Column, Percutaneous Endoscopic Approach

ØRGEØ4Z   Fusion of Right Sternoclavicular Joint with Internal Fixation Device, Open Approach

ØRGEØ7Z   Fusion of Right Sternoclavicular Joint with Autologous Tissue Substitute, Open Approach

ØRGEØJZ   Fusion of Right Sternoclavicular Joint with Synthetic Substitute, Open Approach

ØRGEØKZ   Fusion of Right Sternoclavicular Joint with Nonautologous Tissue Substitute, Open Approach

ØRGE34Z   Fusion of Right Sternoclavicular Joint with Internal Fixation Device, Percutaneous Approach

ØRGE37Z   Fusion of Right Sternoclavicular Joint with Autologous Tissue Substitute, Percutaneous Approach

ØRGE3JZ   Fusion of Right Sternoclavicular Joint with Synthetic Substitute, Percutaneous Approach

ØRGE3KZ   Fusion of Right Sternoclavicular Joint with Nonautologous Tissue Substitute, Percutaneous Approach

ØRGE44Z   Fusion of Right Sternoclavicular Joint with Internal Fixation Device, Percutaneous Endoscopic Approach

ØRGE47Z   Fusion of Right Sternoclavicular Joint with Autologous Tissue Substitute, Percutaneous Endoscopic Approach

ØRGE4JZ   Fusion of Right Sternoclavicular Joint with Synthetic Substitute, Percutaneous Endoscopic Approach

ØRGE4KZ   Fusion of Right Sternoclavicular Joint with Nonautologous Tissue Substitute, Percutaneous Endoscopic Approach

ØRGFØ4Z   Fusion of Left Sternoclavicular Joint with Internal Fixation Device, Open Approach

ØRGFØ7Z   Fusion of Left Sternoclavicular Joint with Autologous Tissue Substitute, Open Approach

ØRGFØJZ   Fusion of Left Sternoclavicular Joint with Synthetic Substitute, Open Approach

ØRGFØKZ   Fusion of Left Sternoclavicular Joint with Nonautologous Tissue Substitute, Open Approach

ØRGF34Z   Fusion of Left Sternoclavicular Joint with Internal Fixation Device, Percutaneous Approach

ØRGF37Z   Fusion of Left Sternoclavicular Joint with Autologous Tissue Substitute, Percutaneous Approach

ØRGF3JZ   Fusion of Left Sternoclavicular Joint with Synthetic Substitute, Percutaneous Approach

ØRGF3KZ   Fusion of Left Sternoclavicular Joint with Nonautologous Tissue Substitute, Percutaneous Approach

ØRGF44Z   Fusion of Left Sternoclavicular Joint with Internal Fixation Device, Percutaneous Endoscopic Approach

ØRGF47Z   Fusion of Left Sternoclavicular Joint with Autologous Tissue Substitute, Percutaneous Endoscopic Approach

ØRGF4JZ   Fusion of Left Sternoclavicular Joint with Synthetic Substitute, Percutaneous Endoscopic Approach

ØRGF4KZ   Fusion of Left Sternoclavicular Joint with Nonautologous Tissue Substitute, Percutaneous Endoscopic Approach

ØRGGØ4Z   Fusion of Right Acromioclavicular Joint with Internal Fixation Device, Open Approach

HAC 12: Surgical Site Infection-Certain Orthopedic Procedures of the Spine, Shoulder, and Elbow (continued)

ØRGGØ7Z Fusion of Right Acromioclavicular Joint with Autologous Tissue Substitute, Open Approach

ØRGGØJZ Fusion of Right Acromioclavicular Joint with Synthetic Substitute, Open Approach

ØRGGØKZ Fusion of Right Acromioclavicular Joint with Nonautologous Tissue Substitute, Open Approach

ØRGG34Z Fusion of Right Acromioclavicular Joint with Internal Fixation Device, Percutaneous Approach

ØRGG37Z Fusion of Right Acromioclavicular Joint with Autologous Tissue Substitute, Percutaneous Approach

ØRGG3JZ Fusion of Right Acromioclavicular Joint with Synthetic Substitute, Percutaneous Approach

ØRGG3KZ Fusion of Right Acromioclavicular Joint with Nonautologous Tissue Substitute, Percutaneous Approach

ØRGG44Z Fusion of Right Acromioclavicular Joint with Internal Fixation Device, Percutaneous Endoscopic Approach

ØRGG47Z Fusion of Right Acromioclavicular Joint with Autologous Tissue Substitute, Percutaneous Endoscopic Approach

ØRGG4JZ Fusion of Right Acromioclavicular Joint with Synthetic Substitute, Percutaneous Endoscopic Approach

ØRGG4KZ Fusion of Right Acromioclavicular Joint with Nonautologous Tissue Substitute, Percutaneous Endoscopic Approach

ØRGH04Z Fusion of Left Acromioclavicular Joint with Internal Fixation Device, Open Approach

ØRGH07Z Fusion of Left Acromioclavicular Joint with Autologous Tissue Substitute, Open Approach

ØRGHØJZ Fusion of Left Acromioclavicular Joint with Synthetic Substitute, Open Approach

ØRGHØKZ Fusion of Left Acromioclavicular Joint with Nonautologous Tissue Substitute, Open Approach

ØRGH34Z Fusion of Left Acromioclavicular Joint with Internal Fixation Device, Percutaneous Approach

ØRGH37Z Fusion of Left Acromioclavicular Joint with Autologous Tissue Substitute, Percutaneous Approach

ØRGH3JZ Fusion of Left Acromioclavicular Joint with Synthetic Substitute, Percutaneous Approach

ØRGH3KZ Fusion of Left Acromioclavicular Joint with Nonautologous Tissue Substitute, Percutaneous Approach

ØRGH44Z Fusion of Left Acromioclavicular Joint with Internal Fixation Device, Percutaneous Endoscopic Approach

ØRGH47Z Fusion of Left Acromioclavicular Joint with Autologous Tissue Substitute, Percutaneous Endoscopic Approach

ØRGH4JZ Fusion of Left Acromioclavicular Joint with Synthetic Substitute, Percutaneous Endoscopic Approach

ØRGH4KZ Fusion of Left Acromioclavicular Joint with Nonautologous Tissue Substitute, Percutaneous Endoscopic Approach

ØRGJ04Z Fusion of Right Shoulder Joint with Internal Fixation Device, Open Approach

ØRGJ07Z Fusion of Right Shoulder Joint with Autologous Tissue Substitute, Open Approach

ØRGJØJZ Fusion of Right Shoulder Joint with Synthetic Substitute, Open Approach

ØRGJØKZ Fusion of Right Shoulder Joint with Nonautologous Tissue Substitute, Open Approach

ØRGJ34Z Fusion of Right Shoulder Joint with Internal Fixation Device, Percutaneous Approach

ØRGJ37Z Fusion of Right Shoulder Joint with Autologous Tissue Substitute, Percutaneous Approach

ØRGJ3JZ Fusion of Right Shoulder Joint with Synthetic Substitute, Percutaneous Approach

ØRGJ3KZ Fusion of Right Shoulder Joint with Nonautologous Tissue Substitute, Percutaneous Approach

ØRGJ44Z Fusion of Right Shoulder Joint with Internal Fixation Device, Percutaneous Endoscopic Approach

ØRGJ47Z Fusion of Right Shoulder Joint with Autologous Tissue Substitute, Percutaneous Endoscopic Approach

ØRGJ4JZ Fusion of Right Shoulder Joint with Synthetic Substitute, Percutaneous Endoscopic Approach

ØRGJ4KZ Fusion of Right Shoulder Joint with Nonautologous Tissue Substitute, Percutaneous Endoscopic Approach

ØRGK04Z Fusion of Left Shoulder Joint with Internal Fixation Device, Open Approach

ØRGK07Z Fusion of Left Shoulder Joint with Autologous Tissue Substitute, Open Approach

ØRGKØJZ Fusion of Left Shoulder Joint with Synthetic Substitute, Open Approach

ØRGKØKZ Fusion of Left Shoulder Joint with Nonautologous Tissue Substitute, Open Approach

ØRGK34Z Fusion of Left Shoulder Joint with Internal Fixation Device, Percutaneous Approach

ØRGK37Z Fusion of Left Shoulder Joint with Autologous Tissue Substitute, Percutaneous Approach

ØRGK3JZ Fusion of Left Shoulder Joint with Synthetic Substitute, Percutaneous Approach

ØRGK3KZ Fusion of Left Shoulder Joint with Nonautologous Tissue Substitute, Percutaneous Approach

ØRGK44Z Fusion of Left Shoulder Joint with Internal Fixation Device, Percutaneous Endoscopic Approach

ØRGK47Z Fusion of Left Shoulder Joint with Autologous Tissue Substitute, Percutaneous Endoscopic Approach

ØRGK4JZ Fusion of Left Shoulder Joint with Synthetic Substitute, Percutaneous Endoscopic Approach

ØRGK4KZ Fusion of Left Shoulder Joint with Nonautologous Tissue Substitute, Percutaneous Endoscopic Approach

ØRGL03Z Fusion of Right Elbow Joint with Sustained Compression Internal Fixation Device, Open Approach

ØRGL04Z Fusion of Right Elbow Joint with Internal Fixation Device, Open Approach

ØRGL05Z Fusion of Right Elbow Joint with External Fixation Device, Open Approach

ØRGL07Z Fusion of Right Elbow Joint with Autologous Tissue Substitute, Open Approach

ØRGLØJZ Fusion of Right Elbow Joint with Synthetic Substitute, Open Approach

ØRGLØKZ Fusion of Right Elbow Joint with Nonautologous Tissue Substitute, Open Approach

ØRGL33Z Fusion of Right Elbow Joint with Sustained Compression Internal Fixation Device, Percutaneous Approach

ØRGL34Z Fusion of Right Elbow Joint with Internal Fixation Device, Percutaneous Approach

ØRGL35Z Fusion of Right Elbow Joint with External Fixation Device, Percutaneous Approach

ØRGL37Z Fusion of Right Elbow Joint with Autologous Tissue Substitute, Percutaneous Approach

ØRGL3JZ Fusion of Right Elbow Joint with Synthetic Substitute, Percutaneous Approach

ØRGL3KZ Fusion of Right Elbow Joint with Nonautologous Tissue Substitute, Percutaneous Approach

ØRGL43Z Fusion of Right Elbow Joint with Sustained Compression Internal Fixation Device, Percutaneous Endoscopic Approach

ØRGL44Z Fusion of Right Elbow Joint with Internal Fixation Device, Percutaneous Endoscopic Approach

ØRGL45Z Fusion of Right Elbow Joint with External Fixation Device, Percutaneous Endoscopic Approach

ØRGL47Z Fusion of Right Elbow Joint with Autologous Tissue Substitute, Percutaneous Endoscopic Approach

ØRGL4JZ Fusion of Right Elbow Joint with Synthetic Substitute, Percutaneous Endoscopic Approach

ØRGL4KZ Fusion of Right Elbow Joint with Nonautologous Tissue Substitute, Percutaneous Endoscopic Approach

ØRGM03Z Fusion of Left Elbow Joint with Sustained Compression Internal Fixation Device, Open Approach

ØRGM04Z Fusion of Left Elbow Joint with Internal Fixation Device, Open Approach

ØRGM05Z Fusion of Left Elbow Joint with External Fixation Device, Open Approach

ØRGM07Z Fusion of Left Elbow Joint with Autologous Tissue Substitute, Open Approach

ØRGMØJZ Fusion of Left Elbow Joint with Synthetic Substitute, Open Approach

ØRGMØKZ Fusion of Left Elbow Joint with Nonautologous Tissue Substitute, Open Approach

ØRGM33Z Fusion of Left Elbow Joint with Sustained Compression Internal Fixation Device, Percutaneous Approach

ØRGM34Z Fusion of Left Elbow Joint with Internal Fixation Device, Percutaneous Approach

ØRGM35Z Fusion of Left Elbow Joint with External Fixation Device, Percutaneous Approach

ØRGM37Z Fusion of Left Elbow Joint with Autologous Tissue Substitute, Percutaneous Approach

ØRGM3JZ Fusion of Left Elbow Joint with Synthetic Substitute, Percutaneous Approach

ØRGM3KZ Fusion of Left Elbow Joint with Nonautologous Tissue Substitute, Percutaneous Approach

ØRGM43Z Fusion of Left Elbow Joint with Sustained Compression Internal Fixation Device, Percutaneous Endoscopic Approach

ØRGM44Z Fusion of Left Elbow Joint with Internal Fixation Device, Percutaneous Endoscopic Approach

ØRGM45Z Fusion of Left Elbow Joint with External Fixation Device, Percutaneous Endoscopic Approach

ØRGM47Z Fusion of Left Elbow Joint with Autologous Tissue Substitute, Percutaneous Endoscopic Approach

ØRGM4JZ Fusion of Left Elbow Joint with Synthetic Substitute, Percutaneous Endoscopic Approach

HAC 12: Surgical Site Infection-Certain Orthopedic Procedures of the Spine, Shoulder, and Elbow (continued)

ØRGM4KZ Fusion of Left Elbow Joint with Nonautologous Tissue Substitute, Percutaneous Endoscopic Approach

ØRQEØZZ Repair Right Sternoclavicular Joint, Open Approach

ØRQE3ZZ Repair Right Sternoclavicular Joint, Percutaneous Approach

ØRQE4ZZ Repair Right Sternoclavicular Joint, Percutaneous Endoscopic Approach

ØRQEXZZ Repair Right Sternoclavicular Joint, External Approach

ØRQFØZZ Repair Left Sternoclavicular Joint, Open Approach

ØRQF3ZZ Repair Left Sternoclavicular Joint, Percutaneous Approach

ØRQF4ZZ Repair Left Sternoclavicular Joint, Percutaneous Endoscopic Approach

ØRQFXZZ Repair Left Sternoclavicular Joint, External Approach

ØRQGØZZ Repair Right Acromioclavicular Joint, Open Approach

ØRQG3ZZ Repair Right Acromioclavicular Joint, Percutaneous Approach

ØRQG4ZZ Repair Right Acromioclavicular Joint, Percutaneous Endoscopic Approach

ØRQGXZZ Repair Right Acromioclavicular Joint, External Approach

ØRQHØZZ Repair Left Acromioclavicular Joint, Open Approach

ØRQH3ZZ Repair Left Acromioclavicular Joint, Percutaneous Approach

ØRQH4ZZ Repair Left Acromioclavicular Joint, Percutaneous Endoscopic Approach

ØRQHXZZ Repair Left Acromioclavicular Joint, External Approach

ØRQJØZZ Repair Right Shoulder Joint, Open Approach

ØRQJ3ZZ Repair Right Shoulder Joint, Percutaneous Approach

ØRQJ4ZZ Repair Right Shoulder Joint, Percutaneous Endoscopic Approach

ØRQJXZZ Repair Right Shoulder Joint, External Approach

ØRQKØZZ Repair Left Shoulder Joint, Open Approach

ØRQK3ZZ Repair Left Shoulder Joint, Percutaneous Approach

ØRQK4ZZ Repair Left Shoulder Joint, Percutaneous Endoscopic Approach

ØRQKXZZ Repair Left Shoulder Joint, External Approach

ØRQLØZZ Repair Right Elbow Joint, Open Approach

ØRQL3ZZ Repair Right Elbow Joint, Percutaneous Approach

ØRQL4ZZ Repair Right Elbow Joint, Percutaneous Endoscopic Approach

ØRQLXZZ Repair Right Elbow Joint, External Approach

ØRQMØZZ Repair Left Elbow Joint, Open Approach

ØRQM3ZZ Repair Left Elbow Joint, Percutaneous Approach

ØRQM4ZZ Repair Left Elbow Joint, Percutaneous Endoscopic Approach

ØRQMXZZ Repair Left Elbow Joint, External Approach

ØRUEØ7Z Supplement Right Sternoclavicular Joint with Autologous Tissue Substitute, Open Approach

ØRUEØJZ Supplement Right Sternoclavicular Joint with Synthetic Substitute, Open Approach

ØRUEØKZ Supplement Right Sternoclavicular Joint with Nonautologous Tissue Substitute, Open Approach

ØRUE37Z Supplement Right Sternoclavicular Joint with Autologous Tissue Substitute, Percutaneous Approach

ØRUE3JZ Supplement Right Sternoclavicular Joint with Synthetic Substitute, Percutaneous Approach

ØRUE3KZ Supplement Right Sternoclavicular Joint with Nonautologous Tissue Substitute, Percutaneous Approach

ØRUE47Z Supplement Right Sternoclavicular Joint with Autologous Tissue Substitute, Percutaneous Endoscopic Approach

ØRUE4JZ Supplement Right Sternoclavicular Joint with Synthetic Substitute, Percutaneous Endoscopic Approach

ØRUE4KZ Supplement Right Sternoclavicular Joint with Nonautologous Tissue Substitute, Percutaneous Endoscopic Approach

ØRUFØ7Z Supplement Left Sternoclavicular Joint with Autologous Tissue Substitute, Open Approach

ØRUFØJZ Supplement Left Sternoclavicular Joint with Synthetic Substitute, Open Approach

ØRUFØKZ Supplement Left Sternoclavicular Joint with Nonautologous Tissue Substitute, Open Approach

ØRUF37Z Supplement Left Sternoclavicular Joint with Autologous Tissue Substitute, Percutaneous Approach

ØRUF3JZ Supplement Left Sternoclavicular Joint with Synthetic Substitute, Percutaneous Approach

ØRUF3KZ Supplement Left Sternoclavicular Joint with Nonautologous Tissue Substitute, Percutaneous Approach

ØRUF47Z Supplement Left Sternoclavicular Joint with Autologous Tissue Substitute, Percutaneous Endoscopic Approach

ØRUF4JZ Supplement Left Sternoclavicular Joint with Synthetic Substitute, Percutaneous Endoscopic Approach

ØRUF4KZ Supplement Left Sternoclavicular Joint with Nonautologous Tissue Substitute, Percutaneous Endoscopic Approach

ØRUGØ7Z Supplement Right Acromioclavicular Joint with Autologous Tissue Substitute, Open Approach

ØRUGØJZ Supplement Right Acromioclavicular Joint with Synthetic Substitute, Open Approach

ØRUGØKZ Supplement Right Acromioclavicular Joint with Nonautologous Tissue Substitute, Open Approach

ØRUG37Z Supplement Right Acromioclavicular Joint with Autologous Tissue Substitute, Percutaneous Approach

ØRUG3JZ Supplement Right Acromioclavicular Joint with Synthetic Substitute, Percutaneous Approach

ØRUG3KZ Supplement Right Acromioclavicular Joint with Nonautologous Tissue Substitute, Percutaneous Approach

ØRUG47Z Supplement Right Acromioclavicular Joint with Autologous Tissue Substitute, Percutaneous Endoscopic Approach

ØRUG4JZ Supplement Right Acromioclavicular Joint with Synthetic Substitute, Percutaneous Endoscopic Approach

ØRUG4KZ Supplement Right Acromioclavicular Joint with Nonautologous Tissue Substitute, Percutaneous Endoscopic Approach

ØRUHØ7Z Supplement Left Acromioclavicular Joint with Autologous Tissue Substitute, Open Approach

ØRUHØJZ Supplement Left Acromioclavicular Joint with Synthetic Substitute, Open Approach

ØRUHØKZ Supplement Left Acromioclavicular Joint with Nonautologous Tissue Substitute, Open Approach

ØRUH37Z Supplement Left Acromioclavicular Joint with Autologous Tissue Substitute, Percutaneous Approach

ØRUH3JZ Supplement Left Acromioclavicular Joint with Synthetic Substitute, Percutaneous Approach

ØRUH3KZ Supplement Left Acromioclavicular Joint with Nonautologous Tissue Substitute, Percutaneous Approach

ØRUH47Z Supplement Left Acromioclavicular Joint with Autologous Tissue Substitute, Percutaneous Endoscopic Approach

ØRUH4JZ Supplement Left Acromioclavicular Joint with Synthetic Substitute, Percutaneous Endoscopic Approach

ØRUH4KZ Supplement Left Acromioclavicular Joint with Nonautologous Tissue Substitute, Percutaneous Endoscopic Approach

ØRUJØ7Z Supplement Right Shoulder Joint with Autologous Tissue Substitute, Open Approach

ØRUJØJZ Supplement Right Shoulder Joint with Synthetic Substitute, Open Approach

ØRUJØKZ Supplement Right Shoulder Joint with Nonautologous Tissue Substitute, Open Approach

ØRUJ37Z Supplement Right Shoulder Joint with Autologous Tissue Substitute, Percutaneous Approach

ØRUJ3JZ Supplement Right Shoulder Joint with Synthetic Substitute, Percutaneous Approach

ØRUJ3KZ Supplement Right Shoulder Joint with Nonautologous Tissue Substitute, Percutaneous Approach

ØRUJ47Z Supplement Right Shoulder Joint with Autologous Tissue Substitute, Percutaneous Endoscopic Approach

ØRUJ4JZ Supplement Right Shoulder Joint with Synthetic Substitute, Percutaneous Endoscopic Approach

ØRUJ4KZ Supplement Right Shoulder Joint with Nonautologous Tissue Substitute, Percutaneous Endoscopic Approach

ØRUKØ7Z Supplement Left Shoulder Joint with Autologous Tissue Substitute, Open Approach

ØRUKØJZ Supplement Left Shoulder Joint with Synthetic Substitute, Open Approach

ØRUKØKZ Supplement Left Shoulder Joint with Nonautologous Tissue Substitute, Open Approach

ØRUK37Z Supplement Left Shoulder Joint with Autologous Tissue Substitute, Percutaneous Approach

ØRUK3JZ Supplement Left Shoulder Joint with Synthetic Substitute, Percutaneous Approach

ØRUK3KZ Supplement Left Shoulder Joint with Nonautologous Tissue Substitute, Percutaneous Approach

ØRUK47Z Supplement Left Shoulder Joint with Autologous Tissue Substitute, Percutaneous Endoscopic Approach

ØRUK4JZ Supplement Left Shoulder Joint with Synthetic Substitute, Percutaneous Endoscopic Approach

ØRUK4KZ Supplement Left Shoulder Joint with Nonautologous Tissue Substitute, Percutaneous Endoscopic Approach

ØRULØ7Z Supplement Right Elbow Joint with Autologous Tissue Substitute, Open Approach

HAC 12: Surgical Site Infection-Certain Orthopedic Procedures of the Spine, Shoulder, and Elbow (continued)

ØRULØJZ Supplement Right Elbow Joint with Synthetic Substitute, Open Approach

ØRULØKZ Supplement Right Elbow Joint with Nonautologous Tissue Substitute, Open Approach

ØRUL37Z Supplement Right Elbow Joint with Autologous Tissue Substitute, Percutaneous Approach

ØRUL3JZ Supplement Right Elbow Joint with Synthetic Substitute, Percutaneous Approach

ØRUL3KZ Supplement Right Elbow Joint with Nonautologous Tissue Substitute, Percutaneous Approach

ØRUL47Z Supplement Right Elbow Joint with Autologous Tissue Substitute, Percutaneous Endoscopic Approach

ØRUL4JZ Supplement Right Elbow Joint with Synthetic Substitute, Percutaneous Endoscopic Approach

ØRUL4KZ Supplement Right Elbow Joint with Nonautologous Tissue Substitute, Percutaneous Endoscopic Approach

ØRUM07Z Supplement Left Elbow Joint with Autologous Tissue Substitute, Open Approach

ØRUMØJZ Supplement Left Elbow Joint with Synthetic Substitute, Open Approach

ØRUMØKZ Supplement Left Elbow Joint with Nonautologous Tissue Substitute, Open Approach

ØRUM37Z Supplement Left Elbow Joint with Autologous Tissue Substitute, Percutaneous Approach

ØRUM3JZ Supplement Left Elbow Joint with Synthetic Substitute, Percutaneous Approach

ØRUM3KZ Supplement Left Elbow Joint with Nonautologous Tissue Substitute, Percutaneous Approach

ØRUM47Z Supplement Left Elbow Joint with Autologous Tissue Substitute, Percutaneous Endoscopic Approach

ØRUM4JZ Supplement Left Elbow Joint with Synthetic Substitute, Percutaneous Endoscopic Approach

ØRUM4KZ Supplement Left Elbow Joint with Nonautologous Tissue Substitute, Percutaneous Endoscopic Approach

ØSG0070 Fusion of Lumbar Vertebral Joint with Autologous Tissue Substitute, Anterior Approach, Anterior Column, Open Approach

ØSG0071 Fusion of Lumbar Vertebral Joint with Autologous Tissue Substitute, Posterior Approach, Posterior Column, Open Approach

ØSG007J Fusion of Lumbar Vertebral Joint with Autologous Tissue Substitute, Posterior Approach, Anterior Column, Open Approach

ØSG00A0 Fusion of Lumbar Vertebral Joint with Interbody Fusion Device, Anterior Approach, Anterior Column, Open Approach

ØSG00AJ Fusion of Lumbar Vertebral Joint with Interbody Fusion Device, Posterior Approach, Anterior Column, Open Approach

ØSG00J0 Fusion of Lumbar Vertebral Joint with Synthetic Substitute, Anterior Approach, Anterior Column, Open Approach

ØSG00J1 Fusion of Lumbar Vertebral Joint with Synthetic Substitute, Posterior Approach, Posterior Column, Open Approach

ØSG00JJ Fusion of Lumbar Vertebral Joint with Synthetic Substitute, Posterior Approach, Anterior Column, Open Approach

ØSG00K0 Fusion of Lumbar Vertebral Joint with Nonautologous Tissue Substitute, Anterior Approach, Anterior Column, Open Approach

ØSG00K1 Fusion of Lumbar Vertebral Joint with Nonautologous Tissue Substitute, Posterior Approach, Posterior Column, Open Approach

ØSG00KJ Fusion of Lumbar Vertebral Joint with Nonautologous Tissue Substitute, Posterior Approach, Anterior Column, Open Approach

ØSG0370 Fusion of Lumbar Vertebral Joint with Autologous Tissue Substitute, Anterior Approach, Anterior Column, Percutaneous Approach

ØSG0371 Fusion of Lumbar Vertebral Joint with Autologous Tissue Substitute, Posterior Approach, Posterior Column, Percutaneous Approach

ØSG037J Fusion of Lumbar Vertebral Joint with Autologous Tissue Substitute, Posterior Approach, Anterior Column, Percutaneous Approach

ØSG03A0 Fusion of Lumbar Vertebral Joint with Interbody Fusion Device, Anterior Approach, Anterior Column, Percutaneous Approach

ØSG03AJ Fusion of Lumbar Vertebral Joint with Interbody Fusion Device, Posterior Approach, Anterior Column, Percutaneous Approach

ØSG03J0 Fusion of Lumbar Vertebral Joint with Synthetic Substitute, Anterior Approach, Anterior Column, Percutaneous Approach

ØSG03J1 Fusion of Lumbar Vertebral Joint with Synthetic Substitute, Posterior Approach, Posterior Column, Percutaneous Approach

ØSG03JJ Fusion of Lumbar Vertebral Joint with Synthetic Substitute, Posterior Approach, Anterior Column, Percutaneous Approach

ØSG03K0 Fusion of Lumbar Vertebral Joint with Nonautologous Tissue Substitute, Anterior Approach, Anterior Column, Percutaneous Approach

ØSG03K1 Fusion of Lumbar Vertebral Joint with Nonautologous Tissue Substitute, Posterior Approach, Posterior Column, Percutaneous Approach

ØSG03KJ Fusion of Lumbar Vertebral Joint with Nonautologous Tissue Substitute, Posterior Approach, Anterior Column, Percutaneous Approach

ØSG0470 Fusion of Lumbar Vertebral Joint with Autologous Tissue Substitute, Anterior Approach, Anterior Column, Percutaneous Endoscopic Approach

ØSG0471 Fusion of Lumbar Vertebral Joint with Autologous Tissue Substitute, Posterior Approach, Posterior Column, Percutaneous Endoscopic Approach

ØSG047J Fusion of Lumbar Vertebral Joint with Autologous Tissue Substitute, Posterior Approach, Anterior Column, Percutaneous Endoscopic Approach

ØSG04A0 Fusion of Lumbar Vertebral Joint with Interbody Fusion Device, Anterior Approach, Anterior Column, Percutaneous Endoscopic Approach

ØSG04AJ Fusion of Lumbar Vertebral Joint with Interbody Fusion Device, Posterior Approach, Anterior Column, Percutaneous Endoscopic Approach

ØSG04J0 Fusion of Lumbar Vertebral Joint with Synthetic Substitute, Anterior Approach, Anterior Column, Percutaneous Endoscopic Approach

ØSG04J1 Fusion of Lumbar Vertebral Joint with Synthetic Substitute, Posterior Approach, Posterior Column, Percutaneous Endoscopic Approach

ØSG04JJ Fusion of Lumbar Vertebral Joint with Synthetic Substitute, Posterior Approach, Anterior Column, Percutaneous Endoscopic Approach

ØSG04K0 Fusion of Lumbar Vertebral Joint with Nonautologous Tissue Substitute, Anterior Approach, Anterior Column, Percutaneous Endoscopic Approach

ØSG04K1 Fusion of Lumbar Vertebral Joint with Nonautologous Tissue Substitute, Posterior Approach, Posterior Column, Percutaneous Endoscopic Approach

ØSG04KJ Fusion of Lumbar Vertebral Joint with Nonautologous Tissue Substitute, Posterior Approach, Anterior Column, Percutaneous Endoscopic Approach

ØSG1070 Fusion of 2 or More Lumbar Vertebral Joints with Autologous Tissue Substitute, Anterior Approach, Anterior Column, Open Approach

ØSG1071 Fusion of 2 or More Lumbar Vertebral Joints with Autologous Tissue Substitute, Posterior Approach, Posterior Column, Open Approach

ØSG107J Fusion of 2 or More Lumbar Vertebral Joints with Autologous Tissue Substitute, Posterior Approach, Anterior Column, Open Approach

ØSG10A0 Fusion of 2 or More Lumbar Vertebral Joints with Interbody Fusion Device, Anterior Approach, Anterior Column, Open Approach

ØSG10AJ Fusion of 2 or More Lumbar Vertebral Joints with Interbody Fusion Device, Posterior Approach, Anterior Column, Open Approach

ØSG10J0 Fusion of 2 or More Lumbar Vertebral Joints with Synthetic Substitute, Anterior Approach, Anterior Column, Open Approach

ØSG10J1 Fusion of 2 or More Lumbar Vertebral Joints with Synthetic Substitute, Posterior Approach, Posterior Column, Open Approach

ØSG10JJ Fusion of 2 or More Lumbar Vertebral Joints with Synthetic Substitute, Posterior Approach, Anterior Column, Open Approach

ØSG10K0 Fusion of 2 or More Lumbar Vertebral Joints with Nonautologous Tissue Substitute, Anterior Approach, Anterior Column, Open Approach

ØSG10K1 Fusion of 2 or More Lumbar Vertebral Joints with Nonautologous Tissue Substitute, Posterior Approach, Posterior Column, Open Approach

ØSG10KJ Fusion of 2 or More Lumbar Vertebral Joints with Nonautologous Tissue Substitute, Posterior Approach, Anterior Column, Open Approach

ØSG1370 Fusion of 2 or More Lumbar Vertebral Joints with Autologous Tissue Substitute, Anterior Approach, Anterior Column, Percutaneous Approach

Appendix K: Hospital Acquired Conditions

HAC 12: Surgical Site Infection-Certain Orthopedic Procedures of the Spine, Shoulder, and Elbow (continued)

ØSG1371   Fusion of 2 or More Lumbar Vertebral Joints with Autologous Tissue Substitute, Posterior Approach, Posterior Column, Percutaneous Approach

ØSG137J   Fusion of 2 or More Lumbar Vertebral Joints with Autologous Tissue Substitute, Posterior Approach, Anterior Column, Percutaneous Approach

ØSG13AØ   Fusion of 2 or More Lumbar Vertebral Joints with Interbody Fusion Device, Anterior Approach, Anterior Column, Percutaneous Approach

ØSG13AJ   Fusion of 2 or More Lumbar Vertebral Joints with Interbody Fusion Device, Posterior Approach, Anterior Column, Percutaneous Approach

ØSG13JØ   Fusion of 2 or More Lumbar Vertebral Joints with Synthetic Substitute, Anterior Approach, Anterior Column, Percutaneous Approach

ØSG13J1   Fusion of 2 or More Lumbar Vertebral Joints with Synthetic Substitute, Posterior Approach, Posterior Column, Percutaneous Approach

ØSG13JJ   Fusion of 2 or More Lumbar Vertebral Joints with Synthetic Substitute, Posterior Approach, Anterior Column, Percutaneous Approach

ØSG13KØ   Fusion of 2 or More Lumbar Vertebral Joints with Nonautologous Tissue Substitute, Anterior Approach, Anterior Column, Percutaneous Approach

ØSG13K1   Fusion of 2 or More Lumbar Vertebral Joints with Nonautologous Tissue Substitute, Posterior Approach, Posterior Column, Percutaneous Approach

ØSG13KJ   Fusion of 2 or More Lumbar Vertebral Joints with Nonautologous Tissue Substitute, Posterior Approach, Anterior Column, Percutaneous Approach

ØSG147Ø   Fusion of 2 or More Lumbar Vertebral Joints with Autologous Tissue Substitute, Anterior Approach, Anterior Column, Percutaneous Endoscopic Approach

ØSG1471   Fusion of 2 or More Lumbar Vertebral Joints with Autologous Tissue Substitute, Posterior Approach, Posterior Column, Percutaneous Endoscopic Approach

ØSG147J   Fusion of 2 or More Lumbar Vertebral Joints with Autologous Tissue Substitute, Posterior Approach, Anterior Column, Percutaneous Endoscopic Approach

ØSG14AØ   Fusion of 2 or More Lumbar Vertebral Joints with Interbody Fusion Device, Anterior Approach, Anterior Column, Percutaneous Endoscopic Approach

ØSG14AJ   Fusion of 2 or More Lumbar Vertebral Joints with Interbody Fusion Device, Posterior Approach, Anterior Column, Percutaneous Endoscopic Approach

ØSG14JØ   Fusion of 2 or More Lumbar Vertebral Joints with Synthetic Substitute, Anterior Approach, Anterior Column, Percutaneous Endoscopic Approach

ØSG14J1   Fusion of 2 or More Lumbar Vertebral Joints with Synthetic Substitute, Posterior Approach, Posterior Column, Percutaneous Endoscopic Approach

ØSG14JJ   Fusion of 2 or More Lumbar Vertebral Joints with Synthetic Substitute, Posterior Approach, Anterior Column, Percutaneous Endoscopic Approach

ØSG14KØ   Fusion of 2 or More Lumbar Vertebral Joints with Nonautologous Tissue Substitute, Anterior Approach, Anterior Column, Percutaneous Endoscopic Approach

ØSG14K1   Fusion of 2 or More Lumbar Vertebral Joints with Nonautologous Tissue Substitute, Posterior Approach, Posterior Column, Percutaneous Endoscopic Approach

ØSG14KJ   Fusion of 2 or More Lumbar Vertebral Joints with Nonautologous Tissue Substitute, Posterior Approach, Anterior Column, Percutaneous Endoscopic Approach

ØSG3Ø7Ø   Fusion of Lumbosacral Joint with Autologous Tissue Substitute, Anterior Approach, Anterior Column, Open Approach

ØSG3Ø71   Fusion of Lumbosacral Joint with Autologous Tissue Substitute, Posterior Approach, Posterior Column, Open Approach

ØSG3Ø7J   Fusion of Lumbosacral Joint with Autologous Tissue Substitute, Posterior Approach, Anterior Column, Open Approach

ØSG3ØAØ   Fusion of Lumbosacral Joint with Interbody Fusion Device, Anterior Approach, Anterior Column, Open Approach

ØSG3ØAJ   Fusion of Lumbosacral Joint with Interbody Fusion Device, Posterior Approach, Anterior Column, Open Approach

ØSG3ØJØ   Fusion of Lumbosacral Joint with Synthetic Substitute, Anterior Approach, Anterior Column, Open Approach

ØSG3ØJ1   Fusion of Lumbosacral Joint with Synthetic Substitute, Posterior Approach, Posterior Column, Open Approach

ØSG3ØJJ   Fusion of Lumbosacral Joint with Synthetic Substitute, Posterior Approach, Anterior Column, Open Approach

ØSG3ØKØ   Fusion of Lumbosacral Joint with Nonautologous Tissue Substitute, Anterior Approach, Anterior Column, Open Approach

ØSG3ØK1   Fusion of Lumbosacral Joint with Nonautologous Tissue Substitute, Posterior Approach, Posterior Column, Open Approach

ØSG3ØKJ   Fusion of Lumbosacral Joint with Nonautologous Tissue Substitute, Posterior Approach, Anterior Column, Open Approach

ØSG337Ø   Fusion of Lumbosacral Joint with Autologous Tissue Substitute, Anterior Approach, Anterior Column, Percutaneous Approach

ØSG3371   Fusion of Lumbosacral Joint with Autologous Tissue Substitute, Posterior Approach, Posterior Column, Percutaneous Approach

ØSG337J   Fusion of Lumbosacral Joint with Autologous Tissue Substitute, Posterior Approach, Anterior Column, Percutaneous Approach

ØSG33AØ   Fusion of Lumbosacral Joint with Interbody Fusion Device, Anterior Approach, Anterior Column, Percutaneous Approach

ØSG33AJ   Fusion of Lumbosacral Joint with Interbody Fusion Device, Posterior Approach, Anterior Column, Percutaneous Approach

ØSG33JØ   Fusion of Lumbosacral Joint with Synthetic Substitute, Anterior Approach, Anterior Column, Percutaneous Approach

ØSG33J1   Fusion of Lumbosacral Joint with Synthetic Substitute, Posterior Approach, Posterior Column, Percutaneous Approach

ØSG33JJ   Fusion of Lumbosacral Joint with Synthetic Substitute, Posterior Approach, Anterior Column, Percutaneous Approach

ØSG33KØ   Fusion of Lumbosacral Joint with Nonautologous Tissue Substitute, Anterior Approach, Anterior Column, Percutaneous Approach

ØSG33K1   Fusion of Lumbosacral Joint with Nonautologous Tissue Substitute, Posterior Approach, Posterior Column, Percutaneous Approach

ØSG33KJ   Fusion of Lumbosacral Joint with Nonautologous Tissue Substitute, Posterior Approach, Anterior Column, Percutaneous Approach

ØSG347Ø   Fusion of Lumbosacral Joint with Autologous Tissue Substitute, Anterior Approach, Anterior Column, Percutaneous Endoscopic Approach

ØSG3471   Fusion of Lumbosacral Joint with Autologous Tissue Substitute, Posterior Approach, Posterior Column, Percutaneous Endoscopic Approach

ØSG347J   Fusion of Lumbosacral Joint with Autologous Tissue Substitute, Posterior Approach, Anterior Column, Percutaneous Endoscopic Approach

ØSG34AØ   Fusion of Lumbosacral Joint with Interbody Fusion Device, Anterior Approach, Anterior Column, Percutaneous Endoscopic Approach

ØSG34AJ   Fusion of Lumbosacral Joint with Interbody Fusion Device, Posterior Approach, Anterior Column, Percutaneous Endoscopic Approach

ØSG34JØ   Fusion of Lumbosacral Joint with Synthetic Substitute, Anterior Approach, Anterior Column, Percutaneous Endoscopic Approach

ØSG34J1   Fusion of Lumbosacral Joint with Synthetic Substitute, Posterior Approach, Posterior Column, Percutaneous Endoscopic Approach

ØSG34JJ   Fusion of Lumbosacral Joint with Synthetic Substitute, Posterior Approach, Anterior Column, Percutaneous Endoscopic Approach

ØSG34KØ   Fusion of Lumbosacral Joint with Nonautologous Tissue Substitute, Anterior Approach, Anterior Column, Percutaneous Endoscopic Approach

ØSG34K1   Fusion of Lumbosacral Joint with Nonautologous Tissue Substitute, Posterior Approach, Posterior Column, Percutaneous Endoscopic Approach

ØSG34KJ   Fusion of Lumbosacral Joint with Nonautologous Tissue Substitute, Posterior Approach, Anterior Column, Percutaneous Endoscopic Approach

ØSG7Ø4Z   Fusion of Right Sacroiliac Joint with Internal Fixation Device, Open Approach

ØSG7Ø7Z   Fusion of Right Sacroiliac Joint with Autologous Tissue Substitute, Open Approach

ØSG7ØJZ   Fusion of Right Sacroiliac Joint with Synthetic Substitute, Open Approach

ØSG7ØKZ   Fusion of Right Sacroiliac Joint with Nonautologous Tissue Substitute, Open Approach

HAC 12: Surgical Site Infection-Certain Orthopedic Procedures of the Spine, Shoulder, and Elbow (continued)

ØSG734Z Fusion of Right Sacroiliac Joint with Internal Fixation Device, Percutaneous Approach

ØSG737Z Fusion of Right Sacroiliac Joint with Autologous Tissue Substitute, Percutaneous Approach

ØSG73JZ Fusion of Right Sacroiliac Joint with Synthetic Substitute, Percutaneous Approach

ØSG73KZ Fusion of Right Sacroiliac Joint with Nonautologous Tissue Substitute, Percutaneous Approach

ØSG744Z Fusion of Right Sacroiliac Joint with Internal Fixation Device, Percutaneous Endoscopic Approach

ØSG747Z Fusion of Right Sacroiliac Joint with Autologous Tissue Substitute, Percutaneous Endoscopic Approach

ØSG74JZ Fusion of Right Sacroiliac Joint with Synthetic Substitute, Percutaneous Endoscopic Approach

ØSG74KZ Fusion of Right Sacroiliac Joint with Nonautologous Tissue Substitute, Percutaneous Endoscopic Approach

ØSG804Z Fusion of Left Sacroiliac Joint with Internal Fixation Device, Open Approach

ØSG807Z Fusion of Left Sacroiliac Joint with Autologous Tissue Substitute, Open Approach

ØSG80JZ Fusion of Left Sacroiliac Joint with Synthetic Substitute, Open Approach

ØSG80KZ Fusion of Left Sacroiliac Joint with Nonautologous Tissue Substitute, Open Approach

ØSG834Z Fusion of Left Sacroiliac Joint with Internal Fixation Device, Percutaneous Approach

ØSG837Z Fusion of Left Sacroiliac Joint with Autologous Tissue Substitute, Percutaneous Approach

ØSG83JZ Fusion of Left Sacroiliac Joint with Synthetic Substitute, Percutaneous Approach

ØSG83KZ Fusion of Left Sacroiliac Joint with Nonautologous Tissue Substitute, Percutaneous Approach

ØSG844Z Fusion of Left Sacroiliac Joint with Internal Fixation Device, Percutaneous Endoscopic Approach

ØSG847Z Fusion of Left Sacroiliac Joint with Autologous Tissue Substitute, Percutaneous Endoscopic Approach

ØSG84JZ Fusion of Left Sacroiliac Joint with Synthetic Substitute, Percutaneous Endoscopic Approach

ØSG84KZ Fusion of Left Sacroiliac Joint with Nonautologous Tissue Substitute, Percutaneous Endoscopic Approach

XRGAØR7 Fusion of Thoracolumbar Vertebral Joint using Customizable Interbody Fusion Device, Open Approach, New Technology Group 7

XRGA3R7 Fusion of Thoracolumbar Vertebral Joint using Customizable Interbody Fusion Device, Percutaneous Approach, New Technology Group 7

XRGA4R7 Fusion of Thoracolumbar Vertebral Joint using Customizable Interbody Fusion Device, Percutaneous Endoscopic Approach, New Technology Group 7

XRGBØR7 Fusion of Lumbar Vertebral Joint using Customizable Interbody Fusion Device, Open Approach, New Technology Group 7

XRGB3R7 Fusion of Lumbar Vertebral Joint using Customizable Interbody Fusion Device, Percutaneous Approach, New Technology Group 7

XRGB4R7 Fusion of Lumbar Vertebral Joint using Customizable Interbody Fusion Device, Percutaneous Endoscopic Approach, New Technology Group 7

XRGCØR7 Fusion of 2 or more Lumbar Vertebral Joints using Customizable Interbody Fusion Device, Open Approach, New Technology Group 7

XRGC3R7 Fusion of 2 or more Lumbar Vertebral Joints using Customizable Interbody Fusion Device, Percutaneous Approach, New Technology Group 7

XRGC4R7 Fusion of 2 or more Lumbar Vertebral Joints using Customizable Interbody Fusion Device, Percutaneous Endoscopic Approach, New Technology Group 7

XRGDØR7 Fusion of Lumbosacral Joint using Customizable Interbody Fusion Device, Open Approach, New Technology Group 7

XRGD3R7 Fusion of Lumbosacral Joint using Customizable Interbody Fusion Device, Percutaneous Approach, New Technology Group 7

XRGD4R7 Fusion of Lumbosacral Joint using Customizable Interbody Fusion Device, Percutaneous Endoscopic Approach, New Technology Group 7

XRGEØ58 Fusion of Right Sacroiliac Joint using Internal Fixation Device with Tulip Connector, Open Approach, New Technology Group 8

XRGE358 Fusion of Right Sacroiliac Joint using Internal Fixation Device with Tulip Connector, Percutaneous Approach, New Technology Group 8

XRGFØ58 Fusion of Left Sacroiliac Joint using Internal Fixation Device with Tulip Connector, Open Approach, New Technology Group 8

XRGF358 Fusion of Left Sacroiliac Joint using Internal Fixation Device with Tulip Connector, Percutaneous Approach, New Technology Group 8

HAC 13: Surgical Site Infection (SSI) Following Cardiac Implantable Electronic Device (CIED) Procedures

Secondary diagnosis not POA:

K68.11 Postprocedural retroperitoneal abscess

T81.40XA Infection following a procedure, unspecified, initial encounter

T81.41XA Infection following a procedure, superficial incisional surgical site, initial encounter

T81.42XA Infection following a procedure, deep incisional surgical site, initial encounter

T81.43XA Infection following a procedure, organ and space surgical site, initial encounter

T81.44XA Sepsis following a procedure, initial encounter

T81.49XA Infection following a procedure, other surgical site, initial encounter

T82.7XXA Infection and inflammatory reaction due to other internal orthopedic prosthetic devices, implants and grafts, initial encounter

AND

Any of the following procedures:

02H43JZ Insertion of Pacemaker Lead into Coronary Vein, Percutaneous Approach

02H43KZ Insertion of Defibrillator Lead into Coronary Vein, Percutaneous Approach

02H43MZ Insertion of Cardiac Lead into Coronary Vein, Percutaneous Approach

02H63JZ Insertion of Pacemaker Lead into Right Atrium, Percutaneous Approach

02H63MZ Insertion of Cardiac Lead into Right Atrium, Percutaneous Approach

02H73JZ Insertion of Pacemaker Lead into Left Atrium, Percutaneous Approach

02H73MZ Insertion of Cardiac Lead into Left Atrium, Percutaneous Approach

02HK3JZ Insertion of Pacemaker Lead into Right Ventricle, Percutaneous Approach

02HL3JZ Insertion of Pacemaker Lead into Left Ventricle, Percutaneous Approach

02HNØJZ Insertion of Pacemaker Lead into Pericardium, Open Approach

02HNØMZ Insertion of Cardiac Lead into Pericardium, Open Approach

02HN3JZ Insertion of Pacemaker Lead into Pericardium, Percutaneous Approach

02HN3MZ Insertion of Cardiac Lead into Pericardium, Percutaneous Approach

02HN4JZ Insertion of Pacemaker Lead into Pericardium, Percutaneous Endoscopic Approach

02HN4MZ Insertion of Cardiac Lead into Pericardium, Percutaneous Endoscopic Approach

02PAØMZ Removal of Cardiac Lead from Heart, Open Approach

02PA3MZ Removal of Cardiac Lead from Heart, Percutaneous Approach

02PA4MZ Removal of Cardiac Lead from Heart, Percutaneous Endoscopic Approach

02PAXMZ Removal of Cardiac Lead from Heart, External Approach

02WAØMZ Revision of Cardiac Lead in Heart, Open Approach

02WA3MZ Revision of Cardiac Lead in Heart, Percutaneous Approach

02WA4MZ Revision of Cardiac Lead in Heart, Percutaneous Endoscopic Approach

ØJH604Z Insertion of Pacemaker, Single Chamber into Chest Subcutaneous Tissue and Fascia, Open Approach

ØJH605Z Insertion of Pacemaker, Single Chamber Rate Responsive into Chest Subcutaneous Tissue and Fascia, Open Approach

ØJH606Z Insertion of Pacemaker, Dual Chamber into Chest Subcutaneous Tissue and Fascia, Open Approach

ØJH607Z Insertion of Cardiac Resynchronization Pacemaker Pulse Generator into Chest Subcutaneous Tissue and Fascia, Open Approach

ØJH608Z Insertion of Defibrillator Generator into Chest Subcutaneous Tissue and Fascia, Open Approach

ØJH609Z Insertion of Cardiac Resynchronization Defibrillator Pulse Generator into Chest Subcutaneous Tissue and Fascia, Open Approach

ØJH60PZ Insertion of Cardiac Rhythm Related Device into Chest Subcutaneous Tissue and Fascia, Open Approach

ØJH634Z Insertion of Pacemaker, Single Chamber into Chest Subcutaneous Tissue and Fascia, Percutaneous Approach

ØJH635Z Insertion of Pacemaker, Single Chamber Rate Responsive into Chest Subcutaneous Tissue and Fascia, Percutaneous Approach

ØJH636Z Insertion of Pacemaker, Dual Chamber into Chest Subcutaneous Tissue and Fascia, Percutaneous Approach

HAC 13: Surgical Site Infection (SSI) Following Cardiac Implantable Electronic Device (CIED) Procedures (continued)

ØJH637Z   Insertion of Cardiac Resynchronization Pacemaker Pulse Generator into Chest Subcutaneous Tissue and Fascia, Percutaneous Approach

ØJH638Z   Insertion of Defibrillator Generator into Chest Subcutaneous Tissue and Fascia, Percutaneous Approach

ØJH639Z   Insertion of Cardiac Resynchronization Defibrillator Pulse Generator into Chest Subcutaneous Tissue and Fascia, Percutaneous Approach

ØJH63PZ   Insertion of Cardiac Rhythm Related Device into Chest Subcutaneous Tissue and Fascia, Percutaneous Approach

ØJH804Z   Insertion of Pacemaker, Single Chamber into Abdomen Subcutaneous Tissue and Fascia, Open Approach

ØJH805Z   Insertion of Pacemaker, Single Chamber Rate Responsive into Abdomen Subcutaneous Tissue and Fascia, Open Approach

ØJH806Z   Insertion of Pacemaker, Dual Chamber into Abdomen Subcutaneous Tissue and Fascia, Open Approach

ØJH807Z   Insertion of Cardiac Resynchronization Pacemaker Pulse Generator into Abdomen Subcutaneous Tissue and Fascia, Open Approach

ØJH808Z   Insertion of Defibrillator Generator into Abdomen Subcutaneous Tissue and Fascia, Open Approach

ØJH809Z   Insertion of Cardiac Resynchronization Defibrillator Pulse Generator into Abdomen Subcutaneous Tissue and Fascia, Open Approach

ØJH80PZ   Insertion of Cardiac Rhythm Related Device into Abdomen Subcutaneous Tissue and Fascia, Open Approach

ØJH834Z   Insertion of Pacemaker, Single Chamber into Abdomen Subcutaneous Tissue and Fascia, Percutaneous Approach

ØJH835Z   Insertion of Pacemaker, Single Chamber Rate Responsive into Abdomen Subcutaneous Tissue and Fascia, Percutaneous Approach

ØJH836Z   Insertion of Pacemaker, Dual Chamber into Abdomen Subcutaneous Tissue and Fascia, Percutaneous Approach

ØJH837Z   Insertion of Cardiac Resynchronization Pacemaker Pulse Generator into Abdomen Subcutaneous Tissue and Fascia, Percutaneous Approach

ØJH838Z   Insertion of Defibrillator Generator into Abdomen Subcutaneous Tissue and Fascia, Percutaneous Approach

ØJH839Z   Insertion of Cardiac Resynchronization Defibrillator Pulse Generator into Abdomen Subcutaneous Tissue and Fascia, Percutaneous Approach

ØJH83PZ   Insertion of Cardiac Rhythm Related Device into Abdomen Subcutaneous Tissue and Fascia, Percutaneous Approach

ØJPTØFZ   Removal of Subcutaneous Defibrillator Lead from Trunk Subcutaneous Tissue and Fascia, Open Approach

ØJPTØPZ   Removal of Cardiac Rhythm Related Device from Trunk Subcutaneous Tissue and Fascia, Open Approach

ØJPT3FZ   Removal of Subcutaneous Defibrillator Lead from Trunk Subcutaneous Tissue and Fascia, Percutaneous Approach

ØJPT3PZ   Removal of Cardiac Rhythm Related Device from Trunk Subcutaneous Tissue and Fascia, Percutaneous Approach

ØJWTØFZ   Revision of Subcutaneous Defibrillator Lead in Trunk Subcutaneous Tissue and Fascia, Open Approach

ØJWTØPZ   Revision of Cardiac Rhythm Related Device in Trunk Subcutaneous Tissue and Fascia, Open Approach

ØJWT3FZ   Revision of Subcutaneous Defibrillator Lead in Trunk Subcutaneous Tissue and Fascia, Percutaneous Approach

ØJWT3PZ   Revision of Cardiac Rhythm Related Device in Trunk Subcutaneous Tissue and Fascia, Percutaneous Approach

HAC 14: Iatrogenic Pneumothorax with Venous Catheterization

Secondary diagnosis not POA:

J95.811   Postprocedural pneumothorax

AND

Any of the following procedures:

02H633Z   Insertion of Infusion Device into Right Atrium, Percutaneous Approach

02HK33Z   Insertion of Infusion Device into Right Ventricle, Percutaneous Approach

02HS33Z   Insertion of Infusion Device into Right Pulmonary Vein, Percutaneous Approach

02HS43Z   Insertion of Infusion Device into Right Pulmonary Vein, Percutaneous Endoscopic Approach

02HT33Z   Insertion of Infusion Device into Left Pulmonary Vein, Percutaneous Approach

02HT43Z   Insertion of Infusion Device into Left Pulmonary Vein, Percutaneous Endoscopic Approach

02HV33Z   Insertion of Infusion Device into Superior Vena Cava, Percutaneous Approach

02HV43Z   Insertion of Infusion Device into Superior Vena Cava, Percutaneous Endoscopic Approach

05H033Z   Insertion of Infusion Device into Azygos Vein, Percutaneous Approach

05H043Z   Insertion of Infusion Device into Azygos Vein, Percutaneous Endoscopic Approach

05H133Z   Insertion of Infusion Device into Hemiazygos Vein, Percutaneous Approach

05H143Z   Insertion of Infusion Device into Hemiazygos Vein, Percutaneous Endoscopic Approach

05H333Z   Insertion of Infusion Device into Right Innominate Vein, Percutaneous Approach

05H343Z   Insertion of Infusion Device into Right Innominate Vein, Percutaneous Endoscopic Approach

05H433Z   Insertion of Infusion Device into Left Innominate Vein, Percutaneous Approach

05H443Z   Insertion of Infusion Device into Left Innominate Vein, Percutaneous Endoscopic Approach

05H533Z   Insertion of Infusion Device into Right Subclavian Vein, Percutaneous Approach

05H543Z   Insertion of Infusion Device into Right Subclavian Vein, Percutaneous Endoscopic Approach

05H633Z   Insertion of Infusion Device into Left Subclavian Vein, Percutaneous Approach

05H643Z   Insertion of Infusion Device into Left Subclavian Vein, Percutaneous Endoscopic Approach

05HM33Z   Insertion of Infusion Device into Right Internal Jugular Vein, Percutaneous Approach

05HN33Z   Insertion of Infusion Device into Left Internal Jugular Vein, Percutaneous Approach

05HP33Z   Insertion of Infusion Device into Right External Jugular Vein, Percutaneous Approach

05HQ33Z   Insertion of Infusion Device into Left External Jugular Vein, Percutaneous Approach

ØJH63XZ   Insertion of Vascular Access Device into Chest Subcutaneous Tissue and Fascia, Percutaneous Approach

Appendix L: Procedure Combination Tables

The tables below were developed to help simplify the relationship between ICD-10-PCS coding and MS-DRG assignment. The Centers for Medicare & Medicaid Services (CMS) has identified in the MS-DRG Definitions Manual certain procedure combinations that must occur in order to assign a specific MS-DRG. There are many factors influencing MS-DRG assignment, including principal and secondary diagnoses, MCC or CC use, sex of the patient, and discharge status. These tables should be used only as a guide. These tables were created based on the proposed, version 40, MS-DRG Grouper software and Definitions Manual files published with the fiscal 2023 IPPS proposed rule. To view the most current files, refer to the following:
https://www.cms.gov/Medicare/Medicare-Fee-for-Service-Payment/AcuteInpatientPPS/MS-DRG-Classifications-and-Software.

DRG 001-002 Heart Transplant or Implant of Heart Assist System

Heart Transplant

Replacement of Right and Left Ventricle 02RK0JZ and 02RL0JZ

Insertion With Removal of Heart Assist System

Type of Heart Assist System	Code as appropriate Insertion by approach	Code also as appropriate Removal of Heart Assist System by approach
Biventricular External	02HA[0,3,4]RS	02PA[0,3,4]RZ
External	02HA[0,4]RZ	02PA[0,3,4]RZ

Revision With Removal of Heart Assist System

Type of Heart Assist System	Code as appropriate Revision by approach	Code also as appropriate Removal of Heart Assist System by approach
Implantable	02WA[0,3,4]QZ	02PA[0,3,4]RZ
External	02WA[0,3,4]RZ	02PA[0,3,4]RZ

DRG 008 Simultaneous Pancreas/Kidney Transplant

Transplanted Body Part	Code Transplant as appropriate by tissue type			Code also Pancreas Transplant as appropriate by tissue type		
	Allogeneic	Syngeneic	Zooplastic	Allogeneic	Syngeneic	Zooplastic
Kidney, Right	0TY00Z0	0TY00Z1	0TY00Z2	0FYG0Z0	0FYG0Z1	0FYG0Z2
Kidney, Left	0TY10Z0	0TY10Z1	0TY10Z2			

DRG 019 Simultaneous Pancreas/Kidney Transplant with Hemodialysis

Transplanted Body Part	Code Transplant as appropriate by tissue type			Code also Pancreas Transplant as appropriate by tissue type			Code also Hemodialysis		
	Allogeneic	Syngeneic	Zooplastic	Allogeneic	Syngeneic	Zooplastic	< 6 Hours	6-18 Hours	> 18 Hours
Kidney, Right	0TY00Z0	0TY00Z1	0TY00Z2	0FYG0Z0	0FYG0Z1	0FYG0Z2	5A1D07Z	5A1D80Z	5A1D90Z
Kidney, Left	0TY10Z0	0TY10Z1	0TY10Z2						

DRG 023-027 Craniotomy

Site of Neurostimulator Lead	Code as appropriate Insertion of Lead by approach	Code also as appropriate Insertion of Device by type and subcutaneous site						
		Neuro-stimulator Generator	Stimulator Multiple Array Code as appropriate by approach			Stimulator Multiple Array, Rechargeable Code as appropriate by approach		
		Skull	Chest	Back	Abdomen	Chest	Back	Abdomen
Brain	00H0[0,3,4]MZ	0NH00NZ	0JH6[0,3]DZ	0JH7[0,3]DZ	0JH8[0,3]DZ	0JH6[0,3]EZ	0JH7[0,3]EZ	0JH8[0,3]EZ
Cerebral Ventricle	00H6[0,3,4]MZ	0NH00NZ	0JH6[0,3]DZ	0JH7[0,3]DZ	0JH8[0,3]DZ	0JH6[0,3]EZ	0JH7[0,3]EZ	0JH8[0,3]EZ

DRG 028-030 Spinal Procedures

Generator Type	Insertion of Generator by Site			Code also as appropriate Insertion of Neurostimulator Lead by approach	
	Chest	Abdomen	Back	Spinal Canal	Spinal Cord
Single Array	0JH6[0,3]BZ	0JH8[0,3]BZ	0JH7[0,3]BZ	00HU[0,3,4]MZ	00HV[0,3,4]MZ
Single Array, Rechargeable	0JH6[0,3]CZ	0JH8[0,3]CZ	0JH7[0,3]CZ	00HU[0,3,4]MZ	00HV[0,3,4]MZ
Multiple Array	0JH6[0,3]DZ	0JH8[0,3]DZ	0JH7[0,3]DZ	00HU[0,3,4]MZ	00HV[0,3,4]MZ
Multiple Array, Rechargeable	0JH6[0,3]EZ	—	0JH7[0,3]EZ	00HU[0,3,4]MZ	00HV[0,3,4]MZ
Multiple Array, Rechargeable	—	0JH8[0,3]EZ	—	00HU[0,3,4]MZ	00HV[0,3,4]MZ

DRG 040-042 Peripheral and Cranial Nerve and Other Nervous System Procedures
Insertion of Neurostimulator Generator and Lead

Insertion Single Array Generator, by Site		Code also Lead Insertion, by Site						
		Cranial Nerve	Peripheral Nerve	Azygos Vein	Innominate Vein, RT	Innominate Vein, LT	Stomach	Vagus Nerve
Chest	0JH6[0,3]BZ							
Back	0JH7[0,3]BZ	00HE[0,3,4]MZ	01HY[0,3,4]MZ	05H0[0,3,4]MZ	05H3[0,3,4]MZ	05H4[0,3,4]MZ	0DH6[0,3,4]MZ	X0HQ3R8
Abdomen	0JH8[0,3]BZ							

Insertion Single Array, Rechargeable Generator, by Site		Code also Lead Insertion, by Site						
		Cranial Nerve	Peripheral Nerve	Azygos Vein	Innominate Vein, RT	Innominate Vein, LT	Stomach	Vagus Nerve
Chest	0JH6[0,3]CZ							
Back	0JH7[0,3]CZ	00HE[0,3,4]MZ	01HY[0,3,4]MZ	05H0[0,3,4]MZ	05H3[0,3,4]MZ	05H4[0,3,4]MZ	0DH6[0,3,4]MZ	X0HQ3R8
Abdomen	0JH8[0,3]CZ							

Insertion Multiple Array Generator, by Site		Code also Lead Insertion, by Site						
		Cranial Nerve	Peripheral Nerve	Azygos Vein	Innominate Vein, RT	Innominate Vein, LT	Stomach	Vagus Nerve
Chest	0JH6[0,3]DZ							
Back	0JH7[0,3]DZ	00HE[0,3,4]MZ	01HY[0,3,4]MZ	05H0[0,3,4]MZ	05H3[0,3,4]MZ	05H4[0,3,4]MZ	0DH6[0,3,4]MZ	X0HQ3R8
Abdomen	0JH8[0,3]DZ							

Insertion Multiple Array, Rechargeable Generator, by Site		Code also Lead Insertion, by Site						
		Cranial Nerve	Peripheral Nerve	Azygos Vein	Innominate Vein, RT	Innominate Vein, LT	Stomach	Vagus Nerve
Chest	0JH6[0,3]EZ							
Back	0JH7[0,3]EZ	00HE[0,3,4]MZ	01HY[0,3,4]MZ	05H0[0,3,4]MZ	05H3[0,3,4]MZ	05H4[0,3,4]MZ	0DH6[0,3,4]MZ	X0HQ3R8
Abdomen	0JH8[0,3]EZ							

Insertion Stimulator Generator, by Site		Code also Lead Insertion, by Site						
		Cranial Nerve	Peripheral Nerve	Azygos Vein	Innominate Vein, RT	Innominate Vein, LT	Stomach	Vagus Nerve
Chest	0JH6[0,3]MZ							
Back	0JH7[0,3]MZ	00HE[0,3,4]MZ	01HY[0,3,4]MZ	05H0[0,3,4]MZ	05H3[0,3,4]MZ	05H4[0,3,4]MZ	0DH6[0,3,4]MZ	X0HQ3R8
Abdomen	0JH8[0,3]MZ							

DRG 242-244 Permanent Cardiac Pacemaker Implant
Insertion of Generator and Lead(s) Only

Generator Type	Insertion of Generator by Site		Code also Insertion of Lead, by Site			
	Chest	Abdomen	Coronary Vein	Right Atrium (6)/Left Atrium (7)	Right Ventricle (K)/Left Ventricle (L)	Pericardium
Single Chamber	0JH6[0,3]4Z	0JH8[0,3]4Z	02H4[0,3,4][J,M]Z	02H[6,7][0,3,4][J,M]Z	02H[K,L][0,3,4][J,M]Z	02HN[0,3,4][J,M]Z
Single Chamber RR	0JH6[0,3]5Z	0JH8[0,3]5Z	02H4[0,3,4][J,M]Z	02H[6,7][0,3,4][J,M]Z	02H[K,L][0,3,4][J,M]Z	02HN[0,3,4][J,M]Z
Dual Chamber	0JH6[0,3]6Z	0JH8[0,3]6Z	02H4[0,3,4][J,M]Z	02H[6,7][0,3,4][J,M]Z	02H[K,L][0,3,4][J,M]Z	02HN[0,3,4][J,M]Z
Cardiac Resynch	0JH6[0,3]7Z	0JH8[0,3]7Z	02H4[0,3,4][J,M]Z	02H[6,7][0,3,4][J,M]Z	02H[K,L][0,3,4][J,M]Z	02HN[0,3,4][J,M]Z
Cardiac Rhythm Related	0JH6[0,3]PZ	0JH8[0,3]PZ	02H4[0,3,4][J,M]Z	02H[6,7][0,3,4][J,M]Z	02H[K,L][0,3,4][J,M]Z	02HN[0,3,4][J,M]Z

DRG 275-277 Cardiac Defibrillator Implant

Insertion of Generator With Insertion of Lead(s) into Coronary Vein, Atrium or Ventricle

Generator Type	Insertion of Generator by Site		Code also as appropriate Insertion of Leads by site				
	Chest	Abdomen	Coronary Vein	Atrium		Ventricle	
				Right	Left	Right	Left
Defibrillator	ØJH6[Ø,3]8Z	ØJH8[Ø,3]8Z	02H4[Ø,4]KZ	02H6[Ø,3,4]KZ	02H7[Ø,3,4]KZ	02HK[Ø,3,4]KZ	02HL[Ø,3,4]KZ
Cardiac Resynch Defibrillator Pulse Generator	ØJH6[Ø,3]9Z	ØJH8[Ø,3]9Z	02H4[Ø,3,4]KZ or 02H43[J,M]KZ	02H6[Ø,3,4]KZ	02H7[Ø,3,4]KZ	02HK[Ø,3,4]KZ	02HL[Ø,3,4]KZ
Contractility Modulation Device	ØJH6[Ø,3]AZ	ØJH8[Ø,3]AZ	—	02H6[Ø,3,4]MZ	—	02HK[Ø,3,4]MZ	—

Insertion of Generator with Insertion of Lead(s) into Pericardium or Chest

Generator Type	Insertion of Generator by Site		Code also as appropriate Insertion of Leads by Site and Type			
	Chest	Abdomen	Pericardium			Chest
			Pacemaker	Defibrillator	Cardiac	Subcutaneous
Defibrillator	ØJH6[Ø,3]8Z	ØJH8[Ø,3]8Z	02HN[Ø,3,4]JZ	02HN[Ø,3,4]KZ	02HN[Ø,3,4]MZ	ØJH6[Ø,3]FZ
Cardiac Resynch Defibrillator Pulse Generator	ØJH6[Ø,3]9Z	ØJH8[Ø,3]9Z	02HN[Ø,3,4]JZ	02HN[Ø,3,4]KZ	02HN[Ø,3,4]MZ	ØJH6[Ø,3]FZ

DRG 326-328 Stomach, Esophageal and Duodenal Procedures

Site	Resection by Open Approach	Code also as appropriate Resection of Pancreas by Open Approach
Duodenum	ØDT9ØZZ	ØFTGØZZ

DRG 344-346 Minor Small and Large Bowel Procedures

Site	Repair by Open Approach	Code also as appropriate Repair by external approach of Abdominal Wall Stoma
Small Intestine	ØDQ8ØZZ	ØWQFXZ2
Duodenum	ØDQ9ØZZ	ØWQFXZ2
Jejunum	ØDQAØZZ	ØWQFXZ2
Ileum	ØDQBØZZ	ØWQFXZ2
Large Intestine	ØDQEØZZ	ØWQFXZ2
Large Intestine, Right	ØDQFØZZ	ØWQFXZ2
Large Intestine, Left	ØDQGØZZ	ØWQFXZ2
Cecum	ØDQHØZZ	ØWQFXZ2
Ascending Colon	ØDQKØZZ	ØWQFXZ2
Transverse Colon	ØDQLØZZ	ØWQFXZ2
Descending Colon	ØDQMØZZ	ØWQFXZ2
Sigmoid Colon	ØDQNØZZ	ØWQFXZ2

DRG 456-458 Spinal Fusion Except Cervical with Spinal Curvature/Malignancy/ Infection or Extensive Fusions

Fusion of Thoracic and Lumbar Vertebra, Anterior Column

2 to 7 Thoracic Vertebra		Code also 2 or more Lumbar Vertebra	
ØRG[Ø,3,4][7,A,J,K]Ø	XRG7ØF3	ØSG1[Ø,3,4][7,A,J,K]Ø	XRGCØF3

Fusion of Thoracic and Lumbar Vertebra, Posterior Column

2 to 7 Thoracic Vertebra			Code also 2 or more Lumbar Vertebra		
Posterior Approach	Anterior Approach	New Technology	Posterior Approach	Anterior Approach	New Technology
ØRG7[Ø,3,4][7,J,K]1	ØRG7[Ø,3,4][7,A,J,K]J	XRG7Ø92 XRG7ØF3	ØSG1[Ø,3,4][7,J,K]1	ØSG1[Ø,3,4][7,A,J,K]J	XRGCØ92 XRGCØF3

DRG 461-462 Bilateral or Multiple Major Joint Procedures of Lower Extremity

For procedures to qualify as bilateral or multiple joint procedures, at least one replacement code or combination removal and replacement code from two different lower extremity sites from the following table(s) must be reported.

Examples: Left hip and right hip codes (bilateral); left hip and left knee codes (multiple); left hip and right ankle codes (multiple); left knee and right knee codes (bilateral); right hip removal and replacement, with right knee replacement

Hip, RT	Hip, LT	Knee, RT	Knee, LT	Ankle, RT	Ankle, LT
ØSR9Ø19	ØSRBØ19	ØSRCØ69	ØSRDØ69	ØSRFØ7Z	ØSRGØ7Z
ØSR9Ø1A	ØSRBØ1A	ØSRCØ6A	ØSRDØ6A	ØSRFØJ9	ØSRGØJ9
ØSR9Ø1Z	ØSRBØ1Z	ØSRCØ6Z	ØSRDØ6Z	ØSRFØJA	ØSRGØJA
ØSR9Ø29	ØSRBØ29	ØSRCØ7Z	ØSRDØ7Z	ØSRFØJZ	ØSRGØJZ
ØSR9Ø2A	ØSRBØ2A	ØSRCØJ9	ØSRDØJ9	ØSRFØKZ	ØSRGØKZ
ØSR9Ø2Z	ØSRBØ2Z	ØSRCØJA	ØSRDØJA		
ØSR9Ø39	ØSRBØ39	ØSRCØJZ	ØSRDØJZ		
ØSR9Ø3A	ØSRBØ3A	ØSRCØKZ	ØSRDØKZ		
ØSR9Ø3Z	ØSRBØ3Z	ØSRCØL9	ØSRDØL9		
ØSR9Ø49	ØSRBØ49	ØSRCØLA	ØSRDØLA		
ØSR9Ø4A	ØSRBØ4A	ØSRCØLZ	ØSRDØLZ		
ØSR9Ø4Z	ØSRBØ4Z	ØSRCØM9	ØSRDØM9		
ØSR9Ø69	ØSRBØ69	ØSRCØMA	ØSRDØMA		
ØSR9Ø6A	ØSRBØ6A	ØSRCØMZ	ØSRDØMZ		
ØSR9Ø6Z	ØSRBØ6Z	ØSRCØN9	ØSRDØN9		
ØSR9Ø7Z	ØSRBØ7Z	ØSRCØNA	ØSRDØNA		
ØSR9ØJ9	ØSRBØJ9	ØSRCØNZ	ØSRDØNZ		
ØSR9ØJA	ØSRBØJA	ØSRTØ7Z	ØSRUØ7Z		
ØSR9ØJZ	ØSRBØJZ	ØSRTØJ9	ØSRUØJ9		
ØSR9ØKZ	ØSRBØKZ	ØSRTØJA	ØSRUØJA		
ØSRAØØ9	ØSREØØ9	ØSRTØJZ	ØSRUØJZ		
ØSRAØØA	ØSREØØA	ØSRTØKZ	ØSRUØKZ		
ØSRAØØZ	ØSREØØZ	ØSRVØ7Z	ØSRWØ7Z		
ØSRAØ19	ØSREØ19	ØSRVØJ9	ØSRWØJ9		
ØSRAØ1A	ØSREØ1A	ØSRVØJA	ØSRWØJA		

Hip, RT	Hip, LT	Knee, RT	Knee, LT	Ankle, RT	Ankle, LT
ØSRAØ1Z	ØSREØ1Z	ØSRVØJZ	ØSRWØJZ		
ØSRAØ39	ØSREØ39	ØSRVØKZ	ØSRWØKZ		
ØSRAØ3A	ØSREØ3A	ØSPCØJZ	ØSPDØJZ		
ØSRAØ3Z	ØSREØ3Z				
ØSRAØ7Z	ØSREØ7Z				
ØSRAØJ9	ØSREØJ9				
ØSRAØJA	ØSREØJA				
ØSRAØJZ	ØSREØJZ				
ØSRAØKZ	ØSREØKZ				
ØSRRØ19	ØSRSØ19				
ØSRRØ1A	ØSRSØ1A				
ØSRRØ1Z	ØSRSØ1Z				
ØSRRØ39	ØSRSØ39				
ØSRRØ3A	ØSRSØ3A				
ØSRRØ3Z	ØSRSØ3Z				
ØSRRØ7Z	ØSRSØ7Z				
ØSRRØJ9	ØSRSØJ9				
ØSRRØJA	ØSRSØJA				
ØSRRØJZ	ØSRSØJZ				
ØSRRØKZ	ØSRSØKZ				
ØSU9ØBZ	ØSUBØBZ				
ØSUAØBZ	ØSUEØBZ				
ØSURØBZ	ØSUSØBZ				
ØSP9ØJZ	ØSPBØJZ				

Hip Procedure Combinations

Open Removal of Hip Spacer with Replacement

Removal of Spacer		Code also as appropriate Replacement by Device Type					
		Metal	Metal on Poly	Ceramic	Ceramic on Poly	Oxidized Zirc on Poly	Synth Subst
Hip, RT	ØSP9Ø8Z	ØSR9Ø1[9,A,Z]	ØSR9Ø2[9,A,Z]	ØSR9Ø3[9,A,Z]	ØSR9Ø4[9,A,Z]	ØSR9Ø6[9,A,Z]	ØSR9ØJ[9,A,Z]
Hip, LT	ØSPBØ8Z	ØSRBØ1[9,A,Z]	ØSRBØ2[9,A,Z]	ØSRBØ3[9,A,Z]	ØSRBØ4[9,A,Z]	ØSRBØ6[9,A,Z]	ØSRBØJ[9,A,Z]

Open Removal of Hip Spacer with Replacement

Removal of Spacer		Code also as appropriate Replacement by Device Type						
		Acetabular Surface				Femoral Surface		
		Poly	Metal	Ceramic	Synthetic	Metal	Ceramic	Synth
Hip, RT	ØSP9Ø8Z	ØSRAØØ[9,A,Z]	ØSRAØ1[9,A,Z]	ØSRAØ3[9,A,Z]	ØSRAØJ[9,A,Z]	ØSRRØ1[9,A,Z]	ØSRRØ3[9,A,Z]	ØSRRØJ[9,A,Z]
Hip, LT	ØSPBØ8Z	ØSREØØ[9,A,Z]	ØSREØ1[9,A,Z]	ØSREØ3[9,A,Z]	ØSREØJ[9,A,Z]	ØSRSØ1[9,A,Z]	ØSRSØ3[9,A,Z]	ØSRSØJ[9,A,Z]

Open Removal of Hip Liner with Replacement

Removal of Liner		Code also as appropriate Replacement by Device Type					
		Metal	Metal on Poly	Ceramic	Ceramic on Poly	Oxidized Zirc on Poly	Synth Subst
Hip, RT	ØSP9Ø9Z	ØSR9Ø1[9,A,Z]	ØSR9Ø2[9,A,Z]	ØSR9Ø3[9,A,Z]	ØSR9Ø4[9,A,Z]	ØSR9Ø6[9,A,Z]	ØSR9ØJ[9,A,Z]
Hip, LT	ØSPBØ9Z	ØSRBØ1[9,A,Z]	ØSRBØ2[9,A,Z]	ØSRBØ3[9,A,Z]	ØSRBØ4[9,A,Z]	ØSRBØ6[9,A,Z]	ØSRBØJ[9,A,Z]

Open Removal of Hip Liner with Replacement

Removal of Liner		Code also as appropriate Replacement by Device Type						
		Acetabular Surface				Femoral Surface		
		Poly	Metal	Ceramic	Synthetic	Metal	Ceramic	Synth
Hip, RT	ØSP9Ø9Z	ØSRAØØ[9,A,Z]	ØSRAØ1[9,A,Z]	ØSRAØ3[9,A,Z]	ØSRAØJ[9,A,Z]	ØSRRØ1[9,A,Z]	ØSRRØ3[9,A,Z]	ØSRRØJ[9,A,Z]
Hip, LT	ØSPBØ9Z	ØSREØØ[9,A,Z]	ØSREØ1[9,A,Z]	ØSREØ3[9,A,Z]	ØSREØJ[9,A,Z]	ØSRSØ1[9,A,Z]	ØSRSØ3[9,A,Z]	ØSRSØJ[9,A,Z]

Open Removal of Hip Resurfacing Device with Replacement

Removal of Resurfacing Device		Code also as appropriate Replacement by Device Type					
		Metal	Metal on Poly	Ceramic	Ceramic on Poly	Oxidized Zirc on Poly	Synth Subst
Hip, RT	ØSP9ØBZ	ØSR9Ø1[9,A,Z]	ØSR9Ø2[9,A,Z]	ØSR9Ø3[9,A,Z]	ØSR9Ø4[9,A,Z]	ØSR9Ø6[9,A,Z]	ØSR9ØJ[9,A,Z]
Hip, LT	ØSPBØBZ	ØSRBØ1[9,A,Z]	ØSRBØ2[9,A,Z]	ØSRBØ3[9,A,Z]	ØSRBØ4[9,A,Z]	ØSRBØ6[9,A,Z]	ØSRBØJ[9,A,Z]

Open Removal of Hip Resurfacing Device with Replacement

Removal of Resurfacing Device		Code also as appropriate Replacement by Device Type						
		Acetabular Surface				Femoral Surface		
		Poly	Metal	Ceramic	Synthetic	Metal	Ceramic	Synth
Hip, RT	ØSP9ØBZ	ØSRAØØ[9,A,Z]	ØSRAØ1[9,A,Z]	ØSRAØ3[9,A,Z]	ØSRAØJ[9,A,Z]	ØSRRØ1[9,A,Z]	ØSRRØ3[9,A,Z]	ØSRRØJ[9,A,Z]
Hip, LT	ØSPBØBZ	ØSREØØ[9,A,Z]	ØSREØ1[9,A,Z]	ØSREØ3[9,A,Z]	ØSREØJ[9,A,Z]	ØSRSØ1[9,A,Z]	ØSRSØ3[9,A,Z]	ØSRSØJ[9,A,Z]

Open Removal of Hip Articulating Spacer with Replacement

Removal of Articulating Spacer		Code also as appropriate Replacement by Device Type					
		Metal	Metal on Poly	Ceramic	Ceramic on Poly	Oxidized Zirc on Poly	Synth Subst
Hip, RT	ØSP9ØEZ	ØSR9Ø1[9,A,Z]	ØSR9Ø2[9,A,Z]	ØSR9Ø3[9,A,Z]	ØSR9Ø4[9,A,Z]	ØSR9Ø6[9,A,Z]	ØSR9ØJ[9,A,Z]
Hip, LT	ØSPBØEZ	ØSRBØ1[9,A,Z]	ØSRBØ2[9,A,Z]	ØSRBØ3[9,A,Z]	ØSRBØ4[9,A,Z]	ØSRBØ6[9,A,Z]	ØSRBØJ[9,A,Z]

Open Removal of Hip Articulating Spacer with Replacement

Removal of Articulating Spacer		Code also as appropriate Replacement by Device Type						
		Acetabular Surface				Femoral Surface		
		Poly	Metal	Ceramic	Synthetic	Metal	Ceramic	Synth
Hip, RT	ØSP9ØEZ	ØSRAØØ[9,A,Z]	ØSRAØ1[9,A,Z]	ØSRAØ3[9,A,Z]	ØSRAØJ[9,A,Z]	ØSRRØ1[9,A,Z]	ØSRRØ3[9,A,Z]	ØSRRØJ[9,A,Z]
Hip, LT	ØSPBØEZ	ØSREØØ[9,A,Z]	ØSREØ1[9,A,Z]	ØSREØ3[9,A,Z]	ØSREØJ[9,A,Z]	ØSRSØ1[9,A,Z]	ØSRSØ3[9,A,Z]	ØSRSØJ[9,A,Z]

Open Removal of Hip Synthetic Substitute with Replacement

Removal of Synthetic Substitute		Code also as appropriate Replacement by Device Type					
		Metal	Metal on Poly	Ceramic	Ceramic on Poly	Oxidized Zirc on Poly	Synth Subst
Hip, RT	ØSP[9,A,R]ØJZ	ØSR9Ø1[9,A,Z]	ØSR9Ø2[9,A,Z]	ØSR9Ø3[9,A,Z]	ØSR9Ø4[9,A,Z]	ØSR9Ø6[9,A,Z]	ØSR9ØJ[9,A,Z]
Hip, LT	ØSP[B,E,S]ØJZ	ØSRBØ1[9,A,Z]	ØSRBØ2[9,A,Z]	ØSRBØ3[9,A,Z]	ØSRBØ4[9,A,Z]	ØSRBØ6[9,A,Z]	ØSRBØJ[9,A,Z]

Open Removal of Hip Synthetic Substitute with Replacement

Removal of Synthetic Substitute		Code also as appropriate Replacement by Device Type						
		Acetabular Surface				Femoral Surface		
		Poly	Metal	Ceramic	Synthetic	Metal	Ceramic	Synth
Hip, RT	ØSP[9,A,R]ØJZ	ØSRAØØ[9,A,Z]	ØSRAØ1[9,A,Z]	ØSRAØ3[9,A,Z]	ØSRAØJ[9,A,Z]	ØSRRØ1[9,A,Z]	ØSRRØ3[9,A,Z]	ØSRRØJ[9,A,Z]
Hip, LT	ØSP[B,E,S]ØJZ	ØSREØØ[9,A,Z]	ØSREØ1[9,A,Z]	ØSREØ3[9,A,Z]	ØSREØJ[9,A,Z]	ØSRSØ1[9,A,Z]	ØSRSØ3[9,A,Z]	ØSRSØJ[9,A,Z]

Percutaneous Endoscopic Removal of Hip Spacer with Open Replacement

Removal of Spacer		Code also as appropriate Replacement by Device Type					
		Metal	Metal on Poly	Ceramic	Ceramic on Poly	Oxidized Zirc on Poly	Synth Subst
Hip, RT	ØSP948Z	ØSR9Ø1[9,A,Z]	ØSR9Ø2[9,A,Z]	ØSR9Ø3[9,A,Z]	ØSR9Ø4[9,A,Z]	ØSR9Ø6[9,A,Z]	ØSR9ØJ[9,A,Z]
Hip, LT	ØSPB48Z	ØSRBØ1[9,A,Z]	ØSRBØ2[9,A,Z]	ØSRBØ3[9,A,Z]	ØSRBØ4[9,A,Z]	ØSRBØ6[9,A,Z]	ØSRBØJ[9,A,Z]

Appendix L: Procedure Combination Tables *(side margin)*

Percutaneous Endoscopic Removal of Hip Spacer with Open Replacement

Removal of Spacer		Code also as appropriate Replacement by Device Type						
		Acetabular Surface				Femoral Surface		
		Poly	Metal	Ceramic	Synthetic	Metal	Ceramic	Synth
Hip, RT	0SP948Z	0SRA00[9,A,Z]	0SRA01[9,A,Z]	0SRA03[9,A,Z]	0SRA0J[9,A,Z]	0SRR01[9,A,Z]	0SRR03[9,A,Z]	0SRR0J[9,A,Z]
Hip, LT	0SPB48Z	0SRE00[9,A,Z]	0SRE01[9,A,Z]	0SRE03[9,A,Z]	0SRE0J[9,A,Z]	0SRS01[9,A,Z]	0SRS03[9,A,Z]	0SRS0J[9,A,Z]

Percutaneous Endoscopic Removal of Hip Synthetic Substitute with Open Replacement

Removal of Synthetic Substitute		Code also as appropriate Replacement by Device Type					
		Metal	Metal on Poly	Ceramic	Ceramic on Poly	Oxidized Zirc on Poly	Synth Subst
Hip, RT	0SP[9,A,R]4JZ	0SR901[9,A,Z]	0SR902[9,A,Z]	0SR903[9,A,Z]	0SR904[9,A,Z]	0SR906[9,A,Z]	0SR90J[9,A,Z]
Hip, LT	0SP[B,E,S]4JZ	0SRB01[9,A,Z]	0SRB02[9,A,Z]	0SRB03[9,A,Z]	0SRB04[9,A,Z]	0SRB06[9,A,Z]	0SRB0J[9,A,Z]

Percutaneous Endoscopic Removal of Hip Synthetic Substitute with Open Replacement

Removal of Synthetic Substitute		Code also as appropriate Replacement by Device Type						
		Acetabular Surface				Femoral Surface		
		Poly	Metal	Ceramic	Synthetic	Metal	Ceramic	Synth
Hip, RT	0SP[9,A,R]4JZ	0SRA00[9,A,Z]	0SRA01[9,A,Z]	0SRA03[9,A,Z]	0SRA0J[9,A,Z]	0SRR01[9,A,Z]	0SRR03[9,A,Z]	0SRR0J[9,A,Z]
Hip, LT	0SP[B,E,S]4JZ	0SRE00[9,A,Z]	0SRE01[9,A,Z]	0SRE03[9,A,Z]	0SRE0J[9,A,Z]	0SRS01[9,A,Z]	0SRS03[9,A,Z]	0SRS0J[9,A,Z]

Knee Procedure Combinations

Removal of Knee Spacer with Replacement

Removal of Spacer		Code also Replacement by Type of Synthetic Substitute					
		Oxidized Zirc on Poly	Synthetic Substitute	Patello-femoral	Femoral Surface	Tibial Surface	Medial (L)/Lateral (M) Meniscus
Knee, RT	0SPC[0,3,4]8Z	0SRC06[9,A,Z]	0SRC0J[9,A,Z]	0SRC0N[9,A,Z]	0SRT0J[9,A,Z]	0SRV0J[9,A,Z]	XRRG0[L,M]8
Knee, LT	0SPD[0,3,4]8Z	0SRD06[9,A,Z]	0SRD0J[9,A,Z]	0SRD0N[9,A,Z]	0SRU0J[9,A,Z]	0SRW0J[9,A,Z]	XRRH0[L,M]8

Removal of Knee Liner with Replacement

Removal of Liner		Code also Replacement by Type of Synthetic Substitute						
		Oxidized Zirc on Poly	Synthetic Substitute	Medial (L)/Lateral (M) Unicondylar	Patello-femoral	Femoral Surface	Tibial Surface	Medial (L)/Lateral (M) Meniscus
Knee, RT	0SPC09Z	0SRC06[9,A,Z]	0SRC0J[9,A,Z]	0SRC0[L,M][9,A,Z]	0SRC0N[9,A,Z]	0SRT0J[9,A,Z]	0SRV0J[9,A,Z]	XRRG0[L,M]8
Knee, LT	0SPD09Z	0SRD06[9,A,Z]	0SRD0J[9,A,Z]	0SRD0[L,M][9,A,Z]	0SRD0N[9,A,Z]	0SRU0J[9,A,Z]	0SRW0J[9,A,Z]	XRRH0[L,M]8

Removal of Knee Articulating Spacer with Replacement

Removal of Articulating Spacer		Code also Replacement by Type of Synthetic Substitute				
		Oxidized Zirc on Poly	Synthetic Substitute	Femoral Surface	Tibial Surface	Medial (L)/Lateral (M) Meniscus
Knee, RT	0SPC0EZ	0SRC06[9,A,Z]	0SRC0J[9,A,Z]	0SRT0J[9,A,Z]	0SRV0J[9,A,Z]	XRRG0[L,M]8
Knee, LT	0SPD0EZ	0SRD06[9,A,Z]	0SRD0J[9,A,Z]	0SRU0J[9,A,Z]	0SRW0J[9,A,Z]	XRRH0[L,M]8

Removal of Knee Patellar Surface with Replacement

Removal of Patellar Surface		Code also Replacement by Type of Synthetic Substitute					
		Oxidized Zirc on Poly	Synthetic Substitute	Patello-femoral	Femoral Surface	Tibial Surface	Medial (L)/Lateral (M) Meniscus
Knee, RT	0SPC[0,4]JC	0SRC06[9,A,Z]	0SRC0J[9,A,Z]	0SRC0N[9,A,Z]	0SRT0J[9,A,Z]	0SRV0J[9,A,Z]	XRRG0[L,M]8
Knee, LT	0SPD[0,4]JC	0SRD06[9,A,Z]	0SRD0J[9,A,Z]	0SRD0N[9,A,Z]	0SRU0J[9,A,Z]	0SRW0J[9,A,Z]	XRRH0[L,M]8

Removal of Knee Synthetic Substitute with Replacement

Removal of Synthetic Substitute		Code also Replacement by Type of Synthetic Substitute						
		Oxidized Zirc on Poly	Synthetic Substitute	Medial (L)/ Lateral (M) Unicondylar	Patello-femoral	Femoral Surface	Tibial Surface	Medial (L)/ Lateral (M) Meniscus
Knee, RT	ØSPC[Ø,4]JZ	ØSRCØ6[9,A,Z]	ØSRCØJ[9,A,Z]	ØSRCØ[L,M][9,A,Z]	ØSRCØN[9,A,Z]	ØSRTØJ[9,A,Z]	ØSRVØJ[9,A,Z]	XRRGØ[L,M]8
Knee, LT	ØSPD[Ø,4]JZ	ØSRDØ6[9,A,Z]	ØSRDØJ[9,A,Z]	ØSRDØ[L,M][9,A,Z]	ØSRDØN[9,A,Z]	ØSRUØJ[9,A,Z]	ØSRWØJ[9,A,Z]	XRRHØ[L,M]8

Removal of Knee Unicondylar Device with Replacement

Removal of Medial (L)/ Lateral (M) Unicondylar Device		Code also Replacement by Type of Synthetic Substitute					
		Oxidized Zirc on Poly	Synthetic Substitute	Medial Unicondylar	Femoral Surface	Tibial Surface	Medial (L)/Lateral (M) Meniscus
Knee, RT	ØSPC[Ø,4][L,M]Z	ØSRCØ6[9,A,Z]	ØSRCØJ[9,A,Z]	ØSRCØL[9,A,Z]	ØSRTØJ[9,A,Z]	ØSRVØJ[9,A,Z]	XRRGØ[L,M]8
Knee, LT	ØSPD[Ø,4][L,M]Z	ØSRDØ6[9,A,Z]	ØSRDØJ[9,A,Z]	ØSRDØL[9,A,Z]	ØSRUØJ[9,A,Z]	ØSRWØJ[9,A,Z]	XRRHØ[L,M]8

Removal of Knee Patellofemoral Device with Replacement

Removal of Patellofemoral Device		Code also Replacement by Type of Synthetic Substitute					
		Oxidized Zirc on Poly	Synthetic Substitute	Medial Unicondylar	Femoral Surface	Tibial Surface	Medial (L)/Lateral (M) Meniscus
Knee, RT	ØSPC[Ø,4]NZ	ØSRCØ6[9,A,Z]	ØSRCØJ[9,A,Z]	ØSRCØL[9,A,Z]	ØSRTØJ[9,A,Z]	ØSRVØJ[9,A,Z]	XRRGØ[L,M]8
Knee, LT	ØSPD[Ø,4]NZ	ØSRDØ6[9,A,Z]	ØSRDØJ[9,A,Z]	ØSRDØL[9,A,Z]	ØSRUØJ[9,A,Z]	ØSRWØJ[9,A,Z]	XRRHØ[L,M]8

Removal of Knee Femoral/Tibial Surface Device with Replacement

Removal of Femoral (T,U)/ Tibial (V,W) Surface		Code also Replacement by Type of Synthetic Substitute						
		Oxidized Zirc on Poly	Synthetic Substitute	Articulating Spacer	Patello-femoral	Femoral Surface	Tibial Surface	Medial (L)/Lateral (M) Meniscus
Knee, RT	ØSP[T,V][Ø,4]JZ	ØSRCØ6[9,A,Z]	ØSRCØJ[9,A,Z]	ØSRCØEZ	ØSRCØN[9,A,Z]	ØSRTØJ[9,A,Z]	ØSRVØJ[9,A,Z]	XRRGØ[L,M]8
Knee, LT	ØSP[U,W][Ø,4]JZ	ØSRDØ6[9,A,Z]	ØSRDØJ[9,A,Z]	ØSRDØEZ	ØSRDØN[9,A,Z]	ØSRUØJ[9,A,Z]	ØSRWØJ[9,A,Z]	XRRHØ[L,M]8

466-468 Revision of Hip or Knee Replacement

Hip Procedure Combinations

Open Removal of Hip Spacer with Replacement

Removal of Spacer		Code also as appropriate Replacement by Device Type						
		Metal	Metal on Poly	Ceramic	Ceramic on Poly	Oxidized Zirc on Poly	Articulating Spacer	Synth Subst
Hip, RT	ØSP9Ø8Z	ØSR9Ø1[9,A,Z]	ØSR9Ø2[9,A,Z]	ØSR9Ø3[9,A,Z]	ØSR9Ø4[9,A,Z]	ØSR9Ø6[9,A,Z]	ØSR9ØEZ	ØSR9ØJ[9,A,Z]
Hip, LT	ØSPBØ8Z	ØSRBØ1[9,A,Z]	ØSRBØ2[9,A,Z]	ØSRBØ3[9,A,Z]	ØSRBØ4[9,A,Z]	ØSRBØ6[9,A,Z]	ØSRBØEZ	ØSRBØJ[9,A,Z]

Open Removal of Hip Spacer with Replacement

Removal of Spacer		Code also as appropriate Replacement by Device Type						
		Acetabular Surface				Femoral Surface		
		Poly	Metal	Ceramic	Synthetic	Metal	Ceramic	Synth
Hip, RT	ØSP9Ø8Z	ØSRAØØ[9,A,Z]	ØSRAØ1[9,A,Z]	ØSRAØ3[9,A,Z]	ØSRAØJ[9,A,Z]	ØSRRØ1[9,A,Z]	ØSRRØ3[9,A,Z]	ØSRRØJ[9,A,Z]
Hip, LT	ØSPBØ8Z	ØSREØØ[9,A,Z]	ØSREØ1[9,A,Z]	ØSREØ3[9,A,Z]	ØSREØJ[9,A,Z]	ØSRSØ1[9,A,Z]	ØSRSØ3[9,A,Z]	ØSRSØJ[9,A,Z]

Open Removal of Hip Spacer with Liner Insertion (supplement)

Removal of Spacer		Code also as appropriate Supplement of Body Part by Site		
		Joint	Acetabular Surface	Femoral Surface
Hip, RT	ØSP9Ø8Z	ØSU9Ø9Z	ØSUAØ9Z	ØSURØ9Z
Hip, LT	ØSPBØ8Z	ØSUBØ9Z	ØSUEØ9Z	ØSUSØ9Z

Open Removal of Hip Liner with Replacement

Removal of Liner		Code also as appropriate Replacement by Device Type						
		Metal	Metal on Poly	Ceramic	Ceramic on Poly	Oxidized Zirc on Poly	Articulating Spacer	Synth Subst
Hip, RT	ØSP9Ø9Z	ØSR9Ø1[9,A,Z]	ØSR9Ø2[9,A,Z]	ØSR9Ø3[9,A,Z]	ØSR9Ø4[9,A,Z]	ØSR9Ø6[9,A,Z]	ØSR9ØEZ	ØSR9ØJ[9,A,Z]
Hip, LT	ØSPBØ9Z	ØSRBØ1[9,A,Z]	ØSRBØ2[9,A,Z]	ØSRBØ3[9,A,Z]	ØSRBØ4[9,A,Z]	ØSRBØ6[9,A,Z]	ØSRBØEZ	ØSRBØJ[9,A,Z]

Open Removal of Hip Liner with Replacement

Removal of Liner		Code also as appropriate Replacement by Device Type						
		Acetabular Surface				Femoral Surface		
		Poly	Metal	Ceramic	Synthetic	Metal	Ceramic	Synth
Hip, RT	ØSP9Ø9Z	ØSRAØØ[9,A,Z]	ØSRAØ1[9,A,Z]	ØSRAØ3[9,A,Z]	ØSRAØJ[9,A,Z]	ØSRRØ1[9,A,Z]	ØSRRØ3[9,A,Z]	ØSRRØJ[9,A,Z]
Hip, LT	ØSPBØ9Z	ØSREØØ[9,A,Z]	ØSREØ1[9,A,Z]	ØSREØ3[9,A,Z]	ØSREØJ[9,A,Z]	ØSRSØ1[9,A,Z]	ØSRSØ3[9,A,Z]	ØSRSØJ[9,A,Z]

Open Removal of Hip Liner with Liner Insertion (supplement)

Removal of Liner		Code also as appropriate Supplement of Body Part by Site		
		Joint	Acetabular Surface	Femoral Surface
Hip, RT	ØSP9Ø9Z	ØSU9Ø9Z	ØSUAØ9Z	ØSURØ9Z
Hip, LT	ØSPBØ9Z	ØSUBØ9Z	ØSUEØ9Z	ØSUSØ9Z

Open Removal of Hip Resurfacing Device with Replacement

Removal of Resurfacing Device		Code also as appropriate Replacement by Device Type						
		Metal	Metal on Poly	Ceramic	Ceramic on Poly	Oxidized Zirc on Poly	Articulating Spacer	Synth Subst
Hip, RT	ØSP9ØBZ	ØSR9Ø1[9,A,Z]	ØSR9Ø2[9,A,Z]	ØSR9Ø3[9,A,Z]	ØSR9Ø4[9,A,Z]	ØSR9Ø6[9,A,Z]	ØSR9ØEZ	ØSR9ØJ[9,A,Z]
Hip, LT	ØSPBØBZ	ØSRBØ1[9,A,Z]	ØSRBØ2[9,A,Z]	ØSRBØ3[9,A,Z]	ØSRBØ4[9,A,Z]	ØSRBØ6[9,A,Z]	ØSRBØEZ	ØSRBØJ[9,A,Z]

Open Removal of Hip Resurfacing Device with Replacement

Removal of Resurfacing Device		Code also as appropriate Replacement by Device Type						
		Acetabular Surface				Femoral Surface		
		Poly	Metal	Ceramic	Synthetic	Metal	Ceramic	Synth
Hip, RT	ØSP9ØBZ	ØSRAØØ[9,A,Z]	ØSRAØ1[9,A,Z]	ØSRAØ3[9,A,Z]	ØSRAØJ[9,A,Z]	ØSRRØ1[9,A,Z]	ØSRRØ3[9,A,Z]	ØSRRØJ[9,A,Z]
Hip, LT	ØSPBØBZ	ØSREØØ[9,A,Z]	ØSREØ1[9,A,Z]	ØSREØ3[9,A,Z]	ØSREØJ[9,A,Z]	ØSRSØ1[9,A,Z]	ØSRSØ3[9,A,Z]	ØSRSØJ[9,A,Z]

Open Removal of Hip Resurfacing Device with Liner Insertion (supplement)

Removal of Resurfacing Device		Code also as appropriate Supplement of Body Part by Site		
		Joint	Acetabular Surface	Femoral Surface
Hip, RT	ØSP9ØBZ	ØSU9Ø9Z	ØSUAØ9Z	ØSURØ9Z
Hip, LT	ØSPBØBZ	ØSUBØ9Z	ØSUEØ9Z	ØSUSØ9Z

Open Removal of Hip Articulating Spacer with Replacement

Removal of Articulating Spacer		Code also as appropriate Replacement by Device Type					
		Metal	Metal on Poly	Ceramic	Ceramic on Poly	Oxidized Zirc on Poly	Synth Subst
Hip, RT	ØSP9ØEZ	ØSR9Ø1[9,A,Z]	ØSR9Ø2[9,A,Z]	ØSR9Ø3[9,A,Z]	ØSR9Ø4[9,A,Z]	ØSR9Ø6[9,A,Z]	ØSR9ØJ[9,A,Z]
Hip, LT	ØSPBØEZ	ØSRBØ1[9,A,Z]	ØSRBØ2[9,A,Z]	ØSRBØ3[9,A,Z]	ØSRBØ4[9,A,Z]	ØSRBØ6[9,A,Z]	ØSRBØJ[9,A,Z]

Open Removal of Hip Articulating Spacer with Replacement

Removal of Articulating Spacer		Code also as appropriate Replacement by Device Type						
		Acetabular Surface				Femoral Surface		
		Poly	Metal	Ceramic	Synthetic	Metal	Ceramic	Synth
Hip, RT	ØSP9ØEZ	ØSRAØØ[9,A,Z]	ØSRAØ1[9,A,Z]	ØSRAØ3[9,A,Z]	ØSRAØJ[9,A,Z]	ØSRRØ1[9,A,Z]	ØSRRØ3[9,A,Z]	ØSRRØJ[9,A,Z]
Hip, LT	ØSPBØEZ	ØSREØØ[9,A,Z]	ØSREØ1[9,A,Z]	ØSREØ3[9,A,Z]	ØSREØJ[9,A,Z]	ØSRSØ1[9,A,Z]	ØSRSØ3[9,A,Z]	ØSRSØJ[9,A,Z]

Open Removal of Hip Articulating Spacer with Liner Insertion (supplement)

Removal of Articulating Spacer		Code also as appropriate Supplement of Body Part by Site		
		Joint	Acetabular Surface	Femoral Surface
Hip, RT	ØSP9ØEZ	ØSU9Ø9Z	ØSUAØ9Z	ØSURØ9Z
Hip, LT	ØSPBØEZ	ØSUBØ9Z	ØSUEØ9Z	ØSUSØ9Z

Open Removal of Hip Synthetic Substitute with Replacement

Removal of Synthetic Substitute		Code also as appropriate Replacement by Device Type						
		Metal	Metal on Poly	Ceramic	Ceramic on Poly	Oxidized Zirc on Poly	Articulating Spacer	Synth Subst
Hip, RT	ØSP[9,A,R]ØJZ	ØSR9Ø1[9,A,Z]	ØSR9Ø2[9,A,Z]	ØSR9Ø3[9,A,Z]	ØSR9Ø4[9,A,Z]	ØSR9Ø6[9,A,Z]	ØSR9ØEZ	ØSR9ØJ[9,A,Z]
Hip, LT	ØSP[B,E,S]ØJZ	ØSRBØ1[9,A,Z]	ØSRBØ2[9,A,Z]	ØSRBØ3[9,A,Z]	ØSRBØ4[9,A,Z]	ØSRBØ6[9,A,Z]	ØSRBØEZ	ØSRBØJ[9,A,Z]

Open Removal of Hip Synthetic Substitute with Replacement

Removal of Synthetic Substitute		Code also as appropriate Replacement by Device Type						
		Acetabular Surface				Femoral Surface		
		Poly	Metal	Ceramic	Synthetic	Metal	Ceramic	Synth
Hip, RT	ØSP[9,A,R]ØJZ	ØSRAØØ[9,A,Z]	ØSRAØ1[9,A,Z]	ØSRAØ3[9,A,Z]	ØSRAØJ[9,A,Z]	ØSRRØ1[9,A,Z]	ØSRRØ3[9,A,Z]	ØSRRØJ[9,A,Z]
Hip, LT	ØSP[B,E,S]ØJZ	ØSREØØ[9,A,Z]	ØSREØ1[9,A,Z]	ØSREØ3[9,A,Z]	ØSREØJ[9,A,Z]	ØSRSØ1[9,A,Z]	ØSRSØ3[9,A,Z]	ØSRSØJ[9,A,Z]

Percutaneous Endoscopic Removal of Hip Spacer with Open Replacement

Removal of Spacer		Code also as appropriate Replacement by Device Type						
		Metal	Metal on Poly	Ceramic	Ceramic on Poly	Oxidized Zirc on Poly	Articulating Spacer	Synth Subst
Hip, RT	ØSP948Z	ØSR9Ø1[9,A,Z]	ØSR9Ø2[9,A,Z]	ØSR9Ø3[9,A,Z]	ØSR9Ø4[9,A,Z]	ØSR9Ø6[9,A,Z]	ØSR9ØEZ	ØSR9ØJ[9,A,Z]
Hip, LT	ØSPB48Z	ØSRBØ1[9,A,Z]	ØSRBØ2[9,A,Z]	ØSRBØ3[9,A,Z]	ØSRBØ4[9,A,Z]	ØSRBØ6[9,A,Z]	ØSRBØEZ	ØSRBØJ[9,A,Z]

Percutaneous Endoscopic Removal of Hip Spacer with Open Replacement

Removal of Spacer		Code also as appropriate Replacement by Device Type						
		Acetabular Surface				Femoral Surface		
		Poly	Metal	Ceramic	Synthetic	Metal	Ceramic	Synth
Hip, RT	ØSP948Z	ØSRAØØ[9,A,Z]	ØSRAØ1[9,A,Z]	ØSRAØ3[9,A,Z]	ØSRAØJ[9,A,Z]	ØSRRØ1[9,A,Z]	ØSRRØ3[9,A,Z]	ØSRRØJ[9,A,Z]
Hip, LT	ØSPB48Z	ØSREØØ[9,A,Z]	ØSREØ1[9,A,Z]	ØSREØ3[9,A,Z]	ØSREØJ[9,A,Z]	ØSRSØ1[9,A,Z]	ØSRSØ3[9,A,Z]	ØSRSØJ[9,A,Z]

Percutaneous Endoscopic Removal of Hip Spacer with Open Liner Insertion (supplement)

Removal of Spacer		Code also as appropriate Supplement of Body Part by Site		
		Joint	Acetabular Surface	Femoral Surface
Hip, RT	ØSP948Z	ØSU9Ø9Z	ØSUAØ9Z	ØSURØ9Z
Hip, LT	ØSPB48Z	ØSUBØ9Z	ØSUEØ9Z	ØSUSØ9Z

Percutaneous Endoscopic Removal of Hip Synthetic Substitute with Open Replacement

Removal of Synthetic Substitute		Code also as appropriate Replacement by Device Type						
		Metal	Metal on Poly	Ceramic	Ceramic on Poly	Oxidized Zirc on Poly	Articulating Spacer	Synth Subst
Hip, RT	ØSP[9,A,R]4JZ	ØSR9Ø1[9,A,Z]	ØSR9Ø2[9,A,Z]	ØSR9Ø3[9,A,Z]	ØSR9Ø4[9,A,Z]	ØSR9Ø6[9,A,Z]	ØSR9ØEZ	ØSR9ØJ[9,A,Z]
Hip, LT	ØSP[B,E,S]4JZ	ØSRBØ1[9,A,Z]	ØSRBØ2[9,A,Z]	ØSRBØ3[9,A,Z]	ØSRBØ4[9,A,Z]	ØSRBØ6[9,A,Z]	ØSRBØEZ	ØSRBØJ[9,A,Z]

Percutaneous Endoscopic Removal of Hip Synthetic Substitute with Open Replacement

Removal of Synthetic Substitute		Code also as appropriate Replacement by Device Type						
		Acetabular Surface				Femoral Surface		
		Poly	Metal	Ceramic	Synthetic	Metal	Ceramic	Synth
Hip, RT	ØSP[9,A,R]4JZ	ØSRAØØ[9,A,Z]	ØSRAØ1[9,A,Z]	ØSRAØ3[9,A,Z]	ØSRAØJ[9,A,Z]	ØSRRØ1[9,A,Z]	ØSRRØ3[9,A,Z]	ØSRRØJ[9,A,Z]
Hip, LT	ØSP[B,E,S]4JZ	ØSREØØ[9,A,Z]	ØSREØ1[9,A,Z]	ØSREØ3[9,A,Z]	ØSREØJ[9,A,Z]	ØSRSØ1[9,A,Z]	ØSRSØ3[9,A,Z]	ØSRSØJ[9,A,Z]

Appendix L: Procedure Combination Tables

Percutaneous Endoscopic Removal of Hip Synthetic Substitute with Open Liner Insertion (supplement)

Removal of Synthetic Substitute		Code also as appropriate Supplement of Body Part by Site		
		Joint	Acetabular Surface	Femoral Surface
Hip, RT	ØSP[9,A,R]4JZ	ØSU9Ø9Z	ØSUAØ9Z	ØSURØ9Z
Hip, LT	ØSP[B,E,S]4JZ	ØSUBØ9Z	ØSUEØ9Z	ØSUSØ9Z

Knee Procedure Combinations

Removal of Knee Spacer with Replacement

Removal of Spacer		Code also Replacement by Type of Synthetic Substitute						
		Oxidized Zirc on Poly	Synthetic Substitute	Articulating Spacer	Patello-femoral	Femoral Surface	Tibial Surface	Medial (L)/ Lateral (M) Meniscus
Knee, RT	ØSPC[Ø,3,4]8Z	ØSRCØ6[9,A,Z]	ØSRCØJ[9,A,Z]	ØSRCØEZ	ØSRCØN[9,A,Z]	ØSRTØJ[9,A,Z]	ØSRVØJ[9,A,Z]	XRRGØ[L,M]8
Knee, LT	ØSPD[Ø,3,4]8Z	ØSRDØ6[9,A,Z]	ØSRDØJ[9,A,Z]	ØSRDØEZ	ØSRDØN[9,A,Z]	ØSRUØJ[9,A,Z]	ØSRWØJ[9,A,Z]	XRRHØ[L,M]8

Removal of Knee Liner with Replacement

Removal of Liner		Code also Replacement by Type of Synthetic Substitute							
		Oxidized Zirc on Poly	Synthetic Substitute	Articulating Spacer	Medial (L)/ Lateral (M) Unicondylar	Patello-femoral	Femoral Surface	Tibial Surface	Medial (L)/Lateral (M) Meniscus
Knee, RT	ØSPCØ9Z	ØSRCØ6[9,A,Z]	ØSRCØJ[9,A,Z]	ØSRCØEZ	ØSRCØ[L,M][9,A,Z]	ØSRCØN[9,A,Z]	ØSRTØJ[9,A,Z]	ØSRVØJ[9,A,Z]	XRRGØ[L,M]8
Knee, LT	ØSPDØ9Z	ØSRDØ6[9,A,Z]	ØSRDØJ[9,A,Z]	ØSRDØEZ	ØSRDØ[L,M][9,A,Z]	ØSRDØN[9,A,Z]	ØSRUØJ[9,A,Z]	ØSRWØJ[9,A,Z]	XRRHØ[L,M]8

Removal of Knee Articulating Spacer with Replacement

Removal of Articulating Spacer		Code also Replacement by Type of Synthetic Substitute				
		Oxidized Zirc on Poly	Synthetic Substitute	Femoral Surface	Tibial Surface	Medial (L)/Lateral (M) Meniscus
Knee, RT	ØSPCØEZ	ØSRCØ6[9,A,Z]	ØSRCØJ[9,A,Z]	ØSRTØJ[9,A,Z]	ØSRVØJ[9,A,Z]	XRRGØ[L,M]8
Knee, LT	ØSPDØEZ	ØSRDØ6[9,A,Z]	ØSRDØJ[9,A,Z]	ØSRUØJ[9,A,Z]	ØSRWØJ[9,A,Z]	XRRHØ[L,M]8

Removal of Knee Patellar Surface with Replacement

Removal of Patellar Surface		Code also Replacement by Type of Synthetic Substitute						
		Oxidized Zirc on Poly	Synthetic Substitute	Articulating Spacer	Patello-femoral	Femoral Surface	Tibial Surface	Medial (L)/Lateral (M) Meniscus
Knee, RT	ØSPC[Ø,4]JC	ØSRCØ6[9,A,Z]	ØSRCØJ[9,A,Z]	ØSRCØEZ	ØSRCØN[9,A,Z]	ØSRTØJ[9,A,Z]	ØSRVØJ[9,A,Z]	XRRGØ[L,M]8
Knee, LT	ØSPD[Ø,4]JC	ØSRDØ6[9,A,Z]	ØSRDØJ[9,A,Z]	ØSRDØEZ	ØSRDØN[9,A,Z]	ØSRUØJ[9,A,Z]	ØSRWØJ[9,A,Z]	XRRHØ[L,M]8

Removal of Knee Synthetic Substitute with Replacement

Removal of Synthetic Substitute		Code also Replacement by Type of Synthetic Substitute							
		Oxidized Zirc on Poly	Synthetic Substitute	Articulating Spacer	Medial (L)/ Lateral (M) Unicondylar	Patello-femoral	Femoral Surface	Tibial Surface	Medial (L)/ Lateral (M) Meniscus
Knee, RT	ØSPC[Ø,4]JZ	ØSRCØ6[9,A,Z]	ØSRCØJ[9,A,Z]	ØSRCØEZ	ØSRCØ[L,M][9,A,Z]	ØSRCØN[9,A,Z]	ØSRTØJ[9,A,Z]	ØSRVØJ[9,A,Z]	XRRGØ[L,M]8
Knee, LT	ØSPD[Ø,4]JZ	ØSRDØ6[9,A,Z]	ØSRDØJ[9,A,Z]	ØSRDØEZ	ØSRDØ[L,M][9,A,Z]	ØSRDØN[9,A,Z]	ØSRUØJ[9,A,Z]	ØSRWØJ[9,A,Z]	XRRHØ[L,M]8

Removal of Knee Unicondylar Device with Replacement

Removal of Medial (L)/ Lateral (M) Unicondylar Device		Code also Replacement by Type of Synthetic Substitute					
		Oxidized Zirc on Poly	Synthetic Substitute	Medial Unicondylar	Femoral Surface	Tibial Surface	Medial (L)/Lateral (M) Meniscus
Knee, RT	ØSPC[Ø,4][L,M]Z	ØSRCØ6[9,A,Z]	ØSRCØJ[9,A,Z]	ØSRCØL[9,A,Z]	ØSRTØJ[9,A,Z]	ØSRVØJ[9,A,Z]	XRRGØ[L,M]8
Knee, LT	ØSPD[Ø,4][L,M]Z	ØSRDØ6[9,A,Z]	ØSRDØJ[9,A,Z]	ØSRDØL[9,A,Z]	ØSRUØJ[9,A,Z]	ØSRWØJ[9,A,Z]	XRRHØ[L,M]8

Removal of Knee Patellofemoral Device with Replacement

Removal of Patellofemoral Device		Code also Replacement by Type of Synthetic Substitute					
		Oxidized Zirc on Poly	Synthetic Substitute	Medial Unicondylar	Femoral Surface	Tibial Surface	Medial (L)/Lateral (M) Meniscus
Knee, RT	ØSPC[Ø,4]NZ	ØSRCØ6[9,A,Z]	ØSRCØJ[9,A,Z]	ØSRCØL[9,A,Z]	ØSRTØJ[9,A,Z]	ØSRVØJ[9,A,Z]	XRRGØ[L,M]8
Knee, LT	ØSPD[Ø,4]NZ	ØSRDØ6[9,A,Z]	ØSRDØJ[9,A,Z]	ØSRDØL[9,A,Z]	ØSRUØJ[9,A,Z]	ØSRWØJ[9,A,Z]	XRRHØ[L,M]8

Removal of Knee Femoral/Tibial Surface Device with Replacement

Removal of Femoral (T,U)/ Tibial (V,W) Surface		Code also Replacement by Type of Synthetic Substitute						
		Oxidized Zirc on Poly	Synthetic Substitute	Articulating Spacer	Patello-femoral	Femoral Surface	Tibial Surface	Medial (L)/Lateral (M) Meniscus
Knee, RT	ØSP[T,V][Ø,4]JZ	ØSRCØ6[9,A,Z]	ØSRCØJ[9,A,Z]	ØSRCØEZ	ØSRCØN[9,A,Z]	ØSRTØJ[9,A,Z]	ØSRVØJ[9,A,Z]	XRRGØ[L,M]8
Knee, LT	ØSP[U,W][Ø,4]JZ	ØSRDØ6[9,A,Z]	ØSRDØJ[9,A,Z]	ØSRDØEZ	ØSRDØN[9,A,Z]	ØSRUØJ[9,A,Z]	ØSRWØJ[9,A,Z]	XRRHØ[L,M]8

DRG 485-489 Knee Procedures

Joint	Removal of Liner by open approach	Code also as appropriate Supplement of Tibial Surface by Site
Knee, RT	ØSPCØ9Z	ØSUVØ9Z
Knee, LT	ØSPDØ9Z	ØSUWØ9Z

DRG 515-517 Other Musculoskeletal System and Connective Tissue Procedures

Site	Reposition of Vertebra by percutaneous approach	Code also as appropriate Supplement With Synthetic Substitute by Percutaneous Approach at site of Repositioned Vertebra
Cervical	ØPS33ZZ	ØPU33JZ
Coccyx	ØQSS3ZZ	ØQUS3JZ
Lumbar	ØQSØ3ZZ	ØQUØ3JZ
Sacrum	ØQS13ZZ	ØQU13JZ
Thoracic	ØPS43ZZ	ØPU43JZ

DRG 518-52Ø Back and Neck Procedures, Except Spinal Fusion, or Disc Devices/Neurostimulators

Generator Type	Insertion of Generator by Site			Code also as appropriate Insertion Neurostimulator Lead by approach and Site	
	Chest	Abdomen	Back	Spinal Canal	Spinal Cord
Single Array	ØJH6[Ø,3]BZ	ØJH8[Ø,3]BZ	ØJH7[Ø,3]BZ	ØØHU[Ø,3,4]MZ	ØØHV[Ø,3,4]MZ
Single Array, Rechargeable	ØJH6[Ø,3]CZ	ØJH8[Ø,3]CZ	ØJH7[Ø,3]CZ	ØØHU[Ø,3,4]MZ	ØØHV[Ø,3,4]MZ
Multiple Array	ØJH6[Ø,3]DZ	ØJH8[Ø,3]DZ	ØJH7[Ø,3]DZ	ØØHU[Ø,3,4]MZ	ØØHV[Ø,3,4]MZ
Multiple Array, Rechargeable	ØJH6[Ø,3]EZ	—	ØJH7[Ø,3]EZ	ØØHU[Ø,3,4]MZ	ØØHV[Ø,3,4]MZ
Multiple Array, Rechargeable	—	ØJH8[Ø,3]EZ	—	ØØHU[Ø,3,4]MZ	ØØHV[Ø,3,4]MZ

DRG 582-583 Mastectomy for Malignancy

Site	Resection by Open approach	Code also as appropriate Resection of Lymph Nodes by Open approach by site			Code also as appropriate Resection of Thorax Muscle by Open approach	
		Axillary	Internal Mammary	Thorax	Right	Left
Breast, Right	ØHTTØZZ	Ø7T5ØZZ	Ø7T8ØZZ	Ø7T7ØZZ	ØKTHØZZ	—
Breast, Left	ØHTUØZZ	Ø7T6ØZZ	Ø7T9ØZZ	Ø7T7ØZZ	—	ØKTJØZZ
Breast, Bilateral	ØHTVØZZ	Ø7T5ØZZ and Ø7T6ØZZ	Ø7T8ØZZ and Ø7T9ØZZ	Ø7T7ØZZ	ØKTHØZZ	ØKTJØZZ

DRG 584-585 Breast Biopsy, Local Excision and Other Breast Procedures

Resection of Breast With Resection of Lymph Nodes and Thorax Muscle

Site	Resection by Open approach	Code also as appropriate Resection of Lymph Nodes by Open approach by site			Code also as appropriate Resection of Thorax Muscle by Open approach	
		Axillary	Internal Mammary	Thorax	Right	Left
Breast, Right	ØHTTØZZ	Ø7T5ØZZ	Ø7T8ØZZ	Ø7T7ØZZ	ØKTHØZZ	—
Breast, Left	ØHTUØZZ	Ø7T6ØZZ	Ø7T9ØZZ	Ø7T7ØZZ	—	ØKTJØZZ
Breast, Bilateral	ØHTVØZZ	Ø7T5ØZZ and Ø7T6ØZZ	Ø7T8ØZZ and Ø7T9ØZZ	Ø7T7ØZZ	ØKTHØZZ	ØKTJØZZ

Replacement of Breast Tissue

Site	Replacement by Percutaneous approach with Autologous Tissue	Code also as appropriate Extraction of Subcutaneous Tissue by Percutaneous approach					
		Abdomen	Back	Buttock	Chest	Leg, Upper, Right	Leg, Upper, Left
Breast, Right	ØHRT37Z	ØJD83ZZ	ØJD73ZZ	ØJD93ZZ	ØJD63ZZ	ØJDL3ZZ	ØJDM3ZZ
Breast, Left	ØHRU37Z	ØJD83ZZ	ØJD73ZZ	ØJD93ZZ	ØJD63ZZ	ØJDL3ZZ	ØJDM3ZZ
Breast, Bilateral	ØHRV37Z	ØJD83ZZ	ØJD73ZZ	ØJD93ZZ	ØJD63ZZ	ØJDL3ZZ	ØJDM3ZZ

DRG 628-630 Other Endocrine, Nutritional and Metabolic Procedures

Hip Procedure Combinations

Open Removal of Hip Spacer with Replacement

Removal of Spacer		Code also as appropriate Replacement by Device Type					
		Metal	Metal on Poly	Ceramic	Ceramic on Poly	Oxidized Zirc on Poly	Synthetic Substitute
Hip, RT	0SP908Z	0SR901[9,A,Z]	0SR902[9,A,Z]	0SR903[9,A,Z]	0SR904[9,A,Z]	0SR906[9,A,Z]	0SR90J[9,A,Z]
Hip, LT	0SPB08Z	0SRB01[9,A,Z]	0SRB02[9,A,Z]	0SRB03[9,A,Z]	0SRB04[9,A,Z]	0SRB06[9,A,Z]	0SRB0J[9,A,Z]

Open Removal of Hip Spacer with Replacement

Removal of Spacer		Code also as appropriate Replacement by Device Type						
		Acetabular Surface				Femoral Surface		
		Poly	Metal	Ceramic	Synthetic	Metal	Ceramic	Synthetic
Hip, RT	0SP908Z	0SRA00[9,A,Z]	0SRA01[9,A,Z]	0SRA03[9,A,Z]	0SRA0J[9,A,Z]	0SRR01[9,A,Z]	0SRR03[9,A,Z]	0SRR0J[9,A,Z]
Hip, LT	0SPB08Z	0SRE00[9,A,Z]	0SRE01[9,A,Z]	0SRE03[9,A,Z]	0SRE0J[9,A,Z]	0SRS01[9,A,Z]	0SRS03[9,A,Z]	0SRS0J[9,A,Z]

Open Removal of Hip Spacer with Liner Insertion (supplement)

Removal of Spacer		Code also as appropriate Supplement of Body Part by Site		
		Joint	Acetabular Surface	Femoral Surface
Hip, RT	0SP908Z	0SU909Z	0SUA09Z	0SUR09Z
Hip, LT	0SPB08Z	0SUB09Z	0SUE09Z	0SUS09Z

Open Removal of Hip Liner with Replacement

Removal of Liner		Code also as appropriate Replacement by Device Type					
		Metal	Metal on Poly	Ceramic	Ceramic on Poly	Oxidized Zirc on Poly	Synthetic Substitute
Hip, RT	0SP909Z	0SR901[9,A,Z]	0SR902[9,A,Z]	0SR903[9,A,Z]	0SR904[9,A,Z]	0SR906[9,A,Z]	0SR90J[9,A,Z]
Hip, LT	0SPB09Z	0SRB01[9,A,Z]	0SRB02[9,A,Z]	0SRB03[9,A,Z]	0SRB04[9,A,Z]	0SRB06[9,A,Z]	0SRB0J[9,A,Z]

Open Removal of Hip Liner with Replacement

Removal of Liner		Code also as appropriate Replacement by Device Type						
		Acetabular Surface				Femoral Surface		
		Poly	Metal	Ceramic	Synthetic	Metal	Ceramic	Synthetic
Hip, RT	0SP909Z	0SRA00[9,A,Z]	0SRA01[9,A,Z]	0SRA03[9,A,Z]	0SRA0J[9,A,Z]	0SRR01[9,A,Z]	0SRR03[9,A,Z]	0SRR0J[9,A,Z]
Hip, LT	0SPB09Z	0SRE00[9,A,Z]	0SRE01[9,A,Z]	0SRE03[9,A,Z]	0SRE0J[9,A,Z]	0SRS01[9,A,Z]	0SRS03[9,A,Z]	0SRS0J[9,A,Z]

Open Removal of Hip Liner with Liner Insertion (supplement)

Removal of Liner		Code also as appropriate Supplement of Body Part by Site		
		Joint	Acetabular Surface	Femoral Surface
Hip, RT	0SP909Z	0SU909Z	0SUA09Z	0SUR09Z
Hip, LT	0SPB09Z	0SUB09Z	0SUE09Z	0SUS09Z

Open Removal of Hip Resurfacing Device with Replacement

Removal of Resurfacing Device		Code also as appropriate Replacement by Device Type					
		Metal	Metal on Poly	Ceramic	Ceramic on Poly	Oxidized Zirc on Poly	Synthetic Substitute
Hip, RT	0SP90BZ	0SR901[9,A,Z]	0SR902[9,A,Z]	0SR903[9,A,Z]	0SR904[9,A,Z]	0SR906[9,A,Z]	0SR90J[9,A,Z]
Hip, LT	0SPB0BZ	0SRB01[9,A,Z]	0SRB02[9,A,Z]	0SRB03[9,A,Z]	0SRB04[9,A,Z]	0SRB06[9,A,Z]	0SRB0J[9,A,Z]

Open Removal of Hip Resurfacing Device with Replacement

Removal of Resurfacing Device		Code also as appropriate Replacement by Device Type						
		Acetabular Surface				Femoral Surface		
		Poly	Metal	Ceramic	Synthetic	Metal	Ceramic	Synthetic
Hip, RT	0SP90BZ	0SRA00[9,A,Z]	0SRA01[9,A,Z]	0SRA03[9,A,Z]	0SRA0J[9,A,Z]	0SRR01[9,A,Z]	0SRR03[9,A,Z]	0SRR0J[9,A,Z]
Hip, LT	0SPB0BZ	0SRE00[9,A,Z]	0SRE01[9,A,Z]	0SRE03[9,A,Z]	0SRE0J[9,A,Z]	0SRS01[9,A,Z]	0SRS03[9,A,Z]	0SRS0J[9,A,Z]

Open Removal of Hip Resurfacing Device with Liner Insertion (supplement)

Removal of Resurfacing Device		Code also as appropriate Supplement of Body Part by Site		
		Joint	Acetabular Surface	Femoral Surface
Hip, RT	ØSP9ØBZ	ØSU9Ø9Z	ØSUAØ9Z	ØSURØ9Z
Hip, LT	ØSPBØBZ	ØSUBØ9Z	ØSUEØ9Z	ØSUSØ9Z

Open Removal of Hip Synthetic Substitute with Replacement

Removal of Synthetic Substitute		Code also as appropriate Replacement by Device Type					
		Metal	Metal on Poly	Ceramic	Ceramic on Poly	Oxidized Zirc on Poly	Synthetic Substitute
Hip, RT	ØSP9ØJZ	ØSR9Ø1[9,A,Z]	ØSR9Ø2[9,A,Z]	ØSR9Ø3[9,A,Z]	ØSR9Ø4[9,A,Z]	ØSR9Ø6[9,A,Z]	ØSR9ØJ[9,A,Z]
Hip, LT	ØSPBØJZ	ØSRBØ1[9,A,Z]	ØSRBØ2[9,A,Z]	ØSRBØ3[9,A,Z]	ØSRBØ4[9,A,Z]	ØSRBØ6[9,A,Z]	ØSRBØJ[9,A,Z]

Open Removal of Hip Synthetic Substitute with Replacement

Removal of Synthetic Substitute		Code also as appropriate Replacement by Device Type						
		Acetabular Surface				Femoral Surface		
		Poly	Metal	Ceramic	Synthetic	Metal	Ceramic	Synthetic
Hip, RT	ØSP9ØJZ	ØSRAØØ[9,A,Z]	ØSRAØ1[9,A,Z]	ØSRAØ3[9,A,Z]	ØSRAØJ[9,A,Z]	ØSRRØ1[9,A,Z]	ØSRRØ3[9,A,Z]	ØSRRØJ[9,A,Z]
Hip, LT	ØSPBØJZ	ØSREØØ[9,A,Z]	ØSREØ1[9,A,Z]	ØSREØ3[9,A,Z]	ØSREØJ[9,A,Z]	ØSRSØ1[9,A,Z]	ØSRSØ3[9,A,Z]	ØSRSØJ[9,A,Z]

Open Removal of Hip Acetabular/Femoral Surface with Replacement

Removal of Acetabular/Femoral Surface		Code also as appropriate Replacement by Device Type					
		Metal	Metal on Poly	Ceramic	Ceramic on Poly	Oxidized Zirc on Poly	Synthetic Substitute
Hip, RT	ØSP[A,R]ØJZ	ØSR9Ø1[9,A,Z]	ØSR9Ø2[9,A,Z]	ØSR9Ø3[9,A,Z]	ØSR9Ø4[9,A,Z]	ØSR9Ø6[9,A,Z]	ØSR9ØJ[9,A,Z]
Hip, LT	ØSP[E,S]ØJZ	ØSRBØ1[9,A,Z]	ØSRBØ2[9,A,Z]	ØSRBØ3[9,A,Z]	ØSRBØ4[9,A,Z]	ØSRBØ6[9,A,Z]	ØSRBØJ[9,A,Z]

Open Removal of Hip Acetabular/Femoral Surface with Replacement

Removal of Acetabular/Femoral Surface		Code also as appropriate Replacement by Device Type						
		Acetabular Surface				Femoral Surface		
		Poly	Metal	Ceramic	Synthetic	Metal	Ceramic	Synthetic
Hip, RT	ØSP[A,R]ØJZ	ØSRAØØ[9,A,Z]	ØSRAØ1[9,A,Z]	ØSRAØ3[9,A,Z]	ØSRAØJ[9,A,Z]	ØSRRØ1[9,A,Z]	ØSRRØ3[9,A,Z]	ØSRRØJ[9,A,Z]
Hip, LT	ØSP[E,S]ØJZ	ØSREØØ[9,A,Z]	ØSREØ1[9,A,Z]	ØSREØ3[9,A,Z]	ØSREØJ[9,A,Z]	ØSRSØ1[9,A,Z]	ØSRSØ3[9,A,Z]	ØSRSØJ[9,A,Z]

Percutaneous Endoscopic Removal of Hip Spacer with Replacement

Removal of Spacer		Code also as appropriate Replacement by Device Type					
		Metal	Metal on Poly	Ceramic	Ceramic on Poly	Oxidized Zirc on Poly	Synthetic Substitute
Hip, RT	ØSP948Z	ØSR9Ø1[9,A,Z]	ØSR9Ø2[9,A,Z]	ØSR9Ø3[9,A,Z]	ØSR9Ø4[9,A,Z]	ØSR9Ø6[9,A,Z]	ØSR9ØJ[9,A,Z]
Hip, LT	ØSPB48Z	ØSRBØ1[9,A,Z]	ØSRBØ2[9,A,Z]	ØSRBØ3[9,A,Z]	ØSRBØ4[9,A,Z]	ØSRBØ6[9,A,Z]	ØSRBØJ[9,A,Z]

Percutaneous Endoscopic Removal of Hip Spacer with Replacement

Removal of Spacer		Code also as appropriate Replacement by Device Type						
		Acetabular Surface				Femoral Surface		
		Poly	Metal	Ceramic	Synthetic	Metal	Ceramic	Synthetic
Hip, RT	ØSP948Z	ØSRAØØ[9,A,Z]	ØSRAØ1[9,A,Z]	ØSRAØ3[9,A,Z]	ØSRAØJ[9,A,Z]	ØSRRØ1[9,A,Z]	ØSRRØ3[9,A,Z]	ØSRRØJ[9,A,Z]
Hip, LT	ØSPB48Z	ØSREØØ[9,A,Z]	ØSREØ1[9,A,Z]	ØSREØ3[9,A,Z]	ØSREØJ[9,A,Z]	ØSRSØ1[9,A,Z]	ØSRSØ3[9,A,Z]	ØSRSØJ[9,A,Z]

Percutaneous Endoscopic Removal of Hip Spacer with Liner Insertion (supplement)

Removal of Spacer		Code also as appropriate Supplement of Body Part by Site		
		Joint	Acetabular Surface	Femoral Surface
Hip, RT	ØSP948Z	ØSU9Ø9Z	ØSUAØ9Z	ØSURØ9Z
Hip, LT	ØSPB48Z	ØSUBØ9Z	ØSUEØ9Z	ØSUSØ9Z

Percutaneous Endoscopic Removal of Hip Synthetic Substitute with Replacement

Removal of Synthetic Substitute		Code also as appropriate Replacement by Device Type					
		Metal	Metal on Poly	Ceramic	Ceramic on Poly	Oxidized Zirc on Poly	Synthetic Substitute
Hip, RT	ØSP94JZ	ØSR901[9,A,Z]	ØSR902[9,A,Z]	ØSR903[9,A,Z]	ØSR904[9,A,Z]	ØSR906[9,A,Z]	ØSR90J[9,A,Z]
Hip, LT	ØSPB4JZ	ØSRB01[9,A,Z]	ØSRB02[9,A,Z]	ØSRB03[9,A,Z]	ØSRB04[9,A,Z]	ØSRB06[9,A,Z]	ØSRB0J[9,A,Z]

Percutaneous Endoscopic of Hip Synthetic Substitute with Replacement

Removal of Synthetic Substitute		Code also as appropriate Replacement by Device Type						
		Acetabular Surface				Femoral Surface		
		Poly	Metal	Ceramic	Synthetic	Metal	Ceramic	Synthetic
Hip, RT	ØSP94JZ	ØSRA00[9,A,Z]	ØSRA01[9,A,Z]	ØSRA03[9,A,Z]	ØSRA0J[9,A,Z]	ØSRR01[9,A,Z]	ØSRR03[9,A,Z]	ØSRR0J[9,A,Z]
Hip, LT	ØSPB4JZ	ØSRE00[9,A,Z]	ØSRE01[9,A,Z]	ØSRE03[9,A,Z]	ØSRE0J[9,A,Z]	ØSRS01[9,A,Z]	ØSRS03[9,A,Z]	ØSRS0J[9,A,Z]

Percutaneous Endoscopic Removal of Hip Synthetic Substitute with Liner Insertion (supplement)

Removal of Synthetic Substitute		Code also as appropriate Supplement of Body Part by Site		
		Joint	Acetabular Surface	Femoral Surface
Hip, RT	ØSP94JZ	ØSU909Z	ØSUA09Z	ØSUR09Z
Hip, LT	ØSPB4JZ	ØSUB09Z	ØSUE09Z	ØSUS09Z

Percutaneous Endoscopic Removal of Hip Acetabular/Femoral Surface with Replacement

Removal of Acetabular/Femoral Surface		Code also as appropriate Replacement by Device Type					
		Metal	Metal on Poly	Ceramic	Ceramic on Poly	Oxidized Zirc on Poly	Synthetic Substitute
Hip, RT	ØSP[A,R]4JZ	ØSR901[9,A,Z]	ØSR902[9,A,Z]	ØSR903[9,A,Z]	ØSR904[9,A,Z]	ØSR906[9,A,Z]	ØSR90J[9,A,Z]
Hip, LT	ØSP[E,S]4JZ	ØSRB01[9,A,Z]	ØSRB02[9,A,Z]	ØSRB03[9,A,Z]	ØSRB04[9,A,Z]	ØSRB06[9,A,Z]	ØSRB0J[9,A,Z]

Percutaneous Endoscopic of Hip Acetabular/Femoral Surface with Replacement

Removal of Acetabular/Femoral Surface		Code also as appropriate Replacement by Device Type						
		Acetabular Surface				Femoral Surface		
		Poly	Metal	Ceramic	Synthetic	Metal	Ceramic	Synthetic
Hip, RT	ØSP[A,R]4JZ	ØSRA00[9,A,Z]	ØSRA01[9,A,Z]	ØSRA03[9,A,Z]	ØSRA0J[9,A,Z]	ØSRR01[9,A,Z]	ØSRR03[9,A,Z]	ØSRR0J[9,A,Z]
Hip, LT	ØSP[E,S]4JZ	ØSRE00[9,A,Z]	ØSRE01[9,A,Z]	ØSRE03[9,A,Z]	ØSRE0J[9,A,Z]	ØSRS01[9,A,Z]	ØSRS03[9,A,Z]	ØSRS0J[9,A,Z]

Percutaneous Endoscopic Removal of Hip Acetabular/Femoral Surface with Liner Insertion (supplement)

Removal of Acetabular/Femoral Surface		Code also as appropriate Supplement of Body Part by Site		
		Joint	Acetabular Surface	Femoral Surface
Hip, RT	ØSP[A,R]4JZ	ØSU909Z	ØSUA09Z	ØSUR09Z
Hip, LT	ØSP[E,S]4JZ	ØSUB09Z	ØSUE09Z	ØSUS09Z

Knee Procedure Combinations

Removal of Knee Liner with Replacement

Removal of Liner		Code also Replacement by Device Type						
		Oxidized Zirc on Poly	Synthetic Substitute	Medial (L)/ Lateral (M) Unicondylar	Patello-femoral	Femoral Surface	Tibial Surface	Medial (L)/ Lateral (M) Meniscus
Knee, RT	ØSPC09Z	ØSRC06[9,A,Z]	ØSRC0J[9,A,Z]	ØSRC0[L,M][9,A,Z]	ØSRC0N[9,A,Z]	ØSRT0J[9,A,Z]	ØSRV0J[9,A,Z]	XRRG0[L,M]8
Knee, LT	ØSPD09Z	ØSRD06[9,A,Z]	ØSRD0J[9,A,Z]	ØSRD0[L,M][9,A,Z]	ØSRD0N[9,A,Z]	ØSRU0J[9,A,Z]	ØSRW0J[9,A,Z]	XRRH0[L,M]8

Removal of Knee Patellar Surface with Replacement

Removal of Patellar Surface		Code also Replacement by Device Type	
		Femoral Surface	Tibial Surface
Knee, RT	ØSPC[0,4]JC	ØSRT0J[9,A,Z]	ØSRV0J[9,A,Z]
Knee, LT	ØSPD[0,4]JC	ØSRU0J[9,A,Z]	ØSRW0J[9,A,Z]

Removal of Knee Synthetic Substitute with Replacement

Removal of Synthetic Substitute		Code also Replacement by Device Type	
		Femoral Surface	Tibial Surface
Knee, RT	ØSPC[Ø,4]JZ	ØSRTØJ[9,A,Z]	ØSRVØJ[9,A,Z]
Knee, LT	ØSPD[Ø,4]JZ	ØSRUØJ[9,A,Z]	ØSRWØJ[9,A,Z]

Removal of Knee Unicondylar Device with Replacement

Removal of Medial (L)/ Lateral (M) Unicondylar Device		Code also Replacement by Device Type	
		Femoral Surface	Tibial Surface
Knee, RT	ØSPC[Ø,4][L,M]Z	ØSRTØJ[9,A,Z]	ØSRVØJ[9,A,Z]
Knee, LT	ØSPD[Ø,4][L,M]Z	ØSRUØJ[9,A,Z]	ØSRWØJ[9,A,Z]

Removal of Knee Patellofemoral Device with Replacement

Removal of Patellofemoral Device		Code also Replacement by Device Type	
		Femoral Surface	Tibial Surface
Knee, RT	ØSPC[Ø,4]NZ	ØSRTØJ[9,A,Z]	ØSRVØJ[9,A,Z]
Knee, LT	ØSPD[Ø,4]NZ	ØSRUØJ[9,A,Z]	ØSRWØJ[9,A,Z]

Removal of Knee Femoral/Tibial Surface Device with Replacement

Removal of Femoral (T,U)/Tibial (V,W) Surface		Code also Replacement by Device Type	
		Femoral Surface	Tibial Surface
Knee, RT	ØSP[T,V][Ø,4]JZ	ØSRTØJ[9,A,Z]	ØSRVØJ[9,A,Z]
Knee, LT	ØSP[U,W][Ø,4]JZ	ØSRUØJ[9,A,Z]	ØSRWØJ[9,A,Z]

DRG 662-664 Minor Bladder Procedure

Repair of Bladder	Code also as appropriate Repair of Abdominal Wall	
	with Stoma	without Stoma
ØTQB[Ø,3,4]ZZ	ØWQFXZ2	ØWQFXZZ

DRG 665-667 Prostatectomy

Site	Resection by approach				Code also as appropriate Resection of Seminal Vesicles, Bilateral by approach	
	Open	Percutaneous Endoscopic	Via Natural or Artificial Opening	Via Natural or Artificial Opening Endoscopic	Open	Percutaneous Endoscopic
Prostate	ØVTØØZZ	ØVTØ4ZZ	ØVTØ7ZZ	ØVTØ8ZZ	ØVT3ØZZ	ØVT34ZZ

DRG 7Ø7-7Ø8 Major Male Pelvic Procedures

Site	Resection by approach				Code also as appropriate Resection of Seminal Vesicles, Bilateral by approach	
	Open	Percutaneous Endoscopic	Via Natural or Artificial Opening	Via Natural or Artificial Opening Endoscopic	Open	Percutaneous Endoscopic
Prostate	ØVTØØZZ	ØVTØ4ZZ	ØVTØ7ZZ	ØVTØ8ZZ	ØVT3ØZZ	ØVT34ZZ

DRG 734-735 Pelvic Evisceration, Radical Hysterectomy and Radical Vulvectomy

Pelvic Evisceration

Resection by Site						
Bladder	Cervix	Fallopian Tubes, Bilateral	Ovaries, Bilateral	Urethra	Uterus	Vagina
ØTTBØZZ	ØUTCØZZ	ØUT7ØZZ	ØUT2ØZZ	ØTTDØZZ	ØUT9ØZZ	ØUTGØZZ

Radical Hysterectomy

Approach	Resection by Site		
	Cervix	Uterus	Uterine Support Structure
Vaginal	ØUTC[7,8]ZZ	ØUT9[7,8]ZZ	ØUT4[7,8]ZZ
Abdominal, Endoscopic	ØUTC4ZZ	ØUT9[4,F]ZZ	ØUT44ZZ
Abdominal, Open	ØUTCØZZ	ØUT9ØZZ	ØUT4ØZZ

Radical Vulvectomy

Resection by Site	Code also as appropriate Excision of Inguinal Lymph Nodes by Approach	
Vulva	Right	Left
ØUTM[Ø,X]ZZ	Ø7BH[Ø,4]ZZ	Ø7BJ[Ø,4]ZZ

Non-OR procedure combinations

Note: The following table identifies procedure combinations that are considered Non-OR even though one or more procedures of the combination are considered valid DRG OR procedures

Insertion With Removal of Intraluminal Device

Code as appropriate Insertion of Intraluminal Device into Hepatobiliary Duct	Code also as appropriate Removal of Intraluminal Device by Approach and Site			
	Via Natural or Artificial Opening		External	
	Hepatobiliary Duct	Pancreatic Duct	Hepatobiliary Duct	Pancreatic Duct
ØFHB7DZ	ØFPB[7,8]DZ	ØFPD[7,8]DZ	ØFPBXDZ	ØFPDXDZ

Appendix M: Coding Exercises and Answers

Using the ICD-10-PCS tables construct the code that accurately represents the procedure performed.

Medical Surgical Section

Procedure	Code
1. Excision of malignant melanoma from skin of right ear	
2. Laparoscopy with excision of endometrial implant from left ovary	
3. Percutaneous needle core biopsy of right kidney	
4. EGD with excisional gastric biopsy	
5. Open endarterectomy of left common carotid artery	
6. Excision of basal cell carcinoma of lower lip	
7. Open excision of tail of pancreas	
8. Percutaneous biopsy of right gastrocnemius muscle	
9. Sigmoidoscopy with sigmoid polypectomy	
10. Open excision of lesion from right Achilles tendon	
11. Open resection of cecum	
12. Total excision of pituitary gland, open	
13. Explantation of left failed kidney, open	
14. Open left axillary total lymphadenectomy	
15. Laparoscopic-assisted vaginal hysterectomy	
16. Right total mastectomy, open	
17. Open resection of papillary muscle	
18. Total retropubic prostatectomy, open	
19. Laparoscopic cholecystectomy	
20. Endoscopic bilateral total maxillary sinusectomy	
21. Amputation at right elbow level	
22. Right below-knee amputation, proximal tibia/fibula	
23. Fifth ray carpometacarpal joint amputation, left hand	
24. Right leg and hip amputation through ischium	
25. DIP joint amputation of right thumb	
26. Right wrist joint amputation	
27. Trans-metatarsal amputation of foot at left big toe	
28. Mid-shaft amputation, right humerus	
29. Left fourth toe amputation, mid-proximal phalanx	
30. Right above-knee amputation, distal femur	
31. Cryotherapy of wart on left hand	
32. Percutaneous radiofrequency ablation of right vocal cord lesion	
33. Left heart catheterization with laser destruction of arrhythmogenic focus, A-V node	
34. Cautery of nosebleed	
35. Transurethral endoscopic laser ablation of prostate	
36. Percutaneous cautery of oozing varicose vein, left calf	
37. Laparoscopy with destruction of endometriosis, bilateral ovaries	
38. Laser coagulation of right retinal vessel, percutaneous	
39. Thoracoscopic pleurodesis, left side	
40. Percutaneous insertion of Greenfield IVC filter	
41. Forceps total mouth extraction, upper and lower teeth	

Procedure	Code
42. Removal of left thumbnail	
43. Extraction of right intraocular lens without replacement, percutaneous	
44. Laparoscopy with needle aspiration of ova for in vitro fertilization	
45. Nonexcisional debridement of skin ulcer, right foot	
46. Open stripping of abdominal fascia, right side	
47. Hysteroscopy with D&C, diagnostic	
48. Liposuction for medical purposes, left upper arm	
49. Removal of tattered right ear drum fragments with tweezers	
50. Microincisional phlebectomy of spider veins, right lower leg	
51. Routine Foley catheter placement	
52. Incision and drainage of external anal abscess	
53. Percutaneous drainage of ascites	
54. Laparoscopy with left ovarian cystotomy and drainage	
55. Laparotomy and drain placement for liver abscess, right lobe	
56. Right knee arthrotomy with drain placement	
57. Thoracentesis of left pleural effusion	
58. Phlebotomy of left median cubital vein for polycythemia vera	
59. Percutaneous chest tube placement for right pneumothorax	
60. Endoscopic drainage of left ethmoid sinus	
61. External ventricular CSF drainage catheter placement via burr hole	
62. Removal of foreign body, right cornea	
63. Percutaneous mechanical thrombectomy, left brachial artery	
64. Esophagogastroscopy with removal of bezoar from stomach	
65. Foreign body removal, skin of left thumb	
66. Transurethral cystoscopy with removal of bladder stone	
67. Forceps removal of foreign body in right nostril	
68. Laparoscopy with excision of old suture from mesentery	
69. Incision and removal of right lacrimal duct stone	
70. Nonincisional removal of intraluminal foreign body from vagina	
71. Right common carotid endarterectomy, open	
72. Open excision of retained sliver, subcutaneous tissue of left foot	
73. Extracorporeal shockwave lithotripsy (ESWL), bilateral ureters	
74. Endoscopic retrograde cholangiopancreatography (ERCP) with lithotripsy of common bile duct stone	
75. Thoracotomy with crushing of pericardial calcifications	
76. Transurethral cystoscopy with fragmentation of bladder calculus	
77. Hysteroscopy with intraluminal lithotripsy of left fallopian tube calcification	
78. Division of right foot tendon, percutaneous	

Procedure	Code		Procedure	Code
79. Left heart catheterization with division of bundle of HIS			122. Craniotomy with clipping of cerebral aneurysm	
80. Open osteotomy of capitate, left hand			123. Nonincisional, transnasal placement of restrictive stent in right lacrimal duct	
81. EGD with esophagotomy of esophagogastric junction			124. Catheter-based temporary restriction of blood flow in abdominal aorta for treatment of cerebral ischemia ·	
82. Sacral rhizotomy for pain control, percutaneous			125. Percutaneous ligation of esophageal vein	
83. Laparotomy with exploration and adhesiolysis of right ureter			126. Percutaneous embolization of left internal carotid-cavernous fistula	
84. Incision of scar contracture, right elbow			127. Laparoscopy with bilateral occlusion of fallopian tubes using Hulka extraluminal clips	
85. Frenulotomy for treatment of tongue-tie syndrome			128. Open suture ligation of failed AV graft, left brachial artery	
86. Right shoulder arthroscopy with coracoacromial ligament release			129. Percutaneous embolization of vascular supply, intracranial meningioma	
87. Mitral valvulotomy for release of fused leaflets, open approach			130. Percutaneous embolization of right uterine artery, using coils	
88. Percutaneous left Achilles tendon release			131. Open occlusion of left atrial appendage, using extraluminal pressure clips	
89. Laparoscopy with lysis of peritoneal adhesions			132. Percutaneous suture exclusion of left atrial appendage, via femoral artery access	
90. Manual rupture of right shoulder joint adhesions under general anesthesia			133. ERCP with balloon dilation of common bile duct	
91. Open posterior tarsal tunnel release			134. PTCA of two coronary arteries, LAD with stent placement, RCA with no stent	
92. Laparoscopy with freeing of left ovary and fallopian tube			135. Cystoscopy with intraluminal dilation of bladder neck stricture	
93. Liver transplant with donor matched liver			136. Open dilation of old anastomosis, left femoral artery	
94. Orthotopic heart transplant using porcine heart			137. Dilation of upper esophageal stricture, direct visualization, with Bougie sound	
95. Right lung transplant, open, using organ donor match			138. PTA of right brachial artery stenosis	
96. Transplant of large intestine, organ donor match			139. Transnasal dilation and stent placement in right lacrimal duct	
97. Left kidney/pancreas organ bank transplant			140. Hysteroscopy with balloon dilation of bilateral fallopian tubes	
98. Replantation of avulsed scalp			141. Tracheoscopy with intraluminal dilation of tracheal stenosis	
99. Reattachment of severed right ear			142. Cystoscopy with dilation of left ureteral stricture, with stent placement	
100. Reattachment of traumatic left gastrocnemius avulsion, open			143. Open gastric bypass with Roux-en-Y limb to jejunum	
101. Closed replantation of three avulsed teeth, lower jaw			144. Right temporal artery to intracranial artery bypass using Gore-Tex graft, open	
102. Reattachment of severed left hand			145. Tracheostomy formation with tracheostomy tube placement, percutaneous	
103. Right open palmaris longus tendon transfer			146. PICVA (percutaneous in situ coronary venous arterialization) of single coronary artery	
104. Endoscopic radial to median nerve transfer			147. Open left femoral-popliteal artery bypass using cadaver vein graft	
105. Fasciocutaneous flap closure of left thigh, open			148. Shunting of intrathecal cerebrospinal fluid to peritoneal cavity using synthetic shunt	
106. Transfer left index finger to left thumb position, open			149. Colostomy formation, open, transverse colon to abdominal wall	
107. Percutaneous fascia transfer to fill defect, right neck			150. Open urinary diversion, left ureter, using ileal conduit to skin	
108. Trigeminal to facial nerve transfer, percutaneous endoscopic			151. CABG of LAD using pedicled left internal mammary artery, open off-bypass	
109. Endoscopic left leg flexor hallucis longus tendon transfer			152. Open pleuroperitoneal shunt, right pleural cavity, using synthetic device	
110. Right scalp advancement flap to right temple			153. Percutaneous placement of ventriculoperitoneal shunt for treatment of hydrocephalus	
111. Resection right breast with TRAM flap reconstruction, open			154. End-of-life replacement of spinal neurostimulator generator, multiple array, in lower abdomen	
112. Skin transfer flap closure of complex open wound, left lower back			155. Percutaneous insertion of spinal neurostimulator lead, lumbar spinal cord	
113. Open fracture reduction, right tibia				
114. Laparoscopy with gastropexy for malrotation				
115. Left knee arthroscopy with reposition of anterior cruciate ligament				
116. Open transposition of ulnar nerve				
117. Closed reduction with percutaneous internal fixation of right femoral neck fracture				
118. Trans-vaginal intraluminal cervical cerclage				
119. Cervical cerclage using Shirodkar technique				
120. Thoracotomy with banding of left pulmonary artery using extraluminal device				
121. Restriction of thoracic duct with intraluminal stent, percutaneous				

Procedure	Code
156. Percutaneous replacement of broken pacemaker lead in left atrium	
157. Open placement of dual chamber pacemaker generator in chest wall	
158. Percutaneous placement of venous central line in right internal jugular, with tip in superior vena cava	
159. Open insertion of multiple channel cochlear implant, left ear	
160. Percutaneous placement of Swan-Ganz catheter in pulmonary trunk	
161. Bronchoscopy with insertion of Low Dose, Pd-103 brachytherapy seeds, right lung	
162. Open insertion of interspinous process device into lumbar vertebral joint	
163. Open placement of bone growth stimulator, left femoral shaft	
164. Cystoscopy with placement of brachytherapy seeds in prostate gland	
165. Percutaneous insertion of Greenfield IVC filter	
166. Full-thickness skin graft to right lower arm, autograft (do not code graft harvest for this exercise)	
167. Excision of necrosed left femoral head with bone bank bone graft to fill the defect, open	
168. Penetrating keratoplasty of right cornea with donor matched cornea, percutaneous approach	
169. Excision of abdominal aorta with Gore-Tex graft replacement, open	
170. Total right knee arthroplasty with insertion of total knee prosthesis	
171. Tenonectomy with graft to right ankle using cadaver graft, open	
172. Mitral valve replacement using porcine valve, open	
173. Percutaneous phacoemulsification of right eye cataract with prosthetic lens insertion	
174. Transcatheter replacement of pulmonary valve using of bovine jugular vein valve	
175. Total left hip replacement using ceramic on ceramic prosthesis, without bone cement	
176. Aortic valve annuloplasty using ring, open	
177. Laparoscopic repair of left inguinal hernia with marlex plug	
178. Autograft nerve graft to right median nerve, percutaneous endoscopic (do not code graft harvest for this exercise)	
179. Exchange of liner in femoral component of previous left hip replacement, open approach	
180. Anterior colporrhaphy with polypropylene mesh reinforcement, open approach	
181. Implantation of CorCap cardiac support device, open approach	
182. Abdominal wall herniorrhaphy, open, using synthetic mesh	
183. Tendon graft to strengthen injured left shoulder using autograft, open (do not code graft harvest for this exercise)	
184. Onlay lamellar keratoplasty of left cornea using autograft, external approach	
185. Resurfacing procedure on right femoral head, open approach	
186. Exchange of drainage tube from right hip joint	
187. Tracheostomy tube exchange	
188. Change chest tube for left pneumothorax	

Procedure	Code
189. Exchange of cerebral ventriculostomy drainage tube	
190. Foley urinary catheter exchange	
191. Open removal of lumbar sympathetic neurostimulator lead	
192. Nonincisional removal of Swan-Ganz catheter from right pulmonary artery	
193. Laparotomy with removal of pancreatic drain	
194. Extubation, endotracheal tube	
195. Nonincisional PEG tube removal	
196. Transvaginal removal of brachytherapy seeds	
197. Transvaginal removal of extraluminal cervical cerclage	
198. Incision with removal of K-wire fixation, right first metatarsal	
199. Cystoscopy with retrieval of left ureteral stent	
200. Removal of nasogastric drainage tube for decompression	
201. Removal of external fixator, left radial fracture	
202. Trimming and reanastomosis of stenosed femorofemoral synthetic bypass graft, open	
203. Open revision of right hip replacement, with readjustment of prosthesis	
204. Adjustment of position, pacemaker lead in left ventricle, percutaneous	
205. External repositioning of Foley catheter to bladder	
206. Taking out loose screw and putting larger screw in fracture repair plate, left tibia	
207. Revision of totally implantable VAD port placement in chest wall, causing patient discomfort, open	
208. Thoracotomy with exploration of right pleural cavity	
209. Diagnostic laryngoscopy	
210. Exploratory arthrotomy of left knee	
211. Colposcopy with diagnostic hysteroscopy	
212. Digital rectal exam	
213. Diagnostic arthroscopy of right shoulder	
214. Endoscopy of maxillary sinus	
215. Laparotomy with palpation of liver	
216. Transurethral diagnostic cystoscopy	
217. Colonoscopy, discontinued at sigmoid colon	
218. Percutaneous mapping of basal ganglia	
219. Heart catheterization with cardiac mapping	
220. Intraoperative whole brain mapping via craniotomy	
221. Mapping of left cerebral hemisphere, percutaneous endoscopic	
222. Intraoperative cardiac mapping during open heart surgery	
223. Hysteroscopy with cautery of post-hysterectomy oozing and evacuation of clot	
224. Open exploration and ligation of post-op arterial bleeder, left forearm	
225. Control of post-operative retroperitoneal bleeding via laparotomy	
226. Reopening of thoracotomy site with drainage and control of post-op hemopericardium	
227. Arthroscopy with drainage of hemarthrosis at previous operative site, right knee	
228. Radiocarpal fusion of left hand with internal fixation, open	
229. Posterior approach spinal fusion at L1-L3 level with BAK cage interbody fusion device, open	

Procedure	Code
230. Intercarpal fusion of right hand with bone bank bone graft, open	
231. Sacrococcygeal fusion with bone graft from same operative site, open	
232. Interphalangeal fusion of left great toe, percutaneous pin fixation	
233. Suture repair of left radial nerve laceration	
234. Laparotomy with suture repair of blunt force duodenal laceration	
235. Perineoplasty with repair of old obstetric laceration, open	
236. Suture repair of right biceps tendon (upper arm) laceration, open	
237. Closure of abdominal wall stab wound	
238. Cosmetic face lift, open, no other information available	
239. Bilateral breast augmentation with silicone implants, open	
240. Cosmetic rhinoplasty with septal reduction and tip elevation using local tissue graft, open	
241. Abdominoplasty (tummy tuck), open	
242. Liposuction of bilateral thighs	
243. Creation of penis in female patient using tissue bank donor graft	
244. Creation of vagina in male patient using synthetic material	
245. Laparoscopic vertical (sleeve) gastrectomy	
246. Left uterine artery embolization with intraluminal biosphere injection	

Obstetrics

Procedure	Code
1. Abortion by dilation and evacuation following laminaria insertion	
2. Manually assisted spontaneous abortion	
3. Abortion by abortifacient insertion	
4. Bimanual pregnancy examination	
5. Extraperitoneal C-section, low transverse incision	
6. Fetal spinal tap, percutaneous	
7. Fetal kidney transplant, laparoscopic	
8. Open in utero repair of congenital diaphragmatic hernia	
9. Laparoscopy with total excision of tubal pregnancy	
10. Transvaginal removal of fetal monitoring electrode	

Placement

Procedure	Code
1. Placement of packing material, right ear	
2. Mechanical traction of entire left leg	
3. Removal of splint, right shoulder	
4. Placement of neck brace	
5. Change of vaginal packing	
6. Packing of wound, chest wall	
7. Sterile dressing placement to left groin region	
8. Removal of packing material from pharynx	
9. Placement of intermittent pneumatic compression device, covering entire right arm	
10. Exchange of pressure dressing to left thigh	

Administration

Procedure	Code
1. Peritoneal dialysis via indwelling catheter	
2. Transvaginal artificial insemination	
3. Infusion of total parenteral nutrition via central venous catheter	
4. Esophagogastroscopy with Botox injection into esophageal sphincter	
5. Percutaneous irrigation of knee joint	
6. Systemic infusion of recombinant tissue plasminogen activator (r-tPA) via peripheral venous catheter	
7. Transabdominal in vitro fertilization, implantation of donor ovum	
8. Autologous bone marrow transplant via central venous line	
9. Implantation of anti-microbial envelope with cardiac defibrillator placement, open	
10. Sclerotherapy of brachial plexus lesion, alcohol injection	
11. Percutaneous peripheral vein injection, glucarpidase	
12. Introduction of anti-infective envelope into subcutaneous tissue, open	

Measurement and Monitoring

Procedure	Code
1. Cardiac stress test, single measurement	
2. EGD with biliary flow measurement	
3. Right and left heart cardiac catheterization with bilateral sampling and pressure measurements	
4. Temperature monitoring, rectal	
5. Peripheral venous pulse, external, single measurement	
6. Holter monitoring	
7. Respiratory rate, external, single measurement	
8. Fetal heart rate monitoring, transvaginal	
9. Visual mobility test, single measurement	
10. Left ventricular cardiac output monitoring from pulmonary artery wedge (Swan-Ganz) catheter	
11. Olfactory acuity test, single measurement	

Extracorporeal or Systemic Assistance and Performance

Procedure	Code
1. Intermittent mechanical ventilation, 16 hours	
2. Intubated patient on mechanical ventilation, positioned prone for 14 hrs	
3. Cardiac countershock with successful conversion to sinus rhythm	
4. IPPB (intermittent positive pressure breathing) for mobilization of secretions, 22 hours	
5. Renal dialysis, 12 hours	
6. IABP (intra-aortic balloon pump) continuous	
7. Intraoperative cardiac pacing, continuous	
8. Intraoperative ECMO (extracorporeal membrane oxygenation), central	
9. Controlled mechanical ventilation (CMV), 45 hours	
10. Pulsatile compression boot with intermittent inflation	

Extracorporeal or Systemic Therapies

Procedure	Code
1. Donor thrombocytapheresis, single encounter	
2. Bili-lite phototherapy, series treatment	
3. Whole body hypothermia, single treatment	
4. Circulatory phototherapy, single encounter	
5. Shock wave therapy of plantar fascia, single treatment	
6. Antigen-free air conditioning, series treatment	
7. TMS (transcranial magnetic stimulation), series treatment	
8. Therapeutic ultrasound of peripheral vessels, single treatment	
9. Plasmapheresis, series treatment	
10. Extracorporeal electromagnetic stimulation (EMS) for urinary incontinence, single treatment	

Osteopathic

Procedure	Code
1. Isotonic muscle energy treatment of right leg	
2. Low velocity-high amplitude osteopathic treatment of head	
3. Lymphatic pump osteopathic treatment of left axilla	
4. Indirect osteopathic treatment of sacrum	
5. Articulatory osteopathic treatment of cervical region	

Other Procedures

Procedure	Code
1. Near infrared spectroscopy of leg vessels	
2. CT computer assisted sinus surgery	
3. Suture removal, abdominal wall	
4. Isolation after infectious disease exposure	
5. Robotic assisted open prostatectomy	
6. CSF extracted from LP shunt	

Chiropractic

Procedure	Code
1. Chiropractic treatment of lumbar region using long lever specific contact	
2. Chiropractic manipulation of abdominal region, indirect visceral	
3. Chiropractic extra-articular treatment of hip region	
4. Chiropractic treatment of sacrum using long and short lever specific contact	
5. Mechanically-assisted chiropractic manipulation of head	

Imaging

Procedure	Code
1. Noncontrast CT of abdomen and pelvis	
2. Intravascular ultrasound, left subclavian artery	
3. Fluoroscopic guidance for insertion of central venous catheter in SVC, low osmolar contrast	
4. Chest x-ray, AP/PA and lateral views	
5. Endoluminal ultrasound of gallbladder and bile ducts	
6. MRI of thyroid gland, contrast unspecified	
7. Esophageal videofluoroscopy study with oral barium contrast	
8. Portable x-ray study of right radius/ulna shaft, standard series	
9. Routine fetal ultrasound, second trimester twin gestation	
10. CT scan of bilateral lungs, high osmolar contrast with densitometry	
11. Fluoroscopic guidance for percutaneous transluminal angioplasty (PTA) of left common femoral artery, low osmolar contrast	

Nuclear Medicine

Procedure	Code
1. Tomo scan of right and left heart, unspecified radiopharmaceutical, qualitative gated rest	
2. Technetium pentetate assay of kidneys, ureters, and bladder	
3. Uniplanar scan of spine using technetium oxidronate, with first-pass study	
4. Thallous chloride tomographic scan of bilateral breasts	
5. PET scan of myocardium using rubidium	
6. Gallium citrate scan of head and neck, single plane imaging	
7. Xenon gas nonimaging probe of brain	
8. Upper GI scan, radiopharmaceutical unspecified, for gastric emptying	
9. Carbon 11 PET scan of brain with quantification	
10. Iodinated albumin nuclear medicine assay, blood plasma volume study	

Radiation Therapy

Procedure	Code
1. Plaque radiation of left eye, single port	
2. 8 MeV photon beam radiation to brain	
3. IORT of colon, 3 ports	
4. HDR brachytherapy of prostate using low dose palladium-103, unidirectional source	
5. Electron radiation treatment of right breast, with custom device	
6. Hyperthermia oncology treatment of pelvic region	
7. Contact radiation of tongue	
8. Heavy particle radiation treatment of pancreas, four risk sites	
9. LDR brachytherapy to spinal cord using iodine	
10. Whole body Phosphorus 32 administration with risk to hematopoietic system	

Physical Rehabilitation and Diagnostic Audiology

Procedure	Code
1. Bekesy assessment using audiometer	
2. Individual fitting of left eye prosthesis	
3. Physical therapy for range of motion and mobility, patient right hip, no special equipment	
4. Bedside swallow assessment using assessment kit	
5. Caregiver training in airway clearance techniques	
6. Application of short arm cast in rehabilitation setting	
7. Verbal assessment of patient's pain level	
8. Caregiver training in communication skills using manual communication board	
9. Group musculoskeletal balance training exercises, whole body, no special equipment	
10. Individual therapy for auditory processing using tape recorder	

Mental Health

Procedure	Code
1. Cognitive-behavioral psychotherapy, individual	
2. Narcosynthesis	
3. Light therapy	
4. ECT (electroconvulsive therapy), unilateral, multiple seizure	
5. Crisis intervention	
6. Neuropsychological testing	
7. Hypnosis	
8. Developmental testing	
9. Vocational counseling	
10. Family psychotherapy	

Substance Abuse Treatment

Procedure	Code
1. Naltrexone treatment for drug dependency	
2. Substance abuse treatment family counseling	
3. Medication monitoring of patient on methadone maintenance	
4. Individual interpersonal psychotherapy for drug abuse	
5. Patient in for alcohol detoxification treatment	
6. Group motivational counseling	
7. Individual 12-step psychotherapy for substance abuse	
8. Post-test infectious disease counseling for IV drug abuser	
9. Psychodynamic psychotherapy for drug dependent patient	
10. Group cognitive-behavioral counseling for substance abuse	

New Technology

Procedure	Code
1. Infusion of terlipressin via peripheral venous catheter	
2. Transcatheter dilation of left peroneal artery with 2 SAVAL stents	
3. Cranial reconstruction using Longeviti ClearFit® cranial implant	

Answers to Coding Exercises

Medical Surgical Section

Procedure	Code
1. Excision of malignant melanoma from skin of right ear	0HB2XZZ
2. Laparoscopy with excision of endometrial implant from left ovary	0UB14ZZ
3. Percutaneous needle core biopsy of right kidney	0TB03ZX
4. EGD with excisional gastric biopsy	0DB68ZX
5. Open endarterectomy of left common carotid artery	03CJ0ZZ
6. Excision of basal cell carcinoma of lower lip	0CB1XZZ
7. Open excision of tail of pancreas	0FBG0ZZ
8. Percutaneous biopsy of right gastrocnemius muscle	0KBS3ZX
9. Sigmoidoscopy with sigmoid polypectomy	0DBN8ZZ
10. Open excision of lesion from right Achilles tendon	0LBN0ZZ
11. Open resection of cecum	0DTH0ZZ
12. Total excision of pituitary gland, open	0GT00ZZ
13. Explantation of left failed kidney, open	0TT10ZZ
14. Open left axillary total lymphadenectomy	07T60ZZ (RESECTION is coded for cutting out a chain of lymph nodes.)
15. Laparoscopic-assisted vaginal hysterectomy	0UT9FZZ
16. Right total mastectomy, open	0HTT0ZZ
17. Open resection of papillary muscle	02TD0ZZ (The papillary muscle refers to the heart and is found in the *Heart and Great Vessels* body system.)
18. Total retropubic prostatectomy, open	0VT00ZZ
19. Laparoscopic cholecystectomy	0FT44ZZ
20. Endoscopic bilateral total maxillary sinusectomy	09TQ8ZZ, 09TR8ZZ
21. Amputation at right elbow level	0X6B0ZZ
22. Right below-knee amputation, proximal tibia/fibula	0Y6H0Z1 (The qualifier *High* here means the portion of the tib/fib closest to the knee.)
23. Fifth ray carpometacarpal joint amputation, left hand	0X6K0Z8 (A *complete* ray amputation is through the carpometacarpal joint.)
24. Right leg and hip amputation through ischium	0Y620ZZ (The *Hindquarter* body part includes amputation along any part of the hip bone.)
25. DIP joint amputation of right thumb	0X6L0Z3 (The qualifier *Low* here means through the distal interphalangeal joint.)
26. Right wrist joint amputation	0X6J0Z0 (Amputation at the wrist joint is considered a complete amputation of the hand.)
27. Trans-metatarsal amputation of foot at left big toe	0Y6N0Z9 (A *partial* amputation is through the shaft of the metatarsal bone.)
28. Mid-shaft amputation, right humerus	0X680Z2
29. Left fourth toe amputation, mid-proximal phalanx	0Y6W0Z1 (The qualifier *High* here means anywhere along the proximal phalanx.)

Procedure	Code
30. Right above-knee amputation, distal femur	0Y6C0Z3
31. Cryotherapy of wart on left hand	0H5GXZZ
32. Percutaneous radiofrequency ablation of right vocal cord lesion	0C5T3ZZ
33. Left heart catheterization with laser destruction of arrhythmogenic focus, A-V node	02583ZZ
34. Cautery of nosebleed	093K7ZZ
35. Transurethral endoscopic laser ablation of prostate	0V508ZZ
36. Percutaneous cautery of oozing varicose vein, left calf	0Y3J3ZZ
37. Laparoscopy with destruction of endometriosis, bilateral ovaries	0U524ZZ
38. Laser coagulation of right retinal vessel, percutaneous	085G3ZZ (The *Retinal Vessel* body-part values are in the *Eye* body system.)
39. Thoracoscopic pleurodesis, left side	0B5P4ZZ
40. Percutaneous insertion of Greenfield IVC filter	06H03DZ
41. Forceps total mouth extraction, upper and lower teeth	0CDWXZ2, 0CDXXZ2
42. Removal of left thumbnail	0HDQXZZ (No separate body-part value is given for thumbnail, so this is coded to *Fingernail*.)
43. Extraction of right intraocular lens without replacement, percutaneous	08DJ3ZZ
44. Laparoscopy with needle aspiration of ova for in vitro fertilization	0UDN4ZZ
45. Nonexcisional debridement of skin ulcer, right foot	0HDMXZZ
46. Open stripping of abdominal fascia, right side	0JD80ZZ
47. Hysteroscopy with D&C, diagnostic	0UDB8ZX
48. Liposuction for medical purposes, left upper arm	0JDF3ZZ (The *Percutaneous* approach is inherent in the liposuction technique.)
49. Removal of tattered right ear drum fragments with tweezers	09D77ZZ
50. Microincisional phlebectomy of spider veins, right lower leg	06DY3ZZ
51. Routine Foley catheter placement	0T9B70Z
52. Incision and drainage of external anal abscess	0D9QXZZ
53. Percutaneous drainage of ascites	0W9G3ZZ (This is drainage of the cavity and not the peritoneal membrane itself.)
54. Laparoscopy with left ovarian cystotomy and drainage	0U914ZZ
55. Laparotomy and drain placement for liver abscess, right lobe	0F9100Z
56. Right knee arthrotomy with drain placement	0S9C00Z
57. Thoracentesis of left pleural effusion	0W9B3ZZ (This is drainage of the pleural cavity)
58. Phlebotomy of left median cubital vein for polycythemia vera	059C3ZZ (The median cubital vein is a branch of the basilic vein)
59. Percutaneous chest tube placement for right pneumothorax	0W9930Z
60. Endoscopic drainage of left ethmoid sinus	099V4ZZ
61. External ventricular CSF drainage catheter placement via burr hole	009630Z

Procedure	Code
62. Removal of foreign body, right cornea	Ø8C8XZZ
63. Percutaneous mechanical thrombectomy, left brachial artery	Ø3C83ZZ
64. Esophagogastroscopy with removal of bezoar from stomach	ØDC68ZZ
65. Foreign body removal, skin of left thumb	ØHCGXZZ (There is no specific value for thumb skin, so the procedure is coded to *Hand*.)
66. Transurethral cystoscopy with removal of bladder stone	ØTCB8ZZ
67. Forceps removal of foreign body in right nostril	Ø9CKXZZ (Nostril is coded to *Nasal mucosa and soft tissue* body-part value.)
68. Laparoscopy with excision of old suture from mesentery	ØDCV4ZZ
69. Incision and removal of right lacrimal duct stone	Ø8CXØZZ
70. Nonincisional removal of intraluminal foreign body from vagina	ØUCG7ZZ (The approach *External* is also a possibility. It is assumed here that since the patient went to the doctor to have the object removed, that it was not in the vaginal orifice.)
71. Right common carotid endarterectomy, open	Ø3CHØZZ
72. Open excision of retained sliver, subcutaneous tissue of left foot	ØJCRØZZ
73. Extracorporeal shockwave lithotripsy (ESWL), bilateral ureters	ØTF6XZZ, ØTF7XZZ (The *Bilateral Ureter* body-part value is not available for the root operation FRAGMENTATION, so the procedures are coded separately.)
74. Endoscopic retrograde cholangiopancreatography (ERCP) with lithotripsy of common bile duct stone	ØFF98ZZ (ERCP is performed through the mouth to the biliary system via the duodenum, so the approach value is *Via Natural or Artificial Opening Endoscopic*.)
75. Thoracotomy with crushing of pericardial calcifications	Ø2FNØZZ
76. Transurethral cystoscopy with fragmentation of bladder calculus	ØTFB8ZZ
77. Hysteroscopy with intraluminal lithotripsy of left fallopian tube calcification	ØUF68ZZ
78. Division of right foot tendon, percutaneous	ØL8V3ZZ
79. Left heart catheterization with division of bundle of HIS	Ø2883ZZ
80. Open osteotomy of capitate, left hand	ØP8NØZZ (The capitate is one of the carpal bones of the hand.)
81. EGD with esophagotomy of esophagogastric junction	ØD948ZZ
82. Sacral rhizotomy for pain control, percutaneous	Ø18R3ZZ
83. Laparotomy with exploration and adhesiolysis of right ureter	ØTN6ØZZ
84. Incision of scar contracture, right elbow	ØHNDXZZ (The skin of the elbow region is coded to *Lower Arm*.)
85. Frenulotomy for treatment of tongue-tie syndrome	ØCN7XZZ (The frenulum is coded to the body-part value *Tongue*.)

Procedure	Code
86. Right shoulder arthroscopy with coracoacromial ligament release	ØMN14ZZ
87. Mitral valvulotomy for release of fused leaflets, open approach	Ø2NGØZZ
88. Percutaneous left Achilles tendon release	ØLNP3ZZ
89. Laparoscopy with lysis of peritoneal adhesions	ØDNW4ZZ
90. Manual rupture of right shoulder joint adhesions under general anesthesia	ØRNJXZZ
91. Open posterior tarsal tunnel release	Ø1NGØZZ (The nerve released in the posterior tarsal tunnel is the tibial nerve.)
92. Laparoscopy with freeing of left ovary and fallopian tube	ØUN14ZZ, ØUN64ZZ
93. Liver transplant with donor matched liver	ØFYØØZØ
94. Orthotopic heart transplant using porcine heart	Ø2YAØZ2 (The donor heart comes from an animal [pig], so the qualifier value is *Zooplastic*.)
95. Right lung transplant, open, using organ donor match	ØBYKØZØ
96. Transplant of large intestine, organ donor match	ØDYEØZØ
97. Left kidney/pancreas organ bank transplant	ØFYGØZØ, ØTY1ØZØ
98. Replantation of avulsed scalp	ØHMØXZZ
99. Reattachment of severed right ear	Ø9MØXZZ
100. Reattachment of traumatic left gastrocnemius avulsion, open	ØKMTØZZ
101. Closed replantation of three avulsed teeth, lower jaw	ØCMXXZ1
102. Reattachment of severed left hand	ØXMKØZZ
103. Right open palmaris longus tendon transfer	ØLX5ØZZ
104. Endoscopic radial to median nerve transfer	Ø1X64Z5
105. Fasciocutaneous flap closure of left thigh, open	ØJXMØZC (The qualifier identifies the body layers in addition to fascia included in the procedure.)
106. Transfer left index finger to left thumb position, open	ØXXPØZM
107. Percutaneous fascia transfer to fill defect, right neck	ØJX43ZZ
108. Trigeminal to facial nerve transfer, percutaneous endoscopic	ØØXK4ZM
109. Endoscopic left leg flexor hallucis longus tendon transfer	ØLXP4ZZ
110. Right scalp advancement flap to right temple	ØHXØXZZ
111. Resection right breast with TRAM flap reconstruction, open	ØHTTØZZ, ØHRTØ76 (Code both the resection and the replacement per guideline B3.18)
112. Skin transfer flap closure of complex open wound, left lower back	ØHX6XZZ
113. Open fracture reduction, right tibia	ØQSGØZZ
114. Laparoscopy with gastropexy for malrotation	ØDS64ZZ
115. Left knee arthroscopy with reposition of anterior cruciate ligament	ØMSP4ZZ
116. Open transposition of ulnar nerve	Ø1S4ØZZ
117. Closed reduction with percutaneous internal fixation of right femoral neck fracture	ØQS634Z
118. Trans-vaginal intraluminal cervical cerclage	ØUVC7DZ
119. Cervical cerclage using Shirodkar technique	ØUVC7ZZ
120. Thoracotomy with banding of left pulmonary artery using extraluminal device	Ø2VRØCZ

Procedure	Code
121. Restriction of thoracic duct with intraluminal stent, percutaneous	Ø7VK3DZ
122. Craniotomy with clipping of cerebral aneurysm	Ø3VGØCZ (The clip is placed lengthwise on the outside wall of the widened portion of the vessel.)
123. Nonincisional, transnasal placement of restrictive stent in right lacrimal duct	Ø8VX7DZ
124. Catheter-based temporary restriction of blood flow in abdominal aorta for treatment of cerebral ischemia	Ø4VØ3DJ
125. Percutaneous ligation of esophageal vein	Ø6L33ZZ
126. Percutaneous embolization of left internal carotid-cavernous fistula	Ø3LL3DZ
127. Laparoscopy with bilateral occlusion of fallopian tubes using Hulka extraluminal clips	ØUL74CZ
128. Open suture ligation of failed AV graft, left brachial artery	Ø3L8ØZZ
129. Percutaneous embolization of vascular supply, intracranial meningioma	Ø3LG3DZ
130. Percutaneous embolization of right uterine artery, using coils	Ø4LE3DT
131. Open occlusion of left atrial appendage, using extraluminal pressure clips	Ø2L7ØCK
132. Percutaneous suture exclusion of left atrial appendage, via femoral artery access	Ø2L73ZK
133. ERCP with balloon dilation of common bile duct	ØF798ZZ
134. PTCA of two coronary arteries, LAD with stent placement, RCA with no stent	Ø27Ø3DZ, Ø27Ø3ZZ (A separate procedure is coded for each artery dilated, since the device value differs for each artery.)
135. Cystoscopy with intraluminal dilation of bladder neck stricture	ØT7C8ZZ
136. Open dilation of old anastomosis, left femoral artery	Ø47LØZZ
137. Dilation of upper esophageal stricture, direct visualization, with Bougie sound	ØD717ZZ
138. PTA of right brachial artery stenosis	Ø3773ZZ
139. Transnasal dilation and stent placement in right lacrimal duct	Ø87X7DZ
140. Hysteroscopy with balloon dilation of bilateral fallopian tubes	ØU778ZZ
141. Tracheoscopy with intraluminal dilation of tracheal stenosis	ØB718ZZ
142. Cystoscopy with dilation of left ureteral stricture, with stent placement	ØT778DZ
143. Open gastric bypass with Roux-en-Y limb to jejunum	ØD16ØZA
144. Right temporal artery to intracranial artery bypass using Gore-Tex graft, open	Ø31SØJG
145. Tracheostomy formation with tracheostomy tube placement, percutaneous	ØB113F4
146. PICVA (percutaneous in situ coronary venous arterialization) of single coronary artery	Ø21Ø3D4
147. Open left femoral-popliteal artery bypass using cadaver vein graft	Ø41LØKL
148. Shunting of intrathecal cerebrospinal fluid to peritoneal cavity using synthetic shunt	ØØ16ØJ6
149. Colostomy formation, open, transverse colon to abdominal wall	ØD1LØZ4
150. Open urinary diversion, left ureter, using ileal conduit to skin	ØT17ØZC

Procedure	Code
151. CABG of LAD using pedicled left internal mammary artery, open off-bypass	Ø21ØØZ9
152. Open pleuroperitoneal shunt, right pleural cavity, using synthetic device	ØW19ØJG
153. Percutaneous placement of ventriculoperitoneal shunt for treatment of hydrocephalus	ØØ163J6
154. End-of-life replacement of spinal neurostimulator generator, multiple array, in lower abdomen	ØJH8ØDZ (Taking out of the old generator is coded separately to the root operation *Removal*)
155. Percutaneous insertion of spinal neurostimulator lead, lumbar spinal cord	ØØHV3MZ
156. Percutaneous replacement of broken pacemaker lead in left atrium	Ø2H73JZ (Taking out the broken pacemaker lead is coded separately to the root operation *Removal*.)
157. Open placement of dual chamber pacemaker generator in chest wall	ØJH6Ø6Z
158. Percutaneous placement of venous central line in right internal jugular, with tip in superior vena cava	Ø2HV33Z
159. Open insertion of multiple channel cochlear implant, left ear	Ø9HEØ6Z
160. Percutaneous placement of Swan-Ganz catheter in pulmonary trunk	Ø2HP32Z (The Swan-Ganz catheter is coded to the device value *Monitoring Device* because it monitors pulmonary artery output.)
161. Bronchoscopy with insertion of Low Dose Pd-103 brachytherapy seeds, right lung	ØBHK81Z, DB11BBZ
162. Open insertion of interspinous process device into lumbar vertebral joint	ØSHØØBZ
163. Open placement of bone growth stimulator, left femoral shaft	ØQHYØMZ
164. Cystoscopy with placement of brachytherapy seeds in prostate gland	ØVH81Z
165. Percutaneous insertion of Greenfield IVC filter	Ø6HØ3DZ
166. Full-thickness skin graft to right lower arm, autograft (do not code graft harvest for this exercise)	ØHRDX73
167. Excision of necrosed left femoral head with bone bank bone graft to fill the defect, open	ØQR7ØKZ
168. Penetrating keratoplasty of right cornea with donor matched cornea, percutaneous approach	Ø8R83KZ
169. Excision of abdominal aorta with Gore-Tex graft replacement, open	Ø4RØØJZ
170. Total right knee arthroplasty with insertion of total knee prosthesis	ØSRCØJZ
171. Tenonectomy with graft to right ankle using cadaver graft, open	ØLRSØKZ
172. Mitral valve replacement using porcine valve, open	Ø2RGØ8Z
173. Percutaneous phacoemulsification of right eye cataract with prosthetic lens insertion	Ø8RJ3JZ
174. Transcatheter replacement of pulmonary valve using of bovine jugular vein valve	Ø2RH38Z
175. Total left hip replacement using ceramic on ceramic prosthesis, without bone cement	ØSRBØ3A
176. Aortic valve annuloplasty using ring, open	Ø2UFØJZ
177. Laparoscopic repair of left inguinal hernia with marlex plug	ØYU64JZ
178. Autograft nerve graft to right median nerve, percutaneous endoscopic (do not code graft harvest for this exercise)	Ø1U547Z

Procedure	Code
179. Exchange of liner in femoral component of previous left hip replacement, open approach	ØSUS09Z (Taking out of the old liner is coded separately to the root operation *Removal*)
180. Anterior colporrhaphy with polypropylene mesh reinforcement, open approach	ØJUCØJZ
181. Implantation of CorCap cardiac support device, open approach	02UAØJZ
182. Abdominal wall herniorrhaphy, open, using synthetic mesh	ØWUFØJZ
183. Tendon graft to strengthen injured left shoulder using autograft, open (do not code graft harvest for this exercise)	ØLU207Z
184. Onlay lamellar keratoplasty of left cornea using autograft, external approach	08U9X7Z
185. Resurfacing procedure on right femoral head, open approach	ØSURØBZ
186. Exchange of drainage tube from right hip joint	ØS2YX0Z
187. Tracheostomy tube exchange	ØB21XFZ
188. Change chest tube for left pneumothorax	ØW2BXØZ
189. Exchange of cerebral ventriculostomy drainage tube	0020X0Z
190. Foley urinary catheter exchange	ØT2BXØZ (This is coded to *Drainage Device* because urine is being drained.)
191. Open removal of lumbar sympathetic neurostimulator lead	01PYØMZ
192. Nonincisional removal of Swan-Ganz catheter from right pulmonary artery	02PYX2Z
193. Laparotomy with removal of pancreatic drain	ØFPGØØZ
194. Extubation, endotracheal tube	ØBP1XDZ
195. Nonincisional PEG tube removal	ØDP6XUZ
196. Transvaginal removal of brachytherapy seeds	ØUPH71Z
197. Transvaginal removal of extraluminal cervical cerclage	ØUPD7CZ
198. Incision with removal of K-wire fixation, right first metatarsal	ØQPN04Z
199. Cystoscopy with retrieval of left ureteral stent	ØTP98DZ
200. Removal of nasogastric drainage tube for decompression	ØDP6X0Z
201. Removal of external fixator, left radial fracture	ØPPJX5Z
202. Trimming and reanastomosis of stenosed femorofemoral synthetic bypass graft, open	04WYØJZ
203. Open revision of right hip replacement, with readjustment of prosthesis	ØSW90JZ
204. Adjustment of position, pacemaker lead in left ventricle, percutaneous	02WA3MZ
205. External repositioning of Foley catheter to bladder	ØTWBXØZ
206. Taking out loose screw and putting larger screw in fracture repair plate, left tibia	ØQWH04Z
207. Revision of totally implantable VAD port placement in chest wall, causing patient discomfort, open	ØJWTØWZ
208. Thoracotomy with exploration of right pleural cavity	ØWJ90ZZ
209. Diagnostic laryngoscopy	ØCJS8ZZ
210. Exploratory arthrotomy of left knee	ØSJD0ZZ
211. Colposcopy with diagnostic hysteroscopy	ØUJD8ZZ
212. Digital rectal exam	ØDJD7ZZ
213. Diagnostic arthroscopy of right shoulder	ØRJJ4ZZ
214. Endoscopy of maxillary sinus	09JY4ZZ
215. Laparotomy with palpation of liver	ØFJ00ZZ
216. Transurethral diagnostic cystoscopy	ØTJB8ZZ
217. Colonoscopy, discontinued at sigmoid colon	ØDJD8ZZ

Procedure	Code
218. Percutaneous mapping of basal ganglia	00K83ZZ
219. Heart catheterization with cardiac mapping	02K83ZZ
220. Intraoperative whole brain mapping via craniotomy	00K00ZZ
221. Mapping of left cerebral hemisphere, percutaneous endoscopic	00K74ZZ
222. Intraoperative cardiac mapping during open heart surgery	02K80ZZ
223. Hysteroscopy with cautery of post-hysterectomy oozing and evacuation of clot	ØW3R8ZZ
224. Open exploration and ligation of post-op arterial bleeder, left forearm	ØX3FØZZ
225. Control of post-operative retroperitoneal bleeding via laparotomy	ØW3HØZZ
226. Reopening of thoracotomy site with drainage and control of post-op hemopericardium	ØW3DØZZ
227. Arthroscopy with drainage of hemarthrosis at previous operative site, right knee	ØY3F4ZZ
228. Radiocarpal fusion of left hand with internal fixation, open	ØRGP04Z
229. Posterior approach spinal fusion at L1-L3 level with BAK cage interbody fusion device, open	ØSG10AJ
230. Intercarpal fusion of right hand with bone bank bone graft, open	ØRGQ0KZ
231. Sacrococcygeal fusion with bone graft from same operative site, open	ØSG507Z
232. Interphalangeal fusion of left great toe, percutaneous pin fixation	ØSGQ34Z
233. Suture repair of left radial nerve laceration	01Q60ZZ (The approach value is *Open*, though the surgical exposure may have been created by the wound itself.)
234. Laparotomy with suture repair of blunt force duodenal laceration	ØDQ90ZZ
235. Perineoplasty with repair of old obstetric laceration, open	ØWQNØZZ
236. Suture repair of right biceps tendon (upper arm) laceration, open	ØLQ30ZZ
237. Closure of abdominal wall stab wound	ØWQFØZZ
238. Cosmetic face lift, open, no other information available	ØW020ZZ
239. Bilateral breast augmentation with silicone implants, open	ØHVØJZ
240. Cosmetic rhinoplasty with septal reduction and tip elevation using local tissue graft, open	090K07Z
241. Abdominoplasty (tummy tuck), open	ØW0FØZZ
242. Liposuction of bilateral thighs	ØJ0L3ZZ, ØJ0M3ZZ
243. Creation of penis in female patient using tissue bank donor graft	ØW4N0K1
244. Creation of vagina in male patient using synthetic material	ØW4M0J0
245. Laparoscopic vertical (sleeve) gastrectomy	ØDB64Z3
246. Left uterine artery embolization with intraluminal biosphere injection	04LF3DU

Obstetrics

Procedure	Code
1. Abortion by dilation and evacuation following laminaria insertion	10A07ZW
2. Manually assisted spontaneous abortion	10E0XZZ (Since the pregnancy was not artificially terminated, this is coded to *Delivery* because it captures the procedure objective. The fact that it was an abortion will be identified in the diagnosis code.)
3. Abortion by abortifacient insertion	10A07ZX
4. Bimanual pregnancy examination	10J07ZZ
5. Extraperitoneal C-section, low transverse incision	10D00Z1
6. Fetal spinal tap, percutaneous	10903ZA
7. Fetal kidney transplant, laparoscopic	10Y04ZS
8. Open in utero repair of congenital diaphragmatic hernia	10Q00ZK (Diaphragm is classified to the *Respiratory* body system in the *Medical and Surgical* section.)
9. Laparoscopy with total excision of tubal pregnancy	10T24ZZ
10. Transvaginal removal of fetal monitoring electrode	10P073Z

Placement

Procedure	Code
1. Placement of packing material, right ear	2Y42X5Z
2. Mechanical traction of entire left leg	2W6MX0Z
3. Removal of splint, right shoulder	2W5AX1Z
4. Placement of neck brace	2W32X3Z
5. Change of vaginal packing	2Y04X5Z
6. Packing of wound, chest wall	2W44X5Z
7. Sterile dressing placement to left groin region	2W27X4Z
8. Removal of packing material from pharynx	2Y50X5Z
9. Placement of intermittent pneumatic compression device, covering entire right arm	2W18X7Z
10. Exchange of pressure dressing to left thigh	2W0PX6Z

Administration

Procedure	Code
1. Peritoneal dialysis via indwelling catheter	3E1M39Z
2. Transvaginal artificial insemination	3E0P7LZ
3. Infusion of total parenteral nutrition via central venous catheter	3E0436Z
4. Esophagogastroscopy with Botox injection into esophageal sphincter	3E0G8GC (Botulinum toxin is a paralyzing agent with temporary effects; it does not sclerose or destroy the nerve.)
5. Percutaneous irrigation of knee joint	3E1U38Z
6. Systemic infusion of recombinant tissue plasminogen activator (r-tPA) via peripheral venous catheter	3E03317
7. Transabdominal in vitro fertilization, implantation of donor ovum	3E0P3Q1
8. Autologous bone marrow transplant via central venous line	30243G0
9. Implantation of anti-microbial envelope with cardiac defibrillator placement, open	3E0102A
10. Sclerotherapy of brachial plexus lesion, alcohol injection	3E0T3TZ

Procedure	Code
11. Percutaneous peripheral vein injection, glucarpidase	3E033GQ
12. Introduction of anti-infective envelope into subcutaneous tissue, open	3E0102A

Measurement and Monitoring

Procedure	Code
1. Cardiac stress test, single measurement	4A02XM4
2. EGD with biliary flow measurement	4A0C85Z
3. Right and left heart cardiac catheterization with bilateral sampling and pressure measurements	4A023N8
4. Temperature monitoring, rectal	4A1Z7KZ
5. Peripheral venous pulse, external, single measurement	4A04XJ1
6. Holter monitoring	4A12X45
7. Respiratory rate, external, single measurement	4A09XCZ
8. Fetal heart rate monitoring, transvaginal	4A1H7CZ
9. Visual mobility test, single measurement	4A07X7Z
10. Left ventricular cardiac output monitoring from pulmonary artery wedge (Swan-Ganz) catheter	4A1239Z
11. Olfactory acuity test, single measurement	4A08X0Z

Extracorporeal or Systemic Assistance and Performance

Procedure	Code
1. Intermittent mechanical ventilation, 16 hours	5A1935Z
2. Intubated patient on mechanical ventilation, positioned prone for 14 hrs	5A09C5K
3. Cardiac countershock with successful conversion to sinus rhythm	5A2204Z
4. IPPB (intermittent positive pressure breathing) for mobilization of secretions, 22 hours	5A09358
5. Renal dialysis, 12 hours	5A1D80Z
6. IABP (intra-aortic balloon pump) continuous	5A02210
7. Intra-operative cardiac pacing, continuous	5A1223Z
8. Intraoperative ECMO (extracorporeal membrane oxygenation), central	5A15A2F
9. Controlled mechanical ventilation (CMV), 45 hours	5A1945Z
10. Pulsatile compression boot with intermittent inflation	5A02115 (This is coded to the function value *Cardiac Output*, because the purpose of such compression devices is to return blood to the heart faster.)

Extracorporeal or Systemic Therapies

Procedure	Code
1. Donor thrombocytapheresis, single encounter	6A550Z2
2. Bili-lite phototherapy, series treatment	6A601ZZ
3. Whole body hypothermia, single treatment	6A4Z0ZZ
4. Circulatory phototherapy, single encounter	6A650ZZ
5. Shock wave therapy of plantar fascia, single treatment	6A930ZZ
6. Antigen-free air conditioning, series treatment	6A0Z1ZZ
7. TMS (transcranial magnetic stimulation), series treatment	6A221ZZ

Procedure	Code
8. Therapeutic ultrasound of peripheral vessels, single treatment	6A750Z6
9. Plasmapheresis, series treatment	6A551Z3
10. Extracorporeal electromagnetic stimulation (EMS) for urinary incontinence, single treatment	6A210ZZ

Osteopathic

Procedure	Code
1. Isotonic muscle energy treatment of right leg	7W06X8Z
2. Low velocity-high amplitude osteopathic treatment of head	7W00X5Z
3. Lymphatic pump osteopathic treatment of left axilla	7W07X6Z
4. Indirect osteopathic treatment of sacrum	7W04X4Z
5. Articulatory osteopathic treatment of cervical region	7W01X0Z

Other Procedures

Procedure	Code
1. Near infrared spectroscopy of leg vessels	8E023DZ
2. CT computer assisted sinus surgery	8E09XBG (The primary procedure is coded separately.)
3. Suture removal, abdominal wall	8E0WXY8
4. Isolation after infectious disease exposure	8E0ZXY6
5. Robotic assisted open prostatectomy	8E0W0CZ (The primary procedure is coded separately.)
6. CSF extracted from LP shunt	8C01X6J

Chiropractic

Procedure	Code
1. Chiropractic treatment of lumbar region using long lever specific contact	9WB3XGZ
2. Chiropractic manipulation of abdominal region, indirect visceral	9WB9XCZ
3. Chiropractic extra-articular treatment of hip region	9WB6XDZ
4. Chiropractic treatment of sacrum using long and short lever specific contact	9WB4XJZ
5. Mechanically-assisted chiropractic manipulation of head	9WB0XKZ

Imaging

Procedure	Code
1. Noncontrast CT of abdomen and pelvis	BW21ZZZ
2. Intravascular ultrasound, left subclavian artery	B342ZZ3
3. Fluoroscopic guidance for insertion of central venous catheter in SVC, low osmolar contrast	B5181ZA
4. Chest x-ray, AP/PA and lateral views	BW03ZZZ
5. Endoluminal ultrasound of gallbladder and bile ducts	BF43ZZZ
6. MRI of thyroid gland, contrast unspecified	BG34YZZ
7. Esophageal videofluoroscopy study with oral barium contrast	BD11YZZ
8. Portable x-ray study of right radius/ulna shaft, standard series	BP0JZZZ
9. Routine fetal ultrasound, second trimester twin gestation	BY4DZZZ

Procedure	Code
10. CT scan of bilateral lungs, high osmolar contrast with densitometry	BB240ZZ
11. Fluoroscopic guidance for percutaneous transluminal angioplasty (PTA) of left common femoral artery, low osmolar contrast	B41G1ZZ

Nuclear Medicine

Procedure	Code
1. Tomo scan of right and left heart, unspecified radiopharmaceutical, qualitative gated rest	C226YZZ
2. Technetium pentetate assay of kidneys, ureters, and bladder	CT631ZZ
3. Uniplanar scan of spine using technetium oxidronate, with first-pass study	CP151ZZ
4. Thallous chloride tomographic scan of bilateral breasts	CH22SZZ
5. PET scan of myocardium using rubidium	C23GQZZ
6. Gallium citrate scan of head and neck, single plane imaging	CW1BLZZ
7. Xenon gas nonimaging probe of brain	C050VZZ
8. Upper GI scan, radiopharmaceutical unspecified, for gastric emptying	CD15YZZ
9. Carbon 11 PET scan of brain with quantification	C030BZZ
10. Iodinated albumin nuclear medicine assay, blood plasma volume study	C763HZZ

Radiation Therapy

Procedure	Code
1. Plaque radiation of left eye, single port	D8Y0FZZ
2. 8 MeV photon beam radiation to brain	D0011ZZ
3. IORT of colon, 3 ports	DDY5CZZ
4. HDR brachytherapy of prostate using low dose palladium-103, unidirectional source	DV10BB1
5. Electron radiation treatment of right breast, with custom device	DM013ZZ
6. Hyperthermia oncology treatment of pelvic region	DWY68ZZ
7. Contact radiation of tongue	D9Y57ZZ
8. Heavy particle radiation treatment of pancreas, four risk sites	DF034ZZ
9. LDR brachytherapy to spinal cord using iodine	D0016B9Z
10. Whole body Phosphorus 32 administration with risk to hematopoietic system	DWY5GFZ

Physical Rehabilitation and Diagnostic Audiology

Procedure	Code
1. Bekesy assessment using audiometer	F13Z31Z
2. Individual fitting of left eye prosthesis	F0DZ8UZ
3. Physical therapy for range of motion and mobility, patient right hip, no special equipment	F07L0ZZ
4. Bedside swallow assessment using assessment kit	F00ZHYZ
5. Caregiver training in airway clearance techniques	F0FZ8ZZ
6. Application of short arm cast in rehabilitation setting	F0DZ7EZ (Inhibitory cast is listed in the equipment reference table under E, *Orthosis*.)
7. Verbal assessment of patient's pain level	F02ZFZZ

Procedure	Code
8. Caregiver training in communication skills using manual communication board	F0FZJMZ (Manual communication board is listed in the equipment reference table under M, *Augmentative/ Alternative Communication*.)
9. Group musculoskeletal balance training exercises, whole body, no special equipment	F07M6ZZ (Balance training is included in the motor treatment reference table under *Therapeutic Exercise*.)
10. Individual therapy for auditory processing using tape recorder	F09Z2KZ (Tape recorder is listed in the equipment reference table under *Audiovisual Equipment*.)

Mental Health

Procedure	Code
1. Cognitive-behavioral psychotherapy, individual	GZ58ZZZ
2. Narcosynthesis	GZGZZZZ
3. Light therapy	GZJZZZZ
4. ECT (electroconvulsive therapy), unilateral, multiple seizure	GZB1ZZZ
5. Crisis intervention	GZ2ZZZZ
6. Neuropsychological testing	GZ13ZZZ
7. Hypnosis	GZFZZZZ
8. Developmental testing	GZ10ZZZ
9. Vocational counseling	GZ61ZZZ
10. Family psychotherapy	GZ72ZZZ

Substance Abuse Treatment

Procedure	Code
1. Naltrexone treatment for drug dependency	HZ94ZZZ
2. Substance abuse treatment family counseling	HZ63ZZZ
3. Medication monitoring of patient on methadone maintenance	HZ81ZZZ
4. Individual interpersonal psychotherapy for drug abuse	HZ54ZZZ
5. Patient in for alcohol detoxification treatment	HZ2ZZZZ
6. Group motivational counseling	HZ47ZZZ
7. Individual 12-step psychotherapy for substance abuse	HZ53ZZZ
8. Post-test infectious disease counseling for IV drug abuser	HZ3CZZZ
9. Psychodynamic psychotherapy for drug dependent patient	HZ5CZZZ
10. Group cognitive-behavioral counseling for substance abuse	HZ42ZZZ

New Technology

Procedure	Code
1. Infusion of terlipressin via peripheral venous catheter	XW03367
2. Transcatheter dilation of left peroneal artery with 2 SAVAL stents	X27U395
3. Cranial reconstruction using Longeviti ClearFit® cranial implant	XNR80D9

Notes

Notes

Notes

Notes